W0043391

Handbook of
Experimental Pharmacology

Continuation of Handbuch der experimentellen Pharmakologie

Vol. 50/II

Anti-Inflammatory Drugs

Contributors

C. G. van Arman · M. E. J. Billingham · D. Brodie · K. Brune
G. E. Davies · P. W. Dodge · S. H. Ferreira · A. W. Ford-Hutchinson
M. Gábor · L. G. Garland · A. F. Green · R. J. Gryglewski
H. F. Hodson · E. W. Holmes · P. L. J. Holt · E. C. Huskisson
M. K. Jasani · P. R. Johnston · J. Kovarsky · D. C. Kvam
D. J. McCarty · B. D. Mitchell · P. J. Piper · M. Di Rosa
C. Rosendorff · J. L. Selph · T. Y. Shen · M. J. H. Smith
K. F. Swingle · R. J. Trancik · J. F. Truax · J. R. Vane
B. B. Vargaftig · R. Vinegar · M. W. Whitehouse · C. J. Woolf

Editors

J. R. Vane · S. H. Ferreira

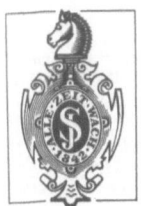

Springer-Verlag Berlin Heidelberg New York 1979

Dr. JOHN R. VANE, The Wellcome Research Laboratories, Langley Court, Beckenham, Kent BR3 3BS, UK

Dr. SERGIO H. FERREIRA, Universidade de São Paulo, Faculdade de Medicina de Ribeirão Preto, CEP 14.100, São Paulo, Brazil

With 101 Figures

ISBN-13: 978-3-642-66893-7   e-ISBN-13: 978-3-642-66891-3
DOI: 10.1007/978-3-642-66891-3

Library of Congress Cataloging in Publication Data. Main entry under title: Anti-inflammatory drugs. (Handbook of experimental pharmacology; v. 50/II). Includes bibliographies and indexes. 1. Anti-inflammatory agents. 2. Inflammation. I. Vane, John R. II. Ferreira, S. H., 1934–. III. Series: Handbuch der experimentellen Pharmakologie: New series: v. 50/II. [DNLM: 1. Antiinflammatory agents. 2. Inflammation-Chemically induced. W1 HA514 new ser. v. 50 pt. II/QV247 A6295] QP905.H3, vol. 50/II. [RM405]. 615.1′08s. [615′.75]. 78–1606

Softcover reprint of the hardcover 1st edition 1979

Contents

Screening and Toxicity of Anti-Inflammatory Drugs

CHAPTER 19

Screening and Assessment of the Potency of Anti-Inflammatory Drugs in vitro.
R. J. GRYGLEWSKI. With 3 Figures

CHAPTER 20

Inhibition of Erythema and Local Hyperthermia. K. F. SWINGLE, R. J. TRANCIK, and D. C. KVAM. With 4 Figures

CHAPTER 21

Oedema and Increased Vascular Permeability. C. G. VAN ARMAN

CHAPTER 22

Short-Term Drug Control of Crystal-Induced Inflammation. D. J. MCCARTY.
With 4 Figures

CHAPTER 23

**Experimental Models of Arthritis in Animals as Screening Tests for Drugs to Treat
Arthritis in Man.** M. E. J. BILLINGHAM and G. E. DAVIES. With 2 Figures

CHAPTER 24

Antagonism of Bradykinin Bronchoconstriction by Anti-Inflammatory Drugs.
P. J. PIPER and J. R. VANE

CHAPTER 25

Interference of Anti-Inflammatory Drugs With Hypotension. B. B. VARGAFTIG.
With 11 Figures

CHAPTER 26

Antagonism of Pain and Hyperalgesia. R. VINEGAR, J. F. TRUAX, J. L. SELPH, and
P. R. JOHNSTON. With 3 Figures

CHAPTER 27

Inhibition of Cell Migration in vivo and Granuloma Formation. M. DI ROSA

CHAPTER 28

Inhibition of Fever. C. ROSENDORFF and C. J. WOOLF. With 3 Figures

CHAPTER 29

Evaluation of the Toxicity of Anti-Inflammatory Drugs. P. W. DODGE, D. BRODIE, and B. D. MITCHELL

Pharmacology of the Anti-Inflammatory Agents

CHAPTER 30

Prostaglandin Synthetase Inhibitors I. T. Y. SHEN. With 1 Figure

CHAPTER 31

Mode of Action of Anti-Inflammatory Agents Which are Prostaglandin Synthetase Inhibitors. S. H. FERREIRA and J. R. VANE. With 2 Figures

CHAPTER 32

Penicillamine and Drugs With a Specific Action in Rheumatoid Arthritis.
E. C. HUSKISSON. With 8 Figures

CHAPTER 33

Antagonists of Histamine, 5-Hydroxytryptamine and SRS—A. A. F. GREEN,
L. G. GARLAND, and H. F. HODSON. With 11 Figures

CHAPTER 34

Inhibitors of the Release of Anaphylatic Mediators. L. G. GARLAND, A. F. GREEN, and H. F. HODSON. With 26 Figures

CHAPTER 35

Cytostats With Effects in Chronic Inflammation. K. BRUNE and M. W. WHITEHOUSE.
With 1 Figure

CHAPTER 36

Control of Hyperuricemia. J. KOVARSKY and E. W. HOLMES. With 2 Figures

CHAPTER 37

Anti-Inflammatory Steroids: Mode of Action in Rheumatoid Arthritis and Homograft Reaction. M. K. JASANI. With 19 Figures

CHAPTER 38

Anti-Inflammatory Agents of Animal Origin. M. J. H. SMITH and A. W. FORD-HUTCHINSON

CHAPTER 39

Anti-Inflammatory Substances of Plant Origin. M. GÁBOR

CHAPTER 40

A Critical Comparison of the Evaluation of Anti-Inflammatory Therapy in Animal Models and Man. P. J. L. HOLT. With 1 Figure

Contents
Part I: Inflammatory

List of Contributors

C. G. VAN ARMAN, Biological Research, Wyeth Laboratories Inc., P. O. Box 8299, Philadelphia, Pennsylvania 19101, USA

M. E. BILLINGHAM, I. C. I. Ltd., Alderley Edge, Macclesfield, Cheshire SK 104TG, UK

D. BRODIE, Pharmacology and Medicinal Chemistry Division, Abbott Research Laboratories, North Chicago, Illinois 60064, USA

K. BRUNE, Biozentrum der Universität Basel, Klingelbergstr. 70, 4056 Basel, Switzerland

G. E. DAVIES, I. C. I. Ltd., Alderley Edge, Macclesfield, Cheshire SK 10 4TG, UK

P. W. DODGE, Scientific Divisions, Pharmacology and Medicinal Chemistry Division, Abbott Laboratories, Abbott Park, North Chicago, Illinois 60064, USA

S. H. FERREIRA, Universidade de São Paulo, Faculdade de Medicina de Ribeirão Preto, CEP 14.100, São Paulo, Brazil

A. W. FORD-HUTCHINSON, Department of Biochemical Pharmacology, King's College Hospital, Medical School, Denmark Hill, London SE5 8RX, UK

M. GABOR, Institute of Pharmacodynamics, University Medical School, P.O. Box 121, 6701 Szeged, Hungary

L. G. GARLAND, The Wellcome Research Laboratories. Langley Court, Beckenham, Kent BR3 3BS, UK

A. F. GREEN, The Wellcome Research Laboratories, Langley Court, Beckenham, Kent BR3 3BS, UK

R. J. GRYGLEWSKI, Department of Pharmacology, School of Medicine, Grzegórzecka 16, 31-531 Cracow, Poland

H. F. HODSON, The Wellcome Research Laboratories, Langley Court, Beckenham, Kent BR3 3BS, UK

E. W. HOLMES, Jr., Division of Rheumatic and Genetic Diseases, Duke University Medical Center, Durham, North Carolina 27710, USA

P. L. J. HOLT, University of Manchester, Department of Rheumatology, Manchester M13 9PT, UK

E. C. HUSKISSON, The Royal Hospital of Bartholomew, West Smithfield, London EC 1A 7BE, UK

M. K. JASANI, Research Division, Ciba Laboratories, Wimblehorst Road Horsham, Sussex RH12 4AB, UK

P. R. JOHNSTON, The Wellcome Research Laboratories, Bourroughs Wellcome Co., 3030 Cornwallis Road, Research Triangle Park, North Carolina 27709, USA

J.KOVARSKY, Rheumatology Service, William Beaumont Army Medical Center, P.O. Box 70302, El Paso, Texas 79920, USA

D.C.KVAM, Riker Laboratories Inc., 3 M Company, Building 218-2, St. Paul, Minnesota 55101, USA

D.J.McCARTY, Department of Medicine, Medical College of Wisconsin, Milwaukee County General Hospital, 8700 West Wisconsin Avenue, Milwaukee, Wisconsin 53226, USA

B.D.MITCHELL, 536 Sheridan Road, Wilmette, Illinois 60091, USA

P.J.PIPER, Department of Pharmacology, Royal College of Surgeons of England, Lincoln's Inn Fields, London WC2A 3PN, UK

M.DI ROSA, Universita di Napoli, Facolta di Farmacia, II Cattedra di Farmacologia e Farmacognosia, Via Leopoldo Rodinó 22, 80138 Napoli, Italy

C.ROSENDORFF, Department of Physiology, University of the Witwatersrand, Medical School, Hospital Street, Johannesburg 2001, South Africa

J.L.SELPH, The Wellcome Research Laboratories, Burroughs Wellcome Co., 3030 Cornwallis Road, Research Triangle Park, North Carolina 27709, USA

T.Y.SHEN, Merck Sharp & Dohme Research Laboratories, P.O. Box 2000 Rahway, New Jersey 07065, USA

M.J.H.SMITH, Department of Biochemical Pharmacology, King's College Hospital, Medical School, Denmark Hill, London SE5 8RX, UK

K.F.SWINGLE, Riker Laboratories Inc., 3 M Company, Building 218-2, St. Paul, Minnesota 55101, USA

R.J.TRANCIK, Riker Laboratories Inc., 3 M Company, Building 218-2, St. Paul, Minnesota 55101, USA

J.F.TRUAX, The Wellcome Research Laboratories, Burroughs Wellcome Co., 3030 Cornwallis Road, Research Triangle Park, North Carolina 27709, USA

J.R.VANE, The Wellcome Research Laboratories, Langley Court, Beckenham, Kent BR3 3BS, UK

B.B.VARGAFTIG, Unité des venins, Institut Pasteur, 28, Rue du Dr. Roux, 75024 Paris Cedex 15, France

R.VINEGAR, The Wellcome Research Laboratories, Burroughs Wellcome Co., 3030 Cornwallis Road, Research Triangle Park, North Carolina 27709, USA

M.W.WHITEHOUSE, Department of Experimental Pathology, The John Curtin School of Medical Research, The Australian National University, P.O. Box 334, Canberra City, A.C.T. 2601, Australia

C.J.WOOLF, Department of Physiology, University of the Witwatersrand, Medical School, Hospital Street, Johannesburg 2001, South Africa

List of Abbreviations

AA	adjuvant arthritis		hypersensitivity
Aa	arachidonic acid	CFC	citrus flavonoid complex
ACI	anti-inflammatory cyclo-oxygenose inhibitors	CH_{50}	haemolytix complement
ACTH	adrenocorticitrophic hormone	CiSLs	circulating sensitized lymphocytes
ADCC	antibody-dependent cellular cytotoxicity	CNDO	complete neglect of differential overlap
ADP	adenosine diphospate	Col	colchicine
AH	anterior hypothalamic	CON-A	concanavallin A
AI	anaphylatoxin inactivator	CP	cyclophosphamide
ALG	antilymphocytic globulin	CPA	N-(Z-carboxyphenyl)-phenoxyacetamides
ALS	antilymphocytic serum	CP-CPK	creatinine phosphokinase
ANTU	alphanaphthyl thiourea	CPPD	calcium pyrophosphate dihydrate
AThP	azothioprine		
ATP	adenosine triphosphate	CR	capillary resistance
		CRF	corticotrophin releasing factor
BAL	dimercaptopropanol		
BaSO4	Barium sulphate	CTL	cytolitically active T-lymphocytes
BCG	Bacille Calmette-Guerin		
BGG	bovine γ globulin	CVF	cobra venom factor
Bk	bradykinin	CVP	citrus vitamin P
BK-A	basophil kallikrein of anaphylaxis	CY	cyclophosphamide
Bkg	bradykininogen	DAS	depressor active substance
BP	bacterial pyrogen	Db-cAMP	dibutyryl derivative of cAMP
BPF	bradykinin potentiating factor	DES	diethylstilboestrol
		DFP	diisopropylphospho-fluoridate
BSA	bovine serum albumin		
BSV	bovine seminal vesicle	DH	delayed hypersensivity
		DHM	dehydromonocrotaline
CB	cytochalasin	DMSO	dimethyl sulphoxide
CBC	chlorambucil	$DNBSO_3$	dinitrobenzene sulphonic acid
C3bI	C3b inactivators		
C3 NeF	C3 nephritic factor	DNCB	2,4,-dinitrochlorobenzene
C3 PA	C3 proactivator	DNP	dinitrophenylated
CBH	cutaneous basophil	DPP	diphloretin phosphate

EACA	epsilon amino caproic acid	LDH	
ECF	eosinophil chemotactic factor	LMW	low molecular weight
ECF-A	eosinophil chemotactic factor of anaphylaxis	LoSLs	locally sensitized lymphocytes
EDTA	ethylene diamine tetra acetic acid	LPF	lymph node permeability factor
EFA	essential fatty acid	LSD	lysergic acid diethylamide
EGTA	ethylene gycol tetra acetic acid	MAF	macrophage activating factor
ER	endoplasmic reticulum	MCDP	mast cell degranulating peptide
ESR	erythrocyte sedimentation rate	MDA	malondialdehyde
ETA	eicostatetraynoic acid	MED	minimal erythemal dose
		MEM	minimal essential medium
FA	fluocinolone acetonide	MF	mitogenic factor
FCA	Freund's complete adjuvant	MIF	migration inhibitory factor
FIA	Freund's incomplete adjuvant	MNI	methylnitroimidazole
		6MP	6-mercaptopurine
GBG	glycene-rich β-glycoprotein	MPGN	membranoproliferative glomerulonephritis
GFR	glomerular filtration rate	MPI	monocyte production inhibitor
HAO	hereditary angio-oedema	MSU	monosodium urate mono-hydrate
HETE	12S-hydroxy-5,8,10,14-eicosatetraenoic acid	MTX	methotrexate
HGPRT	hypoxanthine-guanine phosphoribosyltransferase	NCF	neutrophil chemotactic factor
HMW	high molecular weight	NEM	n-ethyl malemide
HNA	heparin-neutralising activity	OAF	osteoclast activating factor
HPF	human plasma factor		
HSA	human serum albumin	P	properdin
5-HT	5-hydroxytryptamine	PAF	platelet-activating factor
HTT	C_{17}-hydroxy acid	PCA	passive cutaneous ana-phylaxis
IAP	intra-articular pressure	pCPA	p-chlorophenyl-alanine
IDS	inhibitor of DNA synthesis	PCZ	procarbazine
IF	initiating factor	PDE	phosphodiesterase
ITAIF	irritated tissue anti-inflammatory factor	PF3	plateled factor 3
		PF/dil	permeability globulin factor
KAF	C3b inactivator	PF/Glob	high molecular permeability factors
KDO	2-beta-3 deoxyoctonic acid	PG	prostaglandin
LASS	labile aggregation stimulating substance	PGD_2	

PGE	prostaglandin E	RES	reticulo-endothelial system
PGE_1	prostaglandin E_1	RF	rheumatoid factor
PGE_2	PGE_2	RPA	reverse passive Arthus reaction
PHA	phytohaemoglutanin		
PHD	(8-(1-hydroxy-3-oxopropyl)-9,-12S-dihydroxy-5cis, 10cis, heptadecadienore)	SBTI	soybean trypsin inhibitor (Garcia Leme-Chapter 14 or SBT, Fig. 1)
PMA	phorol myristate acetate	SGOT	serum glutamic oxaloacetic transaminase
PMN	polymorphonuclear leucocytes	SGPT	serum glutamic-pyruvic transaminase
PNP	pyroninophilic	SLE	systemic lupus erythmatosus
PPD	protein-purified derivative of tuberculin	SPD	storage pool deficient
PPG	C-mucopolysaccharide-peptidoglycan	SRS	slow-reacting substance
		SRS-A	SRS of anaphylaxis
PPLO	mycoplasmas	SRS-C	SRS from cobra venom
PPP	polyphloretin phosphate	SSV	sheep seminal vesicle
PPS	pain-producing substance		
PVP	polyvinylpyrrolidone	TAMe	p-tosyl-arginine methyl ester
PVPNO	polyvinyl pyridine N-oxide	TBA	thiobarbituric acid
R	rectus	THFN	tetrahydrofurfuryl nicotinate
RA	rheumatoid arthritis	TNP	trinitrophenylated
RCS	rabbit aorta contrasting substance	UDPG	uridine diphosphate glucose
RCS-RF	RCS-releasing factor	UPD	uridine diphosphate

Screening and Toxicity
of Anti-Inflammatory Drugs

CHAPTER 19

Screening and Assessment of the Potency of Anti-Inflammatory Drugs in vitro

R. J. GRYGLEWSKI

A. Introduction

Many in vitro models have been developed to predict the anti-inflammatory potency of newly synthesized compounds, but none of these methods is satisfactory. GLENN et al. (1973) stated bluntly: "All of these in vitro methods are virtually useless for a predictive assessment of drugs in vivo. They are useful only after drugs are discovered in other systems." The above statement was justified when in vitro methods relied entirely on non-specific interactions between non-steroid anti-inflammatory agents (NSAID) and a variety of proteins. However, it has been discovered that the target biomolecule for NSAID is fatty acid cyclo-oxygenase, a component of the prostaglandin (PG) synthetase system (VANE, 1971; SMITH and WILLIS, 1971; FERREIRA et al., 1971; see also Section C.III). Consequently, in vitro assessment of the inhibition of PG synthetase seems to be the rational approach for screening of compounds for their anti-inflammatory activity. The search for new NSAID of various chemical structures has been extensively reviewed (SHEN, 1972; SCHERRER and WHITEHOUSE, 1974). In this chapter, the in vitro screening procedures for acidic NSAID will mainly be discussed.

B. Interaction With Non-Enzymic Proteins

I. Binding to Plasma Proteins

Several reviews have been published on the character of drug-protein interactions (BRODIE and HOGBEN, 1957; MEYER and GUTTMAN, 1968; SETTLE et al., 1971) and on methods for studying them (CHIGNELL, 1971). The binding of NSAID to proteins is usually assessed by methods of equilibrium dialysis and frontal analysis chromatography (KERESZTES-NAGY et al., 1972; ZAROSLINSKI et al., 1974), circular dichroism (CHIGNELL, 1969; PERRIN and NELSON, 1972; SJÖHOLM and SJÖDIN, 1972) and displacement of a probe from the probe-protein complex (WHITEHOUSE et al., 1971; CHAPLIN et al., 1973; ROBAK et al., 1975b).

Acidic NSAID are strong ligands to enzymic and non-enzymic proteins. Their anionic radicals interact with the surface polar groups of proteins (WHITEHOUSE, 1965a, b; WHITEHOUSE and SKIDMORE, 1965; SKIDMORE and WHITEHOUSE, 1966), whereas their lipophilic moieties are anchored into hydrophobic clefts of protein molecules (CHIGNELL, 1969, 1971; DUNN, 1973). Both sites of binding are essential for a distortion of the tertiary structure of proteins by NSAID (CHIGNELL, 1969, 1971), and that leads to a variety of easily measurable physico-chemical effects

(GRANT et al., 1970). Some of these in vitro effects were thought to be essential for anti-inflammatory activity in vivo and thus proposed for prediction of anti-inflammatory properties of new compounds.

1. Displacement Reactions

NSAID compete with several low-molecular substances for binding sites to proteins. Thus, NSAID either displace or prevent binding to serum albumin of aldehydes (SKIDMORE and WHITEHOUSE, 1965), coumarin anti-coagulants (AGGELER et al., 1967; SOLOMON and SCHROGIE, 1967), tryptophan (McARTHUR and DAWKINS, 1969), long-chain fatty acids (DAWKINS et al., 1970), urate (WHITEHOUSE et al., 1971), dansylamide (WHITEHOUSE et al., 1971; DUNN, 1973), thiopental (CHAPLIN et al., 1973), 8-anilino-1-naphthalene sulphonate (GRYGLEWSKI, 1974; ROBAK et al., 1975b) and PGs (ATTALLAH et al., 1974). NSAID can also displace each other from albumin (MASON and McQUEEN, 1974), but do not affect binding sites for corticosteroids (STENLAKE et al., 1971).

The aldehyde and urate displacement models were proposed for the prediction of anti-inflammatory and uricosuric activities of drugs. Unfortunately, the displacement models produce an abundance of false positive results (PHILLIPS et al., 1967; GRANT et al., 1971).

2. Disulphide Interchange Reactions

GERBER et al. (1967) have shown that NSAID accelerate disulphide interchange reaction between serum protein sulphydryl groups and 5,5'-dithiobis-(2-nitrobenzoic) acid (DTNB) in vitro. A similar effect has been found for NSAID using ovalbumin and β-hydroxyethyl-2,4-dinitrophenyl disulphide (HEDD) (GRYGLEWSKI and PANCZENKO, 1968). NSAID also accelerate the reaction between DTNB and protein sulphydryl groups in lymphocyte and mitochondrial membranes (FAMAEY and WHITEHOUSE, 1975).

These effects of NSAID are attributed to their ability to unmask sulphydryl groups which are normally hidden inside the tertiary structure of proteins (GERBER et al., 1967; GRYGLEWSKI and PANCZENKO, 1968; GRYGLEWSKI, 1970; WALZ and DI-MARTINO, 1972). Some of the exposed protein sulphydryl groups may be a regulatory factor in inflammatory response (FAMAEY and WHITEHOUSE, 1975). Actually, in rats with adjuvant arthritis, the number of serum sulphydryl groups is reduced and can be normalised by NSAID (BUTLER et al., 1969). There is also a strikingly good correlation between the results of GERBER et al.'s test and the protective potencies of various NSAID against the ultraviolet induced erythema in guinea pigs (SWINGLE et al., 1970). Furthermore, sulphydryl agents inhibit the release of endogenous pro-inflammatory substances from aggregating platelets (VARGAFTIG et al., 1974). However, the disulphide interchange reaction and the displacement reaction are influenced by NSAID at a range of concentrations which are not likely to be met in vivo.

3. Protection Against Protein Denaturation

NSAID protect serum albumin (Cohn fraction F V) against denaturation induced by heat and several physical and chemical agents (MIZUSHIMA, 1964; MIZUSHIMA and

SUZUKI, 1965; MIZUSHIMA et al., 1975). Nephelometric assay of the NSAID-sensitive thermal denaturation of serum albumin is known as Mizushima's test (WAGNER-JAUREGG et al., 1969). Mizushima's test was used to predict the anti-inflammatory potencies of drugs (WAGNER-JAUREGG et al., 1969; GRANT et al., 1970; WAGNER-JAUREGG, 1972; KALBHEN, 1972; MÖRSDORF and WOLF, 1972; GLENN et al., 1973). This test provides us with another method for measuring NSAID-protein interaction, as clearly demonstrated by GRANT et al. (1971), who analysed the in vitro and in vivo potencies of 370 compounds. They found a significant association between of the results of Mizushima's test with aldehyde displacement (see Section B.I.1) and disulphide interchange reactions (see Section B.I.2) but no such association with four anti-inflammatory tests in vivo.

4. Fibrinolytic Activity

When tested by the von Kaulla method (1965) NSAID dissolve human plasma clots in vitro (GRYGLEWSKI, 1966; GRYGLEWSKI and GRYGLEWSKA, 1966; ROUBAL and NĚMEČEK, 1966; VON KAULLA, 1970; CEPELAK et al., 1972; ROUBAL et al., 1972). This in vitro activity is not a peculiar property of NSAID, for fibrinolysis is also induced by a number of large asymmetric organic anions devoid of anti-inflammatory action (VON KAULLA, 1970; HANSCH and VON KAULLA, 1970; DESNOYERS et al., 1972), including biarylcarboxylates with hypocholesterolemic properties (GRYGLEWSKI and ECKSTEIN, 1967). On the other hand suprofen, a potent acidic NSAID, has no fibrinolytic activity (DE CLERCK et al., 1975). Nonetheless a rough correlation between fibrinolytic and anti-inflammatory potencies for several known NSAID has been reported (GRYGLEWSKI, 1966, 1970). The fibrinolytic assay is less sensitive than other in vitro assays which rely on the interaction of NSAID with proteins (Fig. 1).

II. Interaction With Biological Membranes

NSAID interact with biological membranes in vitro. Those interactions result in either stabilization (MILLER and SMITH, 1966) or labilization (BROWN and SCHWARTZ, 1969) of lysosomal membrane, swelling of mitochondria (FAMAEY, 1973), changes in mitochondrial membrane permeability (FAMAEY et al., 1975), changes in neuronal membrane permeability (LEVITAN and BARKER, 1972, 1973), swelling of lymphocytes (FAMAEY and WHITEHOUSE, 1973), stabilisation of erythrocyte membrane (BROWN et al., 1967), decrease in adhesiveness of platelets, erythrocytes and leucocytes (KOVÁCS and GÖRÖG, 1972), and possibly cytotoxic effects in cultured cells (KARZEL, 1967). It is generally believed that proteins are the main binding sites for NSAID in biological membranes (MIZUSHIMA and SAKAI, 1969; KALBHEN and LOYEN, 1973; FAMAEY and WHITEHOUSE, 1975; MIZUSHIMA et al., 1975), although their interaction with membrane lipids (GULICK-KRZYWICKY et al., 1970), or more precisely with the phospholipid bilayer membranes (MCLAUGHLIN, 1973) cannot be excluded.

1. Effects on Erythrocyte Membrane

Millimolar concentrations of NSAID stabilise the dog erythrocyte membranes (BROWN et al., 1967; BROWN and MACKEY, 1968) and the rat erythrocyte membranes

(GLENN and BOWMAN, 1969) against heat-induced haemolysis. A similar protective action of NSAID has been described for human erythrocytes against hypotonic haemolysis (INGLOT and WOLNA, 1968). Several new potent NSAID are claimed to stabilise erythrocyte membranes at 100-fold lower concentrations than those reported for classic NSAID (MIZUSHIMA et al., 1975). The erythrocyte stabilizing effect of NSAID is pH-dependent (INGLOT and WOLNA, 1968; BROWN et al., 1971) and temperature-dependent (TANAKA et al., 1973). Indeed, at 0° C NSAID inhibit, whereas at 37° C they stimulate, hypotonic haemolysis of rat erythrocytes (TANAKA et al., 1973).

Several authors have reported a similar order of potencies for anti-inflammatory effects and for stabilisation of erythrocyte membranes by NSAID (GLENN and BOWMAN, 1969; KALBHEN et al., 1970; WOLNA et al., 1973b; MIZUSHIMA et al., 1975). However, the erythrocyte stabilising effect is not an inherent property of NSAID, since aspirin, phenylbutazone (TANAKA et al., 1973) and meclofenamic acid (KALBHEN and LOYEN, 1973) are hardly effective in this respect. On the other hand, the erythrocyte stabilising effects are also displayed by corticosteroids (BROWN and MACKEY, 1968), local anaesthetics (SEEMAN, 1966), anti-histamine agents, tranquilizers, neuroleptics (SEEMAN and WEINSTEIN, 1966; TANAKA et al., 1973), β-adrenoceptor blocking agents (WIETHOLD et al., 1973) and a number of commonly used drugs (MIKIKITIS et al., 1970).

The erythrocyte stabilising effect of anionic NSAID differs from that of cationic drugs in being temperature-dependent (TANAKA et al., 1973). Moreover, acidic NSAID selectively quench the fluorescence of the probe-erythrocyte membrane complex (ROBAK et al., 1975a).

NSAID also inhibit erythrocyte sedimentation and aggregation induced by various biological agents (GÖRÖG and KOVÁCS, 1970a; GLENN et al., 1972; KOVÁCS and GÖRÖG, 1972) and suppress the adhesiveness of leucocytes to plasma-coated glass beads (KOVÁCS and GÖRÖG, 1972). NSAID do not protect leucocytes against heat-induced lesions of their membranes (KALBHEN and HABIB-MAHMOUD, 1973).

2. Effects on Lysosomal Membrane

Extensive reviews have been published on the methods of isolation of lysosomes and assessment of the fragility of their membranes (DINGLE, 1972), as well as on the pharmacological regulation of the lysosomal enzymes secretion (IGNARRO, 1974). Steroid anti-inflammatory drugs stabilize rat and rabbit liver lysosomes and lysosomes from human leucocytes against labilisation induced by numerous chemical and physical agents (WEISSMANN and DINGLE, 1961; WEISSMANN and THOMAS, 1962, 1963; WEISSMANN, 1964; LEWIS et al., 1970, 1974; POLLOCK and BROWN, 1971; IGNARRO, 1972, 1974; ALHO, 1973). The in vivo and in vitro studies have shown that a stabilising effect of corticosteroids on the lysosomal membrane occurs at concentrations which can readily be achieved therapeutically, and it seems likely that this is a major factor in the anti-inflammatory action of corticosteroids (POLLOCK and BROWN, 1971).

NSAID have been reported variously to decrease the release of marker enzymes and hence to stabilise hepatic lysosomes (MILLER and SMITH, 1966; TANAKA and IIZUKA, 1968; IGNARRO, 1971a, b; PHILLIPS and MUIRDEN, 1972; MIGNE et al., 1975), to exert no effect (WEISSMANN, 1968; HARFORD and SMITH, 1970; LEWIS, 1970) or to enhance the liberation of the lysosomal enzymes (BROWN and SCHWARTZ, 1969; WEISSMANN et al., 1971). The type of action of NSAID on lysosomal membranes depends on the drug concentration (LEWIS, 1970; LEWIS et al., 1971) as well as on the temperature (IGNARRO, 1971a), pH (HARFORD and SMITH, 1970; IIZUKA et al., 1972) and composition of the incubation medium (IGNARRO, 1973). Possibly because of this capricious behaviour the lysosomes obtained from the NSAID-pretreated rats were reported either to be protected (IGNARRO, 1972; COPPI et al., 1973; MIGNE et al., 1975) or not protected (POLLOCK and BROWN, 1971) against the labilisation procedures.

Unlike corticosteroids and chloroquine, NSAID do not stabilise lysosomes from rabbit peritoneal leucocytes (IGNARRO, 1971b), but stabilise lysosomes from guinea pig peritoneal leucocytes (IGNARRO and COLOMBO, 1972) and from zymozan-treated human neutrophilic granulocytes (IGNARRO, 1974). Indomethacin suppresses the immunologically induced release of lysosomal enzymes from human leucocytes, but no such effect was found in cultured mice macrophages phagocytosing zymozan (RINGROSE et al., 1975). Aspirin retards the labilising effect of histamine on epidermal lysosomes (CHAYEN et al., 1972). On the other hand, CARRANO and MALBICA (1972) have shown that NSAID enhance the labilizing properties of N,N,N',N'-tetrahydro-methylazoformamide on rat liver lysosomes. These authors have suggested their in vitro test as a screening procedure for NSAID. These confusing reports leave little doubt that, in contrast to the lysosome stabilizing properties of corticosteroids, the effects of NSAID on lysosomal membrane cannot be the fundamental part of their anti-inflammatory action, and therefore there is no rational basis for the employment of isolated lysosomes to predict the pharmacological activity of NSAID in vivo.

3. Cytotoxic Properties

NSAID inhibit multiplication of mammalian cells cultured in vitro (KARZEL, 1967), cause changes in the mean volume and the volume distribution of cells (KARZEL et al., 1973), stimulate lactate production and glucose uptake by cells (WOLNA and INGLOT, 1973; WOLNA et al., 1973a) and exert a number of other metabolic effects (KARZEL et al., 1971a,b), which can be at least partially dependent on the membrane effects of NSAID. Ehrlich ascites tumour cells (KARZEL et al., 1973), mastocytoma cells, fibroblasts (KARZEL, 1967), chick embryonal cells (WOLNA and INGLOT, 1973), human HeLa cells (LECHAT et al., 1970) and human synovial cells (YARON et al., 1972) were all used for studying the cytotoxic properties of NSAID and sometimes for prediction of anti-inflammatory potencies of NSAID (INGLOT et al., 1973). However, there is no clear correlation between cytotoxic in vitro and anti-inflammatory in vivo potencies of NSAID (KARZEL et al., 1973).

NSAID were claimed to be anti-viral in vitro (INGLOT et al., 1966, 1973; SKWAREK and SZCZYGIELSKA, 1973) and in vivo (INGLOT and WOYTOŃ, 1971), as well as to inhibit bacterial growth in vitro (WAGNER-JAUREGG and FISCHER, 1968; SCHWARTZ and MANDEL, 1972). Cytototxic properties of NSAID might be of interest for studying the mechanism of drug action (LECHAT et al., 1970; WAGNER-JAUREGG et al., 1970; KARZEL et al., 1971a,b) but are of minor relevance for prediction of the anti-inflammatory potencies of new NSAID.

4. Effects on Leucocyte Migration

NSAID inhibit polymorphonuclear leucocyte migration into inflammatory exudates in vivo (BLACKHAM and OWEN, 1975; FORD-HUTCHINSON et al., 1975). The mechanism of this effect is disputed (HIGGS et al., 1975; SMITH et al., 1975). The chemotactic PGE_1 (KALEY and WEINER, 1971; HIGGS et al., 1975) is generated by phagocytosing leucocytes (HIGGS and YOULTEN, 1972; McCALL and YOULTEN, 1973; HIGGS et al., 1975). NSAID have been shown to inhibit PG generation by phagocytosing leucocytes (HIGGS et al., 1975), to suppress random motility of leucocytes (PHELPS and McCARTY, 1967; PHELPS, 1969; DI ROSA, 1974) and to inhibit phagocytosis (CHANG, 1972), but not the liberation of leucocytic pyrogen (VAN MIERT et al., 1972; BODEL et al., 1973). The chemotactic behaviour of leucocytes in Boyden chambers was either not influenced (KELLER and SOROKIN, 1965; BOREL, 1973) or was suppressed (HIGGS et al., 1975) by NSAID. Interestingly enough, colchicine influences neither the chemotaxis of leucocytes in response to immune complex-activated chemotactic factors, nor the motility of these cells (CHANG, 1975), although colchicine stimulates the generation of PGs in the inflamed area in vivo (GLATT et al., 1975) and in the synovial tissue in vitro (ROBINSON et al., 1975). At present, any in vitro model involving leucocytic chemotaxis, motility or phagocytosis cannot be recommended as the standard screening procedure for assessment of anti-inflammatory activity of drugs.

C. Interaction With Enzymic Proteins

I. General Considerations

NSAID at millimolar concentrations inhibit a great number of enzymes in vitro. It is thought that NSAID interact with enzymes and other proteins in a similar way (WHITEHOUSE, 1965a, 1965b; WHITEHOUSE and SKIDMORE, 1965; see also Section B.I). Thus, impairment of enzymic activity by NSAID is caused by a non-specific distortion of the tertiary structure of an enzyme, i.e. its denaturation. However, the conformational structure of enzymic proteins is more complex than that of albumin, and it might be that NSAID fit much better to some enzymic molecules than to others (GRYGLEWSKI, 1974), thus gaining a certain degree of specifity for their anti-enzymic action. The sophisticated, hypothetical anti-inflammatory receptor site for NSAID was laboriously designed (SCHERRER and WHITEHOUSE, 1974); this receptor might be built into a few or even into a single enzymic protein. The following data support this concept. Millimolar concentrations of NSAID do not inhibit kallikrein (HEBBORN and SHAW, 1963; DAVIES et al., 1966), lysosomal acid phosphatase (HARFORD and SMITH, 1970; PHILLIPS and MUIRDEN, 1972), hyaluronidase (DINNENDAHL and KALBHEN, 1971) and DNA-synthetase (KLEIN et al., 1974), whereas many other enzymes need more than 0.1 mM of indomethacin to be inhibited (Fig. 1). On the other hand the affinity of indomethacin, fenamates and pirprofen for the PG synthetase system is so high that their K_i values are comparable to those for the specific substrate analogues (KU and WASVARY, 1975). In this respect, acidic NSAID can be considered as the 'specific' inhibitors of the PG synthetase system, although the interference of NSAID with peroxidase-hydroperoxide interaction has been proposed (SAEED and WARREN, 1973).

II. Interaction With Enzymes Involved in Carbohydrate, Protein, and Nucleic Acid Metabolism

1. Carbohydrate, Protein, and Amino Acid Metabolism

NSAID are inhibitors of enzymes that affect the metabolism of carbohydrates and mucopolysaccharides (BRYANT et al., 1963; WOLNA et al., 1969; McCOUBREY et al., 1970; SCHÖNHÖFER and ANSPACH, 1967; NAKAGAWA and BENTLEY, 1971; AKAMATSU and MIURA, 1972; DAWSON, 1975), as well as the metabolism of amino acids, peptides and proteins (GOULD et al., 1963; MÖRSDORF, 1965; BERTELLI et al., 1965; SKIDMORE and WHITEHOUSE, 1966, 1967; RADWAN and WEST, 1968; GRYGLEWSKI, 1970; BURLEIGH and SMITH, 1971; AALTO and KULONEN, 1972; ROSENIOR and TONKS, 1974; WOJTECKA-ŁUKASIK and DANCEWICZ, 1974; REINICKE, 1975). These enzymic reactions are inhibited by indomethacin or by other NSAID at concentrations higher than 0.1 mM (Fig. 1). In most cases, these in vitro effects have not been demonstrated in vivo. Some enzymic reactions which have been inhibited in vitro are stimulated in vivo by NSAID (REINICKE, 1975). Five randomly chosen enzymic and non-enzymic tests were found to be of no value, either singly or in combination, as the screening procedure for anti-inflammatory activity of NSAID (McCOUBREY et al., 1970).

2. Nucleic Acid and Nucleotide Metabolism

NSAID inhibit enzymic reactions that affect nucleic acid turnover (WHITEHOUSE, 1965B; JANAKIDEVI and SMITH, 1969, 1970a,b; GAUT and SOLOMON, 1971; SCHWARTZ and MANDEL, 1972; WESTWICK et al., 1972). Two reactions closely related to the nucleotide metabolism will be discussed below.

a) Uncoupling of Oxidative Phosphorylation

Millimolar concentrations of salicylates (BRODY, 1956; ADAMS and COBB, 1958) and of other NSAID (WHITEHOUSE and HASLAM, 1962; WHITEHOUSE, 1964a, b; 1967) uncouple oxidative phosphorylation in isolated mitochondria, i.e. suppress the generation of ATP without depressing oxygen consumption. The uncoupling effect was also observed in mitochondria taken from aspirin-treated animals (MEHLMAN et al., 1972). The mechanism of the uncoupling effect of NSAID is not known, but it has been intensively investigated (VAINIO et al., 1971; MEHLMAN et al., 1972; FAMAEY, 1973; FAMAEY and MOCKEL, 1973; FAMAEY et al., 1975). The uncoupling effect of NSAID in vitro was thought to be causally related to their metabolic (DAWSON, 1975), toxic (BRODY, 1956; MEHLMAN et al., 1972) or therapeutic (ADAMS and COBB, 1958; WHITEHOUSE, 1965a,b) effects in vivo.

There is no correlation between uncoupling and anti-inflammatory potencies of sodium salicylate and indomethacin (SAEKI et al., 1972), fenamates (SAEKI et al., 1972; TERADAet al., 1974) and arylindandiones (VAN DEN BERG and NAUTA, 1975). On the other hand the uncoupling potencies of NSAID correlate very well with their potencies for binding to albumin (WHITEHOUSE, 1967; LEWIS et al., 1972; TERADA et al., 1974).

b) Inhibition of Cyclic AMP Phosphodiesterase

Indomethacin at a low concentration (Fig. 1) inhibits the activity of AMP phosphodiesterase (PDE) from rat brain and cat heart (WEINRYB et al., 1972), bovine heart

(MOFFAT et al., 1972; ROY and WARREN, 1974; STEFANOVICH, 1974), toad bladder (FLORES and SHARP, 1972) and human lungs (ROY and WARREN, 1974). Indomethacin and fenamates (STEFANOVICH, 1974), unlike disodium cromoglycate (ROY and WARREN, 1974), are not competitive inhibitors of PDE, whereas aspirin is ineffective as an inhibitor of PDE (STEFANOVICH, 1974). NSAID were also reported to influence the activity of adenyl cyclase (WEINRYB and MICHEL, 1974) and AMP-dependent protein kinases (DINNENDAHL et al., 1973), as well as to impair the interaction of ATP with actomyosin (GÖRÖG and KOVÁCS, 1970 B, 1972).

III. Inhibition of Prostaglandin Synthetase

In three pioneering papers, NSAID were shown to inhibit PG biosynthesis in guinea pig lung homogenates (VANE, 1971), perfused dog spleen (FERREIRA et al., 1971) and in human platelets (SMITH and WILLIS, 1971). This inhibition was confirmed in other biological systems both in vivo and in vitro (VANE, 1974; FLOWER and VANE, 1974 a, b; FLOWER, 1974). VANE (1971, 1972 a, b; 1973 a, b; 1974) has postulated that NSAID exert their pharmacological actions through inhibition of PG biosynthesis in tissues. This concept has been supported by numerous experiments from different laboratories, as reviewed by FLOWER (1974) and FERREIRA et al. (1974). Owing to VANE'S discovery, the rationally motivated in vitro tests for prediction of anti-inflammatory action of drugs are at present being developed.

1. Prostaglandin Synthetase System

The enzymic generation of PGE_2 from arachidonic acid was originally demonstrated in sheep seminal vesicle homogenates (BERGSTRÖM et al., 1964; VAN DORP et al., 1964). Though complex, the main pathways of PG biosynthesis were soon elucidated (BERGSTRÖM et al., 1968; VAN DORP, 1969, 1971; SAMUELSSON, 1972; SAMUELSSON and HAMBERG, 1974). The proposed route of PG biosynthesis was confirmed by the isolation of two hypothetical endoperoxide intermediates (HAMBERG and SAMUELSSON, 1973; NUGTEREN and HAZELHOF, 1973). Recently, a new enzymic transformation of arachidonic acid to non-PG thromboxanes has been discovered (HAMBERG and SAMUELSSON, 1974; MALMSTEN et al., 1975; SAMUELSSON et al., 1975; see Fig. 1). Other non-PG products can also be formed from unsaturated fatty acid by microsomal 'PG synthetase system' (FLOWER et al., 1973; HAMBERG and SAMUELSSON, 1974; NUGTEREN, 1975).

The multi-enzymic complex of PG synthetase is membrane bound and is found in the microsomal fraction of tissue homogenates. The biochemical separation of its components is in progress (MIYAMOTO et al., 1974). The substrates for PG synthetase are 20-carbon unsaturated fatty acids, having three, four or five all-cis double bonds. Eicosa-5,8,11,14-tetraenoic acid (arachidonic acid) is the most frequently used for biochemical studies (Fig. 1). The activity of PG synthetase depends on the availability of the substrate, oxygen and heat-stable cytoplasmic cofactors (LANDS et al., 1971; LEE and LANDS, 1972; SIH and TAKEGUCHI, 1973; MYIAMOTO et al., 1974). The cofactors can be replaced by reduced glutathione and by phenolic compounds, e.g. phenol, hydroquinone or catecholamines. The rate and the preferential pathway of PG biosynthesis (Fig. 1) is also influenced by pH, concentrations of Cu^{++} ions, thiol

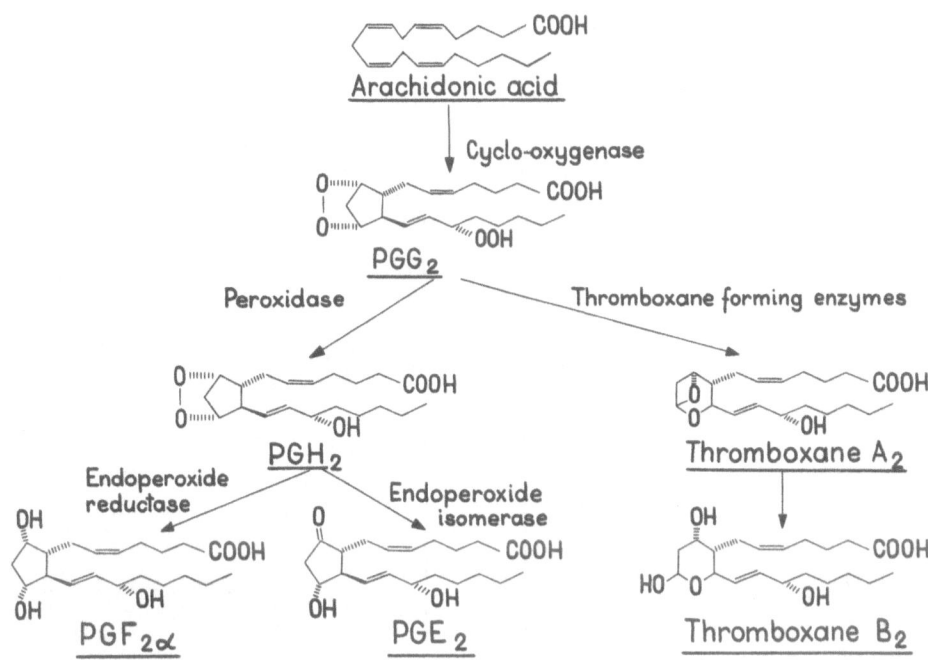

Fig. 1. A simplified scheme of enzymic transformations of arachidonic acid by the microsomal "prostaglandin/thromboxane synthetase system" (HAMBERG and SAMUELSSON, 1974; SAMUELSSON et al., 1975)

compounds and endogenous inhibitors and activators (LANDS et al., 1971, 1974, 1975; WALLACH and DANIELS, 1971; ROSE and COLLINS, 1974). Adenine nucleotides were claimed to control PG biosynthesis in brain (ABDULLA and MCFARLANE, 1972). The biochemical characteristics of PG synthetases derived from various organs are usually different for each microsomal preparation (FLOWER and VANE, 1972; VANE, 1972a; FLOWER, 1974; FLOWER and VANE, 1974a,b; EAKINS, 1974; ROSE and COLLINS, 1974).

2. Assay of Prostaglandin Synthetase Activity

a) Seminal Vesicle Microsomes

Ram (SAMUELSSON et al., 1967; SMITH and LANDS, 1971) and bovine (TAKEGUCHI et al., 1971; TAKEGUCHI and SIH, 1972) seminal vesicle microsomes are most frequently used as the source of the enzyme (Table 1). Fresh and lyophilized microsomes as well as the aceton pentane powders of vesical glands can be employed (WALLACH and DANIELS, 1971). The incubation mixture usually contains arachidonic acid, gluta-thione, a phenolic compound and the enzyme in 0.05–0.1 M buffer of pH 8.0–8.3. Tris-HCl, Tris-acetate, Na-EDTA, glycine-NaOH and phosphate buffers are used. At a low substrate concentration, and in the presence of reduced glutathione, the predominantly formed PG is PGE_2 (FLOWER et al., 1973; GRYGLEWSKI, 1974). This is extracted with organic solvents from the acidified incubation mixture and separated

Table 1. Inhibition of PG biosynthesis in vitro by aspirin and indomethacin. IC_{50} is a micromolar concentration of either drug which inhibits the enzymic activity by a half. Molar ratio represents the relative anti-enzymic potency of indomethacin as compared to that of aspirin. NT = not tested. Figures marked with asterisks refer to K_i values

Approximate IC_{50} (µM)		Molar ratio	Source of enzyme	References
Aspirin	Indomethacin			
9000	10.0	900	Sheep seminal vesicle microsomes	Smith and Lands (1971)
83	0.45	184	Sheep seminal vesicle microsomes	Ham et al. (1972)
200	2.0	100	Sheep seminal vesicle microsomes	Raz et al. (1973)
230	0.35	657	Sheep seminal vesicle microsomes	Young et al. (1974)
5500*	6.5*	846	Sheep seminal vesicle microsomes	Ku and Wasvary (1975)
NT	0.5	—	Sheep seminal vesicle microsomes	Gaut et al. (1975)
820	2.0	410	Bovine seminal vesicle microsomes	Takeuchi and Sih (1972)
15000	7.0	2143	Bovine seminal vesicle microsomes	Tomlinson et al. (1972)
9000	38.0	237	Bovine seminal vesicle microsomes	Flower et al. (1973)
NT	0.8	—	Bovine seminal vesicle microsomes	Burstein et al. (1973)
600	1.0	600	Bovine seminal vesicle microsomes	Collier (1974)
NT	0.5*	—	Bovine seminal vesicle microsomes	Ho and Esterman (1974)
162	0.1	1620	Bovine seminal vesicle microsomes	Gryglewski (1974)
60	1.4	43	Bovine seminal vesicle microsomes	Horodniak et al. (1974)
330	21.0	16	Bovine seminal vesicle microsomes	Deby et al. (1975)
37	0.17	218	Dog spleen microsomes	Flower et al. (1972)
2620	3.7	708	Rabbit kidney microsomes	Flower (1974)

			Preparation	Reference
188	0.15	1253	Rabbit kidney medulla microsomes	DEMBIŃSKA-KIEĆ et al. (1975)
NT	1.6	—	Rabbit kidney medulla microsomes	BHATTACHERJEE and EAKINS (1974)
NT	0.14	—	Rabbit spleen microsomes	BHATTACHERJEE and EAKINS (1974)
>2750	24.0	—	Rabbit conjunctiva microsomes	BHATTACHERJEE and EAKINS (1974)
>2750	140.0	—	Rabbit retina microsomes	BHATTACHERJEE and EAKINS (1974)
>2750	52.0	—	Rabbit anterior uvea microsomes	BHATTACHERJEE and EAKINS (1974)
60	6.0	10	Human epidermal microsomes	ZIBOH et al. (1972)
10000	610.0	16	Rat skin microsomes	GREAVES et al. (1975)
100	0.4	250	Human synovial microsomes	CROOK and COLLINS (1975)
35	0.75	47	Guinea pig lung homogenates	VANE (1971)
NT	0.3	—	Guinea pig lung homogenates	SYKES and MADDOX (1972)
150	3.6	42	Guinea pig lung homogenates	LEE (1974)
25	0.61	41	Guinea pig lung homogenates	TOLMAN and PARTRIDGE (1975)
61	3.6	17	Rabbit brain homogenates	FLOWER and VANE (1972)
NT	0.1	—	Rabbit kidney medulla homogenates	BLOCK et al. (1975)
NT	2.5	—	Rabbit polymorphonuclear sonicates	HIGGS et al. (1975)
60	0.003	≥ 2000	Mouse tumour cells	LEVINE (1972)
NT	0.008	—	Guinea pig macrophages	GORDON and BRAY (1975)
14	2.8	5	Human epidermal cells	FÖRSTRÖM et al. (1974)
1,7	0.17	10	Human blood platelets	SMITH and WILLIS (1971)
16	2.2	7	Rat blood platelets	PATRONO et al. (1975)
28.8	1.3	22	Human blood platelets	PATRONO et al. (1976)
172	1.1	156	Human synovial slices	PATRONO et al. (1976)
210	2.1	100	Rabbit spleen slices	GRYGLEWSKI and VANE (1972a)
≥ 100	0.4	≥ 250	Guinea pig chopped lung	FJALLAND (1974)

by thin-layer chromatography. Then PGE_2 can be quantified either biologically (VANE, 1971; FLOWER et al., 1972) or radiometrically (TOMLINSON et al., 1972; FLOWER et al., 1973). In the latter case, a radioactive substrate has to be used. PGs also can be quantified radioimmunologically (LEVINE, 1972; FÖRSTRÖM et al., 1974; BAUMINGER et al., 1973) and by gas chromatography—mass spectrometry (HAMBERG, 1972; HORODNIAK et al., 1974). Indirect assays of PG synthetase activity are based on measuring oxygen uptake (LANDS et al., 1971), formation of adrenochrome from adrenaline (TAKEGUCHI and SIH, 1972) or formation of malonyldialdehyde from arachidonic acid (FLOWER et al., 1973). Other methods have been reviewed by SIH and TAKEGUCHI (1973).

Fatty acid cyclo-oxygenase is a component of PG synthetase which is sensitive to the inhibitory action of NSAID (see Section C.III.3.a). This enzyme has two unusual features that influence its interaction with NSAID: an accelerative positive feedback, thus allowing the maximal velocity of the enzymic reaction to be is reached quickly and a negative feedback due to self-catalyzed destruction of the enzyme (LANDS et al., 1971, 1974, 1975). These unique properties of cyclo-oxygenase result in the divergence of the kinetic parameters for an inhibitor from those expected for traditional enzyme formulation (LANDS et al., 1975). This divergence seems to be the greatest with arachidonic acid concentrations close to its K_m value. Therefore, the concentration of arachidonic acid in the incubation mixture dramatically influences the rate of reaction, the ratio of products formed and the inhibitory potency of NSAID (FLOWER et al., 1973; GRYGLEWSKI, 1974; HO and ESTERMAN, 1974; see also Table 1). Unfortunately, in various laboratories arachidonic acid was used at a wide range of concentrations varying from 0.1 μM (HO and ESTERMAN, 1974) to 1000 μM (FLOWER et al., 1973). The reported K_m values also varied from 1 to 100 μM (see ROBAK et al., 1975b). KU and WASVARY (1975) have recommended for NSAID studies the use of low substrate concentrations (0.2–2.0 μM), and low temperature (25° C) and short duration (10 min) of incubation. The optimal concentrations for glutathione and reducing agents (adrenaline or hydroquinone) seem to be 1–2 mM (HAM et al., 1972; FLOWER et al., 1973; KU and WASVARY, 1975). An inhibitor (e.g. indomethacin) can be preincubated (SMITH and LANDS, 1971) or not preincubated (KU and WASVARY, 1975) with the enzyme. In the first case, the inhibitory action of indomethacin hardly depends on the substrate concentration (ROBAK et al., 1975b).

Presently, PG synthetases from seminal vesicle glands are available as crude multi-enzymic preparations and might contain variable quantitities of unknown substances that influence their enzymic properties. The calculated kinetic data for the enzymic activity and for the inhibitory action of NSAID differ considerably from one laboratory to another (Table 1). Therefore, these data are mainly of comparative value in the same laboratory. A generally accepted unification of the assay procedure for PG synthetase activity is badly needed.

b) Other Sources of Prostaglandin Synthetase

Other microsomal systems in which PG synthesis is inhibited by NSAID have been reviewed by FLOWER (1974) and some of them are listed in Table 1. Full homogenates are not recommended as the source of the enzyme because of the presence of cytoplasmic enzymes, which metabolize PGs. The cultured cells, macrophages, platelets, epidermal cells and various tissue slices (see Table 1) were also proposed as PG generators. A cellular or tissue preparation can be conveniently employed in screening for anti-PG synthetase activity; its advantage is that it does not require the exogenous substrate and co-factors, and thus operates in more 'physiological' conditions than isolated microsomes. The disadvantage of this model is that highly potent NSAID may be bound to cell membranes and do not reach microsomes (RAZ et al., 1973); however, this is not true for every preparation (FJALLAND, 1974).

3. Prostaglandin Synthetase Inhibitors

a) Non-Steroid Anti-Inflammatory Drugs

NSAID inhibit prostaglandin biosynthesis at a very early stage of the cyclo-oxygenase activity (SMITH and LANDS, 1971; LANDS et al., 1975; FLOWER et al., 1973). Therefore, NSAID also suppress the formation of cyclic endoperoxides and thromboxanes (SAMUELSSON et al., 1975; see Fig. 1). This last effect was observed in biological experiments (PIPER and VANE, 1969; VARGAFTIG and DAO HAI, 1971; GRYGLEWSKI and VANE, 1972a, b; VARGAFTIG and ZIRNIS, 1973; WILLIS, 1974; FJALLAND, 1974) before the identity of a rabbit aorta contracting substance (RCS) with thromboxane A_2 was established (SAMUELSSON et al., 1975; SVENSSON et al., 1975). Most NSAID seem to be equipotent inhibitors of the release of RCS and PG from chopped guinea pig lungs (FJALLAND, 1974).

The Mechanism of inhibition of PG synthetase by NSAID is complex and might differ for various NSAID (FLOWER et al., 1973; HORODNIAK et al., 1974; KU and WASVARY, 1975). The anti-enzymic effect of indomethacin is time-dependent, substrate-dependent (competitive) and irreversible. Most NSAID behave like indomethacin (KU and WASVARY, 1975; ROBAK et al., 1975a). It might well be that this type of inhibition is similar to the "active site-directed irreversible inhibition", which has been described for other enzymes and other inhibitors (SCHAEFFER, 1971).

Inhibitory action on PG synthetase is a common feature for all acidic NSAID (see Table 2); however, some non-acidic NSAID, e.g. indoxole (HAM et al., 1972), benzydamine (FLOWER et al., 1973), isoquinoline derivatives (YOUNG et al., 1974) and indol derivatives (DEBY et al., 1971, 1975) have also been reported to inhibit PG synthesis. Several acidic NSAID have an asymmetric carbon atom in their molecules; in each case, the in vivo active enantiomer has been found to be a more potent PG synthetase inhibitor than its partner (HAM et al., 1972; TAKEGUCHI and SIH, 1972; TOMLINSON et al., 1972; SHEN et al., 1974; GAUT et al., 1975). This stereospecific effect could not be detected in other in vitro tests (MIZUSHIMA et al., 1975). Non-narcotic analgesics, 4-acetamidophenol (FLOWER and VANE, 1972) and dipyrone (DEMBIŃSKA-KIEĆ et al., 1975) selectively inhibit PG synthetase in brain. On the other hand, narcotic analgesics, anti-inflammatory steroids, anti-histamine agents, disodium cromoglycate and a number of other commonly used drugs are not PG synthetase inhibitors (see FLOWER, 1974).

b) Other Prostaglandin Synthetase Inhibitors

A number of substrate analogues and other fatty acids are 'competitive-irreversible' inhibitors of PG synthetase (see FLOWER, 1974). The most potent inhibitors are eicosa-8 *cis*, 12 *trans*,14 cis-trienoic acid (NUGTEREN, 1970) and eicosa-5,8,11,14-

Table 2. Inhibition of PG biosynthesis in vitro by acidic anti-inflammatory drugs. Molar ratios represent the relative anti-enzymic potencies of the drugs as compared to the inhibitory potency of aspirin in the same assay system. Most of these assay systems are presented in Table 1. The others are: sheep seminal vesicle microsomes (Ku et al., 1975) and bovine seminal vesicle microsomes (KRUPP et al., 1975). The data of PATRONO et al. (1976) refer to the superfused slices of human synovium. The data of DEMBIŃSKA-KIEĆ et al. (1975) include the unpublished results from our laboratory

Drugs	IC_{50} (µM)	Molar ratio	References
Niflumic acid	0.1	370	FLOWER et al. (1972)
	1.2	69	HAM et al. (1972)
	3.8	49	DEMBIŃSKA-KIEĆ et al. (1975)
Arylalkanoic acids			
Ibuprofan	1.5	55	HAM et al. (1972)
	1200	0.7	TAKEGUCHI and SIH (1972)
	2000	4.5	FLOWER et al. (1973)
	42	4.5	DEMBIŃSKA-KIEĆ et al. (1975)
Metiazinic acid	3	28	HAM et al. (1972)
Fenclozic acid	3	28	HAM et al. (1972)
Naproxen	6	14	HAM et al. (1972)
	220	3.7	TAKEGUCHI and SIH (1972)
	100	150	TOMLINSON et al. (1972)
	370	24	FLOWER et al. (1973)
	0.4	1500	COLLIER (1974)
	48	3.9	DEMBIŃSKA-KIEĆ et al. (1975)
Fenoprofen	4	4	PATRONO et al. (1975)
	2.2	78	PATRONO et al. (1976)
	73	2.6	DEMBIŃSKA-KIEĆ et al. (1975)
	0.5	—	HO and ESTERMAN (1974)
Pirprofen	1.2	4580	KU and WASVARY (1975)
Fluribiprofen	0.05	2000	CROOK and COLLINS (1975)
Diclofenac	2.4	2290	KU et al. (1975)
	1.0	—	KRUPP et al. (1975)
d-1,6-chloro-α-methyl-carbazole-2-acetic acid	31	—	GAUT et al. (1975)
Salicylates			
Aspirin	2–15000	1	See Table 1
Sodium salicylate	750	0.05	VANE (1971)
	8000	0.08	COLLIER (1974)
	500	0.20	FJALLAND (1974)
	312	0.05	TOLMAN and PARTRIDGE (1975)
Flufenisal	40	2.0	HAM et al. (1972)
Pyrazolones			
Phenylbutazone	7	5.3	FLOWER et al. (1972)
	12	6.9	HAM et al. (1972)
	420	2.0	TAKEGUCHI and SIH (1972)
	1400	6.4	FLOWER et al. (1973)
	88	1.8	GRYGLEWSKI (1974)
	24	9.6	YOUNG et al. (1974)
	88	2.1	DEMBIŃSKA-KIEĆ et al. (1975)
	5	5.0	TOLMAN and PARTRIDGE (1975)
	3	33.0	FJALLAND (1974)
	98	56.0	KU and WASVARY (1975)

Table 2 (continued)

Drugs	IC_{50} (μM)	Molar ratio	References
Oxphenbutazone	50	1.7	HAM et al. (1972)
	730	7.5	KU and WASVARY (1975)
Azapropazone	1	83.0	HAM et al. (1972)
Amidopyrine	100	0.8	HAM et al. (1972)
	> 10000	< 0.9	FLOWER et al. (1973)
	> 1000	< 0.2	GRYGLEWSKI (1974)
	2950	0.06	DEMBIŃSKA-KIEĆ et al. (1975)
Fenamates			
Mefenamic acid	0.7	53	FLOWER et al. (1972)
	2.0	42	HAM et al. (1972)
	15.0	55	TAKEGUCHI and SIH (1972)
	0.4	405	GRYGLEWSKI (1974)
	0.3	625	DEMBIŃSKA-KIEĆ et al. (1975)
	3.2	1720	KU and WASVARY (1975)
	0.05	500	TOLMAN and PARTRIDGE (1975)
Meclofenamic acid	0.1	370	FLOWER et al. (1972)
	10.0	900	FLOWER et al. (1973)
	0.1	6000	COLLIER (1974)
	0.5	375	DEMBIŃSKA-KIEĆ et al. (1975)
	2.6	2110	KU and WASVARY (1975)
Flufenamic acid	2.5	33	HAM et al. (1972)
	48.0	17	TAKEGUCHI and SIH (1972)
	4.0	47	DEMBIŃSKA-KIEĆ et al. (1975)
	0.1	370	FLOWER et al. (1972)
	0.25	400	FJALLAND (1974)

tetraynoic acid (TYA) (AHERN and DOWNING, 1970) with K_i values 0.12 and 2.5 μM respectively. PG synthetase is also inhibited by anti-oxidants, including α-tocopherol (NUGTEREN et al., 1966), santoquin, α-naphthol (VANDERHOEK and LANDS, 1973) and 2,7-naphthalendiol (TAKEGUCHI and SIH, 1972). This last is a potent noncompetitive inhibitor of the enzyme (KU and WASVARY, 1975).

Some metal ions (Cu^{++}, Ca^{++}, Zn^{++}) are inhibitory at concentrations of 50–100 μM (NUGTEREN et al., 1966). Inhibition of PG biosynthesis by copper ions in sheep seminal vesicle microsomes is accompanied by an increase in PGF formation (LEE and LANDS, 1972). Gold and silver preparations (1 μM) have been reported to inhibit PG biosynthesis (DEBY et al., 1973). WALLACH and DANIELS (1971) investigated PG synthetase activity from ram seminal vesicle microsomes in six different buffers of the same molarity and the same pH. The highest enzymic activity was observed in Na-EDTA buffer. This finding indicates that the removal of divalent ions is favourable for the well-being of the enzyme.

Psychotropic drugs were reported to inhibit PG synthetase in guinea pig lung homogenates (LEE, 1974) and in bovine seminal vesicle microsomes (KRUPP and WESP, 1975). The most active PG synthetase inhibitors were found in the group of monoamino-oxidase inhibitors (IC_{50} value for phenelzine is 0.37 μM). Neuroleptics inhibited PG synthetase at concentrations higher than 100 μM. However, inhibition

Table 3. Comparison of anti-PG synthetase and anti-inflammatory potencies of psychotropic and anti-inflammatory drugs

Drugs	Anti-inflammatory activity in vivo[a]		Anti-prostaglandin synthetase activity in vitro[b]
	Oral dose (mg/kg)	Percent inhibition of edema	IC_{50} (µM)
Aspirin	100	18	150
Indomethacin	5	50	3.6
Chlorpromazine	100	65	170
Tranylcypromine	10	38	3.9

[a] Anti-inflammatory activities in the carrageenin rat paw oedema (CARRANO and MALBICA, 1972)
[b] Anti-PG synthetase activities in guinea pig lung homogenates (LEE, 1974)

of PG synthetase by psychotropic drugs seems to be of minor relevance for their central effect, since such potent psychotropic drugs as haloperidol and imipramine do not inhibit PG biosynthesis (KRUPP and WESP, 1975). On the other hand, the inhibition of PG synthetase by chlorpromazine and tranylcypromine correlates with their anti-inflammatory side-effects (Table 3), which are frequently overlooked. Tetrahydrocannabinol (BURSTEIN and RAZ, 1972), naturally occurring cannabinoids (BURSTEIN et al., 1973) and essential oil components of marijuana (BURSTEIN et al., 1975) all are fairly potent PG synthetase inhibitors, but their anti-enzymic potencies in vitro are not correlated with their psychoactive potencies in vivo.

Some anti-thrombotic, hypocholesterolemic and anti-hypertensive agents are moderate inhibitors of PG synthetase (FLOWER et al., 1972; BLOCK et al., 1975; DEBY et al., 1975; PATRONO et al., 1975).

c) Design of Prostaglandin Synthetase Inhibitors

When an anti-enzymic test is employed it is essential to know that the drug concentrations which are used in vitro are likely to be met in vivo. Indomethacin inhibits PG synthetase at micromolar concentrations (Table 1), which are within the plasma levels achieved by the drug during normal therapy, even allowing for its plasma binding (Fig. 2). The same is true for other NSAID (FLOWER et al., 1972; FLOWER, 1974). Furthermore, the inhibition of PG generation was conclusively demonstrated in vivo after ingestion of therapeutic doses of NSAID (COLLIER and FLOWER, 1971; SMITH and WILLIS, 1971; HAMBERG, 1972; HORTON et al., 1973; SAMUELSSON, 1974).

There exists a rough correlation between anti-PG synthetase and anti-inflammatory potencies of acidic NSAID (VANE, 1971; FLOWER et al., 1972, 1973; HAM et al., 1972; LEVINE, 1972; TAKEGUCHI and SIH, 1972; TOMLINSON et al., 1972; COLLIER, 1974; FJALLAND, 1974; GRYGLEWSKI, 1974, 1975; SHEN, 1974; KU and WASVARY, 1975; TOLMAN and PARTRIDGE, 1975). This correlation seems to wane (SHEN, 1974) or even to disappear (VAN DER BERG et al., 1975) for non-acidic NSAID, and therefore the PG synthetase-directed design of anti-inflammatory agents should be restricted to acidic compounds, although the anionic chemical structure is not a firm requirement either for anti-inflammatory action (WHITEHOUSE and FAMAEY, 1973;

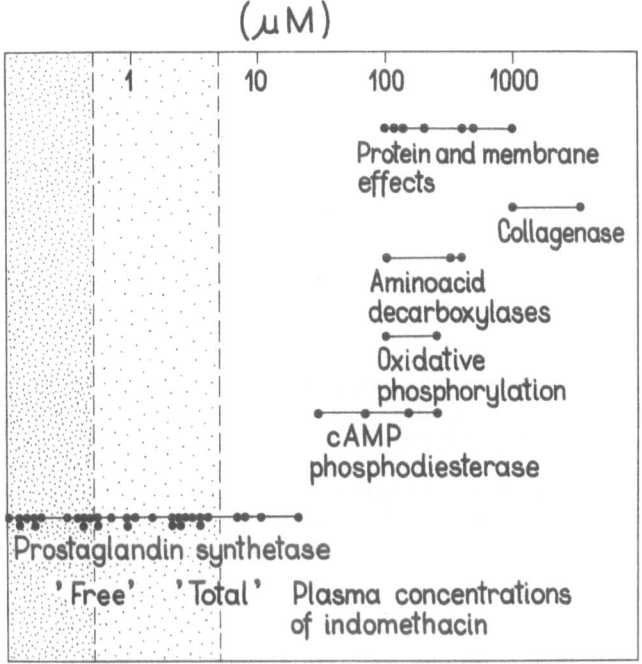

Fig. 2. Interactions of indomethacin with non-enzymic and enzymic proteins. Effective concentrations of indomethacin are presented in increasing order of potency for the following protein and membrane effects: fibrinolytic activity (GRYGLEWSKI, 1970), stabilisation of lysosomal membranes (IGNARRO, 1971 a), stabilisation of erythrocyte membranes BROWN et al., 1971), stabilisation of albumin (GRANT et al., 1970), inhibition of urate binding to albumin (WHITEHOUSE et al., 1971), displacement of 8-anilino-1-naphthalene sulphonate from albumin (ROBAK et al., 1975 b), inhibition of adhesiveness of leucocytes to plasma coated glass beads (KOVÁCS and GÖRÖG, 1972), protection against heat-induced denaturation of albumin (MIZUSHIMA et al., 1975), stabilisation of erythrocyte membranes (MIZUSHIMA et al., 1975). The inhibitory action of indomethacin on enzymic activities is also given in an increasing order of potency for the following enzymes: collagenase (BROWN and POLLOCK, 1970; WOJTECKA-LUKASIK and DANCEWICZ, 1974), histidine decarboxylase (SKIDMORE and WHITEHOUSE, 1966; RADWAN and WEST, 1968), 5-hydroxytryptophan decarboxylase (SKIDMORE and WHITEHOUSE, 1967), uncoupling of oxidative phosphorylation (WHITEHOUSE and HASLAM, 1962; SAEKI et al., 1972) and AMP phosphodiesterase (ROY and WARREN, 1974—two results; STEFANOVICH, 1974; FLORES and SHARP, 1972). The anti-PG synthetase potencies of indomethacin are those which are presented in Table 1. Four values (two lowest and two highest) are omitted, as well as those referring to the ocular microsomal preparations, which are apparently not sensitive to the inhibitory action of indomethacin (BHATTACHERJEE and EAKINS, 1974). 'Total' and 'free' plasma concentrations of indomethacin in human beings treated with therapeutic doses of the drug are cited after PALMÉER et al. (1974) and FLOWER (1974)

SCHERRER and WHITEHOUSE, 1974) or for PG synthetase inhibition (see Section C.III.3.a).

The general structural requirements for acidic NSAID have been proposed (SHEN, 1972, 1974; GRYGLEWSKI, 1974; SCHERRER and WHITEHOUSE, 1974). Most known NSAID are arylalkanoic acids or double-ring aromatic acids. In our laboratory, over 350 compounds having the above structures have been tested for inhibition of PG synthetase and for binding to albumin. Only a few compounds exerted

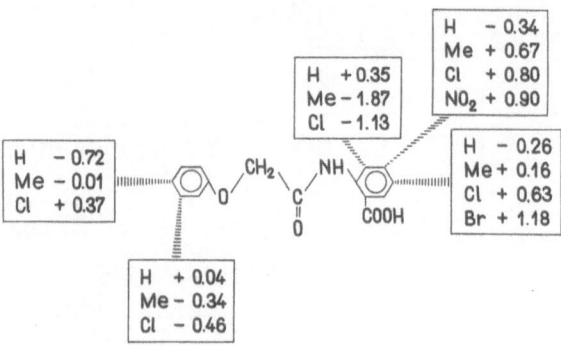

Fig. 3. Activity contribution of the substituents to PG synthetase inhibition by derivatives of N-(2-carboxyphenyl)-phenoxyacetamide. The observed anti-enzymic activities of 21 synthetised derivatives were analysed using the model of FREE and WILSON (1964). Results of statistical tests ($R = 0.9552$, $R^2 = 0.9124$, $F = 10.42$, $df_1 = df_2 = 10$, $p < 0.01$) allowed calculation of activity of parent structure ($\log(1/C) = 4.98$) and indicated activity contributions of fixed substituents. Thus, the anti-PG synthetase activities of over 250 non-existing compounds have been predicted (GRYGLEWSKI et al., 1976)

anti-enzymic action at concentrations lower than 300 µM, but all of them were appreciably bound to albumin. We consider that the capability of a compound to bind to non-enzymic proteins is a prerequisite but not sufficient requirement for its binding to the target enzymic molecule, i.e. to PG synthetase (GRYGLEWSKI, 1974). This explains an abundance of false positive results when the protein-binding tests were singly used to assess the anti-inflammatory potency of newly synthetized compounds (PHILLIPS et al., 1967; GRANT et al., 1971; see also Section B). However, binding of a potential NSAID to albumin should not be overlooked, even when the anti-PG synthetase assay is employed. An exact correlation between the potencies of NSAID to inhibit the enzyme in vitro and to exert anti-inflammatory action in vivo cannot be expected for many reasons (SHEN et al., 1974; GRYGLEWSKI, 1974), one of which is the different degree of binding to plasma albumin for various PG synthetase inhibitors. Therefore we propose to use two in vitro tests for the design of new anti-inflammatory agents. These tests are inhibition of PG synthetase in bovine seminal vesicle microsomes and binding to bovine serum albumin. We have reported (GRYGLEWSKI et al., 1976) that the difference between anti-enzymic and albumin-ligand potencies of a compound is a relatively good denominator for its anti-inflammatory potency in the rat carageenin oedema test. A tentative explanation for this fact is that only that portion of a PG synthetase inhibitor which remains unbound by plasma proteins has a chance to inhibit the enzyme in vivo and thus to suppress acute inflammation.

Let me give an example. Within a series of N-(2-carboxyphenyl)-phenoxyacetamides (CPA) we found potent inhibitors of PG synthetase (GRYGLEWSKI et al., 1976). Positional isomers of CPA derivatives have shown a remarkable difference in their anti-PG synthetase potencies, whereas their potencies to bind to albumin were more or less the same. Therefore it seems that binding sites for CPA in molecules of the enzymic protein are far more stereospecific than those in albumin. In vitro anti-enzymic potency of several CPA derivatives approached that of indomethacin; however, their in vivo anti-inflammatory potency was close to that of aspirin. It was not the anti-enzymic potency of CPA derivatives, but the ratio of that potency to their albumin-ligand potency which correlated with the anti-inflammatory activity in vivo.

We found it rewarding to use de novo models for the design of chemical structures for new PG synthetase inhibitors. A computer assisted programme (PURCELL et al., 1973) employing the additive mathematical model of FREE and WILSON (1964) has been successfully used. The observed anti-enzymic activities of 21 CPA derivatives allowed calculation of the biological activities of over 250 non-existing CPA (Fig. 3). One of the most active compounds, N-(2-carboxy-4-bromophenyl)-4'-chloro-phenoxyacetamide had the calculated anti-PG synthetase activity $\log(1/C) = 6.53$ and its observed activity of $\log(1/C) = 6.38$. Because of its avid binding to albumin ($\log(1/C) = 4.60$), this compound had a weak anti-inflammatory activity equal to that of aspirin, in spite of the fact that its anti-enzymic potency was only 4 times lower than that of indomethacin and 390 times higher than that of aspirin (GRYGLEWSKI et al., 1976). It is suggested that the general chemical character of acidic PG synthetase inhibitors lends itself to a wide application of the additive mathematical model of FREE and WILSON (1964) for the design of anti-inflammatory drugs.

4. Inhibition of Platelet Aggregation

a) Structural Features of Platelets

Platelet structure, physiology and function have recently been reviewed (WEISS, 1975a, b). The blood platelets have a trilaminar plasma membrane covered with an amorphous coat. Their disc-shape is maintained by a microtubular system. Deep invaginations of plasma membrane form the surface-connecting system closely associated to a dense tubular system. Platelets have no nuclei but mitochondria and two types of granules. These are dense-body granules which are the storage pool for adenine nucleotides, 5-hydroxytryptamine (5-HT) and calcium ions and α-granules which more or less resemble lysosomes.

b) Platelet Adhesion and Aggregation

Platelets adhere to broken vascular endothelium and to subendothelial tissues. Platelet adhesion is associated with the release of platelet constituents from granules (see CAPRINO and ROSSI, 1974; HENSON, 1974; MUSTARD and PACKHAM, 1975; WEISS, 1975a). Among the substances released is adenosine diphosphate (ADP), which directly aggregates platelets. Exogenous ADP, adrenaline, 5-HT and thrombin can also initiate platelet aggregation, which primarily does not involve the release reaction. This type of reversible aggregation is also known as the primary or first-phase aggregation. The irreversible aggregation mediated through the release of endogenous ADP is referred to as the second-phase aggregation. Aggregation induced by collagen (SHIO and RAMWELL, 1972; FLOWER et al., 1975) and by arachidonic acid (SILVER et al., 1973; VARGAFTIG and ZIRINIS, 1973; SMITH et al., 1974a; FLOWER et al., 1975) are thought to be purely of the second-phase type. Recently, it has been demonstrated (MALMSTEN et al., 1975; SAMUELSSON et al., 1975) that the release reaction is always triggered by PG endoperoxides and by thromboxane A_2 (see Fig. 2). Therefore, an appearance of the second phase of aggregation depends on the efficiency of the NSAID-sensitive PG/thromboxane synthesizing system in platelets.

c) Principles of the Methods in vitro

Platelet aggregation can be assessed in several types of commercially available aggregometers, according to the principle described by BORN (1962a, b). Light is passed through citrated platelet rich plasma (PRP) being stirred at 37° C. A pro-aggregatory agent is added to PRP and then an increase in light transmission is measured. Special techniques allow evaluation of the shape of platelets. The anti-aggregatory effects of NSAID can be studied either by addition to PRP or by administration of a drug to the PRP donor. Several methods for evaluation of platelet adhesiveness were critically reviewed (DESNOYERS and VERRY, 1972). Various drugs which influence platelet adhesiveness, aggregation and the release reaction have been extensively reviewed (MUSTARD and PACKHAM, 1970, 1975; DE GAETANO et al., 1971b; CAPRINO and ROSSI, 1974).

d) Pro-Aggregatory Agents and Non-Steroid Anti-Inflammatory Drugs

Most NSAID inhibit only second-phase aggregation (O'BRIEN, 1968; WEISS et al., 1968; ZUCKER and PETERSON, 1968, 1970) and therefore collagen is most frequently used as the pro-aggregatory agent in the NSAID studies. The responsiveness of human platelets to the pro-aggregatory effect of collagen is highly variable. To obtain meaningful results for the anti-aggregatory potency of NSAID, the threshold pro-aggregatory concentration of collagen for each individual PRP should be established (GREEN et al., 1973).

Adrenaline-induced aggregation has two distinct phases and only the second one is suppressed by NSAID (MACMILLAN, 1968; O'BRIEN, 1968; WEISS et al., 1968).

NSAID do not inhibit the primary-phase aggregation induced by ADP (PACKHAM et al., 1967; EVANS et al., 1968; WEISS et al., 1968; ARFORS et al., 1972); however, when low concentrations of ADP (2–4 µM) are used, there is an antiaggregatory effect of NSAID on the second-phase aggregation (O'BRIEN, 1968; ZUCKER and PETERSON, 1968; SHIO and RAMWELL, 1972; GAUT et al., 1975). Cationic NSAID, e.g. benzydamine or chloroquine, inhibit the primary-phase aggregation, whereas anti-inflammatory corticosteroids are totally ineffective as anti-aggregatory agents (KOVÁCS and GÖRÖG, 1972).

Arachidonic acid, thrombin, thromboplastin, immune complexes and endotoxin are sometimes used as the pro-aggregatory agents in studying the influence of NSAID on platelet function (DE GAETANO et al., 1972; KOVÁCS and GÖRÖG, 1972; VARGAFTIG and ZIRNIS, 1973; DE CLERCK et al., 1975).

e) Anti-Aggregatory Effect of Aspirin

The inhibitory potency of aspirin against collagen-induced aggregation of rabbit platelets increases during the time of incubation of the drug with PRP (ROSENBERG et al., 1971). It is likely that aspirin, in contrast to other NSAID (DE GAETANO et al., 1971a; CONSTANTINE and PURCELL, 1973; FENICHEL et al., 1974) irreversibly interacts with platelets (WEISS et al., 1968; AL-MONDHIRY et al., 1970; ROSENBERG et al.,

1971) and therefore its anti-aggregatory potency in vitro is high and its effect on platelet function in vivo is long lasting (O'BRIEN, 1968; WEISS et al., 1968; ZUCKER and PETERSON, 1968; ATAC et al., 1970; STUART, 1970; BOLOGNA, 1972; SMITH et al., 1974a) Recently, ROTH et al. (1975) have reported that the catalytic subunit of human platelet PG cyclo-oxygenase (a protein of m.w. 85000) is irreversibly acetylated by aspirin. Arachidonic acid blocks this active site directed effect of aspirin. It is still unknown whether any other NSAID act in an analogous fashion, but at least the finding of ROTH et al., (1975) explains the persistent action of aspirin on platelets (see Section C.III.4.h). Aspirin also inhibits the adhesive behaviour of platelets in response to various surface stimuli (EVANS et al., 1967; KÓVACS and GÖRÖG, 1972).

f) Anti-Aggregatory Effects of Other Non-Steroid Anti-Inflammatory Drugs

A great number of acidic NSAID inhibit collagen-induced platelet aggregation in various species including human beings. One of the most potent anti-aggregatory NSAID is sudoxicam, being active at a concentration of $1 \mu M$ (CONSTANTINE and PURCELL, 1973). The following NSAID need 5–1000 times higher concentrations than sudoxicam to inhibit platelet aggregation in vitro: aspirin (WEISS and ALEDORT, 1967; GORDON and MACINTYRE, 1974), indomethacin (O'BRIEN et al., 1970, DE GAETANO, 1971a; FLOWER et al., 1975), pyrazoles (PACKHAM and MUSTARD, 1969), pyrazolidines (ROUBAL et al., 1972), phenylbutazone (PACKHAM et al., 1967; FLEMING et al., 1970), fenamates (O'BRIEN, 1968; ČEPELAK et al., 1972), fenoprofen (HERRMANN et al., 1972), ditizole (CAPRINO et al., 1973b), suprofen (DE CLERCK et al., 1975), 2-(p-chlorphenyl)-4-thiazoleacrylic acid (Wy-23,049) (FENICHEL et al., 1974), 6-chloro-α-methylcarbazole-2-acetic acid (GAUT et al., 1975) and some other NSAID (MARMO et al., 1974).

There is little correlation between the anti-aggregatory in vitro and anti-inflammatory in vivo potencies of NSAID (DE GAETANO et al., 1971a; FLEMING et al., 1970; Caprino et al., 1973a,b), although such a correlation has been reported for sudoxicam and the reference NSAID (CONSTANTINE and PURCELL, 1973).

g) Effects of Non-Steroid Anti-Inflammatory Drugs on the Platelet Release Reaction

Aspirin (EVANS et al., 1968; WEISS et al., 1968), phenylbutazone (O'BRIEN, 1968), pyrazole compounds (PACKHAM and MUSTARD, 1969), indomethacin (GLENN et al., 1972; DE CLERCK et al., 1975), sudoxicam (CONSTANTINE and PURCELL, 1973) and suprofen (DE CLERCK et al., 1975) inhibit the release of ADP, 5-HT and acid hydrolases from aggregating platelets. NSAID also suppress the generation by platelets of PGs (SMITH and WILLIS, 1971; GLENN et al., 1972; SMITH et al., 1974a; PATRONO et al., 1976), PG endoperoxides and thromboxanes (HAMBERG et al., 1974; SAMUELSSON et al., 1975). These last two are triggers of the release reaction in platelets (MALMSTEN et al., 1975).

The involvement of cyclic nucleotides in the release reaction has not been elucidated. Many compounds that inhibit both platelet aggregation and the release reaction also increase cAMP concentration in platelets (SALZMAN, 1972; SHIO and RAMWELL, 1972; BRUNO et al., 1974; McDONALD and STUART, 1974). On the other hand, collagen-induced aggregation is associated with an increase in cGMP concentration in platelets (HASLAM and McCLENAGHAN, 1974). The effects of NSAID on the concentration of both nucleotides in platelets are not equivocal (BALL et al., 1970; HASLAM and McCLENAGHAN, 1974).

h) Mode of Action

HAMBERG and SAMUELSSON (1974) and SAMUELSSON et al. (1975) have shown that arachidonic acid in addition to its lipoxygenation in platelets (HAMBERG and SAMUELSSON, 1974; NUGTEREN, 1975) is also converted via PGG_2 and PGH_2 to thromboxane A_2 (Fig. 2). These substances initiate the release reaction and thus trigger second-phase aggregation (MALMSTEN et al., 1975; SAMUELSSON et al., 1975). Their pro-aggregatory effects contrast with the potent anti-aggregatory effects of PGE_1 and PGD_2 (SMITH et al., 1974c; NISHIZAWA et al., 1975) and small or ambiguous effects of other PGs (KLOEZE, 1967; WEEKS et al., 1969; CHANDRA SEKHAR, 1970; BRUNO et al., 1974; McDONALD and STUART, 1974).

Thromboxane A_2 (SAMUELSSON et al., 1975) is biologically similar to RCS (PIPER and VANE, 1969). A labile aggregation-stimulating substance (LASS) of WILLIS and KUHN (1973) and an unidentified factor with aggregatory properties of VARGAFTIG (1973) might be the mixtures of PGG_2, PGH_2, and thromboxane A_2. These substances are generated from arachidonic acid by the NSAID-sensitive enzymic system, which is also inhibited by the substrate analogue tetraynoic acid (WILLIS et al., 1974a). Recently, BUNTING et al. (1975) and MONCADA et al. (1976) have identified an enzyme in platelet microsomes which selectively converts PGG_2 and PGH_2 into thromboxane A_2. This thromboxane synthetase is not sensitive to most NSAID which are cyclooxygenase inhibitors.

The discovery by the Swedish scientists offers a direct biochemical explanation for the mechanism of arachidonic acid-induced platelet aggregation and its inhibition by NSAID (SILVER et al., 1973, 1974a; VARGAFTIG and ZIRINIS, 1973; WILLIS and KUHN, 1973; SMITH et al., 1974a, b). There is also substantial evidence that collagen-induced aggregation, as well as the second-phase aggregation induced by adrenaline, thrombin and ADP are mediated by generation of PGG_2, PGH_2, and thromboxane A_2 in platelets (VARGAFTIG and ZIRINIS, 1973; HORNSTRA and HODDEMAN, 1974; SMITH et al., 1974b; WILLIS et al., 1974a, b; FLOWER et al., 1975; GAUT et al., 1975; MALMSTEN et al., 1975; SAMUELSSON et al., 1975).

It might well be that a pro-aggregatory agent, e.g. collagen, induces release of phospholipase A from platelet α-granules (SMITH et al., 1973), and subsequently the digested phospholipids liberate arachidonic acid for the generation of PGG_2, PGH_2, and thromboxane A_2 (FLOWER et al., 1975). These substances liberate ADP from dense-body granules and the released ADP is responsible for the induction of second-phase aggregation (MALMSTEN et al., 1975). Thus, the suppressive effects of NSAID on the second-phase aggregation have a common denominator, that is the inhibition of arachidonic acid cyclo-oxygenase activity in platelets.

i) Relevance of in vitro Anti-Aggregatory Effects of Non-Steroid Anti-Inflammatory Drugs to Their in vivo Activity

Platelet aggregation is believed to play an important role in initiation of microthrombi and vascular inflammation (MUSTARD and PACKHAM, 1970). During the haemostatic process, pro-inflammatory agents are released from platelets (SILVER et al., 1974b; VARGAFTIG et al., 1974). Thus, anti-aggregatory effects of NSAID may contribute to their anti-inflammatory action. On the other hand, platelet cyclo-oxygenase has distinctly different susceptibility to NSAID than cyclo-oxygenases from other tissues (VAGAFTIG and DAO HAI, 1973; PATRONO et al., 1975, 1976; GAUT et al., 1975). This opens the possibility for development of a selective inhibitor of fatty acid cyclo-oxygenase in platelets, which would have anti-thrombotic activity in vivo. The theoretically substantiated objection against this reasoning is that such an inhibitor will also suppress the generation of anti-aggregatory PGE_1 and PGD_2 (see Section C.III.4.h). However, animal studies on fenoprofen (HERRMANN et al., 1972) aspirin (BOUSSER and LECRUBIER, 1973) and sudoxicam (CONSTANTINE and PURCELL, 1973) revealed a good correlation between their in vitro anti-aggregatory and in vivo anti-thrombotic potencies. Unfortunately, it is not the case with all NSAID (FLEMING et al., 1970). Also, aspirin has little or no anti-thrombotic activity in post operative venous thrombosis in man (M.R.C. Steering Committee, 1972), and its effectiveness in prevention of arterial thrombosis is has not yet been ascertained.

5. Effects on Smooth Muscle

The maintenance of the resting tone and/or spontaneous activity of certain smooth muscle organs (e.g. rat fundic stomach strip, rat uterus, rabbit jejunum) depend on the intramural generation of PG. NSAID at low concentrations depress both the muscular tone and the PG release from these organs (AIKEN, 1972, 1974; ECKENFELS and VANE, 1972; FERREIRA et al., 1972; VANE and WILLIAMS, 1973; BOTTING and SALZMANN, 1974). NSAID also inhibit the nerve-mediated contractions of guinea pig ileum, and this effect can be reversed by small amounts of PG (CHONG and DOWNING, 1973; 1974; EHRENPREIS et al., 1973; KADLEC et al., 1974; BENNETT et al., 1975). PG antagonists lower the basal tone of smooth muscle (BENNETT and POSER, 1971), and stomach strips taken from rats deficient in essential fatty acid do not maintain their basal tone (FRANKHUIJZEN and BONTA, 1975). Therefore, a modulatory role of PG in the maintaining of tone and contractility of smooth muscles has been suggested. There are no tissue stores for PG and the release of PGs equals their biosynthesis de novo (PIPER and VANE, 1971; VANE, 1972a, 1972b, 1973a, 1973b), and so smooth muscle preparations can be used to assess the anti-PG synthetase activity of drugs. Indeed, it has been shown that potencies of NSAID which produce tonal inhibition of the rat fundic strip (COLLIER, 1974) and inhibition of rat uterine contractions (AIKEN, 1972, 1974) correspond with those for inhibition of PG synthetase in vitro. Suppression of PG release (PATRONO et al., 1974) and inhibition of spontaneous activity (LEWIS et al., 1975) of the isolated rat uterus have been proposed for the assessment of anti-enzymic and anti-inflammatory potencies of NSAID.

NSAID at relatively high concentrations inhibit contractions of smooth muscles produced by a variety of agents (JAQUES and DEMENJOZ, 1950; STARR and WEST, 1966; COLLIER et al., 1966; NORTHOVER, 1967, 1971; SORRENTINO et al., 1972). Anti-bradykinin activity (COLLIER, 1965; COLLIER et al., 1966; GRYGLEWSKI et al., 1969; BERGER et al., 1973), as well as anti-PG activity (SORRENTINO et al., 1972; BURKA and EYRE, 1974; PANCZENKO et al., 1975; SMITH et al., 1975; TOLMAN and PARTRIDGE, 1975) are the most consistent among NSAID. The antagonistic effects of NSAID on contractile actions of slow reacting substance of anaphylaxis (SRS-A) (COLLIER et al.,

1966) and arachidonic acid hydroperoxide (HELFER and JAQUES, 1974; VAN NEUEN et al., 1975) have been also reported.

The mechanisms for antagonistic actions of NSAID against contractile agents are not highly specific and probably are different for each smooth muscle organ and for each agonist. The following mechanisms have been considered: a) impairment of the PG link in contractile response (ECKENFELS and VANE, 1971; BENNETT et al., 1975; BURNSTOCK et al., 1975); b) binding of NSAID to active sites for agonists (COLLIER et al., 1966; PANCZENKO et al., 1975; TOLMAN and PARTRIDGE, 1975; see also SCHERRER and WHITEHOUSE, 1974); c) inhibition of transmembrane calcium transport (NORTHOVER, 1971, 1973); d) impairment of the interaction between ATP and actomyosin (GÖRÖG and KOVÁCS, 1970b, 1972).

Anti-bradykinin action of NSAID on tracheo-bronchial muscle (COLLIER et al., 1966) and on the guinea pig ileum (COLLIER, 1965; BERGER et al., 1973), as well as anti-PG action of NSAID on the gerbil colon (TOLMAN and PARTRIDGE, 1975) have been used as complementary procedures for assessment of anti-inflammatory activity of drugs.

D. Conclusions

Inhibition of prostaglandin generation in vivo accounts for the therapeutic effectiveness of acidic NSAID. Inhibition of PG biosynthesis in vitro is, therefore, the most promising and rational approach to predict anti-inflammatory activity for new compounds. However, several factors dissociate the concordance of the in vitro and in vivo data. These are mainly individual pharmacokinetic properties of anti-inflammatory agents and their differential inhibitory actions on PG synthetases from various tissues.

All potent acidic NSAID are strongly bound to albumin. Their in vivo anti-PG synthetase potencies and consequently their anti-inflammatory potencies can be attributed to their plasma unbound fractions. Therefore, the in vitro anti-enzymic activity of a compound should be corrected for its binding to albumin in order to obtain a better approximation of the in vitro index for prediction of anti-inflammatory activity in vivo. The direct evaluation of the effects of NSAID on PG generation by microsomal preparations and by cellular preparations may be complemented by the indirect methods consisting of the evaluation of the effects of NSAID on platelet aggregation and smooth muscle tone in vitro.

The potencies of known NSAID which stabilise proteins and biological membranes in vitro are occasionally indicative of their anti-inflammatory potencies in vivo. To obtain these in vitro effects relatively high concentrations of NSAID are required. Furthermore, within series of compounds of unknown anti-inflammatory activities the above in vitro tests very often produce false positive results. Perhaps strong binding of a compound to non-enzymic proteins is a prerequisite but not a sufficient requirement for its strong anti-PG synthetase activity. There are precise (though still unknown) steric, electronic and lipophilic requirements for transforming the chemical structure of a plain 'protein-stabilizer' into that of a PG synthetase inhibitor and thus an anti-inflammatory drug.

Although there are many gaps in our understanding of the interrelationship between the anti-PG synthetase activity in vitro and the anti-inflammatory, analgesic and antipyretic activities in vivo, the 'PG synthetase test' has a better chance of becoming a useful tool for designing new anti-inflammatory drugs than any other test which has been employed until now.

References

Aalto, M., Kulonen, E.: Effects of serotonin, indomethacin, and other antirheumatic drugs on the synthesis of collagen and other proteins in granulation tissues slices. Biochem. Pharmacol. **21**, 2835—2840 (1972)

Abdulla, Y. H., McFarlane, E.: Control of prostaglandin biosynthesis in rat brain homogenates by adenine nucleotides. Biochem. Pharmacol. **21**, 2841—2847 (1972)

Adams, S. S., Cobb, R.: A possible basis for the anti-inflammatory activity of salicylates and other non-hormonal anti-rheumatic drugs. Nature (Lond.) **181**, 773—774 (1958)

Aggeler, P. M., O'Reilly, R. A., Leong, L., Kowitz, P. E.: Potentiation of anti-coagulant effect of warfarin by phenylbutazone. New Engl. J. Med. **276**, 496—501 (1967)

Ahern, D. G., Downing, D. T.: Inhibition of prostaglandin biosynthesis by eicosa-5,8,11,14-tetraynoic acid. Biochim. biophys. Acta **210**, 456—461 (1970)

Aiken, J. W.: Aspirin and indomethacin prolong parturition in rats: Evidence that prostaglandins contribute to expulsion of foetus. Nature (Lond.) **240**, 21—25 (1972)

Aiken, J. W.: Prostaglandin and prostaglandin synthetase inhibitors: Studies on uterine motility and function. In: Robinson, H. J., Vane, J. R. (Eds.): Prostaglandin Synthetase Inhibitors, pp. 289—301. New York: Raven Press 1974

Akamatsu, N., Miura, Y.: Inhibition of aminosugar formation by several non-steroid anti-inflammatory agents. Biochem. Pharmacol. **21**, 1991—1993 (1972)

Alho, A.: Effects of vasoactive drugs on lysosomal stability in vitro. Biochem. Pharmacol. **22**, 2521—2527 (1973)

Al-Mondhiry, H., Marcus, A. J., Spaet, T. H.: On the mechanism of platelet-function inhibition by acetylsalicylic acid. Proc. Soc. exp. Biol. (N.Y.) **133**, 632—636 (1970)

Arfors, K. E., Bygdeman, S., McKenzie, F. N., Svensjö, E.: Effect of acetylsalicylic acid on platelet behaviour in vitro and in vivo. Acta Univ. Carol. [Med.] (Praha) **52**, 75—78 (1972)

Atac, A., Spagnuolo, M., Zucker, M. B.: Long term inhibition of platelet function by aspirin. Proc. Soc. exp. Biol. (N.Y.) **133**, 1331—1333 (1970)

Attallah, A. A., Duchesne, M. J., Lee, J. B.: The effect of salycylic acid on plasma PGA binding and metabolism in the rat. Prostaglandins **6**, 547—548 (1974)

Ball, G., Brereton, G. G., Fulwood, M., Ireland, D. M., Yates, P.: Effect of prostaglandin E_1 alone and in combination with theophylline or aspirin on collagen-induced platelet aggregation and on platelet nucleotides including adenosine 3'5'-cyclic monophosphate. Biochem. J. **120**, 709—718 (1970)

Bauminger, S., Zor, U., Lindner, H. R.: Radioimmunological assay of prostaglandin synthetase activity. Prostaglandins **4**, 313—324 (1973)

Bennett, A., Eley, K. G., Stockley, H. L.: Modulation by prostaglandins of contractions in guinea pig ileum. Prostaglandins **9**, 377—384 (1975)

Bennett, A., Posner, J.: Studies on prostaglandin antagonists. Brit. J. Pharmacol. **42**, 584—594 (1971)

Berger, F. M., Bates, H. M., Diamantis, W., Kletzkin, M., Plekss, O. J., Sofia, R. D., Spencer, H. J.: The pharmacological properties of seclazone (7-chloro-3,3-a-dihydro-2H, 9H-isooxazolo 3,2-b 1,3 benzoxazin-9-one) a new anti-inflammatory agent. Pharmacology **9**, 164—176 (1973)

Bergström, S., Carlson, L. A., Weeks, J. R.: The prostaglandins: a family of biologically active lipids. Pharmacol. Rev. **20**, 1—48 (1968)

Bergström, S., Danielsson, H., Samuelsson, B.: The enzymatic formation of prostaglandin E_2 from arachidonic acid. Biochim. biophys. Acta **90**, 207—210 (1964)

Bertelli, A., Donati, L., Rossano, M. A.: Possible relationship between antiprotease and antiphlogistic activity. In: Garattini, S., Dukes, M. N. G. (Eds.): Nonsteroidal Anti-inflammatory Drugs, pp. 98—102. Amsterdam-New York-London-Milan-Tokyo-Buenos Aires: Excerpta Medica Foundation 1965

Bhattacherjee, P., Eakins, K. E.: Inhibition of the prostaglandin synthetase systems in ocular tissues by indomethacin. Brit. J. Pharmacol. **50**, 227—230 (1974)

Blackham, A., Owen, R. T.: Prostaglandin synthetase inhibitors and leucocytic emigration. J. Pharm. (Lond.) **27**, 201—203 (1975)

Block, H. U., Taube, C., Förster, W.: Einfluß blutdrucksenkender Pharmaka auf die in vitro-Biosynthese der Prostaglandine E und $F_{2\alpha}$ im Kaninchennierenmark. Arch. int. Pharmacodyn. **216**, 160—164 (1975)

Bodel, P., Reynolds, C. F., Atkins, E.: Lack of effect of salicylate on pyrogen release from human blood leucocytes in vitro. Yale J. biol. Med. **46**, 190—195 (1973)

Bologna, E.: Influence of some drugs on platelet aggregation: a study in hypertensive patients. Acta Univ. Carol. [Med.] (Praha) **52**, 87—92 (1972)

Borel, J. F.: Effect of some drugs on the chemotaxis of rabbit neutrophils in vitro. Experientia (Basel) **29**, 676—678 (1973)

Born, G. V. R.: Quantitative investigations into aggregation of blood platelets. J. Physiol. (Lond.) **162**, 67 P—68 P (1962 a)

Born, G. V. R.: Aggregation of blood platelets by adenosine diphosphate and its reversal. Nature (Lond.) **194**, 927—929 (1962 b)

Botting, J. H., Salzmann, R.: The effect of indomethacin on the release of prostaglandin E_2 and acetylocholine from guinea pig isolated ileum at rest and during field stimulation. Brit. J. Pharmacol. **50**, 119—124 (1974)

Bousser, M. G., Lecrubier, C.: Agrégation plaquettaire expérimentale et thrombose artérielle. Action de l'aspirine. Nouv. Presse méd. **25**, 1687—1692 (1973)

Brodie, B. B., Hogben, C. A. M.: Some physico-chemical factors in drug action. J. Pharm. (Lond.) **9**, 345—380 (1957)

Brody, T. M.: Action of sodium salicylate and related compounds on tissue metabolism in vitro. J. Pharmacol. exp. Ther. **117**, 39—51 (1956)

Brown, J. H., Mackey, H. K.: Further studies on the erythrocyte anti-inflammatory assay. Proc. Soc. exp. Biol. (N.Y.) **128**, 504—509 (1968)

Brown, J. H., Mackay, H. K., Rigillo, D. A.: A novel in vitro assay for anti-inflammatory agents based on stabilization of erythrocytes. Proc. Soc. exp. Biol. (N.Y.) **125**, 837—843 (1967)

Brown, J. H., Pollock, S. H.: Inhibition of elastase and collagenase by anti-inflammatory drugs. Proc. Soc. exp. Biol. (N.Y.) **135**, 792—795 (1970)

Brown, J. H., Schwartz, N. L.: Interaction of lysosomes and anti-inflammatory drugs. Proc. Soc. exp. Biol. (N.Y.) **131**, 614—620 (1969)

Brown, J. H., Taylor, J. L., Waters, I. W.: Effect of pH on erythrocyte stabilization by anti-inflammatory drugs. Proc. Soc. exp. Biol. (N.Y.) **136**, 137—140 (1971)

Bruno, J. J., Taylor, L. A., Droller, M. J.: Effects of prostaglandin E_2 on human platelet adenyl cyclase and aggregation. Nature (Lond.) **251**, 721—723 (1974)

Bryant, C., Smith, M. J. H.: Effects of salicylate and γ-resorcylate on the metabolism of radioactive succinate and fumarate by rat liver mitochondria and on dehydrogenase enzymes. Biochem. J. **86**, 391—396 (1963)

Bunting, S., Moncada, S., Needleman, P., Vane, J. R.: Formation of prostaglandin endoperoxides and rabbit aorta contracting substance (RCS) by coupling two enzymes. Proc. Brit. pharmacol. soc. 17—15 Dec., 6—7 (1975)

Burka, J. F., Eyre, P.: Studies on prostaglandins and prostaglandin antagonists on bovine pulmonary vein in vitro. Prostaglandins **6**, 333—343 (1974)

Burleigh, M., Smith, M. J.: The site of the inhibitory action of salicylate on protein biosynthesis in vitro. J. Pharm. (Lond.) **23**, 518—527 (1971)

Burnstock, G., Cocks, T., Paddle, B., Staszewska-Barczak, J.: Evidence that prostaglandin is responsible for the "rebound contraction" following stimulation of non-adrenergic, non-cholinergic ("purinergic") inhibitory nerves. Europ. J. Pharmacol. **31**, 360—362 (1975)

Burstein, S., Levin, E., Varanelli, C.: Prostaglandins and cannabis. II. Inhibition of biosynthesis by the naturally occuring cannabinoids. Biochem. Pharmacol. **22**, 2905—2910 (1973)

Burstein, S., Raz, A.: Inhibition of prostaglandin E_2 biosynthesis by Δ^1-tetrahydrocannabinol. Prostaglandins 2, 369—374 (1972)

Burstein, S., Varanelli, C., Slade, L.: Prostaglandins and cannabis. III. Inhibition of biosynthesis by essential oil components of marihuana. Biochem. Pharmacol. 24, 1053—1054 (1975)

Butler, M., Giannina, T., Cargill, D. I., Popick, F., Steinetz, B. G.: Abnormal sulfhydryl-disulfide interchange in serum of rats with adjuvant arthritis: Correction by anti-inflammatory drugs. Proc. Soc. exp. Biol. (N.Y.) 132, 484—488 (1969)

Caprino, L., Borelli, F., Falchetti, R.: Pharmacological research on 4,5-diphenyl-2-bis(2-hydroxy-ethyl)-aminoxazol (Ditazol), a new synthetic oxazole derivative as an anti-inflammatory agent. Arzneimittel-Forsch. 23, 1272—1277 (1973a)

Caprino, L., Borelli, F., Falchetti, R.: Effect of 4,5-diphenyl-2-bis-(2-hydroxyethyl)-aminoxazol (Ditazol) on platelet aggregation, adhesiveness and bleeding time. Arzneimittel-Forsch. 23, 1277—1283 (1973b)

Caprino, L., Rossi, E. C.: Platelet aggregation and drugs. Proceedings of the Serono Symposia, vol. 3, London-New York-San Francisco: Academic Press 1974

Carrano, R. A., Malbica, J. O.: Primary screening approach for anti-inflammatory agents utilizing an in vivo and a new in vitro method. J. pharm. Sci. 61, 1450—1453 (1972)

Čepelák, V., Roubal, Z., Čepeláková, H., Němeček, O.: Chemical induction of fibrinolysis and inhibition of platelet aggregation (with special respect to effect of nonsteroid antiinflammatory drugs). Acta Univ. Carol. [Med.] (Praha) 52, 41—47 (1972)

Chandra Sekhar, N.: Effect of eight prostaglandins on platelet aggregation. J. med. Chem. 13, 39—44 (1970)

Chang, Y. H.: Studies on phagocytosis. II. The effect of non-steroidal anti-inflammatory drugs on phagocytosis and on urate crystal-induced canine joint inflammation. J. Pharmacol. exp. Ther. 183, 235—244 (1972)

Chang, Y. H.: Mechanism of action of colchicine. II. Effects of colchicine and its analogs on phagocytosis and chemotaxis in vitro. J. Pharmacol. exp. Ther. 194, 159—164 (1975)

Chaplin, M. D., Roszkowski, A. P., Richards, R. K.: Displacement of thiopental from plasma proteins by non-steroidal anti-inflammatory agents. Proc. Soc. exp. Biol. (N.Y.) 143, 667—671 (1973)

Chayen, J., Bitensky, L., Ubhi, G. S.: The experimental modification of lysosomal dysfunction by anti-inflammatory drugs acting in vitro. Beitr. path. Anat. 147, 6—20 (1972)

Chignell, C. F.: Optimal studies of drug-protein complexes III. Interaction of flufenamic acid and other N-aryl-anthranilates with serum albumin. Molec. Pharmacol. 5, 455—462 (1969)

Chignell, C. F.: Physical methods for studing drug-protein binding. In: Handbook of experimental Pharmacology. Concepts in Biochemical Pharmacology, Vol. XXVIII/1, pp. 187—212. Berlin-Heidelberg-New York: Springer 1971

Chong, E. K. S., Downing, O. A.: Selective inhibition of angiotensin-induced contractions of smooth muscle by indomethacin. J. Pharm. (Lond.) 25, 170—172 (1973)

Chong, E. K. S., Downing, O. A.: Reversal by prostaglandin E_2 of the inhibitory effect of indomethacin on contractions of guinea pig ileum induced by angiotensin. J. Pharm. (Lond.) 26, 729—730 (1974)

Collier, H. O. J.: Some pharmacological correlates of anti-inflammatory activity: a study on non-steroidal anti-inflammatory drugs as antagonists of local hormones. In: Non-steroidal Anti-inflammatory Drugs, pp. 139—150. Amsterdam-New York-London-Milan-Tokyo-Buenos Aires: Excerpta Medica Foundation 1965

Collier, H. O. J.: Prostaglandin synthetase inhibitors and the gut. In: Prostaglandin Synthetase Inhibitors, pp. 121—133. New York: Raven Press 1974

Collier, H. O. J., James, G. W. L., Schneider, C.: Antagonism by aspirin and fenamates of bronchoconstriction and nociception induced by adenosine-5'-triphosphate. Nature (Lond.) 212, 411—412 (1966)

Collier, J. G., Flower, R. J.: Effect of aspirin on human seminal prostaglandins. Lancet 1971, II, 852—853

Constantine, J. W., Purcell, I. M.: Inhibition of platelet aggregation and of experimental thrombosis by sudoxicam. J. Pharmacol. exp. Ther. 187, 653—665 (1973)

Coppi, G., Bonardi, G., Vidi, A.: Effects of 4-prenyl-1,2-diphenyl-3,5-pyrazolidinedione (DA 2370, fenilprenazone) on lysosomes. Biochem. Pharmacol. 22, 1237—1239 (1973)

Crook, D., Collins, A. J.: Prostaglandin synthetase activity from human rheumatoid synowial tissue and its inhibition by non-steroidal anti-inflammatory drugs. Prostaglandins **9**, 857—865 (1975)

Davies, G. E., Holman, G., Johnston, T. P., Lowe, J. S.: Studies on kallikrein: failure of some anti-inflammatory drugs to affect release of kinin. Brit. J. Pharmacol. **28**, 212—217 (1966)

Dawkins, P. D., McArthur, J. N., Smith, M. J. H.: The effect of sodium salicylate on the binding of long-chain fatty acids to plasma proteins. J. Pharm. (Lond.) **22**, 405—410 (1970)

Dawson, A. G.: Effects of acetylsalicylate on gluconeogenesis in isolated rat kidney tubules. Biochem. Pharmacol. **24**, 1407—1411 (1975)

Deby, C., Bacq, Z. M., Simon, D.: In vitro inhibition of the biosynthesis of a prostaglandin by gold and silver. Biochem. Pharmacol. **22**, 3141—3143 (1973)

Deby, C., Descamps, M., Binon, F., Bacq, Z. M.: Inhibition de la biosynthése in vitro de la prosta-glandine E_2 par des substances anti-inflamatoires. C.R. Soc. Biol. (Paris) **165**, 2465—2468 (1971)

Deby, C., Descamps, M., Binon, F., Bacq, Z. M.: Correlation between anti-inflammatory proper-ties and inhibition of prostaglandin biosynthesis in vitro. Biochem. Pharmacol. **24**, 1089—1092 (1975)

De Clerck, F., Vermylen, J., Reneman, R.: Effects of suprofen, an inhibitor of prostaglandin bio-synthesis, on platelet function, plasma coagulation and fibrynolysis. I. In vitro experiments. Arch. int. Pharmacodyn. **216**, 263—279 (1975)

De Gaetano, G., Donati, M. B., Vermylen, J.: Some effects of indomethacin an platelet function, blood coagulation and fibrynolysis. Int. J. clin. Pharmacol. **5**, 196—199 (1971 a)

De Gaetano, G., Vermylen, J., Verstraete, M.: L'inhibition de l'agrégation plaquettaire: données expérimentales et perspectives cliniques. Nouv. Rev. franc. Hémat. **11**, 339—364 (1971 b)

De Gaetano, G., Vermylen, J., Verstraete, M.: Platelet aggregation by Thrombofax. Acta Univ. Carol. Med. (Praha) **53/54**, 391—398 (1972)

Dembińska-Kieć, A., Krupińska, J., Sobański, H., Gryglewski, R.: Selective inhibitors of prosta-glandin synthetase from rabbit brain. Abstracts of International Conference on Prosta-glandins, Florence, p. 39, 1975

Desnoyers, P., Labume, J., Conrad, J., Samama, M.: Research on the mechanism of synthetic thrombolytic agents. Acta Univ. Carol. [Med.] (Praha) **52**, 33—40 (1972)

Desnoyers, P., Verry, M.: Measure of platelet stickness: the glaaa beads retention test in animal and human being. Acta Univ. Carol. [Med.] (Praha) **53/54**, 381—389 (1972)

Dingle, J. T.: Lysosomes: a laboratory handbook. Amsterdam-London: North-Holland 1972

Dinnendahl, V., Kalbhen, D. A.: Pharmakologische Studien zur Beeinflussung des Chondroitin-sulfat-Abbaus in vitro. Arch. int. Pharmacodyn. **192**, 302—320 (1971)

Dinnendahl, V., Peters, H. D., Schönhöfer, P. S.: Effects of sodium salicylate and acetylsalicylic acid on cyclic $3',5'$-AMP-dependent protein kinase. Biochem. Pharmacol. **22**, 2223—2228 (1973)

DiRosa, M.: Prostaglandins, leucocytes and non-steroidal anti-inflammatory drugs. Pol. J. Phar-macol. Pharm. **26**, 25—36 (1974)

Dunn, W. J.: III. Binding of certain non-steroidal anti-inflammatory agents and uricosuric agents to human serum albumin. J. med. Chem. **16**, 484—486 (1973)

Eakins, K. E.: Prostaglandins and prostaglandin synthetase inhibitors: action in ocular disease. In: Prostaglandin Synthetase Inhibitors, pp. 343—352. New York: Raven Press 1974

Eckenfels, A., Vane, J. R.: Prostaglandins: oxygen tension and smooth muscle tone. Brit. J. Phar-macol. **45**, 451—462 (1972)

Ehrenpreis, S., Greenberg, J., Belman, S.: Prostaglandins reverse inhibition of electrically-induced contractions of guinea pig ileum by morphine, indomethacin and acetylsalicyclic acid. Na-ture (Lond.) **245**, 280—282 (1973)

Evans, G., Packham, M. A., Nishizawa, E. E., Mustard, J. F.: The effect of acetylsalicylic acid (aspi-rin) on platelet function. J. exp. Med. **128**, 877—894 (1968)

Evans, G., Packham, M. A., Nishizawa, E. E., Mustard, J. F., Murphy, E. A.: The effect of acetysali-cylic acid on platelet function. J. exp. Med. **128**, 877—894 (1968)

Famaey, J. P.: Interactions between non-steroidal anti-inflammatory drugs and biological mem-branes. I. High amplitude pseudoenergized mitochondrial swelling and membrane perme-ability changes induced by various non-steroidal anti-inflammatory drugs. Biochem. Phar-macol. **22**, 2693—2705 (1973)

Famaey, J. P., Mockel, J.: Importance of sulfhydryl groups for the uncoupling activity of non-steroidal acidic anti-inflammatory drugs and valionomycin in oxidative phosphorylation. Biochem. Pharmacol. **22**, 1487—1498 (1973)

Famaey, J. P., Whitehouse, M. W.: Interactions between non-steroidal antiinflammatory drugs and biological membranes. II. Swelling and membrane permeability changes induced in some immuno-competent cells by various non-steroidal anti-inflammatory drugs. Biochem. Pharmacol. **22**, 2707—2717 (1973)

Famaey, J. P., Whitehouse, M. W.: Interaction between non-steroidal anti-inflammatory drugs and biological membranes. IV. Effects of non-steroidal anti-inflammatory drugs and various ions on the availability of sulfhydryl groups and lymphoid cells and mitochondrial membranes. Biochem. Pharmacol. **24**, 1609—1615 (1975)

Famaey, J. P., Whitehouse, M. W., Dick, W. C.: Interactions between non-steroidal anti-inflammatory drugs and biological membranes. III. Effect of non-steroidal anti-inflammatory drugs on bound mitochondrial bromothymol blue and possible intramitochondrial pH variations induced by these drugs. Biochem. Pharmacol. **24**, 267—275 (1975)

Fenichel, R. L., Dougherty, J. A., Alburn, H. E.: Inhibition of platelet aggregation by 2-(p-chloro-phenyl)-4-thiazoleacrylic acid (Wy-23,049)—comparison with acetylsalicylic acid. Biochem. Pharmacol. **23**, 3273—3282 (1974)

Ferreira, S. H., Herman, A., Vane, J. R.: Prostaglandin generation maintains the smooth muscle tone of the rabbit isolated jejunum. Brit. J. Pharmacol. **44**, 328P—329P (1972)

Ferreira, S. H., Moncada, S., Vane, J. R.: Indomethacin and aspirin abolish prostaglandin release from the spleen. Nature (New Biol.) **231**, 237—239 (1971)

Ferreira, S. H., Moncada, S., Vane, I. R.: Prostaglandin and signs and symptoms of inflammation. In: Prostaglandin Synthetase Inhibitors, pp. 175—187. New York: Raven Press 1974

Fjalland, B.: Inhibition by non-steroidal anti-inflammatory agents of the release of rabbit aorta contracting substance and prostaglandins from chopped guinea pig lungs. J. Pharm. (Lond.) **26**, 448—451 (1974)

Fleming, J. S., Bierwagen, M. E., Campbell, J. A., King, S. P.: The effect of new anti-inflammatory agent (5-cyclohexylindan-1-carboxylic acid, BL-2365) on platelet aggregation. Arch. int. Pharmacodyn. **199**, 164—171 (1972)

Fleming, J. S., Bierwagen, M. E., Losada, M., Campbell, J. A. L., King, S. P., Pindell, M. H.: The effect of three anti-inflammatory agents on platelet aggregation, in vitro and in vivo. Arch. int. Pharmacodyn. **186**, 120—128 (1970)

Flores, A. G. A., Sharp, G. W. G.: Endogenous prostaglandins and osmotic water flow in the toad bladder. Amer. J. Physiol. **223**, 1392—1397 (1972)

Flower, R. J.: Drugs which inhibit prostaglandin biosynthesis. Pharmacol. Rev. **26**, 33—67 (1974)

Flower, R. J., Blackwell, G. J., Parsons, M. F.: Mechanism of collagen induced platelet aggregation. Abstracts VI. International Congress Pharmacology p. 292. Helsinki 1975

Flower, R. J., Cheung, H. S., Cushman, D. W.: Quantitative determination of prostaglandins and malonyldialdehyde formed by arachidonate oxygenase system in bovine seminal vesicles. Prostaglandins **4**, 325—341 (1973)

Flower, R. J., Gryglewski, R., Herbaczynska-Cedro, K., Vane, J. R.: The effect of anti-inflammatory drugs on prostaglandin biosynthesis. Nature (New Biol.) **238**, 104—106 (1972)

Flower, R. J., Vane, J. R.: Inhibition of prostaglandin synthetase in brain explains the antipyretic activity of paracetamol (4-acetamidophenol). Nature (Lond.) **240**, 410—411 (1972)

Flower, R. J., Vane, J. R.: Inhibition of prostaglandin biosynthesis. Biochem. Pharmacol. **23**, 1439—1450 (1974a)

Flower, R. J., Vane, J. R.: Some pharmacologic and biochemical aspects of prostaglandin biosynthesis. In: Prostaglandin biosynthesis inhibitors, pp. 1—18. New York: Raven Press 1974b

Ford-Hutchinson, A. W., Smith, M. J. H., Elliot, P. N. C., Bolam, J. G., Walker, J. R., Lobo, A. A., Badcock, J. K., Colledge, A. J., Billimoria, F. J.: Effects of human plasma fraction on leucocyte migration into inflammatory exudates. J. Pharm. (Lond.) **27**, 106—112 (1975)

Förström, L., Goldyne, M. E., Winkelmann, R. K.: Prostaglandin production by human epidermal cells in vitro: a model for studing pharmacological inhibition of prostaglandin synthesis. Prostaglandins **8**, 107—115 (1974)

Frankhuijzen, A. L., Bonta, I. L.: Role of prostaglandins in tone and effector reactivity of the isolated rat stomach preparation. Europ. J. Pharmacol. **31**, 44—52 (1975)

Free, S. M., Jr., Wilson, J. W.: A mathematical contribution to structure-activity studies. J. med. Chem. **7**, 395—399 (1964)

Gaut, Z. N., Baruth, H., Randall, L. O., Ashley, C., Paulsrud, J. R.: Stereometric relationships among anti-inflammatory activity, inhibition of platelet aggregation, and inhibition of prostaglandin synthetase. Prostaglandins **10**, 59—66 (1975)

Gaut, Z. N., Solomon, H. M.: Inhibition of nicotinate phosphoribosyl transferase by non-steroidal anti-inflammatory drugs. J. pharm. Sci. **60**, 1887—1888 (1971)

Gerber, D. A., Cohen, N., Giustra, R.: The ability of nonsteroidal anti-inflammatory compounds to accelerate a disulfide interchange reaction of serum sulfhydryl groups and 5',5'-dithio-bis-(2-nitrobenzoic) acid. Biochem. Pharmacol. **16**, 115—123 (1967)

Glatt, M., Graf, P., Brune, K.: Anti-inflammatory doses of colchicine increase prostaglandin content in inflamed tissue. Abstracts of International Conference on Prostaglandins, Florence, 1975, p. 40

Glenn, E. M., Bowman, B. J.: In vitro effects of non-steroidal anti-inflammatory drugs. Proc. Soc. exp. Biol. (N.Y.) **130**, 1327—1332 (1969)

Glenn, E. M., Rohloff, N., Bowman, B. J., Lyster, S. C.: The pharmacology of 2-(2-fluoro-4-biphenylyl)propionic acid (flurbiprofen), a potent non-steroidal anti-inflammatory drug. Agents Actions **3/4**, 210—216 (1973)

Glenn, E. M., Wilks, J., Bowman, B. J.: Platelets, prostaglandins, red cells, sedimentations rates, serum and tissue proteins and non-steroidal anti-inflammatory drugs. Proc. Soc. exp. Biol. (N.Y.) **141**, 879—886 (1972)

Gordon, D., Bray, M. A.: Macrophage prostaglandin synthesis: a screen for non-steroidal anti-inflammatory drugs relevant to inflammation. Abstracts VI International Congress Pharmacology, p. 425, Helsinki 1975

Gordon, J. L., MacIntyre, D. E.: Inhibition of collagen-induced platelet aggregation by aspirin. Brit. J. Pharmacol. **50**, 469P (1974)

Görög, P., Kovàcs, I. B.: The inhibitory effect of non-steroidal anti-inflammatory agents on aggregation of red cells in vitro. J. Pharm. (Lond.) **22**, 86—92 (1970a)

Görög, P., Kovàcs, I. B.: Effect of anti-inflammatory compounds on actomyosin-adeno-sinetriphosphate interaction. Biochem. Pharmacol. **19**, 2289—2294 (1970b)

Görög, P., Kovàcs, I. B.: Superprecipitation of vascular actomyosin. Effect of vasoactive compounds and anti-inflammatory agents on the process. Biochem. Pharmacol. **21**, 1713—1723 (1972)

Gould, B. J., Huggins, A. K., Smith, M. J. K.: Effects of salicylate on glutamate dehydrogenase and glutamate decarboxylase. Biochem. J. **88**, 346—349 (1963)

Grant, N. H., Alburn, H. E., Kryzanavskas, C.: Stabilization of serum albumin by anti-inflammatory drugs. Biochem. Pharmacol. **19**, 715—722 (1970)

Grant, N. H., Alburn, H. E., Singer, A. C.: Correlation between in vitro and in vivo models in anti-inflammatory drug studies. Biochem. Pharmacol. **20**, 2137—2140 (1971)

Greaves, M. W., Kingston, W. P., Pretty, K.: Action of series of non-steroidal and steroid anti-inflammatory drugs on prostaglandin synthesis by microsomal fraction of rat skin. Brit. J. Pharmacol. **53**, 470 (1975)

Green, D., Dunne, B., Schmid, F. R., Rossi, E. C., Louis, G.: A study of the variable response of human platelets to collagen Relation to aspirin-induced inhibition of aggregation. Amer. J. clin. Path. **60**, 920—926 (1973)

Gryglewski, R.: The fibrynolytic activity of anti-inflammatory drugs. J. Pharm. (Lond.) **18**, 474 (1966)

Gryglewski, R.: On the mechanism of fibrynolysis induced by anti-inflammatory drugs. In: Chemical control of fibrynolysis, thrombolysis. pp. 44—72. New York-London-Sidney-Toronto: Wiley-Interscience 1970

Gryglewski, R.: Structure-activity relationships of some prostaglandin synthetase inhibitors. In: Prostaglandin synthetase inhibitors. pp. 33—52. New York: Raven Press 1974

Gryglewski, R.: Prostaglandins and prostaglandin synthesis inhibitors in etiology and treatment of inflammation. Abstracts VIth International Congress Pharmacology, p. 482. Helsinki 1975

Gryglewski, R.: Eckstein, M.: Fibrinolytic activity of some biarylcarboxylic acids. Nature (Lond.) **214**, 626—627 (1967)

Gryglewski, R., Gryglewska, T.: The fibrinolytic activity of N-arylanthranilates. Biochem. Pharmacol. 15, 1171—1175 (1966)

Gryglewski, R., Panczenko, B.: The influence of sodium flufenamate an the reaction of protein sulfhydryl groups with beta-hydroxyethyl-2,4-dinitrophenyldisulfide (HEDD). Diss. pharm. (Krakow) 20, 479—488 (1968)

Gryglewski, R., Panczenko, B., Górka, Z., Chytkowski, A., Zmuda, A.: Antibradykinin activity of flufenamic acid. Diss. pharm. (Kraków) 21, 1—14 (1969)

Gryglewski, R., Ryznerski, Z., Gorczyca, M., Krupińska, J.: Design of new prostaglandin synthetase inhibitors in a group of N-(2-carboxyphenyl)phenoxyacetamides and their anti-inflammatory activity. In: Advances in Prostaglandin and thromboxane Research, pp. 117—120. New York: Raven Press 1976

Gryglewski, R., Vane, J. R.: The release of prostaglandins and rabbit aorta contracting substance (RCS) from rabbit spleen and its antagonism by anti-inflammatory drugs. Brit. J. Pharmacol. 45, 37—47 (1972a)

Gryglewski, R., Vane, I. R.: The generation from arachidonic acid of rabbit aorta contracting substance (RCS) by microsomal enzyme preparation which also generates prostaglandins. Brit. J. Pharmacol. 46, 449—457 (1972b)

Gulick-Krzywicky, T., Schechter, E., Iwataobu, M., Rank, I. L., Luzati, V.: Correlation between structure and spectroscopic properties in membrane systems: tryptophane and 1-anilino-8-naphtalene sulphonate fluorescence in protein-lipid-water phases. Biochim. biophys. Acta 219, 1—10 (1970)

Ham, E. A., Cirillo, K. J., Zanetti, M., Shen, T. Y., Kuehl, F. A.: Studies on the mode of action of non-steroidal anti-inflammatory agents. In: Prostaglandins in cellular biology, pp. 345—352. New York: Plenum Press 1972

Hamberg, M.: Inhibition of prostaglandin synthesis in man. Biochem. biophys. Res. Commun. 49, 720—726 (1972)

Hamberg, M., Samuelsson, B.: Detection and isolation of and endoperoxide intermediate in prostaglandin biosynthesis. Proc. nat. Acad. Sci. (Wash.) 70, 899—903 (1973)

Hamberg, M., Samuelsson, B.: Prostaglandin endoperoxides. Novel transformations of arachidonic acid in human platelets. Proc. nat. Acad. Sci. (Wash.) 71, 3400—3404 (1974)

Hamberg, M., Svenson, J., Wakabayashi, T., Samuelsson, B.: Isolation and structure of two prostaglandins endoperoxides that cause platelet aggregation. Proc. nat. Acad. Sci. (Wash.) 71, 345—449 (1974)

Hansch, C., von Kaulla, K. N.: Fibrinolytic congeners of benzoic and salicylic acid. A mathematical analysis of correlation between structure and activity. Biochem. Pharmacol. 19, 2193—2200 (1970)

Harford, D. J., Smith, M. J. H.: The effect of sodium salicylate on the release of acid phosphatase activity from rat liver lysosomes in vitro. J. Pharm. (Lond.) 22, 587—583 (1970)

Haslam, R. J., McClenagham, M. D.: Effects of collagen and of aspirin on the concentration of guanosine 3′5′-cyclic monophosphate in human blood platelets: measurent by prelabelling technique. Biochem. J. 138, 317—320 (1974)

Hebborn, P., Shaw, B.: The action of sodium salicylate and aspirin on some kallikrein systems. Brit. J. Pharmacol. 20, 254—263 (1963)

Helfer, H., Jaques, R.: Vasotropic activity of arachidonic acid peroxide on the isolated murine portal vein and its modification by anti-inflammatory substances. Experientia (Basel) 30, 172—173 (1974)

Henson, P. M.: Mechanism of mediator release from inflammatory cells. In: Mediators of Inflammation, pp. 9—50. New York-London: Plenum Press 1974

Herrmann, R. G., Marshall, W. S., Crowe, V. G., Frank, J. D., Marlett, D. L., Lacefield, W. B.: Effect of a new anti-inflammatory drug, fenoprofen, on platelet aggregation and thrombus formation. Proc. Soc. exp. Biol. (N.Y.) 139, 548—552 (1972)

Higgs, G. A., McCall, E., Youlten, L. J. F.: A chemotactic role of prostaglandins released from polymorphonuclear leucocytes during phogocytosis. Brit. J. Pharmacol. 53, 539—546 (1975)

Higgs, G. A., Youlten, L. J. F.: Prostaglandin production by rabbit peritoeal polymorphonuclear leucocytes in vitro. Brit. J. Pharmacol. 44, 330P (1972)

Ho, P. P., Esterman, M. A.: Fenoprofen: inhibition of prostaglandin synthesis. Prostaglandins 6, 107—113 (1974)

Hornstra, G., Haddeman, E.: Prostaglandins, essential free fatty acids, platelet function and thrombosis. Thromb. Res. **4** Suppl. I, 91—92 (1974)

Horodniak, J. W., Julius, M., Zarembo, J. E., Bender, D.: Inhibitory effects of aspirin and indomethacin in the biosynthesis of PGE_2 and $PGF_{2\alpha}$. Biochem. biophys. Res. Commun. **57**, 539—545 (1974)

Horton, E. W., Jones, R. L., Marr, G. G.: Effects of aspirin on prostaglandin and fructose levels in human semen. J. Reprod. Fertil. **33**, 385—392 (1973)

Ignarro, L. J.: Effects of anti-inflammatory drugs on the stability of rat liver lysosomes in vitro. Biochem. Pharmacol. **20**, 2847—2860 (1971 a)

Ignarro, L. J.: Dissimilar effects of anti-inflammatory drugs on stability of lysosomes from peritoneal and circulating leukocytes and liver. Biochem. Pharmacol. **20**, 2861—2870 (1971 b)

Ignarro, L. J.: Lysosomal membrane stabilization in vivo: effects of steroidal and non-steroidal anti-inflammatory drugs on the intergrity of rat liver lysosomes. J. Pharmacol. exp. Ther. **182**, 179—188 (1972)

Ignarro, L. J.: Preservation of structural integrity of liver lysosomes and membrane-stabilizating action of anti-inflammatory drugs, catecholamines and cyclic adenosine monophosphate in isotonic salt media. Biochem. Pharmacol. **22**, 1269—1282 (1973)

Ignarro, L. J.: Regulation of lysosomal enzyme secretion: role in inflammation. Agents Actions **4**, 241—258 (1974)

Ignarro, L. J., Colombo, C.: Enzyme release from guinea pig polymorphonuclear leukocyte lysosomes inhibited in vitro by anti-inflammatory drugs. Nature (New Biol.) **239**, 155—157 (1972)

Inglot, A. D., Kochman, M., Mastalerz, P.: Aktiwnost salicylatow kak ingibitorov virusnoj replikacii in vitro i sposob ich diejstvia. Acta virol. **10**, 185—194 (1966)

Inglot, A. D., Machon, Z. D., Wolna, E., Wilimowski, M., Prandota, J.: New isothiazole derivatives. II. Cytotoxicity and antiviral activity in tissue cultures. Arch. Immunol. Ther. exp. **21**, 891—902 (1973)

Inglot, A. D., Wolna, E.: Reactions of non-steroidal anti-inflammatory drugs with the erythrocyte membrane. Biochem. Pharmacol. **17**, 269—279 (1968)

Inglot, A. D., Woyton, A.: Topical treatment of cutaneous Herpes simplex in humans with the non-steroidal anti-inflammatory drugs: mefenamic acid and indomethacin in dimethylsulfoxide. Arch. Immunol. Ther. exp. **19**, 555—566 (1971)

Izuka, Y., Kobayashi, K., Tanaka, K.: Anti-inflammatory effect of bimetopyrol. IV. Stabilizing effect on rat liver lysosomes. Yakugaku Zasshi **92**, 311—315 (1972)

Janakidevi, K., Smith, M. J. H.: Inhibition of nucleic acid polimerases by salicylate in vitro. J. Pharm. (Lond.) **21**, 401—402 (1969)

Janakidevi, K., Smith, M. J. H.: Differential inhibition of RNA polymerase activities by salicylate in vitro. J. Pharm. Pharmacol. **22**, 58—59 (1970a)

Janakidevi, K., Smith, M. J. H.: Effects of salicylate on RNA polymerase activity and on the incorporation of orotic acid and thymidine into the nucleic acid of rat foetuses in vitro. J. Pharm. (Lond.) **22**, 249—252 (1970 b)

Jaques, R., Domenjoz, R.: Histaminantagonistische Wirkung bei Pyrazolen und Antihistaminen. Naunyn-Schmiedeberg's Arch. exp. Path. Pharmak. **212**, 124—134 (1950)

Kadlec, O. K., Mašek, K., Šeferna, I.: A modulating role of prostaglandins in contractions of the guinea pig ileum. Brit. J. Pharmacol. **51**, 565—570 (1974)

Kalbhen, D. A.: Hemmung der Hitzedenaturierung ono Albumin durch Antiphlogistika/Antirheumatica. Dtsch. med. Wschr. **97**, 918—919 (1972)

Kalbhen, D. A., Gelderblom, P., Domenjoz, R.: Effect of antirheumatic drugs on human erythrocyte membranes. Pharmacology **3**, 353—366 (1970)

Kalbhen, D. A., Habib-Mahmoud, A.: Einfluß entzündungshemmender Pharmaka auf die hitzeinduzierte Schädigung menschlicher Leukozyten in vitro. Arzneimittel-Forsch. **23**, 1016—1020 (1973)

Kalbhen, D. A., Loyen, R.: Wirkung neuer Antirheumatica/Antiphlogistika auf die hitzeinduzierte Hämolyse menschlicher Erythrozyten in vitro. Arzneimittel-Forsch. **23**, 945—949 (1973)

Kaley, G., Weiner, R.: Prostaglandin E_1: A potential mediator of the inflammatory response. Ann. N.Y. Acad. Sci. **180**, 338—350 (1971)

Karzel, K.: Der Einfluß von Antiphlogistica auf Lebens- und Vermehrungsfähigkeit normaler und neoplastischer Zellen in vitro. Arch. int. Pharmacodyn. **169**, 70—82 (1967)

Karzel, K., Aulepp, H., Hack, G.: Effects of recently developed antiphlogistic drugs on viability, reduplication, mean volume and volume distribution of mammalian cells cultured in vitro. Pharmacology **10**, 272—290 (1973)

Karzel, K., Peters, H. D., Hack, G.: Zum Nachweis von Antiphlogistikawirkungen auf die Vermehrung und den Vermehrungsstoffwechsel teilungsfähiger Zellen in vitro. Int. J. clin. Pharmacol. **5**, 203—205 (1971 a)

Karzel, K., Peters, H. D., Hack, G.: Untersuchungen zum Mechanismus der cytostatischen Wirkung einiger Antiphlogistica. Naunyn-Schmiedebergs Arch. Pharmacol. **269**, 485 (1971 b)

Keller, H. U., Sorkin, E.: The effect of anti-inflammatory drugs on chemotaxis of granulocytes. In: Non-steroidal Anti-inflammatory Drugs, pp. 134—135. Amsterdam-New York-London-Milan-Tokyo-Buenos Aires: Excerpta Medica Foundation 1965

Keresztes-Nagy, S., Mais, R. F., Oester, Y. T., Zaroslinski, J. F.: Protein binding methodology: comparison of equilibrium dialysis and frontal analysis chromatography in the study of salicylate binding. Analyt. Biochem. **48**, 80—89 (1972)

Klein, G., Altmann, H., Wottawa, A., Eberl, R.: Über den Einfluß von Naproxen auf die DNS-Synthese und DNS-Reparatur menschlicher Lymphozyten. Arzneimittel-Forsch. **24**, 960—961 (1974)

Kloeze, J.: Influence of prostaglandins on platelet adhessivenes and platelet aggregation. In: Second Nobel Symposium, pp. 241—252. Stockholm: Almquist and Wiksell 1967

Kovács, I. B., Görög, P.: The effect of anti-inflammatory drugs on the aggregation and adhesiveness of platelets, red cells an leukocytes. Acta Univ. Carol. [Med.] (Praha) **52**, 69—73 (1972)

Krupp, P., Exer, B., Menassé, R., Ziel, R.: Neue Aspekte der Entzündungshemmung durch nichtsteroide Antiphlogistica: Wirkung von Voltaren. Schweiz. med. Wschr. **105**, 646—652 (1975)

Krupp, P., Wesp, M.: Inhibition of prostaglandin synthetase by psychotropic drugs. Experientia (Basel) **31**, 330—331 (1975)

Ku, E. C., Wasvary, J. M.: Inhibition of prostaglandin synthetase by pirprofen. Studies with sheep seminal vesicle enzyme. Biochim. biophys. Acta **384**, 360—368 (1975)

Ku, E. C., Wasvary, J. M., Cash, W. D.: Diclofenac sodium (GP 45840, Voltaren), a potent inhibitor of prostaglandin synthetase. Biochem. Pharmacol. **24**, 641—643 (1975)

Lands, W. E. M., Cook, H. W., Rome, L. H.: Prostaglandin biosynthesis: consequences of oxygenase mechanism upon in vitro assays of drug effectiveness. Abstracts International Conference on Prostaglandins, p. 3. Florence, 1975

Lands, W. E. M., Lee, R., Smith, W.: Factors regulating the biosynthesis of various prostaglandins. Ann. N.Y. Acad. Sci. **180**, 107—122 (1971)

Lands, W. E. M., LeTellier, P. R., Rome, L. H., Vanderhoek, J. Y.: Regulation of prostaglandin synthesis. In: Prostaglandin Synthetase Inhibitors, pp. 1—7. New York: Raven Press 1974

Lechat, P., Giroud, J. P., Fontagné Deysson, G., Adolphe, M.: Essai de différenciation pharmacologique de certains antiinflammatoires et immunodépresseurs. J. Pharmacol. (Paris) **1**, 255—265 (1970)

Lee, R. E.: The influence of psychotropic drugs on prostaglandin biosynthesis. Prostaglandins **5**, 63—68 (1974)

Lee, R. E., Lands, W. E. M.: Cofactors in the biosynthesis of prostaglandin $F_{1\alpha}$ and $F_{2\alpha}$. Biochim. biophys. Acta **260**, 203—211 (1972)

Levine, L.: Prostaglandin production by mouse fibrosarcoma cells in culture: inhibition by indomethacin and aspirin. Biochem. biophys. Res. Commun. **47**, 888—896 (1972)

Levitan, H., Barker, J. L.: Salicylate: A structure-activity study of its effects on membrane permeability. Science **176**, 1423—1424 (1972)

Levitan, H., Barker, J. L.: Membrane permeability: cation selectively reversibly altered by salicylate. Science **178**, 63—64 (1973)

Lewis, A. J., Cottney, J., Sugrue, M. F.: The spontaneously contracting pregnant rat uterus as a model for anti-inflammatory drug activity. J. Pharm. (Lond.) **27**, 375—376 (1975)

Lewis, D. A.: The actions of some non-steroidal drugs on lysosomes. J. Pharm. (Lond.) **22**, 909—912 (1970)

Lewis, D. A., Capstick, R. B., Ancill, R. J.: The action of azapropazone, oxyphenbutazone and phenylbutazone on lysosomes. J. Pharm. (Lond.) **23**, 931—935 (1971)

Lewis, D. A., Capstick, R. B., Ancill, R. J.: Biochemical properties of azapropazone and other anti-inflammatory drugs. Biochem. Pharmacol. **21**, 2531—2533 (1972)

Lewis, D. A., Symons, A. M., Ancill, R. J.: The stabilization-lysis action of anti-inflammatory steroida on lysosomes. J. Pharm. (Lond.) **22**, 902—908 (1970)

Lewis, D. A., Symons, A. M., Ancill, R. J.: Action of anti-inflammatory steroids on the lytic action of phospholipase C and 2,4,6-trinitrobenzene sulphonic acid on lysosomes. Biochem. Pharmacol. **23**, 467—470 (1974)

McArthur, J. N., Dawkins, P. D.: The effect of sodium salicylate on the binding of L-tryptophan to serum proteins. J. Pharm. (Lond.) **21**, 744—750 (1969)

McCall, E., Youlten, L. J. F.: Prostaglandin E_1 synthesis by phagocytosing rabbit polymorphonuclear leucocytes: its inhibition by indomathacin and its role in chemotaxis. J. Physiol (Lond.) **234**, 98P—100P (1973)

McCoubrey, A., Smith, M. H., Lane, A. C.: Inhibition of enzymes by alkylsalicylic acids. J. Pharm. (Lond.) **22**, 333—337 (1970)

McDonald, J. W. D., Stuart, R. K.: Interaction of prostaglandins E_1 and E_2 in regulation of cyclic-AMP and aggregation in human platelets: evidence for a common prostaglandin receptor. J. Lab. clin. Med. **84**, 111—121 (1974)

McLaughlin, S.: Salicylates and phospholipid bilayer membranes. Nature (Lond.) **243**, 234—236 (1973)

MacMillan, D. C.: Effect of salicylates on human platelets. Lancet 1968, **1**, 1151

Malmsten, C., Hamberg, M., Svensson, J., Samuelsson, B.: Physiological role an endoperoxide in human platelet: hemostatic defect due to platelet cyclo-oxygenase deficiency. Proc. nat. Acad. Sci. (Wash.) **72**, 1446—1450 (1975)

Marmo, E., Caputi, A. P., Vacca, C., Cazzola, M.: Interferenze tra alcuni antiflogistici e aggregazione delle piastrine. Riv. Farmacol. Ter. **5**, 279 a—294 a (1974)

Mason, R. W., McQueen, E. G.: Protein binding of indomethacin: binding of indomethacin to human plasma albumin and its displacement from binding by ibuprofen, phenylbutazone and salicylate, in vitro. Pharmacology **12**, 12—19 (1974)

Mehlman, M. A., Tobin, R. B., Sporn, E. M.: Oxidative phosphorylation and respiration by rat liver mitochondria from aspirin-treated rats. Biochem. Pharmacol. **21**, 3279—3285 (1972)

Meyer, M. C., Guttman, D. E.: The binding of drugs by plasma proteins. J. pharm. Sci. **57**, 895—917 (1968)

Migne, J., Védrine, Y., Muller, G.: Lysosome membrane stabilization by a new anti-inflammatory drugs ketoprofane. Abstracts VI. International Congress Pharmacology Helsinki, 1975, p. 241

Mikikits, S., Mortara, A., Spector, R. G.: Effect of drugs on red cell fragility. Nature (Lond.) **225**, 1150—1151 (1970)

Miller, W. S., Smith, J. G.: Effect of acetylsalicylic acid on lysosomes. Proc. Soc. exp. Biol. (N.Y.) **122**, 634—636 (1966)

Miyamoto, T., Ymamoto, S., Hayashi, O.: Prostaglandin synthetase system-resolution into oxygenase and isomerase components. Proc. nat. Acad. Sci. (Wash.) **71**, 3645—3648 (1974)

Mizushima, Y.: Inhibition of protein denaturation by anti-rheumatic or antiphlogistic agents. Arch. int. Pharmacodyn. **149**, 1—7 (1964)

Mizushima, Y., Ishi, Y., Masumoto, S.: Physico-chemical properties of potent non-steroidal anti-inflammatory drugs. Biochem. Pharmacol. **24**, 1589—1592 (1975)

Mizushima, Y., Sakai, S.: Stabilization of erythrocyte membranes by non-steroidal anti-inflammatory drugs. J. Pharm. (Lond.) **21**, 327—327 (1969)

Mizushima, Y., Suzuki, H.: Interaction between plasma proteins and antirheumatic or new antiphlogistic drugs. Arch. int. Pharmacodyn. **157**, 115—124 (1965)

Moffat, A. C., Patterson, D. A., Curry, A. S., Gwen, P.: Inhibition in vitro of cyclic 3'5'-nucleotide phosphodiesterase activity by drugs. Europ. J. Toxicol. **5**, 160—162 (1972)

Moncada, S., Needleman, P., Vane, J. R., Bunting, S.: Thromboxane synthesis and inhibition. Difference with an endoperoxide generating system. 1976, To be published

Mörsdorf, K.: The influence of anti-phlogistics on tissue proteases. In: Non-steroidal Anti-inflammatory Drugs. Amsterdam-New York-London-Milan-Tokyo-Buenos Aires: Excerpta Medica Foundation 1965, pp. 85—89

Mörsdorf, K., Wolf, G.: Vergleichende Untersuchungen zur Wirkungspotenz neuerer Antiphlogistica. Arzneimittel-Forsch. **22**, 2105—2110 (1972)

M.R.C. Steering Committee: Effect of aspirin on post-operative venous thrombosis. Lancet **1972 II**, 441—445

Mustard, J. F., Packham, M. A.: Factors influencing platelet function: adhesion, release, and aggregation. Pharmacol. Rev. **22**, 97—187 (1970)

Mustard, J. F., Packham, M. A.: Platelets, thrombosis and drugs. Drugs **9**, 1976 (1975)

Nakagawa, H., Bentley, J. P.: Salicylate-induced inhibition of collagen and mucopolysaccharide biosynthesis by a chick embryo cell-free system. J. Pharm. (Lond.) **23**, 399—406 (1971)

Nishizawa, E. E., Miller, W. L., Gorman, R. R., Bundy, G. L., Svensson, J., Hamberg, M.: Prostaglandin D_2 as a potential antithrombotic agent. Prostaglandins **9**, 109—121 (1975)

Northover, B. J.: The effect of anti-inflammatory drugs on vascular smooth muscle. Brit. J. Pharmacol. **31**, 483—493 (1967)

Northover, B. J.: Mechanism of inhibitory action of indomethacin on smooth muscles. Brit. J. Pharmacol. **41**, 540—551 (1971)

Northover, B. J.: Effect of anti-inflammatory drugs on the binding of calcium to cellular membranes in various human and guinea-pig tissues. Brit. J. Pharmacol. **48**, 496—504 (1973)

Nugteren, D. H.: Inhibition of prostaglandin biosynthesis by 8cis, 12trans, 14cis-eicosatrienoic acid. Biochem. biophys. Acta **210**, 171—176 (1970)

Nugteren, D. H.: Arachidonate lipoxygenase in blood platelets. Biochem. biophys. Acta **380**, 299—307 (1975)

Nugteren, D. H., Beerthius, R. K., Van Dorp, D. A.: The enzymic conversion of all-cis 8,11,14-eicosatrienoic acid into prostaglandin E_1. Rec. Trav. chim. Pays-Bas **85**, 405—419 (1966)

Nugteren, D. H., Hazelhof, E.: Isolation and properties of intermediates in prostaglandin biosynthesis. Biochim. biophys. Acta **326**, 448—461 (1973)

O'Brien, J. R.: Effect of anti-inflammatory agents on platelets. Lancet **1**, 894—895 (1968)

O'Brien, J. R., Finch, W., Clark, E.: A comparison of an effect of different anti-inflammatory drugs on human platelets. J. clin. Path. **23**, 522—525 (1970)

Packham, M. A., Mustard, J. F.: The effect of pyrazole compounds on thrombin-induced platelet aggregation. Proc. Soc. exp. Biol. (N.Y.) **130**, 72—75 (1969)

Packham, M. A., Warrior, E. S., Glynn, M. F., Senyi, A. S., Mustard, J. F.: Alteration of the response of platelets to surface stimuli by pyrazole compounds. J. exp. Med. **126**, 171—188 (1967)

Palmér, L., Bertilsson, L., Alván, G., Orme, M., Sjöqvist, F., Holmstedt, B.: Indomethacin: quantitative determination in plasma by mass fragmentography including pilot pharmacokinetics in man. In: Prostaglandin Synthetase Inhibitors, pp. 91—97. New York: Raven Press 1974

Panczenko, B., Grodzinska, L., Gryglewski, R.: The dual action of meclofenamate on the contractile response to $PGF_{2\alpha}$ in the guinea pig trachea. Pol. J. Pharmacol. Pharm. **27**, 273—276 (1975)

Patrono, C., Ciabattoni, G., Greco, F., Grossi-Belloni, D.: Comparative evaluation of the inhibitory effects of aspirin-like drugs on prostaglandin production by human platelets and synovial tissue. In: Advances in Prostaglandin and Thromboxane Research, Vol. 1, pp. 125—131. New York: Raven Press 1976

Patrono, C., Ciabattoni, G., Grossi-Belloni, D.: In vitro and in vivo inhibition of prostaglandin synthesis by fenoprofen, a non-steroidal anti-inflammatory drug. Pharmacol. Res. Commun. **6**, 509—518 (1974)

Patrono, C., Ciabattoni, G., Grossi-Belloni, D.: Release of prostaglandin $F_{1\alpha}$ and $F_{2\alpha}$ from superfused platelets: quantitative evaluation of the inhibitory effects of some aspirin-like drugs. Prostaglandins **9**, 557—568 (1975)

Perrin, J. H., Nelson, D. A.: Induced optical activity following the binding of warfarin, indomethacin, 4-hydroxycoumarin and salicylic acid to human serum albumin. Life Sci. **11**, 277—283 (1972)

Phelps, P.: Polymorphonuclear leukocyte motility in vitro. II. Stimulatory effect of monosodium urate crystals and urate in solution; partial inhibition by colchicine and indomethacin. Arthr. and Rheum. **12**, 189—196 (1969)

Phelps, P., McCarty, D. J.: Supressive effects of indomethacin on crystal-induced inflammation in canine joints and on neutrophilic motility in vitro. J. Pharmacol. exp. Ther. **158**, 546—553 (1967)

Phillips, B. M., Sancilio, L. F., Kurchacova, E.: In vitro assessment of antiinflammatory activity. J. Pharm. (Lond.) **19**, 696—697 (1967)

Phillips, M.L., Muirden, K.D.: An effect of ibuprofen and prednisolone on lysosomes. J. Pharm. (Lond.) **24**, 653—654 (1972)

Piper, P.J., Vane, J.R.: Release of additional factors in anaphylaxis and its antagonism by anti-inflammatory drugs. Nature (Lond.) **233**, 29—35 (1969)

Piper, P.J., Vane, J.R.: The release of prostaglandins from lungs and other tissues. Ann. N.Y. Acad. Sci. **180**, 363—383 (1971)

Pollock, S.H., Brown, J.H.: Studies on the acute inflammatory response. III. Glucocorticoids and vitamin E (in vivo) attenuate thermal labilization of isolated hepatic lysosomes. J. Pharmacol. exp. Ther. **178**, 609—615 (1971)

Purcell, W.P., Bass, G.E., Clayton, J.M.: Strategy of Drug Design: a Guide to Biological Activity. New York: Wiley Interscience 1973

Radwan, A.G., West, G.B.: The effect of non-steroidal anti-inflammatory drugs on histamine formation in the rat. Brit. J. Pharmacol. **33**, 193—198 (1968)

Raz, A., Stern, H., Kenig-Wakshal, R.: Indomethacin and aspirin inhibition of prostaglandin E_2 synthesis by sheep seminal vesicles microsome powder and seminal vesicle slice. Prostaglandins **3**, 337—352 (1973)

Reinicke, C.: Influence of non-steroid anti-inflammatory drugs (NSAIDs) on hepatic tyrosine aminotransferase (TA) activity in rats in vitro and in vivo. Biochem. Pharmacol. **24**, 193—198 (1975)

Ringrose, P.S., Parr, M.A., McLaren, M.: Effects of anti-inflammatory and other compounds on the release of lysosomal enzymes from macrophages. Biochem. Pharmacol. **24**, 607—614 (1975)

Robak, J., Dembinska-Kiec, A., Gryglewski, R.: The influence of saturated fatty acids on prostaglandin synthetase activity. Biochem. Pharmacol. **24**, 2075—2060 (1975 a)

Robak, J., Panczenko, B., Gryglewski, R.: Binding of the membrane active drugs to bovine serum albumin and human erythrocyte membranes. Biochem. Pharmacol. **24**, 571—574 (1975 b)

Robinson, D.R., Smith, H., McGuire, M.B., Levine, L.: Prostaglandin synthesis by rheumatoid synovium and its stimulation by colchicine. Prostaglandins **10**, 67—85 (1975)

Rose, A.J., Collins, A.J.: The effect of pH on the production of prostaglandins E_2 and $F_{2\alpha}$, and a possible pH dependent inhibitor. Prostaglandins **8**, 271—283 (1974)

Rosenberg, F.J., Gimber-Phillips, P.E., Groblewski, G.E., Davison, C., Phillips, D.K., Goralnick, S.J., Cahill, E.D.: Acetylsalicylic acid: inhibition of platelet aggregation in the rabbit. J. Pharmacol. exp. Ther. **179**, 410—418 (1971)

Rosenior, J.C., Tonks, R.S.: Salicylate inhibition of in vitro plasminogen activation by saline extracts of rat tissue. Biochem. Pharmacol. **23**, 2339—2341 (1974)

Roth, G.T., Stanford, N., Majerus, P.W.: Acetylation of prostaglandin synthetase by aspirin. Proc. nat. Acad. Sci. (Wash.) **72**, 3073—3076 (1975)

Roubal, Z., Čepelák, V., Němeček, O.: Newly synthetized pyrazolidine derivatives as potential activators of fibrynolysis and anti-aggregating agents. Acta Univ. Carol. [Med.] (Praha) **52**, 49—54 (1972)

Roubal, Z., Němeček, O.: Activation of fibrinolysis by derivatives of diphenyldioxopyrazolidine. Nature (Lond.) **212**, 861—862 (1966)

Roy, A.C., Warren, B.T.: Inhibition of c-AMP phosphodiesterase by disodium cromoglycate. Biochem. Pharmacol. **23**, 917—920 (1974)

Saeed, S.A., Warren, B.T.: On the mode of action and biochemical properties of anti-inflammatory drugs. J. Biochem. Pharmacol. **22**, 1965—1969 (1973)

Saeki, K., Muraoka, S., Yamasaki, H.: Anti-inflammatory properties of N-phenylanthranilic acid derivatives in relation to uncoupling of oxidative phosphorylation. Jap. J. Pharmacol. **22**, 187—199 (1972)

Salzman, E.W.: Cyclic cAMP and platelet function. New Engl. J. Med. **286**, 358—363 (1972)

Samuelsson, B.: Biosynthesis of prostaglandins. Fed. Proc. **31**, 1442—1450 (1972)

Samuelsson, B.: Endogenous synthesis of prostaglandins in guinea pig and man: effects of inhibitors. In: Prostaglandin Synthetase Inhibitors, pp. 99—106. New York: Raven Press 1974

Samuelsson, B., Granström, E., Hamberg, M.: On the mechanism of biosynthesis of prostaglandins. In: Nobel Symposium 2, Prostaglandins, pp. 31—44. Stockholm: Almqvist and Wiksell 1967

Samuelsson, B., Hamberg, M.: Role of endoperoxides in the biosynthesis and action of prostaglandins. In: Prostaglandin Synthetase Inhibitors, pp. 99—119. New York: Raven Press 1974

Samuelsson, B., Hamberg, M., Svensson, J., Malmsten, C.: The role of prostaglandin endoperoxides in human platelets. Abstracts VI. International Congress Pharmacology, p. 480. Helsinki 1975

Schaeffer, H. J.: Factors in the design of reversible and irreversible enzyme inhibitors. In: Drug design, Vol. II, pp. 129—160. New York-London: Academic Press 1971

Scherrer, R. A., Whitehouse, M. W.: Anti-inflammatory agents. Medicinal Chemistry. A Series of Monographs, Vol. 13. New York-San Francisco-London: Academic Press 1974

Schönhöfer, P., Anspach, K. F.: Die Aktivität der 1-Glutamin-D-Fructose-6-Phosphat-Aminotransferase im Verlauf einer durch Carageenin induzierten Entzündung und ihre Hemmbarkeit durch Phenylbutazon. Arch. int. Pharmacodyn. 166, 382—389 (1967)

Schwartz, C. S., Mandel, H. G.: The selective inhibition of microbial RNA synthesis by salicylate. Biochem. Pharmacol. 21, 771—785 (1972)

Seeman, P.: II. Erythrocyte membrane stabilization by local anaesthetic and tranquilizers. Biochem. Pharmacol. 15, 1753—1766 (1966)

Seeman, P., Weinstein, J.: I. Erythrocyte membrane stabilization by tran-quilizers and antihistaminics. Biochem. Pharmacol. 15, 1737—1752 (1966)

Settle, W., Hegeman, S., Featherstone, R. M.: The nature of drug-protein interaction. In: Handbook of experimental Pharmacology, Vol. 28/I, Concepts in Biochemical Pharmacology, pp. 175—186. Berlin-Heidelberg-New York: Springer 1971

Shen, T. Y.: Neuere nichtsteroidatige entzündungshemmende Wirkstoffe (Antiphlogistica). Angew. Chem. 84, 512—526 (1972)

Shen, T. Y., Ham, E. A., Cirillo, V. J., Zanetti, M.: Structure-activity relationship of certain prostaglandin synthetase inhibitors. In: Prostaglandin Synthetase Inhibitors, pp. 19—31. New York: Raven Press 1974

Shio, H., Ramwell, P.: Effect of prostaglandin E_2 and aspirin an the secondary aggregation of human platelets. Nature (New Biol.) 236, 45—46 (1972)

Sih, C. J., Takeguchi, C. A.: Biosynthesis. In: The Prostaglandins, Vol. I, pp. 83—100. New York-London: Plenum Press 1973

Silver, M. J., Hoch, W., Kocsis, J. J., Ingerman, C., Smith, J. B.: Arachidonic acid causes sudden death in rabbits. Science 183, 1085—1087 (1974a)

Silver, M. J., Smith, J. B., Ingerman, C. M.: Blood platelets and the inflammatory precess. Agents Actions 4, 233—240 (1974b)

Silver, M. J., Smith, J. B., Ingerman, C. M., Kocsis, J. J.: Arachidonic acid-induced human platelet aggregation and prostaglandin formation. Prostaglandins 4, 863—875 (1973)

Sjöholm, I., Sjödin, T.: Binding of drugs to human serum albumin. I. Circular dichroism studies on the binding of some analgesics, sedative and anti-depressive agents. Biochem. Pharmacol. 21, 3041—3052 (1972)

Skidmore, I. F., Whitehouse, M. W.: Effect of non-steroidal anti-inflammatory drugs on aldehyde binding to plasma albumen: a novel in vitro assay for potential anti-inflammatory activity. J. Pharm. (Lond.) 17, 671—673 (1965)

Skidmore, I. F., Whitehouse, M. W.: Concerning the regulation of some diverse biochemical reactions underlying the inflammatory response by salicylic acid, phenylbutazone and other acidic antirheumatic drugs. J. Pharm. (Lond.) 18, 558—560 (1966)

Skidmore, I. F., Whitehouse, M. W.: Biochemical properties of anti-inflammatory drugs. X: The inhibition of serotonin formation in vitro and inhibition of the esterase activity of α-chymotrypsin. Biochem. Pharmacol. 16, 737—751 (1967)

Skwarek, Szczygielska, J.: Wplyw nowych pochodnych tiosemikarbazonu oraz kilku leków przeciwzapalnych na rozwój wirusów grupy A_2 i B. Farm. Pol. 29, 789—795 (1973)

Smith, I. D., Temple, D. M., Shearman, R. P.: The antagonism by anti-inflammatory analgesics of prostaglandin $F_{2\alpha}$-induced contractions human and rabbit myometrium in vitro. Prostaglandins 10, 41—57 (1975)

Smith, J. B., Ingerman, C. M., Kocsis, J. J., Silver, M. J.: Studies on platelet aggregation: synthesis of prostaglandins and effects of synthetase inhibitors. In: Prostaglandin Synthetase Inhibitors, pp. 229—239. New York: Raven Press 1974a

Smith, J. B., Ingerman, C. M., Kocsis, J. J., Silver, M. J.: Formation of an intermediate in prostaglandin biosynthesis and its association with the platelet release reaction. J. clin. Invest. **53**,
1468—1472 (1974b)

Smith, J. B., Silver, M. J., Ingerman, C. M., Kocsis, J. J.: Prostaglandin D_2 inhibits the aggregation
of human platelets. Thromb. Res. **5**, 291—299 (1974c)

Smith, J. B., Silver, M. J., Webster, G. R.: Phospholipase A_1 of human blood platelets. Biochem. J.
131, 615—616 (1973)

Smith, J. B., Willis, A. L.: Aspirin selectively anhibits prostaglandin production in human platelets. Nature (New Biol.) **231**, 235—237 (1971)

Smith, M. J. H., Ford-Hutchinson, A. W., Elliott, P. N. C.: Prostaglandins and the anti-inflammatory activities of aspirin and sodium salicylate. J. Pharm. (Lond.) **27**, 473—478 (1975)

Smith, W. L., Lands, W. E. M.: Stimulation and blockade of prostaglandin biosynthesis. J. biol.
Chem. **246**, 6700—6702 (1971)

Solomon, H. M., Schrogie, J. J.: The effect of various drugs on the binding of warfarin—^{14}C to
human albumin. Biochem. Pharmacol. **16**, 1219—1226 (1967)

Sorrentino, L., Capasso, F., DiRosa, M.: Indomethacin and prostaglandins. Europ. J. Pharmacol.
17, 306—308 (1972)

Starr, M. S., West, G. B.: The effect of bradykinin and anti-inflammatory agents on isolated arteries. J. Pharm. (Lond.) **18**, 838—840 (1966)

Stefanovich, V.: Inhibition of 3',5'-cyclic AMP phosphodiesterase with anti-inflammatory agents.
Res. Commun. chem. Path. Pharmacol. **7**, 573—582 (1974)

Stenlake, J. B., Williams, W. D., Davidson, A. G., Downie, W. W.: The effect of anti-inflammatory
drugs on the protein-binding of 1,2-^{3}H cortisol in human plasma in vitro. J. Pharm. (Lond.)
23, 145—146 (1971)

Stuart, R. K.: Platelet function studies in human being receiving 300 mg aspirin per day. J. Lab.
clin. Med. **75**, 463—471 (1970)

Svensson, J., Hamberg, M., Samuelsson, B.: Prostaglandin endoperoxides IX. Characterization of
rabbit aorta contracting substance (RCS) from guinea pig lung and human platelets. Acta
physiol. scand. **94**, 222—228 (1975)

Swingle, K. F., Jaques, L. W., Grant, T. J., Kvam, D. C.: Apparent association of activity of anti-
inflammatory drugs in a sulfhydryl exchange reaction in vitro and in the guinea pig erythema
assay. Biochem. Pharmacol. **19**, 2995—2999 (1970)

Sykes, J. A. C., Maddox, I. S.: Prostaglandin production by experimental tumours and effects of
anti-inflammatory compounds. Nature (New Biol.) **237**, 59—60 (1972)

Takeguchi, C., Kohono, E., Sih, C. J.: Mechanism of prostaglandin biosynthesis. I. Characterization and assay of bovine prostaglandin synthetase. Biochemistry **10**, 2372—2376 (1971)

Takeguchi, C., Sih, C. J.: A rapid spectrophotometric assay for prostaglandin synthetase: application to the study of non-steroidal anti-inflammatory agents. Prostaglandins **2**, 169—184
(1972)

Tanaka, K., Iizuka, Y.: Supression of enzyme release from isolated rat liver lysosomes by non-
steroidal anti-inflammatory drugs. Biochem. Pharmacol. **17**, 2023—2032 (1968)

Tanaka, K., Kobayashi, K., Kazui, S.: Temperature dependent reaction of flufenamic acid with
rat erythrocyte membrane. Biochem. Pharmacol. **22**, 879—886 (1973)

Terada, H., Muroaka, S., Fujita, T.: Structure-activity relationship of fenamic acids. J. med.
Chem. **17**, 330—334 (1974)

Tolman, E. L., Partridge, R.: Multiple sites of interaction between prostaglandins and non-steroidal anti-inflammatory agents. Prostaglandins **9**, 349—359 (1975)

Tomlinson, R. V., Ringold, H. J., Quershi, M. C., Forchielli, E.: Relationship between inhibition of
prostaglandin synthesis and drug efficacy: support for the current theory on mode of action
of aspirin-like drugs. Biochem. biophys. Res. Commun. **46**, 552—559 (1972)

Vainio, H., Hänninen, O., Puukka, R.: Mitochondrial toxicity of ulcerogenic cinchophen and its
derivatives in vitro. Biochem. Pharmacol. **20**, 1589—1597 (1971)

Van den Berg, G., Bultsma, T., Nauta, W. T.: Inhibition of prostaglandin biosynthesis by 2-aryl-
1,3-indandiones. Biochem. Pharmacol. **24**, 1115—1119 (1975)

Van den Berg, G., Nauta, W. T.: Effects of anti-inflammatory 2-aryl-1,3-indandiones on oxydative
phosphorylation in rat liver mitochondria. Biochem. Pharmacol. **24**, 815—821 (1975)

Vanderhoek, J. Y., Lands, W. E. M.: The inhibition of the fatty acid oxygenase of sheep vascular
gland by anti-oxydants. Biochim. biophys. Acta **296**, 382—385 (1973)

Van Dorp, D. A.: Essentielle Fettsäuren und Prostaglandine. Naturwissenschaften **56**, 124 (1969)
Van Dorp, D. A.: Essentielle Fettsäuren und Prostaglandine. In: Fettstoffwechselstörungen, ihre Erkennung und Behandlung, pp. 152—177. Stuttgart: Georg Thieme 1971
Van Dorp, D. A., Beerthius, R. K., Nugteren, D. H., Vonkeman, H.: The biosynthesis of prostaglandins. Biochim. biophys. Acta **90**, 204—207 (1964)
Vane, J. R.: Inhibition of prostaglandin synthesis as a mechanism of action for aspirin-like drugs. Nature (New Biol.) **231**, 232—235 (1971)
Vane, J. R.: Prostaglandins in inflammation. In: Inflammation, Mechanism and Control, pp. 261—279. New York-London: Academic Press 1972a
Vane, J. R.: Prostaglandins and aspirin-like drugs. Hosp. Pract. **7**, 61—71 (1972b)
Vane, J. R.: Prostaglandins and aspirin-like drugs. In: Proceedings of the V. International Congress Pharmacology, San Francisco, Vol. V, pp. 352—377. Basel: Karger 1973a
Vane, J. R.: Inhibition of prostaglandin biosynthesis as the mechanism of action of aspirin-like drugs. In: Advances in Biosciences, Vol. IX, pp. 395—412. Braunschweig: Pergamon Press-Vieweg 1973b
Vane, J. R.: Mode of action of aspirin and similar compounds. In: Prostaglandin Synthetase Inhibitors, pp. 155—163 New York: Raven Press 1974
Vane, J. R., Williams, K. I.: The contribution of prostaglandin production to contractions of the isolated uterus of the rat. Brit. J. Pharmacol. **48**, 629—639 (1973)
Van Miert, A. S. J., Van Essen, J. A., Tropm, G. A.: The antipyretic effect of pyrazolone derivatives and salicylates on fever induced with leukocytic or bacterial pyrogen. Arch. int. Pharmacodyn. **197**, 388—391 (1972)
Van Neuten, J. M., Hoebeke, J., Fontaine, J.: Suprofen, a specific inhibitor of the biosynthesis of prostaglandins. Effect on the peristaltic effect in vitro. Abstracts VI. International Congress Pharmacology, p. 292. Helsinki 1975
Vargaftig, B. B.: The pharmacology of slow reacting substance C and of arachidonic acid. Agents Actions **3**, 357—365 (1973)
Vargaftig, B. B., Dao Hai, N.: Inhibition by acetamidophenol of the production of prostaglandin-like material from blood platelets in vitro in relation to some in vitro actions. Europ. J. Pharmacol. **24**, 283—288 (1973)
Vargaftig, B. B., Tranier, Y., Chignard, M.: Inhibition by sulfhydryl agents of arachidonic acid induced platelet aggregation and release of potential inflammatory substances. Prostaglandins **8**, 133—156 (1974)
Vargaftig, B. B., Zirinis, P.: Arachidonic acid induced platelet aggregation is accompanied by release of potential inflammatory mediators distinct from PGE_2 and $PGF_{2\alpha}$. Nature (New Biol.) **244**, 114—116 (1973)
Von Kaulla, K.: A simple test tube arrangement for screening activity of synthetic organic compounds. J. med. Chem. **8**, 164—171 (1965)
Von Kaulla, K.: On the in vitro mechanism of synthetic fibrinolytic agents. In: Chemical Control of Fibrynolysis-Thrombolysis. New York-London-Sidney-Toronto: Wiley-Interscience 1970, pp. 3—41
Wagner-Jauregg, T.: Zur Bedeutung des Mizushima-Tests (Mt) für die Beurteilung der Antirheumatika. Int. J. clin. Pharmacol. **6**, 391—396 (1972)
Wagner-Jauregg, T., Bürlimann, W., Fischer, J.: Vergleich antiphlogistischer Substanzen im Plasmaeiweiß-Trübungstest nach Mizushima. Arzneimittel-Forsch. **19**, 1532—1536 (1969)
Wagner-Jauregg, T., Fischer, J.: Über Hemmung des Wachstums von Lactobacillus casei durch einige Antiphlogistika. Experientia (Basel) **24**, 1029—1031 (1968)
Wagner-Jauregg, T., Fischer, J., Jahn, U.: Cytostatische Antiphlogistica. Arzneimittel-Forsch. **20**, 831—838 (1970)
Wallach, D. P., Daniels, E. G.: Properties of a novel preparation of prostaglandin synthetase from sheep semina vesicles. Biochim. biophys. Acta **231**, 445—457 (1971)
Walz, D. T., Dimartino, M. J.: Effect of antiarthritic drugs on sulfhydryl reactivity of rat serum. Proc. Soc. exp. Biol. (N.Y.) **140**, 263—268 (1972)
Weeks, J. R., Chandra Sekhar, N., Ducharme, D. W.: Relative activity of prostaglandins E_1, A_1, E_2 and A_2 on lypolysis, platelet aggregation, smooth muscle and the cardiovascular system. J. Pharm. (Lond.) **21**, 103—108 (1969)
Weinryb, I., Michel, I. M.: Interactions of α-metylfluorene-2-acetic acid with adenyl cyclase. Biochem. Pharmacol. **23**, 2411—2419 (1974)

Weinryb, I., Chasin, M., Free, C. A., Harris, D. M., Goldenberg, H., Michel, I. M., Raik, V. S., Phillips, M., Samamiego, S., Hess, S.: Effects of therapeutic agents on cyclic AMP metabolism in vitro. J. pharm. Sci. **61**, 1556—1567 (1972)

Weiss, H. J.: Platelets: physiology and abnormalities of function. New Engl. J. Med. **293**, 531—541 (1975a)

Weiss, H. J.: Platelets: physiology and abnormalities of function. New Engl. J. Med. **293**, 580—588 (1975b)

Weiss, H. J., Aledort, L. M.: Impaired platelet (connective-tissue reaction in man after aspirin ingestion). Lancet **1967II**, 495—497

Weiss, H. J., Aledort, L. M., Kochwa, S.: The effect of salicylates on the hemostatic roperties of platelets in man. J. clin. Invest. **47**, 2169—2180 (1968)

Weissmann, G.: Labilization and stabilization of lysosomes. Fed. Proc. **23**, 1038—1044 (1964)

Weissmann, G.: The Interaction of Drugs and Subcellular Components in Animal Cells, pp. 203—212. London: Churchill 1968

Weissmann, G., Dingle, J. T.: Release of lysosomal protease by ultraviolet irradiation and inhibition by hydrocortisone. Exp. Cell Res. **25**, 207—210 (1961)

Weissmann, G., Dukor, P., Zurier, R. B.: Effect of cyclic AMP on release of lysosomal enzymes from phagocytes. Nature (New Biol.) **231**, 131—135 (1971)

Weissmann, G., Thomas, L.: Studies on lysosomes. I. Effects of endotoxin, endotoxin tolerance and cortisone on release of acid hydrolases from granular fraction of rabbit liver. J. exp. Med. **116**, 433—450 (1962)

Weissmann, G., Thomas, L.: Studies on lysosomes. II. Effect of cortisone on release of acid hydrolases from large granule fraction of rabbit liver induced by excess of vitamin A. J. clin. Invest. **42**, 661—669 (1963)

Westwick, W. J., Allsop, J., Watts, R. W. E.: A study of the effect of some drugs which cause agranulocytosis on the biosynthesis of pyrimidines in human granulocytes. Biochem. Pharmacol. **21**, 1955—1966 (1972)

Wiethold, G., Hellenbrecht, D., Lemmer, R., Palm, D.: Membrane effects of beta-adrenergic blocking agents: investigation with the fluorescence probe 1-anilino-8-naphtalene sulphonate (ANS) and antihemolytic activities. Biochem. Pharmacol. **22**, 1437—1449 (1973)

Whitehouse, M. W.: Biochemical properties of anti-inflammatory drugs—III. Uncoupling of oxidative phosphorylation in a connective tissue (cartilage) and liver mitochondria by salicylate analogues: relationship of structure to activity. Biochem. Pharmacol. **13**, 319—336 (1964a)

Whitehouse, M. W.: Uncoupling of oxidative phosphorylation by some arylacetic acids (anti-inflammatory or hypocholesterolemic drugs). Nature (Lond.) 201, 629—630 (1964b)

Whitehouse, M. W.: Some biochemical properties of non-steroidal anti-inflammatory drugs which may determine their clinical activity. In: Non-steroidal Anti-inflammatory Drugs, pp. 52—57. Amsterdam-New York-London-Milan-Tokyo-Buenos Aires: Excerpta Medica Foundation 1965a

Whitehouse, M. W.: Some biochemical and pharmacological properties of anti-inflammatory drugs. In: Progress in Drugs Research. Vol. VIII, pp. 321—429. Basel-Stuttgart: Birkhäuser Verlag 1965b

Whitehouse, M. W.: Biochemical properties on anti-inflammatory drugs. XI. Structure-action relationship for the uncoupling of oxidative phosphorylation and inhibition of chymotrypsin by N-substituted anthranilates and related compounds. Biochem. Pharmacol. **16**, 753—760 (1967)

Whitehouse, M. W., Famaey, J. P.: Concerning the pharmacological activity of nonsteroid anti-inflammatory drugs: is the acidic function essential? Agents Actions **3**, 217—220 (1973)

Whitehouse, M. W., Haslam, J. M.: Ability of some antirheumatic drugs to uncouple oxidative phosphorylation. Nature (Lond.) **196**, 1323—1324 (1962)

Whitehouse, M. W., Kippen, I., Klinenberg, J. R.: Biochemical properties of anti-inflammatory drugs. XII. Inhibition of urate binding to human albumin by salicylate and phenylbutazone analogues and some novel anti-inflammatory drugs. Biochem. Pharmacol. **20**, 3309—3320 (1971)

Whitehouse, M. W., Skidmore, I. F.: Concerning the regulation of some diverse biochemical reactions, underlying the inflammatory response, by salicylic acid, phenylbuthazone and other acidic antirheumatic drugs. J. Pharm. (Lond.) **17**, 668—670 (1965)

Willis, A. L.: Isolation of chemical trigger for thrombosis. Prostaglandins **5**, 1—25 (1974)

Willis, A. L.: An enzymic mechanism for the antithrombotic and antihemostatic actions of aspirin. Science **183**, 325—327 (1974)

Willis, A. L., Kuhn, D. C.: A new potential mediator of arterial thrombosis whose biosynthesis is inhibited by aspirin. Prostaglandins **4**, 127—129 (1973)

Willis, A. L., Kuhn, D. C., Weiss, H. J.: Acetylenic analog of arachidonate that acts like aspirin on platelets. Science **183**, 327—330 (1974a)

Willis, A. L., Vane, F. M., Kuhn, D. C., Scott, C. G., Petrin, M.: An endoperoxide aggregator (LASS), formed in platelets in response to thrombotic stimuli, purification, identification and unique biological significance. Prostaglandins **8**, 453—507 (1974b)

Wojtecka-Łukasik, E., Dancewicz, A. M.: Inhibition of human leukocyte collagenase by some drugs used in the therapy of rheumatic diseases. Biochem. Pharmacol. **23**, 2077—2081 (1974)

Wolna, E., Inglot, A. D.: Non-steroidal anti-inflammatory drugs: effects on the utilization of glucose and production of lactic acid in tissue culture. Experientia (Basel) **29**, 69—71 (1973)

Wolna, E., Inglot, A. D., Machon, Z.: New isothiazole derivatives. III. Influence on glucose consumption and lactic acid production in tissue cultures. Arch. Immunol. Ther. exp. **21**, 903—908 (1973a)

Wolna, E., Inglot, A. D., Machon, Z., Piatek, K.: New isothiazole derivatives. IV. Stabilization of human erythrocyte membranes. Arch. Immunol. Ther. exp. **21**, 909—914 (1973b)

Wolna, E., Wolny, M., Inglot, A. D.: Inhibition of some enzymes by non-steroidal anti-inflammatory compounds at high temperature. Arch. Immunol. Ther. exp. **17**, 795—805 (1969)

Yaron, M., Yaron, I., Allalouf, D.: Model for evaluating the effect of drugs on the inflammatory process (in Hebrew). Harefuah **82**, 111—114 (1972)

Young, P. R., Dodge, P. W., Carter, G. W., Kimura, E. T.: Experimental anti-inflammatory and analgesic studies with 3-trifluoromethyl-s-triazolo(3,4-α)-isoquinoline. Arch. int. Pharmacodyn. **212**, 205—213 (1974)

Zaroslinski, J. wF., Keresztes-Nagy, S., Mass, R. wF., Oester, Y. T.: Effect of temerature on the binding of salicylate by human serum albumin. Biochem. Pharmacol. **23**, 1767—1776 (1974)

Ziboh, V. A., McElligott, T., Hsia, S. L.: Prostaglandin E_2 biosynthesis in human skin: subcellular localization and inhibition by unsaturated fatty acids and anti-inflammatory agents. In: Advances in Bioscences, Vol. IX, pp. 457—460. Oxford-Edinburgh-New York-Toronto-Sidney-Braunschweig: Pergamon Press-Vieweg 1972

Zucker, M. B., Peterson, J.: Inhibition of adenosine diphosphate-induced secondary aggregation and other platelet functions by acetylsalicylic acid ingestion. Proc. Soc. exp. Biol. (N.Y.) β127, 547—551 (1968)

Zucker, M. B., Peterson, J.: Effect of acetylsalicylic acid, other non-steroidal anti-inflammatory agents, and dipyridamole on human blood platelets. J. Lab. clin. Med. **76**, 66—75 (1970)

CHAPTER 20

Inhibition of Erythema and Local Hyperthermia

K. F. SWINGLE, R. J. TRANCIK, and D. C. KVAM

A. Introduction

Each of the four cardinal signs of inflammation (rubor, calor, tumor, dolor), as recorded by CELSUS in the first century A.D., has been used by pharmacologists to establish methods for the detection and definition of anti-inflammatory substances (SWINGLE, 1974). The inhibition of an induced oedema, usually in the paw of the rat, has been the preferred method (WHITEHOUSE, 1965; WINTER, 1966; SWINGLE, 1974). Inhibition of the appearance of erythema in guinea pigs after exposure of depilated skin to ultraviolet (UV) ligth (WILHELMI, 1949, 1950; WINDER et al., 1958) has also been a popular method, particularly for the detection of drugs which may properly be classified as anti-inflammatory/analgesic/antipyretic. Procedures utilizing the human for assessment of antierythemic activity of substances include the erythema induced by UV irradiation and that induced by topical application of tetrahydrofurfuryl nicotinate (THFN) (TRUELOVE and DUTHIE, 1959; ADAMS and COBB, 1963). The development and availability of thermometers capable of recording skin temperature accurately and rapidly have led to the use of this parameter by some investigators to evaluate inflammatory and anti-inflammatory effects.

The anatomical, physiological and biochemical considerations in the development of erythema and local hyperthermia are discussed in Chapters 2 and 16 of this volume. Erythema and local hyperthermia are a consequence of the increased blood flow which occurs in an inflamed area (LEWIS, 1927). These two manifestations of the acute inflammatory response seem to be independent of the important event in the acute response, i.e. increased permeability of the micro-vasculature. The time course of development of erythema and that of increased vascular permeability after UV irradiation of guinea pig skin were shown to differ (GUPTA and LEVY, 1973). Early changes in vascular permeability after UV irradiation could be inhibited in the rat and guinea pig by antagonists of 5-hydroxytryptamine (S-HT) and histamine, respectively. However, these agents had no effect on the intensity of erythema (LOGAN and WILHELM, 1966a). Oedema and local hyperthermia in yeast-injected paws of rats were separate phenomena (PIRCIO and GROSKINSKY, 1966). Temperature increases in paws of rats injected with Freund's adjuvant preceded swelling of the paws (WALZ et al., 1970; COLLINS and RING, 1972). Oedema and erythema could be separated after thermal burns of guinea pigs (SEVITT, 1964). Erythema (LOGAN and WILHELM, 1966b) and local hyperthermia (PIRCIO and GROSKINSKY, 1966) have in common with increased permeability of the microvasculature a biphasic pattern in their development after the introduction of certain inflammatory stimuli: an initial transitory increase in each of these parameters is followed by a second more prolonged increase. There is, however, no strict correlation between the time courses of development of hyper-aemia and increased permeability. One must suspect that different mechanisms exist for the induction of hyperaemia and increased permeability of the microvasculature at inflammatory foci, and the evaluation of substances for antagonistic activity to the acute inflammatory response should properly include an assessment of their effects on both phenomena.

B. Ultraviolet (UV) Light and the Erythematous Response

UV and visible light are comprised of wavelengths from 200 to 760 nm. Infrared radiation continues from 760 to 5000 nm. The inclusive wavelengths of variously designated light, as used in this chapter, are provided in Table 1. Solar radiation reaching the earth's surface ranges in wavelength from 290 nm, in the uv, to 1000 nm, in the near-infrared region. Approximately 75% of the sun's energy is in the 290–700 nm range (ERICKSON, 1975). Oxygen in the outer level of the atmosphere absorbs uv radiation of wavelengths less than 240 nm to form ozone (O_3) which becomes an effective agent in blocking almost all radiation below 290 nm (WILLIS, 1971). Thus, UV-C light does not reach the earth's surface. Water vapour in the atmosphere effectively filters radiation greater than 1000 nm and as a consequence very little infrared radiation reaches the earth. Less than 1% of the solar radiation reaching the earth lies in the UV spectrum and under optimal conditions, only about 0.2% of this radiation (that in the range 290–320 nm) will produce sunburn (WILLIS, 1971). Some of the factors known to influence the amount and type of solar radiation reaching the earth's surface are time of day, latitude, season, ozone layer and altitude. Regional atmospheric variations such as cloudiness, haze, smoke, fog, dust and humidity are also important determinants. Latitude is the most important of these factors and the lower the latitude, the greater the risk of harmful solar effects. The hours of greatest risk of UV-induced injury to skin at all latitudes are between 1000 and 1500 h, solar time (WILLIS, 1971).

Responses of the skin to UV irradiation depend upon the dose, the amount of pre-existing melanin and the thickness of the epidermis. Skin reacts only to the energy to which it is exposed (dose) and not to the rate of delivery (flux) (BERGER, 1969). Short

Table 1. Radiation definitions

Radiation	Wavelength
Ultraviolet (UV)	200– 400 nm
UV-C	200– 280 nm
UV-B	280– 320 nm
UV-A	320– 400 nm
Visible	400– 760 nm
Blue	$\approx$450 nm
Green	$\approx$530 nm
Red	$\approx$700 nm
Infrared (IR)	760–5000 nm
Solar	290–1000 nm

intense periods of irradiation produce the same effect as weaker continuous irradiation of the same spectral energy. The latency, time to reach maximal response and duration of erythema and pigmentation vary considerably with the dosage and type of UV irradiation (i.e. UV-A, UV-B or UV-C) (BACHEM, 1955).

Protection against actinic damage to human skin is due largely to the ability of the stratum corneum to absorb and scatter UV light. Wavelengths greater than 300 nm may be transmitted by the stratum cornea to the extent of 50% (SAYRE, 1973). Hyperaemia can be induced in the subcutaneous tissues by 400 to 1400 nm radiation and wavelengths of 320 to 400 nm penetrate to the Malpighian and basal cell layers of skin. Only a small fraction of UV-B light (280–320 nm) reaches the Malpighian layer and dermis (FITZPATRICK et al., 1963). It has been estimated that 15% of UV-B light penetrates to the dermis whereas 60% of the visible spectrum of light reaches the superficial blood vessels of the dermis (HARBER, 1975). The minimal transmission of light by skin occurs at the wavelengths at which the aromatic amino acids present in proteins of the skin absorb maximally (270–280 nm). Light in the wavelength range 260–280 nm reaches the stratum granulosum and that in the range 200–260 nm can penetrate no further than the stratum corneum. These relationships are summarized in Table 2. The sunburn-producing spectrum of UV light comprises those wavelengths between 250 and 320 nm and the maximal effect is induced by UV-B irradiation (HAUSSER and VAHLE, 1927). UV-A light is weakly erythemogenic. The production of erythema by UV-A light requires 200–300 times more energy than that of UV-B light (PATHAK and EPSTEIN, 1971). UV-A light, however, has been implicated in many light-induced phenomena including melanogenesis, photosensitivities to drugs and other photobiological reactions (YING et al., 1974), and appears to be photoaugmentative (WILLIS et al., 1973) or photoadditive (PARRISH et al., 1974) with shorter wavelength UV light. In general, the erythemogenic and melanogenic effects of UV light increase with increasing wavelength (BREIT and KLIGMAN, 1969). Exposure to increasing wavelengths of UV light tends to increase the latency of onset of the response and decrease the duration of the effect (HAUSSER and VAHLE, 1927). These qualitatively different effects of the various types of UV light may be related to the depth of penetration (Table 2). It is also suspected that different mechanisms are involved in the damage produced by different types of UV light. Thus, the longer wavelengths which can penetrate deeply may exert at least part of their effect by a direct action on the dermal blood vessels, while it has been proposed that poorly

Table 2. Skin penetration of light of different wavelengths

Structure	Penetrating wavelengths, nm
Epidermis	
Stratum corneum	200– 260
Stratum granulosum	260– 280 (UV-C)
Stratum malpighii	280– 320 (UV-B)
Basal cell layer	320– 400 (UV-A)
Dermis	400–1400

penetrating shorter wavelength light induces the epidermal release of endogenous vasoactive mediators which diffuse to the dermal blood vessels and produce vasodilatation (BREIT and KLIGMAN, 1969). In addition to a possible direct effect of UV light on blood vessels (SAMS and WINKELMANN, 1969), proposed mediators of the erythematous response induced by UV irradiation include hydrolytic and proteolytic enzymes of lysosomes whose membranes are susceptible to damage after exposure to UV light (JOHNSON and DANIELS, 1969; OLSON and EVERETT, 1969), histamine released as a result of injury to mast cells (VALTONEN, 1961; VALTONEN et al., 1964; GRÓF and KÓVACS, 1967), kinins (EPSTEIN and WINKELMANN, 1967), unidentified factors released from leucocytes and prostaglandins (GREAVES and SONDERGAARD, 1970; MATHUR and GANDHI, 1972; SNYDER and EAGLSTEIN, 1974a).

C. Instrumentation

I. Light Sources for Induction of Erythema

Commercially available UV light sources are listed in the reviews by MONASH (1965), SCHÄFER (1969), and HARBER et al., (1974a, 1974b) and in Table 3. The UV component of sunlight which reaches the earth's surface is comprised of approximately 40% UV-B and 60% UV-A light. Many unfiltered, artificial light sources have significant output in the UV-C range which includes wavelengths not present in natural sunlight at the earth's surface. To study the effects of more limited ranges of wavelengths of UV light, various filters may be employed (Table 4). A solar simulator is also available (Table 3).

II. Measurement of Erythema and Local Hyperthermia

1. Erythema

TRONNIER (1969) has summarized the methods used to assess erythema. These include subjective observation, photography and reflectometry. Subjective evaluation is probably the most widely used method and appears adequate for a pharmacological screening programme. For more precise characterization of the response of skin to UV light, assessment by the eye is inadequate (BREIT and KLIGMAN, 1969; DANIELS and IMBRIE, 1958). According to BREIT and KLIGMAN (1969), a recording spectrophotometer adapted for reflectance measurements is the definitive instrument.

2. Skin Temperature

The measurement of skin temperature may be accomplished by several techniques and each has its own advantages and disadvantages. A commonly employed contact thermometer is the thermistor-type Tele-thermometer (Model 43TA, Yellow Springs Instrument Company, Yellow Springs, OH, U.S.A.). SNYDER and EAGLSTEIN (1974b) and CHIMOSKEY and FLANAGAN (1974) utilized this instrument in their measurements of inflammatory hyperthermia. Contact thermometers have a number of disadvantages and COLLINS and RING (1972) felt them to be less reliable than an infrared radiometer because of their slower response time.

Table 3. Commercially available UV light sources

Source	Type	Emission spectrum (UV + visible)	Approximate erythemal dose (human)	Disadvantages	Advantages	Manufacturer (U.S.A.)
Sun	Black body	Continuous ≃290→760 nm max. ≃330→760 nm	≃20 min	Difficult to control, UV-A content varies	Economical, high intensity, availability	—
Carbon arc	Open arc atm. pressure	Continuous ≃250→760 nm max. 360→500 nm	5–20 s	Variable output, electrode deterioration, gaseous waste products	Approximates sunlight	Union Carbide, National Carbon Div., Cleveland, OH
Fluorescent 'sun lamp'	Hg° arc low pressure	Continuous 280→380 nm max. 313 nm	90–120 s (25.4 cm)	Negligible energy > 340 nm	Economical, good source of erythemogenic radiation, easy to obtain and standardize	Westinghouse, Pittsburgh, PA
Fluorescent 'black light'	Hg° arc low pressure	Continuous 320→450 nm max. 360 nm	Not suitable	Poor source of erythemogenic radiation, negligible energy < 340 nm	Economical, easy to obtain and standardize	Westinghouse, Pittsburgh, PA; Sylvania, New York, NY General Electric, Stanford, CT
Solar simulator	Xe° arc high pressure	Continuous 295→450 nm max. 320→390 nm	60–120 s (25.4 cm)	Expensive, bulky	Very close to sunlight, standard source	Solar Light Company, Philadelphia, PA
Hot quartz (Alpine)	Hg° arc high pressure	Discontinuous, major peaks: 254 nm 265 nm 297 nm 303 nm 313 nm 365 nm	30–60 s (46 cm)	Significant output < 290 nm lamp deterioration	Convenience	Hanovia, Newark, NJ

Hot quartz (Krohmayer)	Hg° arc high pressure	Discontinuous, major peaks: 254 nm 265 nm 297 nm 303 nm 313 nm 365 nm	2–6 s (contact)	Expensive, small field, significant output <290 nm	Convenience	Hanovia, Newark, NJ
Cold quartz	Hg° arc low pressure	Discontinuous, major peak 254 nm	30 s (25 cm)	>90% emission at 254 nm	Economical	R. A. Fischer, Glendale, CA
Woodlight	Hg° arc high pressure	Discontinuous, major peak at 365 nm	Not suitable	Emission >350 nm, unsuitable research tool	Economical	UV Products Inc., San Gabriel, CA

Table 4. Filters for UV light sources

Filter	Transmission
Window glass	>320 nm
Pyrex glass	>290 nm
Mylar film (Dupont)	>310 nm
Schott WG 5	>300 nm
Corning 9863	<420 nm
Schott WG 3	>320 nm

A more sophisticated, and expensive, method of measuring temperatures of the skin is infrared thermography (KARPMAN, 1970). The infrared emission from a human or animal body can be collected optically, transformed and recorded. Descriptions of available equipment may be found in the review by GERSHON-COHEN et al. (1965). A commonly used instrument is the Barnes Medical Thermograph (Barnes Engineering Company, Stanford, Connecticut, U.S.A.). This instrument has a sensitivity of about 0.1° C and an accuracy of about 0.5° C. Infrared thermography appears to be used more in diagnostic medicine than in laboratory research.

D. Procedures

I. Erythema

1. UV-Induced

a) Guinea Pig

The method, originally described by WILHELMI (1949, 1950) and WILHELMI and DOMENJOZ (1951), was critically examined by WINDER et al. (1958), and the reader is referred to their articles for a detailed description of the procedure. Albino guinea pigs are depilated 12 to 24 h prior to the assay. Chemical depilators[1] are preferred to clipping of the hair to provide a smooth, more easily assessable area of skin. Chemical depilation (or clipping) may occasionally produce a mild local dermatitis but the 12 to 24 h interval between removal of the hair and the assay minimizes any interference with the grading of the erythemas that this might produce. There may be some influence on the assay by the location of skin that is used. WINDER et al. (1958) noted that the erythema was easier to see on the ventro-lateral than on the dorsolateral areas, and LOGAN and WILHELM (1966 b) observed that the intensity of erythema decreased "slightly but progressively from the cervical toward the lumbar levels (of the dorsal trunk)." Guinea pigs of either sex may be used and the weight range does not appear to be critical except for ease of handling. Animals ranging from 250 to 800 g have been used with apparently no large discrepancies in the results achieved among different laboratories. Most investigators utilize guinea pigs which have been fasted overnight, but the effects of the presence of food in the gut on the response of the erythema to drugs are not always predictable (WINDER et al., 1962). The unanaesthetized animals are restrained and circumscribed areas (usually three circles, 6–10 mm in diameter) of skin are exposed to the UV light source. Some investigators use more than three exposed sites, but because of the cervical-lumbar gradient in erythematous response (above) and the diminution of radiation density toward the margins of the filter (WINDER et al., 1958), there is a limit to the number of sites which may be exposed without introducing another variable into the assay.

The most popular light source for the routine assessment of nonsteroid antiinflammatory drugs has been the Krohmayer hot quartz lamp (Table 3), equipped with a type of heat filter to minimize the complication of concomitant thermal injury.

---

[1] See WINDER et al. (1958) for the composition of one depilatory preparation.

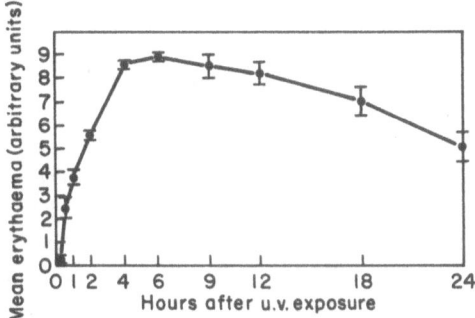

Fig. 1. Time course of development of UV-induced erythema of the guinea pig skin. Each point represents mean of 12 observations; the vertical bars represent standard error of the mean. (From GUPTA and LEVY, 1973; with permission)

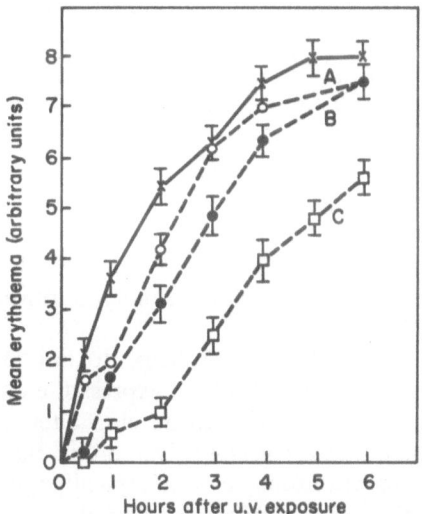

Fig. 2. Development of UV erythema in control and drug-treated animals. Drugs were administered intragastrically 30 min before UV exposure. Controls received the vehicle alone. Each point is the mean of at least 8 observations; *vertical bars* represent the standard error of the mean. ——— control; ––– indomethacin. A — 1 mg/kg; B — 2 mg/kg; C — 4 mg/kg. (From GUPTA and LEVY, 1973; with permission)

This lamp is not suitable for the assessment of sunscreening preparations because it is not a "solar simulator". However, it does produce an erythema which is inhibited by "reasonable" doses of conventional nonsteroid anti-inflammatory drugs. Exposure times of 20–120 s at a distance of 3–20 cm are required to produce erythema. If the shorter wavelengths are filtered out, a longer exposure time is required to produce erythema. The erythemas are usually rated 2 h after irradiation, which is not the time of maximal response (Fig. 1) but rather a time when most nonsteroid anti-inflammatory drugs may be relied on to produce a definite inhibitory effect (Fig. 2).

The erythemas are usually rated on a three or four point scale according to their completeness within the exposed area. Although some investigators have incorporated a grading of the intensity of the erythema in their scoring systems, WINDER et al. (1958) point out that the variability in response among animals treated alike makes this parameter rather unreliable. Using each animal as its own control may help reduce such variability (NAVARRO et al., 1974). These investigators irradiated one side of the nonmedicated animal and recorded the erythematous score. The next day the other side was irradiated after administering the test drug to the animal. The difference in scores between the two sides was used to determine the percent inhibition of the response. A disadvantage of this method, however, would be the regrowth of hair by the 2nd day which is claimed to interfere with irradiation (LOGAN and WILHELM, 1966 b). Because of the subjective nature of the scoring of erythema, it is imperative that the scorer be unaware of the treatments the animals have received and that randomization is employed. A more objective measurement of the response is suggested by the data of LAMBELIN et al. (1971) who demonstrated a close correlation between cutaneous temperature and development of erythema in the exposed sites. The data are usually treated quantally and those animals showing less than half the maximal erythematous response are scored as 'protected'. Such data may then be conveniently handled by probit analysis. WINDER et al. (1958) found that the numerical scores of individual animals were not suitably distributed for variance analysis. These same authors also demonstrated that a homogeneous binomial distribution existed for the quantal responses of 526 control five-animal samples. Other ways of expressing the data include the pharmacologically sound method of determining areas under the time-response curve (KOSERSKY et al., 1973), which assists in making valid comparisons between drugs which have different onsets and durations of action.

Because nonsteroid anti-inflammatory drugs do not prevent, but only delay, the development of erythema it is possible to express the data in terms of the time required for the erythematous response to develop after administration of drugs (GUPTA and LEVY, 1973). Drugs are usually given orally, but parenteral routes have also been used. Drug preparations may also be topically applied and, if this route is used, they should be applied after irradiation unless the UV-screening ability of the preparations is being assessed. Drugs were administered in the original descriptions of the method in two doses. One-half of the desired dosage was given 1 h before, and the other half immediately after, UV exposure. Others have opted for a single dose (30–60 min prior to irradiation), but this regimen may decrease the sensitivity of the assay. For example, ADAMS and COBB (1958) and SWINGLE et al. (1971 and Fig. 3) estimate ED_{50} values for phenylbutazone, after administration of a single dose, which are about twice those estimated by WINDER et al. (1958) who utilized the divided dosage regimen.

b) Other Species

α) Rat

First utilized by SCHIKORR (1932) in evaluating the effect of anti-inflammatory drugs on UV-induced erythema, the use of this species has since received little or no attention and the guinea pig is the laboratory species preferred for this type of assay.

β) Mouse

The response of mouse skin to acute UV irradiation has been used by some laboratories to evaluate anti-inflammatory drugs or sunscreen preparations. VALTONEN (1966) utilized the erythematous response of the mouse ear to UV irradiation. Depilated mouse skin is pink and this interferes with the scoring of erythema but the use of the ear as the irradiated site circumvents this problem. SIM (1965) measured both accumulation of protein and increased vascular permeability at the site of irradiation in this species. These events, however, appear to be phenomena discrete from the erythematous response.

The UV-induced erythematous response in the skin of the hairless mouse, a variant strain requiring no depilation, was used by WOLSKA et al. (1974) to evaluate sunscreen preparations. SIM (1965), however, reported this more convenient strain to be somewhat less sensitive than various haired strains in its response to UV radiation.

Evaluation of drugs using UV light-induced erythema in this species does not appear to offer any advantage over the frequently used and much better characterized assay in the guinea pig.

γ) Man

UV light-induced erythema in man has been utilized for the assay of anti-inflammatory drugs. Steroids (JARVINEN, 1951; SCOTT and KALZ, 1956; BURDICK et al., 1973; SNYDER and EAGLSTEIN, 1974a, 1974b) and nonsteroids (SCHNEIDER and TRONNIER, 1957; MILLER et al., 1967; GRUBER et al., 1972; SNYDER and EAGLSTEIN, 1974a, 1974b) have been reported to suppress the reaction in man. As in the guinea pig, effective agents delay, rather than prevent, the erythematous response (GRUBER et al., 1972).

To conduct a well-controlled assay in humans, the variables that apply to the assay in guinea pigs (see above) should be considered. The site to be irradiated should be untanned and relatively free of body hair. The abdomen, the buttocks and the volar surface of the forearms are the most commonly used areas of skin. When one is evaluating sunscreens or antisunburn agents, the light source must be one which simulates sunlight.

The time of exposure is that which produces a minimal erythematous response (minimal erythemal dose, MED) or some multiple of that value for that individual. The method of scoring the erythema varies considerably. Certain investigators recorded scores cumulatively during a period of time (GRUBER et al., 1972), but most score the erythema at one predetermined time which is commonly between 4 and 24 h.

Variability in the assay can be reduced by using each individual as his own control. For the assay of topical preparations, this is easily accomplished by assessing treated and untreated areas of skin in the subject. Randomization of treatment and control sites should be used. Such a protocol is described by TRONNIER (1969). For studies in which the drugs are administered systemically, determinations of the MED for each subject should be determined prior to administration of the drug.

An assessment of the efficacy of a prospective anti-inflammatory agent against UV-induced erythema in man is obviously desirable because this, in most cases, is the species for which the drug is intended. It also provides the pharmacologist an opportunity to ensure that his screening procedures can be extrapolated to man.

2. Thurfyl Nicotinate-Induced

Several different esters of nicotinic acid have been utilized to produce a localized erythema (STOUGHTON et al., 1960; EMDEN et al., 1971). The most popular compound for the evaluation of certain nonsteroid agents is the tetrahydro-furfuryl ester of nicotinic acid (thurfyl nicotinate, THFN, Trafuril). The hyperaemic properties of this agent were first described by GROSS and MERZ (1948).

a) Guinea Pig

This method for evaluating anti-inflammatory substances was used in the guinea pig after its use in man for that purpose (TRUELOVE and DUTHIE, 1959). As described by HAINING (1963), a 5% aqueous solution of the THFN is applied to sites on one side of the depilated backs of guinea pigs. In these studies, the other side was irradiated with UV light for comparison. Erythema induced by the THFN solution reaches its maximum at approximately 15 min and begins to subside at about 1 h. In general, the dose of drug required to inhibit the response to THFN is less than that required to inhibit the response to UV light. However, the erythema resulting from the topical application of THFN is fainter and more difficult to read than that which occurs after UV irradiation.

An advantage of this method, as of UV erythema, is that it allows the estimation of the relative effectiveness of drugs in man and animals by the same means.

b) Man

The inflammation which results from the topical application of THFN has been used for the evaluation of nonsteroid anti-inflammatory compounds (TRUELOVE and DUTHIE, 1959). A 5% cream or ointment of THFN is applied to the volar surface of the forearm for about 20 min and then usually removed. The erythema is then assessed at 45–60 min intervals.

In this assay, a control erythematous response is determined first. The test drug is administered and at an appropriate time thereafter the erythemal challenge is repeated. The response is determined from the difference between the scores before and after administration of the drug.

3. Miscellaneous Procedures for Producing Erythema

a) Tetrahydrofurfuryl Alcohol

The method has been described by SCHLAGEL and NORTHAM (1959) and BRUNNER and FINKELSTEIN (1960) as a procedure for evaluating the efficacy of topically applied steroids on human skin. The compounds to be evaluated are dissolved in the irritant alcohol and applied to the skin in small volumes (0.25 ml) under an occlusive dressing. The dressings are left in place from late afternoon until the following morning and then removed. The erythema is scored visually. Topically applied steroids inhibit the erythematous response to this irritant.

b) Retinoic Acid

Treatment of depilated skin of guinea pigs twice daily with 0.05% retinoic acid results in development of an erythema which is maximal at 3 days (ZIBOH et al., 1975). The development of erythema was suppressed by the topical application of indomethacin.

c) Tuberculin Reaction

The delayed hypersensitivity reaction, produced by injection of tuberculin into sensitized guinea pigs, produces erythema in addition to other inflammatory changes (FLOERSHEIM, 1965; WALTERS and WILLOUGHBY, 1965). Both steroid and nonsteroid anti-inflammatory drugs suppress the early erythema but have no effect on the other phases. The erythema associated with the tuberculin reaction in man is well documented and may be suppressed by steroids (LONG and FAVOUR, 1950; DOUGH-ERTY et al., 1954). A nonsteroid anti-inflammatory drug, ibuprofen, was reported to be ineffective (BROOKS et al., 1973).

d) Thermally Induced Erythema

Thermal injury of the skin of animals produces an inflammatory response which is accompanied by erythema. A thermal stimulus of 50–60° C will produce the response in rats (SPECTOR and WILLOUGHBY, 1958), guinea pigs (SEVITT, 1958) and rabbits (WILHELM and MASON, 1960). Erythema is part of the immediate response to injury which is followed by a delayed oedematous response. Suppression of the erythema per se by anti-inflammatory agents apparently has not been determined.

e) Lipopolysaccharide-Induced Erythema

Subcutaneous injection of a highly purified lipopolysaccharide from *Salmonella* (pyrexal) (HEILMEYER and HIEMEYER, 1965) or *Pseudomonas* (piromen) (HIEMEYER, 1968) into the forearm of man produces an erythema which persists for an average of 37–41 h. Both steroids and nonsteroids shorten the duration of the erythema.

f) Other

Erythemas produced by X-ray (HIRABAYASHI and GRAHAM, 1969), bacterial infection (BURKE and MILES, 1958), mustard oil or nitric acid (SCOTT and KALZ, 1956) and skin stripping with cellophane tape (WELLS, 1957) have been used for assessing the anti-inflammatory activity of substances.

Immediate hypersensitivity reactions induced in the skin of various species include an erythematous phase but this has seldom been utilized in the evaluation of anti-inflammatory agents.

II. Local Hyperthermia

There is no widely accepted standard experimental technique which utilizes the increased temperature of an inflamed site for the assessment of the anti-inflammatory activity of substances. Increased blood flow, erythema, and elevated temperature are strictly correlated (e.g. CHIMOSKEY et al., 1974) and, although inherently the measurement of temperature would appear to be more objective than the grading of degrees of redness, there have been relatively few attempts by pharmacologists to utilize local hyperthermia as the measured response. Some of the studies utilizing local hyperthermia as the measured response may be found in Section C.II. of this chapter.

1. Local Hyperthermia in Paws of Rats Injected With Irritants

a) Yeast

PIRCIO and GROSKINSKY (1966) describe a method for evaluating the effects of anti-inflammtory drugs on the local hyperthermia occurring in yeast-injected hind paws of rats. These investigators utilized an infrared thermometer for determining skin temperature. After the injection of an aqueous suspension of brewer's yeast into the plantar tissues of rats, a biphasic response was observed. The initial temperature rise in the paw (the maximal response occurred around the tibiotarsal joint) was apparent approximately 2 min after the injection of yeast and reached its maximum at 12–14 min. A decrease in the temperature of the paw occurred in the next 40 min and was followed by a second phase of local hyperthermia which reached its maximum about 3–4 h after the injection. In contradistinction to the local temperature changes occurring in paws of rats injected with carrageenin (see below), there was no significant rise in temperature of the noninjected paw nor of body temperature during the test period. PIRCIO and GROSKINSKY (1966), however, followed the response for only $2\frac{1}{2}$ h and the possibility of a systemic hyperthermia developing after this time cannot be ruled out because this is approximately the time that rises in body temperature (SOBANSKI et al., 1974) and skin temperature of the noninflamed paw (VINEGAR et al., 1969) occur in carrageenin-injected rats.

The method of PIRCIO and GROSKINKSY (1966) is sufficiently defined to serve as a standard procedure for assessing the activity of substances on the local hyperthermic component of the inflammatory response. These investigators established that the skin temperatures of hind paws of rats not injected with yeast were normally distributed but the equally important distribution, i.e. the temperatures of yeast-injected paws, was not reported. This local hyperthermia can be inhibited by nonsteroid anti-inflammatory drugs (Section E.IV.) which suggests that the method would be a useful adjunct to the battery of tests used to screen for anti-inflammatory activity of compounds of this type.

b) Carrageenin

Inhibition of the oedema produced in the paw of the rat after injection of the polysaccharide, carrageenin, into the plantar tissues is widely used for assessing anti-inflammatory activity of substances (Chapter 21). In addition to measuring the oedematous response, a few investigators have also determined changes in skin temperature of the inflamed paw. VINEGAR et al. (1969), using a contact thermometer, described the biphasic development of hyperthermia in the carrageenin-injected paw. There occurred an immediate increase in temperature (ca. 6° C) which lasted approximately 30 min. By 45 min the temperature of the inflamed paw had returned to its normal value. The second phase of hyperthermia began at about 1 h and steadily increased during the next 4 h. Temperatures were apparently not determined after this time. COLLINS and RING (1972), utilizing a noncontact infrared thermometer, demonstrated the persistence of the hyperthermia for at least 48 h following the injection of carrageenin. VINEGAR et al. (1969) reported that the temperature of the noninflamed paw also rose between 2 and 4 h after injection of the irritant and the rate of rise equalled that of the inflamed paw. These investigators attributed this to the rats resting their bodies on their hindlimbs between measurements. This would appear to be an important variable in methods using rats. They could eliminate the increase in temperature of the noninjected paw by taking more frequent measurements, but observed that such repeated manipulations of the animals resulted in a diminution of the *oedematous* response in the paw. This decrease in swelling was presumably due to the release of endogenous anti-inflammatory corticosteroids. Another explanation for the increase in temperature of both paws after the injection of carrageenin into one is suggested by the data of SOBANSKI et al. (1974). After the injection of carrageenin into the plantar tissues, a sustained *systemic* hyperthermia ensued. This increase in body temperature coincides with the second phase of *local* hyperthermia described by VINEGAR et al. (1969).

c) Freund's Adjuvant

Many parameters of adjuvant-induced arthritis in the rat have been used to assess the anti-inflammatory activity of substances (SWINGLE, 1974). One of these is the local hyperthermia which occurs in the arthritic paw. WALZ et al. (1970), who injected adjuvant into one hind paw, demonstrated a biphasic hyperthermia in this paw. The maximal paw temperature occurred on the 1st day after injection of the adjuvant. The other paw which also becomes oedematous in this model after a delay of approximately 8–10 days (Chapter 23) became hyperthermic on day 7. These investigators found no correlation between the volumes of the paws (oedema) and the local hyperthermia, which once again points out the apparent independence of these two phenomena at inflammatory loci. COLLINS and RING (1972) confirmed the findings of WALZ et al. (1970) for the local hyperthermic changes occurring in the adjuvant arthritic rat.

2. Local Hyperthermia in UV-Irradiated Skin

a) Guinea Pig

LAMBELIN et al. (1970, 1971), using a contact thermometer, determined the effect of topically applied anti-inflammatory agents on the local hyperthermia resulting from UV-irradiation of guinea pig skin. These investigators established the time course of temperature rises in exposed and unexposed skin. The maximal temperature increase at UV-irradiated sites occurred about 5–6 h after exposure. Elevated temperatures at the exposed sites were still apparent at 24 h. A slight increase in temperature of nonexposed skin was also apparent. These investigators chose to use each animal as its own control because of significant between-group interaction of skin temperatures in untreated animals. This was accomplished by recording the difference in temperature between untreated and treated exposed sites on each animal. Skin temperature of the erythematous sites appears to be closely correlated with the subjective assessment of redness as reported by GUPTA and LEVY (1973 and Figure 1).

Because of this apparently close and expected correlation between erythema and skin temperature, the measurement of cutaneous temperature seems a priori to be a more suitable parameter for assessing the response than the subjective evaluation of erythema in the guinea pig.

b) Man

SNYDER and EAGLSTEIN (1974b) and SNYDER (1975) determined cutaneous temperature in addition to a subjective evaluation of erythema of UV-irradiated skin in humans with or without treatment with the anti-inflammatory drug, indomethacin. These investigators, using a contact thermometer, reported a difference in temperature between irradiated and nonirradiated sites of 0.83–1.1° C.

E. Inhibition of Erythema and Local Hyperthermia

I. UV-Induced Erythema

1. Systemic Administration of Drugs

Nonsteroidal anti-inflammatory drugs which are acidic will, with few exceptions, delay the appearance of UV-induced erythema in the skin of guinea pigs (Fig. 2). Ranges of ED_{50} values reported by various laboratories for six common anti-inflammatory drugs are given in Table 5. There occurs for certain drugs an eightfold difference in estimates of the ED_{50}. The most obvious explanation for this discrepancy is the lack of uniformity in the method employed by various laboratories. Differences in the conditions of irradiation (amount of energy delivered, wavelengths of light used, presence or absence of heat filters, etc.) would be expected to be

Table 5. Ranges of ED_{50} values determined for certain anti-inflammatory drugs on UV-induced erythema of guinea pig skin

Drug	Oral ED_{50}, mg/kg	References[a]
Acetylsalicylic acid	52 –86	3, 9, 15, 18
Aminopyrine	43 –80	5, 11, 18
Phenylbutazone	3.5–23	1, 2, 3, 4, 5, 6, 7, 8, 9, 10, 15, 18, 19, 20
Indomethacin	0.9–10.2	1, 2, 3, 7, 12, 19, 20
Mefenamic acid	8 –65	1, 6, 7, 13, 17, 18
Ibuprofen	4 – 6.8	14, 16

[a] 1. ALPERMANN (1970)
2. YAMAMOTO et al. (1969)
3. BARRON et al. (1968)
4. GÖRÖG and SZPORNY (1966)
5. WINDER et al. (1958)
6. JAHN and ADRIAN (1969)
7. KOSERSKY et al. (1973)
8. ROSENKILDE (1964)
9. SWINGLE et al. (1971)
10. NAVARRO et al. (1974)
11. ADAMS (1960)
12. JULOU et al. (1971)
13. SWINGLE et al. (1970)
14. JAHN and WAGNER-JAUREGG (1974)
15. ADAMS and COBB (1958)
16. ADAMS et al. (1969)
17. WINDER et al. (1962)
18. WINDER et al. (1965)
19. RIEDEL and SCHOETENSACK (1973)
20. BIRNIE et al. (1967).

important variables in the assay (VALTONEN, 1966). Lower doses of irradiation will not induce the first phase of increased vascular permeability in the skin of guinea pigs (LOGAN and WILHELM, 1966b) or mice (SIM, 1965), demonstrating the importance of controlling the amount of energy delivered in the assay. EAGLSTEIN and MARSICO (1975) showed in UV-irradiated humans that doses of indomethacin (given i.d.), which were effective antagonists of erythema induced by UV-B, had little effect on that induced by UV-C light. The physical form of the dosage (suspension-solution, particle size in suspension) and the condition of the guinea pigs (fed or fasted) were found to alter dramatically the ED_{50} of mefenamic acid (WINDER et al., 1962). These investigators reported independent estimates of the ED_{50} for this drug ranging from about 7–32 mg/kg depending on the above cited variables, with all other conditions of the assay remaining constant. In addition to the expected physicochemical interactions of drug with food in the gut, another influence of fasting on the assay is possible. Fasted animals normally reduce their intake of water and, if such animals are in a state of partial dehydration, a lesser response to UV light might be expected because hydration of the skin promotes injury induced by UV light (OWENS et al., 1975). SIM (1965) attributed the reduced accumulation of protein in irradiated mouse skin to the reduction of water intake by the fasted animals.

Because most laboratories tend to modify procedures, a better point of comparison for data between laboratories is probably the determination of relative potencies of drugs versus some common standard (e.g. phenylbutazone). Although the range of ED_{50} values for indomethacin in Table 5 is 0.9–10.2 mg/kg, when the relative potencies to phenylbutazone are calculated (in those cases where both drugs were used), the values range from 2.0–3.3.

WINDER et al. (1958, 1962) showed that the test could be used for the comparative bioassay of drugs and such a bioassay is shown in Figure 3. Some investigators were unable to use the procedure for comparative bioassay because of nonparallelism of

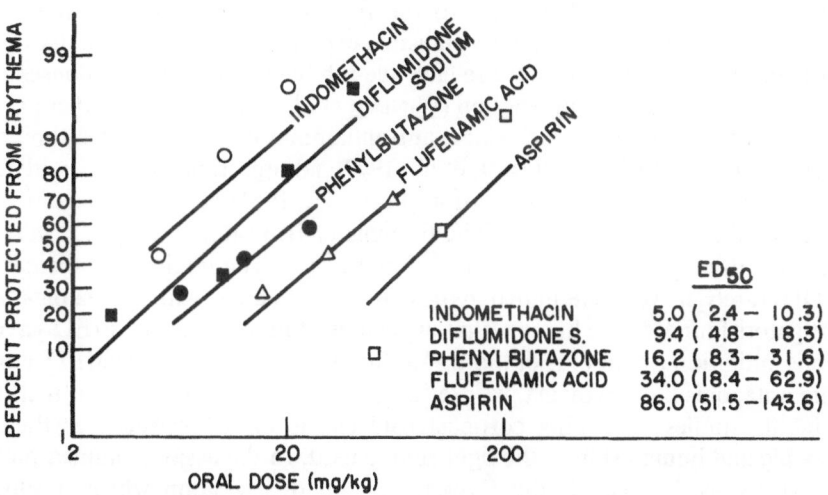

Fig. 3. Effect of anti-inflammatory drugs on UV-induced erythema of guinea pig skin. (From SWINGLE et al., 1971; with permission)

dose-response curves for certain drugs (ADAMS et al., 1969; KOSERSKY et al., 1973). The estimates of relative potencies obtained in this assay for acidic nonsteroid anti-inflammatory drugs are, in general, similar to those obtained in the more widely used assay for drugs of this type, i.e. carrageenin-induced oedema of the rat's paw (SWINGLE, 1974).

As pointed out by ADAMS and COBB (1958) and WINDER et al. (1958, 1965), the ability of a drug to delay the appearance of UV-induced erythema in guinea pig skin is closely correlated with its potency as an anti-inflammatory drug in man. The fact that such a correlation exists is surprising since the delay of UV-induced erythema in skin would superficially appear to bear no resemblance or relevance to the human inflammatory conditions for which such drugs are prescribed. WINDER et al. (1965) preferred to use the term 'antipreinflammatory' to describe the action of this class of drugs and, if true, then the antagonism of some early common event in inflammation (for example the inhibition of prostaglandin synthetase) might explain the correlation.

Effective drugs, even after repeated doses, do not inhibit but only delay the appearance of erythema (WILHELMI, 1949, 1950; WINDER et al., 1958; GUPTA and LEVY, 1973). Such an effect by the nonsteroid anti-inflammatory drugs on the erythema suggests that whatever component of the response is antagonized is not a prerequisite for the final expression of erythema. Perhaps the inflammatory response proceeds via pathways different from those normally used by the animal when such drugs are present.

The assay in guinea pigs is quite selective for drugs of the acidic nonsteroid anti-inflammatory type (WINDER et al., 1958). The inactivity of the anti-inflammatory glucocorticosteroids, even in massive doses and with a variety of treatment regimens, has been shown many times (BAVIN et al., 1955; WINDER et al., 1958; ROSENKILDE, 1964). Cortisone also fails to potentiate the antierythemic effect of phenylbutazone (WINDER et al., 1958) or hydrocortisone that of aspirin (SWINGLE, unpublished data). Although guinea pigs (and humans) are described as "steroid-resistant", particularly with respect to the lymphocytolytic effect of these compounds, this does not appear to be a plausible explanation for the inactivity of these compounds in the assay. Steroids are effective inhibitors of certain responses in the guinea pig, e.g. the tuberculin reaction (WINDER et al., 1957). Although there is some controversy regarding the conclusions, anti-inflammatory steroids after topical application under occlusion (BURDICK et al., 1973), i.d. injection (SNYDER and EAGLSTEIN, 1974a) or systemic administration (JARVINEN, 1951) partially antagonize UV-induced erythema in human skin. The findings of BURDICK et al. (1973) may help explain the discrepancy between man and guinea pig. The minimal erythemal dose (MED) is rarely, if ever, determined in the conventional assay with guinea pigs. These investigators found, in the human, that exposures of more than one MED gave less obvious inhibition by steroids of the UV-induced erythema. At three MED, corticosteroid antagonism of erythema was not apparent. Another difference in methodology in the studies examining corticosteroid effects on UV-induced erythema in guinea pig and human skin, is the light source used. In the assay in guinea pigs, the most widely used source is the Krohmayer hot quartz lamp which produces a significant amount of UV-C light (Table 3). In the human studies, the radiation is generally filtered so as to produce only UV-B light.

The inactivity of corticosteroids in the assay in guinea pigs is not necessarily a disadvantage in the routine screening of potential nonsteroid anti-inflammatory drugs since the possibility that a new compound is anti-inflammatory by virtue of stimulating the hypothalamic-pituitary-adrenal axis may be excluded.

The relative ineffectiveness of the clinically effective anti-inflammatory drug, oxyphenbutazone, against UV-induced erythema of guinea pig skin is the exception to the apparent selectivity of the assay for acidic nonsteroid anti-inflammatory drugs (WHITEHOUSE, 1965). Some investigators have shown activity at nontoxic doses for the drug although of a potency much less than would be predicted from clinical experience (JAHN and ADRIAN, 1969; YAMAMOTO et al., 1969), while others have reported it to be essentially inactive at high doses (WILHELMI, 1965; SWINGLE et al., 1970). JAHN and WAGNER-JAUREGG (1974) suggest that the relative ineffectiveness of oxyphenbutazone is due to unsatisfactory peroral absorption of the drug in guinea pigs. WEINER and PILIERO (1970) also point out that because of species differences in the size, anatomy and motility of the gut, it is not safe to assume that absorption of drugs by different species is equivalent.

The antimalarials (e.g. chloroquine) and basic nonsteroidal drugs, which have been used as antirheumatic agents in man, fail to influence UV-induced erythema in the guinea pig (WINDER et al., 1958; ROSENKILDE, 1964).

WINDER et al. (1958) tested the effects of over a hundred drugs or chemicals from diverse pharmacological classes on UV-induced erythema of guinea pig skin. In 1958, the only acidic nonsteroid anti-inflammatory agents which had been identified and reported were the pyrazolones (e.g. phenylbutazone, antipyrine, aminopyrine), the salicylates and the cincophens. These were the only drugs tested that were found to have significant erythema-delaying activity at nontoxic doses and prompted the designation of the assay as selective for clinically useful nonsteroid antirheumatic agents. ADAMS (1960) also showed that the pyrazolones and salicylates were effective in delaying UV-induced erythema and, as WINDER et al. (1958), also reported, that the p-aminophenol derivatives (acetanilide, phenacetin, acetaminophen) were ineffective. On the basis of his findings, ADAMS suggested that the pharmacological group which was (and still is, in certain textbooks) classified as 'analgesic-antipyretic' be subdivided into two classes: viz., those which also possess anti-inflammatory activity (salicylates, pyrazolones, subsequently discovered agents) and those which do not (p-aminophenols). Drugs effective in delaying UV-induced erythema of guinea pig skin (an 'anti-inflammatory' effect), in most cases, also can be shown experimentally to have antipyretic and analgesic activities. ADAMS et al. (1969) believe that all three properties '...must be present if a compound is to show nonsteroid antirheumatic activity." WINDER et al. (1962) felt that "There may be some fundamental meaning in the circumstance that anti-inflammatory agents are also antipyretic". Because of the consistent association of the three activities in many compounds, it is tempting to propose a common mechanism of action to explain the correlation. An attractive hypothesis is that all three activities may be explained by the ability of compounds of this type to inhibit prostaglandin synthetase (see Chapters 30 and 31 of this volume).

An indication of the selectivity of the assay in guinea pigs for the anti-inflammatory/analgesic/antipyretic acidic nonsteroid anti-inflammatory drugs may be appreciated by the ineffectiveness of other pharmacological classes of compounds

Table 6. Drugs which do not inhibit UV-induced erythema of guinea pig skin

Drug	References [a]
Salicyl agents (salicylamide, gentisic acid, resorcylic acid, *p*-aminosalicylic acid)	1, 3
p-Aminophenol analgesics/antipyretics (acetanilide, acetaminophen, phenacetin)	1, 3
Xanthines (aminophylline, theobromine, caffeine)	1
Hormones (cortisone, hydrocortisone, dexamethasone, paramethasone, aldosterone, ACTH)	1, 2, 4, 6
Antimalarials (chloroquine, amodiaquine, quinacrine, primaquine, quinine)	1, 4
Antihistamines (except certain phenothiazines)	1, 4, 5
Local anesthetics-antiarrhythmics (procaine, procainamide, quinidine)	1
Barbiturates	1
Narcotic analgesics (codeine, morphine, meperidine, methadone)	1
Chemotherapeutic antimicrobial, immunosuppressive, antineoplastic agents (chloramphenicol, streptomycin, diethylcarbamazine, pyrazinamide, isoniazid, busulfan, 6-MP)	1, 6
Vitamins (niacinamide, pantothenic acid, pyridoxine, riboflavin, thiamine, ascorbic and dehydroascorbic acid, flavonoids)	1
Parasympathomimetics (methacholine, pilocarpine)	1, 4
Sympathomimetics (amphetamine, methamphetamine, ephedrine)	1, 4
Antimuscarinics (atropine)	1, 4
Adrenergic blocking agents (yohimbine, chlorpromazine)	1, 4
Vasodilators (hydralazine, nicotinic acid, papverine)	1
Miscellaneous (2,4-dinitrophenol, disulfiram, heparin, trypsin, fibrinolysin, colchicine, diphenylhydantoin, urethane)	1

[a] 1. WINDER et al. (1958)
2. BAVIN et al. (1955)
3. ADAMS (1960)
4. ROSENKILDE (1964)
5. WILHELMI and DOMENJOZ (1951)
6. KOSERSKY et al. (1973).

(Table 6). There are instances of *apparently* nonanti-inflammatory agents which will delay UV-induced erythema of guinea pig skin, but most of these drugs can be excluded on the basis of the doses used which are toxic and thus lead one to suspect that nonspecific actions of the drugs are involved in the inhibition. The effectiveness of carbachol (WINDER et al., 1958) and the postganglionic adrenergic blocking agents, bretylium and guanethidine, (ROSENKILDE, 1964) in the assay requires clarification.

The delay of UV-induced erythema of guinea pig skin by drugs must be included as one of the most selective pharmacological bioassays which utilizes a crude and ill-defined response in the whole animal.

2. Topically or Intradermally

Those acidic nonsteroid anti-inflammatory drugs which are effective in delaying UV-induced erythema after systemic administration will also delay the erythema when applied topically or injected i.d. at the irradiated sites (Table 7). Although conflicting reports exist, the steroid anti-inflammatory agents appear to be ineffective in inhibiting UV-induced erythema when applied topically, as they are when administered systemically (Table 8). KAIDBEY and KLIGMAN (1974) as well as BURDICK et al. (1973) reported that topically applied corticosteroids would diminish the erythema produced by one MED, but not at multiples of the MED. At one MED, it is conceivable that the vasoconstrictor property of the corticosteroids may account for their activity against UV-induced vasodilatation. Those nonsteroid anti-inflammatory drugs which have been tested after topical application will inhibit UV-induced erythema whether applied before or after irradiation. For certain compounds, however, there is a possibility that they (or the vehicle in which they are contained) will absorb a significant amount of the UV light if they are applied prior to irradiation. Such compounds may not be truly anti-inflammatory but rather UV light screening agents. For example, GRAEME et al. (1975) found that hydrocortisone would delay UV-induced erythema in guinea pigs when applied before, but not after, irradiation. Hydrocortisone has an absorption maximum of 242 nm and, depending upon the light source used in the study, can act as an effective UV light-screening agent (KANOF, 1955).

II. Tetrahydrofurfuryl Nicotinate (THFN) Erythema

Using this compound to produce erythema in the guinea pig, HAINING (1963) found that several nonsteroid anti-inflammatory agents reduced the response. Oral doses of drugs found to reduce the erythemic response by 30% were as follows: phenylbutazone, 5 mg/kg; aspirin, 50 mg/kg; sodium salicylate, 100 mg/kg. These doses were about half of those required for equivalent protection against UV erythema in this study.

A quantitative comparison of results obtained in man from different laboratories is somewhat difficult because of procedural differences. However, THFN erythema in man is inhibited by aspirin (ADAMS and COBB, 1963; TRUELOVE and DUTHIE, 1959), ibufenac (ADAMS et al., 1968; BROOKS et al., 1973) and ibuprofen (ADAMS et al., 1969). These latter two agents are newer nonsteroid anti-inflammatory drugs which resemble aspirin in their pharmacological activity in the laboratory. Effective doses in man of the above three agents were reported to be: aspirin, 225 mg; ibufenac, 960 mg; ibuprofen, 300 mg (ADAMS et al., 1968, 1969).

Sodium salicylate, phenylbutazone, and oxyphenbutazone have all been reported to be inactive against this model of inflammation in man (ADAMS and COBB, 1963).

III. Other Erythemas

Some anti-inflammatory drugs which inhibit erythematous responses induced by other means are given in Table 9.

IV. Local Hyperthermia

PIRCIO and GROSKINSKY (1966) demonstrated the inhibition by aspirin (200 mg/kg) of the hyperthermic response occurring in yeast-injected paws of rats (Fig. 4). This dose of aspirin had no effect on the oedema of the paw. The first phase of local hyperthermia was not as sensitive to aspirin as was the second phase. These investigators

Table 7. Inhibition of UV-induced erythema and hyperthermia by local nonsteroid antiinflammatory agents

Compound	Route[a]		Species[b]		Parameters		UV light source	Results	References
	T	ID	Man	GP	Ery-thema	Hyper-thermia			
Aspirin	X		X	X		X	Hanau lamp high pres. Hg° (predominantly UV-C)	Aspirin ≈ phenylbutazone < bufexamac	LAMBELIN et al., 1971
Aspirin		X	X	X	X		Westinghouse FS 20	Aspirin ≪ indomethacin	SNYDER and EAGLSTEIN, 1974a
Aspirin	X			X	X		Hanovia high pres. Hg° (predominantly UV-C)	Aspirin ≪ indomethacin = diflumidone	TRANCIK and SWINGLE, unpublished
Indomethacin		X	X	X	X		Westinghouse FS 20	Indomethacin ≫ aspirin	SNYDER and EAGLSTEIN, 1974a
Indomethacin	X		X	X	X	X	Sunlight and Westinghouse FS 20	Indomethacin ≫ fluocinonide	SNYDER and EAGLSTEIN, 1974b
Indomethacin	X		X	X	X	X	Westinghouse FS 20	Marked decrease in UV light-induced erythema and hyperthermia	SNYDER, 1975

				Light source	Result	Reference
Indomethacin	X	X	X	Westinghouse FS 20 (UV-B) & Westinghouse sterilamp 782L-30 (UV-C)	Decrease in UV-B-induced erythema but not UV-C-induced erythema	EAGLSTEIN and MARSICO, 1975
Indomethacin	X	X	X	Hanovia high pres. Hg° (predominantly UV-C)	Indomethacin = diflumidone ≫ aspirin	TRANCIK and SWINGLE, unpublished
Phenylbutazone	X	X	X	Hanau lamp high pres. Hg° (predominantly UV-C)	Phenylbutazone ≈ aspirin < bufexamac	LAMBELIN et al., 1971
Bufexamac	X	X	X	Hanau lamp high pres. Hg° (predominantly UV-C)	Bufexamac > phenylbutazone ≈ aspirin	LAMBELIN et al., 1971
Diflumidone	X	X	X	Hanovia high pres. Hg° (predominantly UV-C)	Diflumidone = indomethacin ≫ aspirin	TRANCIK and SWINGLE, unpublished

[a] T = Topical, ID = Intradermal.
[b] GP = Guinea pig.

Table 8. Inhibition of UV-induced erythema and hyperthermia by local steroid antiinflammatory agents

Compound	Route[a]		Species[b]		Parameters		UV-light source	Results	References
	T	ID	Man	GP	Ery-thema	Hyper-thermia			
Fluocinonide	X		X		X	X	Sunlight and Westinghouse FS 20	Fluocinonide = vehicle ≪ indomethacin	SNYDER and EAGLSTEIN, 1974b
Fluocinolone Acetonide	X			X		X	Hanau lamp high pres. Hg° (predominantly UV-C)	Ineffective	LAMBELIN et al., 1971
Fluocinolone Acetonide	X		X			X	Westinghouse RS	Ineffective	CHIMOSKEY et al., 1974
Triamcinolone Acetonide		X	X	X	X		Westinghouse FS 20	Effective in man but not in guinea pigs	SNYDER and EAGLSTEIN, 1974a
Hydrocortisone		X		X	X		Westinghouse FS 20	Ineffective	SNYDER and EAGLSTEIN, 1974a
Hydrocortisone	X			X	X		Hanovia high pres. Hg° (predominantly UV-C)	Ineffective	TRANCIK and SWINGLE, unpublished
Hydrocortisone	X		X		X		"Hot quartz generator"	Ineffective	KANOF, 1955

[a] T = Topical, ID = Intradermal.
[b] GP = Guinea pig.

Table 9. Inhibition by antiinflammatory drugs of erythema induced by various stimuli

Stimulus	Species	Drug	Route[a] T	p.o.	Minimal effective dose or concentration	Reference
Tetrahydrofurfuryl alcohol	Man	Hydrocortisone	X		1.0%	SCHLAGEL and NORTHAM (1959)
		Prednisolone	X		0.5%	
		6 α-methylprednisolone	X		0.25%	
		9 α-fluorohydrocortisone	X		0.1%	
Retinoic acid, 0.05%	Guinea pig	Indomethacin	X		1.0%	ZIBOH et al. (1975)
Tuberculin	Guinea pig	Aminopyrine		X	15 mg/kg × 2	FLOERSHEIM (1965)
		Phenylbutazone		X	15 mg/kg × 2	
		Prednisolone		X	30 mg/kg × 2	
		Chloroquine		X	45 mg/kg × 2	
		Indomethacin		X	10 mg/kg × 2	
Bacterial lipopolysaccharide	Man	Prednisone		X	10 mg × 2 days	WALTERS and WILLOUGHBY (1965) HEILMEYER and HIEMEYER (1965)
		Salicylamide		X	4 g × 4 days	
		Phenylbutazone		X	600 mg × 2 days	
		Oxyphenbutazone		X	400 mg × 5 days	
Mustard oil, 80%	Man	Hydrocortisone	X		1.0%	SCOTT and KALZ (1956)
		Fluorocortisone	X		0.25%	
Nitric acid, 15%	Man	Hydrocortisone	X		1.0%	SCOTT and KALZ (1956)
		Fluorocortisone	X		0.25%	
Skin stripping with cellophane tape	Man	Hydrocortisone	X		1.0%	WELLS (1957)
		Fluorohydrocortisone	X		0.1%	

[a] T = Topical, p.o. = per os.

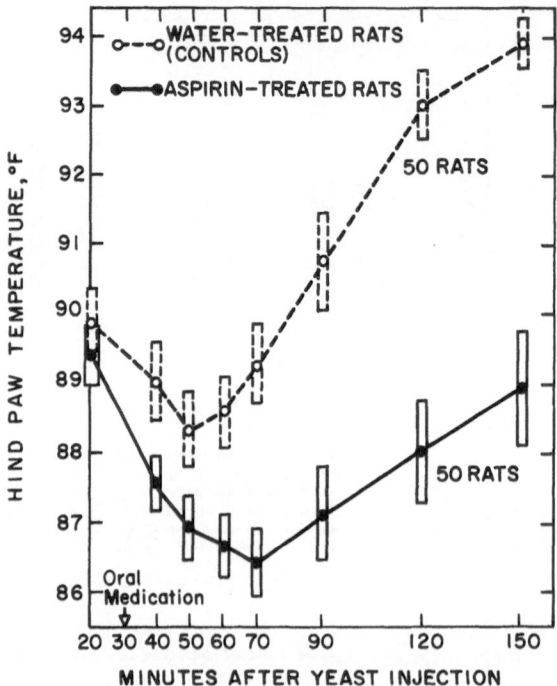

Fig. 4. Mean paw temperatures at various time periods with 95% confidence limits after plantar injection of yeast. (From PIRCIO and GROSKINSKY, 1966; with permission)

proposed that histamine was one of the mediators involved in the hyperthermic response because of partial inhibition of the response by chlorpheniramine (10 mg/ kg, p.o.). Because of the sensitivity of, particularly, the second phase of hyperthermia to aspirin and the only partial inhibition of the response by chlorpheniramine, these investigators suspected that other chemical mediators were involved in the response. Likely candidates are the prostaglandins (Chapter 31).

VINEGAR et al. (1969), using carrageenin-induced inflammation of the rat's paw, reported that adrenaline (2.5 μg) injected into the hyperthermic plantar tissues reduced the temperature to normal values. Since local hyperthermia is a result of inflammatory hyperaemia, such an effect by adrenaline is not unexpected. COLLINS and RING (1972) demonstrated a dose-related inhibition of the hyperthermia which occurred in carrageenin-injected paws of rats after oral administration of the nonsteroidal drug, azapropazone. SWINGLE (unpublished data) found that chlorpromazine and the nonsteroidal anti-inflammatory drug, diflumidone, administered orally, produced dose-related reductions in the hyperthermia of carrageenin-injected paws of rats.

WALZ et al. (1971a) assessed the effects of repeated doses of aspirin, indomethacin, prednisolone, cyclophosphamide and methotrexate on a number of parameters of adjuvant arthritis of the rat. Measurements of paw temperatures on day 16 after injection of the adjuvant showed that at certain doses all the drugs except cyclophosphamide significantly reduced the temperature of one or both of the arthritic hind paws. The reductions were not impressive, however, and of all the parameters measured, these investigators felt that the assessment of the secondary inflammatory response (i.e. the volume on day 16 of the paw not injected with adjuvant) was the most sensitive and appropriate for evaluation of drugs. MARTEL et al. (1974) demonstrated some reduction in the hyperthermia of the arthritic paws on day 16 after injection of the adjuvant for rats treated with prodilic acid. As WALZ et al. (1971a) reported, the secondary inflammatory response appeared to be the most sensitive parameter for assessing drug action. WALZ et al. (1971b) delivered either aspirin or hydrocortisone as hydroalcoholic solutions transcutaneously through arthritic paws of rats and compared this with the oral route of administration of these drugs. One of the parameters assessed was local hyperthermia. Aspirin, by both routes, produced a significant reduction in the temperature while hydrocortisone did so after local administration but not at the oral dose used (10 mg/kg).

LAMBELIN et al. (1970, 1971) studied the effects of topically applied steroid and nonsteroid anti-inflammatory drugs on the local hyperthermia produced in guinea pig skin by UV-irradiation. Phenylbutazone, aspirin, alclofenac, and bufexamac all inhibited significantly the local hyperthermia when applied as 5% creams. The preparations were equally effective whether applied before or after UV-irradiation which rules out the possibility that certain of them might be acting as UV-screening agents. The inability of topically applied fluocinolone acetonide (0.025%) to inhibit hyperthermia is in agreement with the known inability of *systemically* administered steroids to modify the development of UV-induced erythema in the guinea pig. As has been shown for erythema in this model, the development of local hyperthermia was not really inhibited but only delayed in its onset.

SNYDER and EAGLSTEIN (1974b) reported that the topical application of a 2.5% solution of indomethacin resulted in lower skin temperatures at UV-irradiated sites in man. Topical fluocinonide (0.05% cream) was ineffective. The results with the steroid might be due to experimental design rather than inherent inactivity of the molecule. BURDICK et al. (1973) reported that at exposures greater than one MED, effects by steroids on UV-induced erythema in human skin were difficult to show and that the site of application of the steroid had to be occluded. SNYDER and EAGLSTEIN (1974b) utilized exposures of three or more MED's and no occlusion in their studies.

F. Conclusion

Erythema and local hyperthermia, two manifestations of the acute inflammatory response, may be used to characterize the anti-inflammatory activity of substances. There is no evidence to assume, however, that such anti-inflammatory substances would be useful for treating chronic inflammatory diseases of man. Erythema and local hyperthermia are easily, although in most cases imperfectly, assessed and procedures utilizing these parameters may be used to provide rapid estimations of the probable anti-inflammatory activity of substances. Because the phenomena occur or are reflected in the skin, they are useful for ascertaining the anti-inflammatory activity of substances after topical application. The most widely used pharmacological screening procedure in animals which employs these parameters is UV light-induced erythema and local hyperthermia in the skin of guinea pigs. This procedure has been carefully described by WINDER et al. (1958) and could serve as the standard method for describing the "anti-acute-inflammatory" (or "antipreinflammatory") activity of substances. The discovery of a drug which would prevent rather than delay the development of erythema in this model could very well be the one that physicians are seeking for the treatment of chronic inflammatory diseases of man.

References

Adams,S.S.: Analgesics-antipyretics. J. Pharm. (Lond.) **12**, 251—252 (1960)
Adams,S.S., Cobb,R.: A possible basis for the anti-inflammatory activity of salicylates and other non-hormonal anti-rheumatic drugs. Nature (Lond.) **181**, 773—774 (1958)
Adams,S.S., Cobb,R.: The effect of salicylates and related compounds on erythema in the guinea-pig and man. In: Dixon,S.St.J., Martin,B.K., Smith,M.J.H., Wood,P.H.N. (Eds.): Salicylates. An International Symposium, pp. 127—140. Boston: Little Brown 1963
Adams,S.S., Hebborn,P., Nicholson,J.S.: Some aspects of the pharmacology of ibufenac, a non-steroidal anti-inflammatory agent. J. Pharm. (Lond.) **20**, 305—312 (1968)
Adams,S.S., McCullough,K.F., Nicholson,J.S.: The pharmacological properties of ibuprofen, an anti-inflammatory, analgesic and antipyretic agent. Arch. int. Pharmacodyn. **178**, 115—129 (1969)
Alpermann,H.G.: Verzögerung des UV-Erythems durch Thiophencarbonsäure-Derivate. Arzneimittel-Forsch. **20**, 293—294 (1970)
Bachem,A.: Time factors of erythema and pigmentation, produced by ultraviolet rays of different wavelengths. J. invest. Derm. **25**, 215—218 (1955)
Barron,D.I., Copley,A.R., Valiance,D.K.: Anti-inflammatory and related properties of 4-(p-biphenylyl)-3-hydroxybutyric acid. Brit. J. Pharmacol. **33**, 396—407 (1968)
Bavin,E.M., Drain,E.J., Seymour,D.E., Waterhouse,P.P.: Anti-inflammatory compounds. Part I. The activity of a series of new compounds compared with phenylbutazone and cortisone. J. Pharm. (Lond.) **7**, 1022—1031 (1955)
Berger,D.S.: Specification and design of solar ultraviolet simulators. J. invest. Derm. **53**, 192—199 (1969)
Birnie,J.H., Sutton,B.M., Zuccarello,M., Rush,J.A.: Some anti-inflammatory properties of 8-trifluoromethylphenothiazine-1-carboxylic acid (SK&F 22908). Med. pharm. exp. (Basel) **17**, 51—59 (1967)
Breit,R., Kligman,A.M.: Measurement of erythemal and pigmentary responses to ultraviolet radiation of different spectral qualities. In: Urbach,F. (Ed.): The Biological Effects of Ultra-violet Radiation, pp. 267—275. Oxford: Pergamon Press Ltd. 1969
Brooks,C.D., Schagel,C.A., Sekhai,N.C., Sobota,J.T.: Tolerance and pharmacology of ibuprofen. Curr. ther. Res. **15**, 180—190 (1973)
Brunner,M.J., Finkelstein,P.: A laboratory method for evaluation of topical anti-inflammatory agents. Arch. Derm. **81**, 453—457 (1960)
Burdick,K.H., Haleblian,J.K., Poulsen,B.J., Cobner,S.E.: Corticosteroid ointments: comparison by two bioassays. Curr. ther. Res. **15**, 233—242 (1973)
Burke,J.F., Miles,A.A.: The sequence of vascular events in early infective inflammation. J. Path. Bact. **76**, 1—19 (1958)
Chimoskey,J.E., Flanagan,W.: Ultraviolet-induced cutaneous hyperemia and steroid-induced cutaneous hyperemia measured by Xenon 133 disappearance in dogs. J. invest. Derm. **63**, 362—364 (1974)
Chimoskey,J.E., Flanagan,W., Holloway,G.A., Jr.: Ultraviolet-induced cutaneous hyperemia measured by Xenon 133 in man. J. invest. Derm. **63**, 367—368 (1974)
Collins,A.J., Ring,E.F.J.: Measurement of inflammation in man and animals by radiometry. Brit. J. Pharmacol. **44**, 145—152 (1972)
Daniels,F., Imbrie,J.D.: Comparison between visual grading and reflectance measurements of erythema produced by sunlight. J. invest. Derm. **30**, 295—304 (1958)

Dougherty, T.F., Appel, B., Fernandez, J.M.: The influence of the local injection of hydrocorti-sone, compound F, on the reaction to tuberculin, leproming Ducrey and Frei antigens. J. invest. Derm. **23**, 237—250 (1954)

Eaglstein, W.H., Marsico, A.R.: Dichotomy in response to indomethacin in UV-C and UV-B induced ultraviolet light inflammation. J. invest. Derm. **65**, 238—240 (1975)

Emden, J., Schaefer, H., Stüttgen, G.: Vergleich physikalischer Parameter von Hautdurchblu-tungsänderungen nach epicutaner Applikation von Nikotinsäurebenzylester. Arch. derm. Forsch. **241**, 353—363 (1971)

Epstein, J.H., Winkelmann, R.K.: Ultraviolet light-induced kinin formation in human skin. Arch. Derm. **95**, 532—536 (1967)

Erickson, K.L.: Sunlight: Its effect on mammalian skin. Primate Newslett. (Oregon) **13**, 3—8 (1975)

Fitzpatrick, T.P., Pathak, M.A., Magnus, I.A., Curwen, W.L.: Abnormal reactions of man to light. Ann. Rev. Med. **14**, 195—214 (1963)

Floersheim, G.L.: The tuberculin reaction as a screening method for anti-rheumatic drugs. In: Garratini, S., Dukes, M.N.G. (Eds.): Non-steroidal anti-inflammatory drugs, International Congress Series 82, pp. 232—235. Milan: Excerpta Medica Foundation 1965

Gershon-Cohen, J., Haberman-Brueschke, J.D., Brueschke, E.E.: Medical thermography: a sum-mary of current status. Radiol. Clin. N. Amer. **3**, 403—431 (1965)

Görög, P., Szporny, L.: Ethylbutyl-malonic acid-di(*m*-amino)-anilide, a new, non-steroid anti-inflammatory compound. Arzneimittel-Forsch. **16**, 1211—1214 (1966)

Graeme, M.L., Peters, P., Maiorana, K., Cooper, C.: The effect of topically applied agents on ultraviolet erythema in guinea pigs. Pharmacologist **17**, 226 (1975)

Greaves, M.W., Sondergaard, J.: Pharmacologic agents released in ultraviolet inflammation stud-ied by continuous skin perfusion. J. invest. Derm. **54**, 365—367 (1970)

Gróf, P., Kovács, A.: On the mode of action of UV-light. Effect of UV-A rays on mast cells in vivo. Acta physiol. Acad. Sci. hung. **32**, 35—44 (1967)

Groß, F., Merz, E.: Pharmakologische Eigenschaften des Trafuril, eines neuen Nikotinsäureester mit hyperämisierender Wirkung. Schweiz. med. Wschr. **78**, 1151—1155 (1948)

Gruber, C.M., Ridolofo, A.S., Nickander, R., Mikulaschek, W.M.: Delay of erythema of human skin by anti-inflammatory drugs after ultraviolet irradiation. Clin. Pharmacol. Ther. **13**, 109—113 (1972)

Gupta, N., Levy, L.: Delayed manifestation of ultraviolet reaction in the guinea pig caused by anti-inflammatory drugs. Brit. J. Pharmacol. **47**, 240—248 (1973)

Haining, C.G.: Effects of antirheumatic compounds and pyridine derivatives on the cutaneous response to thurfyl nicotinate in the guinea pig. Brit. J. Pharmacol. **21**, 104—112 (1963)

Harber, L.C.: Practical aspects of the electromagnetic spectrum as applied to the skin. American Medical Association Conference on Sunlight and Health, New York, 1975

Harber, L.C., Bickers, D.R., Epstein, J.H., Pathak, M.A., Urbach, F.: Report on ultraviolet light sources. Arch. Derm. **109**, 833—839 (1974a)

Harber, L.C., Bickers, D.R., Epstein, J.H., Pathak, M.A., Urbach, F.: Light sources used in photo-patch testing. In: Fitzpatrick, T.B., Patrick, M.A., Pathak, M.A., Harber, L.C., Seiji, M., Kuki-ta, A. (Eds.): Sunlight and Man, pp. 559—568. Tokyo: University of Tokyo Press 1974b

Hausser, K.W., Vahle, W.: Sunburning and suntanning. Wissenschaftliche Veröffentlichungen des Siemens Konzerns **6**, 101—120 (1927) Translated and published. In: Urbach, F. (Ed.): The Biological Effects of Ultraviolet Radiation, pp. 3—21. Oxford: Pergamon Press 1969

Heilmeyer, L., Hiemeyer, V.: Studies on the anti-inflammatory effect of drugs in man using the pyrexal skin test-method. In: Garratini, S., Dukes, M.N.G. (Eds.): Non-steroidal anti-inflam-matory drugs, International Congress Series 82, pp. 324—334. Milan: Excerpta Medica Foundation 1965

Hiemeyer, V.: Studies on the regulation of inflammation in man. In: Silvestrini, B., Tura, S. (Eds.): Inflammation, International Congress Series **163**, pp. 87—96. Amsterdam: Excerpta Medica Foundation 1968

Hirabayashi, K., Graham, J.: Mediation of radiation erythema. Int. J. Radiat. Biol. **16**, 85—91 (1969)

Jahn, U., Adrian, R.W.: Pharmakologische und toxikologische Prüfung des neuen Antiphlogisti-cums Azapropazon. 3-Dimenthylamino-7-methyl-1, 2-(*n*-propylmalonyl)-1,2-dihydro-1,2,4-Benzotriazen. Arzneimittel-Forsch. **19**, 36—52 (1969)

Jahn, U., Wagner-Jauregg, T. H.: Wirkungsvergleich saurer Antiphlogistika im Bradykinin-, UV-Erythem- und Rattenpfotenödem-Test. Arzneimittel-Forsch. **24**, 494—499 (1974)

Järvinen, K. A. J.: Effect of cortisone on reaction of skin to ultraviolet light. Brit. med. **1951 II**, 1377—1378

Johnson, B. E., Daniels, F.: Lysosomes and the reactions of skin to ultraviolet radiation. J. invest. Derm. **53**, 85—94 (1969)

Julou, L., Guyonnet, J. C., Ducrot, R., Garret, C., Bardone, M. C., Maignan, G., Pasquet, J.: Etude des propriétés pharmacologiques d'un nouvel anti-inflammatoire, l'acide (benzoyl-3 phenyl)-2 propionique (19583 R.P.). J. Pharmacol. (Paris) **2**, 259—286 (1971)

Kaidbey, K. H., Kligman, A. M.: Assay of topical corticosteroids by suppression of experimental inflammation in humans. J. invest. Derm. **63**, 292—297 (1974)

Kanof, N. B.: Observations on the effects of local application of hydrocortisone upon thermal burns and ultraviolet erythema. J. invest. Derm. **25**, 329—334 (1955)

Karpman, H. L.: Current status of thermography. Angiology **21**, 103—109 (1970)

Kosersky, D. S., Watson, W. C., Malone, M. H.: Effects of cryogenine and selected other anti-inflammatory agents on ultraviolet-induced erythema. Proc. W. Pharmacol. Soc. **16**, 249—251 (1973)

Lambelin, G., Vassart-Thys, D., Roba, J.: Pharmacological studies of bufexamac topically applied on the skin. Arch. int. Pharmacodyn. **187**, 401—414 (1970)

Lambelin, G., Vassart-Thys, D., Roba, J.: Cutaneous thermometry for topical therapy evaluation of U.V. erythema in the guinea-pig. Arzneimittel-Forsch. **21**, 44—47 (1971)

Lewis, T.: The blood vessels of the human skin and their responses. London: Shaw and Sons 1927

Logan, G., Wilhelm, D. L.: Vascular permeability changes in inflammation: I. The role of endogenous permeability factors in ultraviolet injury. Brit. J. exp. Path. **47**, 300—314 (1966 a)

Logan, G., Wilhelm, D. L.: The inflammatory reaction in ultraviolet injury. Brit. J. exp. Path. **47**, 286—299 (1966 b)

Long, J. B., Favour, C. B.: The ability of ACTH & cortisone to alter delayed type of bacterial sensitivity. Bull. Johns Hopk. Hosp. **87**, 186—202 (1950)

Martel, R. R., Klicius, J., Herr, F.: Investigations of 1,3,4,9-tetrahydro-1-propylpyrano [3,4-bΔ indole-1-acetic acid (prodilic acid), a new non-steroidal anti-inflammatory agent, in rats. Agents Actions **4**, 370—376 (1974)

Mathur, G. P., Gandhi, V. M.: Prostaglandin in human and albino rat skin. J. invest. Derm. **58**, 291—295 (1972)

Miller, W. S., Rudeiman, F. R., Smith, J. G., Jr.: Aspirin and ultraviolet light-induced erythema in man. Arch. Derm. **95**, 357—358 (1967)

Monash, S.: Composition of sunlight and of a number of ultraviolet lamps. Arch. Derm. **91**, 495—496 (1965)

Navarro, J., Stoliaroff, M., Savy, J. M., Berny, C., Brunaud, M.: Etude des propriétés pharmacologiques d'un nouvel anti-inflammatoire non-steroidique, l'acide bucloxique (804 CB). Arzneimittel-Forsch. **24**, 1368—1378 (1974)

Olson, R. L., Everett, M. A.: Alterations in epidermal lysosomes following ultraviolet light exposure. In: Urbach, F. (Ed.): The Biologic Effects of Ultraviolet Radiation, pp. 473—476. Oxford: Pergamon Press 1969

Owens, D. W., Knox, J. M., Hudson, H. T., Troll, D.: Influence of humidity on ultraviolet injury. J. invest. Derm. **64**, 250—252 (1975)

Parrish, J. A., Ying, C. Y., Pathak, M. A., Fitzpatrick, T. B.: Erythemogenic properties of long-wave ultraviolet light. In: Fitzpatrick, T. B., Pathak, M. A., Harber, L. C., Seiji, M., Kukita, A. (Eds.): Sunlight and Man, pp. 131—141. Tokyo: Tokyo University Press 1974

Pathak, M. A., Epstein, J. H.: Normal and abnormal reactions of man to light. In: Fitzpatrick, T. B., Arndt, K. A., Eisen, D. F., Van Scott, E. J., Vaughans, J. H. (Eds.): Dermatology in Clinical Medicine, pp. 993—995. New York: McGraw-Hill 1971

Pircio, A. W., Groskinsky, E. J.: Radiometric measurement of paw temperature changes associated with local inflammation. J. Pharmacol. exp. Ther. **154**, 103—109 (1966)

Riedel, R., Schoetensack, W.: Zur Pharmakologie von butyl-malonsäure-mono-(1,2-diphenylhydrazid)-calcium (bumadizon-calcium). Arzneimittel-Forsch. **23**, 1215—1225 (1973)

Rosenkilde, H.: Animal techniques for evaluating anti-inflammatory drugs. In: Nodine, J. H., Siegler, P. E. (Eds.): Animal and Clinical Pharmacologic Techniques in Drug Evaluation, Vol. I, pp. 492—501. Chicago: Year Book Medical Publications Inc. 1964

Sams, W. M., Jr., Winkelmann, R. K.: The effect of ultraviolet light on isolated cutaneous blood vessels. J. invest. Derm. **53**, 79—83 (1969)

Sayre, R.: The influence of ultraviolet light on skin. Thesis, State Univ. N.Y., Buffalo 1973

Schäfer, V.: Artificial production of ultraviolet radiation, introduction and historical review. In: Urbach, F. (Ed.): The Biologic Effects of Ultraviolet Radiation, pp. 93—105. Oxford: Pergamon Press 1969

Schikorr, R.: The inhibition of inflammation by cinchophen and calcium. Naunyn-Schmiedeberg's Arch. exp. Path. Pharmak. **168**, 190—205 (1932)

Schlagel, C. A., Northam, J. I.: Comparative anti-inflammatory efficacy of topically applied steroids on human skin. Proc. Soc. exp. Biol. (N.Y.) **101**, 629—632 (1959)

Schneider, W., Tronnier, H.: Zur Prüfung anti-phlogistisch wirkender Substanzen am Menschen. Arzneimittel-Forsch. **7**, 659—662 (1957)

Scott, A., Kalz, F.: The effect of the topical application of corticotrophin, hydrocortisone and fluorocortisone on the process of cutaneous inflammation. J. invest. Derm. **26**, 361—378 (1956)

Sevitt, S.: Early and delayed oedema and increase in capillary permeability after burns of the skin. J. Path. Bact. **75**, 27—37 (1958)

Sevitt, S.: Inflammatory changes in burned skin: reversible and irreversible effects and their pathogenesis. In: Thomas, L., Uhr, J. W., Grant, L. (Eds.): Injury, Inflammation and Immunity, pp. 183—210. Baltimore: Williams and Wilkins 1964

Sim, M. F.: The response of mouse skin to ultra-violet irradiation and its modification by drugs. In: Garratini, S., Dukes, M. N. G. (Eds.): Non-steroidal Anti-inflammatory Drugs, International Congress Series **82**, pp. 207—213. Milan: Excerpta Medica Foundation 1965

Snyder, D. S.: Cutaneous effects of topical indomethacin, an inhibitor of prostaglandin synthesis, on UV-damaged skin. J. invest. Derm. **64**, 322—325 (1975)

Snyder, D. S., Eaglstein, W. H.: Intradermal anti-prostaglandin agents and sunburn. J. invest. Derm. **62**, 47—50 (1974a)

Snyder, D. S., Eaglstein, W. H.: Topical indomethacin and sunburn. Brit. J. Derm. **90**, 91—93 (1974b)

Sobanski, H., Krupinska, J., Gryglewski, R. J.: Carrageenin hyperthermia in rats. Experientia (Basel) **30**, 1326—1328 (1974)

Spector, W. G., Willoughby, D. A.: Experimental suppression of increased capillary permeability in thermal burns in rats. Nature (Lond.) **182**, 949—950 (1958)

Stoughton, R. B., Clendenning, W. E., Kruse, D.: Percutaneous absorption of nicotinic acid and derivatives. J. invest. Derm. **35**, 337—341 (1960)

Swingle, K. F.: Evaluation for antiinflammatory activity. In: Scherrer, R. A., Whitehouse, M. W. (Eds.): Anti-inflammatory agents, Vol. II, pp. 33—122. New York: Academic Press 1974

Swingle, K. F., Hamilton, R. R., Harrington, J. K., Kvam, D. C.: 3-Benzoyl-difluoromethanesulfonanilide, sodium salt (diflumidone sodium, MBR 4164-8): A new anti-inflammatory agent. Arch. int. Pharmacodyn. **189**, 129—144 (1971)

Swingle, K. F., Jaques, L. W., Grant, T. J., Kvam, D. C.: Apparent association of activity of anti-inflammatory drugs in a sulfhydryl exchange reaction in vitro and in the guinea pig erythema assay. Biochem. Pharmacol. **19**, 2995—2999 (1970)

Tronnier, H.: Evaluation and measurement of ultraviolet erythema. In: Urbach, F. (Ed.): The Biologic Effects of Ultraviolet Radiation, pp. 255—266. Oxford: Pergamon Press 1969

Truelove, L. H., Duthie, J. J. R.: Effect of aspirin on cutaneous response to the local application of an ester of nicotinic acid. Ann. rheum. Dis. **18**, 137—141 (1959)

Valtonen, E. J.: An experimental study on mice. Acta path. microbiol. scand. Suppl. **151**, 1—6 (1961)

Valtonen, E. J.: Studies of the mechanism of ultra-violet erythema formation. 3. A method for biological testing of ultra-violet radiation sources and substances affecting the degree of erythema. Acta derm.-venereol. (Stockh.) **46**, 292—300 (1966)

Valtonen, E. J., Jänne, J., Siimes, M.: The effect of the erythemal reaction caused by ultraviolet irradiation on mast cell degranulation, in the skin. Acta derm.-venereol. (Stockh.) **44**, 269—272 (1964)

Vinegar, R., Schreiber, W., Hugo, R.: Biphasic development of carrageenin edema in rats. J. Pharmacol. exp. Ther. **166**, 96—103 (1969)

Walters, M. N.-I., Willoughby, D. A.: Indomethacin, a new anti-inflammatory drug: its potential use as a laboratory tool. J. Path. Bact. **90**, 641—648 (1965)

Walz, D. T., Dimartino, M. J., Kuch, J. H., Zuccarello, W.: Adjuvant-induced arthritis in rats. I. Temporal relationship of physiological, biochemical, and hematological parameters. Proc. Soc. exp. Biol. (N.Y.). **136**, 907—910 (1970)

Walz, D. T., Dimartino, M. J., Misher, A.: Adjuvant-induced arthritis in rats. II. Drug effects on physiologic, biochemical and immunologic parameters. J. Pharmacol. exp. Ther. **178**, 223—231 (1971 a)

Walz, D. T., Dolan, M. M., Dimartino, M. J., Yankell, S. L.: Effects of topical hydrocortisone and acetylsalicylic acid on the primary lesion of adjuvant-induced arthritis. Proc. Soc. exp. Biol. (N.Y.). **137**, 1466—1469 (1971 b)

Weiner, M., Piliero, S. J.: Nonsteroid anti-inflammatory agents. Ann. Rev. Pharmacol. **10**, 171—198 (1970)

Wells, G. C.: The effect of hydrocortisone on standardized skin trauma. Brit. J. Derm. **69**, 11—18 (1957)

Whitehouse, M. W.: Some biochemical and pharmacological properties of anti-inflammatory drugs. Fortschr. Arzneimittel-Forsch. **8**, 321—429 (1965)

Wilhelm, D. L., Mason, B.: Vascular permeability changes in inflammation: the role of endogenous permeability factors in mild thermal injury. Brit. J. exp. Path. **41**, 487—506 (1960)

Wilhelmi, G.: Über die pharmakologischen Eigenschaften von Irgapyrin, einem neuen Präparat aus der Pyrazolreihe. Schweiz. med. Wschr. **79**, 577—582 (1949)

Wilhelmi, G.: Über die antiphlogistische Wirkung von Pyrazolen, speziell von Irgapyrin. Bei peroraler und parenteraler Verabreichung. Schweiz. med. Wschr. **80**, 936—942 (1950)

Wilhelmi, G.: Newer pharmacological data on oxyphenbutazone. Jap. J. Pharmacol. **15**, 187—198 (1965)

Wilhelmi, G., Domenjoz, R.: Vergleichende Untersuchungen über die Wirkung von Pyrazolen und Antihistaminen bei verschiedenen Arten der experimentellen Entzündung. Arch. int. Pharmacodyn. **85**, 129—143 (1951)

Willis, I.: Sunlight and the skin. J. Amer. med. Ass. **217**, 1088—1093 (1971)

Willis, I., Kligman, A., Epstein, J.: Effects of long ultraviolet rays of human skin: photoprotective or photoaugmentative? J. invest. Derm. **59**, 416—420 (1973)

Winder, C. V., Sarber, R. W., Hemans, M., Wax, J., Bratton, A. C., Jr.: A comparison of the effects of cortisone and phenylbutazone on the tuberculin reaction. Arch. int. Pharmacodyn. **112**, 212—220 (1957)

Winder, C. V., Wax, J., Burr, V., Been, M., Rosiere, C. E.: A study of pharmacological influences on ultraviolet erythema in guinea pigs. Arch. int. Pharmacodyn. **116**, 261—292 (1958)

Winder, C. V., Wax, J., Scotti, L., Scherrer, R. A., Jones, E. M., Short, F. W.: Anti-inflammatory, antipyretic and antinociceptive properties of N-(2,3-xylyl)anthranilic acid (mefenamic acid). J. Pharmacol. exp. Ther. **138**, 405—413 (1962)

Winder, C. V., Wax, J., Welford, M.: Anti-inflammatory and antipyretic properties of N-(2,6-dichloro-m-tolyl)anthranilic acid (CI-583). J. Pharmacol. exp. Ther. **148**, 422—429 (1965)

Winter, C. A.: Nonsteroid antiinflammatory agents. Fortschr. Arzneimittel-Forsch. **10**, 139—203 (1966)

Wolska, H., Langner, A., Marzulli, F. N.: The hairless mouse as an experimental model for evaluating the effectiveness of sunscreen preparations. J. Soc. Cosmetic Chemists **25**, 639—644 (1974)

Yamamoto, H., Saito, C., Okamoto, T., Awata, H., Inukai, T., Hirohashi, A., Yukawa, Y.: Synthesis and pharmacology of a new potential anti-inflammatory drug, 1-3(3',4'-methylenedioxybenzoyl)-2-methyl-5-methoxy-3-indolylacetic acid (ID-955). Arzneimittel-Forsch. **19**, 981—984 (1969)

Ying, C. Y., Parrish, J. A., Pathak, M. A.: Additive erythemogenic effects of middle-(280—320 nm), and long-(320—400 nm) wave ultraviolet light. J. invest. Derm. **63**, 273—278 (1974)

Ziboh, V. A., Price, B., Fulton, J.: Effects of retinoic acid on prostaglandin biosynthesis in guinea-pig skin. J. invest. Derm. **65**, 370—374 (1975)

CHAPTER 21

Oedema and Increased Vascular Permeability

C.G. VAN ARMAN

A. General Principles of Assays

No laboratory model using animals can be a perfect duplicate of a human disease. There are always differences of some kind. For a practical result to be achieved, however, such as finding a drug for clinical use, it is not required that the animal model should even remotely resemble the human disease in its superficial aspects. As examples, morphine can be assayed by the curling of a mouse's tail; digitalis by the vomiting of a pigeon; anesthetics by the membrane resistance of isolated cells; and anti-epileptic drugs by antagonism of electroshock-induced convulsions. Practically, it does not matter whether one measures a *side-effect* in an assay rather than the *desired* effect, so long as these vary together in a known manner.

Indomethacin was detected in the laboratory because it prevented granuloma formation around a cotton pellet implanted under the skin of the rat (WINTER et al., 1963). This finding carried no obvious implication that the drug would alleviate the pain of a human gouty attack; yet it does. In order to understand why, one needs an overall view of the complete inflammatory process—or processes, because there are many. This chapter is especially concerned with oedema and vascular permeability, but these phenomena do not exist by themselves. We shall refer to other chapters, therefore, which are particularly apropos for other phenomena that are inextricably related.

Oedema formation is not simply the result of increased vascular permeability, because oedema can result from a simple elevation of capillary pressure (KEELE and NEIL, 1965). It seems that increased permeability of blood vessels without oedema should be possible if circulatory and lymphatic sufficiency is maintained in the inflamed area (SWINGLE, 1974). Many other investigators have also shown that oedema and increased permeability are separate phenomena (GÖZSY and KATO, 1956; COTRAN and MAJNO, 1964; BROWN and ROBSON, 1964; PAPADIMITRIOU et al., 1967). When we discuss increased vascular permeability, we should specify what kind of permeability we mean. HURLEY (Chapter 2) defines increased vascular permeability as pertaining to plasma protein. Water is only one substance that permeates; also passing through are molecules and ions such as salts, peptides, proteins and hormones, and entire cells. All of these may react with each other as well as with the new interstitial environment into which they have arrived from the circulating blood.

Notwithstanding that oedema and vascular permeability are different and can be so demonstrated in the laboratory, most assay procedures involve both phenomena, each to greater or less extent, and in fact also involve other phenomena without attention usually being paid to this fact. For example, carrageenin in a rat's foot causes not only oedema and increased permeability of blood vessels, but also immigration of leucocytes and increase of paw temperature. Both of these latter effects could conceivably be used as measurements, although less reliable (see Chapters 3, 4, 16, and 27).

Validity[1] and reliability[2] are separate concepts which must be clear before one studies details of the several laboratory assay methods, if one is interested in their applications to human medicine. *Validity* requires that drugs proved effective clinically should be effective in the laboratory model, and that drugs not effective clinically should not be effective in the model. For inflammatory diseases, such requirements cannot be met at present; there is no single method in vitro or in vivo that correlates well with clinical experience over an extensive range of different chemical structures (see also Chapter 19). With a compound from a new area of structure, therefore, one should not trust any single laboratory method, nor even several, to predict results in the clinic.

The point is illustrated by Table 1, which shows data obtained in a single laboratory (Van Arman and Bohidar, 1978).

The seven compounds tested in the six assay methods illustrate that indeed there is a general trend of the data, even across methods as different as those depending upon oedema and increased vascular permeability (the first two), upon a reflex response to inflammatory pain (the third), fever (the fourth), longer-term fibrin deposition (the fifth), and delayed hypersensitivity (the sixth). Of the seven compounds, all but one are used clinically; the remaining one merely illustrates how one can fit an experimental drug into its likely proper place for purposes of study. Lombardino et al. (1975) have similarly shown correlation between doses effective against carrageenin-induced foot oedema in the rat and daily clinical anti-arthritic doses of fifteen different anti-inflammatory agents, all of acidic structure.

Despite the general trend of Table 1, there are irregularities and other difficulties. Certain other drugs accepted as clinically active (for example, D-penicillamine in rheumatoid arthritis) can hardly be shown active in these tests at any dose. Drugs such as the alkylating agents (cyclophosphamide), purines (6-mercaptopurine) and dihydrofolate reductase inhibitors (methotrexate)—all of which have been used clinically—do not have any anti-inflammatory effect in short-term assays like carrageenin oedema, unless they are given several days before the test in doses sufficient to lower the circulating white cell count to a very small fraction of normal (Van Arman, 1974). Phelps and McCarty (1966) and Chang and Gralla (1968), using pressure in the dog's knee-joint as a criterion, found a similar requirement of polymorphonuclear leucocytes for acute inflammation to occur, by depletion of these cells from the general circulation.

Potency, of course, is not always important, but it is one measurement the pharmacologist must make, so that it may be compared with the inevitable unwanted side-effects and toxicity. Every substance, even water, has side-effects and toxicity if given in sufficient amount in a suitable way.

---

[1] The term 'accuracy' as customarily used for chemical assays means the same as 'validity' used here.
[2] The term 'precision' as customarily used for chemical assays means the same as 'reliability' used here.

Table 1. Comparison of seven drugs tested in each of six different assays. Figures in body of table are ED$_{50}$'s in mg/kg given orally

Assay	Indomethacin	Sulindac	Diflunisal	Phenyl-butazone	2,5-Bis(ethylamino)-1,3,4-thiadiazole	Aspirin	Thiabendazole
Carrageenin foot oedema	2.7	5.5	9.8	27.7	22.4	89.2	200
Topical, mouse's ear	1.65	6.1	3	4.3	inact.	5.5	12.4
Dog's knee joint	1.57	45	24	12	8.4	72	>150
Yeast fever	1.31	2.9	24	24	5.7	45	83
Granuloma, cotton pellet	0.35	5.4	74	40	30	115	inact.
Adjuvant arthritis	0.25	0.55	9.8	14	~50	67	217

Table 2. Rank order of potencies of seven drugs in each of six assays

Assay	Indomethacin	Sulindac	Diflunisal	Phenyl-butazone	2,5-Bis(ethylamino)-1,3,4-thiadiazole	Aspirin	Thiabendazole
Carrageenin foot oedema	1	2	3	5	4	6	7
Topical, mouse's ear	1	5	2	3	7	4	6
Dog's knee joint	1	5	4	3	2	6	7
Yeast fever	1	2	4$^{1}/_{2}$	4$^{1}/_{2}$	3	6	7
Granuloma, cotton pellet	1	2	5	4	3	6	7
Adjuvant arthritis	1	2	3	4	5	6	7
Sum of rank orders of potency of each drug in above 6 assays	6	18	21$^{1}/_{2}$	23$^{1}/_{2}$	24	34	41
Rank order of potency of drug in laboratory within the group of 7.	1	2	3	4	5	6	7
Rank order of potency of drug in several clinical situations (see text)	1	2	3	4	not used	5	6

Reliability means to what extent a given assay method is reproducible in the laboratory: if an assay has high variability, it has low reliability. For completeness with any compound, one should show the dose-response line, measure the slope of it, give the confidence limits at certain doses (usually at the median effective dose required for a stated degree of effect), state the potency with respect to some standard drug, and give the confidence limits of this relative potency. It is important for the pharmacologist to know quantitatively how reliable is the method he uses, not only as used in his own laboratory but also as used in other laboratories.

Up to the present, relatively few investigators have published those statistics necessary to compare results from one laboratory with another. It is the rule, rather than the exception, that each laboratory develops its own methods or variations of standard methods; and even slight procedural changes affect the ED_{50}'s. Therefore, it seems best at present that comparisons across laboratories should be made not by ED_{50} values but by ranking lists. The rank order of a drug in a list of standards seems likely to agree across laboratories despite the often large discrepancies in absolute ED_{50}'s. Another difficulty is that it seems to be the general practice, when information is published on new drugs, that few comparisons are made directly with standard drugs; also, when several assay methods are used in a publication, the same standard drugs are not used in all of them. To illustrate the usefulness of rank orders, Table 2 shows the improvement in perspective that can result by merely transforming the data from Table 1 into rank orders.

The bottom line of this table shows the estimated rank order of potency in clinical use, arbitrarily given here, assigned on the basis of general information across a number of clinical situations as different as gout, osteoarthritis, dracunculosis, headache, ankylosing spondylitis and rheumatoid arthritis. In the present state of the art of medicine, which is qualitative rather than quantitative, opinions vary about potency, so that there can hardly be a rigorous proof of such assigned rank orders. In any case, *potency*—that is, effect per unit weight of drug—is not of great importance. More important (for both laboratory and clinical evaluation) is the maximum achievable effect without toxicity. This value needs to be determined experimentally for each drug, and compared with the value found for the minimum chronic dose causing some intolerable side-effect. For inflammatory diseases, the ratio of these two values in the laboratory must be at least several-fold for new drugs. Certain useful old drugs like gold sodium thiomalate and steroids, in a large fraction of patients, have a ratio near unity, and surely less than two. New drugs, however, with the present severe regulatory scrutiny, will need a ratio much better than two. Laboratory results with new drugs generally give a more optimistic picture than the actual clinical long-term experience; whatever ratio the laboratory finds is likely to be decreased in the clinic.

Most new drugs are found initially by screening methods in research laboratories of pharmaceutical companies. The most important feature of any screening method should be its validity for clinical purposes, but unfortunately in inflammatory diseases there is as yet no certain validity of any known laboratory method. Reliability in the laboratory, however, is a different matter; it can readily be known for any assay by gathering enough data. Certain statistical criteria must be employed, and these will be described below.

I. Statistical Considerations in Assay Work

The reader can find more detailed expositions of these concepts in the first 5 chapters of FINNEY (1964).

1. Relationship of Dose to Effect

In almost all biological assays, the relationship of the dose x to the effect y is

$$y = m \log x + b$$

This equation describes a straight line on semilogarithmic graph paper. In most assays, the results deviate from the straight line below about 15% of the maximum response and above 85% of it. The slope of the line is m; this measures the rate of change in response for a unit change in the logarithm of the dose. For many anti-inflammatory assays, it is convenient to express the results y as a percentage of the inflammatory response without any drug treatment. It is more meaningful to compare dimensionless percentages across different assays than to compare ml of oedema in one assay, for example, with mg weight gain of a cotton pellet or with degrees of fever in another assay.

If two drugs have identical slopes, then the relative potencies are inversely proportional to the doses of each required to produce equal effects, anywhere along the dose-response lines; but if the slopes are different, one must specify the effect that is wanted, before the relative potencies can be stated. For more details of these calculations, as well as the calculation of the combined effects of two drugs, see VAN ARMAN et al. (1973).

2. Definition of ED$_{50}$

The symbol ED$_{50}$ means a certain *dose* at which half the animals have a drug effect greater than a certain fixed measurement, and half have less. In some assays the drug *effect* is an inhibition of a certain response to a certain inflammatory agent, but this inhibition may never amount to as much as 50%. It is important not to confuse these concepts. In Table 1, 50% inhibition is used with certain measurements shown in parentheses, with carrageenin oedema (swelling), topical mouse's ear (increase in weight), dog's knee joint (behavioral scale), and adjuvant arthritis (swelling); but in contrast, with granuloma, only 25% inhibition, and with yeast fever, 1° C reduction in fever.

3. Confidence Limits

The 95% confidence limits are an estimate that the true ED$_{50}$ will prove eventually to lie between these limits, on the average 19 times out of 20 experiments. With hundreds of animals, the limits tend to converge so that after enough experiments there is no practical value in any better definition. For indomethacin in the carrageenin assay, the limits of 2.54 and 2.92 mg/kg are close enough, so that further refinement would be a waste of time. Slight changes in procedure would of course alter such values.

4. Coefficient of Variation

The variability of an assay is expressed by its standard deviation, and when this value is divided by the mean and multiplied by 100, one has a dimensionless number. This is very useful for comparisons across assays that may be expressed in different units—for example, degrees of fever in a rat and pressure exerted by a dog's foot.

5. The g Value

An important concept for measuring the precision (reliability) of an assay is the g value. The lower it is, the better. It is defined as

$$g = \frac{t^2 s^2}{b^2 [X^2]}$$

in which t is the usual familiar number found in statistical tables. The tabular t decreases as the number of animals (or readings of some kind) increases, and of course for significance, the experimental t found must be greater than that listed in the table.

s is the pooled standard deviation, that represents variability among the readings in a given test. If a procedure is reliable it will have a small s, and if it is complicated, each step will increase s.

b is the slope of the dose-response line. It is the change in response per unit increase in the logarithm of the dose. A good assay has a steeper dose-response line than a poor one, and therefore a greater b.

$[X^2]$ stands for the spread of doses in an assay. It is best to have this spread as large as possible while still keeping the response in the linear region. This is the corrected sum of squares for doses, calculated as $\Sigma x^2 - (\Sigma x)^2/n$, in which n is the number of observations.

Changes in any of these four values will change g. A biological assay with a g value near 0.05 is considered to be of high precision, but 0.10 or 0.15 is still useful. Values above 0.7 should hardly be used. The width of the confidence limits of the ED_{50} depends upon g, which is therefore very important. As g becomes smaller, the confidence limits become narrower.

6. The Lambda Value, λ

This is a simpler concept than the g value but it is similar. It is merely the standard deviation of the slope, divided by the slope. It can be interpreted as follows for most animal assays: 0.05 or less is excellent, 0.1–0.2 is acceptable, and 0.5 and higher should not be used—one should look for another kind of assay.

7. Errors of Types I and II

There are two dangers to watch for in screening assays. Type I error happens when one accepts as active a compound that in fact is not. This is a common error, but it can be tolerated, because it will become obvious in subsequent tests that the compound really is inactive. Type II error, however, is more serious. This can occur if the test fails to detect activity that a compound really has. This error is serious because usually a supposedly inactive compound will not be tested again, and will thus be lost. Such errors must be minimized. The probability of detecting an active compound is called 'the power of a test.' This means how *unlikely* the test is to have Type II errors. If an assay detects 99 compounds of 100 having a certain degree of activity, it has a 'power' of 0.99.

B. Methods for Producing and Measuring Oedema and Increased Vascular Permeability

There are more methods for causing and measuring oedema and capillary permeability than it is useful to cite here. One may be sure that at least a few different mechanisms are involved among these various methods, but because the mechanisms are poorly known, it is better to list the methods according to the test object and inflammatory agent, rather than by the supposed mechanisms.

I. Oedemas of the Rat's Paw

1. Measurement

One direct method of measuring oedema is to remove the rat's injected hind paw and weigh it. The weight is compared with that of the other hind paw. This method is simple and precise, but it is relatively slow, and only a single datum is obtainable from each rat. One can also measure the thickness of the paw with calipers or the equivalent; repeated readings may be taken, but the reliability does not compare well with that of other methods.

It was realized 40 years ago that objective methods for volume were required (SELYE, 1937), but even as late as 1950 quantification was made by a mere visual score (GROSS, 1950). WILHELMI and DOMENJOZ (1951) introduced a plethysmometric method in which the rat was anaesthetized, an inflammatory agent was injected into the paw, and the paw was sealed with grease in a bulb of an oncometer connected with a microburette; the increase in volume was measured by the water displacement caused by the slight change in air pressure. HILLEBRECHT (1954) improved on this by dipping the foot into a water-alcohol solution; WINDER et al. (1957) improved the system further and used it with unanaesthetized rats. BUTTLE (1957) also described a simple glass apparatus capable of measuring the volume of water displaced to the nearest 1%. These methods were precise, but relatively slow. In 1955, ENDERS and HEIDBRINCK used a mercury pool into which the foot was dipped; a side-arm carried an iron float that moved a lever indicator across a calibrated scale. Many variations of the mercury-displacement idea have appeared since then. Among the simple but slow modifications are those of BARAN and MOSKOVIC (1970), who used a small cylinder filled up to a side-arm with mercury; the rat's foot displaced mercury into a burette, in which the volume was measured. SINGH and MOURYA (1972) used a 1-metre horizontal capillary tube connected to a mercury pool in which the foot was dipped; movement in the tube was converted to volume. NETTI et al. (1972) observed the rise of dyed ethanol in a tube connected with the mercury surface.

In order to obtain large amounts of data in screening operations, however, it is necessary to use automatic recording devices. In certain industrial laboratories there can be immediate ('on-line') digital print-out of the foot volumes and of the statistics thereby generated comparing various treated groups. Such methods are based on mercury displacement as described by Winter et al. (1962) and Van Arman et al. (1965), with the further required interface equipment being individually developed or applied by specialists in instrumentation in the various laboratories (Wong et al., 1973). It is often very useful to have frequent serial measurements on the same rats. Apparently there is no disturbing effect upon the course of the inflammation if the rats are handled quickly and gently. Automatic recording methods enable one person to take readings every few minutes on a group of perhaps 10 rats.

2. Agents Causing Paw Oedema; Characteristics of Oedemas Caused by Several Agents

a) Carrageenin and the Role of White Cells

Carrageenin is a mucopolysaccharide from Irish sea moss, *Chondrus crispus*. Di Rosa (1972) has reviewed the biological properties of carrageenin and refers to chemical studies on it. The first report of its use in causing fibrous tissue formation seems to be that of Robertson and Schwartz (1953), but Winter et al. (1962) were the first to apply it to the acute and easily quantifiable paw oedema. There are differences among the various fractions and suppliers; the experimenter is advised to read Moore and Trottier (1974).

The carrageenin assay as usually carried out, is slightly modified from that of Winter et al.: The compound to be assayed is given orally in saline or 1% methylcellulose suspension. One hour later, 0.10 ml (rather than 0.05 ml as in Winter et al., op. cit.) of 1% carrageenin suspension in normal saline solution is injected into the plantar tissue of one hind paw, and the paw volume is recorded. Three hours later, the volume is measured. The swelling in the treated rats is calculated as a percentage of that in the control rats. For indomethacin, the following data obtained in the author's laboratory illustrate the kind of results obtainable also with other nonsteroid anti-inflammatory drugs:

Median effective dose for 50% inhibition of swelling: 2.73 mg/kg.

95% confidence limits: 2.54—2.92 mg/kg.

Number of rats used: 139 groups of 6 rats each, over doses of 1, 3, and 9 mg/kg.

Coefficient of variation (standard deviation of mean/mean): 17.9%.

g value ($t^2 s^2 / b^2 [X]^2$): 0.0058.

λ value (standard deviation of slope/slope): 0.0384.

Dose-response line for indomethacin: $y = 38.0 \log x + 33.4$, in which y is percent inhibition and x is the oral dose in mg/kg.

Dose-response line for oedema by carrageenin: $s = 0.52 \log C + 0.76$, in which s is ml swelling and C is mg carrageenin (Viscarin, Marine Colloids, RE 6573) in 0.1 ml injected.

Vinegar et al. (1969, 1974) have demonstrated that there are two phases of oedema formation over the first few hours: the first phase begins within a few minutes and is complete by one hour, while the second phase begins at about one hour and continues through at least three hours. All laboratories do not report the same relative magnitudes of these phases. WINTER and VAN ARMAN have not observed a clear first phase, but only the second—even after exchanging carrageenin samples with the laboratories of VINEGAR and of ROSENTHALE. These latter two investigators, however, as well as DI ROSA et al., have always seen a clearly demarcated first phase. Since VINEGAR et al. (1969) showed that the first phase is not inhibited by chlorpheniramine or cyproheptadine, it cannot be mediated by histamine or 5-hydroxytryptamine (5-HT). The second phase measured at 3 hours is not inhibited by cyproheptadine either (WINTER et al., 1962; VAN ARMAN et al., 1965; VINEGAR et al., 1974); one thus infers that neither histamine nor 5-HT plays a significant role in carrageenin oedema in the rat. That bradykinin does so is suspected but not clearly established (VAN ARMAN et al., 1968; VAN ARMAN and NUSS, 1969; FERREIRA et al., 1974; MONCADA et al., 1973).

GARCIA LEME et al. (1973) injected carrageenin into the paw and Evans blue dye i.v., and observed a peak oedema at 4–5 hours, while the dye leakage into the paw was maximum after 1 h. Diphenhydramine hydrochloride and methysergide had no influence, but aspirin and indomethacin reduced both phenomena. DOHERTY and ROBINSON (1975), however, using ^{125}I-labelled human serum albumin instead of Evans blue dye as a marker of protein leakage, found that the protein leaked into the inflamed area at a rate parallel with the increase in volume, over 5 hours. They also found that if they subtracted the volume of a saline-injected foot from the carrageenin-injected one, the first phase was reduced, although not entirely. However, intrapleural injection of carrageenin into rats, with collection of the oedema fluid at intervals, gave no first phase at all, as VINEGAR et al. found (1974). The authors concluded that the first phase seen in the paw must be due to trauma of injection, since it is seen after saline injection, is independent of the amount of carrageenin, and is not seen after intrapleural injection. Their findings with regard to protein excretion apparently agree with the views of HURLEY (Chapter 2).

Carrageenin-induced inflammation apparently depends upon white blood cells. Cyclophosphamide and 6-mercaptopurine, given orally to rats once daily for 3 days, reduced the circulating white cell count to a varying extent in different rats (VAN ARMAN et al., 1971; VAN ARMAN, 1974). In 46 untreated rats the total white count was 11,940/cu. mm. When carrageenin was injected into the paws, the swelling in the 46 control rats was 0.67 ml, and in the 76 treated rats the swelling y as a function of white count x was given by

$$y = 0.31 \log x - 0.55,$$

in which y is ml of oedema and x is the white count per cu. mm. The correlation coefficient r was 0.81, which is highly significant. One may infer that if there are no white cells, there can be no inflammation by carrageenin. It is probable that carrageenin is inflammatory for reasons different from those to be found with thermal injury or turpentine pleurisy, since WILLOUGHBY and SPECTOR (1968) found no relationship between cell count and swelling in these latter procedures.

b) Nystatin Oedema

ARRIGONI-MARTELLI et al. (1971) have used a polyene antibiotic, nystatin (Mycostatin, Squibb) by injection into the hind paw of rats to induce a swelling to approximately double the normal size, peaking at the 15th hour and decreasing only slowly through 4 days. This assay is of interest because of its long duration, and because it differs from the carrageenin assay in that standard drugs are just as effective when given after the swelling has reached its maximum, as when given 1 hour before the nystatin. Very small doses (5 mg/kg orally) of cyclophosphamide given daily for 5 days caused 40% inhibition of the oedema. This result compares very well with the 67% inhibition seen in carrageenin-induced oedema after 3 days' dosage with high doses of cyclophosphamide (100 mg/kg orally), or with the 50% inhibition after 5 days' dosage with 25 mg/kg, reported by Van Arman et al. (1971, 1974). Possibly both of these inflammatory agents depend upon the white cells to cause the oedema.

c) Yeast Oedema

The Randall-Selitto assay procedure (1957) consists of applying pressure by an air-driven plunger to the yeast-inflamed hind paw of the rat, and noting the pressure at which the rat reacts by squeaking. This is an assay for analgesic compounds, since it can quantify the potencies of the strong analgesics (morphine-like) as well as the weaker ones like aspirin; but in general among the non-steroid anti-inflammatory agents, analgesia to yeast is parallel with other anti-inflammatory effects, especially with suppression of oedema. When drugs like indomethacin are given before the yeast injection, they prevent the oedema; when given after oedema has developed, they do not reduce it. Whether given early or later, however, they restore the pressure threshold to normal (Winter and Flataker, 1965a). It should be noted that there is nothing unique about yeast in this regard, because other agents such as carrageenin and mustard also cause both hypersensitivity and swelling; the ratios of these effects may vary from one agent to another. Winter and Flataker (1965a) with an improved technique have shown simultaneous measurements of decreased pressure thresholds and paw swelling for six different agents. 5-HT, egg white and dextran caused swelling but not hyperesthesia. Indomethacin raised the threshold in circumstances in which oedema volume was not affected, i.e. after the oedema had become established. This fact, therefore, probably represents an inhibition of the release of lysosomal enzymes from the polymorphonuclear leucocytes that have arrived into the area of inflammation (Van Arman et al., 1970; Van Arman, 1974).

d) Thermal Oedema

Application of heat over the entire body causes a fall in the bradykininogen level of the plasma, a rise in free kinins in peritoneal fluid and blood, and circulatory collapse (De Souza and Rocha e Silva, 1973). When heat is applied to limited areas of skin, many investigators have found interesting phenomena. Hoene (1954), in Selye's laboratory, showed that previous brief heating of a rabbit's ear or a rat's foot (48° C) would protect against a slightly longer second heating (49° C) 2 or 3 days later, which caused severe oedema and necrosis in the previously untreated contralateral ear or foot. Wilhelm and Mason (1960) presented clear evidence for biphasic reactions to moderate local heat in the skin of the trunk of unanesthetized guinea pigs, rats and rabbits with blue dye in their blood. The first phase (5 min) is mediated by histamine or 5-HT; the delayed phase is not affected by antihistamine drugs, but probably is mediated largely by kinins and other materials.

ARMSTRONG et al. (1966a) have shown that human plasma contains a kinin-forming system that is activated when the plasma temperature is increased to 50° C and then brought back to 37°, or when plasma is cooled to 0° C for several hours. The reason seems to be that normally Hageman factor is inhibited by C'l esterase inhibitor in plasma, but that this inhibitor is removed by heating or cooling, so that Hageman factor becomes active. Patients with hereditary angioneurotic oedema have a very low titre of free C'l esterase inhibitor (DONALDSON, 1968). The plasma of parturient women is especially sensitive in that it quickly forms bradykinin upon being cooled and the kininogen content of the plasma is depleted (ARMSTRONG et al., 1966b). It is possibly of considerable importance that kinins may be formed not only by cooling of serum but also by its contact with heat-aggregated human gamma globulin (ARMSTRONG and DÍAS DA SILVA, 1970), and with antigen-antibody complexes (MOVAT, 1967).

ROCHA E SILVA and ANTONIO (1960) have described a technique by which a perfusate is collected from a rat's paw immersed in water at 45° C. With this technique applied to both hind paws, one of which had been injected with various substances, GARCIA LEME et al. (1970) found that soya-bean trypsin inhibitor and certain preparations of inhibitors of kallikrein or pancreatic trypsin would prevent the appearance of active kinins. It is known that soya-bean trypsin inhibitor will also prevent carrageenin-induced oedema of the rat's paw (VAN ARMAN et al., 1965); such evidence, as well as certain other facts, supports the concept that oedema caused by heat and also by other mediators may be at least partly mediated by kinins.

On the other hand, STARR and WEST (1967) agree with others that histamine and 5-HT are not important at 46° C, and do agree that bradykinin is involved in thermal injury, but nevertheless suggest that there are yet other factors to be identified. GOODWIN et al. (1963) observed histamine and kinins, including bradykinin and other peptides, in the urine of human patients with burns of the skin. It is significant that these authors also observed substances that potentiated the effect of histamine on the isolated test organs (guinea pig ileum, rat duodenum and rat uterus), which observation suggests that several mediators such as bradykinin, 5-HT and certain prostaglandins could have been present. HORAKOVA and BEAVEN (1974) found that compound 48/80, which depletes rats of mast cells and therefore of histamine, prevented the paw-swelling usually induced by 53° C or 56° C. They failed to find swelling at 48° C, however, in contrast to results of many other workers. Those planning research in this area should note that not all strains of rats behave alike (SALMON and WEST, 1973).

e) Miscellaneous Paw Oedemas

OH-ISHI and SAKUMA (1970) derived equations from very simple assumptions that fit moderately well the swellings found as a function of time, caused by 5-HT, dextran, carrageenin, bradykinin, histamine, hot water and acetic acid. Of course, the fact that a mathematical model fits the data does not show that the assumptions are correct; the complexities of inflammation are still beyond the mathematician's craft.

Bentonite gel injected into the paw (0.05 ml of 5%) causes an oedema beginning within 1 h and lasting for 10 days (MAREK, 1969). Protease activity rapidly appears in the serum.

Trauma can also be used to cause paw oedema of the rat (SUCKERT, 1967; RIESTERER and JAQUES, 1970). The latter authors established conditions such that maximum oedema occurred 3 hours after contusion with a 50-g metal rod falling through 50 cm. Aminopyrine, phenylbutazone and other drugs given before injury reduced the oedema. Adrenalectomy reduced the anti-inflammatory effects of these drugs. Crush injury evoked increased vascular permeability (CUMMINGS and LYKKE, 1970), which was suppressed by a 5-HT antagonist.

Urate crystals in the rat's paw are inflammatory (WEBSTER et al., 1972), and probably cause oedema by formation of kinins, histamine and the activation of complement; however, it would appear unlikely that these represent the full story.

II. Increased Vascular Permeability

Since the discussion by HURLEY (Chapter 2) deals with this subject in detail, little more need be said than to point out the review by WILHELM (1962) and also the findings by GARCIA LEME et al. (1973) and DOHERTY and ROBINSON (1975) as they pertain to carrageenin oedema. An excellent review by ROCHA E SILVA (1966) covers the literature through the early 1960s. A technique applicable to many species used in inflammation is that described by WILLIAMS and MORLEY (1974), in which there is continuous recording of extravasated ^{125}I-labelled albumin in a fold of skin. There were differences in time-response curves with thermal injury, histamine, prostaglandin E_1, kallikrein, and lymphokine. Vascular permeability cannot be divorced in a practical sense from the other phenomena of inflammation. Suppression of the initial immediate response in thermal or ultraviolet lesions in the guinea pig has no effect whatsoever on the ensuing delayed phase. On the other hand, there is evidence that delayed exudation in the rat is partly suppressed with kinin-antagonists in heat-, cold-, crush- and chemically-induced injury (WILHELM, 1973).

For those interested in setting up laboratory assays involving permeability to dyes, a helpful discussion may be found in ROCHA E SILVA and GARCIA LEME (1972).

III. Oedema in the Pleural Space

Apparently the first of the various methods using inflammation of the pleural cavity of the rat was described in a doctoral thesis by MERITS (1955). LADEN et al. (1958) employed this technique with Evans blue dye and gum arabic, by injecting 5 ml of the suspension into the pleural cavity, and removing the fluid at various times. They injected the hind knee-joint at the same time with silver nitrate, and found that this resulted not only in swelling of the injected leg but also in a decreased pleural exudate, even when the injected leg was enclosed in a plaster cast to prevent oedema. The anti-inflammatory effect of the silver nitrate was attributed to some unidentified anti-inflammatory substance. It has since then become fairly common knowledge that simultaneous inflammation in two sites will result in less oedema at one site than if the second injection is not made. Chapter 37 of this volume considers agents of animal origin that may be formed in response to inflammation. Also, in a short-term experiment the number of polymorphonuclear leucocytes that can be mobilized is limited, and the inflammation caused by certain substances depends entirely or largely upon these cells (VAN ARMAN et al., 1971; VINEGAR et al., 1973). The numbers of cells involved at the two sites may thus explain the inhibition observed, but more precise data are needed with two-site injections. WINTER and FLATAKER (1965b) showed, by using the pain threshold of the yeast-injected paw of the rat, that if an intraperitoneal injection of some irritant is given there is a dose-related inhibition of the expected lowering of the pain threshold. This is what one would expect on the basis of competition for white cells by the two sites.

HOLTKAMP et al. (1958) found with the technique of LADEN et al. (1958) that hydrocortisone, aspirin and phenylbutazone were effective, but remarked that the assay was a qualitative one. SANCILIO and RODRIGUEZ (1966) developed the Evans blue method into a roughly quantitative one, showing lambda values of 0.32–1.42 (not very good) for 6-rat groups with usual standard drugs. After 3 years' more work, SANCILIO (1969) by adding carrageenin to the Evans blue, obtained much better reliability with respectable lambda values of 0.27–0.45 and g values of 0.06–0.14. VINEGAR et al. (1973), using only 500 µg of carrageenin intrapleurally, obtained excellent standard errors. By counting the infiltrating cells, identifying the types and recording the volumes of exudate, they were able to show that in this model of inflammation there was no early phase (40 min) that many workers (including VINE-GAR) have found with paw oedema. DOHERTY and ROBINSON (1975) confirmed this finding. VINEGAR et al. demonstrated the same sequence of cellular events for the pleural space that has been shown in other sites and by other authors, i.e. that there is a sharp increase in the neutrophilic infiltration between $1^1/_2$ and 3 hours, while the monocytes have a slower rise peaking after the 7th hour.

SPECTOR (1956) used turpentine to cause pleural oedema in the rat. In 1968, WILLOUGHBY and SPECTOR found that in such pleural oedema reduction of the polymorphonuclear leukocyte count by methotrexate had no effect on the volume of exudate. They suggested that perhaps depletion of complement might be responsible for the failure of other workers to find inflammatory vascular changes after giving inflammatory agents to polymorph-depleted animals.

C. Conclusion

One who studies oedema and increased vascular permeability may be interested not only in the phenomena themselves, but also in developing drugs against clinical inflammatory diseases. The state of knowledge, however, has not advanced far enough that one can deliberately design anti-inflammatory drugs. There are no entirely valid laboratory models. The reliability, fortunately, is a statistical matter that can be known for any method. The laboratory models mentioned in Table 1 have proved to be well-enough correlated with clinical results so that all the useful new anti-inflammatory drugs of the past two decades have been found by these or other animal models more or less similar. All are imperfect copies of human inflammatory diseases, and it is therefore best to use a number of different models. After drugs have been found, they may be used as research tools (for example, as indomethacin has been used) to uncover their own mechanisms of action, and thus to shed light on the entire inflammatory process. Oedema and increased vascular permeability are more characteristic of acute inflammation than of chronic; it is noteworthy that drugs active against laboratory models such as carrageenin oedema may be quite active against acute gouty attacks, but are less effective against chronic syndromes such as rheumatoid arthritis. It is not known what the mediators may be that are important for acute inflammations, but thus far no single mediator has been proved responsible. Most likely several mediators play certain roles at various times, and potentiation has been demonstrated among some of them. Some of the mediators appear to be brought by white cells to the site of certain inflammations and released there. There must surely be mediators and phenomena not yet known that contribute to the overall inflammation.

References

Armstrong, D., Días da Silva, W.: Kinin formation in human blood serum induced by cooling and by heat aggregated human gamma globulin preparations. In: Bradykinin and Related Kinins: Cardiovascular, Biochemical and Neural Actions, pp. 31—37, New York: Plenum Press 1970

Armstrong, D., Mills, G. L., Sicuteri, F.: Physiological influence on the liberation of human plasma kinin at low temperatures. In: Hypotensive Peptides, Proceedings of Symposium, Florence 1965, pp. 139—148. Berlin-Heidelberg-New York: Springer 1966a

Armstrong, D. A. J., Mills, G. L., Stewart, J. W.: Thermally induced effects on the kinin-forming system of native human plasma, 37–0° C and 37–50° C. In: International Symposium on Vasoactive Polypeptides: Bradykinin and Related Kinins, p. 167. Edart, Sao Paulo: Ribeirao Preto 1966b

Arrigoni-Martelli, E., Schiatti, P., Selva, D.: The influence of anti-inflammatory and immunosuppressant drugs on nystatin induced oedema. Pharmacology 5, 215—224 (1971)

Baran, L., Moskovic, S.: Un simple dispositivo para el estudio de anti-inflamatorios. Acta physiol. lat.-amer. 20, 81—83 (1970)

Brown, D. M., Robson, R. D.: Effect of antiinflammatory agents on capillary permeability and oedema formation. Nature (Lond.) 202, 812—813 (1964)

Buttle, G. A. H., D'Arcy, P. F., Howard, E. M., Kellett, D. N.: Plethysmographic measurement of swelling in the feet of small laboratory animals. Nature (Lond.) 179, 629 (1957)

Chang, Y.-H., Gralla, E. H.: Suppression of urate crystal-induced canine joint inflammation by heterologous antipolymorphonuclear-leukocyte serum. Arthr. Rheum. 11, 145—150 (1968)

Cotran, R. S., Majno, G.: A light and electron microscopic analysis of vascular injury. Ann. N.Y. Acad. Sci. 116, 750—764 (1964)

Cummings, R., Lykke, A. W. J.: Increased vascular permeability evoked by crush injury in the rat. Brit. J. exp. Path. 51, 19—27 (1970)

De Souza, J. M., Rocha e Silva, M.: Release of kinin-like material in rats submitted to hyperthermia (40—43° C). Agents Actions 3, 382 (1973)

Di Rosa, M.: Review. Biological properties of carrageenan. J. Pharm. (Lond.) 24, 89—102 (1972)

Doherty, N. S., Robinson, B. V.: The inflammatory response to carrageenan. J. Pharm. (Lond.) 27, 701—702 (1975)

Donaldson, V. H.: Mechanisms of activation of C'l esterase in hereditary angioneurotic oedema plasma in vitro. The role of Hageman Factor, a clot-promoting agent. J. exp. Med. 127, 411—429 (1968)

Enders, A., Heidbrinck, W.: Volumetrische Messung des Rattenpfotenödems durch Verdrängung von Quecksilber. Z. ges. exp. Med. 126, 79—81 (1955)

Ferreira, S. H., Moncada, S., Parsons, M., Vane, J. R.: The concomitant release of bradykinin and prostaglandin in the inflammatory response to carrageenan. C. 2, Proc. Brit. Pharmacol. Soc. 11—12 July (1974)

Finney, D. J.: Statistical Methods in Biological Assay, 2nd Ed. New York: Hafner Publishing Co. 1964

Garcia Leme, J., Hamamura, L., Leite, M. P., Rocha e Silva, M.: Pharmacological analysis of the acute inflammatory process induced in the rat's paw by local injection of carrageenan and heating. Brit. J. Pharmacol. **48**, 88—96 (1973)

Garcia Leme, J., Hamamura, L., Rocha e Silva, M.: Effects of antiproteases and hexadimethrine bromide on the release of a bradykinin-like substance on heating (46° C) of rat paws. Brit. J. Pharmacol. **40**, 294—309 (1970)

Goodwin, L. G., Jones, C. R., Richards, W. H. G., Kohn, J.: Pharmacologically active substances in the urine of burned patients. Brit. J. Path. **44**, 551—560 (1963)

Gözsy, B., Kato, L.: Oedema formation in rat's skin. Nature (Lond.) **178**, 1352 (1956)

Gross, F.: Unspezifische Beeinflussung entzündlicher Reaktionen. Schweiz. med. Wschr. **80**, 697—701 (1950)

Hillebrecht, J.: Zur routinemäßigen Prüfung antiphlogistischer Substanzen in Rattenpfotentest. Arzneimittel-Forsch. **4**, 607—614 (1954)

Hoene, R.: Acquisition of topical resistance to thermal injury. Proc. Soc. exp. Biol. (N.Y.) **85**, 56—61 (1954)

Holtkamp, D. E., Wang, R., Doggett, M.: Rapid method for the measurement of antiinflammatory activity utilizing fluid volume of experimentally inflamed pleural cavity of the rat. Fed. Proc. **17**, 379 (1958)

Horakova, Z., Beaven, M. A.: Time course of histamine release and edema formation in the rat paw after thermal injury. Europ. J. Pharmacol. **27**, 305—312 (1974)

Keele, C. A., Neil, E.: Oedema. In: Samson Wright's Applied Physiology, 11th Ed., pp. 44—46. London-New York: Oxford University Press 1965

Laden, C., Blackwell, R. Q., Fosdick, L. S.: Antiinflammatory effects of counterirritants. Amer. J. Physiol. **195**, 712—718 (1958)

Lombardino, J. G., Otterness, I. G., Wiseman, E. H.: Acidic inflammatory agents—correlations of some physical, pharmacological and clinical data. Arzneimittel-Forsch. **25**, 1629—35 (1975)

Marek, J.: A contribution to the mechanism of bentonite-induced oedema in the rat paw. In: Inflammation Biochemistry and Drug Interaction, pp. 76—82. Baltimore: Williams and Wilkins 1969

Merits, I.: Chemical studies of inflammatory edema, experimentally induced. Northwestern University thesis (Ph.D.), Evanston, Illinois 1955

Moncada, S., Ferreira, S. H., Vane, J. R.: Prostaglandins, aspirin-like drugs and the oedema of inflammation. Nature (Lond.) **246**, 217—219 (1973)

Moore, E., Trottier, R. W., Jr.: Comparison of various types of carrageenan in promoting pedal edema in the rat. Res. Commun. chem. path. Pharmacol. **7**, 625—628 (1974)

Movat, H. Z.: Activation of the kinin system by antigen-antibody complexes. In: International Symposium on Vaso-active Polypeptides: Bradykinin and Related Kinins, pp. 177—188. Sao Paulo: Edart Livraria Editora 1967

Netti, C., Bandi, G. L., Pecile, A.: Antiinflammatory action of proteolytic enzymes of animal, vegetable or bacterial origin administered orally compared with that of known antiphlogistic compounds. Farmaco, Ed. prat. **27**, 453—466 (1972)

Oh-Ishi, S., Sakuma, A.: A model for rat paw edema. I. Fitness of the model to some types of edema. Jap. J. Pharmacol. **20**, 337—348 (1970)

Papadimitriou, J. M., Shilkin, K. B., Archer, J. M., Walters, M. N. I.: Inflammation induced by dimethylsulfoxide (DMSO). II. Ultrastructural investigation of the inflammatory phase. Exp. molec. Path. **6**, 347—360 (1967)

Phelps, P., McCarty, D. J., Jr.: Crystal-induced inflammation in canine joints. II. Importance of polymorphonuclear leukocytes. J. exp. Med. **124**, 115—126 (1966)

Randall, L. O., Selitto, J. J.: A method for measurement of analgesic activity on inflamed tissue. Arch. int. Pharmacodyn. **111**, 409—419 (1957)

Riesterer, L., Jaques, R.: The influence of antiinflammatory drugs on the development of an experimental traumatic paw oedema in the rat. Pharmacology **3**, 243—251 (1970)

Robertson, W. van B., Schwartz, B.: Ascorbic acid and the formation of collagen. J. biol. Chem. **201**, 698—696 (1953)

Rocha e Silva, M.: Increased capillary permeability in inflammation. In: Histamine and Antihistaminics. Part I. Histamine. Its Chemistry, Metabolism and Physiological and Pharmacological Actions, Vol. XVIII/I, pp. 274—278. Berlin-Heidelberg-New York: Springer 1966

Rocha e Silva, M., Antonio, A.: Release of bradykinin and the mechanism of production of a "thermic edema (45° C)" in the rat's paw. Med. exp. (Basel) **3**, 371—382 (1960)

Rocha e Silva, M., Garcia Leme, J.: Chemical Mediators of the Acute Inflammatory Reaction, pp. 65—73. Oxford-New York: Pergamon Press 1972

Salmon, G. K., West, G. B.: Variation in the response of rats to chemical and thermal injury. Brit. J. Pharmacol. **47**, 625 P—626 P (1973)

Sancilio, L. F.: Evans blue-carrageenan pleural effusion as a model for the assay of nonsteroidal antiinflammatory drugs. J. Pharmacol. exp. Ther. **168**, 199—204 (1969)

Sancilio, L. F., Rodriguez, R.: Effect of non-steroidal antiinflammatory drugs in the Evans blue pleural effusion. Proc. Soc. exp. Biol. (N.Y.) **123**, 707—710 (1966)

Selye, H.: Studies on adaptation. Endocrinology **21**, 169—188 (1937)

Singh, R. H., Mourya, S. P.: Development and standardization of a new apparatus for accurate measurement of swelling in paw of small laboratory animals. Indian J. med. Res. **60**, 488—490 (1972)

Spector, W. G.: The mediation of altered capillary permeability in acute inflammation. J. Path. Bact. **72**, 367—380 (1956)

Starr, M. S., West, G. B.: Bradykinin and oedema formation in heated paws of rats. Brit. J. Pharmacol. **31**, 178—187 (1967)

Suckert, R.: Experimentelle Modelle für traumatische Rattenpfotenoedeme. Med. Pharmacol. exp. (Basel) **17**, 43—50 (1967)

Swingle, K. F.: Evaluation for antiinflammatory activity. In: Antiinflammatory Agents, Chemistry and Pharmacology, pp. 92—107. New York: Academic Press 1974

Van Arman, C. G.: Antiinflammatory drugs. Clin. Pharmacol. Ther. **16**, 900—904 (1974)

Van Arman, C. G., Begany, A. J., Miller, L. M., Pless, H. H.: Some details of the inflammations caused by yeast and carrageenan. J. Pharmacol. exp. Ther. **150**, 328—334 (1965)

Van Arman, C. G., Bohidar, N. R.: Antiarthritics. In: Rubin, A. A. (Ed.): New Drugs—Discovery and Development, Vol. 5 of the series Drugs and the Pharmaceutical Sciences. New York: Marcel Dekker, Inc. 1978

Van Arman, C. G., Carlson, R. P., Brown, W. R., Itkin, A.: Indomethacin inhibits the Shwartzman reaction. Proc. Soc. exp. Biol. (N.Y.) **134**, 163—168 (1970)

Van Arman, C. G., Nuss, G. W.: Plasma bradykininogen levels in adjuvant arthritis and carrageenan inflammation. J. Path. **99**, 245—250 (1969)

Van Arman, C. G., Nuss, G. W., Risley, E. A.: Interactions of aspirin, indomethacin and other drugs in adjuvant-induced arthritis in the rat. J. Pharmacol. exp. Ther. **187**, 400—414 (1973)

Van Arman, C. G., Nuss, G. W., Winter, C. A., Flataker, L.: Proteolytic enzymes as mediators of pain. In: Proceedings 3rd International Pharmacology Meeting. Pharmacology of Pain, Vol. IX, pp. 25—32. Oxford-New York: Pergamon Press 1968

Van Arman, C. G., Risley, E. A., Kling, P. J.: Correlation between white cell count and inflammatory swelling induced by carrageenan in the rat's foot. Pharmacologist **13**, 284 (1971)

Vinegar, R., Macklin, A. W., Truax, J. F., Selph, J. L.: Formation of pedal edema in normal and granulocytopenic rats. In: White Cells in Inflammation, pp. 111—138. Illinois: Charles C. Thomas 1974

Vinegar, R., Schreiber, W., Hugo, R.: Biphasic development of carrageenan edema in rats. J. Pharmacol. exp. Ther. **166**, 96—103 (1969)

Vinegar, R., Truax, J. F., Selph, J. L.: Some quantitative temporal characteristics of carrageenan-induced pleurisy in the rat. Proc. Soc. exp. Biol. (N.Y.) **143**, 711—714 (1973)

Webster, M. E., Maling, H. M., Zweig, M. H., Williams, M. A., Anderson, W., Jr.: Urate crystal induced inflammation in the rat: evidence for the combined actions of kinins, histamine, and components of complement. Immunol. Commun. **1**, 185—198 (1972)

Wilhelm, D. L.: The mediation of increased vascular permeability in inflammation. Pharmacol. Rev. **14**, 251—280 (1962)

Wilhelm, D. L.: Mechanisms responsible for increased capillary permeability in acute inflammation. Agents Actions **3**, 297—306 (1973)

Wilhelm, D. L., Mason, B.: Vascular permeability changes in inflammation: the role of endogenous permeability factors in mild thermal injury. Brit. J. exp. Path. **41**, 487—506 (1960)

Wilhelmi, G., Domenjoz, R.: Die Beeinflussung des Hühnereiweiß-Oedems an der Rattenpfote durch Pyrazole sowie Cortison und ACTH; plethysmographische Registrierung des Schwellengrades. Arzneimittel-Forsch. **1**, 151—154 (1951)

Williams, T. J., Morley, J.: Measurement of rate of extravasation of plasma protein in inflammatory responses in guinea pig skin using a continuous recording method. Brit. J. exp. Path. **55**, 1—12 (1974)

Willoughby, D. A., Spector, W. G.: Inflammation in agranulocytic rats. Nature (Lond.) **219**, 1258 (1968)

Winder, C. V., Wax, J., Been, M. A.: Rapid foot volume measurements on unanesthetized rats and the question of a phenylbutazone effect on anaphylactoid edema. Arch. int. Pharmacodyn. **112**, 174—182 (1957)

Winter, C. A., Flataker, L.: Reaction thresholds to pressure in edematous hind-paws of rats and responses to analgesic drugs. J. Pharmacol. exp. Ther. **150**, 165—171 (1965a)

Winter, C. A., Flataker, L.: Nociceptive thresholds as affected by parenteral administration of irritants and of various antinociceptive drugs. J. Pharmacol. exp. Ther. **148**, 373—379 (1965b)

Winter, C. A., Risley, E. A., Nuss, G. W.: Carrageenan-induced edema in hind paw of the rat as an assay for antiinflammatory drugs. Proc. Soc. exp. Biol. (N.Y.) **111**, 544—547 (1962)

Winter, C. A., Risley, E. A., Nuss, G. W.: Antiinflammatory and antipyretic activities of indomethacin, 1-(p-chlorobenzoyl)-5-methoxy-2-methylindole-3-acetic acid. J. Pharmacol. exp. Ther. **141**, 369—376 (1963)

Wong, S., Gardocki, J. F., Pruss, T. P.: Pharmacologic evaluation of Tolectin (tolmetin, McN-2559) and McN-2891, two antiinflammatory agents. J. Pharmacol. (Kyoto) **185**, 127—138 (1973)

CHAPTER 22

Short-Term Drug Control
of Crystal-Induced Inflammation*

D. J. McCarty

A. Historical Aspects

The constant presence of microcrystalline monosodium urate monohydrate (MSU) in joint fluid from acute gout was first documented in 1961 (McCarty and Hollander, 1961). MSU needles can be seen by ordinary light microscopy, but the strongly negative birefringence with axial extinction by compensated polarized light microscopy is a much more sensitive test that is quite specific. Van Leeuwenhoek (b. 1633) was the first to describe urate crystals, having obtained them from a draining tophus (McCarty, 1970a). He was unaware of their chemical composition, as uric (lithic) acid was not discovered until a century later (Scheele, 1776). It is of historic interest that A. B. Garrod had used polarized light microscopic inspection of fresh tissue sections cut by hand with a razor blade to identify urate crystals (Garrod, 1876). He wrote that "... in the *constancy* of such deposition lies the clue that has long been wanting; the occurrence of the deposit is at once pathognomonic and separates gout from every other disease which at first sight may appear allied to it." Phagocytosis of MSU crystals by both polymorphonuclear and mononuclear cells was first described in recently erupted human skin tophi by the Viennese dermatologist Gustav Riehl (Riehl, 1897), a phenomenon re-discovered later in gouty joint fluid (McCarty, 1962).

An acute inflammatory response associated with crystal phagocytosis was induced by injection of synthetic urate crystals and control crystals composed of other substances into normal human and canine joints (Faires and McCarty, 1962) or into the joints of gouty patients (Seegmiller et al., 1962). Crystal-induced inflammation was characterized as dose related, completely reversible, and non-specific with reference both to host species and to chemical composition of the crystal. Crystals such as diamond dust and cholesterol were not phlogistic. Inflammation induced in both human and canine joints by injection of adrenocorticosteroid esters was thought to be responsible for the "post steroid injection flare" (McCarty and Hogan, 1964).

Earlier, the Swiss investigators Wilhelm His Jr. and Max Freudweiler had described an inflammatory response to injected synthetic MSU and other crystals in man and several other species, including dog and rabbit (His, 1900; Freudweiler, 1899; Freudweiler, 1901; Brill and McCarty, 1964; Brill and McCarty, 1965). Such lesions were followed by serial biopsy and eventuated in a tophus with histologic criteria indistinguishable from those of a natural human gouty tophus.

* From the Rheumatology Section, Department of Medicine, Medical College of Wisconsin, 8700 West Wisconsin Avenue, Milwaukee, Wisconsin 53226. Supported in part by grants AM 13069 and AM 05621.

B. Mechanism of Crystal-Induced Inflammation

I. Phagocytosis

Phase contrast and polarized light microscopic study of supravitally stained joint fluid leucocytes from inflamed gouty joints, and of buffy-coat leucocytes that had engulfed MSU crystals in vitro, failed to show the expected phagosome (sac) around the ingested particles (McCarty, 1962). Calcium pyrophosphate dihydrate (CPPD) crystals in joint fluid leucocytes from patients with the newly discovered disease *pseudogout* were often inside phagosomes and such sacs were seen in nearly all buffy-coat leucocytes that had ingested CPPD (McCarty et al., 1962). Polymorphonuclear leucocytes rapidly disintegrated after ingestion of MSU, releasing crystals into the ambient medium, often with shreds of adherent cytoplasm; CPPD crystal phagocytosis also resulted in death and disintegration of the phagocyte, sometimes releasing phagosomes with crystals still inside (McCarty, 1962; McCarty et al., 1965).

Electron microscopic (EM) studies confirmed that the MSU crystals in polymorphonuclear leucocytes in gouty exudates had no surrounding membranous sac, leading to speculation that they had formed intracellularly (Riddle et al., 1967; Bluhm et al., 1969). Sequential EM studies of phagocytes exposed to synthetic MSU crystals for varying times, showed that a phagosome was formed initially by inversion of the plasma membrane, but that breaks in the sac soon occurred (Schumacher and Phelps, 1971). MSU crystals were often liberated into the cytoplasm. The plasma membrane of the polymorph also fragmented eventually and the crystal was again extracellular. Similar study of synthetic CPPD crystal phagocytosis, with incubation periods up to 2 h, showed phagolysosome formation but relatively few breaks in their integrity, although cell death was greater (23%) than in cells incubated without crystals (8%) (Schumacher, 1972). EM examination of leucocytes from acutely inflamed pseudogouty joints confirmed that most, although not all, crystals were inside membranous sacs. EM inspection of the synovium from patients with pseudogout revealed CPPD crystals both free in the synoviocyte cytoplasm and within sacs (Schumacher, 1968).

Characterization of MSU and CPPD crystals from patients with gout and pseudogout, synthesis of crystals with identical properties and production of inflammation in the normal joints of man and several species of experimental animals, fulfill Koch's postulates in a metabolic disease. Polymorphonuclear leucocytes are an absolute requirement of the host response to crystals for the following reasons: (1) they are constantly associated with crystals during the acute attack (McCarty, 1962; McCarty et al., 1962); (2) depletion of these cells in experimental animals with drugs (Phelps and McCarty, 1966; Chang and Gralla, 1968) completely inhibits the inflammatory response; (3) restoration of leucocytes by perfusion of the crystal-containing limb of a leucopenic dog with fresh dog blood restores the inflammatory response (Phelps and McCarty, 1966).

II. Membranolysis

Previous studies by several groups of investigators showed that silica crystals haemolyzed erythrocytes and, after phagocytosis, induced rupture of macrophage phagolysosomes (Charache et al., 1962; Nash et al., 1965; Allison et al., 1966). Such lysis was blocked by potent hydrogen acceptors such as polyvinyl pyridine N-oxide

(PVPNO) which was thought to be due to the formation of pre-emptive hydrogen bonds with the surface of silica crystals. PVPNO was absorbed by both MSU and silica crystals but not by erythrocytes or CPPD crystals. MSU crystals were found to behave much like silica, producing brisk haemolysis of washed erythrocytes (WAL-LINGFORD and McCARTY, 1971). CPPD crystals induced a much slower red cell destruction, significantly exceeding control values only after 2 h, but reaching 50% of MSU-induced haemolysis after 21 h. The haemolytic effects of silica and MSU were blocked completely by PVPNO and were greatly inhibited by normal plasma. That actual physical contact with crystals, rather than with ions, was responsible for cell breakdown was shown by the absence of haemolysis when cells and crystals were separated by dialysis membranes.

These observations, coupled with the EM findings described above, led us to the following hypothesis (WALLINGFORD and McCARTY, 1971):

> Protein coated crystals are phagocytosed, and subsequent fusion of lysosomes with the phagosome produces a phagolysosome that contains enzymes. These digest the protein coat on the crystal, allowing hydrogen bond mediated membranolysis to occur. Phagolysosome lysis is accompanied by the release of hydrolytic enzymes into the cytoplasm, resulting in cellular autolysis, increased permeability of the outer membrane and release of enzymes into the extracellular medium.

MSU and silica crystals are polymerized weak acids (pKa of both approximately = 10) and therefore present an ordered array of positively charged hydrogens at their surface—available for bonding with a complementary array of negatively charged groups, such as occur in proteins and phospholipids of cell membranes and in anionic polymers such as PVPNO. Hydrogen bonds are extremely weak (2–10 KCal/mole), but the combined energy of thousands of such bonds could conceivably produce a strong union between complementary surfaces. How this leads to breaks in membrane continuity is not known. The mechanism of the much slower membranolytic effect of CPPD is also unknown. No damage to leucocyte membranes occurs when MSU or silica crystals are incubated with these cells in the presence of fluoride which blocks phagocytosis (WALLINGFORD and TREND, 1971). Why is this same membrane vulnerable when it is turned outside in to form a phagosome? Perhaps adsorbed serum proteins are digested away by lysosomal proteases and the membrane becomes vulnerable to hydrogen bonding, or the areas of lysosomal membrane incorporated into the phagosome during merger of the 2 sacs *are* the areas of vulnerability, the 'Achilles heel' of the phagolysosome. Definition of the mechanism of this reaction depends on the precise characterization of the reaction between the crystal and the inner side of the phagolysosome. A direct relationship between the solubility of urate crystals prepared with different mono and divalent cations and their membranolytic potential has been reported recently (LUSSIER and DE MEDICIS, 1974). They postulate an osmotic effect on membranes due to rapid crystal dissolution.

The single crystal (lattice) structures of both MSU and triclinic CPPD, the most common of the 2 crystals found in pseudogout, have recently been solved (MANDEL, 1975; MANDEL and MANDEL, 1976). Both of these crystals, as well as silicon dioxide crystals, have irregular surfaces at the atomic level, as opposed to non-phlogistic crystals such as diamond and several rarer types of silica crystals that show a flat lattice structure. MANDEL believes that an ionic mechanism of binding is at least as likely on theoretical grounds as is hydrogen bonding, and that the irregular lattice structure of the inflammation-producing crystals results in forces that cause deformity in the bound phospholipid polar head groups. Alternatively, such bound phospholipids may be rendered vulnerable to the action of phospholipases such as lysolecithin. The presence on the crystal surface of discontinuities due to uneven growth might further accentuate the membrane-breaking ability of the phlogistic crystals.

Although the generalization relating crystal surface characteristics at the level of the atomic lattice to inflammatory potency is still highly speculative, because relatively few crystals whose lattice structure is completely solved have been characterized as to such potency and *vice versa*, it is useful both as a testable hypothesis and as an example of reductionism in science!

The pattern of release of polymorphonuclear lysosomal enzymes and the cytoplasmic marker enzyme lactate dehydrogenase after ingestion of MSU or CPPD crystals, has been studied by several groups (WALLINGFORD and TREND, 1971; WEISSMANN et al., 1971; ANDREWS and PHELPS, 1971). Both crystals induced release of lysosomal enzymes into the extracellular medium, but only MSU crystals caused release of LDH marker enzyme, indicating loss of integrity of the cell membrane. Lactic acid dehydrogenase (LDH) release peaked 5 h after MSU crystals had been incubated with the leucocytes.

Synthetic MSU and CPPD have been tested against: isolated heavy granule fraction of rabbit liver cells, containing both mitochondria and lysosomes; isolated human polymorph lysosomes; artificial lipid membranes (liposomes) which have a precisely defined composition and which contained marker anions (WEISSMANN and RITA, 1972). MSU crystals produced a dose related release of lysosomal but not mitochondrial marker enzymes, MSU (20 mg/ml) causing a twofold increase in enzyme release over control after a 60 min incubation; CPPD crystals failed to release enzymes from either lysosomes or mitochondria. Isolated human leucocyte lysosomes released acid phosphatase into the supernatant upon contact with MSU crystals; 40 mg/ml caused a 40% increase in liberated enzyme over control after a 15 min incubation. The lack of release of marker enzyme from the cholesterol-poor membranes of mitochondria suggested a requirement for this molecule for membrane vulnerability. Marker anion release from liposomes by MSU crystals was doubled when cholesterol was incorporated into the membrane and essentially no anion release over control was found when cholesterol was omitted. Liposomes were made 'female' with 1% 17-estradiol, or 'male' with 1% testosterone. MSU crystals (20 mg/ml) incubated for 4 h with liposomes of each 'sex,' showed release of only 20% more marker over control from the 'female' liposomes, but 100% increase over control from the 'male' liposomes.

'Packing' of membrane phospholipid controlled by steroid 'spacer' was suggested by these authors, who speculated that the observed 'sex' difference may account for the markedly increased incidence of clinical gouty arthritis in men (WEISSMANN and RITA, 1972).

The evidence suggesting a cholesterol requirement for membrane vulnerability to MSU appears stronger than that for oestrogen protection, as at least one natural cholesterol-poor membrane (mitochondrial) was spared in addition to the demonstrated lack of effect on cholesterol-free liposomes. There is no evidence yet that natural membranes are protected by oestrogen from MSU crystals, and the oestrogen effect even in liposomes is not specific for crystals, but also stabilizes them against other types of perturbation.

However, the sensitivity of the erythrocyte system is considerably greater than systems using lysosome or liposome suspensions. MSU crystal haemolysis was consistently 6 times greater than control lysis in the RBC system compared with a maximum of 2 times control for the smaller particles, even though greater crystal concentrations were used in the latter experiments. The much longer incubation periods used with the red cell incubations showed unequivocal haemolysis with synthetic CPPD crystals, although the *rate* of lysis was 8 times slower than that of MSU, and 42 times slower than that of silica! Moreover, the finding of CPPD crystals free, as well as membrane bound, in the cytoplasm of synovial cells and synovial fluid polymorphs by EM suggests that CPPD crystal membranolysis may actually occur in vivo. Hydrogen bonding can hardly be the mechanism, as there was no protection by PVPNO over that afforded control erythrocytes incubated without crystals (Wᴀʟʟɪɴɢꜰᴏʀᴅ and MᴄCᴀʀᴛʏ, 1971).

Further studies have demonstrated direct visual disruption of phagosome after MSU crystal ingestion by dogfish leucocytes, and by EM peroxidase staining material was shown escaping into the adjacent cytoplasm of human polymorphs through breaks in the phagosome, affording direct evidence in support of the 'suicide sac' hypothesis outlined above (Hᴏꜰꜰꜱᴛᴇɪɴ and Wᴇɪꜱꜱᴍᴀɴɴ, 1975).

III. Inflammatory Mediators

Sodium urate crystals, like nearly all colloids and suspensoids, are electronegative (Kᴇʟʟᴇʀᴍᴇʏᴇʀ and Bʀᴇᴄᴋᴇɴʀɪᴅɢᴇ, 1965). Like glass surfaces, MSU crystals bind and denature Hageman factor (clotting factor XII) which, then activated, sets in motion the clotting cascade, the kinin system and the plasmin system. Hageman factor has been identified in synovial fluid, and factors that increase vascular permeability have been induced by adding Hageman factor to normal joint fluid (Kᴇʟʟᴇʀ-ᴍᴇʏᴇʀ and Bʀᴇᴄᴋᴇɴʀɪᴅɢᴇ, 1966; Kᴇʟʟᴇʀᴍᴇʏᴇʀ, 1967). An acute inflammatory response in chicken joints injected with MSU crystals has been demonstrated; as chickens lack Hageman factor, this substance is obviously not a sine qua non for the inflammatory response (Sᴘɪʟʙᴇʀɢ, 1974).

Kinin levels were shown by bioassay to be elevated in the synovial fluid in both natural gout and in inflammation induced in man by synthetic MSU crystals (Mᴇʟ-ᴍᴏɴ et al., 1967). However, there was no difference in the severity of MSU crystal-induced inflammation in the canine joint model, when carboxypeptidase B (which hydrolyzes the terminal arginine from the nonapeptide bradykinin, converting it into an impotent octapeptide) was injected into the joint along with the crystals (Pʜᴇʟᴘꜱ et al., 1966). About half of this enzyme was recovered from the joint at the end of the experiment, enough to completely block the effects of intrasynovially injected synthetic bradykinin. An anti-inflammatory effect of trypsin-kallikrein inhibitor on urate crystal induced inflammation in rabbits has been demonstrated (Sᴘɪʟʙᴇʀɢ and Oꜱᴛᴇʀʟᴀɴᴅ, 1970); but no increase in ornithokinin activity was found in chicken synovial fluid (Sᴘɪʟʙᴇʀɢ, 1974). Kinins do not appear to be a sine qua non for crystal synovitis, at least not in dogs or chickens.

Pretreatment of dogs (PHELPS and McCARTY, 1969 a) and rabbits (SPILBERG, 1973; SPILBERG and OSTERLAND, 1970) with cobra venom factor (CVF) resulted in greatly lowered total haemolytic complement ($C'H_{50}$) levels but did not detectably suppress urate or CPPD (SPILBERG, 1973) crystal induced inflammation.

We had always heated MSU and CPPD crystals to 180–200° C for 2 h to destroy pyrogens that may have been trapped in the crystal from the mother liquor during its growth. Such treatment will totally destroy bacterial pyrogen deliberately added to the solution from which we prepared crystals. The pyrogen *is* taken up by the crystals and such crystals are extraordinarily potent when tested in the dog model (PHELPS and McCARTY, unpublished data). Joints are exquisitely sensitive to pyrogen, and amounts of pyrogen not detected by the usual i.v. test in the rabbit will produce a marked synovitis (HOLLINGSWORTH and ATKINS, 1965).

Unheated MSU crystals exposed to normal serum (4 mg/ml) will result in a lowering of $C'H_{50}$ levels, but the same crystals, after heat treatment, will not (PHELPS and McCARTY, 1969 a). Similar results on total $C'H_{50}$ have been found by others, who also measured the individual components (NAFF and BYERS, 1973; BYERS et al., 1973). Unheated crystals lowered the levels of C'_2 and C'_4 which argues against entrapped pyrogen which, if present, should activate the complement system through the properdin (shunt) pathway, bypassing these early components. Also there was little activation of C'_1, so that these crystals were presumably not activating the system through the classical pathway either. It is possible that complement activation by unheated synthetic MSU crystals is by an unique mechanism beginning with C'_4. Recent data have shown that heating synthetic MSU crystals to 200° C for 2 h may drive off the water of hydration and change the lattic structure of the crystal (MANDEL, 1976). A synergistic effect of i.v. administered bacterial pyrogen and MSU crystals given intra-articularly has been demonstrated (VAN ARMAN et al., 1974).

The striking complete suppression of tenderness, out of proportion to effects on swelling, local heat and volume of local effusion in MSU crystal induced synovitis in normal human volunteers pretreated with aspirin (STEELE and McCARTY, 1966), suggests that prostaglandins may play a role as mediators of the pain. A report has been published showing that rats on a diet deficient in prostaglandin precursors had a diminished response to injected MSU crystals that was restored by the addition of PGE_1 (DENKO, 1974).

IV. Chemotactic Factors

A nondialyzable chemotactic factor with a molecular weight of about 8500 daltons, released from human, dog or rabbit polymorphonuclear leucocytes after MSU or CPPD crystal phagocytosis, has been found (PHELPS, 1970; TSE and PHELPS, 1970). Diamond crystals were phagocytosed but did not release this chemotactic factor nor, as mentioned above, do they induce an inflammatory response. Colchicine, in concentrations of 10^{-6} M, a level approximating that obtained with the usual therapeutic doses given to patients (ERTEL and WALLACE, 1971) predictably blocks the release of this factor by at least 50% after MSU crystal phagocytosis, but its effects on chemotactic factor release after CPPD crystal phagocytosis is much less predictable (TSE and PHELPS, 1970). These in vitro observations parallel the effects of colchicine clinically in the treatment of gout and pseudogout. In gout, the drug is nearly always effective in control of inflammation, whereas in pseudogout the effects range from dramatic to none at all (McCarty, 1972a).

Colchicine has been measured in human serum, urine and peripheral blood polymorphonuclear leucocytes after the intravenous administration of usual therapeutic doses (Wallace et al., 1970; Ertel and Wallace, 1971). The highest plasma concentration (zero time extrapolation of decay curve) was found to be 7×10^{-7} M. Drug concentration in peripheral blood leucocytes was much greater, ranging from $1-2 \times 10^{-5}$ M; at 72 h colchicine levels approximated 5×10^{-6} M, and detectable levels were still found in cells isolated from the blood 10 days later. The increased concentration in leucocytes is probably related to their content of labile microtubules, each dimer subunit of which specifically binds one molecule of colchicine (Borisy and Taylor, 1967). Numerous parameters of neutrophilic leucocyte function are altered by colchicine (for review see McCarty, 1970b).

Another leucocyte-derived chemotactic factor released from rabbit or horse polymorphs that have phagocytosed aggregated gamma globulin, has been described more recently (Zigmond and Hirsch, 1973). As urate crystals bind IgG predominantly, and as binding may partially denature the bound molecules, these two factors might prove to be related (Kozin and McCarty, 1976). However, MSU crystal-released factor is heat labile, whereas the Hirsch factor is heat stable. Although experiments showing "cell derived" chemotactic factors are performed in serum-free systems, the possibility remains that serum protein molecules adsorbed to the cell membrane may become incorporated into the phagolysosome during phagocytosis.

Others have confirmed and extended Phelps' observations, finding that the generation of chemotactic factor is inhibited by actinomycin D (Spilberg et al., 1974), and that the newly formed chemotactic factor is present in the lysosomal fraction of the cell in addition to being released extracellularly. That synthesis of new polypeptide is needed is surprising, as Phelps found chemotactic factor release into the ambient medium within 7 min after urate crystal phagocytosis, which seems a rather rapid action for protein synthetic machinery (Phelps, 1970).

If natural sodium urate crystals activate complement as the unheated synthetic crystals do, then complement-derived chemotactic factors may be involved in the genesis of crystal induced inflammation. Such factors have been shown for synthetic crystals (Byers et al., 1973). The lack of suppressive effect of C_3 depletion by CVF in studies cited above argue against this possibility.

C. Experimental Models

I. Animal

After the initial demonstration of urate crystal induced synovitis in man, a similar reaction was found in unanesthetized dogs, using the time of onset of a 3-legged gait as a sharply defined end point (Faires and McCarty, 1962). As it was our intention to dissect the mechanism of the host response, we developed a model in the dog that permitted serial measurement of a number of physiologically meaningful parameters simultaneously. Such parameters had not been described in 1961 and were developed so that we could apply them to our purposes.

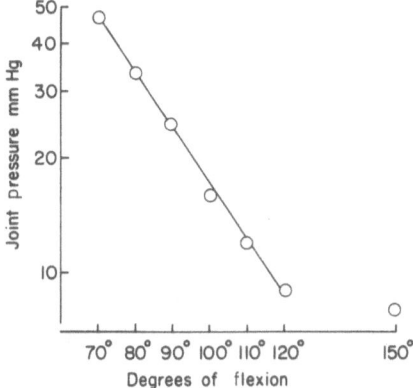

Fig. 1. Change in intra-articular pressure in a catheterized dog joint is shown as a function of its degree of flexion. See text for details

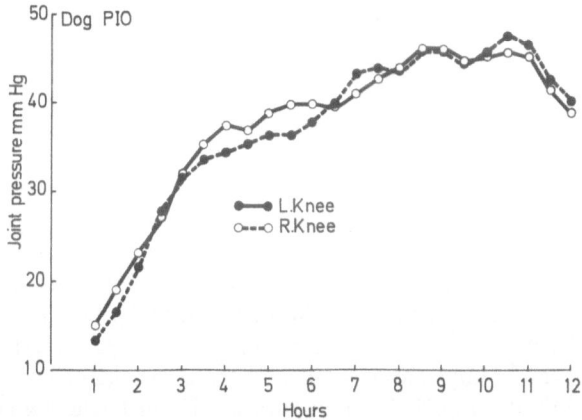

Fig. 2. Intra-articular pressure, reflecting the fluid phase of exudation, is derived by exudation from blood plasma and may approximate diastolic blood pressure. It is quite reproduceable, as shown in measurements on both knee joints of a single dog injected with the same crystal dose (20 mg). The reaction began to subside in both joints 10 h after crystal injection

Mongrel dogs of medium to large size were lightly anesthetized with barbiturates. A stifle (knee) joint was catheterized with a polyethelyene catheter which was attached via a three-way stop cock to a pressure transducer (McCarty et al., 1966). The joint was fixed with tape in 90° of flexion as intra-articular pressure (IAP) varied with the position of the joint (Fig. 1). Normal IAP is approximately atmospheric. Change in IAP, once position of the joint is constant, reflects volume change in the joint, and is an *index of the fluid phase of the exudative inflammatory response.* The IAP rise is driven by the hydrodynamic pressure within the arterial circulation and in a joint at rest tends to equilibrate with the diastolic blood pressure (Fig. 2). When the joint is flexed, the pressure often rises to several hundred mm Hg pressure, and the articular capsule may even rupture, emptying joint contents into the tissue spaces of the leg. The IAP response to injected crystals is dose related and quite reproduceable in the same animal, using the same dose (Fig. 2). In experiments of such long dura-

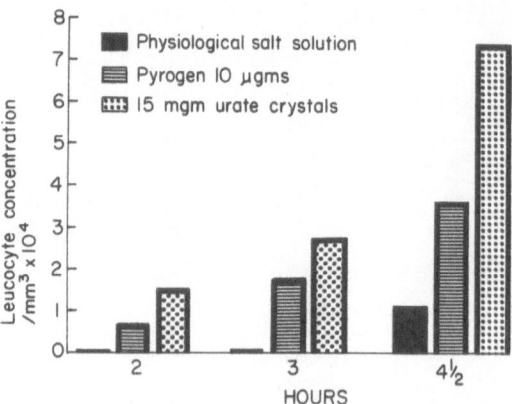

Fig. 3. Leucocyte concentration in a catheterized dog joint rises gradually for several hours after ingestion of urate crystals. A similar increased concentration occurs after bacterial pyrogen ingestion, or even after physiologic saline, which may contain minute quantities of pyrogen. No comparable rise in leucocyte concentration followed injection of even large amounts of bradykinin (PHELPS et al., 1966)

tion, a thermistor probe was inserted into the rectum and hypothermia avoided by use of a heated table and/or an electric blanket.

The gradual fall in synovial fluid pH is entirely due to leucocytic exudation and represents an *index of the cellular phase* of the exudative inflammatory response. The leucocytic concentration can be determined serially in small samples obtained through the indwelling catheter; estimated total synovial exudative response often can be calculated by aspiration of the joint to zero (atmospheric) pressure with direct measurement of volume. The rate of increase in leucocyte concentration is similar after injection of sterile physiologic saline, bacterial pyrogen or urate crystals, differing only in magnitude (Fig. 3). No comparable rise in leucocyte concentration occurred after injection of even large amounts of bradykinin. Concentrations of enzymes have also been measured serially in joint fluid (PHELPS et al., 1966). Drug concentrations could easily be measured also, although to my knowledge, the model has never been used for this purpose.

Although it is unlikely that true synovial membrane blood flow can be measured because of the many assumptions that must be made (PHELPS et al., 1972), ^{133}Xenon clearance from the joint does provide an index of such flow, and does increase after urate crystal injection.

Other advantages of this model are the ability to perform concurrent histologic studies (PHELPS and McCARTY, 1966), and as the animal is not sacrificed, the opposite limb can be used as control. Furthermore, because the inflammation is completely reversible, control experiments can be performed on the *same joint*, after 4 or more weeks have elapsed.

We have tested intravenous indomethacin using this model and found it efficacious in lowering the leucocyte and pressure responses to MSU crystals (PHELPS and McCARTY, 1969 b). The same dose of indomethacin given directly into the joint was not irritating in itself, but failed to block the inflammatory response as efficiently as when the drug was given by the intravenous route. As the leucocytic response was suppressed by i.v. indomethacin out of proportion to the suppression of the fluid phase of exudation and to the suppression of ^{133}Xenon clearance, the drug was tested in vitro where a suppressant effect on leucocytic motility was demonstrated (PHELPS and McCARTY, 1967). The relatively weaker local anti-inflammatory effect could not be explained, but as concentrations of indomethacin above 10^{-6} M were

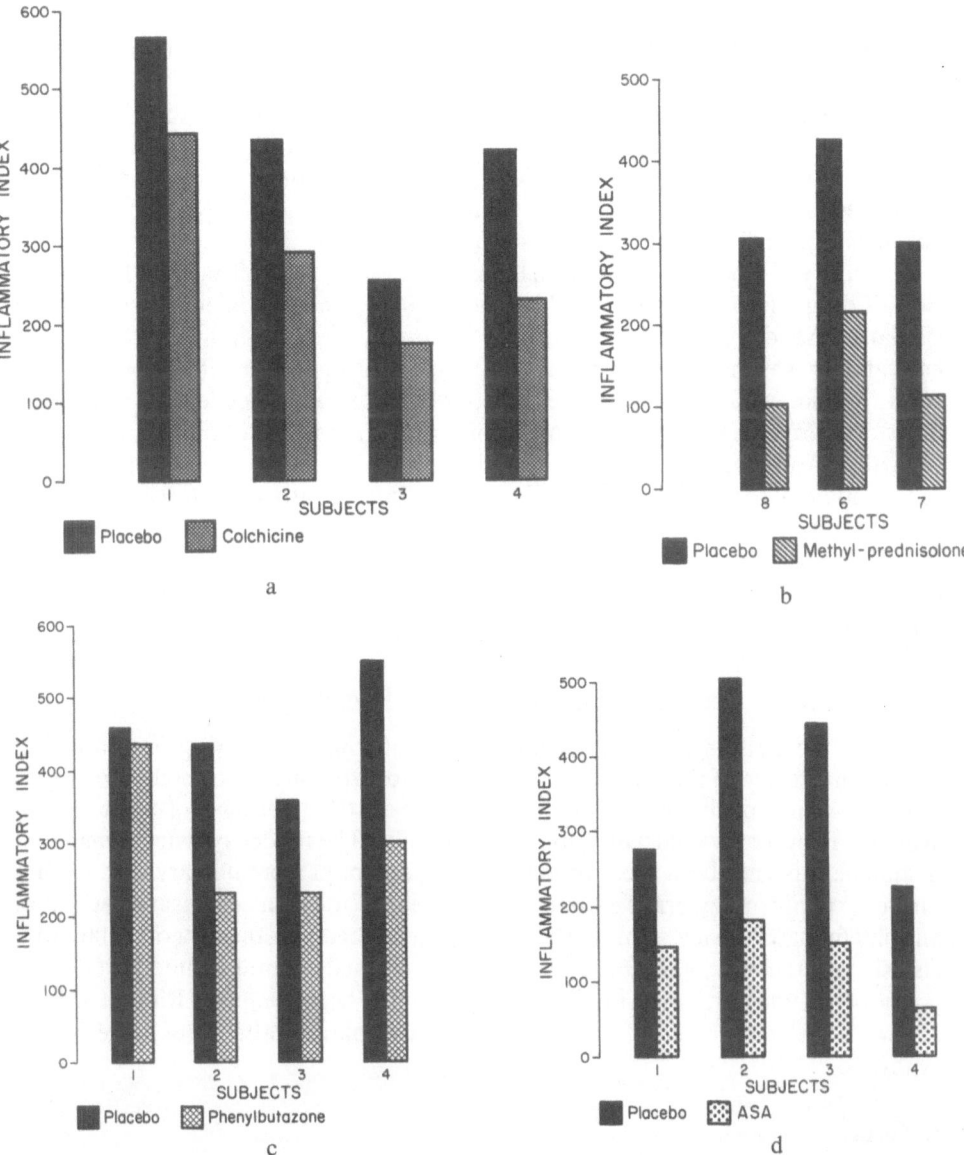

Fig. 4a–d. Effectiveness of four drugs known to be anti-inflammatory in the treatment of patients with acute gouty arthritis on an "inflammatory index" is illustrated. Subjects received either placebo or (a) colchicine, (b) methyl-prednisolone, (c) phenylbutazone, or (d) aspirin. Evaluations were performed by an observer who was unaware of the treatment received and each patient served as his own control. (Reproduced with permission, Arthritis and Rheumatism)

less effective in suppressing leucocyte motility, it is conceivable that the local joint tissue drug concentrations achieved in vivo were actually too high! The model has been used to determine the effects of exercise on the inflammatory response (AGU-DELO et al., 1972). No other studies using this model have been published.

II. Man

Crystal-induced inflammation was first used in 1965 as an experimental model testing for drug effectiveness in humans (MALAWISTA and SEEGMILLER, 1965). The response to subcutaneous injection of crystals was evaluated by measurement of the diameter of induration and erythema; the response to intra-articular crystals was gauged by an inflammatory index arrived at by clinical rating of local heat, swelling, tenderness and erythema on a 0–4+ scale. The effectiveness of pretreatment with colchicine, phenylbutazone or corticosteroids was shown.

Urate crystal-induced synovitis in humans proved to be a safe method for evaluation of drug efficacy (STEELE and McCARTY, 1966). An experimental arrangement similar to that described above for canine joints was used. An indwelling polyethylene catheter was inserted into normal knee joints through a small skin wound and sewn in place with a single suture. Intra-articular volume, tenderness of selected areas of the overlying skin, skin temperature over the joint and joint circumference were all measured in standard fashion and all proved useful as empirical parameters of the inflammatory response. The effect of anti-inflammatory drugs was invariably detectable if the changes in each parameter were added to provide an inflammatory index. The indices for four drugs known to be effective in treating patients with clinical gout are shown in Figures 4 a–d. Efficacy of a single new drug was proven by this technique (STEELE and McCARTY, 1967).

D. Therapy of Acute Attacks of Gout and Pseudogout

Although the model systems of crystal-induced inflammation have proved useful in dissection of some of the critical features of the host response to crystals, the precise mode of action of drugs known to be effective in the treatment of acute crystal synovitis in everyday clinical practice is not known. The model systems in man and in animals have not been used for this purpose, except in a preliminary way. Even if further experimental work is carried out with regard to the mechanism of action of anti-inflammatory drugs, it must always be remembered that the experimental models using synthetic crystals are at best *analogues* of their natural counterparts, acute gouty or pseudogouty arthritis. This review would be incomplete without a brief review of the empiric use of drugs in treatment of natural attacks of acute crystal synovitis.

I. Gout

The aims of therapy are: (1) to alleviate the pain, which is often excruciating; and (2) to restore the inflamed joint to useful function (SMYTHE, 1972). After protection of the joint by splinting, and after analgesics are given, a choice of effective drugs is at hand. Thorough aspiration of the joint, often possible at the time of diagnostic arthrocentesis necessary to obtain fluid for crystal identification, may be accompanied by local injection of microcrystalline adrenocorticosteroid esters. Such therapy is ideal for an attack in a single large joint; inflammation subsides predictably within 12 h of treatment, regardless of the prior duration of the acute attack.

Colchicine remains the drug of choice in the average case, especially when small joints are involved or in polyarticular attacks. The drug may be given orally, 0.5 mg every hour until relief or side effects occur. About 10 tablets are generally required. Diarrhoea is almost always produced. Signs and symptoms of inflammation subside in 12 to 24 h and pain is gone in over 90% of patients with in 24–48 h. Electrolyte imbalances in the elderly may be severe, the bone marrow may be fatally depressed especially in persons with haematologic malignancies receiving chemotherapy. The drug often cannot be given orally in persons with postoperative acute gout. The intravenous route must be used in these instances. Here, 1–3 mg is given with care to avoid extravasation because of the marked irritating properties of the drug. Subsequent doses of 1 mg every 6–8 h are given. Gastrointestinal effects are avoided completely and the anti-inflammatory effects are more rapid, with noticeable effects in 6 to 8 h and complete relief in 24 h.

Phenylbutazone and its derivative oxyphenbutazone are as effective as i.v. colchicine and are regarded by many as the drugs of choice in acute gout. About 600 mg is given in the first 24 h, followed by 100 mg four times daily for about 1 week. Nearly all attacks of acute gout can be controlled with these drugs. Side effects of fluid retention or gastritis are common.

Indomethacin is very effective. In studies using initial doses of 400 mg in the first 24 h and 100 mg in divided doses over the next 4–5 days, it is as effective as phenylbutazone. Side effects are also similar to those of phenylbutazone. (Indomethacin causes sodium retention by the kidney—this was inadvertently discovered by me when marked oedema was produced during treatment of a patient with Addison's Disease!)

ACTH and corticosteroids are reportedly effective agents in acute gout, although the latter may control pain while inflammation simmers at a subdued level. Corticosteroids are often given chronically by clinicians for poylarticular gout wrongly diagnosed as rheumatoid arthritis. Additional joints become inflamed and the patient looks more and more as though he has the disease for which he is being treated! I have never used either ACTH or corticosteroids for the treatment of acute gout and I doubt if there is any indication for their use in this disease.

II. Pseudogout

Supportive measures are useful as outlined above. Thorough aspiration of a large joint is often very effective in reversing acute inflammation, even without local corticosteroid injection (McCARTY, 1972b). This effect is presumably due to removal of sufficient crystals to control what is an experimentally demonstrable dose-related response. Concomitant use of local steroid esters is 100% effective in control of acute pseudogout in a single large joint.

Phenylbutazone, oxyphenbutazone, and indomethacin are effective, used in doses outlined above for the treatment of acute gout. Colchicine effectiveness is unpredictable and this might be related to its variable effects on release of the cell-derived chemotactic factor discussed above (PHELPS, 1970; TSE and PHELPS, 1970).

E. Summary

The concepts of crystal induced inflammation and of the crystal deposition diseases is only 15 years old. Much has been learned about the cellular and molecular mechanisms of interaction between sodium urate and calcium pyrophosphate and host tissues. There has been little exploitation of model systems of crystal-induced inflammation in man and animals with regard to effectiveness, or to the mechanism of action of anti-inflammatory drugs. Empirical therapy in both acute gout and acute pseudogout is entirely satisfactory. New drugs for the treatment of the inflammation associated with these diseases should be directed at the removal of the asymptomatic crystal and not at the inflammation itself. Such removal has been accomplished in gout, but remains the chief therapeutic challenge in pseudogout.

References

Agudelo, C. A., Schumacher, H. R., Phelps, P.: Effect of exercise on urate crystal-induced inflammation in canine joints. Arthr. Rheum. **15**, 609—616 (1972)

Allison, A. C., Harington, J. S., Birbeck, M.: An examination of the cytotoxic effects of silica on macrophages. J. exp. Med. **124**, 141—153 (1966)

Andrews, R., Phelps, P.: Release of lysosomal enzymes from polymorphonuclear leukocytes (PMN) after phagocytosis of monosodium urate (MSU) and calcium pyrophosphate dihydrate (CPPD) crystals: effect of colchicine and indomethacin. Arthr. Rheum. **14**, 368 (abs.) (1971)

Bluhm, G. B., Riddle, J. M., Barnhart, L.: Intracellular formation of urate crystals. Arthr. Rheum. **12**, 283 (abs.) (1969)

Borisy, G. G., Taylor, E. W.: The mechanism of action of colchicine binding of colchicine-^{3}H to cellular protein. J. Cell Biol. **34**, 525—533 (1967)

Brill, J. M., McCarty, D. J.: (Studies on the nature of gouty tophi. Freudweiler, M. Dtsch. Arch. klin. Med. 1899) An abridged translation with comments. Ann. intern. Med. **60**, 486—505 (1964)

Brill, J. M., McCarty, D. J.: (Experimental investigations into the origin of gouty tophi. Freudweiler, M. Dtsch. Arch. klin. Med. 1901) An abridged translation with comments. Arthr. Rheum. **8**, 267—288 (1965)

Byers, P. H., Ward, P. H., Kellermeyer, R. W., Naff, G. B.: Complement as a mediator of inflammation in acute gouty arthritis. II. Biological activities generated from complement by the interaction of serum complement and sodium urate crystals. J. Lab. clin. Med. **81**, 761—769 (1973)

Chang, Y., Gralla, E. J.: Suppression of urate crystal induced joint inflammation by heterologous antipolymorphonuclear leukocyte serum. Arthr. Rheum. **11**, 145—150 (1968)

Charache, P., MacLeod, C. M., White, P.: Effects of silicate polymers on erythrocytes in the presence and absence of complement. J. gen. Physiol. **45**, 1117—1143 (1962)

Denko, C. W.: Phlogistic action of prostaglandins in urate crystal inflammation. J. Rheum. **1**, 24 (abs.) (1974)

Ertel, N. H., Wallace, S. L.: Measurement of colchicine in urine and peripheral blood leukocytes. Clin. Res. **19**, 348 (1971)

Faires, J. S., McCarty, D. J.: Acute arthritis in man and dog after intrasynovial injection of sodium urate crystals. Lancet **1962 II**, 682—685

Freudweiler, M.: Studies on the nature of gouty tophi. Dtsch. Arch. klin. Med. **63**, 266—335 (1899)

Freudweiler, M.: Experimental investigations into the origin of gouty tophi. Dtsch. Arch. klin. Med. **69**, 155—205 (1901)

Garrod, A. B.: A treatise on Gout and Rheumatic Gout (Rheumatoid Arthritis) 3rd ed. London: Longmans, Green and Co. 1876

His, W., Jr.: Fate and effects of the acid uric acid sodium in the abdominal and joint cavities of the rabbit. Dtsch. Arch. klin. Med. **67**, 81—108 (1900)

Hoffstein, S., Weissmann, G.: Mechanisms of lysosomal enzyme release from leukocytes. IV. Interaction of monosodium urate crystals with dogfish and human leukocytes. Arthr. Rheum. **18**, 153—166 (1975)

Hollingsworth, J. W., Atkins, E.: Synovial inflammatory response to bacterial endotoxin. Yale J. Biol. Med. **38**, 241—256 (1965)

Kellermeyer, R. W.: The inflammatory process in acute gouty arthritis. III. Vascular permeability enhancing activity in normal human synovial fluid; induction by Hageman factor activators; and inhibition by Hageman factor antiserum. J. Lab. clin. Med. **70**, 372—383 (1967)

Kellermeyer, R. W., Breckenridge, R. T.: The inflammatory process in acute gouty arthritis. I. Activation of Hageman factor by sodium urate crystals. J. Lab. clin. Med. **65**, 307—315 (1965)

Kellermeyer, R. W., Breckenridge, R. T.: The inflammatory process in acute gouty arthritis. II. The presence of Hageman factor and plasma thromboplastin antecedent in synovial fluid. J. Lab. clin. Med. **67**, 455—460 (1966)

Kozin, F., McCarty, D. J.: Protein adsorption to monosodium urate, calcium pyrophosphate dihydrate and silica crystals: relationship to the pathogenesis of crystal-induced inflammation. In: McCarty, D. J. (Ed.): Symposium on Pseudogout and Pyrophosphate Metabolism. Arthr. Rheum. Suppl. **19**, 433—438 (1976)

Kozin, F., McCarty, D. J.: Unpublished data

Lussier, A., de Medicis, R.: Mechanism of phagolysosome membranolysis by urate crystals. J. Rheum. **1** (suppl.), 23 (abs.) (1974)

Malawista, S. E., Seegmiller, J. E.: The effect of pretreatment with colchicine on the inflammatory response to microcrystalline urate. Ann. intern. Med. **62**, 648—657 (1965)

Mandel, N. S.: The crystal structure of calcium pyrophosphate dihydrate. Acta crystallogr. **B 31**, 1730—1734 (1975)

Mandel, N. S.: The structural basis of crystal-induced membranolysis. In: Symposium on Pseudogout and Pyrophosphate Metabolism. McCarty, D. J. (ed.). Arthr. Rheum. Suppl. **19**, 439—445 (1976)

Mandel, N. S., Mandel, G. S.: Monosodium urate monohydrate: the gout culprit. J. Amer. chem. Soc. **98**, 2319—2323 (1976)

McCarty, D. J.: Phagocytosis of urate crystals in gouty synovial fluid. Amer. J. med. Sci. **243**, 288—295 (1962)

McCarty, D. J.: A historical note: Leeuwenhoek's description of crystals from a gouty tophus. Arthr. Rheum. **13**, 414—418 (1970a)

McCarty, D. J.: Pathogenesis and treatment of the acute attack of gout. Clin. Orthop. **71**, 28—39 (1970b)

McCarty, D. J.: Urate crystal phagocytosis by polymorphonuclear leukocytes and the effects of colchicine. In: Williams, R. C., Fudenberg, H. H. (Eds.): Phagocytic Mechanisms in Health and Disease. Intercontinental Medical Book Corporation, pp. 107—121. New York-London: Grune and Stratton 1972a

McCarty, D. J.: Pseudogout; articular chondrocalcinosis. Calcium pyrophosphate crystal deposition disease. In: Hollander, J. L., McCarty, D. J. (Eds.): Arthritis and Allied Conditions, 8th Ed., pp. 1140—1159. Philadelphia: Lea and Febiger 1972b

McCarty, D. J., Gatter, R. A., Brill, J. M., Hogan, J. M.: Crystal deposition diseases. Sodium urate (gout) and calcium pyrophosphate (chondrocalcinosis, pseudogout). J. Amer. med. Ass. **193**, 129—132 (1965)

McCarty, D. J., Hogan, J. M.: Inflammatory reaction after intrasynovial injection of microcrystalline adrenocorticosteroid esters. Arthr. Rheum. **7**, 359—367 (1964)

McCarty, D. J., Hollander, J. L.: Identification of urate crystals in gouty synovial fluid. Ann. intern. Med. **54**, 452—460 (1961)

McCarty, D. J., Kohn, N. N., Faires, J. S.: The significance of calcium phosphate crystals in the synovial fluid of arthritic patients: The "pseudogout syndrome." I. Clinical aspects. Ann. intern. Med. **56**, 711—737 (1962)

McCarty, D. J., Phelps, P., Pyenson, J.: Crystal induced inflammation in canine joints I. An experimental model with quantification of the host response. J. exp. Med. **124**, 99—114 (1966)

Melmon, K. L., Webster, M. E., Goldfinger, S. E., Seegmiller, J. E.: The presence of a kinin in inflammatory synovial effusion from arthritides of varying etiologies. Arthr. Rheum. **10**, 13—20 (1967)

Naff, G. B., Byers, P. H.: Complement as a mediator of inflammation in gout I. Studies on the reaction between human serum complement and sodium urate crystals. J. Lab. clin. Med. **81**, 747—760 (1973)

Nash, T., Allison, A. C., Harington, J. S.: Physicochemical properties of silica in relation to its toxicity. Nature (Lond.) **207**, 874 (1965)

Phelps, P.: Polymorphonuclear leukocyte motility in vitro. IV. Colchicine inhibition of chemotactic activity formation after phagocytosis of urate crystals. Arthr. Rheum. **13**, 1—9 (1970)

Phelps, P., McCarty, D. J.: Unpublished data

Phelps, P., McCarty, D. J.: Crystal-induced inflammation in canine joints. II. Importance of polymorphonuclear leukocytes. J. exp. Med. **124**, 115—126 (1966)

Phelps, P., McCarty, D. J.: Suppressive effects of indomethacin on crystal-induced inflammation in canine joints and on neutrophilic motility in vitro. J. Pharmacol. exp. Ther. **158**, 546—553 (1967)

Phelps, P., McCarty, D. J.: Crystal induced arthritis. Postgrad. Med. **45**, 87—94 (1969 a)

Phelps, P., McCarty, D. J.: Animal techniques for evaluating anti-inflammatory agents. In: Siegler, P., Moyer, J. H. (Eds.): Animal and Clinical Pharmacologic Techniques in Drug Evaluation, Vol. II, pp. 742—747. Chicago: Yearbook Publishers 1969 b

Phelps, P., Prockop, D. J., McCarty, D. J.: Crystal induced inflammation in canine joints. III. Evidence against bradykinin as a mediator of inflammation. J. Lab. clin. Med. **68**, 433—444 (1966)

Phelps, P., Steele, A. D., McCarty, D. J.: Significance of Xenon-133 clearance rate from canine and human joints. Arthr. Rheum. **15**, 360—370 (1972)

Riddle, J. M., Bluhm, G. B., Barnhart, M. L.: Ultrastructural study of leukocytes and urates in gouty arthritis. Ann. rheum. Dis. **26**, 389—401 (1967)

Riehl, G.: Zur Anatomie der Gicht. Wien. klin. Wschr. **10**, 761 (1897)

Scheele, C. W.: Analysis of the calculus vesicae, 1776. In: The Chemical Essays of Charles William Scheele, p. 199. Translated from the transaction of the Academy of Sciences of Stockholm. London: J. Murray 1787

Schumacher, H. R.: The synovitis of pseudogout: electron microscopic observations. Arthr. Rheum. **11**, 426—435 (1968)

Schumacher, H. R.: Phagocytosis of calcium pyrophosphate crystals by polymorphonuclear leukocytes: sequential electron microscopic observations. Arthr. Rheum. **15**, 453 (abs.) (1972)

Schumacher, H. R., Phelps, P.: Sequential changes in human polymorphonuclear leukocytes after urate crystal phagocytosis: an electron microscopic study. Arthr. Rheum. **14**, 513—526 (1971)

Seegmiller, J. E., Howell, R. R., Malawista, S. E.: The inflammatory reaction to sodium urate. J. Amer. med. Ass. **180**, 469—475 (1962)

Smythe, C. J.: Diagnosis and treatment of gout. In: Hollander, J. L., McCarty, D. J. (Eds.): Arthritis and Allied Conditions, pp. 1112—1139. Philadelphia: Lea and Febiger 1972

Spilberg, I.: Studies on the mechanism of inflammation induced by calcium pyrophosphate crystals. J. Lab. clin. Med. **82**, 86—91 (1973)

Spilberg, I.: Urate crystal arthritis in animals lacking Hageman factor. Arthr. Rheum. **17**, 143—148 (1974)

Spilberg, I., Mandell, B., Wochner, R. D.: Studies on crystal-induced chemotactic factor. I. Requirement for protein synthesis and neutral protease activity. J. Lab. clin. Med. **83**, 56—63 (1974)

Spilberg, I., Osterland, C. K.: Anti-inflammatory effect of the trypsin-kallikrein inhibitor in acute arthritis induced by urate crystals in rabbits. J. Lab. clin. Med. **76**, 472—479 (1970)

Steele, A. D., McCarty, D. J.: An experimental model of inflammation in man. Arthr. Rheum. **9**, 430—442 (1966)

Steele, A. D., McCarty, D. J.: Suppressive effects of indoxole in crystal-induced synovitis in man. Ann. rheum. Dis. **26**, 39—42 (1967)

Tse, R. L., Phelps, P.: Polymorphonuclear leukocyte motility in vitro. V. Release of chemotactic activity following phagocytosis of calcium pyrophosphate crystals, diamond dust, and urate crystals. J. Lab. clin. Med. **76**, 403—415 (1970)

Van Arman, C. G., Carlson, R. P., Kling, P. J., Allen, D. J., Bondi, J. V.: Experimental gouty synovitis caused by bacterial endotoxin adsorbed onto urate crystals. Arthr. Rheum. **17**, 439—450 (1974)

Wallace, S. L., Omokoku, B., Ertel, N. H.: Colchicine plasma levels—Implications as to pharmacology and mechanisms of action. Amer. J. Med. **48**, 443—448 (1970)

Wallingford, W. R., McCarty, D. J.: Differential membranolytic effects of microcrystalline sodium urate and calcium pyrophosphate dihydrate. J. exp. Med. **133**, 100—112 (1971)

Wallingford, W. R., Trend, B.: Phagolysosome rupture after monosodium urate (MSU) but not calcium pyrophosphate dihydrate (CPPD) phagocytosis in vitro. Arthr. Rheum. **14**, 420 (abs.) (1971)

Weissmann, G., Rita, G.: Molecular basis of gouty inflammation: interaction of monosodium urate crystals with lysosomes and liposomes. Nature (New Biol.) **240**, 167—172 (1972)

Weissmann, G., Zurier, R. B., Spieler, P. G., Goldstein, I. M.: Mechanisms of lysosomal enzyme release from leukocytes exposed to immune complexes and other particle. J. exp. Med. **134**, Suppl., 149s+ (1971)

Zigmond, S. H., Hirsch, J. G.: Leukocyte locomotion and chemotaxis. New methods for evaluation, and demonstration of a cell-derived chemotactic factor. J. exp. Med. **137**, 387—410 (1973)

Experimental Models of Arthritis in Animals as Screening Tests for Drugs to Treat Arthritis in Man

M. E. J. BILLINGHAM and G. E. DAVIES

A. Introduction

There is a growing feeling of dissatisfaction with the methods used to screen compounds for activity against arthritic diseases in man. In 1968, SPECTOR and WILLOUGHBY alluded to "the temptation to select the present, inadequate drugs, design tests that give positive results and then with the aid of these tests to search for further compounds giving positive results. Such methodology may lead only to 'old' anti-inflammatory agents instead of 'new'." More recently, PAULUS and WHITEHOUSE (1973) pointed out the lack of any breakthrough in the search for drugs to be used in the treatment of human arthritic disease.

It is apparent that the ideal drug for the treatment of rheumatoid arthritis (RA) still awaits discovery. CONSTABLE et al. in 1975 gave a succinct and pertinent view of the situation in the clinic: "Rheumatoid arthritis is usually badly treated. In our experience there are two common mistakes, either patients are kept on aspirin-like drugs for long periods in the face of obvious and marked deterioration, or corticosteroids are given early with considerable immediate effect but at greater cost later on."

This state of affairs is current despite the continued search for new drugs which is being carried out with an increasing intensity, as may be judged from the two-volume monograph edited by SCHERRER and WHITEHOUSE (1974) and from the present volumes. In general, two classes of drugs are available: a large number which exert symptomatic control of the disease (mainly non-steroidal anti-inflammatory agents) and a much smaller number which appear to affect the disease fundamentally (penicillamine, gold salts and chloroquine). The current screening methods appear capable of selecting only the first group and it is difficult to escape the conclusion that better methods are desirable.

It would be expected a priori that the best screening test for anti-arthritic drugs would be based on an experimental model of arthritis in animals and in this chapter we set out to appraise the available models. Overwhelmingly, attention has been directed to adjuvant arthritis (AA) in the rat, and this bias is reflected in the contents of the chapter, but we have also discussed a number of other models which seem to merit more attention than has so far been paid to them by workers primarily interested in drug discovery.

B. Advantages and Disadvantages of Models of Arthritis—Comparison With Acute Models

Broadly speaking, one of the main considerations in a screening programme for any kind of drug is the ability to screen the maximum number of chemical types and individual compounds with maximum economy in the use of compound, experimental animals and technical assistance. With such limitations it is understandable, in our present context, that tests involving acute inflammation are far more frequently used than are experimental models of arthritis. A typical approach might start with carrageenin-induced oedema of the rat hind paw as an initial screen, followed by a second confirmatory acute model such as ultraviolet erythema in guinea pig skin. Further evaluation of the compound in a more chronic model, for example AA, may then be undertaken or a proliferative model such as the cotton-pellet granuloma test may be used.

Such approaches have been adopted widely and have led to the introduction of a number of very useful drugs, but it is becoming increasingly apparent that such drugs are effective inhibitors of the symptoms of the underlying disease process but do not influence the progress of human arthritic disease (CONSTABLE et al., 1975). One of the main advantages of using an experimental model of arthritis as an initial screen is the attendant degree of chronic inflammatory change which renders it likely to detect useful activity in compounds which would not be manifest in an acute model of inflammation, e.g. the thiazolidinone of NEWBOULD (1965).

On the debit side, the use of experimental models of arthritis as initial screens would be more expensive in time and materials than screens of an acute nature. A more serious criticism is that the few drugs regarded by clinicians fundamentally to affect arthritic disease in man have not been shown conclusively to be active in any experimental model of inflammation, be it acute or chronic.

The major challenge remains with the biologist, to devise means for the discovery of drugs with value in the treatment of human arthritic disease. This would be easier to achieve if more were known about the aetiology of human disease, but in the absence of such knowledge the task is difficult. Although the available models of arthritis represent, more or less, some aspects of the human disease, none does so completely, and it may not even be reasonable to expect that they should, considering the many anatomical, physiological and immunological differences between man and laboratory animals.

The remainder of this chapter is devoted to the appraisal of models of arthritis which have been used in the search for drugs. In our view, improved models of arthritis are more likely to demonstrate novel activity and a new generation of drugs than any test involving acute inflammation. It is recognised that to date they have not done so, but it is also apparent that very few of the available models have been used to evaluate the activity of novel compounds.

C. Adjuvant-Induced Arthritis

The most widely used model of experimental arthritis which has been used for screening purposes is the disease produced in the rat by the injection of Freund's complete adjuvant into certain dermal and subdermal tissue sites. No other model has been investigated to the same extent, possibly because adjuvant disease of the rat is so very reproducible and lends itself readily to screening programmes. In fact, the very success of this model of arthritis in the hands of most investigators, and the facility with which it can be utilised, has probably been a major reason why additional models have not been developed as screening tests for anti-inflammatory/

antirheumatic drugs. This model has been reviewed recently by SWINGLE (1974) and ROSENTHALE (1974).

I. First Observation. First Use as a Screen for Anti-Inflammatory/Antirheumatic Drugs

STOERK et al. (1954) were the first to observe the appearance of a polyarthritis in rats injected with Freund's complete adjuvant. Whilst studying immunity against homologous tissue in the rat, they injected extracts of spleen as an emulsion in Freund's complete adjuvant subcutaneously into a large group of rats. Three weeks later, about half of the rats developed red, painful swellings in one or several joints which were seen to develop and persist in the presence of large amounts of antibiotics (penicillin, streptomycin). The polyarthritic lesions persisted for some months although there was some tendency for individual lesions to subside and reappear. It was concluded that the polyarthritis was not due to the presence of a pathogen but may have been due to sensitization against an 'organ-specific' antigen. These observations were extended by PEARSON (1956) who demonstrated that it was not necessary to incorporate extracts of tissues in the emulsion and that Freund's adjuvant alone was capable of inducing the polyarthritis.

The first use of adjuvant-induced polyarthritis as a screening test was by NEWBOULD (1963) although the inhibitory effects of steroids on the syndrome were described a little earlier by PEARSON and WOOD (1959) and by HOUSSAY and FRANGIONE (1961). NEWBOULD (1963) pointed out that the then "inadequacy in the understanding of the aetiology and pathogenesis of rheumatoid arthritis seriously impaired the development of laboratory tests for compounds with specific anti-arthritis activity ... clearly better methods are desirable." AA has now been very widely adopted since its first use as a screening test, but it has only partially fulfilled the need for better methods, since it has been the only model extensively used and it may be wrong to assume that it is an appropriate model of RA in man.

The original method of NEWBOULD (1963) serves as a useful starting point for a discussion of AA as a screening test. Over the years, modifications have been made, but essentially the test remains the same, although preferences exist for various methods of induction and measurement of the polyarthritis produced.

In his original paper, NEWBOULD induced the arthritis syndrome "by an intradermal injection of 0.05 ml of a 5 mg/ml fine suspension of dead tubercle bacilli (human strains PN, DT, and C) in liquid paraffin B.P. into the plantar surface of the right hind foot." The development of the arthritic syndrome was measured in terms of foot thickness increase and secondary lesion development.

"The injection of dead tubercle bacilli in liquid paraffin into the right hind-foot produced an inflamed swelling which reached its maximum size during the first 3 days. Thereafter, the swelling slowly subsided until the 8th day when the foot began to swell again. Ten days after injection, inflamed lesions (which we call secondary lesions) were detected on the left hind-foot, which began to increase in thickness and in the fore-paws, ears and tail. Little further swelling of the feet or joints occurred after the 13th day, and by the 30th day the inflammation had started to subside leaving pale granulomatous swellings around the joints. Ear lesions, which were first seen on the 10th day as small patches of dilated capillaries, had developed into inflamed red nodules up to 3 mm in diameter by the 13th day and had begun to subside by the 30th day. Numerous

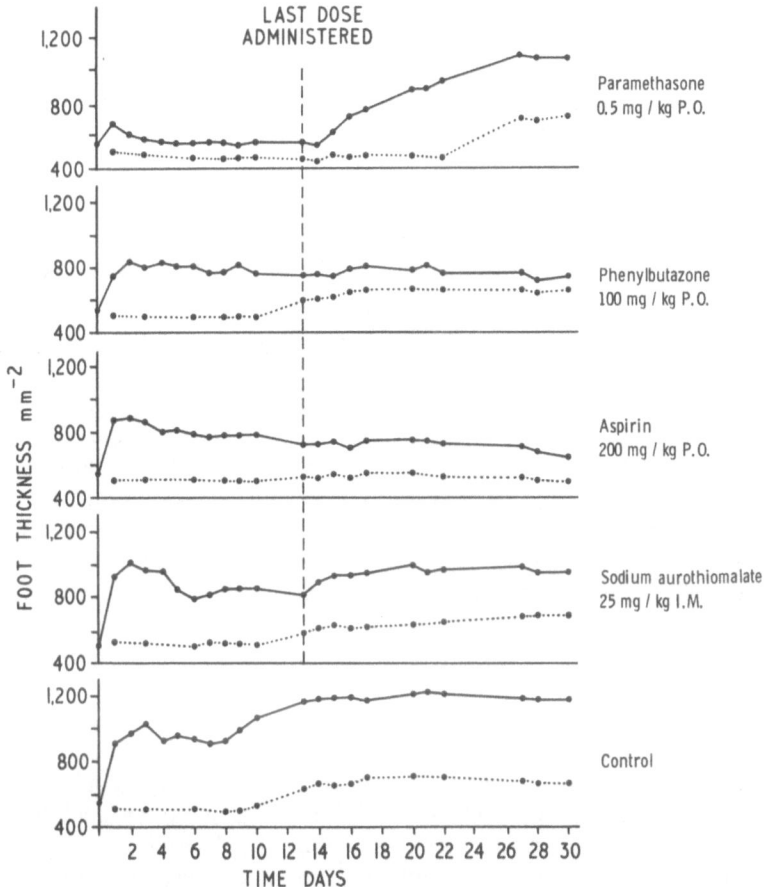

Fig. 1. Effect of paramethasone, phenylbutazone, aspirin and gold on adjuvant arthritis in rats —
after NEWBOULD (1963). Effect measured as inhibition of foot thickness increase in treated
animals, compared with untreated controls

inflamed lesions on the tail, which were also first detected on the 10th day, had also started to
subside by the 30th day. By this time the tail had become noticeably thicker and in some rats
spondylitis had developed. During the development of the arthritic syndrome the rats invariably
lost weight. The heavier the rat at the time of injection, the greater was the weight loss in absolute
terms."

The effect of the then well-known antirheumatic agents, steroids, phenylbutazone, acetyl salicylic acid and sodium aurothimalate is shown in Figure 1 which is
based on NEWBOULD's (1963) original experiments. Measurement of the increase in
thickness of the injected right hind foot was found to be a simple and adequate
indicator of drug effect. In addition, visual assessment of secondary lesion development as nil, mild, moderate or severe and weight change were noted to be useful
parameters of drug effect.

II. Production

Although AA can be readily induced in rats, careful attention to detail is essential for the production of a model sufficiently reproducible for use as a screening test. In this section we have reviewed briefly those aspects of technique which govern the development of a suitable model.

1. Adjuvant

A variety of species of dead mycobacteria (usually *M. tuberculosis*, *M. butyricum* or *M. phlei*), suspended in vegetable or mineral oil may be used. PARONETTO (1970) has induced arthritis with *Corynebacterium rubrum* and FLAX and WAKSMAN (1963) have used *Nocardia asteroides*.

Attempts have been made to identify the fraction of the bacterial cell responsible for inducing the arthritis. It appears to reside in the wax D fraction of the mycobacterial cell wall (PEARSON and WOOD, 1959; WAKSMAN et al., 1960) and was characterized as a peptidoglycan by JOLLÈS et al. (1964) and MIGLIORE and JOLLÈS (1968). WOOD et al. (1969) found that the incidence of arthritis was determined by a component of wax D characterized as a mycolic acid ester of a peptide-linked polysaccharide, resembling the mucopeptides of mycobacterial cell walls. When acetylated, the fraction lost its arthritogenicity. AZUMA et al. (1972) examined fractions from mycobacteria, corynebacteria, and nocardia and identified the active material of mycobacterial wax D as a mycolic acid-arabinogalactan-mucopeptide. A similarly structured active fragment was found in the cell walls of corynebacteria and nocardia; the difference between the various bacteria was in the number of carbon atoms in the acid portion with mycolic acid (70–90) > nocardic acid (50–58) > corynemycolic acid (32–34). Removal of the acid portion and arabinogalactan by acid treatment or removal of the acid by alkali treatment resulted in loss of activity.

It would appear that the intact triplet is essential for activity and the occurrence of similar triplets in mycobacteria, corynebacteria and nocardia would explain why they are all capable of inducing arthritis. More recent work on the peptidoglycan component of Wax D from tubercle bacilli (KOGA et al., 1976a; KOHASHI et al., 1976) has shown it to be water soluble and that it can also be obtained from Lactobacillus plantarum, several Streptococcus species, Staphlococcus aureus and Clostridium botulinum. Digestion with glycan-degrading enzymes destroyed anany arthritogenic activity. Unlike AZUMA et al. (1972) however, KOGA et al. (1976b) found that removal of the arabinogalactan portion of the water soluble arthritogen component did not result in loss of activity.

KOHASHI et al. (1976; 1977) were able to obtain arthritogenic water soluble peptidoglycans from both arthritogenic and non-arthritogenic bacterial cell walls and it is reasonable to assume that a common peptidoglycan within bacterial cell walls is responsible for producing adjuvant disease. Careful extraction procedures are needed however to obtain it from cell walls which are not normally arthritogenic.

The suitability of the vehicle for suspending the mycobacteria has been studied by a number of workers (WARD and JONES, 1962; GLENN and GRAY, 1965; KEITEL et al., 1969), but probably the most extensive study has been that of WHITEHOUSE et al. (1974) who examined over a hundred synthetic compounds and natural materials for their ability to induce arthritis when mixed with heat-killed, delipidated *M. tubercu-*

losis (Strains C, DT, PN, human) in four separate strains of rat. Forty of the compounds were capable of inducing arthritis in conjunction with the mycobacteria. They include normal hydrocarbons greater than C_{10}, especially tridecane through to octadecane, certain cyclic hydrocarbons, branched hydrocarbons, e.g. squalene (C_{30} H_{50}), squalane (C_{70} H_{62}), pristane and related natural products such as vitamin K_1 and tocopherol, many oils and triglycerides, e.g. olive oil, corn oil. Other compounds related to cholesterol and fatty acid esters such as butyl palmitate and butyl stearate and lipids extracted from rat tissues were also found to be effective. Obviously a whole host of substances possess the ability to induce arthritis in rats when mixed with *M. tuberculosis*. WHITEHOUSE et al. (1974) comment that in effect squalane, pristane and hexadecane make excellent substitutes for mineral oil in the preparation of arthritogenic adjuvants from various mycobacteria and also from *C. rubrum* and *N. asteroides*.

The concentration of mycobacteria in the suspending vehicle can influence the incidence of arthritis. WARD and JONES (1962) obtained 100% incidence with 0.6 mg per rat, 80% with 0.3 mg and 30% with 0.1 mg and similar dose-related effects accord with our own experience although GLENN and GRAY (1965) found no difference in incidence or severity with amounts of bacteria from 0.1 to 10 mg per rat.

Probably the most important technical consideration for the preparation of a suitable adjuvant is the degree of dispersion. NEWBOULD (1963) emphasized the need for a *fine* suspension of bacilli in oil and, more recently, LIYANAGE et al. (1975) have determined the optimal aggregate size for inducing polyarthritis. They showed that aggregates of heat-killed *M. tuberculosis* in the range 45–90 µm were essential, aggregates in excess of 90 µm being much less effective: the degree of cell-mediated immunity to mycobacterial antigens was similarly correlated but antibody production was not influenced by aggregate size.

For screening purposes, refined preparations, such as wax D, are not easy to reproduce and a properly prepared suspension of mycobacteria is adequate. Preparation of the suspension is best done simply with a pestle and mortar. When using a new strain of rat, we have found it useful initially to try various concentrations of tubercle bacilli in light paraffin to find the concentration which gives an incidence of arthritis of more than 95% without too great a degree of severity. The Sprague Dawley strain from Charles River (U.K.) is a good example, for at a concentration of 3 mg/ml of mycobacteria in light paraffin (0.1 ml into the right foot pad) a 95–100% incidence was obtained coincident with a weight gain only 20% below that of normal control rats. At lower concentrations the incidence fell, as was also found by WARD and JONES (1962) and above this concentration, although the incidence remained the same, the severity of the arthritis increased and was associated with a much poorer gain in weight. WINDER et al. (1969) avoided the problem of weight loss in their experiments by using the tail as the site of injection. They found that injection into the foot pad was followed by severe weight loss of the rats, although this was also seen to a lesser extent following tail injection depending on the volume of adjuvant, i.e. the amount of mycobacteria injected. WINDER et al. (1969) regard the weight loss as a serious affront to the animals' welfare; we would agree and suggest the use of preliminary experiments to find a suitable concentration of mycobacteria that is consistent with a high incidence and reasonable weight gain. It may, however, be necessary to select a suitable strain of rat to achieve these ends. WHITEHOUSE and

Beck (1974) have suggested the use of a standardised adjuvant mixture which can be used in different laboratories around the world. This would be used for comparative purposes and not necessarily supplant the 'in-house' formulations, the aim being to facilitate data comparisons between individual laboratories. This seems a good idea, and a further suggestion might be that if and when the responsible antigen is isolated, as Azuma et al. (1972) have been attempting, it may be possible to obtain a truly standard formulation.

2. Route of Injection

The most commonly used routes of injection of the adjuvant mixture are into the footpad or tail of the rat. Winder et al. (1969) prefer the tail since they consider loss of weight to be unacceptable, as mentioned above. Swingle (1974) shares this view, pointing out that if the initial primary swelling in the injected paw is to be used as a measure of acute inflammation then there are better acute models. We have seen, however, that it is possible to overcome the problem of weight loss following footpad injection if a suitable strain of rat and a suitable dose of adjuvant are found. Perper et al. (1971) consider that tail injection leads to a poorer incidence of arthritis, although Swingle's results (1974) would refute this.

Koga et al. (1976c) regard injection directly into the inguinal lymph node to be superior to injection into the foot pad in terms of both higher incidence and earlier onset of adjuvant arthritis.

3. Species Variation and Strain Variation

Adjuvant disease is essentially restricted to the rat. Attempts to establish the disease in other species have not been successful. Glenn and Gray (1965) were unable to produce adjuvant disease in the hamster, mouse, gerbil, guinea pig, rabbit, pig, dog, and chicken. The guinea pig and mouse were also found by Graeme et al. (1966) to be resistant to adjuvant disease, although both species exhibited a profound acute swelling following injection of the adjuvant mixture. Keitel et al. (1971), however, appear to have had limited success in mice and hamsters; although the incidence was small and variability considerable.

The disease in the rat varies with the strain of rat used and many groups of workers have discussed the phenomenon of strain variation, with regard to incidence and severity of the adjuvant disease.Swingle (1974) has pointed out that improper production of the adjuvant mixture may well account for some of the disparities seen between laboratories but there is considerable evidence of varying degrees of resistance to induction of the disease from strain to strain. An extreme example is the study by Zidek and Perlik (1971) who demonstrated an apparently total resistance to adjuvant disease in one rat strain; when this strain was subjected to backcross studies with a highly susceptible strain the progeny were resistant, and this led to the conclusion that resistance to the disease was genetically dominant. Freeman and West (1972) and Eisen et al. (1973) have also reported a strain of rat which is resistant to AA. Whilst rat strains which are apparently resistant to adjuvant disease appear to be the exception rather than the rule, susceptible strains vary quite widely in their response (Swingle et al., 1969; Ryzewska et al., 1969; Rosenthale, 1970; Zidek and Perlik, 1971; Baumgartner et al., 1974a).

It is virtually impossible to choose from the literature which of the many strains is most appropriate for screening purposes, although the inbred Lewis strain appears to be the most favoured. In an imperfect world, however, local problems of supply and expense will no doubt dictate the choice of rat strain; nevertheless, by varying the amount of mycobacteria injected and the site of injection, many problems with regard to incidence, severity and debilitation can be overcome.

4. Time Course of the Disease

The course of adjuvant disease has been described frequently (PEARSON, 1956; PEARSON and WOOD, 1959; PEARSON et al., 1961; NEWBOULD, 1963) and the description by NEWBOULD (1963) of the initial use of AA as a screening test for potential anti-inflammatory/antirheumatic drugs has been given in Section I. It appears from the literature that although the syndrome is essentially the same in each laboratory, many slight differences do exist. This is especially true of the way in which various strains of rat recover from the later phases of the disease after day 21.

The time of onset of adjuvant disease occurs from about day 9 onwards after the injection of the mycobacterial adjuvant, although reports vary: PEARSON (1956) described the appearance of the disease 22 days after adjuvant injection, NEWBOULD (1963) describes the appearance of symptoms at 10 days, GLENN and GRAY (1965) give 13–19 days and SWINGLE (1974) states 9–12 days as the time of onset. As discussed previously, other factors such as method of preparation of the adjuvant, site of injection and rat strain will influence the rate of onset of the disease. There is more general agreement that the disease approaches its maximum intensity between days 18–21 after adjuvant injection (GLENN and GRAY, 1965; SWINGLE, 1974; BILLINGHAM and GORDON, 1976a, 1976b).

BAUMGARTNER et al. (1974a) have described five phases in the course of AA largely in terms of changes in plasma protein levels, fibrinogen and α2-macroglobulin (plasma inflammation units—see below in this review), plasma albumin, serum thiols, hepatic drug metabolism and changes in paw size. The biochemical changes provided considerably more information than the change in paw size, "since it was evident that measurements of paw swelling alone are insufficient for determining the extent of ongoing (chronic) active inflammation."

Table 1. Phases of adjuvant arthritis (after BAUMGARTNER et al., 1974a)

Phase	Time after adjuvant inoculation (days)	General characteristics
a	1–4	Acute local inflammation—slight fall in thiol titre and fall in plasma albumin
b	7–12	Remission of acute inflammation—rise in albumin levels
c	12–28	Very extensive inflammation—marked fall in thiol titre and albumin level—secondary lesion development
d	21 onwards	Residual inflammation with osteogenesis
e	35 onwards	Permanent attendant deformity with minimal burnt out inflammation—albumin levels and thiol titre return to normal values

The use of plasma albumin levels and certain other plasma proteins for studying time course has been described (LOWE, 1964; GLENN et al., 1968; BILLINGHAM and GORDON, 1976a, 1976b) and will be discussed at greater length in Section IV.

III. Aetiology

1. Role of Lymphatic System

Two of the most striking features of AA are: (1) that it is apparently restricted to rats and (2) that certain routes of injection of adjuvant are better than others. It is probable that the two features are related since it may be speculated that the anatomy of the rat lymphatic system may be conducive to the dissemination of adjuvant.

Intradermal injections of adjuvant into the foot pad, tail or flank are superior to subcutaneous or intramuscular injections for producing the syndrome (PEARSON, 1956; WAKSMAN et al., 1960; WARD and JONES, 1962). The intradermal route gives ready access to the lymphatic system (HUDACK and McMASTER, 1933) and it might, therefore, be supposed that ready access to the lymphatic system is an essential feature. WARD and JONES (1962) were able to prevent the development of secondary lesions by removal of the depot within 2 h of injecting antigen into the tail. However, WAKSMAN et al. (1960) were unable to affect progress of the disease by removal of homolateral or contralateral popliteal nodes either 5 days before or 7 days after injection of adjuvant into the foot pad. The situation was resolved by NEWBOULD (1964a, 1964b) who demonstrated the presence of adjuvant in several lymph nodes after injection by routes favouring development of the syndrome and showed that to inhibit the syndrome it was essential to remove all draining lymph within 5 days of injection. If the same nodes were removed on day 7, development of the syndrome was unimpaired.

AKAMATSU et al. (1966) demonstrated the presence of intact tubercle bacilli in lymph nodes remote from the site of injection. Transfer of the disease using thoracic duct lymph and lymphocytes requires the presence of mycobacterial components, according to QUAGLIATA and PHILLIPS-QUAGLIATA (1972). Furthermore VERNON-ROBERTS et al. (1976) have demonstrated rapid and extensive dissemination of rhodamine labelled tubercle bacilli following foot pad injection. Rhodamine labelled material was found in the synovial lining cells of joints distant to the injection site. Dissemination of the tuberculous material to these sites occurred either in the free form or within macrophages and VERNON-ROBERTS et al. (1976) concluded that the wider distribution, after passage through draining lymph nodes, must have been via the thoracic duct and blood stream, though they were unable to observe fluorescent material 'in transit'.

2. Immunological Mechanisms

There is little doubt that immune mechanisms are involved in the development of secondary lesions, but two problems remain unresolved: (1) the identity of the antigen and (2) the nature of the immunocompetent cells responsible for the lesions. The bulk of the published evidence appears to be in favour of a delayed hypersensitivity (i.e. T cell mediated) response to a disseminated antigen which is probably derived from the tubercle bacillus (WAKSMAN et al., 1960; PEARSON and WOOD, 1959; FLAX and WAKSMAN, 1963; WAKSMAN and WENNERSTEN, 1963; GERY and WAKSMAN, 1967). BERRY et al. (1973) were able to inhibit in vitro migration of leucocytes from arthritic rats with an extract of paws inflamed by injection of carrageenin and suggested that an endogenous antigen produced by inflammatory damage is involved. Much of this evidence, however, would apply equally well to an antibody-dependent mechanism. Passive transfer of the disease in inbred animals (WAKSMAN and WENNERSTEN, 1963) would transfer B cells as well as T cells and antigen, and there is no reason why antibody production should not continue in the recipients. QUAGLIATA and PHILLIPS-QUAGLIATA (1972) have in fact demonstrated that myco-bacterial components are necessary for the successful transfer of the disease. Pre-treatment of rats with mycobacteria (the presumed source of antigen) in saline inhibits the development of arthritis but leaves tuberculin sensitivity unaffected (GERY and WAKSMAN, 1967). Treatment of rats with the immunosuppressive drugs methotrexate and 6-mercaptopurine inhibited the development of arthritis but left hypersensitivity to tuberculin unaffected (WARD et al., 1964). Other authors (KALLIOMÄKI et al., 1964) with a much lower dose were able to inhibit both tuberculin sensitivity and arthritis.

A more telling argument against the delayed hypersensitivity theory is the demonstration that neonatal thymectomy does not impair the animal's ability to develop arthritis (LENNON and BYRD, 1973; HOLLINGSWORTH et al., 1976; KAYASHIMA et al., 1976). In view of these apparent discrepancies, and the failure so far to identify the antigen, it is pertinent to enquire whether these immunological phenomena are really essential to the development of arthritis; AKAMATSU et al. (1966) have suggested that a direct toxic effect might be produced by materials leaking out of adjuvant droplets such as they demonstrated in lymph nodes distant from the injection site. The argument is of more than academic interest in our present context. Immunosuppressive drugs inhibit the syndrome and other drugs have been detected in the first place by their effect on AA (DAVIES, 1968; NEWBOULD, 1965); if the model is to be used to screen for immunosuppressant activity, it is important to clarify the mechanisms involved.

3. Histology

The histological changes which accompany the development of AA are obviously germane to a model used to screen drugs for their effects on RA. Detailed descriptions are provided by PEARSON and WOOD (1959), GLENN and GRAY (1965), SILVER-STEIN and SOKOLOFF (1960), JONES and WARD (1963) and BURSTEIN and WAKSMAN (1964). PEARSON (1963) and MUIRDEN and PEACE (1969) came to the conclusion that although AA resembles RA in many respects, the human condition most closely matched is Reiter's disease.

Of special interest to pharmacologists is the finding by GRYFE et al. (1971) that mast cells appear to play an important role in the development of arthritis. They are the first cells to appear in increased numbers, reaching a peak incidence on the 6th day. On the 11th day, coincident with the arrival of extravascular polymorphs, the mast cells degranulate—a finding consistent with the authors' suggestion that degranulation is mediated by lysosomal enzymes and cationic protein released from polymorphs. A histochemical investigation of adjuvant disease has been undertaken by NUSBICKEL and TROYER (1976) showing increased alkaline phosphatase, acid phosphatase and ATPase activity in the articular cartilage and osteochondral junction.

4. Lysosomal Enzymes

The potential for damage possessed by lysosomal enzymes has led naturally to a study of their role in adjuvant-induced arthritis. Anderson (1970) found that the increased lysosomal enzyme activity (β-glucuronidase, acid phosphatase and colla-genase) in homogenates of adjuvant-injected hind paws paralleled the increase in paw volume. Treatment with phenylbutazone or hydrocortisone inhibited increases in both paw volume and enzyme activity. Ignarro and Slywka (1972) demon-strated a correlation between the state of the disease and changes in liver lysosome fragility and plasma β-glucuronidase and acid phosphatase activity. Paramethasone, phenylbutazone and indomethacin given from day 14 reduced both the oedema in the foot and the fragility of liver lysosomes, whereas aspirin (200 mg/kg) and chloro-quine phosphate were ineffective. Correlation of increased enzyme activity (amino acid naphthylamidase, acid phosphatase and β-glucuronidase) in liver, lung and testes with histological damage was reported by Velo et al. (1972). From a histo-chemical study, Pearse (1974) concluded that acid phosphatase, alkaline phospha-tase and leucine naphthylamidase play an active role in cartilage and bone erosion whereas β-glucuronidase remains localized in inflammatory and synovial cells and does not appear to participate actively in the destructive process. Lowe and Tur-ner (1973) used, as lysosomes, isolated granules from rabbit polymorphs and found that plasma taken from rats with developing arthritis was less able than normal plasma to protect the granules against lysis induced by Triton X-100. Fenclozic acid, whilst reducing the severity of arthritis, did not prevent the fall in stabilizing activity. In contrast, paramethasone increased the stabilizing activity of plasma, not only in arthritic rats but also in normal animals.

Further studies on the role of lysosomal enzymes in AA are desirable. It would seem obvious that an inflammatory reaction which causes an increased influx of polymorphs would ipso facto result in an increased local concentration of lysosomal enzymes, and it would follow that release of these enzymes would lead to further tissue damage. However, it is not clear how drugs can be used to interfere with this process or whether any of the available drugs exert their beneficial effects by interfer-ing with the process, and if so, at what stage. In particular, the nature of the lysoso-mal stabilizing factor in plasma studied by Lowe and Turner (1973) merits further attention.

IV. Assessment

The progress and severity of adjuvant-induced arthritis has been assessed by param-eters which fall into two main categories: (1) the gross physical changes which occur in the affected joints and limbs and (2) the biochemical changes which Glenn et al. (1968) aptly refer to as part of the systemic response to inflammation. Two minor categories include certain physiological changes such as grip function, temperature change and anatomical changes as demonstrated by X-radiography. Swingle (1974) has tabulated many of the parameters used to assess AA and the effects of therapy, and pointed out that apart from erythema all the other cardinal signs of inflamma-tion have been used for assessing AA.

1. Physical Assessment—Gross Measurements

These methods are based on the incidence and/or severity of the arthritic lesion.

a) Scoring Systems

PEARSON and WOOD (1959) described a numerical grading system involving each peripheral joint and the tail for evaluation of the severity of the disease; the maximum possible score for any given animal on any given day being 180. With this system, they demonstrated the inhibitory effect of hydrocortisone on AA.

Other scoring systems of a simpler nature based on the degree of joint involvement in the four paws, ears and tail have been described (WARD and CLOUD, 1966; GRAEME et al., 1966; JESSOP and CURREY, 1968; CURREY and ZIFF, 1968; BROWN et al., 1970; ROSENTHALE, 1970). Essentially, each limb, ear and tail (when used) is included and figures are based on a subjective assessment of the severity of the arthritis at that site. The total score for an animal or group of animals can then be compared with other animals or groups and the efficacy of treatment established.

b) Size of Hind Paws

This has been measured in various ways in terms of volume by mercury displacement (WINTER and NUSS, 1966; BARRON et al., 1968; PERPER et al., 1971), the thickness between the upper and lower surface (NEWBOULD, 1963; GRAEME et al., 1966), the circumference of the tibiotarsal (ankle) joint (ASPINALL and CAMMARATA, 1969) and the weight (DI PASQUALE et al., 1975). The method we use at present is a fully automated assessment of the thickness of the injected hind paws (DAVIES et al., 1971). Essentially, the apparatus consists of a micrometer which, when activated by a foot switch, accurately measures the thickness of the hind paws of the rat. The data is automatically recorded and fed via punched tape directly into a computer for statistical analysis of the results. Additionally, the spread and severity of the adjuvant disease at sites remote from the injection site is scored on a 0–4 scale and correlated with weight gain. Weight gain has frequently been used as an additional parameter for assessing drug effectiveness (NEWBOULD, 1963; WINDER et al., 1969; WALZ et al., 1971 a; DI PASQUALE et al., 1975) and allows the distinction to be made between compounds which, by virtue of being grossly toxic, interfere with the ability of the rat to mount an inflammatory response and those which are active.

c) X-Ray Analysis

X-ray analysis of the hind feet of rats with adjuvant arthritis has been described (BLACKHAM et al., 1977). The main changes were osteoporosis of tarsals and metatarsals, erosions of the tarsals and periosteal reactions in the metatarsals which occurred from day 10 onwards and progressed up to days 21–24. Cystic fibrosis also occurred in the above sites from day 14 and increased to involve the tibia and fibula by day 21, becoming the most dominant abnormality by day 35. Cystic fibrosis and calcification were the main features of the disease at day 50. Scoring of the individual X-ray changes was found to be a useful method of assessing drug activity and was considered by BLACKHAM et al. (1977) to offer a means of identifying antirheumatoid activity.

2. Physiological/Functional Parameters

a) Paw Temperature

Walz et al. (1971 a, 1971 b) have used paw temperature to assess the inflammation in the hind paws of rats with AA. The study of Walz et al. (1971 b) included a comparison of paw temperature change with hind paw volume and serum lysozyme activity as additional parameters for assessing the degree of inflammation. Although it was concluded that the hind paw volume was the most sensitive indicator, paw temperature and serum lysozyme, especially, were also useful for determining the effectiveness of drug treatment.

b) Grip Function

Grip function (Walz et al., 1971 a) has been compared in rats at day 14 of AA (measured as the time they managed to stay on a vertical screen) with hind paw volume, serum lysozyme levels and the temperature of the inflamed hind paws. Oedema formation, as measured by the paw volume changes correlated well with the serum lysozyme levels, which increased biphasically with the primary and secondary phases of the disease. There was no significant correlation, however, between oedema formation, the changes in paw temperature and grip function and it was concluded that these parameters represented independent expressions of the inflammation of AA.

Perrine and Takesue (1968) have used a rotaod for determining grip strength in rats with adjuvant-induced arthritis. A good correlation existed between paw volume increase and .the ability of rats to stay on a rotating rod, i.e. the greater the paw volume increase and severity of arthritis, the less able the rats were to stay on the rotarod. Anti-inflammatory and certain analgesic agents both produced an increase in grip strength indicating that grip strength may be a measure of pain tolerance as well as an anti-inflammatory effect.

3. Biochemical Parameters

An extensive inflammatory reaction, or disease process, such as AA of the rat involves not only the obvious inflammatory changes at the sites of the individual lesions but also produces a host of other changes in a variety of haematological and biochemical systems. Many of these have been used to supplement the more easily measurable parameters of the disease such as paw size change, and several authors have indicated the usefulness of such measurements for defining the profiles of activity of pharmacological agents (Glenn et al., 1968; Walz et al., 1971 b; Baumgartner et al., 1974 a). Others, however, have questioned the advantage of such parameters over the more traditional methods of assessment (Swingle, 1974).

The many biochemical parameters which have been followed during the course of AA have, in the main, been monitored from the changes occurring in the serum or plasma of the arthritic rats (Table 2).

A number of the biochemical parameters in Table 2 involve measurement of liver-synthesized plasma proteins, and both the serum 'turbidity' and plasma 'inflammation units' reflect changes of the plasma protein pattern. Those plasma proteins which increase in concentration are known collectively as 'acute phase proteins' and they increase after many kinds of inflammatory injury. Koj (1975) has recently

Table 2. Biochemical parameters used to assess the course, severity and/or effect of drugs on AA

Parameter measured	Reference	Comment
Erythrocyte sedimentation	PILIERO et al. (1966) GLENN et al. (1965) GRALLA and WISEMAN (1968)	Good correlation with severity and demonstrates effective drug treatment
Serum 'turbidity'	PILIERO and COLOMBO (1969)	
Plasma 'inflammation units'—heat induced coagulability of plasma proteins	GLENN et al. (1965) GLENN and KOOYERS (1966) GRALLA and WISEMAN (1968) BAUMGARTNER et al. (1974a)	Reflects severity of disease and decreases with effective drug treatment
Albumin/globulin ratios and albumin levels in plasma or serum	LOWE (1964) GLENN et al. (1965) PILIERO et al. (1966) GLENN et al. (1968) WEIMER et al. (1968) KATZ and PILIERO (1969) BAUMGARTNER et al. (1974a) BILLINGHAM and GORDON (1976a, 1976b)	Fall in albumin levels show a good correlation with severity of the disease— successful drug treatment normalizes the plasma protein pattern
Plasma fibrinogen	PILIERO et al. (1966) GLENN et al. (1968) WEIMER et al. (1968) GLENN (1969) BILLINGHAM and GORDON (1976a)	Fibrinogen levels increase during AA and this is prevented by effective treatment
Serum $\alpha 2$-glycoprotein	LOWE (1964) BOGDEN et al. (1967) WEIMER et al. (1968) GLENN et al. (1968) BILLINGHAM and GORDON (1976a)	Reflects disease activity and falls to normal levels with effective drug therapy—normally absent from serum
Serum $\alpha 1$-acid glycoprotein	BILLINGHAM and GORDON (1976a, 1976b)	Reflects disease activity
Plasma sialic acid	GRALLA and WISEMAN (1968) BHARGAVA (1971)	
Plasma copper	GRALLA and WISEMAN (1968)	
Lysosomal enzyme levels/ activity in paws	ANDERSON (1970)	Enzyme levels in paw homogenates correlate with paw volume increase— both respond to drug treatment
Lysozyme activity in serum	PILIERO and COLOMBO (1969) WALZ et al. (1971b)	Lysozyme activity correlated well with other parameters of disease assessment and with effective drug treatment
Serum sulphhydryl activity	BUTLER et al. (1969)	
Serum macromolecular thiols	BAUMGARTNER et al. (1974a)	
Protease and antiprotease activity	PARROTT and LEWIS (1977)	

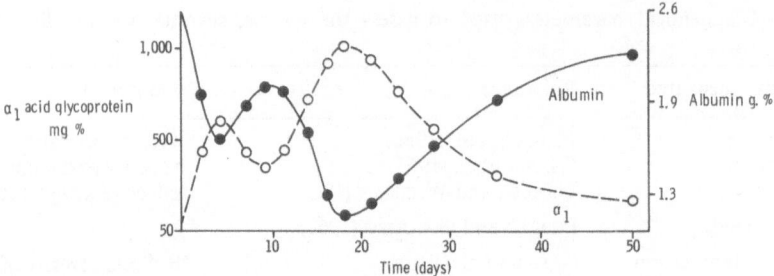

Fig. 2. Changes in the plasma concentration of albumin and α_1 acid glycoprotein during adjuvant arthritis in a hooded rat strain. Levels of albumin and α_1 acid glycoprotein were determined by radial immunodiffusion (MANCINI et al., 1965). A total of 120 rats ($\male$ hooded strain from the National Institute of Medical Research, Mill Hill, London, England) were used for the determinations

reviewed this subject very extensively, especially the relationship between degree of injury and the increase in synthesis rate and concentration of individual proteins in the plasma; it is generally concluded that fluctuations in the concentration of the acute phase protein reflect the changes in severity of inflammation and tissue damage.

The introduction of the technique of radial immunodiffusion (MANCINI et al., 1965) provided a simple means of measuring individual antigens, such as plasma proteins, using very small samples. Albumin, fibrinogen, α_2-glycoprotein and α_1-acid glycoprotein (Table 2) have all been measured throughout AA by this technique and as an example Figure 2 shows the levels of α_1-acid glycoprotein and albumin during AA, as measured by radial immunodiffusion. We prefer the use of α_1-acid glycoprotein for following the progress of AA since it is the major acute phase reactant in the rat (BILLINGHAM and GORDON, 1976a) and is a relatively small molecule compared with fibrinogen and α_2-glycoprotein.

Small samples of blood can be taken from the tail throughout the arthritis with little difficulty, and since only a few microlitres of serum are necessary for a given measurement by radial immunodiffusion, the trauma to the rat is negligible. The main advantage of this approach is the ability to follow the progress of the disease; this can be important, for as Figure 2 shows, the disease process in this particular strain of rat stopped quite rapidly at about day 19–20, as shown by the sudden drop of α_1-acid glycoprotein and the rise in the level of albumin. Many assays for anti-inflammatory activity in AA involve administration of compound after the disease is 'established,' i.e. from day 16–20 onward; a strain of rat which 'switches off' at day 21 could give a misleading result for activity in circumstances where the disease is regressing naturally.

All the various biochemical parameters which have been measured correlate more or less with physical measurements of disease severity and with effective drug treatment. The value of measuring these additional biochemical parameters may be questioned in such circumstances; as SWINGLE (1974) points out, the essential question to be answered when screening is: 'does treatment either prevent development or reduce severity of the disease?' and this is most easily answered by gross examination and measurement of the hind paws.

Biochemical parameters do, however, provide valuable information concerning the underlying disease process in the rat, i.e. whether the disease is active or quiescent, and some of these parameters have also been measured in the human disease situation. Plasma proteins patterns in RA have been established (MINCHIN-CLARKE et al., 1970) and are being used to monitor progress of the disease and drug effectiveness (McCONKEY et al., 1972; McCONKEY et al., 1973; CONSTABLE et al., 1975). The use of objective biochemical measurements of disease activity in human RA, such as those plasma proteins called acute phase proteins, should assist the search for drugs which slow down the disease process. The drugs considered by clinicians as most able to alter and slow RA, e.g. gold, steroids, chloroquine, do in fact produce a fall in the acute phase proteins coincident with the remission of disease (McCONKEY et al., 1972, 1973), whereas the non-steroidal anti-inflammatory drugs of the aspirin type have not as yet been shown to do so.

4. Period of Dosing of Compounds

AA has been used as a screen for anti-inflammatory/anti-arthritic compounds in essentially two ways. Compounds are administered either prophylactically during the first 14–21 days of the development of the disease, or they are given once the disease is established, i.e. from day 14 onwards, for a period of at least 7 days. In clinical practice, the inflammatory arthritic conditions are always present as active ongoing conditions and therefore more closely simulated by the preexisting disease of established rat arthritis. Most investigators, however, use the prophylactic assay, as we do, but invariably ensure that compounds of interest are tested in established rat arthritis. Another advantage of the prophylactic assay is that it is capable of demonstrating not only the activity of anti-inflammatory compounds but also of a number of immunosuppressive drugs (for review, see ROSENTHALE, 1974); immunosuppressive agents are not usually active against the established disease. On balance we prefer the prophylactic assay as it avoids the problem of keeping animals for longer than is essential and as such is probably more humane; it also has the advantage of demonstrating more than one type of drug activity. Certain variations on this general theme, mainly in terms of shortening the period of dosing, have been described from time to time.

A number of investigators, using the foot pad as the route of adjuvant injection, have utilised the swelling in the injected foot occurring at day 3–4 as a measure of acute inflammation for determining drug activity (NEWBOULD, 1963; WARD and CLOUD, 1966; GRAEME et al., 1966). PERPER et al. (1971) used a 12 day dosing schedule, with measurement of the arthritis at day 21, to differentiate between the standard anti-inflammatory compounds, which were not active in such circumstances, and immunosuppressive agents which were. For similar purposes, BROWN et al. (1970) dosed the immunosuppressive agent cyclophosphamide for only the first 5 days of AA; steroidal drugs were not active under such circumstances. A useful variation using only a 4 day dosing period has been described by SWINGLE (1974); the method involves the random distribution of those rats, 14 days after adjuvant injection, with paw volumes between 2–4 ml. Compounds were administered for 4 days and paw volumes and body weights recorded after this period. The known anti-inflammatory agents were active in such circumstances. Interestingly, the Holtzman strain used by SWINGLE (1974) undergoes a natural remission of its disease from about day 21 onwards, as was the case with the hooded strain in Figure 2. The use of alternate day dosing has been described (DI PASQUALE et al., 1975) as a useful means of demonstrating the activity of longer acting anti-inflammatory compounds.

V. Effect of Drugs

AA was originally shown to be responsive to drug treatment by PEARSON and WOOD (1959). Subsequently, NEWBOULD (1963) developed the disease model as a tool in the search for antiarthritic drugs and since then, many groups have demonstrated the effectiveness of a host of agents. Not only are both steroid and nonsteroid anti-inflammatory agents active, but immunosuppressive agents and treatments as diverse as non-specific irritants and highly potent pharmacological agents, such as the prostaglandins, inhibit this experimental model of disease. In fact, a comprehensive account of the treatments which have been reported to be effective in AA would embrace a good proportion of available classes of drug, thus indicating the complexity of this model.

1. Non-Steroid Anti-Inflammatory Drugs

The term 'nonsteroid anti-inflammatory drug' was originally taken to mean drugs of the aspirin, phenylbutazone, indomethacin type, all of which are acidic but may be extended to cover non-acidic molecules (SHEN, 1974).

The very size of the literature reporting activity of such compounds is a tribute to the ingenuity of both chemists and biologists, but it is not our intention to list it here since there is general agreement that 'non-steroid anti-inflammatory drugs' inhibit all phases of AA.

Quantitative determination of potency has, however, presented some problems. WINDER et al. (1969) emphasized the need for strict statistical treatment of data, involving logarithmic conversion of paw volume and body weight for the construction of parallel, linear dose-response lines, but WINTER and NUSS (1966) achieved such lines without conversion of data. In our experience a 'glance in the cage' is all that is needed to detect an active compound but we recognise that more elaborate treatment of data is needed for determination of ED_{50} values and potency ratios.

There are variations between laboratories in ED_{50} values for given compounds. For example, GLENN (1966), using an arthritic score as measure of effectiveness obtained an ED_{50} value of 0.2 mg/kg for indomethacin, given twice daily, whereas the corresponding value in our tests, which measure foot thickness, is 2 mg/kg, once daily—a value similar to that obtained by DI PASQUALE et al. (1975), who measured paw volume. Possible sources of variability are discussed in Section A.II., and WHITEHOUSE and BECK (1974) have pointed out the difficulty of comparing results from different laboratories, in view of the heterogeneity of rat strain, adjuvant mixture, route and timing of dosing used.

Although the mode of action of these non-steroid agents is not fully understood, they are undoubtedly very good inhibitors of AA, and allow the animals to gain weight at a rate comparable to that of normal, non-arthritic rats. The biochemi-

Table 3. Steroids found effective in AA

Drug	Effective dose mg/kg	Route admin.	Reference
Paramethasone	1	Oral	NEWBOULD (1963)
Dexamethasone	1	Oral	
Betamethasone	1	Oral	
Triamcinolone	10	Oral	
Prednisolone	10	Oral	
Cortisone	50	Oral	
Hydrocortisone	2.5–20	S.c.	GLENN (1966)
Prednisolone	4	Oral	WARD and CLOUD (1966)
Dexamethasone	.005–.02	Oral	WINTER and NUSS (1966)
Paramethasone	0.5	Oral	GRAEME et al. (1966)
Cortisone	8.5	S.c.	ROSENTHALE and NAGRA (1967)
Paramethasone	0.5	Oral	PILIERO and COLOMBO (1969)
Cortisone	30	I.p.	BROWN et al. (1971)
Triamcinolone	0.4	I.p.	
Hydrocortisone	10–100	I.p.	CURREY (1971)
Triamcinolone	1	Oral	ROSENTHALE et al. (1972)
Hydrocortisone	2% × 4 daily	Topically or injected foot	WALZ et al. (1971c)

cal changes associated with adjuvant disease are invariably returned to normal or near normal levels by successful treatment with non-steroid anti-inflammatory agents, in contrast with many non-specific inhibitors of the syndrome.

2. Steroid Anti-Inflammatory Drugs

There is general agreement that the clinically effective steroids inhibit all phases of AA including the established disease (Table 3), although they may exacerbate the reduced weight gain of the animals and cause atrophy of lymphoid tissue, the spleen and adrenals (NEWBOULD, 1963; GLENN, 1966; ROSENTHALE and NAGRA, 1967). Cessation of treatment usually results in a rapid reappearance of active disease (NEWBOULD, 1963; WARD and CLOUD, 1966; GRAEME et al., 1966). WALZ et al. (1971 c) found that topical application of 2% hydrocortisone in alcohol, 4 times daily, produced a marked inhibition of the primary lesion, but our own experience would suggest that this effect was a consequence of systemic absorption since similar effects could be obtained by steroids applied to areas of the skin remote from the site of injection.

3. Gold, Chloroquine, and Penicillamine

A small group of compounds has come to be regarded by clinicians as doing more than merely treating the symptoms of RA; this group includes gold, chloroquine, and penicillamine. Consequently, many investigators have looked at the effect of these compounds in AA, albeit with conflicting results.

Gold has been studied on several occasions. NEWBOULD (1963), administering sodium aurothiomalate (25 mg/kg) daily intramuscularly, achieved a 38% inhibition of foot thickness increase 14 days after adjuvant injection, and the spread and severity of the disease were reduced. At doses of 12.5, 25, and 50 mg/kg given on alternative days by subcutaneous administration, JESSOP and CURREY (1968) found sodium aurothiomalate to be without effect against AA, and administration of gold further aggravated the failure to gain weight by the arthritic rats. JESSOP and CURREY (1968) were 'unable to reconcile' their results with those of NEWBOULD (1963).

Later studies by WALZ et al. (1971 d) and SOFIA and DOUGLAS (1973) corroborated the earlier findings of NEWBOULD (1963) and demonstrated that intramuscular sodium aurothiomalate produced a dose dependent inhibition of the 'primary' lesion and secondary polyarthritis during AA; the dose used was between 5 and 10 mg/kg daily. WALZ et al. (1971 d) also demonstrated that the effect on AA was related to the serum gold level achieved.

The studies of SOFIA and DOUGLAS (1973), however, included a comparison of gold therapy with indomethacin, aspirin and hydrocortisone and involved measurements of erythrocyte sedimentation rate (ESR) and albumin/globulin ratios in the experimental evaluation of disease activity. Whereas the effectiveness of therapy with aspirin, indomethacin and hydrocortisone was associated with a decrease in paw volumes and a return towards normal values for ESR and albumin/globulin ratios, that with gold was only seen against paw volume, the ESR and albumin/globulin ratio being unaffected. Further, SOFIA and DOUGLAS (1973) found gold to have little effect against established disease. MCCONKEY et al. (1973) have shown that successful treatment with gold in human rheumatoid patients is associated with a marked fall in both ESR and elevated globulin levels. It would appear therefore that the effect of intramuscular gold in rat AA is difficult to interpret; the dosage is very high compared with the human regime and the effect very rapid in onset. Furthermore, parenteral administration of many materials, especially irritants, produces an inhibition of AA (ATKINSON, 1971); the phenomenon of counterirritation may have influenced the studies with gold.

Such a criticism cannot be made, however, with the studies of WALZ et al. (1972) with SKF 36914, a gold compound which was administered orally. At a daily dose of 5 or 10 mg/kg it produced a significant inhibition of paw swelling at day 3 and also at day 16, and was associated with a body weight gain greater than that of control arthritic animals. The beneficial effect was related to the serum level of gold. No experiments on the effect of this compound on established arthritis were reported and it is still an open question as to whether the effects obtained with gold compounds in AA reflect the beneficial effects seen in human disease. Another noble metal, platinum (as cis-dichlorodiamminoplatinum), inhibits AA, but the doses used (0.75 and 1.0 mg/kg, intraperitoneally) were associated with toxic manifestations (BOWEN and GALE, 1974). A later study of WALZ et al. (1976) demonstrated that SKF 39162 given orally was more effective against adjuvant arthritis than an equivalent intramuscular treatment with gold sodium thiomelate and was less toxic.

Chloroquine produced significant reductions in the paw volume of arthritic rats (WINTER and NUSS, 1966) although the doses used had an adverse effect on body weight. In the main, however, chloroquine and hydroxychloroquine have been found inactive by most workers (NEWBOULD, 1963; WARD and CLOUD, 1966; GRAEME et al., 1966; PÈRRINE and TAKESUE, 1968).

Very little work has been reported on the effect of penicillamine in rat AA. Some recently reported multicentre controlled trials have demonstrated the effectiveness of

D-penicillamine in the clinic (MULTICENTRE TRIAL GROUP, 1973; DIXON et al., 1975), but KLAMER et al. (1968) and LIYANAGE and CURREY (1972) were unable to show an effect against AA, even at a daily dose of 200 mg/kg. The effective human dose is rarely above 1.2 g daily and it is claimed that much lower doses are effective (DIXON et al., 1975). Interestingly, an effect has been reported in pyridoxine deficient rats but the relevance is not clear (BAUMGARTNER et al., 1974 b).

In conclusion, the effects obtained with gold, chloroquine and penicillamine have not been dramatic, and some doubt exists as to the relevance and specificity of such effects considering the dosages used and the poor gain in weight so often encountered.

4. Immunosuppressant Drugs

The effect of immunosuppression on AA has been reviewed by ROSENTHALE (1974) (see also Chapter 35). In general, cytotoxic-immunosuppressant drugs exert their main effect on the development of secondary lesions and are less effective on the primary inflammation or on the established disease (WARD et al., 1964; KALLIOMÄKI et al., 1964; NEWBOULD, 1965; GRAEME et al., 1966; PILLIERO et al., 1966; GLENN, 1966 and many others). ROSENTHALE and NAGRA (1967), however, found that 6-mercaptopurine inhibited the primary lesion, and BROWN et al. (1970) showed cyclophosphamide to be similarly active, suggesting that both of these drugs show anti-inflammatory properties in addition to their immunosuppressant effect.

Immunosuppressive activity can be differentiated from anti-inflammatory effects, the former being characterized by (1) frequent failure to inhibit the primary swelling, (2) effective when given only during the first 5 days, (3) lack of effect on established disease and (4) an aggravation of weight loss (NEWBOULD, 1965; BROWN et al., 1971; ROSENTHALE et al., 1969, 1972; PERPER et al., 1971; ROSENTHALE, 1974).

5. Antilymphocytic Serum, Antigens

a) Antilymphocytic Serum

The effect of antilymphocytic serum (ALS) on AA has been studied (CURREY and ZIFF, 1966, 1968; JASIN and ZIFF, 1970; POSSANZA and STEWART, 1970; CURREY, 1971) and, as with other immunosuppressant agents, there is some question as to whether ALS exerts its inhibitory effect on AA entirely by an immunosuppressant action or whether it also has a direct anti-inflammatory effect.

Administration of ALS or the purified globulin fraction (CURREY and ZIFF, 1968) throughout the development of the arthritis produced a profound inhibition of the arthritis without any evidence of a 'rebound' phenomenon when treatment was stopped. As with the cytotoxic-immunosuppressant drugs, treatment with ALS for only the first few days of AA, up to day 4 (CURREY and ZIFF, 1968; JASIN and ZIFF, 1970), prevented the development of the arthritis, demonstrating an immunosuppressant activity of the ALS. The exact nature of the immunosuppression is not clear.

CURREY and ZIFF (1968) concluded from their study that antilymphocytic globulin (ALG) prevented the initial sensitization of the lymphocytes to the arthritogenic antigen in M. tuberculosis. DENMAN (1969) questioned this conclusion by indicating that the skin reaction to tuberculoprotein in the arthritic rats of CURREY and ZIFF (1968) was not suppressed. A later study (CURREY, 1971), however, did demonstrate a reduction of tuberculoprotein sensitivity in arthritic rats. Since a limited administration (day −1 to 4) of ALS prevented the development of AA, it is possible to conclude that the lymphocyte is heavily involved in the early induction phase of the arthritis.

ALS also inhibits the primary lesion of AA (POSSANZA and STEWART, 1970; JASIN and ZIFF, 1970; CURREY, 1971). In addition, CURREY and ZIFF (1968) showed that ALG administered in the later, established stages of the disease produced a fall in the severity of the arthritis. This was confirmed (JASIN and ZIFF, 1970) by the demonstration of an inhibition of foot swelling when ALG was administered during the established disease. The general conclusion was that these effects demonstrated an anti-inflammatory action of the ALS or ALG. Indeed the anti-inflammatory properties of ALS have often been described (STEVENS and WILLOUGHBY, 1969; WILLOUGHBY et al., 1969; PERPER et al., 1969; POSSANZA and STEWART, 1970). The precise manner in which ALS exerts its anti-inflammatory effect is not known. BILLINGHAM et al. (1970) demonstrated that both the IgG fraction of ALS and an alphaglobulin fraction, containing an anti-inflammatory, acute phase protein (BILLINGHAM et al., 1971) markedly inhibited carrageenin-induced oedema. The observation of depression of complement levels during acute inflammation following administration of ALS (WILLOUGHBY et al., 1969) is quite relevant, and perhaps the activation of some 'counterirritant' mechanism may also be involved in the anti-inflammatory activity of ALS (see Chapter 15).

b) Antigens

Prior injection of immunologically immature rats with mycobacteria (WAKSMAN et al., 1960) or wax D (WOOD and PEARSON, 1962; BONHOMME et al., 1968) induces tolerance to the induction of arthritis, as does subcutaneous or intraperitoneal injection of adult animals with mycobacteria in oil or saline (CURREY, 1970; COZINE et al., 1972; FLAX and WAKSMAN, 1963; GERY and WAKSMAN, 1967). FLAX and WAKSMAN (1963) also showed that prior injection of *N. asteroides* in oil induced tolerance to both nocardia and mycobacteria. Attempts to transfer tolerance by means of immune sera have given conflicting results: FLAX and WAKSMAN (1963) and GERY and WAKSMAN (1967) were unable to do so, but successful transfer was claimed by PERPER and ORONSKY (1972). Induction of arthritis can be prevented by prior injection of other bacteria which themselves are non-arthritogenic (PEARSON and WOOD, 1962; WOOD and PEARSON, 1962).

The incorporation of a second non-bacterial antigen into the adjuvant mixture also inhibits the development of AA (FLAX and WAKSMAN, 1963; ISAKOVIC and WAKSMAN, 1965; PEARSON and WOOD, 1969). A number of antigens do this, including bovine serum albumin, hen egg albumin, bovine γ-globulin, rat γ-globulin and rat serum albumin; the degree of inhibition appears to be dependent on the amount of the second antigen (PEARSON and WOOD, 1969). Prior injection of such second antigens in saline, or simultaneously at a site remote to the adjuvant site, did not inhibit the development of the arthritis (PEARSON and WOOD, 1964); this is in contrast to the effect of mycobacteria.

The mechanism of this inhibition of adjuvant disease is unclear but it has been suggested that prior inoculation of mycobacteria induces specific tolerance (GERY and WAKSMAN, 1967), whereas that seen with a second antigen is due to antigenic competition (ISAKOVIC and WAKSMAN, 1965; GERY and WAKSMAN, 1967). An alternative suggestion (PEARSON and WOOD, 1969) is that a combination between the protein antigen and the mycobacteria occurs in vitro during mixing, thereby nullifying its arthritogenicity.

6. Non-Specific Inhibition

A number of drugs, compounds, treatments and bizarre phenomena have been reported to inhibit AA. These have been placed in a 'non-specific' category since in many instances either the mode of action is unknown or the relevance not clearly understood. It is convenient simply to list these in the form of a table and to comment afterwards on the implications. Table 4 is not exhaustive but is intended to give an impression of the diversity of 'treatments' which have been stated to influence AA.

Table 4. Miscellany of non = specific factors which influence AA

Treatment	Effect on AA	Reference
Bee venom	Inhibition	ZURIER et al. (1973a)
Peptide 401 (from bee venom)	Inhibition	BILLINGHAM et al. (1973)
Hepatic injury	Inhibition	PINALS (1973)
Antispermatic agent (U 29409)	Inhibition	GLENN et al. (1971)
Prostaglandins E_1, E_2	Inhibition	GLENN and ROHLOFF (1972)
		ASPINALL and CAMMARATA (1969)
		ZURIER and QUAGLIATA (1971)
		ZURIER and BALLAS (1973)
		ZURIER et al. (1973b)
Antipsoriatic agents	Inhibition	WALZ and BERKOFF (1970)
Irritants, Mustard, dextran	Inhibition	ATKINSON (1971)
Yeast, α-chymotrypsin, Formol saline		
Chlorpromazine	Inactive	GLENN (1966)
	Aggravation	GRAEME et al. (1966)
	Inhibition	WALZ et al. (1971b)
Antihistamines – adrenaline combination	Inhibition	BARBIERI et al. (1973)
Dried mussel extract	Inhibition	CULLEN et al. (1975)
Alloxan diabetes	Inhibition	BEST and SPENCER (1968)
		KELLETT (1965)
Salmon calcitonin	Inhibition	BOBALIK et al. (1974)
Neurological deficiency and trauma	Inhibition	COURTRIGHT and KUZELL (1965)
Phytohaemaglutinin	Inhibition	DELBARRE et al. (1968)
Human plasma fraction	Inhibition	ELLIOTT et al. (1974)
Histidine decarboxylase inhibition (hypostamine)	Inhibition	PELCZARSKA (1969)
Somatotrophic hormone, insulin	Inhibition	ROSZKOWSKI-SLIZ (1973)
Cysteine	Inhibition	RYSEWSKI (1966)
Thyroidectomy	Inhibition	STEINETZ et al. (1970)
Oestrogen	Inhibition	TOIVANEN et al. (1967)
Epsilon aminocaproic acid	Inhibition	TOIVANEN and TOIVANEN (1964)
Histamine and Sinomenine (histamine releaser)	Inhibition	SAEKI et al. (1967)

The number of non-specific inhibitors of AA appears quite extensive. However, WALZ et al. (1971b) concluded that AA had a greater pharmacological specificity than acute anti-inflammatory assays even though certain examples of CNS stimulants, diuretics, nephrotoxic agents, tranquilisers and antidepressants inhibited the secondary lesions of the disease. GLENN and GRAY (1965) had reported earlier that non-specific stress reduced the incidence and severity of AA.

Interestingly, both WALZ et al. (1971b) and GLENN and ROHLOFF (1972) demonstrated that non-specific inhibition of AA, in terms of increase in paw volume and secondary lesion development, was not correlated in their studies with an effect on biochemical parameters such as 'inflammation units' and serum lysozyme. The importance of a biochemical, second assessment in such circumstances is easily seen since specific anti-inflammatory agents invariably reduced both the inflammation and the biochemical changes associated with AA.

Before leaving this aspect, however, the relevance of the influence of 'counterirritant' phenomena in both acute and chronic inflammation is often overlooked, and perhaps is an area which deserves a deeper investigation and understanding than it is presently accorded (see chapter 15). The inhibition of AA with prostaglandins obtained by ZURIER and QUAGLIATA (1971) is almost identical to our experience with peptide 401 (BILLINGHAM et al., 1973) in both effectiveness and side effects. In fact, many of the diverse treatments listed in Table 4 may have a common final pathway and some effort directed towards its understanding may well be worthwhile.

7. The Effect of Adjuvant Arthritis on Drugs

AA causes profound changes in a number of biochemical systems (Table 2). One of the major changes is the alteration of the pattern of plasma protein synthesis by the liver, resulting in a pronounced fall in albumin levels and rise in plasma glycoprotein (Fig. 2) especially at the height of secondary lesion development. Recently, the changes in the plasma concentration of several proteins was correlated with changes in the synthetic rate by the liver (BILLINGHAM and GORDON, 1976a, 1976b); evidently the liver exercises considerable control over the plasma concentration of the individual proteins.

One consequence of the fall in albumin which has been discussed by PAULUS and WHITEHOUSE (1973) is the reduction in available binding sites for highly albumin bound drugs, such as the non-steroid anti-inflammatory agents. The amount of free, unbound drug species is much increased in such circumstances and since it is this species of drug which is generally regarded as the active, and no doubt toxic form of a drug (BRODIE, 1965), an assay based on established arthritis, when albumin concentrations are generally below 40–50% of their normal level, may show an optimistic level of activity of a compound. In such circumstances, a compound may also appear more toxic than in healthy rats with normal albumin levels.

A second problem which has been highlighted is the considerable reduction in drug metabolising capacity by the liver of animals with AA (QUEVAUVILLER et al., 1968; MORTON and CHATFIELD, 1970; BECK and WHITEHOUSE, 1973, 1974; WHITEHOUSE, 1973; DI PASQUALE et al., 1974; BAUMGARTNER et al., 1974a; CAWTHORNE et al., 1976), although this appears to be a general problem with severe inflammatory stress and not restricted to arthritic conditions (BECK and WHITEHOUSE, 1974). The action of barbiturates in rats with AA is considerably prolonged; at the height of the arthritis, days 14–20, sleeping times induced by hexobarbital (WHITEHOUSE, 1973) and pentabarbitone (DI PASQUALE et al., 1974) are many times that seen in control rats. MORTON and CHATFIELD (1970) showed that the levels of cytochrome P450 in the rat liver microsomes, at day 15 of the arthritis, were only 16% of the normal healthy control levels. At this time, N-demethylase activity was reduced to 7% and NADPH$_2$-oxidase activity to 43% of control levels. Phenobarbitone, which normally induces microsomal enzyme formation in the livers of healthy rats was unable to reverse the fall in metabolising capacity seen at day 15 of AA (MORTON and CHATFIELD, 1970), although BECK and WHITEHOUSE (1973) concluded from their study that phenobarbitone could reverse the fall in metabolising activity. A difference in the severity of the arthritis in the different strains of rat used may account for the discrepancy in these findings.

It is obvious from the above that AA has a very profound effect on the liver both in terms of the change in plasma protein synthesis pattern and metabolising enzyme activity. The synthesis of albumin may fall to as little as one-fifth of its normal rate, to be replaced largely by the synthesis of a variety of plasma glycoproteins (BILLINGHAM and GORDON, 1976a). Drug metabolising activity can be very severely reduced with unpredictable consequences. As BECK and WHITEHOUSE (1973) pointed out, drugs may be overrated by virtue of being 'undermetabolised;' conversely, drugs which need to be metabolised in vivo to generate an active metabolite may be underrated in circumstances where the metabolising capacity is severely embarrassed.

The relationship between the altered pattern of plasma protein synthesis and the fall in metabolising activity (and presumably the levels of metabolising enzymes) is unclear. It appears that the level of albumin falls in order to allow the rise of the acute phase proteins (KOJ, 1975; BILLINGHAM and GORDON 1976a, 1976b), the acute phase reaction being a part of the body defence mechanisms. Perhaps the fall in metabolising enzymes is also a consequence of the commitment of the liver to produce acute phase proteins at times of severe inflammatory stress.

D. Arthritis Produced by Intra-Articular Injection of Antigens and Antibodies

It is widely accepted that immune mechanisms play an important role in RA and many attempts have been made to induce chronic arthritis by injection of a variety of antigens into the joints of animals. One of the most successful of these is that described by DUMONDE and GLYNN (1962) who produced a chronic arthritis by injection of fibrin into the joints of rabbits previously immunized by intradermal injection of fibrin in Freund's complete adjuvant. Other antigens apart from fibrin may be used including egg albumin (CONSDEN et al., 1971), bovine serum albumin (COOKE et al., 1972) and autologous inflammatory exudates (PHILLIPS et al., 1966). An analogous model in the guinea pig was described by LOEWI (1968, 1969), and in a series of papers (BRACKERTZ et al., 1977a, 1977b, 1977c) the development of the model in the mouse is fully described. The histological features of the arthritis bore many resemblances to human arthritis (GLYNN, 1968) and unlike many other models a single intra-articular injection was sufficient to produce an arthritis lasting for over a year. It is probable that the long-lasting nature of the arthritis reflects prolonged persistence of antigen (CONSDEN et al., 1971; WEBB et al., 1971; MENARD and DION, 1976). COOKE et al. (1972) identified antigen (bovine serum albumin) on the surface of collagenous tissue from arthritic joints and suggested that the antigen was present in the form of an immune complex since they were also able to show the presence of rabbit Ig and C3. Fox and GLYNN (1975) however concluded that the persistence of antigen may not fully explain the chronicity of allergic rabbit arthritis since persistent antigen could also be found after intra-articular injection in joints which showed no inflammatory symptoms; other factors are also necessary. Evidence that a delayed hypersensitivity response is more important than humoral immunity was presented by GOLDBERG et al. (1974) who used autologous and homologous rabbit IgG as antigen. Delayed-type skin reactions were produced by intradermal injection of antigen into arthritic animals and leucocyte migration in vitro was inhibited by antigen. The arthritis did not correlate with circulating antibody levels: treatment with ALS inhibited the arthritis, delayed skin reactions and leucocyte migration inhibition and was associated with increasing antibody titre. Conversely, cyclophosphamide prevented the production of circulating antibody but had no effect on the arthritis, delayed skin reactions or leucocyte migration. The mouse arthritis described by BRACKERTZ et al. (1977a, 1977b, 1977c) has also been shown to be T-cell dependent and can be transferred by lymphoid cells and interestingly, also by serum though to a much lesser extent.

Only a few detailed studies of the effect of anti-inflammatory compounds on this chronic arthritis have been published. In the experiments described by DAVIS (1971), prednisolone (1 mg/kg daily orally) was given to rabbits rendered arthritic by intra-articular injection of ovalbumin after prior sensitization with this antigen in Freund's complete adjuvant. The joint diameters were measured at intervals and a biphasic response was noticed in control animals not given prednisolone, the first peak swelling appearing on the 3rd to 7th day and a secondary swelling starting on day 70 and reaching a maximum on about day 160. Treatment with prednisolone from day 0 suppressed both swellings but histological examination revealed that protection was only partial and the rate of damage and destruction increased when dosing was stopped. Prednisolone had little effect on the arthritis when dosing was started on days 51 or 101. In the other study, BLACKHAM et al. (1974) treated arthritic rabbits with indomethacin at a dose of 7.5 mg/kg, orally, the first dose being given 1 h before intra-articular injection of antigen and then twice daily. The size of the knee joints were measured with calipers and the skin temperature recorded. At intervals varying from 6 h to 46 days, groups of animals were killed and the synovial fluid collected. Total and differential cell counts were made, and the free and bound acid phosphatase content of the cells determined. The fluids were also assayed for prostaglandins, which were found (mainly as PGE_1) only at 19 h. Although indomethacin treatment prevented this early rise in prostaglandin content of the synovial fluid and reduced the rise in body and articular temperature, it had no effect on the number of leucocytes in the challenged joints, the free acid phosphatase level or the histopathological changes. The coincident appearance of peak levels of free acid phosphatase activity, the large increase in polymorphonuclear cell content and the maximum joint swelling at 47 h suggested that lysosomal enzymes derived from polymorphonuclear cells are important mediators of this inflammation.

D(-) penicillamine, which is known to affect human rheumatoid arthritis, has now been shown to diminish antigen-induced arthritis in the rabbit as assessed by both measurement of joint circumference and histological examination (HUNNEYBALL et al., 1977). The study involved treatment with penicillamine at the equivalent human dosage, but very few animals were involved in the study and confirmation is needed of these interesting preliminary observations.

In addition to this truly chronic model, there are reports describing the production of acute synovitis in rabbits following intra-articular injection of antigen antibody complexes (RAWSON and TORRALBA, 1967) or lymphokine (ANDREIS et al., 1974), and of a reversed passive Arthus reaction resulting from the injection of antibody into the joint of animals previously injected intravenously with antigen (DE SHAZO et al., 1972), but none appears to be entirely suitable for drug studies.

Finally, TRENTHAM et al. (1977) have recently described a model in the rat produced by immunising with type II (cartilage) collagen from the rat, chick or human. Types I and III collagen, from skin and parenchyma, were incapable of inducing the arthritis. Most interestingly the arthritis was induced by injection of type II collagen in either complete or incomplete Freund's adjuvant; very few models of antigen-induced arthritis avoid the use of the mycobacterial component of Freund's. The arthritis produced resembles adjuvant arthritis but there may be subtle differences which could be utilised for screening purposes; this however remains to be determined.

E. Arthritis Produced by Intra-Articular Injection of Lysosome Labilisers

WEISSMAN et al. (1965) have studied the effect of injecting streptolysin S into the knee joints of rabbits. Streptolysin S is water soluble and non-antigenic—and, at least in vitro, disrupts lysosomes at concentrations well below those required to affect other organelles such as mitochondria. Within 4 to 6 h after the injection of 65 µg of streptolysin S into the knee joint, the joint was swollen and erythematous. The arthritis became severe after 18–20 h and a cloudy synovial exudate could be removed. By 72 h the joint had returned to normal but further injections of streptolysin S led to a chronic, apparently self-perpetuating, arthritis. WEISSMAN et al. (1967) compared the ability of a series of polyene antibiotics to lyse lysosomal membrane in vitro with their capacity to induce joint damage when injected into the joints of rabbits—the activities paralleled one another. COOK and FINCHAM (1966) have repeated and extended the experiments of WEISSMAN and his group. They injected streptolysin S into the knee joints of goats and rabbits at weekly intervals, different groups receiving 2, 6, or 9 injections. The rabbits which received the longer courses of injections developed joint swellings which did not subside between the later injections. The histological changes consisted of synovial proliferation and dense infiltration of the synovium with lymphocytes and plasma cells, increased vascularity, deposition of fibrin and, in most animals, pannus formation with erosion of articular cartilage. Similar changes were observed in goats. WEISSMANN et al. (1965) found that the serum from streptolysin-treated rabbits contained a complement-fixing antibody directed against lysosomes obtained from homologous liver homogenation. COOK and FINCHAM (1966), using a purer preparation of lysosomes, were unable to detect such antibody.

It is noteworthy that COOK and FINCHAM (1966) reported that the remaining cartilage matrix did not lose its metachromasia and that fibrin was present in the tissues. It is therefore difficult to account for the pathological changes in terms of a simple lysosomal hypothesis since, if the changes were due solely to lysosomal enzymes, it might be anticipated that a loss of metachromasia would have occurred and fibrin would have been absent.

PAGE THOMAS (1969) prepared liver lysosomal extract from one rabbit of a litter and injected it into the knee joint of a litter mate. Changes at 7 days included a proliferative synovitis in the injected joint and at 2 weeks synovial proliferation, focal round cell accumulation and marked plasma cell infiltration. Surprisingly, identical changes of comparable severity appeared in the uninjected contralateral knee joint. The same author has also produced arthritis by injection of a variety of materials, including diazo dyes, polysaccharides, polystyrene and diamond dust.

F. Arthritis Induced by Infectious Agents

There are a large number of reports in the literature of arthritis produced in animals by infectious agents (for review, see GARDNER, 1960). Recent publications, which merit further attention, include: arthritis caused by a type of *Diplococcus agalactiae* (SVARTZ, 1972); *Mycoplasma arthritidis* (DELBARRE et al., 1964a, 1964b; COLE et al., 1971; HANNAN and HUGHES, 1971); *Mycoplasma pulmonis* (BARDEN and TULLY, 1969; HARWICK et al., 1973) Salmonella enteritidis (VOLKMAN and COLLINS, 1976); cell walls from several bacteria and two Streptomyces species (KOGA et al., 1973); substances derived from RA synovial tissue (WARREN et al., 1972); a cell-free extract of group A streptococci (STEIN et al., 1973); herpes simplex virus (WEBB et al., 1972, 1973); streptoccal L forms (COOK et al., 1969).

G. Conclusions

The models of experimental arthritis currently available, when considered from the viewpoint of the 'drug hunter', can be grouped under three headings (1) adjuvant disease in the rat, (2) chronic monoarticular arthritis induced by intra-articular injection of antigens, and (3) arthritides caused by infectious agents.

From two aspects, adjuvant disease stands alone: it is restricted to the rat and it is the only model that has been used extensively for screening purposes as can be easily judged from the bias in the content of this chapter. There is little doubt that it is a useful model for the detection of certain kinds of drug activity, but its real value as a model of RA remains to be justified. Although it detects compounds active against acute inflammation and also immunosuppressive agents, there are simpler models available for both purposes. In common with other models of inflammation, it is liable to demonstrate spurious activity, especially with irritant compounds administered intraperitoneally. Also in common with other models, it does not appear to detect the activity of those drugs (like penicillamine, gold salts and chloroquine) which seem to affect the human arthritic process fundamentally. In spite of these drawbacks, it will no doubt continue to be useful, if only because it is the only currently available model of inflammation (of immune origin) exhibiting a degree of chronicity, the progress of which can be serially monitored by simple measurements without sacrifice of the animal.

Antigen-induced chronic arthritis, as exemplified by the model of DUMONDE and GLYNN (1962), closely mirrors several aspects of RA but its major drawback is that the only reliable methods of assessment appear to be based on histological examination after sacrifice of the animal and such a procedure is unsuitable for large-scale drug screening. The large-scale use of the rabbit, frequently employed for this model, is also generally impractical. The recent demonstration however that antigen-induced arthritis can be produced in the mouse may enable a screening test to be developed.

Similarly, arthritis caused by infectious agents may represent a closer approximation of the human disease than does adjuvant disease, but there is very little information available on the effect of drug treatment and again assessment of the disease activity is difficult.

It is pertinent to ask the question 'what type of drug do we need?' There are large numbers of steroid and 'conventional' non-steroid anti-inflammatory drugs available, and doubtless others in various stages of development. As we stated in our opening remarks to this chapter, a major target is a drug which slows down or halts the progress of RA, and it is possible that the commonly used parameters, such as foot volume or joint size, do not fully represent the disease that we really want to treat.

Several groups of workers are now emphasizing the importance of the biochemical changes which accompany chronic tissue damage and some promise might be found in this direction. Even in this respect, however, there are problems, for although successful treatment of adjuvant disease with non-steroidal anti-inflammatory agents can be seen as an improvement both in clinical signs and symptoms and a return to near normal of the many altered biochemical parameters (ESR, plasma protein changes, serum lysozyme, etc.), a similar effect has not been demonstrated for these agents in man. In contrast, the few drugs, such as gold and penicillamine, thought to affect fundamentally the disease in man do produce a clinical benefit accompanied by a reversal of a number of the associated biochemical changes: this beneficial effect has not as yet been unequivocally demonstrated in experimental models of arthritis. All the currently available models used for screening anti-arthritic agents may thus lack an element of chronicity which is necessary for detection of the activity of those drugs whose onset of action in man is slow; more effort to find a suitable model for detecting these drugs would undoubtedly be worthwhile.

It is our opinion that *no* really suitable model for screening compounds for anti-arthritic activity is available at present and this challenge to the biologist remains. So far he appears to have been rather conservative and perhaps it would be better to reexamine Cinderella's foot in order to design a shoe which will fit perfectly, than to be continually trying on shoes that fit only part of the foot.

References

Akamatsu,Y., Nishizawa,H., Watanabe,S., Kumagai,A.: Adjuvant induced polyarthritis in rats—its histogenesis. Acta path. jap. **16**, 131—140 (1966)

Anderson,A.J.: Lysosomal enzyme activity in rats with adjuvant-induced arthritis. Ann. rheum. Dis. **29**, 307—313 (1970)

Andreis,M., Stastny,P., Ziff,M.: Experimental arthritis produced by injection of mediators of delayed hypersensitivity. Arthr. Rheum. **17**, 537—551 (1974)

Aspinall, R. L., Cammarata, P. S.: Effect of prostaglandin E_2 on adjuvant arthritis. Nature (Lond.) **224**, 1320—1321 (1969)

Atkinson, D. C.: A comparison of the systemic anti-inflammatory activity of three different irritants in the rats. Arch. int. Pharmacodyn. **193**, 391—396 (1971)

Azuma, I., Kanetsuna, F., Kada, Y., Takashima, T., Yamamura, Y.: Adjuvant-polyarthritogenicity of cell walls of mycobacteria, nocardia and corynebacteria. Jap. J. Microbiol. **16**, 333—336 (1972)

Barbieri, E. J., Rossi, G. V., Orzechowski, R. F.: Effects of antihistamine-epinephrine combinations on adjuvant arthritis in rats. J. pharm. Sci. **62**, 648—651 (1973)

Barden, J. A., Tully, J. G.: Experimental arthritis in mice with mycoplasma pulmonis. J. Bact. **100**, 5—10 (1969)

Barron, D. I., Copley, A. R., Vallance, D. K.: Anti-inflammatory and related properties of 4-(p-biphenylyl)-3 hydroxybutyric acid. Brit. J. Pharmacol. **33**, 396—407 (1968)

Baumgartner, W. A., Beck, F. W. J., Lorber, A., Pearson, C. M., Whitehouse, M. W.: Adjuvant disease in rats: biochemical criteria for distinguishing several phases of inflammation and arthritis. Proc. Soc. exp. Biol. (N.Y.) **145**, 625—630 (1974 a)

Baumgartner, R., Obenaus, H., Stoerk, H. C.: Suppression of adjuvant arthritis by penicillamine in pyridoxine deficient rats. Proc. Soc. exp. Biol. (N.Y.) **146**, 241—244 (1974 b)

Beck, F. J., Whitehouse, M. W.: Effect of adjuvant disease in rats on cyclophosphamide and isophosphamide metabolism. Biochem. Pharmacol. **22**, 2453—2468 (1973)

Beck, F. J., Whitehouse, M. W.: Impaired drug metabolism in rats associated with acute inflammation: a possible assay for anti-injury agents. Proc. Soc. exp. Biol. (N.Y.) **145**, 135—140 (1974)

Berry, H., Willoughby, D. A., Giroud, J. P.: Evidence for an endogenous antigen in the arthritic rat. J. Path. **111**, 229—238 (1973)

Best, R., Spencer, P. S.: The effect of alloxan diabetes upon adjuvant induced arthritis in the rat. J. Pharm. (Lond.) **20** Suppl., 1265—1295 (1968)

Bhargava, A. S.: Effect of anti-inflammatory agents on adjuvant-induced edema modified for primary test. Pharmacol. Res. Commun. **3**, 83—91 (1971)

Billingham, M. E. J., Gordon, A. H.: Changes in concentration and synthesis rates of plasma proteins during experimental arthritis. In: Peeters, H. (Ed.): Protides of the Biological Fluids, Vol. XXIII. Amsterdam: Elsevier 1976 a (in press)

Billingham, M. E. J., Gordon, A. H.: The role of the acute phase reaction in inflammation. In: Giroud, J. P., Willoughby, D. A., Velo, G. P. (Eds.): Future Trends in Inflammation, Vol. II. Basel: Birkhäuser Verlag 1976 b (in press)

Billingham, M. E. J., Gordon, A. H., Robinson, B. V.: Role of the liver in inflammation. Nature (New Biol.) **231**, 26—27 (1971)

Billingham, M. E. J., Morley, J., Hanson, J. M., Shipolini, R. A., Vernon, C. M.: An anti-inflammatory peptide from bee-venom. Nature (Lond.) **245**, 163—164 (1973)

Billingham, M. E. J., Robinson, B. V., Gaugas, J. M.: Two anti-inflammatory components in anti-lymphocytic serum. Nature (Lond.) **227**, 276—277 (1970)

Blackham, A., Burns, J. W., Farmer, J. B., Radziwonik, H., Westwick, J.: An X-ray analysis of adjuvant arthritis in the rat. The effect of prednisolone and indomethacin. Agents Actions **7**, 145—151 (1977)

Blackham, A., Farmer, J. B., Radziwonik H., Westwick, J.: The role of prostaglandins in rabbit monoarticular arthritis. Brit. J. Pharmacol. **51**, 35—44 (1974)

Bobalik, G. R., Aldred, J. P., Kleszynski, R. R., Stubbs, R. K., Zeedyk, R. A., Bastian, J. W.: Effects of salmon calcitonin and combination drug therapy on rat adjuvant arthritis. Agents Actions **4**, 364—369 (1974)

Bogden, A. E., Glenn, E. M., Koslowske, T., Rigiero, C. S.: α-2-GP response in adjuvant-induced polyarthritis: an immunoassay for anti-inflammatory activity. Life Sci. Part 1 **6**, 965—973 (1967)

Bonhomme, F., Boucheron, C., Migliore, D., Jolles, P.: Arthritogenicity and protective effect against adjuvant arthritis of wax DS fractions (glycolipids without a nitrogen-containing moiety) of *Mycobaterium tuberculosis var. hominis and bovis.* Experientia (Basel) **24**, 716—717 (1968)

Bowen, J. R., Gale, G. R.: CIS-Dichlorodiamminoplatinum (II) suppression of adjuvant-induced arthritis in rats. Agents Actions **4**, 108—112 (1974)

Brackertz, D., Mitchell, G. F., Mackay, I. R.: Antigen-induced arthritis in mice. 1. Induction of arthritis in various strains of mice. Arthritis Rheum. **20**, 841—850 (1977a)

Brackertz, D., Mitchell, G. F., Vadas, M. A., Mackay, I. R., Miller, J. F. A. P.: Studies on antigen-induced arthritis in mice. II. Immunologic correlates of arthritis susceptibility in mice. J. Immunol. **118**, 1639—1644 (1977b)

Brackertz, D., Mitchell, G. F., Vadas, M. A., Mackay, I. R.: Studies on antigen-induced arthritis in mice. III. Cell and serum transfer experiments. J. Immunol. **118**, 1645—1648 (1977c)

Brodie, B. B.: Displacement of one drug by another from carrier or receptor sites. Proc. roy. Soc. Med. **58**, 946—955 (1965)

Brown, J. H., Schwartz, N. L., MacKey, H. K., Murray, H. L.: Prophylactic effects of cyclophosphamide in adjuvant-induced arthritis. Arch. int. Pharmacodyn. **183**, 1—11 (1970)

Brown, J. H., Taylor, J. L., Pollock, S. H.: Effect of duration of administration of cyclophosphamide and steroidal anti-inflammatory drugs on the severity of polyarthritis. Arch. int. Pharmacodyn. **194**, 381—386 (1971)

Burstein, N. A., Waksman, B. H.: The pathogenesis of adjuvant disease in the rat. I. A histological study of early lesions in the joints and skin. Yale J. Biol. Med. **37**, 177—194 (1964)

Butler, M., Giannina, T., Cargill, D. I., Popick, F., Steinetz, B. G.: Abnormal sulfhydryl-disulfide interchange in serum of rats with adjuvant arthritis: correction by anti-inflammatory agents. Proc. Soc. exp. Biol. (N.Y.) **132**, 484—488 (1969)

Cawthorne, M. A., Palmer, E. D., Green, J.: Adjuvant-induced arthritis and drug-metabolising enzymes. Biochem. Pharmacol. **25**, 2683—2688 (1976)

Cole, B. C., Golightly-Rowland, L., Ward, J. R.: Arthritis of mice induced by Mycoplasma arthritidis. Humoral antibody and lymphocyte responses of CBA mice. Ann. Rheum. Dis. **35**, 14—22 (1976)

Cole, B. C., Ward, J. R., Jones, R. S., Cahill, J. F.: Chronic proliferative arthritis of mice induced by mycoplasma arthritidis, I. Induction of disease and histopathological characteristics. Infect. Immun. **4**, 344—355 (1971)

Cook, J., Fincham, W. J.: Arthritis produced by intra-articular injections of Streptolysin S in rabbits. J. Path. Bact. **92**, 461—470 (1966)

Cook, J., Fincham, W. J., Lack, C. H.: Chronic arthritis produced by Streptococcal L-Forms. J. Path. Bact. **99**, 283—297 (1969)

Cooke, T. D., Hurd, E. R., Ziff, M., Jasin, H. E.: The pathogenesis of chronic inflammation in experimental antigen-induced arthritis. II. Preferential localization of antigen-antibody complexes to collagenous tissues. J. exp. Med. **135**, 323—338 (1972)

Consden, R., Doble, A., Glynn, L. E., Nind, A. P.: Production of a chronic arthritis with ovalbumin. Its retention in the rabbit knee joint. Ann. rheum. Dis. **30**, 307—315 (1971)

Constable, T. J., Crockson, R. A., Crockson, A. P., McConkey, B.: Drug treatment of rheumatoid arthritis: a systematic approach. Lancet **1975 II**, 1176—1179

Courtright, L. J., Kuzell, W. C.: Sparing effect of neurological deficit and trauma on the course of adjuvant arthritis in the rat. Ann. rheum. Dis. **24**, 360—368 (1965)

Cozine, W. S., Stanfield, A. B., Stephens, C. A. L., Mazur, M. T.: Adjuvant disease. The paradox of prevention and induction with complete Freund's adjuvant. Proc. Soc. exp. Biol. (N.Y.) **141**, 911—914 (1972)

Cullen, J. C., Flint, M. H., Leider, J.: The effect of dried mussel extract on an induced polyarthritis in rats. N. Z. med. J. **81**, 260—261 (1975)

Currey, H. L. F.: Adjuvant arthritis in the rat: effect of intraperitoneal injections of either whole dead mycobacteria or tuberculin. Ann. rheum. Dis. **29**, 314—320 (1970)

Currey, H. L. F.: A comparison of immunosuppressive and anti-inflammatory agents in the rat. Clin. exp. Immunol. **9**, 879—887 (1971)

Currey, H. L. F., Ziff, M.: Suppression of experimentally induced polyarthritis in the rat by heterologous anti-lymphocyte serum. Lancet **1966 II**, 889—891

Currey, H. L. F., Ziff, M.: Suppression of adjuvant disease in the rat by heterologous anti-lymphocyte globulin. J. exp. Med. **127**, 185—203 (1968)

Davies, G. E.: Immunosuppressive activity of 3-acetyl-5-(4-fluorobenzylidene)-4-hydroxy-2-oxo-2:5-dihydrothiophen (I.C.I. 47,776). Immunology **14**, 393—399 (1968)

Davies, G. E., Evans, D. P., Horsfall, G. B.: An automatic device for the measurement of oedema in the feet of rats and guinea pigs. Med. biol. Engng. **9**, 567—570 (1971)

Davis, B.: Effects of prednisolone in an experimental model of arthritis in the rabbit. Ann. rheum. Dis. **30**, 509—520 (1971)

Delbarre, F., Brouilhet, H., Kahan, A.: Atténuation de la polyarthrite à adjuvant du Rat par une phytohémagglutinine. C.R. Soc. Biol. (Paris) **162**, 58—62 (1968)

Delbarre, F., Kahan, A., Amor, B., Kahn, M. F.: Polyarthrite du Rat à *Mycoplasma arthritidis*. I. Reproduction experimentale. C.R. Soc. Biol. (Paris) **158**, 1006—1008 (1964a)

Delbarre, F., Kahan, A., Amor, B.: La polyarthrite du Rat à *Mycoplasma arthritidis*. II. Rôle de différentes facteurs. C.R. Soc. Biol. (Paris) **158**, 1043—1046 (1964b)

Denman, A. M.: Anti-lymphycytic antibody and autoimmune disease: a review. Clin. exp. Immunol. **5**, 217—249 (1969)

De Shazo, C. V., Henson, P. M., Cochrane, C. G.: Acute immunologic arthritis in rabbits. J. clin. Invest. **51**, 50—57 (1972)

Di Pasquale, G., Rassaert, C., Richter, R., Welas, P., Gingold, J., Singer, R.: The anti-inflammatory properties of Isoxicam (4-hydroxy-2-methyl-N-[5-methyl-3-]Isoxolyl-2 H-1,2-benzothiazine-3-carboxamide 1,1-dioxide). Agents Actions **5**, 256—263 (1975)

Di Pasquale, G., Welaj, P., Rassaert, C. L.: Prolonged Pentobarbital sleeping time in adjuvant induced polyarthritic rats. Res. Commun. chem. path. Pharmacol. **9**, 253—264 (1974)

Dixon, A. St. J., Davies, J., Dormandy, T. L., Hamilton, E. B. D., Holt, P. J. L., Mason, R. M., Thompson, M., Weber, J. C. P., Zutshi, D. W.: Synthetic D(-) penicillamine in rheumatoid arthritis. Ann. rheum. Dis. **34**, 416—421 (1975)

Dumonde, D. C., Glynn, L. E.: The production of arthritis in rabbits by an immunological reaction to fibrin. Brit. J. exp. Path. **43**, 373—383 (1962)

Edwards, C. Q., Deiss, A., Cole, B. C., Ward, J. R.: Haematologic changes in chronic arthritis of mice induced by Mycoplasma arthritidis. Proc. Soc. Exp. Biol. Med. **150**, 664—668 (1975)

Eisen, V., Freeman, P. C., Loveday, C., West, G. B.: Blood changes in experimental arthritis in two types of genetically different rats. Brit. J. Pharmacol. **49**, 688—695 (1973)

Elliott, P. N., Bolam, J. P., Ford-Hutchinson, A. W., Smith, M. J. H.: The effects of a human plasma fraction on adjuvant arthritis and granuloma pellet reactions in the rat. J. Pharm. (Lond.) **26**, 751—752 (1974)

Flax, M. H., Waksman, B. H.: Further immunologic studies of adjuvant disease in the rat. Int. Arch. Allergy **23**, 331—347 (1963)

Fox, A., Glynn, L. E.: Persistence of antigen in non-arthritic joints. Ann. Rheum. Dis. **34**, 431—437 (1975)

Freeman, P. C., West, G. B.: Resistance of rats to carrageenan and to adjuvant-induced arthritis. Brit. J. Pharmacol. **44**, 327P—328P (1972)

Gardner, D. L.: The experimental production of arthritis: a review. Ann. rheum. Dis. **19**, 297—317 (1960)

Gery, I., Waksman, B. H.: Studies of the mechanism whereby adjuvant disease is suppressed in rats pretreated with mycobacteria. Int. Arch. Allergy **31**, 57—68 (1967)

Glenn, E. M.: Adjuvant-induced arthritis: effects of certain drugs on incidence, clinical severity and biochemical changes. Amer. J. vet. Res. **27**, 339—352 (1966)

Glenn, E. M.: Fibrinogen and experimental inflammation. Biochem. Pharmacol. **18**, 317—326 (1969)

Glenn, E. M., Bowman, B. J., Koslowske, T. C.: The systemic response to inflammation. Biochem. Pharmacol. Suppl. 27—47 (1968)

Glenn, E. M., Gray, J.: Adjuvant-induced polyarthritis in rats: biologic and histologic background. Amer. J. vet. Res. **26**, 1180—1194 (1965)

Glenn, E. M., Gray, J., Kooyers, W.: Chemical changes in adjuvant-induced polyarthritis of rats. Amer. J. vet. Res. **26**, 1195—1203 (1965)

Glenn, E. M., Kooyers, W. M.: Plasma inflammation units: an objective method for investigating effects of drugs on experimental arthritis. Life Sci. **5**, 619—628 (1966)

Glenn, E. M., Lyster, S. C., Rohloff, N. A.: Antiarthritic effects of the antispermatogic agent 2,3 dihydro-(1-naphthyl)-4-(IH)-quinazolinone (U-29,409). Proc. Soc. exp. Biol. (N.Y.) **138**, 244—248 (1971)

Glenn, E. M., Rohloff, N.: Antiarthritic and antiinflammatory effects of certain prostaglandins. Proc. Soc. exp. Biol. (N.Y.) **139**, 290—294 (1972)

Glynn, L. E.: The chronicity of inflammation and its significance in rheumatoid arthritis. Ann. rheum. Dis. **27**, 105—121 (1968)

Goldberg, V. M., Lance, E. M., Davis, P.: Experimental immune synovitis in the rabbit. Relative roles of cell mediated and humoral immunity. Arthr. Rheum. **17**, 993—1005 (1974)

Graeme, M. L., Fabry, E., Sigg, E. B.: Mycobacterial adjuvant periarthritis in rodents and its modification by anti-inflammatory agents. J. Pharmacol. exp. Ther. **153**, 373—380 (1966)

Gralla, E. J., Wiseman, E. H.: The adjuvant arthritic rat: inflammatory parameters during development and regression of gross lesions. Proc. Soc. exp. Biol. (N.Y.) **128**, 493—495 (1968)

Gryfe, A., Sanders, P. M., Gardner, D. L.: The mast cell in early rat adjuvant arthritis. Ann. rheum. Dis. **30**, 24—30 (1971)

Hannan, P. C. T., Hughes, B. C.: Reproducible polyarthritis in rats caused by *Mycoplasma arthritidis*. Ann. rheum. Dis. **30**, 316—321 (1971)

Harwick, H. J., Kalmanson, G. M., Fox, M. A., Guze, L. B.: Arthritis in mice due to infection with *Mycoplasma pulmonis*. J. infect. Dis. **128**, 533—540 (1973)

Hollingsworth, J. W., Greenberg, D. S., Dawson, M.: Adjuvant arthritis in T lymphocyte depleted rats. Proc. Soc. Exp. Biol. Med. **152**, 183—185 (1976)

Houssay, R. H., Frangione, B.: On the pathogenicity of the arthropathy induced with Freund's adjuvant. In: Atti Del X Congresso della Lega Internazionale Contro il Reumatismo. Vol. II, p. 950. Turin: Tipografia Edizione Minerva Medica 1961

Hudack, S. S., McMaster, P. D.: Lymphatic participation in human cutaneous phenomena; study of minute lymphatics of living skin. J. exp. Med. **57**, 751—774 (1933)

Hunneyball, I. M., Stewart, G. A., Stanworth, D. R.: Effect of D(-) penicillamine on chronic experimental arthritis in rabbits. Ann. Rheum. Dis. **36**, 378—380 (1977)

Ignarro, L. J., Slywka, J.: Changes in liver lysosome fragility, erythrocyte membrane stability, and local and systemic lysosomal enzyme levels in adjuvant-induced polyarthritis. Biochem. Pharmacol. **21**, 875—886 (1972)

Isakovic, K., Waksman, B. H.: Effect of sensitization to BSA on adjuvant disease in normal and neonatally thymectomized rats. Proc. Soc. exp. Biol. (N.Y.) **119**, 676—678 (1965)

Jasin, H. E., Ziff, M.: Influence of anti-lymphycytic serum on auto-immune processes. Fed. Proc. **29**, 177—180 (1970)

Jessop, J. D., Currey, H. L.: Influence of gold salts on adjuvant arthritis in the rat. Ann. rheum. Dis. **27**, 577—581 (1968)

Jollès, P., Samour-Migliore, D., Wijs, H. De., Lederer, E.: Correlation of adjuvant activity and chemical structure of mycobacterial wax D fractions. The importance of amino sugars. Biochim. biophys. Acta **83**, 361—363 (1964)

Jones, R. S., Ward, J. F.: Studies on adjuvant induced polyarthritis in rats. II. Histogenesis of joint and visceral lesions. Arthr. Rheum. **6**, 23—35 (1963)

Kalliomäki, J. L., Saarimmaa, H. A., Toivanen, P.: Inhibition by 6-mercaptopurine of polyarthritis induced by Freund's adjuvant. Ann. rheum. Dis. **23**, 78—80 (1964)

Katz, L., Piliero, S. J.: A study of adjuvant-induced polyarthritis in the rat with special reference to associated immunological phenomena. Ann. N.Y. Acad. Sci. **147**, 515—536 (1969)

Kayashima, K., Koga, T., Onoue, K.: Role of T lymphocytes in adjuvant arthritis. I. Evidence for the regulatory function of thymus-derived cells in the induction of the disease. J. Immunol. **117**, 1878—1882 (1976)

Keitel, W., Rudolph, W., Kroning, G., Kretschmar, B., Jambor, S.: Studies of adjuvant arthritis of rats. 1. Dosage, composition, and administration forms of the adjuvant. Z. Rheumaforsch. **28**, 212—218 (1969)

Keitel, W., Wille, R., Franke, A., Ziegeler, J.: Adjuvant arthritis in mice and hamsters. Acta rheum. scand. **17**, 31—34 (1971)

Kellett, D. N.: Suppression of adjuvant arthritis in alloxan-diabetic rats. J. Pharm. (Lond.) **17**, 184—185 (1965)

Klamer, B., Kimura, E. T., Makstenieks, M.: Effects of oral cysteine, penicillamine and N-acetyl-penicillamine on adjuvant arthritis in rats. Pharmacology (Basel) **1**, 283—288 (1968)

Koga, T., Kotani, S., Narita, T., Pearson, C. M.: Induction of adjuvant arthritis in the rat by various bacterial cell walls and their water-soluble components. Int. Arch. Allergy Appl. Immunol. **51**, 206—213 (1976 a)

Koga, T., Kato, K., Kotani, S., Tanaka, Pearson, C. M.: Effect of degradation of the arabinogalactan portion of a water soluble component from Mycobacterium tuberculosis wax D on polyarthritis induction in the rat. Int. Arch. Allergy Appl. Immunol. **51**, 395—400 (1976b)

Koga, T., Pearson, C. M., Narita, T., Kotani, S.: Polyarthritis induced in the rat with cell walls from several bacteria and two *Streptomyces* species. Proc. Soc. exp. Biol. (N.Y.) **143**, 824—827 (1973)

Koga, T., Sande, B. V., Yeaton, R., Pearson, C. M.: Reevaluation of inguinal lymph node injection for production of adjuvant arthritis in the rat. Int. Arch. Allergy Appl. Immunol. **51**, 359—367 (1976c)

Kohashi, O., Pearson, C. M., Watanabe, Y., Kotani, S., Koga, T.: Structural requirements for arthitogenicity of peptidoglycans from Staphlococcus aureus and Lactobacillus plantarum and analogous synthetic compounds. J. Immunol. **116**, 1635—1639 (1976)

Kohashi, O., Pearson, C. M., Watanabe, Y., Kotani, S.: Preparation of arthritogenic hydrosoluble peptidoglycans from both arthritogenic and non-arthritogenic bacterial cells walls. Infect. Immunity **16**, 861—866 (1977)

Koj, A.: Acute-phase reactants. Their synthesis, turnover and biological significance. In: Allison, A. C. (Ed.): Structure and Function of Plasma Proteins, Vol. I, pp. 73—131. New York: Plenum Press 1975

Lennon, V. A., Byrd, W. J.: Experimental arthritis in thymectomised rats with an impaired humoral immune response. Nature (Lond.) **244**, 38—40 (1973)

Liyanage, S. P., Currey, H. L. F.: Failure of oral D-Penicillamine to modify adjuvant arthritis or immune response in the rat. Ann. rheum. Dis. **31**, 521 (1972)

Liyanage, S. P., Currey, H. L. F., Vernon-Roberts, B.: Influence of Tubercle aggregate size on the severity of adjuvant arthritis in the rat. Ann. rheum. Dis. **34**, 49—53 (1975)

Loewi, G.: Experimental immune inflammation in the synovial membrane. I. The immunological mechanism. Immunology **15**, 417—427 (1968)

Loewi, G.: Experimental immune inflammation in the synovial membrane. II. The origin and local activity of inflammatory cells. Immunology **17**, 489—498 (1969)

Lowe, J. S.: Serum protein changes in rats with arthritis induced by mycobacterial adjuvant. Biochem. Pharmacol. **13**, 633—641 (1964)

Lowe, J. S., Turner, E. H.: The effect of adjuvant arthritis and drugs on the ability of rat plasma to inhibit the Triton X-100 induced lysis of rabbit polymorphonuclear leucocyte granules. Biochem. Pharmacol. **22**, 2069—2078 (1973)

Mancini, G., Carbonara, A. O., Heremans, J. F.: Immunochemical quantitation of antigens by single radial immunodiffusion. Immunochemistry 2 235—254 (1965)

McConkey, B., Crockson, R. A., Crockson, A. P.: The assessment of rheumatoid arthritis. Quart. J. Med. **41** N.S., 115—125 (1972)

McConkey, B., Crockson, R. A., Crockson, A. P., Wilkinson, A. R.: The effects of some anti-inflammatory drugs on the acute phase proteins in rheumatoid arthritis. Quart. J. Med. **42** N.S., 785—791 (1973)

Ménard, H. A., Dion, J.: Is local antigen persistence responsible for the chronicity of the experimental immune arthritis of the rabbit? Experientia **32**, 1474—1475 (1976)

Migliore, D., Jollès, P.: Contribution to the study of the structure of adjuvant active waxes D from Mycobacteria; isolation of a peptidoglycan. FEBS Lett. **2**, 7—9 (1968)

Minchin-Clarke, H. G., Freeman, T., Pryse-Phillips, W. E. M.: Serum protein changes in Still's disease, rheumatoid arthritis and gout. Brit. J. exp. Path. **51**, 441—447 (1970)

Morton, D. M., Chatfield, D. H.: The effects of adjuvant-induced arthritis on the liver metabolism of drugs in rats. Biochem. Pharmacol. **19**, 473—481 (1970)

Muirden, K. D., Peace, G.: Light and electron microscope studies in carragheenin, adjuvant and tuberculin-induced arthritis. Ann. rheum. Dis. **28**, 392—401 (1969)

Multicentre Trial Group: Controlled trial of D-penicillamine in severe rheumatoid arthritis. Lancet **1973** I, 275—280

Newbould, B. B.: Chemotherapy of arthritis induced in rats by injection of mycobacterial adjuvant. Brit. J. Pharmacol. **21**, 127—136 (1963)

Newbould, B. B.: Lymphatic drainage and adjuvant induced arthritis in rats. Brit. J. exp. Path. **45**, 375—383 (1964a)

Newbould, B. B.: Role of lymph nodes in adjuvant-induced arthritis in rats. Ann. rheum. Dis. **23**, 392—396 (1964b)

Newbould, B. B.: Suppression of adjuvant-induced arthritis in rats with 2-butoxycarbon-ylmethylene-4-oxothiazolidine. Brit. J. Pharmacol. **24**, 632—640 (1965)

Nusbickel, F. R., Troyer, H.: Histochemical investigation of adjuvant-induced arthritis. Arthritis Rheum. **19**, 1339—1346 (1976)

Page Thomas, D. P.: Lysosomal enzymes in experimental and rheumatoid arthritis. In: Dingle, J. T., Fell, H. B. (Eds.): Lysosomes in Biology and Pathology, pp. 87—110. Amsterdam: North Holland 1969

Paronetto, F.: Adjuvant arthritis induced by *Corynebacterium rubrum*. Proc. Soc. exp. Biol. (N.Y.) **133**, 296—298 (1970)

Parrott, D. P., Lewis, D. A.: Protease and antiprotease levels in blood of arthritic rats. Ann. Rheum. Dis. **36**, 166—169 (1977)

Paulus, H. E., Whitehouse, M. W.: Nonsteroid anti-inflammatory agents. Ann. Rev. Pharmacol. **13**, 107—125 (1973)

Pearse, A. D.: The histochemical demonstration of hydrolytic enzymes in adjuvant-induced arthritis in rats. Histochem. J. **6**, 431—446 (1974)

Pearson, C. M.: Development of arthritis, periarthritis and periostitis in rats given adjuvants. Proc. Soc. exp. Biol. (N.Y.) **91**, 95—101 (1956)

Pearson, C. M.: Experimental joint disease. Observations on adjuvant-induced arthritis. J. chron. Dis. **16**, 863—874 (1963)

Pearson, C. M., Waksman, B. H., Sharp, T. J.: Studies on arthritis and other lesions induced in rats by injection of mycobacterial adjuvant. V. Changes affecting the skin and mucous membranes. Comparison of the experimental process with human disease. J. exp. Med. **113**, 485—509 (1961)

Pearson, C. M., Wood, F. D.: Studies of polyarthritis and other lesions induced in rats by injection of mycobacteria adjuvant. 1. General clinical and pathologic characteristics and some modifying factors. Arthr. Rheum. **2**, 440—459 (1959)

Pearson, C. M., Wood, F. D.: Factors which modify adjuvant arthritis. Arthr. Rheum. **5**, 654 (1962)

Pearson, C. M., Wood, F. D.: Passive transfer of adjuvant arthritis by lymph node or spleen cells. J. exp. Med. **120**, 547—560 (1964)

Pearson, C. M., Wood, F. D.: Inhibition of adjuvant arthritis by protein antigens. 1. Inhibitory capacities and dose relationships of different proteins. Immunology **16**, 157—165 (1969)

Pelczarska, A.: Treatment of adjuvant arthritis in rats with the histidine decarboxylase inhibitor hypostamine. J. Pharm. (Lond.) **21**, 692—693 (1969)

Perper, R. J., Alvarez, B., Colombo, C., Schroder, H.: The use of a standardized adjuvant arthritis assay to differentiate between anti-inflammatory and immunosuppressive agents. Proc. Soc. exp. Biol. (N.Y.) **137**, 506—512 (1971)

Perper, R. J., Glenn, E. M., Monovich, R. E.: Separation of anti-inflammatory and immunosuppressive activities in heterologous anti-lymphocyte serum. Nature (Lond.) **223**, 86—87 (1969)

Perper, R. J., Oronsky, A. L.: Serum factor protecting against experimental arthritis. Nature (New Biol.) **238**, 23—25 (1972)

Perrine, J. W., Takesue, E. I.: Use of the rotarod in determining grip strength in rats with adjuvant-induced arthritis. Arch. int. Pharmacodyn. **174**, 192—198 (1968)

Phillips, J. M., Kaklamanis, P., Glynn, L. E.: Experimental arthritis associated with auto-immunization. Ann. rheum. Dis. **25**, 165—174 (1966)

Piliero, S. J., Colombo, C.: Action of anti-inflammatory drugs on the lysozyme activity and turbidity of serum from rats with adjuvant arthritis or endocrine deficiency. J. Pharmacol. exp. Ther. **165**, 294—299 (1969)

Piliero, S. J., Graeme, M. C., Sigg, E. B., Chinea, G., Colombo, C.: Action of anti-inflammatory agents upon blood and histopathologic changes induced by periarthritis in rats. Life Sci. **5**, 1057—1069 (1966)

Pinals, R. S.: Effect of hepatic injury on adjuvant arthritis. Ann. rheum. Dis. **32**, 471—474 (1973)

Possanza, G. J., Stewart, P. B.: Suppressant effect of procarbazine and its comparison with anti-lymphocytic serum in adjuvant-induced polyarthritis in rats. Clin. exp. Immunol. **6**, 291—297 (1970)

Quagliata, F., Phillips-Quagliata, J. M.: Competence of thoracic duct cells in the transfer of adjuvant disease and delayed hypersensitivity. Evidence that Mycobacterial components are required for the successful transfer of the disease. Cellular Immunol. **3**, 78—87 (1972)

Quevauviller, A., Chalchat, M. A., Brouichet, H., Delbarre, F.: Action des barbituriques chez le rat atteint d'une polyarthrite a adjuvant. C.R. Soc. Biol. (Paris) **162**, 618—621 (1968)

Rawson, A. J., Torralba, T. P.: Induction of proliferative synovitis in rabbits by intra-articular injection of immune complexes. Arthr. Rheum. **10**, 44—52 (1967)

Rosenthale, M. E.: A comparative study of the Lewis and Sprague Dawley rat in adjuvant arthritis. Arch. int. Pharmacodyn. **188**, 14—22 (1970)

Rosenthale, M. E.: Evaluation for immunosuppressive and anti-allergic activity. In: Scherrer, R. A., Whitehouse, M. W. (Eds.): Anti-inflammatory Agents, Chemistry and Pharmacology, Vol. II, pp. 123—192. New York: Academic Press 1974

Rosenthale, M. E., Datko, L. J., Kassarich, J., Rosanoff, E.: Immunopharmacologic effects of cycloleucine. J. Pharmacol. exp. Ther. **180**, 501—513 (1972)

Rosenthale, M. E., Datko, L. J., Kassarich, J., Schneider, F.: Chemotherapy of experimental allergic encephelomyelitis. Arch. int. Pharmacodyn. **179**, 251—275 (1969)

Rosenthale, M. E., Nagra, C. L.: Comparative effects of some immunosuppressive and anti-inflammatory drugs on allergic encephalomyelitis and adjuvant arthritis. Proc. Soc. exp. Biol. (N.Y.) **125**, 149—154 (1967)

Roszkowski-Sliz, W.: Effect of the somatotrophic hormone, insulin and duration on post-adjuvant arthritis in rats. Acta physiol. pol. **24**, 371—376 (1973)

Ryzewska, A. G., Ryzewski, J., Dabrowski, M.: Influence of specific and non-specific agents on the inflammatory process in the adjuvant-induced polyarthritis in rats. In: Bertelli, A., Houck, J. C. (Eds.): Inflammation Biochemistry and Drug Interaction, pp. 275—282. Amsterdam: Excerpta Medica Foundation 1969

Ryzewski, J.: Effect of cysteine on the generalisation and course of adjuvant polyarthritis in rats. Reumatologia (Warsz.) **4**, 227—234 (1966)

Saeki, K., Wake, K., Yamasaki, H.: Inhibition of adjuvant arthritis by histamine. Arch. Int. Pharmacodyn. Ther. **222**, 132—140 (1975)

Scherrer, R. A., Whitehouse, M. W. (Eds.): Anti-inflammatory agents, chemistry and pharmacology, Vol. I and II. New York: Academic Press 1974

Shen, T. Y.: Non acidic antiarthritic agents and the search for new classes of agents. In: Scherrer, R. A., Whitehouse, M. W. (Eds.): Antiinflammatory Agents, Vol. I, pp. 180—207. New York: Academic Press 1974

Silverstein, E., Sokoloff, L.: Periarthritis produced in rats with Freund's adjuvants. Arthr. Rheum. **3**, 485—495 (1960)

Sofia, R. D., Douglas, J. F.: The prophylactic and therapeutic effects of gold sodium thiomalate against adjuvant-induced polyarthritis in rats. Agents Actions **3**, 335—343 (1973)

Spector, W. G., Willoughby, D. A.: The pharmacology of inflammation. New York: Grune and Stratton 1968, p. 116

Stein, H., Yarom, R., Levin, S., Dishon, T., Ginsburg, I.: Chronic self-perpetuating arthritis induced in rabbits by a cell-free extract of Group streptococci. Proc. Soc. exp. Biol. (N.Y.) **143**, 1106—1112 (1973)

Steinetz, B., Giannina, T., Butler, M., Popick, F.: Influence of thyroidectomy and thyroidal hormones on adjuvant arthritis in rats. Proc. Soc. exp. Biol. (N.Y.) **133**, 401—403 (1970)

Stevens, J. E., Willoughby, D. A.: The anti-inflammatory effect of some immunosuppressive agents. J. Path. Back. **97**, 367—373 (1969)

Stoerk, H. C., Bielinski, T. C., Budzilovich, T.: Chronic polyarthritis in rats injected with spleen in adjuvants. Amer. J. Path. **30**, 616 (1954)

Svartz, N.: The primary cause of rheumatoid arthritis is an infection — the infectious agent exists in milk. Acta med. scand. **192**, 231—239 (1972)

Swingle, K. F.: Evaluation for anti-inflammatory activity. In: Scherrer, R. A., Whitehouse, M. W. (Eds.): Anti-inflammatory Agents, Chemistry and Pharmacology, Vol. II, pp. 33—122. New York: Academic Press 1974

Swingle, K. F., Jaques, L. W., Kvam, D. C.: Differences in the severity of adjuvant arthritis in four strains of rats. Proc. Soc. exp. Biol. (N.Y.) **132**, 608—612 (1969)

Toivanen, P., Siikala, H., Laiho, P.: Suppression of adjuvant arthritis by estrone in adrenalectomised and ovariectomised rats. Experientia (Basel) **23**, 560—561 (1967)

Toivanen, P., Toivanen, A.: Effect of epsilon-aminocaproic acid on adjuvant arthritis in rats. Experientia (Basel) **20**, 579—580 (1964)

Trentham, D. E., Townes, A. S., Kang, A. H.: Autoimmunity to type II collagen: an experimental model of arthritis. J. Exp. Med. **146**, 857—868 (1977)

Velo, G. P., Bertoni, F., Capelli, A., Martinelli, G.: Lysosomes as mediators of paranchymal lesions in adjuvant-induced arthritis in rats. J. Path. Bact. **106**, 201—205 (1972)

Vernon-Roberts, B., Liyanage, S. P., Currey, H. L.: Adjuvant arthritis in the rat. Distribution of fluorescent material after footpad injection of rhodamine-labelled tubercle bacilli. Ann. Rheum. Dis. **35**, 389—397 (1975)

Volkman, A., Collins, F. M.: Role of host factors in the pathogenesis of Salmonella-associated arthritis in rats. Infect. Immun. **13**, 1155—1160 (1976)

Waksman, B. H., Pearson, C. M., Sharp, J. T.: Studies of arthritis and other lesions induced in rats by injection of mycobacterial adjuvant. II. Evidence that the disease is a disseminated immunologic response to exogenous antigen. J. Immunol. **85**, 403—417 (1960)

Waksman, B. H., Wennersten, C.: Passive transfer of adjuvant arthritis in rats with living lymphoid cells of sensitized animals. Int. Arch. Allergy **23**, 129—139 (1963)

Walz, D. T., Berkoff, C. E.: Arthritis and psoriasis: the effects of antipsoriatic agents in the adjuvant-induced arthritis rat. Proc. Soc. exp. Biol. (N.Y.) **135**, 760—762 (1970)

Walz, D. T., DiMartino, M. J., Chakrin, L. W., Sutton, B. M., Misher, A.: Anti-arthritic properties and unique pharmacologic profile of a potential chrysotherapeutic agent: SK & F D-39162. J. Pharmacol. Exp. Ther. **197**, 142—152 (1976)

Walz, D. T., DiMartino, K. J., Koch, J. H., Zuccarello, W.: Adjuvant induced arthritis in rats. 1. Temporal relationship of physiological, biochemical and haematological parameters. Proc. Soc. exp. Biol. (N.Y.) **136**, 907—910 (1971)

Walz, D. T., DiMartino, M. J., Misher, A.: Adjuvant-induced arthritis in rats. II. Drug effects on physiologic, biochemical and immunologic parameters. J. Pharmacol. exp. Ther. **178**, 223—231 (1971 a)

Walz, D. T., Di Martino, M. J., Misher, A.: Suppression of adjuvant induced arthritis in the rat by gold sodium thiomalate. Ann. rheum. Dis. **30**, 303—306 (1971 b)

Walz, D. T., Di Martino, B., Sutton, B., Misher, A.: SK&F 36914 — an agent for oral chrysotherapy. J. Pharmacol. exp. Ther. **181**, 292—297 (1972)

Walz, D. T., Dolan, M. M., Di Martino, M. J., Yankell, S. L.: Effects of topical hydrocortisone and acetylsalicyclic acid on the primary lesion of adjuvant induced arthritis. Proc. Soc. exp. Biol. (N.Y.) **137**, 1466—1469 (1971 c)

Ward, J. R., Cloud, R. S.: Comparative effect of anti-rheumatic drugs on adjuvant-induced polyarthritis in rats. J. Pharmacol. exp. Ther. **152**, 116—121 (1966)

Ward, J. R., Cloud, R. S., Krawitt, E. L., Jones, R. S.: Studies on adjuvant-induced polyarthritis in rats. III. The effect of "immunosuppressive agents" on arthritis and tuberculin hypersensitivity. Arthr. Rheum. **1**, 644—661 (1964)

Ward, J. R., Jones, R. S.: Studies on adjuvant induced polyarthritis in rats. 1. Adjuvant composition, route of injection and removal of depot site. Arthr. Rheum. **5**, 557—564 (1962)

Warren, S. L., Marmor, L., Liebes, D. M., Rosenblatt, H. M.: An active agent from rheumatoid arthritis synovial tissue: transmission by injection or ingestion in mice and rats. Arch. intern. Med. **130**, 899—903 (1972)

Webb, F. W. S., Bluestone, R., Goldberg, L. S., Douglas, S. D., Pearson, C. M.: Experimental viral arthritis induced with Herpes simplex. Arthr. Rheum. **16**, 241—250 (1973)

Webb, F. W. S., Bluestone, R., Goldberg, L. S., Pearson, C. M.: Experimental viral arthritis induced with Herpes Simplex. Clin. Sci. **42**, 12 (1972)

Webb, F. W. S., Ford, P. M., Glynn, L. E.: Persistence of antigen in rabbit synovial membrane. Brit. J. exp. Path. **52**, 31—35 (1971)

Weimer, H. E., Wood, F. D., Pearson, C. M.: Serum protein alterations in adjuvant-induced arthritis. Canad. J. Biochem. **46**, 743—748 (1968)

Weissmann, G., Becher, B., Wiederman, G., Bernheimer, A. W.: Studies on lysosomes. VII. Acute and chronic arthritis produced by intra-articular injections of streptolysin S in rabbits. Amer. J. Path. **46**, 129—147 (1965)

Weissmann, G., Pras, M., Rosenberg, L.: Arthritis induced by filipin in rabbits. Arthr. Rheum. **10**, 325—336 (1967)

Whitehouse, M. W.: Abnormal drug metabolism in rats after an inflammatory insult. Agents Actions **3**, 312—316 (1973)

Whitehouse, M. W., Beck, F. W.: Standardisation of arthritogenic adjuvants for evaluating anti-inflammatory and immunosuppressant drugs. Agents Actions 4, 227—229 (1974)

Whitehouse, M. W., Orr, K. J., Beck, F. W., Pearson, C. M.: Freund's adjuvants: relationship of arthritogenicity and adjuvanticity in rats to vehicle composition. Immunology 27, 311—330 (1974)

Willoughby, D. A., Coote, E., Turk, J. L.: Complement in acute inflammation J. Path. Bact. 97, 295—305 (1969)

Winder, C. V., Lembke, L. A., Stephens, M. D.: Comparative bioassay of drugs in adjuvant-induced arthritis in rats: flufenamic acid, mefenamic acid, and phenylbutazone. Arthr. Rheum. 12, 472—482 (1969)

Winter, C. A., Nuss, G. W.: Treatment of adjuvant arthritis in rats with anti-inflammatory drugs. Arthr. Rheum. 9, 394—404 (1966)

Winter, C. A., Risley, E. A., Nuss, G. W.: Carrageenin-induced oedema in hind paw of the rat as an assay for anti-inflammatory drugs. Proc. Soc. exp. Biol. (N.Y.) 111, 544—547 (1962)

Wood, F. D., Pearson, C. M.: Protection of rats against adjuvant arthritis by bacterial lipopolysaccharide. Science 137, 544—545 (1962)

Wood, F. D., Pearson, C. M., Ranaka, A.: Capacity of mycobacterial wax D and its subfractions to induce adjuvant arthritis in rats. Int. Arch. Allergy 35, 456—467 (1969)

Zidek, Z., Perlik, F.: Genetic control of adjuvant induced arthritis in rats. J. Pharm. (Lond.) 23, 389—390 (1971)

Zurier, R. B., Ballas, M.: Prostaglandin El (PGEl) suppression of adjuvant arthritis. Arthr. Rheum. 16, 251—258 (1973)

Zurier, R. B., Hoffstein, S., Weissmann, G.: Suppression of acute and chronic inflammation in adrenalectomized rats and pharmacologic amounts of prostaglandins. Arthr. Rheum. 16, 606—618 (1973 b)

Zurier, R. B., Mitnick, H., Bloomgarden, D., Weissmann, G.: Effect of bee venom on experimental arthritis. Ann. rheum. Dis. 32, 466—470 (1973 a)

Zurier, R. B., Quagliata, F.: Effect of prostaglandin El on adjuvant arthritis. Nature (Lond.) 234, 304—305 (1971)

Chapter 24

Antagonism of Bradykinin Bronchoconstriction by Anti-Inflammatory Drugs

P. J. PIPER and J. R. VANE

A. Introduction

Bradykinin (Arg-Pro-Pro-Gly-Phe-Phe-Ser-Pro-Phe-Arg) (Bk) is the most widely studied of a group of kinins which includes lys-bradykinin (kallidin), met-lys-bradykinin and gly-arg-met-lys-bradykinin. Bk is thought to be an inflammatory mediator; kallidin and met-lys-bradykinin also occur in mammalian tissues. In general, there are only qualitative differences between the activities of this group of substances (ROCHA E SILVA and GARCIA LEME, 1972).

Bk has both direct and indirect actions on mammalian lungs, reducing the inspiratory volume in several species during spontaneous or artificial respiration in vivo. Bk also increases the rate and depth of respiration. In isolated perfused lungs of guinea pig in vitro Bk contracts tracheal and bronchial smooth muscle and increases pulmonary arterial pressure. The vascular or bronchial smooth muscle of the lung may be affected by exogenous or endogenous kinins since the generating enzyme, kallikrein, is released in the lung during anaphylaxis and possibly other pathological conditions. The half-life of kinins in the circulation approximates one circulation time, due to inactivation in blood and during passage through the pulmonary circulation.

Several of the actions of Bk in the lungs are inconsistent. For instance, kinins are bronchoconstrictor in the guinea pig in vitro and in vivo but not in other species. Bk given by aerosol causes bronchoconstriction in some asthmatics but not in others or in normal patients. Bk is as active as histamine in guinea pig isolated lungs in vitro but less active on the isolated trachea of this species. In the guinea pig in vivo the threshold bronchoconstrictor dose for Bk is less than that for histamine, but the dose response curve for Bk is less steep and reaches a lower maximum. Antagonism of the action of Bk in the lung is also far from straightforward. Aspirin-like drugs are potent inhibitors of the bronchoconstrictor effects of Bk in the artificially ventilated guinea pig in vivo, even after destruction of the CNS and blockade of β-adrenoceptors, but are less active against the action of Bk on isolated trachea in vitro. Catecholamines released by Bk in vivo lessen its bronchoconstrictor effects. This chapter discusses these effects in detail and develops the proposal (VANE and FERREIRA, 1976) that the effects of kinins are modulated or amplified by a local release of prostaglandins (PGs) induced by Bk through activation of phospholipase A_2.

B. Production of Kinins and Other Mediators of Anaphylaxis in the Lungs

I. In vitro

In species where the lungs are the "target organ" of anaphylaxis, anaphylactic shock is accompanied by the release of a number of potent biologically active substances. These mediators are either synthesised de novo in response to antigen challenge or released from stores of preformed material. Histamine (MOTA and VUGMAN, 1956) and eosinophil chemotactic factor of anaphylaxis (ECF-A) (GOETZL and AUSTEN, 1975) are stored preformed in mast cell granules of lung tissue. The release of PGs, thromboxanes, their precursors and metabolites and slow-reacting substance of ana-phylaxis (SRS-A) involves biosynthetic and secretory phases (PIPER and VANE, 1969a, 1971; ORANGE, 1974; MATHÉ and LEVINE, 1973). The kinin-forming enzyme kallikrein is liberated from guinea pig isolated perfused lungs by anaphylaxis (BROCKLEHURST and LAHIRI, 1962; JONASSON and BECKER, 1966). The site of origin of the lung kallikrein is unknown but it may be the secretory cells of the bronchial tree by analogy with salivary kallikrein.

II. In vivo

In 1950, BERALDO showed that blood from an anaphylactic dog contained Bk. BROCKLEHURST and LAHIRI (1962, 1963) showed that kallikrein and Bk are released into the circulation of guinea pigs, rats and rabbits during anaphylaxis and could account for the levels of Bk found in the circulation of intact animals. COLLIER and JAMES (1967) found that anaphylactic bronchoconstriction in the guinea pig in vivo could be lessened by first rendering the guinea pig tachyphylactic to Bk, indicating that kinins probably contribute to this response. EYRE and LEWIS (1972) found greatly increased levels of kinins in blood during anaphylaxis in calves.

Although anaphylactic shock in animals differs from asthma in man, there are similarities between the two conditions which are worth consideration. There is evidence that human lungs can produce kinins in asthma and other disease states. Thus, during severe bronchial asthma, a raised kinin concentration occurs in blood (ABE et al., 1967). Kinin has also been found in secretions from the airways of sufferers from hay fever, asthma and bronchitis, and in extracts of human lung adenocarcinoma (COLLIER, 1970).

III. Release of Catecholamines in vivo

FELDBERG and LEWIS (1964) and STASZEWSKA-BARCZAK and VANE (1967) showed that Bk released catecholamines from the adrenal medulla in the cat and dog in vivo. β-adrenoceptor blockade by pronethalol greatly intensified bronchoconstriction in-duced by intravenous injection of Bk or by anaphylactic shock in the Konzett-Rössler preparation of the guinea pig (COLLER and JAMES, 1966; COLLIER, et al., 1967). This was indirect evidence that Bk and perhaps other mediators of anaphy-laxis released catecholamines in the guinea pig. PIPER et al. (1967), using bioassay techniques, directly showed that, when sensitized guinea pigs were challenged by intravenous injection of antigen, catecholamines were released into the circulation.

The catecholamine was mainly adrenaline and was released from the adrenal medulla. In unsensitized, anaesthetised guinea pigs, the mediators of anaphylaxis, histamine, SRS-A (partially purified) and Bk when given intravenously all caused bronchoconstriction and a release of catecholamines from the adrenal medulla (PIPER et al., 1967). Although Bk also released adrenaline from the adrenals when administered into the arch of the aorta, the release of catecholamines by histamine and SRS-A appeared to be associated with the ability of the latter to cause bronchoconstriction, possibly reflexly via hypoxia (GRAY and DIAMOND, 1957). Antagonism of bronchoconstriction caused by Bk and by SRS-A of histamine by aspirin-like drugs or mepyramine also inhibited the release of adrenaline produced by these substances, although the release of adrenaline by anaphylaxis was unaffected (PIPER, 1969). A similar release of catecholamines may occur in humans during bronchoconstriction since asthmatics are very sensitive to β-adrenoceptor blocking agents which can cause intense bronchoconstriction (MCNEILL, 1964).

C. Action of Bradykinin on Lung Function

I. Bronchial Smooth Muscle in vitro and in vivo

The actions of Bk in the lungs have been described as "capricious" (COLLIER, 1969): there are species differences in responses to Bk and differences between reactions of bronchial smooth muscles in vivo and in vitro. In spontaneously breathing guinea pigs, Bk causes tachypnoea (GJURIS and WESTERMAN, 1963) but, when given to anaesthetised or spinalised guinea pigs prepared for use in the Kònzett-Rössler preparation, Bk given intravenously causes a marked increase in air overflow volume (COLLIER et al., 1959, 1960, 1968). This is mainly due to a decrease in lung compliance (WIDDICOMBE, 1963) and may be explained by the fact that Bk selectively narrows the smaller airways and constricts the respiratory bronchioles (JÄNKÄLÄ and VIRTAMA, 1963). It is difficult to cause bronchoconstriction in guinea pigs with Bk administered by aerosol, although histamine is effective by this route. Bk also increases air overflow volume on the Konzett-Rössler preparation of the cat (KONZETT and STÜRMER, 1960), rabbit and rat (BHOOLA et al., 1962). In the rabbit, the potency of Bk was approximately equivalent to that in the guinea pig; it was less active in the cat and even less potent in the rat.

Bradykinin constricts the airways of guinea pig isolated lungs and contracts tracheal muscle. However it does not contract rabbit tracheal or dog bronchial muscle. Occasionally, human bronchus is contracted by Bk. Inhalation of Bk aerosol causes respiratory embarrassment to some asthmatics but not to others (HERXHEIMER and STRESEMAN, 1963). With increasing doses, the response to bradykinin increases less than does the response to other bronchoconstrictor agents, and it never reaches as high a maximum. Aspirin and other anti-inflammatory acids block the increase in airway resistance brought about by kinins in the artificially ventilated lungs of guinea pigs in vivo, yet show a weaker effect in preparations of isolated lung and tracheal muscle, and are inactive against the actions of Bk in rabbit lung. The effects of Bk on guinea pig or rabbit lung readily show tachyphylaxis (COLLIER et al., 1959, 1960, 1968; ELLIOT et al., 1960; HAUG et al., 1966).

Another feature of Bk-induced bronchoconstriction in the guinea pig is its very long duration of action, despite the speed at which kinin is destroyed in vivo (Ferreira and Vane, 1967a, b, d). This prolonged bronchoconstriction can be overcome by increasing the inflation pressure (Holgate, unpublished), so that the prolonged action was not due to lung oedema. The reversal by over-inflation might be due to the release of a bronchodilator E-type PG (Piper and Vane, 1971). Bk is more potent as a bronchoconstrictor agent in vivo than in vitro and its action is antagonised by aspirin-like drugs (Collier et al., 1959, 1960, 1968), later shown to be PG synthetase inhibitors (Vane, 1971). This suggests that part of its bronchoconstrictor action is due to the release of a product of the cyclo-oxygenase system which is inhibited by aspirin-like drugs. Indeed, Bk has been shown to release rabbit aorta contracting substance (RCS) and PGs from guinea pig isolated perfused lungs, and RCS in vivo (Piper and Vane, 1969a, b, Palmer et al., 1973). Bk, given intravenously, first causes bronchoconstriction and then releases catecholamines (from the adrenal medulla) which antagonise the bronchoconstriction (Piper et al., 1967). Paradoxically, Bk decreases intratracheal pressure in the guinea pig, probably by adrenergic stimulation (James, 1969). When Bk is administered on to the exposed pleural surface in the open-chested, artificially respired guinea pig in vivo it causes bronchoconstriction (Bhoola et al., 1962). In the conscious intact guinea pig, Bk injected intracardially causes severe long-lasting dyspnoea but when given by intraperitoneal injection, does not affect respiration (Herxheimer and Streseman, 1961).

II. Pulmonary Circulation

Although Bk is hypotensive in the systemic circulation, it constricts the pulmonary vein in guinea pig and decreases perfusion of isolated lungs (Greef and Moog, 1964). It also restricts the pulmonary circulation of dog in vivo (Hyman, 1968). Capillary permeability is increased by Bk and, although this was demonstrated in skin (Bhoola and Schachter, 1959; Elliott et al., 1960) a similar increase in vascular permeability may also apply in the lungs.

D. Release of Prostaglandins and Precursors From Lungs by Bradykinin

The first evidence that Bk could release other vasoactive substances from tissues came from Piper and Vane. They used guinea pig isolated lungs perfused with Krebs' solution and measured the release of active substances from the lungs by a cascade bioassay system (Vane, 1964, 1969). When lungs from sensitized guinea pigs were challenged, they demonstrated release of histamine, SRS-A, PGE_2 and $PGF_{2\alpha}$ (Piper and Vane, 1969a, b) and a previously unknown substance which contracted the rabbit aorta. This rabbit aorta contracting substance (RCS) disappeared very rapidly from the Krebs' solution, with a half-life of 1–2 min. Gryglewski and Vane (1972) suggested that RCS was a PG intermediate, possibly an unstable cyclic endoperoxide. The suggestion was supported by the fact that arachidonic acid, the PG precursor, causes a continuous generation of RCS from guinea pig lungs (Var-

GAFTIG and DAO HAI, 1972; PALMER et al., 1973). Furthermore, aspirin or indomethacin, which interfere with PG biosynthesis by substrate competition at the active site of the cyclo-oxygenase enzyme (LANDS et al., 1974) also prevent the generation of RCS (PIPER and VANE, 1969a, b). Several groups have shown that the cyclic endoperoxide intermediates in PG biosynthesis, which HAMBERG and SAMUELSSON (1974a) have named PGG_2 and PGH_2, also contract the rabbit aorta. These substances, too, are short lived but their half-lives are longer than that of RCS. Recently, HAMBERG et al. (1975b) have characterized a non-prostaglandin metabolite of PGG_2 or PGH_2 which they have called thromboxane A_2 (TXA_2). This has a half-life of 30 s and it is now evident that the activity of RCS is mainly due to TXA_2, along with some endoperoxides (HAMBERG et al., 1975b). An enzyme that generates TXA_2 from the endoperoxides has been isolated from platelets (NEEDLEMAN et al., 1976). TXA_2 (or RCS) can also be formed by lungs and spleen; indeed, it is now apparent that in these tissues, TXA_2 generation is the major pathway and formation of PGE_2 and $PGF_{2\alpha}$ accounts for only a small percentage of the total arachidonic acid metabolism. It should be remembered, however, that aspirin-like drugs act as inhibitors of the cyclo-oxygenase enzyme: aspirin itself acetylates the cyclo-oxygenase protein at the active site (ROTH et al., 1975). Thus, the production of endoperoxides and all their derivatives, including TXA_2, will be inhibited by aspirin-like drugs.

There is another enzyme which is involved in arachidonic acid transformation which is not inhibited by aspirin-like drugs. This is a lipoxygenase, isolated from human platelets and guinea pig lung by HAMBERG and SAMUELSSON (1974a, b). This enzyme generates a 12-hydroperoxide derivative of arachidonic acid (HPETE) and 12-S-hydroxy-5,8,10,14-eicosatetraenoic acid (HETE). The importance of HETE in the function of the lung has yet to be determined.

PG endoperoxides (PGG_2 and PGH_2) exert pronounced biological effects. They cause contraction of strips of rabbit aorta (80–200 times more potent than PGE_2), guinea pig trachea (8 times more potent than $PGF_{2\alpha}$) and rat stomach ($^1/_3$–$^1/_2$ as potent as PGE_2). They also contract tracheal muscle from guinea pigs and aggregate human platelets (HAMBERG et al., 1974, 1975a). It has therefore been proposed that endoperoxides are of importance in various physiopathological processes such as anaphylaxis and thrombosis. Some or all of these actions of the endoperoxides may be due to the enzymic formation of TXA_2. Certainly, platelet aggregation by the endoperoxides is thought to be due to TXA_2 formation. Furthermore, stable analogues of the endoperoxides (which exhibit thromboxane-like activity) are amongst the most powerful pulmonary pressor agents encountered in the dog (KADOWITZ, 1976)

An infusion of Bk into isolated lungs of the guinea pig also causes release of RCS (PIPER and VANE, 1969b) and of PGE_2 and $PGF_{2\alpha}$ (PIPER and VANE, 1969a, 1971; PALMER et al., 1973). It is not yet clear whether the PGs are released as such from the lung tissue or whether they are formed from the endoperoxides after they have been released into the perfusion fluid. SRS-A (charcoal purified) and histamine also release PGs and RCS from perfused lungs.

"RCS-RF" (rabbit aorta contracting substance—releasing factor) was the name given by PIPER and VANE (1969b) to an unidentified factor distinct from SRS-A found in the perfusate of immunologically shocked lungs from sensitized guinea pig. RCS-RF injected into the pulmonary artery of perfused lungs from unsensitized guinea pigs induced release of RCS. FLOWER and BLACKWELL (1976) have now partially purified RCS-RF. The preparation was chromatographically free of fatty acids and PGs, but traces of phospholipid material remained. There was no PG-like activity when tested on a PG-sensitive system, the rat fundus strip, rat colon and chick rectum (FERREIRA and VANE, 1967c). High doses (5.0 U) contracted the guinea pig ileum and rat stomach strip. RCS-RF activity was not destroyed by incubation with the enzyme arylsulphatase which selectively inactivates SRS-A (ORANGE et al., 1974). Indeed, RCS-RF activity was often increased by incubation with arylsulphatase.

An intravenous injection of Bk in anaesthetised guinea pigs released RCS into the arterial circulation (PALMER et al., 1973). PGs may also have been released but were not assayed at the time. MATHÉ and LEVINE (1973) and LIEBIG et al. (1974) have shown that PG metabolites are released during anaphylaxis in isolated perfused guinea pig lungs and only small amounts of PGE_2 and $PGF_{2\alpha}$. CRUTCHLEY and PIPER (1975) have shown that these metabolites have biological activity and that a distinction cannot be made by bioassay between a low dose of parent PG or high doses of metabolites. Since the release of PGs from perfused lungs by Bk was detected by bioassay (PALMER et al., 1973), PG metabolites may have accounted for some of the activity detected.

The fact that Bk induces PG biosynthesis in several different tissues (lung, kidney, ileum, blood vessels), irrespective of whether it contracts or relaxes smooth muscle, suggests that a common biochemical mechanism underlies the process. The first clue to such a mechanism came from the work of VARGAFTIG and DAO HAI (1972). They used guinea pig isolated lungs to demonstrate the release of RCS by Bk and arachidonic acid. The release induced by Bk was suppressed by mepacrine, whereas that caused by arachidonic acid was not. Because mepacrine has been described as an inhibitor of phospholipase A (MARKUS and BALL, 1969), VARGAFTIG suggested that Bk activates an acylhydrolase and causes release of PG precursors. FLOWER and BLACKWELL (1976) have shown that mepacrine does indeed inhibit the release of PG precursors from phospholipid pools in slices of guinea pig spleen.

STONER et al. (1973) measured concentrations of cyclic nucleotides in slices of guinea pig lung. With concentrations of Bk varying from 1–100 µg/ml, they found a rapid rise in both cGMP and cAMP. Indomethacin or aspirin prevented the rise in cAMP but did not affect the rise in cGMP, and because of this it was concluded that release of a PG mediated the rise in cAMP. STONER et al. (1973) suggested that in lung and probably in other tissues, Bk enhances the synthesis and release of PGs as one of the consequences of its effect on cGMP metabolism. However, another possibility is that the cGMP effects are unrelated to PG formation and it would be interesting to find whether mepacrine interfered with stimulation of cGMP formation by Bk.

E. Actions of Prostaglandins in the Lungs

I. Bronchial Smooth Muscle

The actions of various PGs have been investigated both in conscious man, anaesthetised experimental animals in vivo and on isolated airway smooth muscle in vitro (Table 1). ROSENTHALE et al. (1970) showed the bronchodilator effects of PGE_2 given

Table 1. Actions of prostaglandins on respiratory smooth muscle in vitro

Prostaglandin	Species	Action	References
RCS	Human	↑	PIPER and WALKER, 1973
E_1	Cat	↓	HORTON, 1969
	Monkey	↓	
	Rabbit	↓	
	Guinea pig	↓	
	Ferret	↓	
	Sheep	↓	
	Pig	↓	
	Human	↓	
	Calf	↓	LEWIS and EYRE, 1972
E_2	Cat	↓	MAIN, 1964
	Human	↓	HORTON, 1969
15-keto-E_2	Guinea pig	↓	CRUTCHLEY and PIPER, 1975
E_2	Cat	↓	MAIN, 1964
$F_{1\alpha}$	Cat	↓	MAIN, 1964
$F_{2\alpha}$	Human	↑	COLLIER and SWEATMAN, 1968
	Calf	—	LEWIS and EYRE, 1972
15-keto-$F_{2\alpha}$	Guinea pig	↑	BENZIE, BOOT and DAWSON, 1973
D_2	Guinea pig	↑	HAMBERG and SAMUELSSON, 1973
G_2	Guinea pig	↑	HAMBERG and SAMUELSSON, 1973
H_2	Guinea pig	↑	HAMBERG and SAMUELSSON, 1974b

by aerosol in guinea pig, dog and monkey in vivo. $PGF_{2\alpha}$ causes bronchocon-striction in the Konzett-Rössler preparation of guinea pig (BERRY and COLLIER, 1964). SMITH and CUTHBERT (1973) have studied the effects of PGE_2 and $PGF_{2\alpha}$ in the lungs of both normal and asthmatic human subjects. When given by aerosol, $PGF_{2\alpha}$ increased fast expired volume (FEV), whereas PGE_2 decreased this function, indicating that $PGF_{2\alpha}$ was a bronchoconstrictor but that PGE_2 was a bronchodila-tor. However, when given intravenously, PGE_2 had variable effects on the airways of asthmatic patients (SMITH, 1974). This was probably due to metabolism of the PG in the pulmonary circulation (JOSE et al., 1976).

MATHÉ et al. (1974) found that asthmatic patients were 8000 times more sensitive to the bronchoconstrictor effects of $PGF_{2\alpha}$ given by aerosol than were normal heal-thy subjects. SMITH and co-workers (1973) confirmed an increased sensitivity to $PGF_{2\alpha}$, but at a level of 160-fold. This discrepancy may be partly explained by different methods of calculation used by the two groups (SMITH, personal communi-cation).

The actions of PGs, their precursors and metabolites have been investigated on isolated smooth muscle from airways, often on extrapulmonary airway smooth mus-cle which had been previously contracted by, for instance, acetylcholine. PG endoper-oxides, TXA_2, PGE_1, PGE_2, and $PGF_{2\alpha}$ are all released from lung tissue (PIPER and VANE, 1969a, b; PIPER and WALKER, 1973; HAMBERG et al., 1975b). BENZIE et al. (1975) showed that lung synthetase was also capable of forming PGD_2, but this PG has not been found in lung effluent. In addition to the parent PGs, the metabolites are also released during anaphylaxis in guinea pig lung. The 15-oxo metabolites are bronchoactive although they have not been detected in lung effluent, possibly be-

Table 2. Actions of prostaglandins on blood vessels of the lung

Prostaglandin	Species	Vessel	Action	Reference
RCS	Rabbit	Pulmonary a	↑	PALMER et al., 1973
		Pulmonary v	↑	
	Man	Intrapulmonary a		
		Intrapulmonary v		
E_1	Calf	Pulmonary a	↓	LEWIS and EYRE, 1972
		Pulmonary v	↓	LEWIS and EYRE, 1972
	Dog	Intrapulmonary a	↓	KADOWITZ et al., 1975
		Intrapulmonary v	↓	KADOWITZ et al., 1975
	Baboon	Intrapulmonary a	↑	
	Sheep	Intrapulmonary a	↓	
		Intrapulmonary v	↓	
E_2	Calf	Pulmonary a	↓	LEWIS and EYRE, 1972
		Pulmonary v	↓	LEWIS and EYRE, 1972
	Dog	Intrapulmonary a	—	KADOWITZ et al., 1975
		Intrapulmonary v	↑	KADOWITZ et al., 1975
$F_{1\alpha}$	Dog	Intrapulmonary a	↑	KADOWITZ et al., 1975
		Intrapulmonary v	↑	KADOWITZ et al., 1975
$F_{2\alpha}$	Calf	Pulmonary a	↑	LEWIS and EYRE, 1972
		Pulmonary v	↑	LEWIS and EYRE, 1972
	Baboon, chimpanzee	Intrapulmonary a	↑	KADOWITZ et al., 1975
		Intrapulmonary v	↑	KADOWITZ et al., 1975
	Man	Intrapulmonary a	↑	KADOWITZ et al., 1975
		Intrapulmonary v	↑	KADOWITZ et al., 1975
	Sheep	Intrapulmonary a	—	KADOWITZ et al., 1975
		Intrapulmonary v	↑	KADOWITZ et al., 1975
A_1	Dog	Intrapulmonary a	—	KADOWITZ et al., 1975
		Intrapulmonary v	↑	KADOWITZ et al., 1975
A_2				
B_1	Dog	Intrapulmonary a	↑	KADOWITZ et al., 1975
B_2		Intrapulmonary a	↑	KADOWITZ et al., 1975

cause they are rapidly metabolised. They may, however, exist long enough to have an action on smooth muscle in the lung. Generally, the E-type PGs relax airway smooth muscle while F-type PGs contract it. 15-oxo PGE_2 is a more potent bronchodilator than PGE_2 (CRUTCHLEY and PIPER, 1975) but reports on 15-oxo $PGF_{2\alpha}$ are controversial.

The actions of PGs on isolated pulmonary blood vessels are shown in Table 2. The blood vessels of the lungs of several species are sensitive to the actions of PGs. Usually, E-type PGs relax pulmonary vascular smooth muscle but there is some species variation in the reaction of intrapulmonary blood vessels. RCS and F-type PGs contract all pulmonary and intrapulmonary blood vessels (PALMER et al., 1973; KADOWITZ et al., 1975). The intrapulmonary vessels will be exposed to the PGs released in the lung by agents such as Bk, SRS-A or histamine.

Bk constricts the pulmonary vein of guinea pig perfused lungs (GREEF and MOOG, 1964) and this could be due to release of either RCS or F-type PG, perhaps from the vessel wall. Bk may also cause vasodilatation partly through PG release from other tissues, as well as from the lungs. The effect may take place locally in the vessel wall, without the released PG entering the circulation. AIKEN (1974) has shown that the Bk-induced relaxations of isolated strips of coeliac artery from the rabbit (maintained in a contracted state by noradrenaline) is completely abolished by indomethacin or fenoprofen. Relaxations induced by PGE_2 were unaffected.

F. Interaction of Bradykinin With Prostaglandins in the Lungs

I. As a Mediator

At low concentrations, substances such as indomethacin and meclofenamate have a selective inhibitory action on PG synthetase. Higher concentrations are needed to inhibit other enzymes. Thus, when the reactions of an organ or a tissue to Bk are modified by low concentrations of indomethacin or other substances which inhibit PG biosynthesis, we can assume that the modification is due to removal of the PG component of the activity of Bk. Those bronchoconstrictor actions of Bk which are suppressed by aspirin-like drugs may be assigned to the PG which is released. In this context, it is interesting to note that both $PGF_{2\alpha}$ and RCS cause contractions of isolated strips of human bronchial muscle (PIPER and WALKER, 1973). Indeed, the cyclic endoperoxide intermediates isolated by NUGTEREN and HAZELHOF (1973), HAMBERG et al. (1974), SAMUELSSON and HAMBERG (1974) have several-fold the potency of $PGF_{2\alpha}$ on isolated bronchial muscle. Thus, the induced local generation of any one of these PGs (but not of PGE_2, which is a bronchodilator) can account for that part of the bronchoconstrictor action of Bk which is abolished by aspirin-like drugs.

IORIO and CONSTANTINE (1969) studied the effects of Bk on guinea pig isolated tracheal muscle. On repeated exposure to Bk, the responses gradually changed from contractions to relaxations. The relaxation induced by Bk was prevented by discontinuing the aeration of the tissues. Phenylbutazone selectively reversed the Bk-induced relaxation. Although the authors postulated that the effects of Bk depended upon the level of tissue tone, it is now evident that the gradual replacement of a contraction by a relaxation can be explained by the induction in the preparation of the synthesis of a PG of the E series. The observation that Bk elicited only contractions in those preparations which were not aerated fits with the fact that PG synthesis depends upon molecular oxygen (SAMUELSSON et al., 1967; NUGTEREN et al., 1967).

II. As a Potentiator

In all of the above reactions, the PG released by Bk contributes to the eventual response through inducing an effect similar to that of Bk. Thus, the PG wholly or partially *mediates* the response to Bk.

FERREIRA (1972) suggested that the main contribution that PGs made to the pain of inflammation was through their ability to sensitize the sensory nerve endings to mechanical or chemical stimulation. PGs may have a similar action in the lung and sensitize the receptors for kinins on the smooth muscle cells and maybe the "lung irritant receptors" (MILLS et al., 1969) to the actions of Bk and other mediators.

III. As a Mediator of Vascular Leakage

The increased vascular leakage brought about by Bk is also potentiated by low concentrations of PGs. In high concentrations, PGs, like Bk, histamine and 5-hydroxytryptamine (5-HT), cause increased vascular permeability by inducing vascular leakage at the post-capillary and collecting venules (KALEY and WEINER, 1971). However, PGs produce more vasodilatation than they do oedema.

From the experiments of MONCADA et al. (1973) with carrageenin-induced oedema in the rat paw, it was concluded that low concentrations of PGs sensitize the blood vessels to the permeability-increasing effects of the other mediators of inflammation. By the use of a specific Bk potentiating factor (BPP_{9a}) (FERREIRA, 1965; GREENE et al., 1972), it was also shown that Bk is continuously involved as one of these mediators in carrageenin oedema (FERREIRA et al., 1977). When given at 0.1, 4 or 6 h in a dose which by itself has no effect, BPP_{9a} significantly increased the oedema formation induced by carrageenin. The rat paw swelling induced by Bk or histamine was also substantially increased when small concentrations of PGE_1 were included.

THOMAS and WEST (1973) found that low concentrations of PGE_1 selectively potentiated the permeability increase in rat skin induced by Bk. WILLIAMS and MORLEY (1973), making use of the little-known fact that PGs do not, by themselves, cause increased vascular permeability on intradermal injection in the guinea pig (HORTON, 1963), studied the potentiating effects of PGs on vascular leakage induced by Bk and other substances. They found that the addition of 1 µg of PGE_1 to a similar dose of Bk produced a nearly 100-fold increase in the potency of Bk in causing vascular leakage. They also showed that the effects of histamine and of three allergic inflammatory reactions (passive cutaneous anaphylaxis, reversed passive Arthus and delayed sensitivity) were potentiated by PGE_1 in concentrations as little as a few nanograms. PGs released by Bk in the lung may similarly potentiate vascular leakage caused by Bk in pulmonary and bronchial vessels.

G. Metabolism of Kinins in the Pulmonary Circulation

Bk is quickly destroyed in blood and its half-life is about 17 s in rats, cats and dogs (FERREIRA and VANE, 1967a, c, d; McCARTHY et al., 1965). FERREIRA and VANE (1967a) showed that when Bk enters the pulmonary circulation it is rapidly inactivated, approximately 80% disappearing during one passage through the lungs of a cat. Similar inactivation of Bk takes place in the pulmonary circulation of rat, guinea pig, dog and sheep (ALABASTER and BAKHLE, 1972a, b; BIRON, 1968; HERBERT et al., 1972; POJDA and VANE, 1971).

Bk does not leave the vascular space in rat lungs and is inactivated in the pulmonary circulation by enzymic hydrolysis of peptide bonds (RYAN et al., 1970). There are several enzymes causing this metabolism of Bk in the lung and they are thought to be on or near the cells of the vascular endothelium. It seems that the peptidase which converts angiotensin I to angiotensin II in the pulmonary circulation also hydrolyses Bk (IGIC et al., 1972), as first suggested by NG and VANE (1968).

H. Inhibition of Bronchoconstriction by Anti-Inflammatory Acids

I. In vivo and in vitro Studies

In 1960, before it was known that non-steroid anti-inflammatory drugs are potent inhibitors of PG synthetase, COLLIER and SHORLEY (1963) found that aspirin was an effective inhibitor of Bk-induced bronchoconstriction in the Konzett-Rössler preparation of guinea pig. Bronchoconstriction caused by acetylcholine or histamine was unaffected. Subsequently, COLLIER and his co-workers found that other anti-inflammatory acids inhibit Bk bronchoconstriction in guinea pig in vivo (Table 3). With aspirin, the antagonism of Bk bronchoconstriction is not truly competitive since the logarithmic dose-response curve has unit slope only for lower concentrations of antagonist (COLLIER and SHORLEY, 1963). The antagonism is long-lasting and does not recover in 5 h. Steroid anti-inflammatory drugs were not active in inhibiting Bk bronchoconstriction. The antagonism of Bk-induced bronchoconstriction by aspirin and meclofenamate was unaffected by vagotomy, destruction of the brain and spinal cord, bilateral adrenalectomy or β-adrenoceptor blockade (COLLIER and SHORLEY, 1963; COLLIER et al., 1968).

In lightly anaesthetised guinea pigs, Bk causes tachypnoea (GJURIS et al., 1964) which is a reflex elicited by bronchoconstriction and is abolished by vagotomy or isoprenaline (MARQUARDT, 1966). The tachypnoea is readily abolished by aspirin and the other anti-inflammatory acids in doses similar to those inhibiting bronchoconstriction (COLLIER, 1965). In perfused and artificially ventilated guinea pig isolated lungs in vitro, bronchoconstriction can be elicited by Bk and this is inhibited by aspirin or phenylbutazone. Bronchoconstriction elicited by histamine or 5-HT in this preparation is not antagonised (GREEF and MOOG, 1964). However, AARSEN (1966) failed to inhibit Bk-induced bronchoconstriction in guinea pig isolated lungs with non-steroid anti-inflammatory drugs.

As mentioned previously, Bk is less active in contracting guinea pig isolated trachea in vitro than in causing bronchoconstriction in vivo. This action is antagonised by aspirin and phenylbutazone but the potency and specificity of these drugs is

Table 3. Minimal effective doses (MED) of antagonists given intravenously in reducing bronchoconstriction induced by bradykinin

Antagonist	MED mg/kg IV	
Acetylsalicylic acid (sodium or calcium salt)	2	
Sodium phenylbutazone	4	
Amidopyrine	8	
Phenazone	8	COLLIER and SHORLEY (1963)
Paracetamol	16	
Sodium mefenamate	1	
Sodium flufenamate	1	
Glafenine	4	
Ibuprofen	8	
Indomethacin	2	COLLIER et al. (1968)
Indoxole	0.25	
Sodium meclofenamate	0.06	

less than in guinea pig isolated perfused lungs in vitro or in the whole animal in vivo (GREEF and MOOG, 1964; COLLIER and SHORLEY, 1960). Bk induces bronchoconstriction when dropped onto the pleural surface of guinea pig lungs in vivo but aspirin is ineffective against bronchoconstriction induced by this means (BHOOLA et al., 1962).

The fact that most of the actions of Bk in the lung are inhibited by PG synthetase inhibitors strongly suggests that these actions of Bk are at least partly mediated by metabolites of arachidonic acid, such as PGs or their precursors. Although some of these drugs also affect other enzymes and cellular functions (PAULUS and WHITE-HOUSE, 1973; SHEN, 1972; SMITH and Dawkins, 1971; COLLIER and GARDINER, 1974), it would be truly remarkable if *all* the PG synthetase inhibitors also similarly affected a different enzyme system.

The order of potency of aspirin-like drugs for antagonism of Bk-induced bronchoconstriction is, in descending order, meclofenamate > mefenamate/flufenamate > indomethacin > aspirin > phenylbutazone > ibuprofen > paracetamol (FLOWER, 1974). However, when making such a generalisation, it must be remembered that the potency of the drugs varies according to the source of PG synthetase. It is interesting that aspirin is a competitive non-reversible inhibitor of PG synthetase (SMITH and LANDS, 1971) and that inhibition of Bk bronchoconstriction in vivo is apparently non-reversible.

II. Comparison With Other Bronchoconstrictor Agents

Agents other than Bk which cause bronchoconstriction in the guinea pig in vivo are listed in Table 4. These include SRS-A, partially purified with charcoal (BERRY and COLLIER, 1964). When injected into guinea pig perfused lungs, the same SRS-A released RCS and PGs and may therefore have contained RCS-RF (PIPER and VANE, 1969 b). SRS-A produced by AUSTEN and his co-workers by a different extraction procedure had little bronchoconstrictor activity in the guinea pig but reduced compliance (DRAZEN et al., 1973). Both the release of mediators from isolated lungs in vitro and the bronchoconstriction in vivo caused by charcoal-purified SRS-A are inhibited by aspirin-like drugs (PIPER and VANE, 1969 a; BERRY and COLLIER, 1964).

Arachidonic acid releases RCS and PGs from guinea pig isolated lungs and causes bronchoconstriction in anaesthetised guinea pigs (VARGAFTIG and DAO HAI, 1972; PALMER et al., 1973; BERRY and COLLIER, 1964). Both of these actions of

Table 4. Effects of aspirin-like drugs on bronchoconstriction induced by substances other than kinins

Agent	Inhibited by aspirin-like drugs	Reference
Histamine	−	COLLIER and SHORLEY, 1963
5-Hydroxytryptamine	−	BERRY and COLLIER, 1964
SRS-A (charcoal purified)	+	BERRY and COLLIER, 1964
Arachidonic acid	+	BERRY, 1966
ATP	+	COLLIER et al., 1966
Prostaglandin $F_{2\alpha}$		BERRY and COLLIER, 1964
Prostaglandin G_2H_2	Not tested	
Thromboxane	Not tested	

arachidonic acid are inhibited by non-steroid anti-inflammatory agents. COLLIER et al. (1966) found that ATP given intravenously in this species causes bronchoconstriction which is antagonised by aspirin.

Thus it appears that, as with Bk, the bronchoconstriction caused by the above agents is mediated, at least in part, by products of arachidonic acid metabolism. The inhibition of bronchoconstriction by aspirin-like drugs is due to antagonism of the formation of these products. Bronchoconstriction by histamine, 5-HT and $PGF_{2\alpha}$ is not blocked by aspirin but there is evidence that PGs are released from tracheal (and maybe bronchial) smooth muscle as it contracts (OREHEK et al., 1973). Histamine and 5-HT, therefore, appear to be strong bronchoconstrictor agents which do not require the potentiating effects of PGs. All the agents causing aspirin-sensitive bronchoconstriction have flatter dose-response curves than, for example, histamine, and are subject to tachyphylaxis. This could be due to failure of repeated doses of agonist to continue to release PGs.

I. Possible Actions and Interactions of Kinins and Prostaglandins in Asthma

Bk certainly contributes to signs of anaphylaxis in the guinea pig, for making the guinea pig tolerant to Bk before challenge lessens the severity of anaphylactic bronchoconstriction (COLLIER and JAMES, 1967). Although there are fundamental differences between asthma and anaphylaxis in the guinea pig, there are some similarities which merit consideration. There is evidence that kinin levels in the blood rise in severe asthma (ABE et al., 1967) and these substances are present in the secretions of the respiratory tract in asthmatics, hay fever sufferers and bronchitics (DOLOVICH et al., 1968). Kinins and kininogen have been found in extracts of human lung adenocarcinoma (DI MATTEI, 1967). Kinins released during anaphylaxis in guinea pig are probably formed by kallikrein released from the lung during anaphylactic shock (JONASSON and BECKER, 1966); a similar release of kallikrein may occur in human lung in asthma thus forming kinins.

PGs E_1, E_2 and $F_{2\alpha}$ are released in anaphylaxis in human lung (PIPER and WALKER, 1973). A PG metabolite, 13,14-dihydro-15-keto $PGF_{2\alpha}$, has been found in peripheral venous blood after asthmatic attack (GRÉEN et al., 1974). Kinins released in vivo may in turn release PGs from lung tissue. Kinins and F-type PGs (also their endoperoxide precursors) will cause bronchoconstriction. The released PGs may sensitize the bronchial smooth muscle to the action of Bk. The physiological function of this constriction of the airways may be to limit further inhalation of antigen. E-type PGs (together with released catecholamines) will tend to reverse bronchoconstriction, but their main function may be to cause vasodilatation, divert blood away from underventilated areas and maintain ventilation/perfusion ratios. There is evidence for increased sensitivity of the "lung irritant receptors" in asthma (GOLD, 1973), possibly due to the action of PGs.

Effective inactivation mechanisms for kinins and PGs exist in the pulmonary circulation of man (BIRON, 1968; JOSE et al., 1976) and animals (FERREIRA and VANE, 1967a, c, d; VANE, 1969). This strongly suggests that kinins and PGs affect lung function, as a mechanism of destruction often exists close to a site of action of local hormones (COLLIER, 1970). However, the fact that non-steroid anti-inflammatory drugs are effective in only a minority of asthmatics, must indicate that kinins and PGs have only a limited role in most asthmatic patients, the most important mediators being either histamine and SRS-A or others, as yet undiscovered.

J. Summary and Conclusions

Bk is one of the mediators released during anaphylactic shock in the guinea pig in vivo and in vitro and probably during asthmatic attack in the human. Bk is released together with histamine, SRS-A, ECF-A, RCS-RF, PGs and RCS (a mixture of TXA_2 and PG endoperoxides).

Bk contracts bronchial smooth muscle of the fine airways, an action which varies in intensity between species. In the guinea pig, Bk is more potent as a bronchoconstrictor agent in vivo than in vitro and induces an asthmatic attack in asthmatic patients but not in normal humans. The overall effect of kinins in guinea pig lung is to lessen lung compliance by constricting airways and contracting smooth muscle in the pleura. Bk releases catecholamines from the adrenal medulla by direct action and as a reflex effect of bronchoconstriction; this tends to reverse the bronchoconstrictor action. Bk is inactivated during passage through the pulmonary circulation but at the same time constricts the pulmonary vein.

PGs and thromboxanes are released from guinea pig lung in vitro and probably in vivo by Bk and other anaphylactic mediators such as SRS-A, RCS-RF and sometimes histamine. Bk appears to initiate arachidonic acid metabolism by activating phospholipase A. It seems that prostaglandins or thromboxanes are essential for at least part of the actions of Bk on lung function since PG synthetase inhibitors are effective antagonists of Bk-induced bronchoconstriction. F-type PGs and PGG_2 and PGH_2 (endoperoxide precursors of PGs) are bronchoconstrictors but they may also act by potentiating the inherent airway smooth muscle-contracting activity of Bk. There must be a greater supply of substrate for PG synthetase in lung tissue in vivo than in vitro which would explain the greater potency of Bk in vivo. The release of PGs by SRS-A (charcoal purified) and arachidonic acid, and the inhibition of bronchoconstriction in vivo by aspirin-like drugs, has been discussed and compared with similar actions of Bk. Kinins may have a role in asthma and the sensitivity of asthmatics to Bk could be explained by the fact that PGs are released more easily from sensitized lung than normal lung (PALMER et al., 1973) and therefore potentiate the action of Bk. This is probably because there is an increased level of PG synthetase in sensitized lungs (BENZIE et al., 1975). However, the lack of effect of aspirin-like drugs in asthma remains unexplained, but this may be due to inability to inhibit an established response.

References

Aarsen, P. N.: The influence of analgesic antipyretic drugs on the responses of guinea pig lungs to bradykinin. Brit. J. Pharmacol. 27, 196—204 (1966)

Abe, K., Watanabe, N., Kumagai, N., Mouri, T., Seki, T., Yoshinaga, K.: Circulating plasma kinin in patients with bronchial asthma. Experientia (Basel) 23, 626—627 (1967)

Aiken, J. W.: Inhibitors of prostaglandin synthesis specifically antagonize bradykinin and angio-tensin-induced relaxations of the isolated coeliac artery from rabbit. Pharmacologist **16**, 295 (1974)

Alabaster, V. A., Bakhle, Y. S.: The inactivation of bradykinin in the pulmonary circulation of isolated lungs. Brit. J. Pharmacol. **45**, 299—309 (1972a)

Alabaster, V. A., Bakhle, Y. S.: Converting enzyme and bradykinase in the lung. Circulat. Res. **30/31**, 72—81 (1972b)

Benzie, R., Boot, J. R., Dawson, W.: A preliminary investigation of prostaglandin synthetase activity in normal, sensitized and challenged sensitized guinea pig lungs. J. Physiol. (Lond.) **246**, 80P (1975)

Beraldo, W. T.: Formation of bradykinin in anaphylactic and peptone shock. Am. J. Physiol. **163**, 283—289 (1950)

Berry, P. A.: Slow reacting substance of anaphylaxis (SRS-A): its release, action and antagonism. Ph. D. Thesis, Council for National Academic Awards, 1966

Berry, P. A., Collier, H. O. J.: Bronchoconstrictor action and antagonism of a slow-reacting substance from anaphylaxis of guinea pig lung. Brit. J. Pharmacol. **23**, 201—216 (1964)

Bhoola, K. D., Schachter, M.: A comparison of serum kallikrein, bradykinin and histamine on capillary permeability in the guinea pig. J. Physiol. (Lond.) **149**, 80P—81P (1959)

Bhoola, K. D., Collier, H. O. J., Schachter, M., Shorley, P. G.: Actions of some peptides on bronchial muscle. Brit. J. Pharmacol. **19**, 190—197 (1962)

Biron, P.: Pulmonary extraction of bradykinin and eledoisin. Rev. Can. Biol. **27**, 75—76 (1968)

Brocklehurst, W. D., Lahiri, S. C.: The production of bradykinin in anaphylaxis. J. Physiol. (Lond.) 15P—16P (1962)

Brocklehurst, W. D., Lahiri, S. C.: Formation and destruction of bradykinin during anaphylaxis. J. Physiol. (Lond.) **165**, 39P—40P (1963)

Collier, H. O. J.: Some pharmacological correlates of anti-inflammatory activity. A study of non-steroidal anti-inflammatory drugs as antagonists of local hormones. In: Garattini, S., Dukes, M. N. G. (Eds.): Non-Steroidal Anti-Inflammatory Drugs, pp. 139—150. Amsterdam: Excerpta Medica Foundation 1965

Collier, H. O. J.: New light on how aspirin works. Nature **223**, 35—37 (1969)

Collier, H. O. J.: Kinins and ventilation of the lungs. In: Erdös, E. G. (Ed.): Handbook of Experimental Pharmacology, Bradykinin, Kallidin and Kallidrein, Vol. XXV, pp. 409—420. Berlin-Heidelberg-New York: Springer 1970

Collier, H. O. J., Gardiner, P. J.: Pharmacology of airways smooth muscle. In: Burley, D. M., Clarke, S. W., Cuthbert, M. F., Paterson, J. W., Shelley, J. H. (Eds.): Evaluation of Bronchodilator Drugs, pp. 17—27. London: Trust for Education & Research in Therapeutics 1974

Collier, H. O. J., James, G. W. L.: Bradykinin and slow-reacting substance in anaphylactic bronchoconstriction in the guinea pig in vivo. J. Physiol. (Lond.) **185**, 71P—72P (1966)

Collier, H. O. J., James, G. W. L.: Humoral factors affecting pulmonary inflation during acute anaphylaxis in the guinea pig in vivo. Brit. J. Pharmacol. **30**, 283—301 (1967)

Collier, H. O. J., Shorley, P. G.: Analgesic antipyretic drugs as antagonists of bradykinin. Brit. J. Pharmacol. **15**, 601—610 (1960)

Collier, H. O. J., Shorley, P. G.: Antagonism by mefenamic and flufenamic acids of the bronchoconstrictor action of kinins in the guinea pig. Brit. J. Pharmacol. **20**, 345—351 (1963)

Collier, H. O. J., Sweatman, W. J. F.: Antagonism by fenamates of prostaglandin $F_{2\alpha}$ and of a slow reacting substance on human bronchial muscle. Nature **219**, 864—865 (1968)

Collier, H. O. J., Holgate, J. A., Schachter, M., Shorley, P. G.: An apparent bronchoconstrictor action of bradykinin and its suppression by some anti-inflammatory drugs. J. Physiol. (Lond.) **149**, 54P—55P (1959)

Collier, H. O. J., Holgate, J. A., Schachter, M., Shorley, P. G.: The bronchoconstrictor action of bradykinin in the guinea pig. Brit. J. Pharmacol. **15**, 290—297 (1960)

Collier, H. O. J., James, G. W. L., Schneider, C.: Antagonism by aspirin and fenamates of bronchoconstriction and nociception induced by adenosine-5'-triphosphate. Nature (Lond.) **212**, 411—412 (1966)

Collier, H. O. J., James, G. W. L., Piper, P. J.: Intensification by adrenalectomy or by β-adrenergic blockade of the bronchoconstriction induced by bradykinin in the guinea-pig. J. Physiol. (Lond.) **180**, 13P—14P (1967)

Collier, H. O. J., James, G. W. L., Piper, P. J.: Antagonism by fenamates and like-acting drugs of bronchoconstriction induced by bradykinin or antigen in the guinea pig. Brit. J. Pharmacol. **34**, 76—87 (1968)

Crutchley, D. J., Piper, P. J.: Comparative bioassay of pulmonary metabolites of prostaglandin E_2. Brit. J. Pharmacol. **54**, 397—399 (1975)

Dawson, W., Lewis, R. L., McMahohn, R. E. Sweatman, W. J. F.: Potent bronchoconstrictor activity of 15-Keto-$PGF_{2\alpha}$. Nature **250**, 331—332 (1974)

Di Mattei: Occurence of bradykinin in human pulmonary carcinoma. Biochem. Pharmacol. **16**, 909—911 (1967)

Dolovich, J., Back, N., Arbesman, C. E.: The presence of bradykinin-like activity in nasal secretions from allergic subjects. J. Allergy Absts. **41**, 103 (1968)

Drazen, J. M., Imming, D. J., Stechschulte, D. J., Amdur, M. O., Austen, K. F., Mead, J.: Effects of intravenous slow-reacting substance of anaphylaxis (SRS-A) on respiratory mechanics. Fed. Proc. **32**, 402 (Abs.) (1973)

Elliott, D. F., Horton, E. W., Lewis, G. P.: Actions of pure bradykinin. J. Physiol. (Lond.) **153**, 473—480 (1960)

Eyre, P. Lewis, A. J.: Production of kinins in bovine anaphylactic shock. Brit. J. Pharmacol. **44**, 311—313 (1972)

Feldberg, W., Lewis, G. P.: The action of peptides on the adrenal medulla. Release of adrenaline by bradykinin and angiotensin. J. Physiol. (Lond.) **171**, 98—108 (1964)

Ferreira, S. H.: A bradykinin potentiating factor (BPF) present in the venom of *Bothrops jararaca*. Brit. J. Pharmacol. **24**, 163—169 (1965)

Ferreira, S. H.: Prostaglandins, aspirin-like drugs and analgesia. Nature [New Biol.] **240**, 200—203 (1972)

Ferreira, S. H., Vane, J. R.: The disappearance of bradykinin and eledoisin in the circulation and vascular beds of the cat. Brit. J. Pharmacol. **30**, 417—424 (1967 a)

Ferreira, S. H., Vane, J. R.: The detection and estimation of bradykinin in the circulating blood. Brit. J. Pharmacol. **29**, 367—377 (1967 b)

Ferreira, S. H., Vane, J. R.: Prostaglandins: their disappearance from and release into the circulation. Nature **216**, 868—873 (1967 c)

Ferreira, S. H., Vane, J. R.: Half-lifes of peptides and amines in the circulation. Nature **215**, 1237—1240 (1967 d)

Ferreira, S. H., Moncada, S., Parsons, M. F., Vane, J. R.: The concomitant release of bradykinin and prostaglandin in the inflammatory response to carrageenin. Brit. J. Pharmacol. **52**, 108P (1974)

Ferreira, S. H., Zanin, M. T., Lorenzetti, B. B.: Relationships between increased vascular permeability, oedema and hyperalgesia. In: Willougby, D. A., Giroud, J. P., Velo, G. P. (Eds.): Perspectives in Inflammation. Future trends and developments, pp. 507—518. MTP Press Ltd, Lancaster

Flower, R. J.: Drugs which inhibit prostaglandin biosynthesis. Pharmacol. Rev. **26**, 33—57 (1974)

Flower, R. J., Blackwell, G. J.: The importance of phospholipase-A_2 in prostaglandin biosynthesis. Biochem. Pharmacol. **25**, 285—291 (1976)

Gjuris, V., Westermann, E.: Zur Frage der bronchoconstrictorischen Wirkung des Bradykinins, Kallidins and Eledoisins. Naunyn Schmiedebergs Arch. Pharmakol. **246**, 17—19 (1963)

Gjuris, V., Heicke, B., Westermann, E.: Über die Stimulierung der Atmung durch Bradykinin and Kallidin. Naunyn Schmiedebergs Arch. Pharmakol. **247**, 429—444 (1964)

Goetzl, E. J., Austen, K. F.: Purification and synthesis of eosinophilotactic tetrapeptides of human lung tissue: Identification as eosinophil chemotactic factor of anaphylaxis. Proc. Nat. Acad. Sci. U.S.A. **72**, 4123—4127 (1975)

Gold, W. M.: Cholinadrenergic Pharmacology in Asthma. In: Austen, J. F., Lichtenstein, L. M. (Eds.): Asthma Physiology, Pharmacology and Treatment, pp. 169—184. New York: Academic Press 1973

Gray, J. A. B., Diamond, J.: Pharmacological properties of sensory receptors. Brit. Med. Bull. **13**, 185—188 (1957)

Greef, K., Moog, E.: Vergleichende Untersuchungen über die bronchoconstriktorische und gefäßconstriktorische Wirkung des Bradykinins, Histamins und Serotonins und isolierten Lungenpräparaten. Naunyn Schmiedebergs Arch. Pharmakol. **248**, 204—215 (1964)

Gréen, K., Hedqvist, P., Svanborg, N.: Increased plasma levels of 15-keto-13, 14-dihydroprostaglandin $F_{2\alpha}$ after allergenprovoked asthma in man. Lancet **1974 II**, 1419—1421

Greene, J. J., Camargo, A. C., Krieg, E., Stewart, J. M., Ferreira, S. H.: Inhibiton of the conversion of angiotensin I to II and potentiation of bradykinin by small peptides present in *Bothrops jararaca* venom. Circ. Res. **31**, 62—71 (1972)

Gryglewski, R., Vane, J. R.: Generation from arachidonic acid of rabbit aorta contracting substance (RCS) by a microsomal enzyme preparation which also generates prostaglandins. Brit. J. Pharmacol. **46**, 449—457 (1972)

Hamberg, M., Samuelsson, B.: Prostaglandin endoperoxides. Novel transformations of arachidonic acid in human platelets. Proc. Natl. Acad. Sci. U.S.A. **71**, 3400—3404 (1974a)

Hamberg, M., Samuelsson, B.: Prostaglandin endoperoxides VII. Novel transformations of arachidonic acid in guinea pig lung. Biochim. Biophys. Res. Commun. **61**, 942—949 (1974b)

Hamberg, M., Hedqvist, P., Strandberg, K., Svensson, J., Samuelsson, B.: Prostaglandin endoperoxides IV. Effects on smooth muscle. Life Sci. **16**, 461—462 (1975a)

Hamberg, M., Svensson, J., Samuelsson, B.: Thromboxane: a new group of biologically active compounds derived from prostaglandin endoperoxides. Proc. Natl. Acad. Sci. U.S.A. **72**, 2994—2998 (1975b)

Hamberg, M., Svensson, J., Wakabayashi, T., Samuelsson, B.: Isolation and structure of two prostaglandin endoperoxides that cause platelet aggregation. Proc. Nat. Acad. Sci. U.S.A. **71**, 345—349 (1974)

Haug, A., Lunde, P. K. M., Waaler, B. A.: The effect of bradykinin, kallidin and eledoisin upon the pulmonary vascular bed of an isolated perfused rabbit lung preparation. Acta Physiol. Scand. **66**, 269—277 (1966)

Hebert, F., Fouron, J. C., Boileau, J. C., Biron, P.: Pulmonary fate of vasoactive peptides in fetal, newborn and adult sheep. Am. J. Physiol. **225**, 20—23 (1972)

Herxheimer, H., Stresemann, E.: The effect of bradykinin aerosol in guinea pigs and in man. J. Physiol. (Lond.) **158**, 38P (1961)

Herxheimer, H., Stresemann, E.: The effect of slow reacting substance (SRS-A) in guinea pigs and asthmatic patients. J. Physiol. (Lond.) **165**, 78P—79P (1963)

Horton, E. W.: Action of prostaglandin E_1 on tissue which responds to bradykinin. Nature **200**, 892—893 (1963)

Horton, E. W.: Hypothesis on physiological roles of prostaglandins. Physiol. Rev. **49**, 122—161 (1969)

Hyman, A. L.: The effects of bradykinin on the pulmonary vein. J. Pharmacol. Exp. Ther. **161**, 78—87 (1968)

Igic, R., Erdos, E. G., Yeh, H. S. J., Sorrells, K., Nakajima, T.: Angiotensin I converting enzyme of the lung. Circ. Res. **31**, 51—61 (1972)

Iorio, L. C., Constantine, J. W.: Bradykinin on isolated guinea pig tracheal muscle. J. Pharmacol. Exp. Ther. **169**, 264—270 (1969)

James, G. W. L.: The use of the in vivo trachea preparation of the guinea pig to assess drug action on lung. J. Pharm. Pharmacol. **21**, 379—386 (1969)

Jänkälä, E. O., Virtama, P.: Bronchographic demonstration of the bronchoconstrictor effect of bradykinin in the guinea pig. Arch. Med. Exp. Fem. **41**, 436—440 (1963)

Jonasson, O., Becker, E. L.: Release of kallikrein from guinea pig lung during anaphylaxis. J. Exp. Med. **123**, 509—522 (1966)

Jose, P., Niederhauser, U., Piper, P. J., Robinson, C., Smith, A. P.: Inactivation of prostaglandin $F_{2\alpha}$ in the human pulmonary circulation. Brit. J. Clin. Pharmacol. **3**, 342P (1976)

Kadowitz, P.: Structure-activity relationships of prostanoate-related compounds. 1976 Winter Prostaglandin Conference Report, Colorado, Session III. Prostaglandins **11**, 437 (1976)

Kadowitz, P. J., Joiner, P. D., Hyman, A. L.: Comparison of the effects of prostaglandins $F_{1\alpha}$, $F_{2\alpha}$, $F_{1\beta}$ and $F_{2\beta}$ on the canine pulmonary vascular bed. Proc. Soc. Exp. Biol. Med. **149**, 356—361 (1975)

Kaley, G., Weiner, R.: Prostaglandin E_1 — a potential mediator of the inflammatory response. Ann. N.Y. Acad. Sci. **180**, 338—350 (1971)

Konzett, H., Stürmer, E.: Biological activity of synthetic polypeptides with bradykinin-like properties. Brit. J. Pharmacol. **15**, 544—551 (1960)

Lands, W., Lee, R., Smith, W.: Factors regulating the biosynthesis of various prostaglandins. Ann. N.Y. Acad. Sci. **180**, 107—122 (1971)

Lands, W. E. M., Le Tellier, P. R., Rome, L., Vandehoek, J. Y.: Regulation of prostaglandin synthesis. In: Prostaglandin Synthetase Inhibitors. Robinson, H., Vane, J. R. (Eds.). New York: Raven Press 1974, pp. 1—8

Lewis, E. J., Eyre, P.: Some cardiorespiratory effects of histamine, 5-hydroxytryptamine, and compound 48—80 in the calf. Can. J. Physiol. Pharmacol. 50, 545—553 (1972)

Liebig, R., Bernauer, W., Peskar, B. A.: Release of prostaglandins, a prostaglandin metabolite, slow-reacting substance and histamine from anaphylactic lungs, and its modification by catecholamines. Naunyn Schmiedebergs Arch. Pharmacol. 284, 279—293 (1974)

Main, I. H. M.: The inhibitory actions of prostaglandins on respiratory smooth muscle. Brit. J. Pharmacol. 22, 511—519 (1964)

Markus, H. B., Ball, E. G.: Inhibition of lipolytic process in rat adipose tissue by antimalarial drugs. Biochim. Biophys. Acta. 187, 486—491 (1969)

Marquardt, H.: Zur Frage der Entstehung der vagal-reflektorischen Bradykinin-Tachypnoe. Naunyn Schmiedebergs Arch. Pharmakol. 253, 207—220 (1966)

Mathé, A. A., Levine, L.: Release of prostaglandins and metabolites from guinea pig lung: inhibition by catecholamines. Prostaglandins 4, 877—890 (1973)

Mathé, A. A., Hedqvist, P., Holmgren, A., Svanborg, N.: Bronchial hyperactivity to $PGF_{2\alpha}$ and histamine in patients with asthma. Brit. Med. J. 1, 193—196 (1974)

McCarthy, D. A., Potter, D. E., Nicolaides, E. D.: Estimation of the potencies and half lives of synthetic bradykinin and kallidin. J. Pharmacol. Exp. Ther. 148, 117—122 (1965)

McNeill, R. S.: Effect of a β-adrenergic-blocking agent, propranolol, on asthmatics. Lancet 1964 II, 1101—1102

Mills, J., Sellick, H., Widdicombe, J. G.: The role of lung irritant receptors in respiratory response to multiple pulmonary embolism anaphylaxis and histamine-induced bronchoconstriction. J. Physiol. (Lond.) 203, 337—357 (1969)

Moncada, S., Ferreira, S. H., Vane, J. R.: Prostaglandins, aspirin-like drugs and the oedema of inflammation. Nature 246, 217—219 (1973)

Mota, I., Vugman, I.: Effects of anaphylactic shock and compound 48/80 on the mast cells of the guinea pig lung. Nature 177, 427—429 (1956)

Neddleman, P., Moncada, S., Bunting, S., Vane, J. R., Hamberg, M., Samuelsson, B.: Identification of an enzyme in platelet microsomes which generates thromboxane A_2 from prostaglandin endoperoxides. Nature 261, 559—560 (1976)

Ng, K. K. F., Vane, J. R.: Fate of angiotensin I in the circulation. Nature 218, 144—150 (1968)

Nijkamp, F. P., Flower, R. J., Moncada, S., Vane, J. R.: Partial purification of rabbit aorta contracting substance-releasing factor and inhibition of its activity by anti-inflammatory steroids. Nature 263, 479—482 (1976)

Nugteren, D. H., Hazelhof, E.: Isolation and properties of intermediates in prostaglandin biosynthesis. Biochim. Biophys. Acta 326, 448—461 (1973)

Nugteren, D. H., Beerthuis, R. K., Van Dorp, D. A.: Biosynthesis of prostaglandins. In: Bergstrom, S., Samuelsson, B. (Eds.): Proceedings 2nd Nobel Symposium, pp. 45—50. New York: Interscience 1967

Orange, R. P.: Formation and release of slow reacting substance of anaphylaxis in human lung tissues. In: Brent, L., Holborow, J. (Eds.): Progress in Immunology II, Vol. IV. North Holland: American Elsevier, pp. 29—39, 1974

Orange, R. P., Murphy, R. C., Austen, K. F.: Inactivation of slow reacting substance of anaphylaxis (SRS-A) by arylsulfatases. J. Immunol. 113, 36—322 (1974)

Orehek, J., Douglas, J. S., Lewis, A. J., Bouhuys, A.: Prostaglandin regulation of airway smooth muscle tone. Nature [New Biol.] 245, 84—85 (1973)

Palmer, M. A., Piper, P. J., Vane, J. R.: Release of rabbit aorta contracting substance (RCS) and prostaglandins induced by chemical stimulation of guinea pig lungs. Brit. J. Pharmacol. 49, 226—242 (1973)

Paulus, H. E., Whitehous, M. W.: Non-steroid anti-inflammatory agents. Annu. Rev. Pharmacol. 13, 107—125 (1973)

Piper, P. J.: Release of catecholamines and other substances by antigen and mediators of the anaphylactic reaction. Ph. D. Thesis: University of London, 1969

Piper, P. J., Vane, J. R.: The release of prostaglandins during anaphylaxis in guinea pig isolated lungs. In: Prostaglandins, Peptides and Amines. Mantegazza, P., Horton, E. W. (Eds.). London: Academic Press 1969 a, pp. 15—19

Piper, P.J., Vane, J.R.: Release of additional factors in anaphylaxis and its antagonism by anti-inflammatory drugs. Nature 223, 29—35 (1969b)

Piper, P.J., Vane, J.R.: The release of prostaglandins from lung and other tissues. Ann. N.Y. Acad. Sci. 180, 363—385 (1971)

Piper, P.J., Walker, J.L.: Release of spasmogenic substances from human chopped lung tissue and its inhibition. Brit. J. Pharmacol. 47, 291—304 (1973)

Piper, P.J., Collier, H.O.J., Vane, J.R.: Release of catecholamines in the guinea pig by substances involved in anaphylaxis. Nature 213, 838—840 (1967)

Pojda, S.M., Vane, J.R.: Inhibitory effects of aprotinin on kallikrein and kininases in dog's blood. Brit. J. Pharmacol. 42, 558—568 (1971)

Rocha E Silva, M., Garcia Leme, J.: Chemical Mediators of the Acute Inflammatory Reaction. New York: Pergamon Press 1972

Rocha E Silva, M., Beraldo, W.T., Rosenfeld, G.: Bradykinin, a hypotensive and smooth muscle stimulating factor released from plasma globulin by snake venoms and by trypsin. Am. J. Physiol. 156, 261—273 (1949)

Rosenthale, M.E., Dervinis, A., Begany, A.J., Lapidus, M., Gluckman, M.I.: Bronchodilator activity of prostaglandin E$_2$ when administered by aerosol to three species. Experientia 26, 119—121 (1970)

Roth, G.J., Stanford, N., Majerus, P.W.: Acetylation of prostaglandin synthetase by aspirin. Proc. Natl. Acad. Sci. U.S.A. 72, 3073—3076 (1975)

Ryan, J.W., Roblero, J., Stewart, J.M.: Inactivation of Bradykinin in rat lung. Adv. Exp. Med. Biol. 8, 263—271 (1970)

Samuelsson, B., Hamberg, M.: Role of endoperoxides in the biosynthesis and action of prostaglandins. In: Robinson, H., Vane, J.R. (Eds.): Prostaglandin Synthetase Inhibitors, pp. 109—119. New York: Raven Press 1974

Samuelsson, B., Granström, E., Hamberg, M.: On the mechanism of biosynthesis of prostaglandins. In: Bergström, S., Samuelsson, B. (Eds.): Proceedings 2nd Nobel Symposium, pp. 31—44. New York: Interscience 1967

Shen, T.Y.: Perspective in non-steroidal, anti-inflammatory agents. Angew. Chem. 11, 460—472 (1972)

Smith, A.P.: Role of prostaglandins in the pathogenesis and treatment of asthma. In: Austen, K.F., Lichtenstein, L.M. (Eds.): Asthma, pp. 267—277. New York: Academic Press 1973

Smith, A.P., Cuthbert, M.F.: Effects of inhaled prostaglandins on bronchial tone in man. In: Bergström, S., Bernhard, S. (Eds.): Advances in the Biosciences. Vol. IX, pp. 213—217. Braunschweig: Pergamon Press Vieweg 1973

Smith, M.J.H., Dawkins, P.D.: Salicylate and enzymes. J. Pharm. Pharmac. 23, 729—744 (1971)

Smith, W., Lands, W.: Stimulation and blockade of prostaglandin biosynthesis. J. Biol. Chem. 246, 6700—6704 (1971)

Staszewska-Barczak, J., Vane, J.R.: The release of catecholamines from the adrenal medulla by peptides. Brit. J. Pharmacol. 30, 655-667 (1967)

Stoner, J., Manganiello, V.C., Vaughan, M.: Effects of bradykinin and indomethacin on cyclic GMP and cyclic AMP in lung slices. Proc. Nat. Acad. Sci. U.S.A. 70, 3830—3833 (1973)

Thomas, G., West, G.B.: Prostaglandins as regulators of bradykinin responses. J. Pharm. Pharmacol. 25, 747—748 (1973)

Vane, J.R.: The use of isolated organs for detecting active substances in the circulating blood. Brit. J. Pharmacol. 23, 360—373 (1964)

Vane, J.R.: Release and fate of vasoactive hormones in the circulation. 2nd Gaddum Memorial Lecture. Brit. J. Pharmacol. 35, 209—243 (1969)

Vane, J.R.: Inhibition of prostaglandin synthesis as a mechanism of action for aspirin-like drugs. Nature [New Biol.] 231, 232—235 (1971)

Vane, J.R., Ferreira, S.H.: Interactions between bradykinin and prostaglandins. Life Sci. 16, 804—805 (1976)

Vargaftig, B.B., Dao Hai, N.: Interference of thiol derivatives with the pharmacological effects of arachidonic acid and slow reacting substance and with the release of rabbit aorta contracting substances. Eur. J. Pharmacol. 18, 43—55 (1972)

Widdicombe, J.G.: Regulation of tracheobronchial smooth muscle. Physiol. Rev. 43, 1—37 (1963)

Williams, T.J., Morley, J.: Prostaglandin as potentiators of increased vascular permeability in inflammation. Nature 246, 215—217 (1973)

CHAPTER 25

Interference of Anti-Inflammatory Drugs With Hypotension

B. B. VARGAFTIG

Introduction

Local inflammation has no characteristic effect on systemic arterial blood pressure, but local vasodilatation is one of the cardinal signs of inflammation. Moreover, the first chemical substance identified as an inflammatory mediator was histamine, which is a powerful vasodilator and hypotensive agent for most animal species. This has justified various hypotheses which stress the role of vasoactive factors in acute and chronic inflammation, but which will not be dealt with in this review. We shall instead concentrate on the specific topic: interference by non-steroid anti-inflammatory drugs (NSAID) with the acute vascular effects of various substances, particularly vasoactive peptides, vasoactive lipids and their potential releasing agents or precursors. There is overwhelming evidence that kinins and prostaglandin (PG)—like substances interact to induce the vascular phase of inflammation (VANE and FERREIRA, 1975, 1976). Moreover, since many of the hypotensive substances, which will be mentioned as subject to antagonism by NSAID, also display marked platelet effects, particular attention will be devoted to platelets as a potential site of action of the referred hypotensive agents (VARGAFTIG, 1974; SILVER et al., 1974)[1].

A. Interference by Non-Steroid Anti-Inflammatory Drugs With Hypotensive Effects of Potential Inflammatory Mediators

I. Kinin Peptides

The exact role of bradykinin (Bk) and similar peptides in inflammatory reactions is still an open question. The demonstration that anti-inflammatory drugs antagonize the effects of Bk in a particular system, can only suggest that it participates in inflammatory conditions. NSAID antagonize bronchoconstriction by Bk in the guinea pig (COLLIER and SHORLEY, 1960), and inhibit bronchoconstriction by other substances such as ATP, slow reacting substances C and A (SRS-C, SRS-A), arachidonic acid (Aa) and collagen (COLLIER et al., 1966; BERRY, 1966; VARGAFTIG et al., 1969; HOLMES, 1977; LEFORT and VARGAFTIG, 1978a and 1978b). Since Bk induces a marked hypotensive response in experimental animals, NSAID were tested as potential antagonists of these effects. Aspirin and its pharmacological analogues did not

[1] Literature survey with a few late exceptions was performed up to December 15th, 1975. Original work was performed in collaboration with MM. J. Lefort and M. Chignard, and will be published in detail. Technical help from Mrs. M. L. Part, J. Kintz and Miss M. Haegeli and secretarial help from Miss A. Muhl, is gratefully acknowledged.

decrease the extent of hypotension due to intravenous Bk (COLLIER and SHORLEY, 1963) but curtailed it markedly in rabbits (VARGAFTIG, 1966) and guinea pigs (COL-LIER et al., 1968). Difficulties may arise in demonstrating this effect in guinea pigs prepared for simultaneous recording of bronchial resistance to inflation by the Konzett-Rössler method, since Bk as well as arachidonic acid may induce hypertensive responses (Fig. 1) resulting from asphyxia due to bronchoconstriction associated with release of catecholamines (COLLIER, 1966). If lungs are by-passed by injecting Bk intra-arterially, the expected hypotension is observed, which is curtailed by NSAID (COLLIER et al., 1968a).

High doses of phenylbutazone may not only curtail the direct effects of Bk on blood pressure but prevent them (LECOMTE, 1960). This effect is probably accounted for by a direct antagonism by NSAID of the venoconstrictor activity of Bk (NORTH-OVER, 1967), rather than by a specific anti-kinin activity. Shortening of hypotensive responses to Bk by NSAID can also be demonstrated in rats (DAMAS and GEIGER, 1973) and in dogs (VARGAFTIG, 1974). In the latter case, in order to obtain a biphasic hypotensive response Bk, and thus to inhibit it with NSAID, inhibition of kininases is required, and can be achieved with 2,3-dimercaptopropranol (40–50 mg/kg, i.p.).

That inhibition of the second phase of Bk-induced hypotension is a specific property of NSAID, is shown by the inability of other drugs, that inhibit to various extents the in vitro spasmogenic effects of Bk on isolated smooth muscle preparations, to affect hypotension. These include 2,2-bis(hydroximethyl)-pyridin-bis-(N-methylcarbamate) (pyridinolcarbamate) (MANTOVANI and IMPICCIATORE, 1970; DA-MAS and LALLEMAND, 1974), 7-chloro-3,3a-dihydro-2H,9H-isoxanolo(3,2-b)(1,3) benz-oxazin-9-one) (Seclazone) (HRDINA and LING, 1973), cryogenine (KOSERSKY, 1971; TROTTIER, 1971), cyproheptadine (GOMAZKOV and SHIMKOVICH, 1975; ROCHA e SILVA and GARCIA LEME, 1965), hydrocortisone, morphine and dexamethasone (VAR-GAFTIG, 1966), methysergide and Iniprol, (VARGAFTIG, 1967). Drugs containing free SH groups and antioxidants such as pyrogallol have been shown to inhibit broncho-constriction and to curtail hypotension due to Bk in the rabbit, without interfering with the effects of another peptide, eledoisin (VARGAFTIG and DAO HAI, 1972a). This has been called a paradoxical effect, since thiol agents are kininase inhibitors (FER-REIRA and ROCHA e SILVA, 1962) and would have been expected to potentiate—as they do in some circumstances—the effects of Bk. Evidence that the effects of Bk which are inhibited by NSAID are due to the release of another mediator in the circulation, is reviewed by COLLIER (1969), VANE (1971), VARGAFTIG (1974), FER-REIRA and VANE (1974) and VANE and FERREIRA (1975, 1976), and are further discussed on page 194.

II. Prostaglandins

Although it is widely accepted that anti-inflammatory activity of NSAID correlates with their ability to inhibit PG synthetase (VANE, 1971), a few of the inhibitors are also known to suppress the direct effect of PGs. Thus, anti-inflammatory agents derived from anthranilic acid ("fenamates") antagonize the contraction of human bronchial muscle induced by $PGF_{2\alpha}$ (COLLIER and SWEATMAN, 1968). One of these derivatives, meclofenamic acid, inhibits the hypotensive response to $PGF_{2\alpha}$ in an-aesthetised rabbits (LEVY and LINDNER, 1971) at doses shown not to interfere with

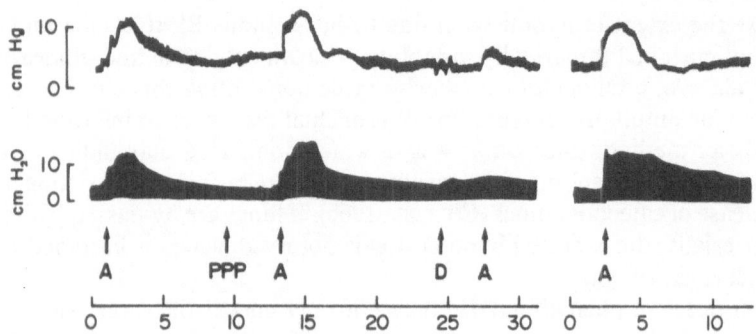

Fig. 1. Failure of polyphloretin phosphate to inhibit in vivo effects of arachidonic acid in the guinea pig; effectiveness of diethyldithiocarbamate. Arterial blood pressure *(upper, in cm Hg)* was measured from the cannulated carotid artery and bronchial resistance to inflation *(lower, in cm H₂O)*, from the trachea by the Konzett-Rössler method. Injections were i.v. as follows: arachidonic acid *(Aa,* 1 mg/kg); before and after polyphloretin phosphate *(PPP,* 100 mg/kg) and, when the latter had no inhibitory activity, after sodium diethyldithiocarbamate *(D,* 100 mg/kg). Last injection of Aa was 30 min after D, and shows quick return of vascular and bronchial effects of Aa. Time scale: minutes

the vascular effects of isoprenaline and of PGE_1. The dose of meclofenamic acid (30 mg/kg) used is much higher than the amounts required to inhibit Bk-induced bronchoconstriction in guinea pigs (COLLIER et al., 1968 a), or to curtail bradykinin-induced hypotension in rabbits (VARGAFTIG and BORD, 1969). High concentrations of indomethacin have likewise been reported to reduce PGE_2-induced contractions of rat uterus or of guinea pig ileum (SORRENTINO et al., 1972). The picture might be clarified to some extent by the hypothesis that natural PGs trigger the formation or the release of a vasodepressor compound, in a process inhibitable by anti-inflammatory drugs. This is suggested by the different haemodynamic responses to PGE and PGA in cats (KANNEGIESSER and LEE, 1971) and by the ability of PGE_1 and PGE_2 to release mast cell histamine in the rat (CRUNKHORN and WILLIS, 1971).

No anti-inflammatory activity can be attributed to the few and unspecific antagonists of PG activity that have been described (SANNER, 1974; EAKINS, 1974; our failure to inhibit carrageenin-induced rat paw oedema with polyphloretin phosphate). It is worth mentioning that polyphloretic phosphate inhibits hypotension by $PGF_{2\alpha}$ in the guinea pig and in the cat (MATHE and STRANDBERG, 1971), but not in the rabbit (LEVY and LINDNER, 1971), and fails to antagonize the vascular effects of arachidonic acid in cats and guinea pigs (Fig. 1).

B. Interference by Non-Steroid Anti-Inflammatory Drugs With the Hypotensive Effects of Agents That Release Potential Inflammatory Mediators

I. Proteolytic Enzymes

Proteolytic enzymes may induce direct and/or indirect release of kinins from plasma (PRADO, 1970; EISEN and VOGT, 1970; Chapt. 13 and 14). When release is direct, the enzyme acts as a kininogenase, and the limiting factors are plasma inhibitors and availability of substrate. When release is indirect, the enzyme acts as a plasma kininogenase activator, and the limiting factors include availability of plasma kininogenase as well. Although substances are known that may deplete quite specifically one or other of these factors (ellagic acid for instance), a clear-cut distinction between sites of action can only be provided by in vitro biochemical assays, and is beyond the purpose of this review.

1. Kininogenases

Activation of trypsin-like enzymes in blood during shock due to peptone and to ascaris extracts has been documented (ROCHA e SILVA and TEIXEIRA, 1946; ROCHA e SILVA and GRANA, 1946a, 1946b; ROCHA e SILVA et al., 1946). The details of the mechanism of this sort of shock have not been unravelled, and even the importance of kinin formation for the final outcome is debatable. Interference by NSAID with these forms of shock is anticipated, because of resemblances with endotoxin shock (p. 188) and because of platelet involvement, demonstrated by reduction of peptone shock in animals rendered thombocytopenic with glycogen (ROCHA e SILVA et al., 1945; ROCHA e SILVA, 1952).

Intravenous administration of proteolytic enzymes in dogs induces hypotension accompanied by characteristic signs of cardiovascular shock (see CORRADO et al., 1966). Mechanisms of action are discussed in ROCHA e SILVA and ROTHSCHILD (1974) and in WERLE (1973), with respect to plasma and urinary kininogenases, and to the venom of *Bothrops jararaca*. Despite the overwhelming evidence that kinin peptides are released after administration of enzymes to animals, or during pathological states such as pancreatitis (OFSTAD, 1970) very little is known concerning the interaction of anti-inflammatory agents with this release. Lack of investigation was probably influenced by the demonstration that NSAID do not inhibit in vitro kinin release by pancreatic kininogenase (pancreatic kallikrein) (DAVIES et al., 1966). We have, nevertheless, shown that hypotension induced by the latter and by the venom of *B. jararaca* is inhibited by NSAID (indomethacin, phenylbutazone, antipyrine, aspirin, isobutylphenylacetic acid and noramidopyrine methanesulphonate (Novalgine), (VARGAFTIG, 1966; VARGAFTIG and BORD, 1969). These NSAID accelerate markedly the rate of recovery of the depressed blood pressure after Bk or trypsin injections in the rabbit (VARGAFTIG, 1966, 1967). Thus, it has been thought that somehow the in vivo kinin release could be influenced by NSAID (VARGAFTIG and BORD, 1969; VARGAFTIG et al., 1970), but this is unlikely because of the in vitro results (DAVIES et al., 1966) that discard a direct interference with the activity of kininogenase upon purified kininogen.

Alternatively, it has been argued (ROCHA e SILVA, personal communication) that inhibition of the activity of kallikrein would occur when the direct effect of Bk is curtailed, since a slow release of kinin in the circulation is equivalent to a slow, easily inhibitable, infusion of Bk. This explanation requires that a similar in vitro inhibition should occur, which is not the case. Another explanation is that kallikrein activates phospholipase A_2 on cells, as it does on mast cells (UVNÄS, 1962), leading to release of PGs and related substances. This would provide a site of action for NSAID that inhibit biosynthesis of PGs. Such on explanation would apply to the effects of *B. jararaca* venom, which contains kininogenases and phospholipase A_2 expected to exert mutual potentiation in releasing histamine (AMUNDSEN et al., 1969). The products of both enzymes, respectively kinins and PGs, also exert a mutual potentiation in their inflammatory effects (VANE and FERREIRA, 1975, 1976).

2. Thrombin

Intravenous administration of thrombin in dogs is followed by hypotension, pulmonary arterial vasoconstriction and by increased intratracheal pressure, accompanied by a major drop in platelet counts (see RÅDEGRAN, 1971). Since thrombin induces platelet aggregation in vitro, which is partially inhibited by aspirin (GRETTE, 1962; DAVEY and LÜSCHER, 1968), the possibility is raised that release of smooth muscle contracting substances from platelets accounts for the effects of thrombin on the pulmonary circulation and on the airways (RÅDEGRAN, 1971). Aspirin inhibited these pulmonary effects, but failed to inhibit hypotension due to intravenous thrombin or the accompanying thrombocytopenia. Indomethacin also failed to inhibit vasodilatation following intra-arterial injection of thrombin into dog paws (JOYNER et al., 1974). Since acute thrombocytopenia that follows intravenous infusions of thrombin is also not blocked by aspirin in rabbits (MORIAU et al., 1974), failure of NSAID to inhibit all the effects of thrombin appears not to be a special case for dogs, but rather to result from an additional effect of thrombin. This does not rule out platelets as the site of in vivo action of thrombin because aspirin only inhibits aggregation by thrombin when threshold amounts of the enzyme are used (see Chap. 5). A direct pulmonary effect of thrombin can be excluded, since thrombin neither increases pulmonary vascular resistance (SWEDENBORG, 1974) nor induces bronchoconstriction in isolated lungs perfused with a cell-free medium. Finally, thrombin, despite being a proteolytic enzyme, does not release kinins or potentiate the kinin effect, as do other enzymes such as chymotrypsin or trypsin (EDERY, 1964). Thus, thrombin appears to have a platelet-mediated in vivo effect, subject to partial inhibition by aspirin. It has not been shown that in vitro PG release from platelets by thrombin (SMITH and WILLIS, 1971) is matched in vivo, nor whether NSAID, apart from aspirin or indomethacin, have antagonistic properties. It has been demonstrated that pretreatment of rabbits with intramuscular ADP prevents thrombocytopenia by thrombin (BUSFIELD and TOMICH, 1968), since it desensitizes platelets to ADP-mediated aggregating stimuli. Similarly, in guinea pigs, infusions of ADP prevent the acute effects of ADP and of ATP, but not those of Bk, or of Aa, both of which exert effects that are platelet-independent.

Polyphloretin phosphate, particularly its high molecular weight fraction, inhibits thrombin and protamine-induced hypotension, increase in pulmonary arterial pressure and the accompanying thrombocytopenia in dogs. No proof is available that release of mediators is also inhibited (SWEDENBORG, 1974). Polyphloretin phosphate is not a specific anti-PG substance, since it displays anti-enzymic properties (DICZFALUZY et al., 1953) and can interfere with haemorrhagic effects of snake venoms (BONTA and VARGAFTIG, 1976). The effectiveness of polyphloretin phosphate in counteracting the activity of thrombin and of protamine in the dog is, moreover, not matched by effectiveness against platelet aggregation by other substances, such as arachidonic acid in the rabbit. Ability of polyphloretin phosphate to inhibit thrombin-induced platelet aggregation in the rabbit is fully accounted for by its anticoagulant activity, since aggregation and clotting of plasma are inhibited by similar concentrations (VARGAFTIG et al., unpublished observations).

3. Other Proteolytic Enzymes

Other kinin releasing enzymes that induce hypotension upon i.v. injection are: venoms from the snake *B. jararaca* (see Chap. 1, and ROCHA e SILVA et al., 1949; HAMBERG and ROCHA e SILVA, 1957; VARGAFTIG, 1967); from *Agkistrodon halys blomhoffii, Trimeresurus flavoviridis* and *T. gramineus* (OSHIMA et al., 1969). Venoms from the elapids *Naja naja* and *N. nigricollis* are devoid of kinin releasing activities; their hypotensive effects result from other mechanisms. Nagarse, a crystalline proteinase from *Bacillus subtilis* also induces what appears to be kinin-dependent hypotension in rats (PRADO et al., 1964). Chymotrypsin, which releases kinin activity only from fresh guinea pig plasma (not from plasma of the dog, hamster, rabbit and man) (ROCHA e SILVA et al., 1967) has no hypotensive effect. Clostripain (clostridiopeptidase B, E.C.3.4.4.20) releases kinins from rat and human plasma because it activates pre-kallikrein (Fletscher factor) by an unknown mechanism, possibly activation of clotting Factor XII (Hageman factor). It also releases kinins directly, either from rat plasma when used at high concentrations, or from dog or rabbit plasma, and from horse and bovine kininogen preparations (PRADO and PRADO, 1962; VARGAFTIG and GIROUX, 1976).

II. Inhibition of Hypotension Due to Substances That Activate Plasma Kininogenase

Activation of plasma kininogenase (plasma kallikrein) should cause kinin release in the circulation, but the relevance of this release to hypotensive responses is uncertain, since kinins are very rapidly metabolized (FERREIRA and VANE, 1967). Activators of plasma kininogenase can be enzymes (trypsin, clostridiopeptidase B in the case of rat plasma, VARGAFTIG and GIROUX, 1976) or substances that display no enzymic activity but trigger activation of plasma enzymes. For example ellagic acid or cellulose sulphate (RATNOFF and CRUM, 1964; ROTHSCHILD, 1967) may induce hypotension subject to a very marked tachyphylaxis, as a second injection fails to display any effect. No results have been reported for antagonism of hypotension induced by these plasma kininogenase activators by NSAID.

1. Carrageenin

Carrageenin is a sulphated polysaccharide extracted from *Chondrus crispus*, which is widely used as a standard oedema-inducing agent (WINTER et al., 1962). It induces hypotension in rabbits (VARGAFTIG et al., 1970), in rats (DI ROSA and SORRENTINO, 1970; NOORDHOEK and BONTA, 1972) and in dogs but has almost no hypotensive effect in cats and in guinea-pigs (LEFORT and VARGAFTIG, 1978b). There is marked desensitization to its effects, and when animals survive a first intravenous injection,

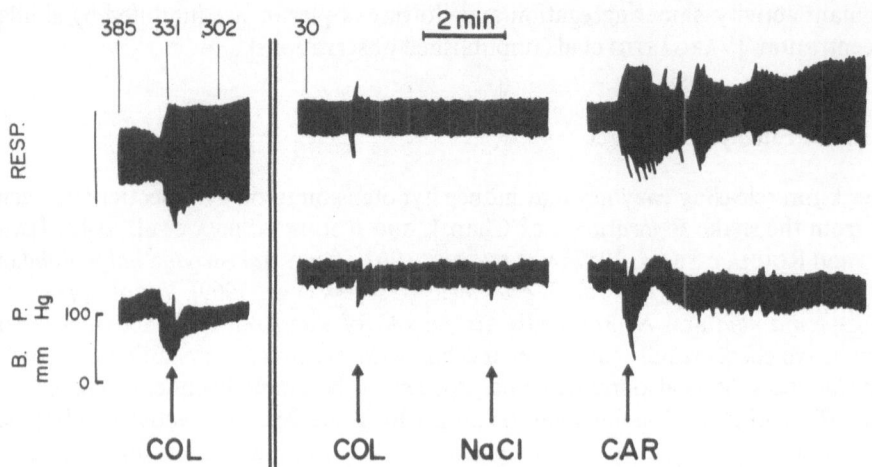

Fig. 2. Inhibition by anti-platelet plasma of hypotension and respiratory stimulation due to collagen. Protection against carrageenin. A pentobarbitone-anaesthetised rabbit was injected i.v. with a collagen suspension (*COL*, 1 ml/kg, prepared according to PACKHAM et al., 1967) before *(left panel)* and after *(right panel)* anti-platelet treatment (LEFORT and VARGAFTIG, 1975). Platelet counts in arterial blood are indicated above the upper tracing (respiration) in cells × 10^3 per mm^3. Effects of collagen after anti-platelet treatment are matched by those of i.v. saline.
Effects of i.v. carrageenin (*CAR*, 10 mg/kg) are markedly reduced as compared with control animals, and in contrast to the occurence in the latter, death is prevented. Upper panel, respiration amplitude. Lower panel, blood pressure (mm HG)

they fail to respond to further injections. Moreover, intraperitoneal administration of carrageenin prevents the intravenous responses (VARGAFTIG et al., 1970). Despite evidence that the protease inhibitor, soybean trypsin inhibitor, fails to inhibit hypotension induced by carrageenin (NOORDHOEK and BONTA, 1972), participation of at least a proteolytic step in its effects is shown by inhibition of hypotension by Trasylol both in rats and in rabbits (VARGAFTIG et al., 1970; DI ROSA and SORRENTINO, 1970). This inhibition, and the fact that kininogen depletion occurs after administration of carrageenin or of other sulphated substances (ROTHSCHILD, 1968; VARGAFTIG et al., 1970), led to the hypothesis that activation of endogenous kinin-releasing mechanisms mediated carrageenin-induced hypotension.

Standard antihistamine or anti-5-hydroxytryptamine (5-HT) agents fail to inhibit hypotension by carrageenin (VARGAFTIG et al., 1970; DI ROSA and SORRENTINO, 1970; NOORDHOEK and BONTA, 1972), but it is suppressed by NSAID in rabbits (VARGAFTIG et al., 1970) (Fig. 2). No information is available for other species.

Since inhibition by NSAID suggested the participation of PGs, and possibly of platelets, which are protected by aspirin-like agents, platelet counts were performed after administration of sublethal and of lethal doses of carrageenin to rabbits (respectively 1 and 10 mg/kg). In both circumstances a marked platelet depletion occurred, apparent, as quickly as 0.5 min after the intravenous injection (see also ANDERSON and DUNCAN, 1965). In vitro assays confirmed these results, for partial platelet aggregation was evoked when carrageenin was added to rabbit platelet-rich plasma (PRP) at 20–350 µg/ml. This aggregation was not inhibited, but was delayed by indomethacin, aspirin and salicylic acid, which were roughly equipotent. This contrasts with their order of activity as inhibitors of PG synthetase (VANE, 1971) or of Aa-induced platelet aggregation (VARGAFTIG and ZIRINIS, 1973). Since anti-inflammatory drugs may interfere with complement activation (GIROUD and TIMSIT, 1972; HARRITY and GOLDLUST, 1974), rabbit platelets were thoroughly washed (VARGAFTIG et al., 1974), and resuspended in Tyrode solution. Under those conditions, platelets were aggregated by concentrations of carrageenin down to 1–2 µg/ml. This aggregation could be inhibited by adenosine, N-ethylmaleimide, Ca^{++} chelating agents and NSAID. The same equi-activity for aspirin and salicylic acid, as seen in PRP, was observed (VARGAFTIG and LEFORT, 1977; VARGAFTIG, 1977a and 1977b).

Bioassay of incubates of rabbit plasma or PRP with carrageenin in the presence of kininase inhibitors (CaEDTA or o-phenanthroline) showed no kinin activity or activation of pre-kallikrein, in contrast to what occurs in rats (GIROUX and VARGAFTIG, 1976). A marked smooth muscle contracting activity was generated from PRP incubated with carrageenin (25–100 µg/ml), showing the presence of 5-HT contained in large amounts in rabbit platelets, and of rabbit aorta contracting substance (RCS) and PG-like substances. Release of RCS and PG-like substances was inhibited by indomethacin and by aspirin (0.05–0.2 mM), whereas salicylic acid was markedly less effective. Carrageenin is thus a powerful platelet aggregating agent in rabbits. Its in vivo and in vitro effects are inhibited by standard anti-inflammatory agents, at doses different from those required to inhibit the effects of Aa, attributed to the activity of PGs and related agents. Carrageenin can precipitate rabbit fibrinogen and thus entrap platelets and blood cells (ANDERSON and DUNCAN, 1965). The role of fibrinogen is probably minor, because platelets from rabbits defibrinated with the extract of malayan pit viper venom Arvin retain their aggregating response to carrageenin, and are as sensitive as control animals to its platelet depleting and lethal in vivo effects. In contrast, platelet depletion reduces markedly the hypotensive effects of carrageenin in rabbits and prevents the otherwise expected death (Fig. 2). For details see VARGAFTIG and LEFORT, 1977; VARGAFTIG, 1977a and 1977b.

2. Other Activators of Plasma Kininogenase

Other activators of the endogenous release of kinins include kaolin, which induces a marked drop in arterial blood pressure of the dog, that is inhibited by Künitz protein protease inhibitor (Iniprol), (VAIREL and HUREAU, 1973). No results have been reported for NSAID. Clostripain (see BI3) can release kinins from rat plasma via activation of the endogenous kinin-generating system at concentrations quite beyond those required to split kininogen directly (VARGAFTIG and GIROUX, 1976). Contamination of commercial collagenase (clostridiopeptidase A) preparations with clostripain probably accounts for its marked hypotensive activity in guinea pigs.

III. Phospholipase A₂

Release of histamine and of other smooth muscle contracting substances by elapid snake venoms were attributed to phospholipase A_2 (phosphatide acyl hydrolase, E.C.3.1.1.4), (FELDBERG and KELLAWAY, 1937, 1938). The subject has been throughly reviewed by VOGT (1957a) and more recent information is provided by FREDHOLM and STRANDBERG (1969) and DAMERAU et al. (1975). Substrates for PG synthetase, i.e. unsaturated fatty acids such as Aa, can be provided after activation of tissue phospholipase A_2 (BARTELS et al., 1970; VOGT, 1967; VOGT et al., 1966, 1969). There is no clear evidence of the mechanism by which phospholipase A_2 itself is activated, but a proteolytic step appears to be required, at least in mast cells (HÖGBERG and UVNAS, 1960) and platelets (VARGAFTIG, 1977b; FEINSTEIN et al., 1977).

Phospholipase A_2 preparations devoid of major contaminants have been studied for their in vivo activity on a limited scale, probably due to non-availability of sufficient amounts of reliable preparations. KLIBANSKY et al., (1962) injected a *Vipera palestinae* phospholipase A_2 lacking lethal, haemorrhagic and neurotoxic activities intravenously into rabbits. Injections were followed by excitation, cyanosis, increased respiratory and heart rate and miosis, all of which cleared within 15 min. Biochemical changes included a marked decrease in plasma lecithin, and an increase in lysolecithin, accompanied by erythrocyte sphering and attachment of lysolecithin to their membranes. No haemolysis was present, but red blood cells became very fragile. No evidence was provided for blood pressure effects, nor for interference by NSAID.

VICK and BROOKS (1972) reported that a phospholipase A_2 preparation extracted from bee venom induces hypotension, respiratory arrest and death of dogs. Since respiratory paralysis was present, purity of phospholipase A_2 is doubtful, and precludes drawing major conclusions as to the mechanism of hypotension.

In another series of experiments using crotoxin, an ionic complex of phospholipase A_2 and of crotactin extracted from the venom of *Crotalus durissus terrificus* (HABERMAN, 1957), VITAL BRAZIL et al. (1966), showed that at equivalent doses in weight, crotoxin had no activity on the dog blood pressure whereas the crude venom induced marked hypotensive effects. Since the study concerned the mechanism of respiratory paralysis due to the venom, no biochemical or drug antagonism assays were performed.

Other vascular effects of phospholipase A_2 include a marked increase in rat skin vascular permeability, which was inhibited in part (not more than 50%) by NSAID, by dexamethasone and by the standard anti-5-HT and antihistamine agent cyproheptadine (ARRIGONI-MARTELLI et al., 1973). In other experiments with crude venoms and partially purified phospholipase A_2 fractions (VARGAFTIG, 1974), local administration of NSAID together with the venom preparations inhibited vascular leakage, but the required concentrations of the inhibitors were very large (0.2–0.5 mg per skin site), which should constrict vessels (NORTHOVER, 1967). Cyproheptadine, as well as a mixture of the antihistamine agent mepyramine with the anti-5-HT agent methysergide, induced total inhibition of leakage, demonstrating that whatever the precise mechanism by which phospholipase A_2 increases the skin vascular permeability, the final mediators are mast-cell contained amines. Effects of snake venoms or of their phospholipase A_2 fractions on platelets in vivo have not been reported.

Pitfalls in such studies are particularly numerous. Thus, it is known that effects of phospholipases on isolated platelets vary according to the source of the enzyme (KIRSCHMANN et al., 1964; KAISER et al., 1972). Moreover, individual venoms contain different phospholipases, some of which are devoid of systemic toxicity, while others are toxic (DELORI, 1973). A further difficulty in studying in vivo activity of phospholipase A_2, even when the enzyme is of recognized purity, concerns pharmacokinetics that profoundly influence the outcome. This includes factors such as protein binding, availability of specific and non-specific antagonists and/or substrates in blood etc. The latter is illustrated by the failure of phospholipase A_2 preparations from bee or from *N. naja* venoms to release RCS or PG-like activity from rabbit PRP, in conditions where large amounts are generated upon addition of Aa. Nevertheless, when lecithin is introduced in the system, thus providing a substrate from which Aa can be split by phospholipase A_2, generation of PGs and of RCS starts immediately. Thus, the tested phospholipases do not split membrane phospholipids under experimental conditions which are optimal for release of PG activity from Aa. As soon as Aa is either introduced from the outside or generated within the system from lecithin by phospholipase A_2, PGs are generated. Indomethacin and Ca^{++} chelating agents inhibit this generation; the former because it blocks PG synthetase irrespective of the underlying activity of phospholipase A_2, and the latter because it inhibits the calcium requiring phospholipase A_2. It is thus completely different to inject phospholipase A_2 intravenously, or to add it to an isolated cell system and to stimulate the endogenous phospholipase A_2. Failure or success in obtaining hypotension upon intravenous administration of phospholipase A_2 will strictly depend on availability of substrate, and cannot be adduced as evidence for or against a phospholipase-dependent mechanism of endogenous formation of PG-related materials. In other systems, such as perfused lungs, phospholipase A_2 can trigger the release of PGs, by splitting available phospholipids, without mast-cell degranulation (DAMERAU et al., 1975).

C. Interference of Anti-Inflammatory Drugs With Hypotensive Responses to Lipid Derivatives

The earliest reported pharmacological experiments on the effects of liposoluble substances in vivo are from DELEZENNE and LEDEBT, (1911) who demonstrated that incubates of egg yolk and snake venoms containing phospholipase A_2 contracted isolated smooth muscle preparations and were very toxic upon intravenous injection. Despite the presence in such incubates of lysolecithin, formed when the unsaturated fatty acid esterified in the β position of lecithin is split by phospholipase A_2, a clear distinction was provided between haemolytic activity and toxicity. FELDBERG and KELLAWAY (1937) studied the effects that follow the injection of crude snake venoms to isolated lungs of various species, and recognized the formation of "slow contracting substances", but did not investigate the in vivo activity of these substances. The whole subject was revised by BOQUET et al. (1950), who demonstrated that the symptoms following intravenous injection of incubates of egg yolk with phospholipase A_2-containing snake venoms markedly resemble those of anaphylactic shock. Thus, rabbits died with pulmonary hypertension, guinea pigs with bronchoconstriction, and dogs with systemic hypotension and splanchnic pooling of blood. A clear demonstration of the liposoluble nature of incubates of egg yolk and phospholipase A_2 was provided by VOGT (1957a), who called the new principle by the now widely accepted name slow reacting substance C (SRS-C), to distinguish it from a pharmacological analogue, SRS-A (BROCKLEHURST, 1963; MIDDLETON and PHILLIPS, 1964). Although studies on the systemic effects of SRS-C and on their

inhibition by NSAID preceded those concerning the hypotensive effects of Aa (Var-
GAFTIG et al., 1969), it appears retrospectively more logical to describe the pharma-
cological properties of Aa, a defined chemical species, before describing those of
SRS-C.

I. Effects of Arachidonic Acid on Arterial Blood Pressure

The first reported observation on acute in vivo effects of Aa was provided by BERRY
(1966), who noted that it induced intense bronchoconstriction in guinea pigs, which
was liable to inhibition by aspirin. The burst of work on PG biosynthesis led to a
rediscovery of the relevance of acute in vivo effects of fatty acids. It is now well
established that Aa induces systemic hypotension in rabbits (LARSSON and
ÄNGGÅRD, 1973), dogs (ROSE et al., 1974), rats (COHEN et al., 1973), and cats (Fig. 3).
Effects on guinea pigs may vary, and hypotension may follow a marked hypertensive
burst (see below).

NSAID inhibit the hypotensive effects of Aa in rabbits, rats, guinea pigs, dogs,
cats, and probably mice (LARSSON and ÄNGGÅRD, 1973; COHEN et al., 1973; ROSE et
al., 1974; see Fig. 3 for cats). Anti-malarial drugs, steroid anti-inflammatory agents,
and anti-5-HT and antihistamin agents are ineffective.

1. Mechanism of Action of Arachidonic Acid on Blood Pressure

Since hypotension by Aa is inhibited by NSAID, it is widely accepted that it results
from activation of PG synthetase. The following aspects have nevertheless not been
fully clarified and deserve further discussion: (a) the site(s) of action of Aa; (b)

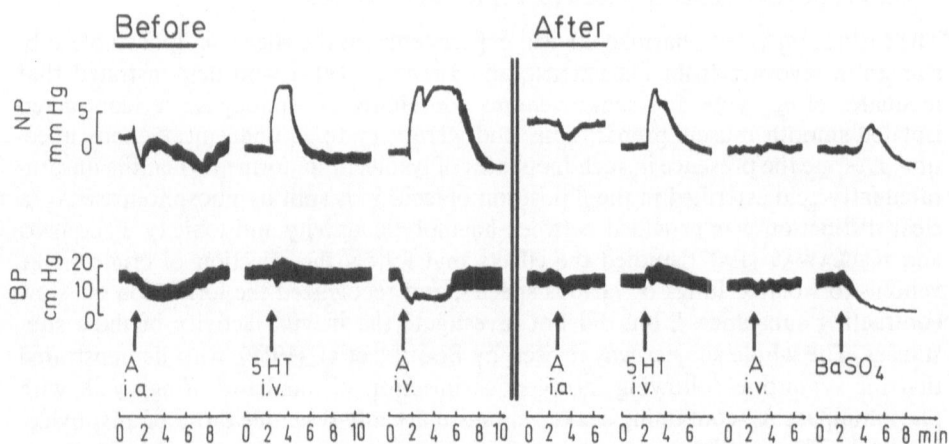

Fig. 3. Inhibition by aspirin of nasal vasodilatation and systemic hypotension due to arachidonic
acid. A pentobarbitone anaesthetised cat was prepared for recording of nasal pressure (NP,
upper tracing, in mm Hg) (VARGAFTIG and LEFORT, 1974) and of carotid blood pressure (BP,
lower tracing, in cm Hg). Injections were as follows: arachidonic acid (Aa) into the lingual artery
towards the nasal cavity (i.a., 0.5 mg total), and i.v. (1 mg/kg); 5-HT (i.v., 40 μg/kg), before and
after 100 mg/kg of aspirin i.v. Effects of Aa are inhibited. Barium sulphate (BaSO₄) (0.3 ml/kg of a
30% solution) was used to kill the animal despite aspirin treatment

differences in species reactivity to Aa; (c) mechanism of Aa-mediated hypotension. The three topics are related and will be discussed together.

a) Effects of Arachidonic Acid on Guinea Pig Blood Pressure

Intravenous injections of Aa to artificially ventilated guinea pigs induce a complex blood pressure response, as may be seen in Figure 4. In some cases an hypertensive burst is followed by secondary hypotension. The latter becomes predominant upon repeated injections of Aa, as if some underlying mechanism accounting for hypertension were exhausted. Bronchoconstriction is induced irrespective of the blood pressure response, and thus the latter appears not to be related to asphyxia. In other cases a slight hypotension is immediately evoked by Aa, followed then by hypertension and hypotensive responses. Neither methysergide nor cyproheptadine, respectively a pure anti-5-HT agent and an anti-5HT and antihistamine agent, interfere

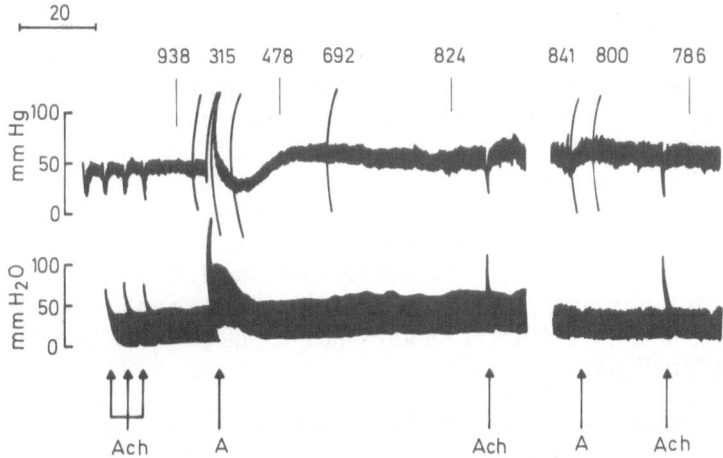

Fig. 4. Aspirin inhibits bronchoconstriction, hypotension and acute thrombocytopenia by arachidonic acid. Acetylcholine *(Ach, 5 μg/kg)* and arachidonic acid (Aa, 0.5 mg/kg) were injected i.v. into an anaesthetised guinea pig before *(left panel)* and after *(right panel)* 10 mg/kg of aspirin which inhibits effects of Aa. Scales as in Figure 1 and platelet counts as in Figure 2.

Table 1. Effect of hypotensive agents on platelet counts in guinea pig arterial blood

Injected agonists	Dose $\mu g \cdot kg^{-1}$	n	% decrease of platelets in arterial blood		
			10 s	60 s	6 min
Bradykinin	0.5	5	12.0 ± 3.8	9.5 ± 3.2	–
ADP	100	22	62.0 ± 4.8	19.7 ± 2.6	–
	250	7	64.4 ± 2.2	21.7 ± 3.2	–
ATP	500	7	50.0 ± 5.0	24.8 ± 5.5	24.5 ± 1.8
	750	24	59.6 ± 3.9	18.9 ± 4.1	–
	1000	8	58.3 ± 3.3	26.5 ± 9.0	–
Arachidonic acid	375	16	–	44.5 ± 5.6	20.7 ± 3.2
	500	11	–	69.6 ± 4.4	20.9 ± 5.0

with bronchoconstriction or with blood pressure responses to Aa, thus ruling out direct amine participation. Arachidonic acid induces in vivo a fall in platelet count (Fig. 4 and Table 1). This platelet effect reflects the platelet-aggregating activity of Aa in vitro, but does not account for bronchoconstriction or hypotension, since thrombocytopenic animals undergo bronchoconstriction and marked hypotension after Aa injections (Fig. 4). Platelet depletion fully inhibits the bronchoconstrictor effect of ADP and of ATP (LEFORT and VARGAFTIG, 1975 and 1978 a) and of collagen (LEFORT and VARGAFTIG, 1978 b), which provides a positive control for the depletion procedure.

All these in vivo effects of Aa are inhibited by NSAID: hypertension, hypotension, bronchoconstriction and the decreased platelet count (Fig. 4). This might suggest participation of $PGF_{2\alpha}$ to account for hypertension and for bronchoconstriction and of PGE_2, to account for hypotension. Failure of the PG antagonist polyphloretin phosphate to inhibit the effects of Aa in guinea pigs (Fig. 1) does not support this possibility. The demonstration that the cyclic endoperoxides PGG_2 and PGH_2 induce bronchoconstriction in guinea pigs (HAMBERG et al., 1975 a) but that their degradative products are inactive, can also be retained as evidence against a causative role of natural PGs. One open possibility is that hypertension following intravenous administration of Aa to guinea pigs results from pulmonary reflexes and/or adrenaline release, hypotension resulting from vasodilatation due to Aa-derived products by PG synthetase at extra-platelet sites such as lungs. The latter are known to be active producers of RCS when injected with Aa (VARGAFTIG and DAO, 1971 a; GRYGLEWSKI and VANE, 1972), and RCS is a mixture of cyclic endoperoxide PG precursors and thromboxane A_2 (VARGAFTIG and DAO HAI, 1972 b; GRYGLEWSKI and VANE, 1972; HAMBERG et al., 1975 a). This is supported by the ability of several thiol agents to inhibit the effects of Aa attributed to endoperoxides (VARGAFTIG and DAO HAI, 1972 b; Fig. 1).

b) Effects of Arachidonic Acid on Dog Blood Pressure

Intra-arterial injections of Aa in dog paws induce vasodilatation (FERREIRA and VARGAFTIG, 1974) and reduce vasoconstriction that follows intra-arterial noradrenaline (RYAN and ZIMMERMAN, 1974). Indomethacin and phenylbutazone prevent these effects of Aa, indicating that at least part of the hypotensive response is explained by peripheral vasodilatation. Since vasoactive substances and PG-like materials are generated in the external circuit of circulating dog blood, i.e. without and before entering the vessels, it has been hypothesised that vasodilatation, and hence hypotension, results from the generation of mediators from platelets (VARGAFTIG, 1973). This hypothesis was reinforced by the demonstration that incubation of Aa with dog PRP, but not with other fractions, is followed by generation of RCS and of PG-like substances similar to these found in incubates of Aa with rabbit or dog blood (FERREIRA and VARGAFTIG, 1974; WILLIS and KUHN, 1973; VARGAFTIG and ZIRINIS, 1973). More recent findings cast some doubt upon the relevance of the platelet effect of Aa to its overall in vivo activity, particularly in dogs.

Aa only induces aggregation of citrated dog PRP when added on the top of a certain (10–20%) spontaneous aggregation. This is particularly clear when the usual 3.8% sodium citrate anticoagulant is replaced by a 2% solution, but does not result directly from Ca^{++} chelation. Non-aggregating dog platelets still generate substances that aggregate rabbit platelets, when incubated with Aa. Formation of these substances is inhibited by metal chelating agents, by thiols and by NSAID (VARGAFTIG et al., 1975; VARGAFTIG and CHIGNARD, 1975; CHIGNARD and VARGAFTIG, 1976).

In line with this observation, intravenous injections of Aa to anaesthetised dogs are usually followed by moderate thrombocytopenia, which is matched by thrombocytopenia induced by a similar dose of the non-PG precursor linoleic acid. At those doses Aa induces hypotension, whereas linoleic acid displays no such effect. Aspirin totally suppresses hypotension at 2 mg/kg, but doses up to 50 mg/kg do not interfere significantly with the drop in platelet count. Similarly, doses of 10 mg/kg of indomethacin i.v. delay rather than inhibit the platelet fall, whereas hypotension is suppressed.

At this stage it appears that in vivo platelet aggregation by Aa in dogs is not related to hypotension, and is probably explained by the same mechanism that accounts for the platelet effect of linoleic acid. Formation of mediators from Aa by PG synthetase and similar enzymes occurs on platelets and on other sites, and is independent of the presence or absence of underlying aggregation. A similar situation prevails in vitro, when Aa is added to dog or to rabbit PRP in the presence of Ca^{++} chelating agents or of thiol reagents (respectively EGTA and EDTA, or N-ethylmaleimide and p-chloromercuribenzoate): aggregation is suppressed, but PG and like substances are abundantly generated (VARGAFTIG et al., 1974).

Hypotension induced by Aa in dogs is still present after thrombocytopenia is obtained with anti-platelet plasma, as is true for rabbits and guinea pigs.

We have developed a new preparation that allows study of the in situ reactivity of the nasal vessels of the dog and of the cat to intra-arterially injected substances. This permits discrimination of the patterns of vascular activity of the various PGs, as compared with other potential mediators and to Aa. The tested substances are injected into the cannulated lingual or auricular artery and reach the nasal vessels. The nasal cavity is occluded at the rear and at the front, and its internal pressure is monitored with an open-tip catheter. When vessels shrink due to vasoconstriction, the internal pressure of the cavity decreases, whereas when vessels dilate, the internal pressure increases. This preparation can be used with one limitation, seen when the injected substances recirculate and display systemic cardiac or vascular effects, that interfere with the local activity. This is the case for high doses of Bk or of histamine that induce systemic hypotension, or for isoprenaline, which moreover induces tachycardia (VARGAFTIG and LEFORT, 1974).

PGE_1, PGE_2 and $PGF_{2\alpha}$ constrict the nasal vessels at ng/kg doses, which contrasts with their overall hypotensive effects, or with the hypotensive effects of Aa when injected intravenously. Aa induces vasodilatation, which is suppressed when the animal is pre-treated with NSAID (Fig.3). When incubates of Aa and of dog or reserpinised rabbit PRP (to avoid interference on the vessels of 5-HT which is present in large amounts in rabbit platelets), are injected into the nasal cavity, vasoconstriction is seen, similar to that due to PGE_2. Generation of the vasoconstrictor activity involves PG synthetase and formation of lipoperoxides, since it can be prevented by indomethacin and catalase, respectively (Fig. 5). When the vasoconstrictor activity is fully inhibited by the presence of either substance, vasodilatation is evoked, similar to that due to Aa itself. This may be interpreted by assuming that upon blockade of

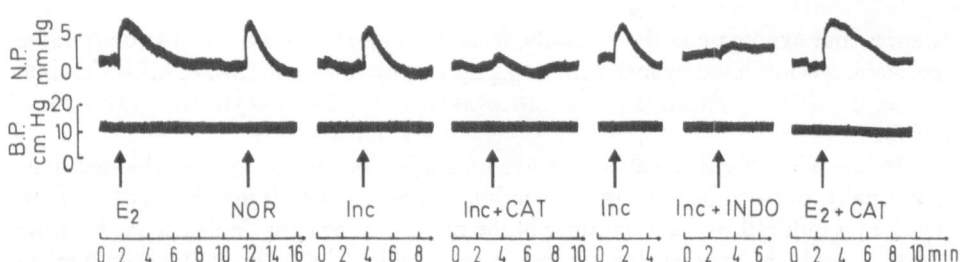

Fig. 5. Inhibition by indomethacin, by catalase and by sodium diethyldithiocarbamate of the generation of nasal vasoconstrictor activity in incubates of dog platelet-rich plasma and arachidonic acid. Recording of the arterial blood pressure of a pentobarbitone-anaesthetised dog *(lower tracing)* and of the internal nasal pressure *(upper tracing)*. Injection procedure and scales according to VARGAFTIG and LEFORT (1974). E_2 (10 ng/kg of PGE_2); Nor (10 ng/kg of noradrenaline); injection of a 5-min incubate of 0.4 ml of autologous platelet-rich plasma with 0.5 mM of arachidonic acid *(INC)* results in nasal vasoconstriction. Generation of this activity is prevented if 375 µg of catalase are added to platelet-rich plasma before arachidonic acid *(INC + CAT)* or if indomethacin (0.1 mM) is added in similar conditions *(INC + INDO)*. Effect of PGE_2 is not affected by a 5-min incubation with catalase *(E_2 + CAT)*

the in vitro generation of PGs, the direct underlying vasodilatation resulting from the interaction of Aa with in vivo structures (blood and/or nasal vessels themselves) is uncovered, since it is not opposed by PG-mediated vasoconstriction. Vasodilatation is inhibited when the animal is treated systemically with a NSAID, indicating involvement of PG synthetase or of like-enzymes. The direct vasodilator effect of Aa on nasal vessels is thus probably due to an intermediate in PG generation which might account for the hypotensive activity. This does not rule out that the latter can be aggravated by PGE_2 formed at the same time, or partially opposed by $PGF_{2\alpha}$, but indicates a major contribution of endoperoxides and/or of thromboxane A_2 to hypotension induced by Aa in the dog. PG endoperoxides (PGG_2 and PGH_2) have not been directly tested on dogs, but analogues have been shown to increase airway resistance, with unspecified alterations of arterial blood pressure and heart rate (WASSERMAN and GRIFFIN, 1975). In fact, the exact nature of the Aa-derived compounds responsible for hypotension has not been unravelled as yet, since there are many candidates for this role. PGG_2, PGH_2, thromboxane A_2, PGE_2, $PGF_{2\alpha}$, are identified Aa-derived substances that are potentially hypotensive. The two natural PGs could well be quantitatively involved, since hypotensive effects of PGE_2 (10–20 µg/kg) and of Aa (250–500 µg/kg) match each other. Prostacyclin is finally another candidate (MONCADA et al., 1976).

Little work has been reported concerning in vivo effects of the precursor of PGE_1, and of $PGF_{1\alpha}$, i.e. dihomo γ-linolenic acid. ROSE et al. (1975) showed that it induces a 30–40% drop in arterial blood pressure when injected to dogs at 2–2.5 mg/kg. This was not influenced by β-adrenoceptor blockade nor by ganglionic blockade. It was better explained by formation of PGE_1 than of $PGF_{1\alpha}$, since the former is hypotensive and the latter is hypertensive in dogs. No effect was seen on platelet counts, but aggregability with ADP was reduced, as might be expected from the known anti-aggregant effects of PGE_1. Aspirin, used at 100 mg/kg, did not fully prevent the hypotensive effects of dihomo γ-linolenic acid, as it did the effects of Aa (ROSE et al., 1974). Dihomo γ-linoleic acid induces bronchoconstriction, slight delayed hypotension and thrombocytopenia in guinea pigs prepared by the Konzett-

Rössler method, but this requires 5–10-fold higher concentrations than in case of Aa. These effects are not inhibited by NSAID (VARGAFTIG et al., unpublished observations). It is noteworthy that dihomo γ-linoleic acid releases RCS and PG-like activity from isolated lungs, which is inhibited by aspirin (PALMER et al., 1973). Failure to aggregate platelets in vivo (ROSE et al., 1974) or in vitro (WILLIS et al., 1974; VARGAFTIG, unpublished) may be accounted for by the ability of PGEs to counteract aggregation due to ADP (SHIO and RAMWELL, 1972) or to Aa (VARGAFTIG and CHIGNARD, 1975), and by the very low ability of dihomo γ-linoleic acid to generate RCS and PG-like activity when incubated with rabbit platelets.

c) Effects of Arachidonic Acid on Rabbit Blood Pressure

Aa decreases the blood pressure of rabbits, and this effect is inhibited by indomethacin (LARSSON and ÄNGGÅRD, 1973). Hypotension can be obtained without any evidence of thrombocytopenia. This contrasts with what occurs with ADP (Fig. 6) which induces transient but marked thrombocytopenia accompanied by smaller hypotensive responses. Another interesting dissociation is that platelets collected from rabbits at different time intervals after intravenous administration of small doses of aspirin (20 mg/kg, for instance) are refractory to aggregation by Aa up to 5 h whereas the hypotensive response to Aa returns within 1 or 2 h. Platelets are irreversibly labelled by aspirin (ROTH et al., 1975) which probably accounts for the irreversible inhibition of Aa-induced aggregation. Aa thus releases hypotensive materials from other sites than platelets, for instance from lungs, where acetylation of PG synthetase as inhibitor mechanism is less critical and/or more reversible.

Heparin and certain amino acids has been reported to potentiate the hypotensive response of rabbits to Aa (DEBY et al., 1974; DAMAS and DEBY, 1974). No simultaneous platelet counts were carried out.

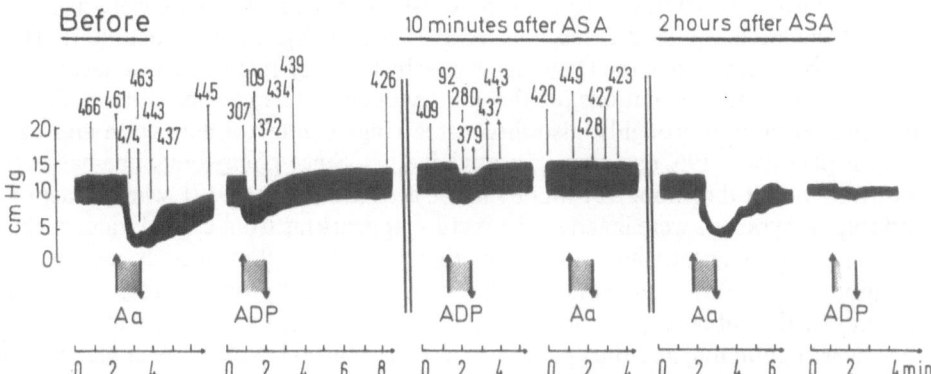

Fig. 6. Interference of aspirin with hypotension induced by arachidonic acid and by ADP in the rabbit. Arterial blood pressure of a pentobarbitone-anaesthetised rabbit. Content of platelets in arterial blood before and at intervals after drug injections was measured. Arachidonic acid (Aa, 50 µg/kg^{-1}·min^{-1}) and ADP (200 µg/kg^{-1}·min^{-1}) were infused i.v. for 2 min, as indicated by hatched signs and inverted arrows. Aspirin (20 mg/kg, i.v.) partially inhibited hypotension due to ADP or to Aa. Figures above tracing are platelet counts at intervals after drug infusion. Arachidonic acid induces hypotension without accompanying drop in platelet counts, whereas the less intense hypotensive response to ADP is accompanied by a marked and transitory drop in platelet counts. Aspirin fails to prevent this drop by ADP, but inhibits hypotension. Time scale in minutes and arterial blood pressure in cm Hg

d) Effects of Arachidonic Acid on Other Animal Species

Aa induces thrombus formation and death upon intravenous injection in mice. This is inhibited by NSAID as well as by ADP antagonists. No information was given about blood pressure (KOHLER et al., 1975). Aa induces hypotension in anaesthetized rats (COHEN et al., 1973). It has also been shown that experimental hypertension in rats is aggravated after oral administration of Aa for 4 weeks to nephrectomised and DOCA-treated rats (LABORIT and VALETTE, 1973). The differences are probably due to sudden generation of hypotensive materials and/or platelet reactions upon acute administration of Aa, as compared with slow metabolic processes expected to follow chronic oral administration. Results of LABORIT and VALETTE (1973), which have been recently republished (1975), should be considered in light of the evidence that PGs provide a negative feedback loop for catecholamine release upon nerve stimulation (HEDQVIST et al., 1970). Aa also lowers the arterial blood pressure of cats, and induces bronchoconstriction and reversible thrombocytopenia. Hypotension and bronchoconstriction are inhibited by 20 mg/kg of aspirin i.v. (Fig. 3).

II. Effects of Fatty Acids Other Than Prostaglandin Precursors

Long-chain saturated fatty acids produced extensive thrombosis and death when given intravenously to dogs (CONNOR et al., 1963), whereas unsaturated fatty acids were inactive. Doses of 10 mg/kg were used and it is surprising that no effect was noted for arachidonate. Haemolysis was not considered as related to the mechanism of action of the fatty acids. The following compounds were active: behenic (C22:0), stearic (C18:0), palmitic (C16:0), and myristic (C14:0) acids. Lauric (C12:0) and capric (C10:0) were inactive. ZBINDEN (1964) has shown that C22:0, C18:0, C16:0, C14:0 but also C12:0 and C10:0 induced thrombocytopenia upon intravenous injection into rabbits. Other fatty acids that displayed such an activity were linolenic (C18:3) and linoleic (C18:2) acids, injected at 1.25–5 mg/kg, and oleic acid (C18:1) at 5–10 mg/kg. Activation of the Hageman factor by the fatty acid as well as haemolysis were discarded as explanations for thrombocytopenia. The case of lauric acid was investigated more thoroughly, also discarding Hageman factor activation and haemolysis (ZBINDEN, 1967) as main causative factors. Since phenylbutazone has been shown to inhibit thrombocytopenia by lauric acid (ZBINDEN, 1967), whereas aspirin and sulphinpyrazone were inactive, the picture appears far from clear. Evidence that a non-PG precursor fatty acid, such as lauric acid, induces thrombocytopenia which is inhibited by a NSAID may indicate that lauric acid (and possibly other fatty acids that induce thrombocytopenia in rabbits) displace Aa from a relatively loose bond, such as with albumin, and thus provide a substrate for PG synthetase in platelets or in other sites. C16:0, C18:0, C22:0 and erucic acid (C22:1) induce aggregation of rabbit platelets in vitro (PROST-DVOJAKOVIC and SAMAMA, 1973, 1974), but failure of oleic acid to display a similar activity makes it difficult to correlate this with the in vivo effects of ZBINDEN (1964). Lack of purity of the sample of oleic acid used by ZBINDEN may be a simple explanation. C22:0, C18:0, C14:0 and arachidic acid (C20:0), induce histamine release from rabbit platelets. This appears not to result from platelet lysis alone, since Ca^{++} and a plasma factor which might be fibrinogen are required, and since keeping platelets at 5° C prevents histamine release (SHORE and ALPERS, 1963). C18:2 and C18:3 were inactive. Aa was not tested.

Linoleic acid induces a transient thrombocytopenia when injected i.v. into dogs at 1 mg/kg. This is not accompanied by hypotension, in contrast to the effect of Aa. It thus appears that platelet aggregation does not cause hypotension by itself. In fact, acute thrombocytopenia by anti-platelet serum in rabbits and in dogs is not followed by any major cardiovascular sign, whereas a similar treatment of guinea pigs leads to bronchoconstriction, followed by lethal hypotension when the injection is performed rapidly. Hypotension by fatty acids other than Aa may either result from the above mentioned displacement of the PG precursor, or from formation of non-PG active substances, like the lipoperoxides. Linoleic and linolenic acids up to 1 mg/kg i.v. do not induce hypotension nor acute thrombocytopenia in guinea pigs.

III. Slow Reacting Substance C

SRS-C induces hypotension in rabbits, dogs, guinea pigs, fowls and monkeys (Fig. 7 and 8). In guinea pigs, hypotension is accompanied by bronchoconstriction, as in the case of Aa. In fact, SRS-C shares with Aa a variety of properties but differs quantita-

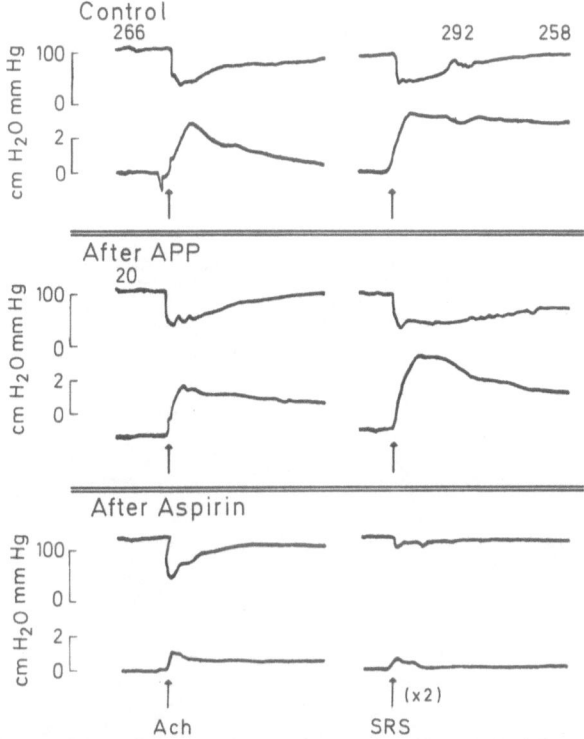

Fig. 7. Inability of anti-platelet plasma to inhibit hypotension and the increase in venous pressure due to slow reacting substance C in a rabbit. Arterial blood pressure and central venous pressure of a pentobarbitone-anaesthetised rabbit were recorded *(upper and lower tracings respectively)*. Acetylcholine *(Ach,* 5 µg/kg) and SRS-C *(SRS,* 0.2 ml/kg and where indicated ×2, 0.4 ml/kg), before *(Control)*, after anti-platelet plasma *(After APP)*, and (since effects of SRS-C were not inhibited by this treatment), after aspirin (10 mg/kg). Number of platelets × 10^3 indicated above tracings, showing that SRS-C does not reduce circulating platelets as expected for Aa, and that only 10% of starting platelets remained after anti-platelet treatment, which failed to prevent effects of SRS-C. Scales as in Figure 6; venous pressure in cm H_2O

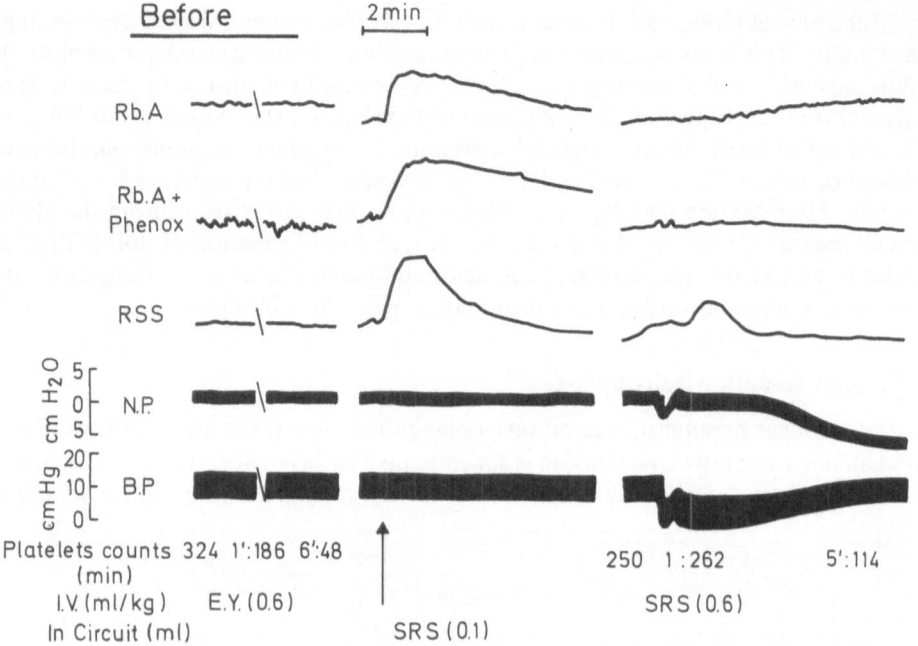

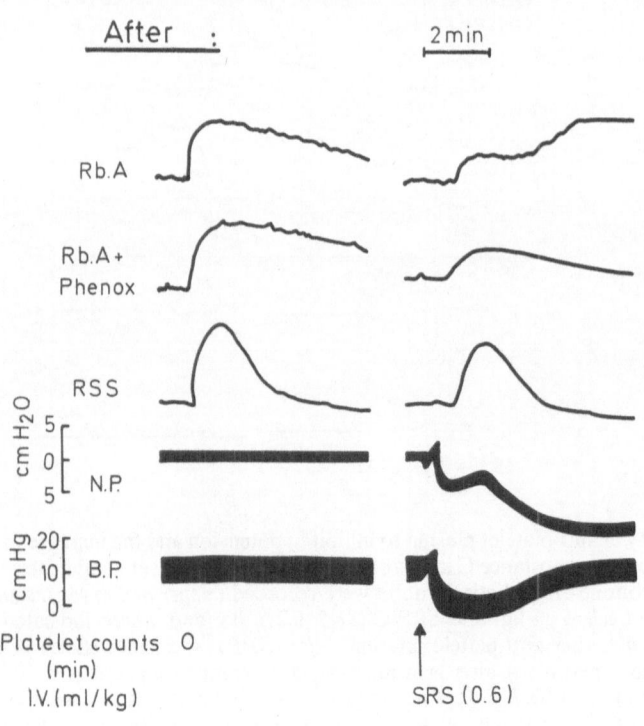

Table 2. Pharmacological properties and antagonism of partially purified slow reacting substance C[a]

In vitro

1. Induces lysis of guinea pig and dog erythrocytes.
2. Contracts isolated rabbit duodenum, rat stomach and guinea pig ileum.
3. Contracts bronchial muscle of isolated perfused guinea pig lungs.
4. Displays no effect on force of contraction and on surface electrocardiogram of isolated perfused rabbit hearts.
5. Does not aggregate rabbit platelets.
6. Induces formation of RCS and of PG-like activities from human, dog, rabbit and guinea pig blood or PRP.

In vivo

1. Induces hypotension in dogs, rabbits, cats, guinea pigs and fowls.
2. Induces bronchoconstriction in guinea pigs and cats.
3. Kills rats and mice upon i.v. injection.
4. Induces no thrombocytopenia in dogs and rabbits.

Inhibitors of effects of slow reacting substance C

1. Non-steroid anti-inflammatory drugs: indomethacin, aspirin, sodium salycilate, amino-pyrine, phenazone, meclofenamic acid, flufenamic acid, phenylbutazone, oxyphenylbutazone, paracetamol, isobutylphenylacetic acid, noramidopyrine methanesulphonate, dl-6-methoxy-1,2,3,4-tetrahydrocarbazole-2-carboxylic acid.
2. Thiol agents:2-mercaptoethanol, 2-thioglycerol, 2,3-dimercaptopropanol, dithiothreitol, sodium diethyldithiocarbamate.
   Note: the following thiols were ineffective in vivo: DL-penicillamine, reduced glutathione, DL-cysteine, thioglycolate and sodium dimethyldithiocarbamate.
3. Other ineffective agents were: CaEDTA, dipyridyl, phenoxybenzamine, phentolamine, atropine, reserpine, kallikrein inhibitors, iodoacetic acid, disodium cromoglycate, ethylmaleimide, ascorbic acid, mepyramine and methysergide.

---

[a] Details in: VARGAFTIG et al. (1969); VARGAFTIG and DAO (1971b); VARGAFTIG and DAO HAI, (1972b); VARGAFTIG and DAO HAI, (1973); VARGAFTIG (1973).

◄ Fig. 8. Failure of platelet depletion to inhibit the hypotensive effects of slow reacting substance in the dog. A pentobarbitone-anaesthetised dog was prepared for recording of arterial blood pressure *(B.P.)* and for detection of potential mediators in the circulation using the blood-bathed organ technique (VANE, 1964). Assay tissues, top to bottom were: rabbit aorta strip *(Rb.A)*, rabbit aorta strip incubated for the overnight with 0.1 µg/ml of the α-adrenoceptor blocking agent phenoxybenzamine *(Rb.A + Phenox)*, and a rat stomach strip *(RSS)*. Nasal pressure *(N.P.)* was recorded according to VARGAFTIG and LEFORT (1974). Platelet counts were performed at intervals, which are indicated as minutes after injections; the latter were either performed i.v., and are indicated as ml of SRS-C/kg of body weight or as total volume when given directly into the tubing transporting blood from animal to assay tissues *(in circuit)*. Control injections are shown in panel "Before", panel "After" indicates that platelet depletion had been obtained (platelet counts: *0*). Observe in panel "Before" that egg yolk alone (*E.Y.*, control for SRS-C) has no effect on the blood pressure, and does not release smooth-muscle contracting substances, whereas a delayed drop in platelet counts occurs. SRS-C (0.1 ml in circuit) leads to marked contractions of the three assay tissues. An i.v. injection of SRS-C (SRS, 0.6 ml/kg) is followed by slight contraction of the smooth muscle preparations, by decreased intranasal pressure, indicating either vasoconstriction or drop in blood flow, by hypotension, and by a decrease of platelet counts, equivalent to that due to egg yolk alone. After platelet depletion is obtained, the responses to SRS 0.1 in the circuit are, equivocally increased, whereas the effects of the i.v. injection are clearly increased. Adrenaline secretion is probably interfering to some extent with the bioassay, since the phenoxybenzamine-treated rabbit aorta strip contracts much less than the untreated one. Arterial blood pressure in cm Hg; nasal (internal) pressure in cm H_2O. Time in minutes

tively when the amount of potential mediators that are released from dog platelets or blood is evaluated (FERREIRA and VARGAFTIG, 1974). It appears that SRS-C also shares with Aa the mechanism of hypotension, since both induce arterial vasodilatation, at least in dogs (FERREIRA and VARGAFTIG, 1974), and they have the same effects on nasal vessels, as discussed above. All vascular effects of SRS-C, as well as bronchoconstriction when apparent, are inhibited by NSAID and by thiol containing agents (Fig. 7 and 8 and Table 2). Threshold doses of NSAID block the effects of Aa better than those of SRS-C, but higher amounts totally suppress effects of SRS-C as well (VARGAFTIG and DAO, 1971 b; VARGAFTIG and DAO HAI, 1972 c). SRS-C has no effect on the force of contraction of rabbit hearts, nor does it affect the surface electrocardiogram.

Intravenous injections of SRS-C do not appear to affect the platelet count in the circulation of dogs or rabbits, in contrast to effects of Aa. Thrombocytopenia (Fig. 8) is also induced by injections of control egg yolk to dogs, and cannot be attributed to SRS-C. Immune platelet depletion does not inhibit the hypotensive effect of SRS-C, or the accompanying increase in venous pressure (Fig. 7), showing that a non-platelet site of action operates in rabbits for SRS-C. Similar results were obtained in platelet-deprived dogs (Fig. 8).

Since RCS (and thus presumably thromboxanes and PGs) are released by SRS-C from isolated perfused guinea pig lungs (VARGAFTIG and DAO, 1971 a), it is hypothesized that at least part of the in vivo activity results from generation by PG synthetase and like enzymes of vasoactive substances in lungs. Inhibition by NSAID, by thiol agents and by pyrogallol of in vitro and in vivo effects of Aa could be explained in this fashion.

1. Mechanism of Action of Slow Reacting Substance C

The procedure currently used partially to purify SRS-C excludes major contamination by saturated fatty acids, but does not eliminate unsaturated fatty acids other than Aa (VARGAFTIG and COIRON, 1971). Crude SRS-C (incubate of egg yolk with phospholipase A_2-containing venom, the latter being neutralised by anti-serum after 1–4 h of incubation) is contaminated with lysolecithin, formed from phospholipids when the esterified acyl residue is hydrolysed (VOGT, 1957 a). The released amounts of lysolecithin appear not to induce in vivo effects, since these are totally inhibited by NSAID, which is not the case for pure lysolecithin. The actual component of the mixture responsible for the pharmacological activity has not been identified. It is quite possible that the main activity is due to Aa, and that the differences between pure Aa and SRS-C result from the modulating effect of other unsaturated fatty acids that accompany Aa in SRS-C. Hydroxy fatty acid (DAKHIL and VOGT, 1962; BABILLI and VOGT, 1965) and PGs have been considered responsible for the activity of SRS-C. Moreover, since addition of pyrogallol or of diethyldithiocarbamate to SRS-C at final concentrations that have no antagonising in vivo effect prevents its subsequent activity (VARGAFTIG and DAO HAI, 1972 b), it may well be that oxidation products present in crude SRS-C are involved. Recent evidence that relatively stable endoperoxide analogues can display intense pharmacological activity (COREY et al., 1975) reinforces the hypothesis that the similarity between the pharmacological properties of SRS-C and of Aa results from the presence in solutions of the former of stable endoperoxide-like materials. If this is the case, inhibition of the effects of SRS-C by NSAID would not be easily explained by their inhibitory activity on PG synthetase. VAN NUETEN et al. (1976) have performed in vitro experiments indicating that both arachidonic acid-hydroperoxide and SRS-C-induced contractions of the guinea pig ileum strip are inhibited by NSAID, as shown previously in other systems (JAQUES, 1959, 1965; VARGAFTIG and DAO, 1971 a). They furthermore observed that the amount of polyunsaturated fatty acids (3 or more double bonds) present in SRS-C could account, on a weight basis, for the contractions obtained with Aa-hydroperoxide. The latter was stated to contain a variety of peroxidized isomers, and the 11-peroxy Aa derivative, a PG precursor. The site of action of SRS-C on rabbits and on dogs does not involve platelet aggregation (Fig. 7 and 8). Incubation of dog or rabbit blood or PRP with SRS-C or injections of the latter into the tubing carrying blood from an anaesthetised animal to assay tissues, lead to rabbit aorta and rat stomach strip contractions, indicating generation of RCS and of PG-like activity (Fig. 8). A similar, but much reduced activity is found when blood is continuously bioassayed after intravenous injections of SRS-C and this activity is not reduced, but in fact increased, after experimental thrombocytopenia (Fig. 8). Hypotensive and smooth muscle contracting substances are thus released by SRS-C from sites other than circulating platelets whether free in blood or trapped in lung vessels.

D. Interference of Non-Steroid Anti-Inflammatory Agents With Effects of Miscellaneous Agents

I. Adenosine Nucleotides

The hypotensive effect of ADP and of ATP is due to direct vasodilatation and to bradycardia that follows atrio-ventricular blockade (CLARKE et al., 1952; THORP and COBBIN, 1959) combined with systemic platelet aggregation (BORN et al., 1965). Intravenous administration of ADP is followed by transient acute thrombocytopenia (ZUCKER, 1967), which is clearly seen 10 s after intravenous injections into guinea pigs and fades within 1 min. Similar effects with a slower onset and longer duration are observed for ATP, suggesting, as occurs in vitro, that ATP must be transformed into ADP to affect platelets. The contribution of platelets to the overall pharmacological activity of ADP and of ATP is more marked in those species in which the former induces an aspirin-sensitive platelet release reaction, as seen in human platelets in vitro. These species include guinea pigs, dogs, and cats. A typical release reaction is not induced by ADP in rabbit platelets (see Chap. 5) as it is by thrombin, collagen or Aa, but a sort of equivalent process is triggered by ADP within the platelet, which can thus be influenced by NSAID. Thus indomethacin and aspirin facilitate disaggregation after ADP, although the height of aggregation is unchanged. The in vivo consequence of this effect is seen in Figure 6, and calls for the following observations:

(a) The hypotensive response to Aa is less marked than that to ADP, but the former does not induce a fall in blood platelet counts, whereas injection of the latter is followed by a marked transient thrombocytopenia (panel *before*).

(b) Hypotension by Aa is completely suppressed within 10 min of administration of 20 mg/kg of aspirin, whereas hypotension by ADP is largely, but not totally, inhibited (panel *10 min after ASA*). Inhibition of hypotension due to ADP is not accompanied by inhibition of thrombocytopenia, which is a direct effect of ADP. This agrees with the above statement that aggregation of rabbit platelets in vitro is not suppressed by NSAID, although one platelet contribution to hypotension is inhibited.

(c) Two hours after the administration of aspirin, the hypotensive effect of Aa is fully restored, whereas ADP is still ineffective. This is evidence that aspirin inhibits hypotension by Aa in a site other than platelets. The demonstration that platelets prepared from blood collected up to 5 h after 2–10 mg/kg of aspirin are fully resistant to the in vitro aggregating effect of Aa, when the hypotensive response is restored within 1 and 2 h reinforces this explanation. Similar experiments have not been performed with ATP, which requires prior transformation to ADP to induce aggregation. Since the effects of ATP appear more slowly, they are better inhibited in vitro by NSAID than those of ADP. This probably explains why NSAID inhibit ATP-induced bronchoconstriction in the guinea pig (COLLIER et al., 1966) and not that due to ADP. Guinea pig lungs are not expected to generate vasodepressor or broncho-constrictor substances after ADP or ATP are injected i.v., since in contrast to Aa or SRS-C, they do not release RCS from perfused guinea pig lungs (VARGAFTIG and DAO, 1971 a). The platelet aggregating effect of the two adenosine derivatives thus probably accounts for all aspirin-sensitive effects.

Adenosine tetraphosphate is also an aggregating nucleotide, and its effects are mediated by ADP, since the enzyme apyrase at 0.5–1 mg/ml, inhibits its effects. Adenosine tetraphosphate induces hypotension, bronchoconstriction and platelet aggregation in guinea pigs (LEFORT and VARGAFTIG, 1978 a), but the actual participation of the release reaction as compared to the direct effect of the compound has not been studied. Cordycepin phosphate, adenosine diphosphate N-oxide, and deoxy ADP are nucleotides that aggregate human platelets (GARADER and LALAND, 1964). The first two nucleotides do not aggregate rabbit or guinea pig platelets in vitro and accordingly, do not induce in vivo platelet falls or bronchoconstriction in guinea pigs, when used i.v. up to 1 mg/kg.

II. Collagen

Since collagen induces aggregation of platelets of most mammalian species (MUS-TARD and PACKHAM, 1970), its in vivo effects have been investigated in the search for methods to induce thromboembolic diseases. A collagen suspension was used to induce thromboembolism in mice, which resulted in death, with platelet aggregates in lung capillaries. This could be prevented by aspirin, by phenylbutazone, and by making animals thrombocytopenic by irradiation or by drug treatment (NISHIZAWA et al., 1972). Collagen induces thrombocytopenia (Fig. 2) and hypotension upon intravenous injection into rabbits, both of which are inhibited by aspirin. Intra-muscular ADP prevents the thrombocytopenic effect of intravenous collagen, point-ing to desensitized action of platelets by the treatment as causally related to the effects of collagen. This is supported by the fact that experimental thrombocytopenia prevents the hypotensive effects of collagen (Fig. 2). Collagen induces bronchocon-striction in guinea pigs which is also inhibited by substances that suppress platelet aggregation, and by thrombocytopenia (LEFORT and VARGAFTIG, 1978 b).

III. Anaphylatoxin

Anaphylatoxin formed in heparinized rat plasma incubated with dextran induces a drop in arterial blood pressure and an increase in the pulmonary blood pressure gradient in cats. A marked reduction of platelet counts and a less marked reduction of leucocyte counts occurs but clears rapidly. Anti-5-HT treatment did not prevent these effects, but experimental (non-immune) thrombocytopenia did, indicating a platelet site of action (SCHUMACHER et al., 1974). The blood pressure response to anaphylatoxin is known to involve a non-histamine component, both in cats and in guinea pigs (BODAMMER, 1969). Since anaphylatoxin releases a substance with PG-like activity from isolated perfused guinea pig lungs (SACKEYFIO, 1972), in a similar fashion to Aa or SRS-C, it is possible that at least part of the hypotensive and non-histamine-dependent activity of anaphylatoxin is inhibited by NSAID.

IV. Depressor Active Substance (DAS)

DAS is a liposoluble substance, generated in bovine serum kept at 28° C for 36 h. It markedly decreases arterial blood pressure and increases pulmonary vascular resistance of cats, leading at the same time to a marked decrease in platelet counts (SCHUMACHER and CLASSEN, 1973). Histological examination of lung tissues after administration of DAS showed massive platelet deposition in the small pulmonary vessels. Interference by anti-5-HT or antihistamine agents has not been reported, but would be logical since cat platelets are the only ones, among other mammal species, to aggregate fully when challenged with 5-HT (TSCHOPP, 1970). The sulphated polysaccharide pentosan sulphate inhibits in vivo and in vitro effects of DAS (SCHUMACHER and CLASSEN, 1973) and has been claimed to display anti-inflammatory effects (KALBHEN, 1973).

V. Platelet Clumping Substance

A platelet clumping substance is generated in heparinised plasma of rabbits given bacterial endotoxin, adrenaline, high molecular substances like agar-agar, or after incubation of plasma with trypsin (YAMAZAKI et al., 1967, 1968; MURASE et al., 1971). There is evidence that this substance is a mucopolysaccharide. Since it is generated in plasma of various species—including man—after weak acidification of plasma, which might occur locally in ischaemic or inflammatory tissues, the relevance to inflammation is obvious. Whether the mechanism of action of this substance is related to that of carrageenin is unclear, since potential antagonists apart from other mucopolysaccharides or related enzymes have not been tested. Moreover, no in vivo work has been reported for formation of this substance for a physiopathological role and for possible antagonism.

VI. Barium Sulphate and Other Particulate Materials

Intravenous barium sulphate ($BaSO_4$) increases pulmonary resistance and decreases pulmonary compliance in various animal species (see NADEL et al., 1964). Few attempts have been made to antagonize these effects. Thus isoprenaline, salbutamol, papaverine and aminophyline reduced the pulmonary effects of $BaSO_4$; this has been attributed to their bronchodilator effect (DALY, 1974). However, the site of action might also be platelets, since these antagonists increase the cyclic AMP content of platelets and thus inhibit aggregation (MILLS and SMITH, 1971).

BaSO4 induces hypotension in cats (Bø et al., 1974) guinea pigs, dogs, and rabbits (NAKANO and MCCLOY, 1973; VARGAFTIG and LEFORT, unpublished results). Since thrombocytopenia with anti-platelet serum prevented the increase in pulmonary arterial pressure by BaSO4 in cats (Bø et al., 1974) we have tried—and failed—to inhibit with aspirin or with indomethacin BaSO4-induced hypotension and the accompanying fall in platelet counts in dogs, rabbits and guinea pigs (Fig. 3). NAKANO and MCCLOY (1973) demonstrated that indomethacin intravenously inhibited bronchoconstriction but not the circulatory responses to embolization with BaSO4, and suggested that this was due to inhibition of generation of PGs. We failed to show release of RCS or of PG-like activity in incubates of rabbit PRP and BaSO4, but this of course does not rule out release from lungs. If only PG generation were involved with effects of BaSO4, it is hard to explain why in the case of dogs only bronchoconstriction and not the increased pulmonary aterial pressure was inhibited by indomethacin.

Injections of other types of particles into dog spleen and rat and guinea pig lungs evokes release of RCS and of PG-like activities (GILMORE et al., 1969; LINDSEY and WYLLIE, 1970; PIPER and VANE, 1971; PALMER et al., 1973). Release was more readily obtained from sensitized than from unsensitized lungs (PALMER et al., 1973). In vivo effects are not reported.

E. Interference of Non-Steroid Anti-Inflammatory Agents With Hypotension in Endotoxin Shock

NSAID inhibit the acute hypotensive response to endotoxin in dogs (NORTHOVER and SUBRAMANIAN, 1962; HINSHAW et al., 1967), cats (GREENWAY and MURTHY, 1971; HALL et al., 1972; PARRATT and STURGESS, 1974, 1975a, 1975b) and sheep (HALL et al., 1972). Since differences have been noted between species and between drugs, it is worth detailing the results, although a study on the pathophysiology of endotoxin shock is beyond the purpose of this review.

I. Dogs

Endotoxin shock in dogs is characterised by an immediate fall in blood pressure, accompanied by a marked increase of portal vein pressure. This is followed by an increase in arterial pressure and by a long-lasting subsequent decrease, with cardiovascular shock and death within 24 h (NORTHOVER and SUBRAMANIAN, 1962). Aspirin, sodium salicylate and γ-resorcylic acid were effective in decreasing order of potency in preventing endotoxin-induced immediate and delayed effects on cardiovascular parameters (NORTHOVER and SUBRAMANIAN, 1962). These effects, as well as the accompanying decrease of blood pH and increase in haematocrit values, were inhibited by aspirin at 100 mg/kg (one quarter to half of the dose used by NORTHOVER and SUBRAMANIAN, 1962), indomethacin (20 mg/kg), phenylbutazone (100 mg/kg) and flufenamic acid (50 mg/kg) (ERDÖS, 1968). Prostaglandins were found in portal and renal blood after endotoxin; their detection was prevented by indomethacin and aspirin, although at the relatively low doses employed as compared to other authors early haemodynamic effects were not inhibited (ANDERSON et al., 1975). Late haemodynamic effects of endotoxin were prevented by indomethacin but not by aspirin. The protocol used by ANDERSON et al. (1975) consisted of administering a low priming dose of the NSAID followed by a slow infusion. This may complicate the comparison of their results with those of other authors. Early suggestions that aspirin inhibits the effects of vasoactive compounds released by endotoxin (histamine, 5-HT, catecholamines, SRS or Bk) (HINSHAW et al., 1967) are less likely, although the doses of aspirin required to inhibit the haemodynamic effects of endotoxin shock are much higher than those required to block the effects of lipidic agonists, such as Aa or SRS-C. Differences between the anti-inflammatory agents should also be considered (ERDÖS et al., 1967; ANDERSON et al., 1975). Acetylsalicylic acid appears to have properties not shared by indomethacin (ROTHSCHILD et al., 1974) which are likely to involve acetylation processes. Moreover, the haemodynamic effects resulting from the injection of live *E. coli* organisms into dogs are partially blocked by NSAID, whereas compounds chemically related but devoid of anti-inflammatory activities are inactive. This includes 4-acetamidophen, sulphinpyrazone, salicylaldoxime and salicylamide (CULP et al., 1970). Sulphinpyrazone is a platelet protecting agent and a complement antagonist (JOBIN and GAGNON, 1970), whereas salicylaldoxime is an antagonist of immune haemolysis (MILLS and LEVINE, 1958). See also JOBIN and TREMBLAY (1969).

Intravenous administration of endotoxin evokes many reactions in plasma and also involves the formed elements of blood. Although these reactions have been studied (see KOVATS, 1972), interference of NSAID at this level is less well established, particularly in the case of dogs (see below, for other animal species). The ability of the protease inhibitor Trasylol (aprotinin) to increase survival of endotoxin-shocked animals, and to reduce depletion of kininogen (ERDÖS et al., 1967), is not direct evidence for involvement of kinin release, since it may be accounted for by inhibition of other proteases by Trasylol. Similar comments can be made with respect to protection against endotoxin shock by ε-amino caproic acid (SPINK and VICK, 1961).

II. Cats

Injection of *E. coli* endotoxin to cats induces a marked rise in pulmonary pressure, accompanied by a transient decrease in systemic arterial blood pressure (acute phase) followed by systemic hypotension, and metabolic acidosis (delayed shock phase) (PARRATT and STURGESS, 1974). The acute phase is abolished by 10–100 mg/kg of aspirin, whereas the delayed phase is unaffected (GREENWAY and MURTHY, 1971), at least for *Salmonella enteritidis* endotoxin. In aspirin-treated cats a marked mesenteric vasoconstriction appears 45–60 min after endotoxin administration, which cannot be inhibited by α-adrenoceptor blocking agents, by hypophysectomy or by nephrectomy, ruling out the participation of catecholamines, vasopressin and angiotensin (GREENWAY and MURTHY, 1971). Indomethacin and meclofenamate inhibit the initial pulmonary hypertension and lung oedema that follow endotoxin administration, and retard rather than block the delayed shock (PARRATT and STUR-

GESS, 1974, 1975a). The suggestion that effects of indomethacin on the acute phase of endotoxin shock are due to interference with release and/or activity of histamine on the lung vessels (the source of histamine being the platelets), and that the effect on the delayed phase results from inhibition of PG synthetase awaits definite proof (PARRATT and STURGESS, 1974). It has nevertheless been shown that histamine depletion and antagonists of H 1 and of H 2 receptors failed to prevent the rise in pulmonary blood pressure upon endotoxin administration, whereas inhibitors of PG synthetase (indomethacin), of PG synthetase and of PG receptors (meclofenamate), or of $PGF_{2\alpha}$ receptors (polyphloretin phosphate) prevented or markedly reduced endotoxin-induced pulmonary vasoconstriction (PARRATT and STURGESS, 1975b). Since indomethacin was not beneficial when administered during bacteraemic or septic shock, it appears that the acute pulmonary changes that occur in the cat within a few minutes of endotoxin administration contribute to the severity of the shock phase (PARRATT and STURGESS, 1975c). This finding, disappointing as it may be, does not mean that NSAID should not be tested in human gram-negative shock, since in this case endotoxins are slowly released and it is important to delay collapse, while symptomatic and antibiotic treatments become effective.

III. Other Animal Species

Although a very large amount of experimental data on cellular reactions to endotoxin (NAGAYAMA et al., 1971) in rabbits has been reported, little work has been performed with anti-inflammatory drugs in vivo. Endotoxin injection into rabbits elicits severe thrombocytopenia, followed by intravascular coagulation (BELLER et al., 1969). Granulocytes appear to be involved in endotoxin-induced activation of intravascular coagulation, but do not influence in vivo thrombocytopenia accompanying endotoxin administration to rabbits (MÜLLER-BERGHAUS and ECKHARDT, 1975), nor the increased fibrinogen synthesis rate. NSAID have not been tested under those circumstances.

F. Mechanism of Action of Hypotensive Agents Liable to Inhibition by Non-Steroid Anti-Inflammatory Drugs

I. Structure-Activity Correlations

Anti-inflammatory activity generally, but not always (VAN DEN BERG et al., 1975), correlates with inhibition of PG synthetase (FLOWER, 1974). A detailed analysis of the deviations from this rule is beyond the scope of this review, except when interactions with hypotension by inflammatory mediators are involved. One interesting case is that of 4-acetamidophenol (paracetamol), which displays feeble anti-inflammatory activity (BIANCHI and DAVID, 1960), does not inhibit PG synthetase from dog spleen (FLOWER et al., 1972), but inhibits brain PG synthetase (WILLIS et al., 1972; FLOWER and VANE, 1972). This has been correlated with the antipyretic activity of paracetamol. Nevertheless, paracetamol also inhibits generation of PGs and of RCS in incubates of Aa and of rabbit platelets, and suppresses the accompanying platelet aggregation (VARGAFTIG and ZIRINIS, 1973; VARGAFTIG and DAO HAI, 1973; VARGAFTIG, 1973). Accordingly, hypotension and bronchoconstriction induced by Aa and by

SRS-C, bronchoconstriction caused by ATP and by Bk, and the second phase of hypotension produced by the latter, are also inhibited by paracetamol. Since platelets are not required for in vivo effects of Aa, of SRS-C or of Bk, paracetamol presumably inhibits PG synthetase from another site. Platelets provide a model for this site, as they provide for brain PG synthetase and for other neurochemical parameters (ABRAMS and SOLOMON, 1969). This example demonstrates the need for determining the source from which PG synthetase should be prepared for inhibitory studies involving predictable anti-inflammatory activity. Interest in this problem is of practical importance for detection of active drugs, and of theoretical interest for identification and understanding of the relevance of mediators involved in acute or chronic inflammation or in related conditions.

1. Thiol and Anti-Oxidant Compounds

Hypotension induced by SRS-C and bronchoconstriction induced by Aa, by ATP and by Bk are inhibited by various thiol agents (Table 2) (VARGAFTIG and DAO HAI, 1972b). These agents also inhibit Aa-induced platelet aggregation, and the accompanying generation of PG-related substances, both in vitro and in vivo (VARGAFTIG and ZIRINIS, 1973; VARGAFTIG et al., 1974). Here again platelets should be considered as a model rather than as an identified site of action, for reasons already outlined. The model is quite reliable, since thiol agents that do not inhibit in vivo effects of SRS-C or of Aa also fail to inhibit platelet aggregation (Table 2).

The in vivo anti-SRS-C effect of thiol agents is reversible with time and can be reproduced in the same animal for various cycles. Inhibition is likewise removed if platelets are washed and resuspended in drug-free plasma, whereas the effects of NSAID are irreversible (VARGAFTIG et al., 1974). Finally, the disulphide reagent 5,5'-dithio-bis (2-nitrobenzoic acid) prevents the in vitro antagonism of Aa-induced platelet aggregation by thiol agents or by pyrogallol, and reverses the in vivo antagonism by at least one thiol agent, i.e. 2-thioglycerol. In contrast, antagonism by indomethacin is unaffected.

Mechanisms of action of thiol and anti-oxidant agents may involve one of the following factors:

1. Chelation of a metal. This could be copper, which stimulated Aa-induced platelet aggregation and generation of RCS and PG-like substances, and reverses inhibition caused by thiol drugs (VARGAFTIG et al., 1974), but not that due to NSAID.

2. Inhibition of formation or stimulation of degradation of endoperoxides like PGG_2 containing a labile O-OH group on carbon 15. This explanation may also account for antagonism by catalase of in vitro effects of Aa (VARGAFTIG et al., 1975), since catalase probably attacks the same O-OH group. Removal of PGG_2 should result in suppression of formation of PGs and of thromboxane A_2 (HAMBERG et al., 1975b) and thus in suppression of rat stomach and rabbit aorta contracting activities as well as of platelet aggregating activity generated in rabbits (VARGAFTIG et al., 1975) or dog PRP (VARGAFTIG et al., 1976; CHIGNARD and VARGAFTIG, 1976).

3. Reduction of disulphide groups. Whereas metal chelation and interference with endoperoxide generation and/or activity are possibly two facets of the same process, reduction of disulphide groups appears to be a less probable mechanism.

Three amino-thiol agents, penicillamine, cysteine and reduced glutathione, do not inhibit the effects of SRS-C in vivo, and in appropriate conditions, potentiate aggregation by Aa. This may be related to generation of free radicals that can trigger lipoperoxidation (Vargaftig et al., 1974). It is thus unlikely that the antirheumatic activity of penicillamine should be explained on the basis of antagonism of lipoperoxide formation, at least from information gathered on the platelet model. The thiol agents reported to inhibit in vivo effects of Aa and of SRS-C also suppress the generation of RCS from isolated perfused guinea pig lungs injected with Bk, SRS-C or Aa (Vargaftig and Dao Hai, 1972a). An interesting exception was sodium diethyldithiocarbamate, inactive in this in vitro model in which lungs are perfused with a plasma-free medium, but active against the effects of SRS-C, of Bk or of Aa, both in vivo and in vitro, when assays are used with plasma present.

Interference with metals has been hypothesised as the mechanism of action of NSAID (Sorenson, 1974), but irreversibility of in vitro anti-aggregating effects distinguished their mechanism of action from that of thiol agents. It is thus expected that thiols and NSAID should display supra-additive effects if the appropriate chemical structures are associated. The in vivo set-up, using Aa, SRS-C or Bk appears particularly appropriate for testing such new structures. This is reinforced by results obtained with stereoisomers of NSAID.

II. Stereospecificity

Anti-inflammatory activity and the ability to inhibit PG synthetase is highly stereospecific, at least in one series of substances (Shen, 1972; Ham et al., 1972; Tomlinson et al., 1972), the d-isomer of arylacetic derivatives being by far more active than the l-isomer in various correlated tests. Such dissociation between stereoisomers has also been reported for a carbazol derivative, equi-active with indomethacin as an antagonist of acute adjuvant arthritis, and less active against PG synthetase, platelet aggregation and Aa-induced diarrhoea in mice (Gaut et al., 1975). The d-isomer was roughly four times as active as the l-isomer, and twice as active as the racemate. No other in vivo information on stereospecificity was provided.

We have correlated the ability of some tetrahydrocarbazole derivatives[2] to suppress experimental inflammation with their ability to inhibit Aa-induced platelet aggregation and hypotension due to SRS-C. The l-isomer (ORG 8259) showed marked anti-inflammatory activity, and inhibited aggregation of rabbit platelets (Table 3). Generation of PG-like and of RCS activities in incubates of Aa and dog blood was also prevented. The d-isomer (ORG 8260) lacked these properties, and only suppressed Aa-induced platelet aggregation at concentrations that also affected aggregation by ADP, i.e. when unspecific membrane effects were probably operating. The potency of the racemate (ORG 8223) was intermediate to the isomers. As seen in

---

[2] Compound ORG 8223 is dl-6-methoxy-1,2,3,4-tetrahydrocarbazole-2-carboxylic acid, sodium salt.

Part of the data contained in Table 3 was kindly provided by Drs. M.F. Sugrue and N. Bhargava (Organon Laboratories Ltd., Great Britain and N.V. Organon, The Netherlands). Active compounds were prepared by Drs. J. Olivie and B. Lacoume (Organon R.D., France) and synthesis was later described independently by Allen (1970). Partial resolution of the mixture was performed by Drs. Olivie and Lacoume and the pure isomers were prepared by Drs. A.C. Campbell and D. Stevenson (Organon Laboratories Ltd., Great Britain).

Table 3. Anti-inflammatory activities of ORG 8223 and of its optical isomers

Compounds	% inhibition of			
	Rat paw oedema[a]	Guinea pig U.V. erythema[b]	Fever[c]	Platelet aggregation by arachidonic acid[d]
ORG 8223 (racemate)	40%	37%	31%	110 ± 36.5^{d}
ORG 8259 (levo isomer)	46%	42%	45%	47.4 ± 41^{c}
ORG 8260 (dextro isomer)	0%	0%	7%	174.4 ± 38^{d}

[a] 0.1 ml of a 10% kaolin suspension was injected into the plantar surface of both hind paws of male Wistar rats grouped by tens. Measurements of change of thickness of the paws were calculated 5 h after administration of 100 mg/kg of potential inhibitors by oral route.
[b] Female Dunkin Hartley guinea pigs were prepared for U.V. exposure according to WINDER et al. (1958). Animals were treated subcutaneously with potential inhibitors (100 mg/kg) 1 h before exposure to U.V. and erythema was scored 4 h thereafter.
[c] Fever was induced in male Wistar rats by sub-cutaneous injection of 15% dried yeast (10 ml/kg). Animals whose body temperature had increased by 1° C from their control values 19 h after dosing were used in groups of eight, potential anti-pyretic drugs being administered orally (200 mg/kg). Rectal temperatures were measured 1, 2, 3 and 4 h thereafter. These values were summed and the mean value calculated for each group, to allow calculation of percentage change in temperature, and thus anti-pyretic activity of each drug.
[d] Aggregation was started by adding arachidonic acid (0.1 mM final concentration) to platelet-rich rabbit plasma (VARGAFTIG et al., 1974, 1975). Potential inhibitors were added 1 min before arachidonic acid, at concentrations between 25 and 1000 µg/ml. Inhibition of aggregation was calculated by comparing the variation in light transmission due to formation of aggregates in samples with and without potential inhibitors.
Figures are concentrations of inhibitors required to block 50% of aggregation $\pm$ SD; numbers in brackets are number of separate assays.

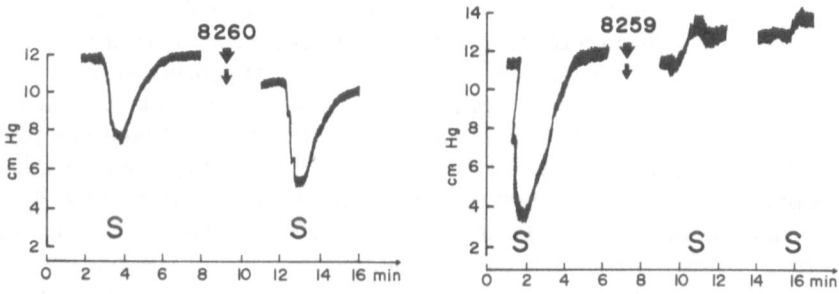

Fig. 9. Stereospecificity of inhibition of hypotension due to slow reacting substance C. Recordings of femoral blood pressure of two dogs injected with 0.4 ml/kg of slow reacting substance C (S), which induces hypotension. This was prevented after 10 mg/kg of ORG 8259 (l-isomer) (right panel, two injections of SRS – C being performed 1 and 60 min after inhibitor), whereas the same dose of ORG 8260 (d-isomer) (left panel) failed to block hypotension by SRS – C. Scales as in Figure 6

Figure 9, these correlations were also found with respect to hypotension induced by SRS-C, since the d-isomer failed to antagonize it while both the l-isomer and the racemate were effective.

III. Mechanism of Action of Hypotensive Agents Subject to Inhibition by Non-Steroid Anti-Inflammatory Drugs

Since NSAID inhibit PG synthetase from all sources that have been explored until now (FERREIRA and VANE, 1974), it is not surprising that they should inhibit the in vivo effects started by a PG precursor such as Aa. Moreover, although the precise structure(s) responsible for the activity of SRS-C have not been unravelled, there is no doubt that SRS-C is a lipid derivative (VOGT, 1957a) and that its activity involves PG synthetase or similar enzymic systems and is thus liable to inhibition by NSAID. Precise mediators of the in vivo effects of Aa and of SRS-C are not known, and we have given evidence earlier that other derivatives than natural PGs, like PGG_2, PGH_2 or thromboxanes, are probably involved.

1. Bradykinin

The effects of Bk cannot be so directly explained. Bk has no platelet effect in vitro in the presence of kininase inhibitors, nor does it induce thrombocytopenia upon intravenous administration (LEFORT and VARGAFTIG, 1975). Bk releases RCS from isolated perfused guinea pig lungs (PIPER and VANE, 1969) and from various other systems (McGIFF et al., 1972; FERREIRA et al., 1973; DAMAS and DEBY, 1974; DAMAS and BOURDON, 1974; NEEDLEMAN et al., 1975; GOLDBERG et al., 1975; MESSINA et al., 1975; there is contradictory evidence in DAMAS and GEIGER, 1973). This release, as well as that of PGs, is inhibited by NSAID. DAMAS and BOURDON (1974) have furthermore shown that Bk triggers release of Aa as well as that of PGs from isolated rat lungs, thus indicating that biosynthesis of PGs after stimulation with Bk may occur not only intracellularly but at the outer part of membranes or even in the circulating fluid.

The mediators of those effects of Bk which are inhibited by NSAID are thus probably PGs or the lipoperoxidized products bioassayed as RCS. A two-step process consisting of activation of membrane phospholipase A_2, followed by release of PG precursors and, in the presence of PG synthetase, of generation of active PG-related substances, would account for aspirin-sensitive effects of Bk. It is thus theoretically possible to inhibit release of PGs by Bk at two sites: the phospholipase A_2 step or the PG synthetase step. This was confirmed since mepacrine, expected to inhibit phospholipase A_2 in certain systems, suppressed release of RCS by Bk, without affecting that due to Aa (VARGAFTIG and DAO, 1972d). Platelets are ruled out as a source of PG-related materials upon Bk administration, since they neither aggregate nor release mediators when challenged with Bk, even in the presence of kininase inhibitors (LEFORT and VARGAFTIG, 1975). Lungs are possibly the main site from which PGs and RCS activity are released. This is indicated by results of PALMER et al. (1973) who have shown that intravenous injections of Bk into guinea pigs is followed by release of RCS. Release was inhibited by aspirin, and could not be shown upon intra-arterial injections, when lungs are by-passed. Evidence for activation of phospholipase A_2 by bradykinin in kidneys was provided by JUAN (1977).

2. Collagen

Since platelet-deprived or ADP-treated animals do not react to collagen with the expected hypotension (Fig. 2) or thrombocytopenia (BUSFIELD and TOMICH, 1968) respectively, it is likely that platelets are the main site of action of collagen in rabbits.

Collagen is administered in the form of a suspension (PACKHAM et al., 1967) and factors such as particle size or microfibril formation may interfere with its activity. Such a suspension is not expected to cross barriers like the vascular endothelium but, until experiments are performed with isolated lungs, a pulmonary origin for RCS and PG-like substances cannot be ruled out. The possibility of a pulmonary release of RCS by collagen is suggested by the ability of other particulate materials to release RCS from lungs (PALMER et al., 1973).

3. Carrageenin

In vivo effects of carrageenin appear to involve a platelet site of action. Since the platelet-depleting technique used involved anti-platelet plasma, which starts complement-dependent lysis, factors other than lack of platelets per se may explain why platelet-deprived animals are less responsive to, and hence survive, intravenous injections of carrageenin. In vitro platelet-aggregating experiments have shown that indomethacin, aspirin and salicylate delay and reduce the height of aggregation due to carrageenin in PRP but do not block it completely. This can be achieved by Ca^{++} chelating agents, thiol scavengers and adenosine (VARGAFTIG, 1977a and 1977b). When platelets are suspended in a plasma-free medium, the amount of carrageenin required to induce aggregation decreases 10–20 fold, and indomethacin, aspirin and salicylate inhibit aggregation completely. At this stage, it is not known whether the response of washed platelets or that of platelets in plasma account better for the in vivo activity of carrageenin. Since aggregation is inhibited by salicylate, which fails to prevent at equivalent concentrations the release of RCS and of PG-like activity started by carrageenin or by Aa, we tend to think that the main causative factor of death by carrageenin is not in vivo aggregation, but the events that follow aggregation, i.e. formation of mediators. Further work should clarify this. Whatever the conclusions turn out to be, one very interesting finding is that a polysaccharide such as carrageenin can induce platelet aggregation quite specifically (cellulose sulphate or dextran sulphate are active at 10–20 times higher concentrations, or inactive, respectively). Since aggregation by carrageenin is accompanied by generation of RCS and PG activities and is inhibited by NSAID, this suggests that activation of phospholipase A_2 is involved which adds further evidence for release of PGs during inflammatory conditions due to carrageenin (WILLIS, 1969), and introduces another step for PG generation. By this we mean that activation of enzymes, such as glycosyltransferases, by polysaccharides, which are involved with collagen-induced aggregation (BARBER and JAMIESON, 1971), may have wider implications and be the missing link for starting and supporting aggregation.

4. Adenosine Nucleotides

ATP and ADP cannot release RCS from isolated guinea pig lungs (VARGAFTIG and DAO HAI, 1972a). Furthermore, since the in vivo effects inhibitable by NSAID are suppressed by platelet depletion, it appears that these effects of adenosine nucleotides are fully accounted for by their interaction with platelets. Although little PG and RCS activity is generated in human PRP challenged with ADP (MONCADA, personal communication), this does not rule out the possibility that PGs and RCS are formed within the cell and are therefore not bioassayed in the suspending fluid.

IV. Conclusions

1. Relevance of Hypotensive Responses to Inflammation and to Study of Inflammatory Events

Figures 10 and 11 summarize what is known for the in vivo activity of agents that display the property of evoking effects subject to inhibition by NSAID. We have concluded that the effects on arterial blood pressure of Aa and of SRS-C, as well as part of those of Bk, of adenosine nucleotides and probably of the effects of other agents, like carrageenin, are due to formation of PG-related hypotensive materials. These materials are probably generated in circulating and/or trapped platelets (in lungs, or in the spleen) and in the lungs, from where they reach the target organs: lung vessels and bronchial smooth muscle (particularly in guinea pigs and cats), the peripheral vessels in all species, leading to hypotension. This suggests that all NSAID should inhibit these responses, each time the general rule of parallelism between anti-PG synthetase and anti-inflammatory activity is confirmed.

Inducer	Bronchial resistance	NSAID	Blood pressure	NSAID	Writhing	NSAID
Arachidonate	▲	+	▼	+	▲	+
SRS–C	▲	+	▼	+		
SRS–A	▲	+	0 or ▼			
Bradykinin	▲	+	▼	+	▲	+
Carrageenin	▲		▼	+		
Collagen	▲	+	▼	+		
ADP/ATP	▲	+	▼	±	▲	+

Fig. 10

Inducer	Interactions with rabbit platelets						Erythrocytes	
	PRP	NSAID	Tyrode solution	NSAID	Mediators	NSAID	Lysis	NSAID
Arachidonate	▲	+	▲	○	▲	+	▲	○
SRS–C	○				▲	+	▲	○
Collagen	▲	+	▲	+	▲	+		
Linolenate	○		○		○		▲	○
Aliphatic lipoperoxides	○		○		○			
Bradykinin	○		○				○	
Carrageenin	▲	+	▲	+	▲	+		

Fig. 11

Figs. 10 and 11. Pharmacological effects liable to blockade by antiinflammatory drugs. Summary of in vivo (Fig. 10) and in vitro (Fig. 11) effects of various hypotensive substances, and of interference of non-steroid anti-inflammatory drugs (*NSAID*). ▼ stands for increase in effect, for aggregation, release of mediators or haemolysis; ▲ stands for hypotension; + stands for inhibition, 0 stands for absence of inhibition and ± stands for partial inhibition. No sign indicates that no results are available. See text for details

There is no proof that platelets directly induce inflammation (VARGAFTIG, 1974; UBATUBA et al., 1975; SILVER et al., 1974), but they certainly can provide inflammatory mediators of various types. Appropriate choice of in vivo models where blood pressure responses are concerned should help to characterize new agents or old drugs. A typical case is that of sodium salicylate, which is a feeble inhibitor of PG synthetase (VANE, 1971), has some anti-aggregating effects, does not inhibit Aa-induced hypotensive responses up to 100 mg/kg, but can at these doses prevent hypotension and death by intravenous carrageenin. The mechanism of action of sodium salicylate as an anti-inflammatory drug may thus be explained by a site of action other than PG synthetase. This leads to the concept of multisequential enzyme activation for acute hypotensive reactions dependent on PG-related products.

2. Multisequential Activation and Acute Hypotensive Responses: Prospects of Research

It has been suggested (VOGT and DISTELKÖTTER, 1967) that activation of phospholipase A_2 leads to PG biosynthesis. This has been supported by other findings, including the observation that during collagen-induced platelet aggregation a loss of Aa from platelet phospholipids occurs unless prevented by mepacrine. Indomethacin only inhibited PG biosynthesis but failed to interfere with the release of Aa (FLOWER et al., 1975). Lack of a specific and highly active phospholipase A_2 inhibitor precluded much further use of the two step concept. This is further accentuated by the difficulties, outlined on page 171, involved in using exogenous phospholipase A_2 preparations in vivo. One possible way of solving the problem is to look for phospholipase A_2 activity or for its direct effects, such as was done by FLOWER et al. (1975), or to investigate, after appropriate pharmacological or pathological stimuli to animals, systems such as the plasma phospholipase A_2 described by DUCHESNE et al. (1972). In the latter case, activators of plasma prophospholipase A_2 are released from platelets, which might help to visualise the complex interaction between platelets, organs such as lungs and spleen where aggregates are trapped, and systemic inflammatory-like stimuli.

The question of what activates phospholipase A_2 is a basic one, and we suggest that polysaccharides such as carrageenin and perhaps vascular mucopolysaccharides display the property of triggering generation of PG-like materials, including thromboxanes because they stimulate phospholipase A_2 activity. This would provide an early entry for the PG generation cascade, that could be outlined, as a process involving at least three steps in circulating platelets:

1. Polysaccharide-platelet interaction, accounting for the role of glycosyl-transferases in aggregation (BARBER and JAMIESON, 1971).

2. Release-reaction, with activation of phospholipase A_2, possibly from lysosomes (ANDERSON et al., 1971).

3. Generation of PGs as soon as Aa is released, since PG synthetase is not in the form of a precursor, but readily available.

This hypothetical "mini"-cascade, if compared with the impressive series of pathways activated during clotting or complement activation, may be a useful concept for unravelling the cellular mechanisms responsible for in vivo and for in vitro release of PGs, thromboxanes and other lipoperoxidized materials. To propose such a scheme amounts to compounding of unanswered questions, such as how to apply these concepts for non-platelet-dependent in vivo effects of agents like Bk. These aspects which need to be clarified already indicate the prospects of research on the in vivo release of mediators affected by NSAID. It is mandatory to refer constantly to biochemical evidence, using appropriate in vitro systems to activity in vivo is indicated by as many findings as possible. This will require use of cross-circulation preparations, more sophisticated methods for in vivo organ exclusion than those usually performed by pharmacologists, use of animals specifically depleted of cells and of precursors, such as employed by VINCENT et al. (1975) with rats deficient in essential fatty acids. A major advance would be the availability of specific antagonists of PGs, active in most experimental animals, without the side-effects of those at present known.

The first results on effects of PG precursors or activators in vivo arrived with this century (DELEZENNE and LEDEBT, 1911). Aa, SRS-C, Bk or carrageenin, and possibly other known and still unknown agents, induce effects in vivo that can be fully accounted for by activation of the multisequential cascade outlined above. Use of these in vivo properties should provide further useful data.

References

Abrams, W. B., Solomon, H. M.: The human platelet as a pharmacologic model for the adrenergic neuron. Clin. Pharmacol. **10**, 702—709 (1969)

Amundsen, E., Ofstad, E., Hagen, P. O.: Histamine release induced by synergistic action of kallikrein and phospholipase A. Arch. int. Pharmacodyn. **178**, 104—114 (1969)

Anderson, A. J., Brocklehurst, W. E., Willis, A. L.: Evidence for the role of lysosomes in the formation of prostaglandins during carrageenin induced inflammation in the rat. Pharmacol. Res. Commun. **3**, 13—19 (1971)

Anderson, W., Duncan, J. G. C.: The anticoagulant activity of carrageenan. J. Pharm. (Lond.) **17**, 647—654 (1965)

Anderson, F. L., Jubiz, W., Tsagaris, T. J., Kuida, H.: Endotoxin-induced prostaglandin E and F release in dogs. Amer. J. Physiol. **228**, 410—414 (1975)

Arrigoni-Martelli, E., Selva, D., Schiatti, P.: Different efficacy of anti-inflammatory drugs in inhibiting the reactions to intradermal phospholipase A and PGE$_2$. J. int. med. Res. **1**, 120—126 (1973)

Babilli, S., Vogt, W.: Nature of the fatty acids acting as "slow reacting substance" (SRS-C). J. Physiol. (Lond.) **177**, 31P—32P (1965)

Barber, A. J., Jamieson, A.: Platelet collagen adhesion characterization of collagen glucosyltransferase of plasma membranes of human blood platelets. Biochim. biophys. Acta **252**, 533—545 (1971)

Bartels, J., Kunze, H., Vogt, W., Wille, G.: Prostaglandin: liberation from and formation in perfused frog intestine. Naunyn-Schmiedeberg's Arch. Pharmacol. **266**, 199—207 (1970)

Beller, F. K., Graeff, H., Gorstein, F.: Disseminated intravascular coagulation during the continuous infusion of endotoxin in rabbits. Amer. J. Obstet. Gynec. **103**, 544—554 (1969)

Berry, P. A.: Slow reacting substance in anaphylaxis (SRS-A): its release, actions and antagonism. In: Thesis for Ph. D. London: Council for National Academic Awards 1966

Bianchi, C., David, A.: Analgesic properties of 4-ethoxycarbonyl-1-(2-hydroxy-3-phenoxypropyl)4-phenylpiperidine (B.D.H. 20) and some related compounds. J. Pharm. (Lond.) **12**, 449—459 (1960)

Bø, G., Hognestad, J., Vaage, J.: The role of blood platelets in pulmonary responses to microembolization with barium sulphate. Acta physiol. scand. **90**, 244—251 (1974)

Bodammer, G.: Untersuchungen über den Mechanismus der Blutdruckwirkung des Anaphylatoxins bei Katzen und Meerschweinchen. Naunyn-Schmiedeberg's Arch. exp. Path. Pharmak. **262**, 197—207 (1969)

Bonta, I. L., Vargaftig, B. B.: Cobra venom induced pulmonary vessel lesion: an unconventional model of acute inflammation. Bull. Inst. Pasteur **74**, 131—136 (1976)

Boquet, P., Dworetzky, M., Essex, H. E.: Physiologic responses of certain animals and isolated preparations to mixtures of snake venom and egg yolk. Amer. J. Physiol. **161**, 561—572 (1950)

Born, G. V. R., Hasma, R. J., Goldman, M., Lowe, R. D.: Comparative effectiveness of adenosine analogues as inhibitors of blood-platelet aggregation and as vasodilators in man. Nature (Lond.) **205**, 678—680 (1965)

Brocklehurst, W. E.: "SRS-A" The slow reacting substance of anaphylaxis. Biochem. Pharmacol. **12**, 431—435 (1963)

Busfield, D., Tomich, E. G.: Inhibition by adenosine diphosphate of the thrombocytopenia induced in rabbits by collagen or thrombin. Nature (Lond.) **217**, 376—378 (1968)

Chignard, M., Vargaftig, B. B.: Dog platelets fail to aggregate when they form aggregating substances upon stimulation with arachidonic acid. Europ. J. Pharmacol. (1976). In press

Clarke, D. A., Davoll, J., Philipps, F. S., Brown, G. B.: Enzymatic deamination and vasodepressor effects of adenosine analogs. J. Pharmacol. exp. Ther. **106**, 291—302 (1952)

Cohen, M., Sztokalo, J., Hinsch, E.: The antihypertensive action of arachidonic acid in the spontaneous hypertensive rat and its antagonism by anti-inflammatory agents. Life Sci. **13**, 317—325

Collier, H. O. J.: Self-antagonism of bronchoconstriction induced by bradykinin and angiotensin. In: Erdös, E. G., Back, N., Sicuteri, F., Wilde, A. (Eds.): Hypotensive Peptides, pp. 305—313, Berlin-Heidelberg-New York: Springer-Verlag 1966

Collier, H. O. J.: New light on how aspirin works. Nature (Lond.) **223**, 35—37 (1969)

Collier, H. O. J., Dinnen, L. C., Perkins, A. C., Piper, P. J.: Curtailment by aspirin and meclofenamate of hypotension induced by bradykinin in the guinea-pig. Naunyn-Schmiedeberg's Arch. exp. Path. Pharmak. **259**, 159—160 (1968)

Collier, H. O. J., James, G. W. L., Schneider, C.: Antagonism by aspirin and fenamates of bronchoconstriction and nociception induced by adenosine-5'-triphosphate. Nature (Lond.) **212**, 411—412 (1966)

Collier, H. O. J., Shorley, P. G.: Analgesic antipyretic drugs as antagonists of bradykinin. Brit. J. Pharmacol. **15**, 601—610 (1960)

Collier, H. O. J., Shorley, P. G.: Antagonism by mefenamic and flufenamic acids of the bronchoconstrictor action of kinins in the guinea-pig. Brit. J. Pharmacol. **20**, 345—351 (1963)

Collier, H. O. J., Sweatman, W. J. F.: Antagonism by fenamates of prostaglandin F2α and of slow reacting substance on human bronchial muscle. Nature (Lond.) **219**, 864—865 (1968)

Connor, W. E., Hoak, J. C., Warner, E. D.: Massive thrombosis produced by fatty acid infusion. J. clin. Invest. **42**, 860—866 (1963)

Corey, E. J., Nicolaou, K. C., Machida, Y., Malmsten, C. L., Samuelsson, B.: Synthesis and biological properties of a 9,11-azoprostanoid: highly active biochemical mimic of prostaglandin endoperoxides. Proc. nat. Acad. Sci. (Wash.) **72**, 3355—3358 (1975)

Corrado, A. P., Reis, M. L., Carvalho, I. F., Diniz, C. R.: Bradykininogen and bradykinin in the cardiovascular shock produced by proteolytic enzymes. Biochem. Pharmacol. **15**, 959—970 (1966)

Crunkhorn, P., Willis, A. L.: Cutaneous reactions to intradermal prostaglandins. Brit. J. Pharmacol. **41**, 49—56 (1971)

Culp, J. R., Erdös, E. G., Hinshaw, L. B., Holmes, D. D.: Effects of anti-inflammatory drugs in shock caused by injection of living *E. coli* cells. Proc. Soc. exp. Biol. (N. Y.) **137**, 219—223 (1970)

Dakhil, T., Vogt, W.: Hydroperoxyde als Träger der darmerregenden Wirkung hochungesättigter Fettsäuren. Naunyn-Schmiedeberg's Arch. exp. Path. Pharmak. **243**, 174—186 (1962)

Daly, M. J.: Pulmonary mechanical effects of experimental lung embolism and their modification by bronchodilator drugs in the guinea-pig. Brit. J. Pharmacol. **51**, 599—601 (1974)

Damas, J., Bourdon, V.: Libération d'acide arachidonique par la bradykinine. C. R. Soc. Biol. (Paris) **168**, 1445—1448 (1974)

Damas, J., Deby, C.: Libération de prostaglandines par la bradykinine chez le rat. C. R. Soc. Biol. (Paris) **168**, 375—378 (1974)

Damas, J., Geiger, R.: Sur la nature des actions cardiovasculaires de la bradykinine chez le rat. C. R. Soc. Biol. (Paris) **167**, 1065—1068 (1973)

Damas, J., Lallemand, G.: Pyridinolcarbamate et bradykinine, chez le rat. C.R. Soc. Biol. (Paris) **168**, 379—382 (1974)

Damerau, B., Lege, L., Oldigs, H. D., Vogt, W.: Histamine release, formation of prostaglandin-like activity (SRS-C) and mast cell degranulation by the direct lytic factor (DLF) and phospholipase A of cobra venom. Arch. Pharmacol. **287**, 141—156 (1975)

Davey, M. G., Lüscher, E. F.: Release reactions of human platelets induced by thrombin and other agents. Biochim. biophys. Acta, **165**, 490—506 (1968)

Davies, G. E., Holman, G., Johnston, T. P., Lowe, J. S.: Studies on kallikrein: failure of some anti-inflammatory drugs to affect release of kinin. Brit. J. Pharmacol. **28**, 212—217 (1966)

Deby, C., Barac, G., Bacq, Z. M.: Action de l'acide arachidonique sur la pression artérielle du lapin avant et après heparine. Arch. int. Pharmacodyn. **208**, 363—364 (1974)

Delezenne, C., Ledebt, S.: Les poisons libérés par les venins aux dépens du vitellus de l'oeuf. C.R. Soc. Biol. (Paris) **71**, 121—124 (1911)

Delori, P. J.: Purification et propriétés physico-chimiques, chimiques et biologiques d'une phospholipase A2 toxique isolée d'un venin de serpent *Viperidae: Vipera berus*. Biochimie **55**, 1031—1045 (1973)

Diczfalusy, E., Fernö, O., Fex, H., Högberg, B., Linderot, R., Rosenberg, T.: Synthetic high molecular weight enzyme inhibitors. I. Polymeric phosphates of phloretin and related compounds. Acta chem. scand. **7**, 913—920 (1953)

Di Rosa, M., Sorrentino, L.: Some pharmacodynamic properties of carrageenin in the rat. Brit. J. Pharmacol. **38**, 214—220 (1970)

Duchesne, M. J., Etienne, J., Grüber, A., Polonovski, J.: Action des plaquettes sur la phophospholipase plasmatique. Biochimie **54**, 257—260 (1972)

Eakins, K. E.: Antagonistes des prostaglandines. Rev. Médecine **15**, 2106—2110 (1974)

Edery, H.: Potentiation of the action of bradykinin on smooth muscle by chymotrypsin, chymotrypsinogen and trypsin. Brit. J. Pharmacol. **22**, 371—379 (1964)

Eisen, V., Vogt, W.: Plasma kininogenases and their activators. In: Erdös, E. G., Wilde, A. (Eds.): Handbook of experimental Pharmacology, Vol. 25. Bradykinin, Kallidin and Kallikrein. Berlin-Heidelberg-New York: Springer 1970

Erdös, E. G.: Effect of nonsteroidal anti-inflammatory drugs in endotoxin shock. Biochem. Pharmacol. Suppl. 283—291 (1968)

Erdös, E. G., Hinshaw, L. B., Gill, C. C.: Effect of indomethacin in endotoxin shock in the dog. Proc. Soc. exp. Biol. (N. Y.) **125**, 916—919 (1967)

Feinstein, M. B., Becker, E. L., Fraser, C.: Thrombin, collagen and A 23187 stimulated endogenous platelet arachidonate metabolism: differential inhibition by PGE 1, local anesthetics and a serine-protease inhibitor. Prostaglandins **14**, 1075—1093 (1977)

Feldberg, W., Kellaway, C. H.: Liberation of histamine from the perfused lung by snake venoms. J. Physiol. (Lond.) **90**, 257—279 (1937)

Feldberg, W., Kellaway, C. H.: Liberation of histamine and formation of lysocithin-like substances by cobra venom. J. Physiol. (Lond.) **94**, 187—226 (1938)

Ferreira, S. M., Rocha e Silva, M.: Potentiation of bradykinin by dimercaptopropanol (BAL) and other inhibitors of its destroying enzyme in plasma. Biochem. Pharmacol. **11**, 1123—1128 (1962)

Ferreira, S. H., Moncada, S., Vane, J. R.: Further experiments to establish that the analgesic action of aspirin-like drugs depends on the inhibition of prostaglandin biosynthesis. Brit. J. Pharmacol. **47**, 629P—630P (1973)

Ferreira, S. H., Vane, J. R.: Detection and estimation of bradykinin in the circulation. Brit. J. Pharmacol. **29**, 367—377 (1967)

Ferreira, S. H., Vane, J. R.: New aspects of the mode of action of nonsteroid anti-inflammatory drugs. Ann. Rev. Pharmacol. **14**, 57—73 (1974)

Ferreira, S. H., Vargaftig, B. B.: Inhibition by non-steroid anti-inflammatory agents of rabbit aorta conctracting activity generated in blood by slow reacting substance C. Brit. J. Pharmacol. **50**, 543—551 (1974)

Flower, R. J.: Drugs which inhibit prostaglandin biosynthesis. Pharmacol. Rev. **26**, 33—67 (1974)

Flower, R. J., Blackwell, G. J., Parsons, M. F.: Mechanism of collagen induced platelet aggregation. In: Abstracts of the Sixth International Congress of Pharmacology, Helsinki, p. 292. 1975

Flower, R., Gryglewski, R., Herbaczynska-Cedro, K., Vane, J. R.: Effects of anti-inflammatory drugs on prostaglandin biosynthesis. Nature (New Biol.) **238**, 104—106 (1972)

Flower, R. J., Vane, J. R.: Inhibition of prostaglandin synthetase in brain explains the anti-pyretic activity of paracetamol (4-acetamidophenol). Nature (Lond.) **240**, 410—411 (1972)

Fredholm, B., Strandberg, K.: Release of histamine and formation of smooth-muscle stimulating principles in guinea-pig lung tissue induced by antigen and bee venom phosphatidase A. Acta physiol. scand. **76**, 446—457 (1969)

Gaarder, A., Laland, S.: Hypothesis for the aggregation of platelets by nucleotides. Nature (Lond.) **202**, 909—910 (1964)

Gaut, Z. N., Baruth, H., Randall, L. O., Ashley, C., Paulsrud, J. R.: Stereoisomeric relationships among anti-inflammatory activity, inhibition of platelet aggregation and inhibition of prostaglandin synthetase. Prostaglandins **10**, 59—66 (1975)

Gilmore, N., Vane, J. R., Wyllie, J. H.: Prostaglandin release by the spleen in response to infusion of particles. In: Mantegazza, P., Horton, E. W. (Eds.): Prostaglandins, Peptides and Amines, pp. 21—29. London: Academic Press 1969

Giroud, J. P., Timsit, J.: Relations entre les propriétés anti-inflammatoires et anticomplémentaires du sulfate de protamine et du bromure d'hexadiméthrine. Thérapie **27**, 297—307 (1972)

Goldberg, M. R., Joiner, P. D., Greenberg, S., Hyman, A. L., Kadowitz, P. J.: Effects of indomethacin on venoconstrictor responses to bradykinin and norepinephrine. Prostaglandins **9**, 385—390 (1975)

Gomazkov, O. A., Shimkovich, M. V.: Ciproheptadin as an inhibitor of the bradykinin effects. Byull. eksp. Biol. Med. **80**, 6—9 (1975)

Greenway, C. V., Murthy, V. S.: Mesenteric vasoconstriction after endotoxin administration in cats pretreated with aspirin. Brit. J. Pharmacol. **43**, 259—269 (1971)

Grette, K.: Studies on the mechanism of thrombin-catalyzed hemostatic reactions in blood platelets. Acta physiol. scand., Suppl. **195**, 1—93 (1962)

Gryglewski, R., Vane, J. R.: The generation from arachidonic acid of rabbit aorta contracting substance (RCS) by a microsomal enzyme preparation which also generates prostaglandins. Brit. J. Pharmacol. **46**, 449—457 (1972)

Habermann, E.: Gewinnung und Eigenschaften von Crotactin, Phospholipase A, Crotamin und „Toxin III" aus dem Gift der brasilianischen Klapperschlange. Biochem. Z. **329**, 405—415 (1957)

Hall, R. C., Hodge, R. L., Irvine, R., Katic, F., Middleton, J. M.: The effect of aspirin on the response to endotoxin. Aust. J. exp. Biol. med. Sci. **50**, 589—601 (1972)

Ham, E. A., Cirillo, V. J., Zanetti, T. Y., Shen, T. Y., Kuehl, F. A. Jr.: Studies on the mode of action of non-steroidal anti-inflammatory agents. In: Ramwell, P. W., Pharriss, B. B. (Eds.): Prostaglandins in Cellular Biology, Vol. I, pp. 345—352. New York-London: Plenum Press 1972

Hamberg, M., Hedqvist, P., Strandberg, K., Svensson, J., Samuelsson, B.: Prostaglandin endoperoxides IV. Effects on smooth muscle. Life. Sci. **16**, 451—462 (1975 a)

Hamberg, M., Svensson, J., Samuelsson, B.: Thromboxanes: A new group of biologically active compounds derived from prostaglandin endoperoxides. Proc. nat. Acad. Sci. (Wash.) **72**, 2994—2998 (1975 b)

Hamberg, U., Rocha e Silva, M.: On the release of bradykinin by trypsin and snake venoms. Arch. int. Pharmacodyn. **110**, 222—238 (1957)

Harrity, T. W., Goldlust, M. B.: Anti-complement effects of two anti-inflammatory agents niflumic and flufenamic acids. Biochem. Pharmacol. **23**, 3107—3120 (1974)

Hedqvist, P., Stjärne, L., Wennmalm, Å.: Inhibition by prostaglandin E_2 of sympathetic neurotransmission in the rabbit heart. Acta physiol. scand. **79**, 139—141 (1970)

Hinshaw, L. B., Solomon, L. A., Erdös, E. G., Reins, D. A., Gunter, B. J.: Effects of acetylsalicylic acid on the canine response to endotoxin. J. Pharmacol. exp. Ther. **157**, 665—671 (1967)

Högberg, B., Uvnas, B.: Further Observations on the disruption of rat mesentery mast cells caused by compound 48/80, antigen-antibody reaction, lecithinase A and decylamine. Acta physiol. scand. **48**, 133—145 (1960)

Holmes, I. B.: A comparison of the effect of proquazone, a new non-steroidal antiinflammatory compound, and acetylsalicylic acid on blood platelet function in vitro and in vivo. Arch. int. Pharmacodyn. **227**, 114—129 (1977)

Hrdina, P. D., Ling, G. M.: The in vivo antibradykinin activity of seclazone (7-chloro-3,3a-dihy-dro-2H,9H-isoxazolo(3,2-b) (1,3)benzoxazin-9-one), a new anti-inflammatory agent. Pharmacology **10**, 136—142 (1973)

Jaques, R.: Arachidonic acid, and unsaturated fatty acid which produces slow contractions of smooth muscle and causes pain. Pharmacological and biochemical characterisation of its mode of action. Helv. Physiol. Acta **17**, 255—267 (1959)

Jaques, R.: Suppression, by morphine and other analgesic compounds, of the smooth-muscle contraction produced by arachidonic acid peroxide. Helv. physiol. Acta **23**, 156—162 (1965)

Jobin, F., Gagnon, F. T.: Platelet reactions and immune processes. IV. The inhibition of complement by pyrazole compounds and other inhibitors of platelet reactions. Canad. J. Microbiol. **16**, 63—67 (1970)

Jobin, F., Tremblay, F.: Platelet reactions and immune processes II. The inhibition of platelet aggregation by complement inhibitors. Thrombs. Diathes. haemorrh. (Stuttg.) **22**, 466—481 (1969)

Joyner, W. L., Iatridis, P. G., Yonce, L. R., Iatridis, S. G.: Influence of a prostaglandin inhibitor on thrombin induced vasodilation. Circulation **50**, Suppl. 3, 287 (1974)

Juan, H.: Mechanism of action of bradykinin-induced release of prostaglandin E. Naunyn-Schmiedeberg's Arch. Pharmacol. **300**, 77—85 (1977)

Kaiser, E., Kramar, R., Lambrechter, R.: The action of direct lytic agents from animal venoms on cells and isolated cell fractions. In: de Vries, A., Kochva, E. (Eds.): Toxins of Animal and Plant Origin, Vol. II, pp. 675—682. New York-London-Paris: Gordon and Breach Science Publishers 1972

Kalbhen, D. A.: Pharmacological studies on the anti-inflammatory effect of a semi-synthetic polysaccharide (pentosan polysulfate). Pharmacology **9**, 74—79 (1973)

Kannegiesser, H., Lee, J. B.: Difference in haemodynamic response to prostaglandins A and E. Nature (Lond.) **229**, 498—500 (1971)

Kirschmann, Ch., Condrea, E., Moav, N., Aloof, S., de Vries, A.: Action of snake venom on human platelet phospholipids. Arch. int. Pharmacodyn. **150**, 372—378 (1964)

Klibansky, C., Condrea, E., de Vries, A.: Changes in plasma phospholipids after intravenous phosphatidase A injection in the rabbit. Amer. J. Physiol. **203**, 114—118 (1962)

Kohler, C., Wooding, W., Ellenbogen, L.: Intravenous arachidonate in mice: a model for evaluating antithrombotic drugs. Pharmacologist **17**, 271 (1975)

Kosersky, D. S.: A pharmacologic investigation of the anti-inflammatory activity of cryogenine. Diss. Abs. **32**, 2904—2905 (1971)

Kovats, T. T.: The role of targets and mediators in endotoxin shock. In: Hinshaw, L. B., Cox, B. G. (Ed.): The fundamental mechanisms of shock, pp. 347—359. New York-London: Plenum Press 1972

Laborit, H., Valette, N.: Action de l'acide arachidonique sur l'hypertension artérielle expérimentale du rat. Agressologie **14**, 387—393 (1973)

Laborit, H., Valette, N.: The action of arachidonic acid on experimental hypertension in the rat. Chem. biol. Interact. **10**, 239—246 (1975)

Larsson, C., Änggård, E.: Arachidonic acid lowers and indomethacin increases the blood pressure of the rabbit. J. Pharm. (Lond.) **25**, 653—655 (1973)

Lecomte, J.: Antagonisme entre bradykinine synthétique et phénylbutazone chez le lapin. C. R. Soc. Biol. (Paris) **154**, 2389—2391 (1960)

Lefort, J., Vargaftig, B. B.: Role of platelet aggregation in bronchoconstriction in guinea-pigs. Brit. J. Pharmacol. **55**, 254P—255P (1975)

Lefort, J., Vargaftig, B. B.: Role of platelets in aspirin-sensitive bronchoconstriction in the guinea-pig: interaction with salicylic acid. Brit. J. Pharmac. **63**, 35—42 (1978a)

Lefort, J., Vargaftig, B. B.: Mechanisms of collagen-induced bronchoconstriction and thrombocytopenia in the guinea-pig. Brit. J. Pharmac. **62**, 422P (1978b)

Lefort, J., Vargaftig, B. B.: Mechanisms of collagen induced bronchoconstriction and thrombocytopenia in the guinea-pig. Brit. J. Pharmac. **62**, 422 P (1978)

Levy, B., Lindner, H. R.: Selective blockade of the vasodepressor response to prostaglandin $F_{2\alpha}$ in the anaesthetized rabbit. Brit. J. Pharmacol. **43**, 236—241 (1971)

Lindsey, H. E., Wyllie, J. H.: Release of prostaglandins from embolized lungs. Brit. J. Surg. **57**, 738—741 (1970)

McGiff, J. C., Terragno, N. A., Malik, K. U., Lonigro, A. J.: Release of a prostaglandin E-like substance from canine kidney by bradykinin. Circulat. Res. **31**, 36—43 (1972)

Mantovani, P., Impicciatore, M.: Osservasioni su alcune azioni farmacologiche del 2,6-bis-(idrossimetil)-piridin-bis-(N-metilcarbammato) (piridinolcarbammato). Farmaco, Ed. sci. **25**, 912—919 (1970)

Mathe, A. A., Strandberg, K.: Antagonism of slow reacting substance by polyphloretin phosphate on isolated human bronchi. Acta physiol. scand. **82**, 460—465 (1971)

Messina, E. J., Weiner, R., Kaley, G.: Inhibition of bradykinin vasodilation and potentiation of norepinephrine and angiotensin vasoconstriction by inhibitors of prostaglandin synthesis in skeletal muscle of the rat. Circulat. Res. **37**, 430—437 (1975)

Middleton Jr., E., Phillips, G. B.: Distribution and properties of anaphylactic and venom-induced slow-reacting-substance and histamine in guinea pigs. J. Immunol. **93**, 220—227 (1964)

Mills, D. C. B., Smith, J. B.: The influence on platelet aggregation of drugs that affect the accumulation of adenosine $3':5'$-cyclic monophosphate in platelets. Biochem. J. **121**, 185—196 (1971)

Mills, S. E., Levine, L.: The inhibition of immune haemolysis by salicylaldoxime. Immunology **2**, 368—383 (1958)

Moncada, S., Gryglewski, R. J., Bunting, S., Vane, J. R.: An enzyme isolated from arteries transforms prostaglandin endoperoxides to an unstable substance that inhibits platelet aggregation. Nature, Lond. **263**, 663—665 (1976)

Moriau, M., Rodhain, J., Noel, H., de Beys-Col, C., Masure, R.: Comparative effects of proteinase inhibitors, plasminogen antiactivators, heparin and acetylsalicylic acid on the experimental disseminated intravascular coagulation induced by thrombin. Thrombos. Diathes. haemorrh. (Stuttg.) **32**, 171—188 (1974)

Müller-Berghaus, G., Eckhardt, T.: The role of granulocytes in the activation of intravascular coagulation and the precipitation of soluble fibrin by endotoxin. Blood **45**, 631—641 (1975)

Murase, H., Ijiri, H., Shimamoto, T., Kobayashi, I., Shimamoto, T., Yamazaki, H.: Acid mucopolysaccharides as cofactor in formation of platelet-clumping substance. Blood **37**, 684—691 (1971)

Mustard, J. F., Packham, M. A.: Factors influencing platelet function: adhesion, release, and aggregation. Pharmacol. Rev. **22**, 97—187 (1970)

Nadel, J. A., Colebatch, H. J. H., Olsen, C. R.: Location and mechanism of airway constriction after barium sulfate microembolism. J. appl. Physiol. **19**, 387—394 (1964)

Nagayama, M., Zucker, M. B., Beller, F. K.: Effects of a variety of endotoxins on human and rabbit platelet function. Thrombos. Diathes. haemorrh. (Stuttg.) **26**, 467—473 (1971)

Nakano, J., McCloy, Jr., R. B.: Effects of indomethacin on the pulmonary vascular and air way resistance responses to pulmonary microembolization. Proc. Soc. exp. Biol. (N. Y.) **143**, 218—221 (1973)

Needleman, P., Key, S. L., Denny, S. E., Isakson, P. C., Marshall, G. R.: Mechanism and modification of bradykinin-induced coronary vasodilation. Proc. nat. Acad. Sci. (Wash.) **72**, 2060—2063 (1975)

Nishizawa, E. E., Wynalda, D. J., Suydam, D. E., Sawa, T. R., Schultz, J. R.: Collagen-induced pulmonary thromboembolism in mice. Thrombos. Res. **1**, 233—242 (1972)

Noordhoek, J., Bonta, I. L.: The mechanism of the anti-inflammatory and hypotensive effect of carrageenin in rats. Arch. int. Pharmacodyn. **197**, 385—386 (1972)

Northover, B. J.: The effect of anti-inflammatory drugs on vascular smooth muscle. Brit. J. Pharmacol. **31**, 483—493 (1967)

Northover, B. J., Subramanian, G.: Analgesic-antipyretic drugs as antagonists of endotoxin shock in dogs. J. Path. Bact. **83**, 463—468 (1962)

Ofstad, E.: Formation and destruction of plasma kinins during experimental acute hemorrhagic pancreatitis in dogs. Scand. J. Gastroent. **5**, Suppl. 5, 9—44 (1970)

Oshima, G., Sato-Ohmori, T., Suzuki, T.: Proteinase, arginineester hydrolase and a kinin releasing enzyme in snake venoms. Toxicon **7**, 229—233 (1969)

Packham, M. A., Warrior, E. S., Glynn, M. F., Senyi, A. S., Mustard, J. F.: Alteration of the response of platelets to surface stimuli by pyrazole compounds. J. exp. Med. **126**, 171—191 (1967)

Palmer, M. A., Piper, P. J., Vane, J. R.: Release of rabbit aorta contracting substance (RCS) and prostaglandins induced by chemical or mechanical stimulation of guinea-pig lungs. Brit. J. Pharmacol. **49**, 226—242 (1973)

Parratt, J.R., Sturgess, R.M.: The effect of indomethacin on the cardiovascular and metabolic responses to *E. coli* endotoxin in the cat. Brit. J. Pharmacol. **50**, 177—183 (1974)

Parratt, J.R., Sturgess, R.M.: The protective effect of sodium meclofenamate in experimental endotoxin shock. Brit. J. Pharmacol. **53**, 466 P (1975a)

Parratt, J.R., Sturgess, R.M.: Evidence that prostaglandin release mediates pulmonary vasoconstriction induced by *E. coli* endotoxin. J. Physiol. (Lond.) **246**, 79 P—80 P (1975b)

Parratt, J.R., Sturgess, R.M.: *E. coli* endotoxin shock in the cat; treatment with indomethacin. Brit. J. Pharmacol. **53**, 485—488 (1975c)

Piper, P.J., Vane, J.R.: Release of additional factors in anaphylaxis and its antagonism by anti-inflammatory drugs. Nature (Lond.) **223**, 29—35 (1969)

Piper, P.J., Vane, J.R.: The release of prostaglandins from lung and other tissues. Ann. N.Y. Acad. Sci. **180**, 363—385 (1971)

Prado, J.L.: Proteolytic enzymes as kininogenases. In: Erdös, E.G., Wilde, A. (Eds.): Handbook of Experimental Pharmacology, Vol. XXV, pp. 156—192. New York: Springer 1970

Prado, J.L., Prado, E.S.: Plasmakinin liberation by clostripaine. An. Acad. bras. Cienc. **34**, 51—55 (1962)

Prado, J.L., Prado, E.S., Jurkiewicz, A.: Crystalline bacterial proteinase from *B. subtilis* (Nagarse) as a new kininogenase. Arch. int. Pharmacodyn. **147**, 53—68 (1964)

Prost-Dvojakovic, R.J., Samama, M.: Clot-promoting and platelet aggregating effects of fatty acids. Haemostasis **2**, 73—84 (1973/74)

Rådegran, K.: Circulatory and respiratory effects of induced platelet aggregation an experimental study in dogs. Acta chir. scand. **420**, Suppl. 1—24 (1971)

Ratnoff, O.D., Crum, J.D.: Activation of Hageman factor by solutions of ellagic acid. J. Lab. clin. Med. **63**, 359—377 (1964)

Rocha e Silva, M.: Concerning the mechanism of anaphylaxis and allergy. Brit. med. J. **1**, 779—784 (1952)

Rocha e Silva, M., Beraldo, W.T., Rosenfeld, G.: Bradykinin, a hypotensive and smooth muscle stimulating factor released from plasma globulin by snake venoms and by trypsin. Amer. J. Physiol. **156**, 261—273 (1949)

Rocha e Silva, M., Garcia Leme, J.: On some antagonists of bradykinin. Naunyn-Schmiedeberg's Arch. exp. Path. Pharmak. **250**, 167—170 (1965)

Rocha e Silva, M., Grana, A.: Anaphylaxis-like reactions produced by ascaris extracts. I. The changes in the histamine content and the coagulability of the blood in guinea pigs and in dogs. Arch. Surg. (Chicago) **52**, 523—537 (1946a)

Rocha e Silva, M., Grana, A.: Anaphylaxis-like reactions produced by ascaris extracts. II. The mechanism of the shock induced in dogs. Arch. Surg. (Chicago) **52**, 713—728 (1946b)

Rocha e Silva, M., Grana, A., Porto, A.: Inhibitory effect of glycogen upon anaphylactic shock in the rabbit. Proc. Soc. exp. Biol. (N.Y.) **59**, 57—61 (1945)

Rocha e Silva, M., Porto, A., Andrade, S.O.: Anaphylaxis-like reactions produced by ascaris extracts. III. The role played by leukocytes and platelets in the genesis of the shock. Arch. Surg. (Chicago) **53**, 199—213 (1946)

Rocha e Silva, M., Reis, M.L., Ferreira, S.H.: Release of kinins from fresh plasma under varying experimental conditions. Biochem. Pharmacol. **16**, 1665—1676 (1967)

Rocha e Silva, M., Rothschild, H.A.: Introduction. In: Rocha e Silva, M., Rothschild, H.A. (Eds.): A Bradykinin Anthology, pp. IX—XXIII. Sao Paulo: Hucitec S.A. 1974

Rocha e Silva, M., Teixeira, R.M.: Role played by leucocytes, platelets and plasma trypsin in peptone shock in the dog. Proc. Soc. exp. Biol. (N.Y.) **61**, 376—382 (1946)

Rose, J.C., Johnson, M., Ramwell, P.W., Kot, P.A.: Effects of arachidonic acid on systemic arterial pressure, myocardial contractility and platelets in the dog. Proc. Soc. exp. Biol. (N.Y.) **147**, 652—655 (1974)

Roth, G.J., Stanford, N., Majerus, P.W.: Acetylation of prostaglandin synthetase by aspirin. Proc. nat. Acad. Sci. (Wash.) **72**, 3073—3076 (1975)

Rothschild, A.M.: Pharmacodynamic properties of cellulose sulfate and related polysaccharides—a group of bradykinin releasing compounds. In: Rocha e Silva, M., Rothschild, H.A. (Eds.): International symposium on vaso-active polypeptides: bradykinin and related kinins, pp. 197—204. Sao Paulo: Edart 1967

Rothschild, A.M.: Some pharmacodynamic properties of cellulose sulphate, a kininogen-depleting agent in the rat. Brit. J. Pharmacol. **33**, 501—512 (1968)

Rothschild, A. M., Castania, A., Cordeiro, R. S. B.: Consumption of kininogen, formation of kinin and activation of arginine ester hydrolase in rat plasma by rat peritoneal fluid cells in the presence of l-adrenaline. Specific sensitivity to acetylsalicylic acid. Arch. Pharmacol. **285**, 243—256 (1974)

Ryan, M. J., Zimmerman, B. G.: Effect of prostaglandin precursors, dihomo-γ-linolenic acid (DLA) and arachidonic acid (AA), on the vasoconstrictor response (VCR) to intraarterial (IA) norepinephrine (NE) in the dog paw. Fed. Proc. **32**, 803 Abst. (1973)

Ryan, M. J., Zimmerman, B. G.: Effect of prostaglandin precursors, dihomo-γ-linolenic acid and arachidonic acid on the vasoconstrictor response to norepinephrine in the dog paw. Prostaglandins **6**, 179—192 (1974)

Sackeyfio, A. C.: Anaphylatoxin-induced release of a substance with prostaglandin-like activity in isolated perfused guinea-pig lungs. Brit. J. Pharmol. **46**, 544 P—545 P (1972)

Sanner, J. H.: Substances that inhibit the actions of prostaglandins. Arch. intern. Med. **133**, 133—146 (1974)

Schumacher, K. A., Classen, H. G.: The preventive effect of a lowmolecular pentosan-polysulphate on DAS-induced increase in pulmonary vascular resistance caused by platelet-aggregation. Arzneimittel-Forsch. **23**, 431—433 (1973)

Schumacher, K. A., Classen, H. G., Hagedorn, M., Benner, K. U., Spaeth, M., Mittermayer, C.: Effects of anaphylatoxin plasma in cats: hemodynamic changes induced by platelet aggregation. Arzneimittel-Forsch. **24**, 122—126 (1974)

Shen, T. Y.: Perspectives in nonsteroidal anti-inflammatory agents. Angew. Chem. **11**, 460—472 (1972)

Shio, H., Ramwell, P.: Effect of prostaglandin E_2 and aspirin on the secondary aggregation of human platelets. Nature (New Biol.) **236**, 45—46 (1972)

Shore, P. A., Alpers, H. S.: Platelet damage induced in plasma by certain fatty acids. Nature (Lond.) **200**, 1331—1332 (1963)

Silver, M. J., Smith, J. B., Ingerman, C. M.: Blood platelets and the inflammatory process. Agents Actions **4**, 233—240 (1974)

Smith, J. B., Willis, A. L.: Aspirin selectively inhibits prostaglandin production in human platelets. Nature (New Biol.) **231**, 235—237 (1971)

Sorenson, J. R. J.: Copper chelates as possible active metabolites of anti-inflammatory agents. In: Medi 73, Abstracts 167th Meeting American Chemical Society, 1973, Abs. No. 001—431, 1974

Sorrentino, L., Capasso, F., Di Rosa, M.: Indomethacin and prostaglandins. Europ. J. Pharmacol. **17**, 306—308 (1972)

Spink, W. W., Vick J. A.: Endotoxin shock and the coagulation mechanism: modification of shock with epsilon-aminocaproic acid. Proc. Soc. exp. Biol. (N. Y.) **106**, 242—247 (1961)

Swedenborg, J.: Inhibitory effect of polyphloretin phosphate upon platelet aggregation and hemodynamic and respiratory changes caused by thrombin and protamine. J. Pharmacol. exp. Ther. **188**, 214—221 (1974)

Thorpe, R. H., Cobbin, L. B.: The cardiovascular actions of 2-chloroadenosine. Arch. int. Pharmacodyn. **118**, 95—106 (1959)

Tomlinson, R. V., Ringold, H. J., Qureshi, M. C., Forchielli, E.: Relationship between inhibition of prostaglandin synthesis and drug efficacy: Support for the current theory on mode of action of aspirin-like drugs. Biochem. biophys. Res. Commun. **46**, 552—559 (1972)

Trottier, R. W. Jr.: Antibradykinin evaluation of cryogenine and selected other agents. Diss. Abs. **32**, 2913—2914 (1971)

Tschopp, Th. B.: Aggregation of cat platelets in vitro. Thrombos. Diathes. haemorrh. (Stuttg.) **23**, 601—620 (1970)

Ubatuba, F. B., Harvey, E. A., Ferreira, S. H.: Are platelets important in inflammation? Agents Actions **5**, 31—34 (1975)

Uvnäs, B.: Mechanism of histamine release in mast cells. Ann. N. Y. Acad. Sci. **103**, 278—284 (1962)

Vairel, E. G., Hureau, J.: Etude du mode d'action de l'inhibiteur de Kunitz dans le choc expérimental au kaolin et comparaison à certains dérivés chimiques utilisés en thérapeutique. Ann. Pharm. franç. **31**, 409—414 (1973)

Van den Berg, G., Bultsma, T., Nauta, W. T.: Inhibition of prostaglandin biosynthesis by 2-aryl-1,3-indandiones. Biochem. Pharmacol. **24**, 1115—1119 (1975)

Vane, J.R.: The use of isolated organs for detecting active substances in the circulating blood. Brit. J. Pharmacol. **23**, 360—373 (1964)

Vane, J.R.: Inhibition of prostaglandin synthesis as a mechanism of action for aspirin-like drugs. Nature (New Biol.) **231**, 232—235 (1971)

Vane, J.R., Ferreira, S.H.: Interactions between bradykinin and prostaglandins. Life Sci. **16**, 804—805 (1975)

Vane, J.R., Ferreira, S.H.: Interactions between bradykinin and prostaglandins. In: Pisano, J.J., Ansten, K.F. (Eds.): Chemistry and Biology of the Kallikrein-kinin System in Health and Disease. Washington: U.S. Government Printing Office 1976. In press

Van Nueten, J.M., Hoebeke, J., de Clerck, F., Awouters, F., Janssen, P.A.J.: Inhibition by suprofen and other non-narcotic analgesic drugs of the effects of prostaglandin precursors on isolated tissues and platelets. Arch. int. Pharmacodyn. (1976) (in press)

Vargaftig, B.B.: Effet des analgesiques non-narcotiques sur l'hypotension due a la bradykinine. Experientia (Basel) **22**, 182—183 (1966)

Vargaftig, B.B.: Antagonisme par les analgesiques non-narcotiques de la liberation de kinines plasmatiques due au venin de *B. jararaca* et la kallikreine pancreatique Med. Pharmacol. exp. **17**, 517—526 (1967)

Vargartig, B.B.: The pharmacology of slow reacting substance C and of arachidonic acid. Agents Actions **3**, 357—365 (1973)

Vargaftig, B.B.: Search for common mechanisms underlying the various effects of putative inflammatory mediators. In: Ramwell, P.W. (Ed.): The Prostaglandins, Vol. II, pp. 205—275. New York-London: Plenum Press 1974

Vargaftig, B.B.: Carrageenan and thrombin trigger prostaglandin synthetase-independent aggregation of rabbit platelets: inhibition by phospholipase A2 inhibitors. J. Pharm. Pharmac. **29**, 222—228 (1977a)

Vargaftig, B.B.: Involvement of mediators in the interaction of platelets and carrageenan. In: Bonta, I.L. (Eds.): Recent developments in the pharmacology of inflammatory mediators, Agent and actions supplements, pp. 9. Basel and Stuttgart: Birkläuser Verlag (1977b)

Vargaftig, B.B., Bhargava, N., de Vos, C.J., Bonta, I.L.: Interference of carrageenin, non-steroidal anti-inflammatory drugs and protease inhibitors with the kallikrein-kinin system. In: Sicuteri, F., Rocha e Silva, M., Back, N. (Eds.): Bradykinin and Related Kinins: Cardiovascular, Biochemical, and Neural Actions, Vol. VIII, pp. 477—485. New York: Plenum Press 1970

Vargaftig, B.B., Bord, M.: Effets de quelques anti-inflammatoires non-steroidiques sur l'action hypotensive de la bradykinine. Thérapie **24**, 513—522 (1969)

Vargaftig, B.B., Chignard, M.: Substances that increase the cyclic AMP content prevent platelet aggregation and the concurrent release of pharmacologically active substances evoked by arachidonic acid. Agents Actions **5**, 137—144 (1975)

Vargaftig, B.B., Coiron, M.: Detection de la phospholipase A de divers venins animaux par ses effets sur la coagulation du jaune d'oeuf et par la formation de "substance a contraction differee C". J. Pharmacol. **2**, 155—174 (1971)

Vargaftig, B.B., Dao, N.: Release of vasoactive substances from guinea-pig lungs by slow-reacting substance C and arachidonic acid. Pharmacology (Basel) **6**, 99—108 (1971a)

Vargaftig, B.B., Dao, N.: Mode d'action et antagoinisme de la »substance a contraction differee C« liberee par la phospholipase A, a partir du jaune d'oeuf. J. Pharmacol. **2**, 287—304 (1971b)

Vargaftig, B.B., Dao Hai, N.: Paradoxical inhibition of the effects of bradykinin by some sulfhydryl reagents. Experientia (Basel) **28**, 59—62 (1972a)

Vargaftig, B.B., Dao Hai, N.: Interference of some thiol derivatives with the pharmacological effects of arachidonic acid and slow reacting substance C and with the release of rabbit aorta contracting substances. Europ. J. Pharmacol. **18**, 43—55 (1972b)

Vargaftig, B.B., Dao Hai, N.: Inhibition by sulfhydryl reagents of the effects of bradykinin, arachidonic acid and "slow reacting substance C". In: Back, N., Sicuteri, F. (Eds.): Vasopeptides, pp. 155—166. New York: Plenum Publishing Corporation 1972c

Vargaftig, B.B., Dao Hai, N.: Selective inhibition by mepacrine of the release of "rabbit aorta contracting substance" evoked by the administration of bradykinin. J. Pharm. (Lond.) **24**, 159—161 (1972d)

Vargaftig, B. B., Dao Hai, N.: Inhibition by acetamidophenol of the production of prostaglandin-like material from blood platelets in vitro in relation to some in vivo actions. Europ. J. Pharmacol. **24**, 283—288 (1973)

Vargaftig, B. B., de Miranda, E. P., Lancoume, B.: Inhibition by non-steroidal anti-inflammatory agents of in vivo effects of "slow reacting substance C". Nature (Lond.) **222**, 883—885 (1969)

Vargaftig, B. B., de Vos, C. J.: Antiinflammatory properties of sulfhydryl and antioxidant reagents. In: Proceedings of the Fifth International Congress on Pharmacology, 1972

Vargaftig, B. B., Giroux, E. L.: Mechanism of clostripain-induced kinin release from human, rat and canine plasma. In: Sicuteri, F., Back, N., Haberland, G. L. (Eds.): Kinins: Pharmacodynamics and Biological Roles. Proceedings of the International Symposium on Vasopeptides 1976, New York: Plenum Press 1976

Vargaftig, B. B., Lefort, J.: Pharmacological evidence for a vasodilator receptor to serotonin in the nasal vessels of the dog. Europ. J. Pharmacol. **25**, 216—225 (1974)

Vargaftig, B. B., Lefort, J.: Acute hypotension due to carrageenan, arachidonic acid and slow reacting substance C in the rabbit: role of platelets and pharmacological antagonism. Europ. J. Pharmacol. **43**, 125—141 (1977)

Vargaftig, B. B., Tranier, Y., Chignard, M.: Inhibition by sulfhydryl agents of arachidonic acid-induced platelet aggregation and release of potential inflammatory substances. Prostaglandins **8**, 133—156 (1974)

Vargaftig, B. B., Tranier, Y., Chignard, M.: Blockade by metal complexing agents and by catalase of the effects of arachidonic acid on platelets: relevance to the study of anti-inflammatory mechanisms. Europ. J. Pharmacol. **33**, 19—29 (1975)

Vargaftig, B. B., Tranier, Y., Chignard, M.: Inhibition by metal-chelating agents and by catalase of arachidonic acid-induced platelet aggregation. In: Samuelsson, B., Paoletti, R. (Eds.): Advances in Prostaglandin and Thromboxane Research, Vol. II, pp. 755—762. New York: Raven Press 1976

Vargaftig, B. B., Zirinis, P.: Platelet aggregation induced by arachidonic acid is accompanied by release of potential inflammatory mediators distinct from PGE_2 and PGF_2. Nature (New Biol.) **244**, 114—116 (1973)

Vick, J. A., Brooks Jr., R. B.: Pharmacological studies of the major fractions of bee venom. Amer. Bee J. **112**, 288—289 (1972)

Vincent, J. E., Zijlstra, F. J., Bonta, I. L.: The effect of nonsteroid anti-inflammatory drugs, dibutyryl cyclic 3′,5′-adenosine monophosphate and phosphodiesterase inhibitors on platelet aggregation and the platelet release reaction in normal and essential fatty acid deficient rats. Prostaglandins **10**, 899—911 (1975)

Vital Brazil, O., Farina, R., Yoshida, L., Oliveira, V. A. de: Pharmacology of crystalline crotoxin. III. Cardiovascular and respiratory effects of crotoxin and *crotalus durissus terrificus* venom. Mem. Inst. Butantan **33**, 993—1000 (1966)

Vogt, W.: Pharmacologically active substances formed in egg yolk by cobra venom. J. Physiol. (Lond.) **136**, 131—147 (1957a)

Vogt, W.: Pharmacologically active lipid-soluble acids of natural occurence. Nature (Lond.) **179**, 300—304 (1957b)

Vogt, W.: Release of prostaglandins by venoms and by endogenous mechanisms. In: Leonardi, A., Walsh, J. (Eds.): Proceedings of the First International Symposium on Drugs of Animal Origin, 1966, pp. 29—33. Milan: Ferro Edizioni 1967

Vogt, W., Distelkötter, B.: Release of prostaglandin from frog intestine. In: Bergström, S., Samuelsson, B. (Eds.): Prostaglandins, Proceedings of the Second Nobel Symposium Stockholm, 1966, pp. 237—240. New York-London-Sydney: Interscience Publishers 1967

Vogt, W., Meyer, U., Kunze, H., Lufft, E., Babilli, S.: Entstehung von SRS-C in der durchströmten Meerschweinchenlunge durch Phospholipase A. Naunyn-Schmiedeberg's Arch. exp. Path. Pharmak. **262**, 124—134

Vogt, W., Suzuki, T., Babilli, S.: Prostaglandins in SRS-C and in a Darmstoff preparation from frog intestinal dialysates. In: Pickles, U. R., Fitzpatrick, R. J. (Eds.): Endogenous Substances Affecting the Myometrium, pp. 137—142. London: Cambridge University Press 1966

Wasserman, M. A., Griffin, R. L.: Prostaglandin endoperoxide analogs: a comparison of bronchopulmonary activity to prostaglandin $F_{2\alpha}$. Pharmacologist **17**, 272 (1975)

Werle, E.: History of kallikrein and some aspects of its chemistry and physiology. In: Haberland, G. L., Rohen, J. W. (Eds.): Kininogenases, pp. 7—22. Stuttgart-New York: F. K. Schattauer Verlag 1973

Willis, A. L.: Release of histamine, kinin and prostaglandins during carrageenin-induced inflammation in the rat. In: Ramwell, P. W., Pharriss, B. B. (Eds.): Prostaglandins, Peptides and Amines, pp. 31—38. London: Academic Press 1969

Willis, A. L., Comai, K., Kuhn, D. C., Paulsrud, J.: Dihomo-γ-linolenate suppresses platelet aggregation when administered in vitro or in vivo. Prostaglandins 8, 509—519 (1974)

Willis, A. L., Davison, P., Ramwell, P. W., Brocklehurst, W. E., Smith, J. B.: Release and actions of prostaglandins in inflammation and fever: inhibition by anti-inflammatory and antipyretic drugs. In: Ramwell, P. W., Pharriss, B. B. (Eds.): Prostaglandins in Cellular Biology, Vol. I, p. 227. New York-London: Plenum Press 1972

Willis, A. L., Kuhn, D. C.: A new potential mediator of arterial thrombosis whose biosynthesis is inhibited by aspirin. Prostaglandins 4, 127—130 (1973)

Winder, C. V., Wax, J., Burr, V., Been, M., Rosiere, C. E.: A study of pharmacological influences on ultraviolet erythema in guinea-pigs. Arch. int. pharmacodyn. 116, 261—265 (1958)

Winter, C. A., Risley, E. A., Nuss, G. W.: Carrageenin-induced edema in hind paw of the rat as an assay for antiinflammatory drugs. Proc. Soc. exp. Biol. (N. Y.) 111, 544—547 (1962)

Yamasaki, H., Saeki, K.: Inhibition of mast-cell degranulation by anti-inflammatory agents. Arch. int. Pharmacodyn. 168, 166—179 (1967)

Yamazaki, H., Murase, H., Shimamoto, T., Shimamoto, T.: Appearance of platelet-clumping substance after acidification of plasma. Blood 31, 348—357 (1968)

Yamazaki, Y., Shimamoto, T., Murase, H., Shimahoto, T.: Appearance of Platelet-clumping substance in plasma of rabbits after intravenous injection of agar solution bacterial endotoxin or adrenaline. Blood 30, 792—795 (1967)

Zbinden, G.: Transient thrombopenia after intravenous injection of certain fatty acids. J. Lipid Res. 5, 378—384 (1964)

Zbinden, G.: Lauric acid-induced thrombocytopenia and thrombosis in rabbits. Thrombos. Diathes. haemorrh. (Stuttg.) 18, 57—65 (1967)

Zucker, M. B.: ADP- and collagen-induced platelet aggregation in vivo and in vitro. Thrombos. Diathes. haemorrh. (Stuttg.) Suppl. 26, 175—184 (1967)

CHAPTER 26

Antagonism of Pain and Hyperalgesia

R. VINEGAR, J. F. TRUAX, J. L. SELPH, and P. R. JOHNSTON

A. Introduction

The purpose of this chapter is to discuss the use of hyperalgesia in the design of assays which quantitatively measure mild analgesic activity. The authors have taken the option not to attempt a comprehensive review of the literature but to comment critically on those contributions which relate directly to this purpose. Broad, comprehensive reviews on pain and analgesic testing are available (WINTER, 1965; SWINGLE, 1974). To achieve their purpose, the authors have relied on their personal experience in the fields of inflammation and analgesic testing. It is their hope that this chapter will provoke new thinking and thus new research into the mechanisms of hyperalgesia and, additionally, lead to the more rational use of hyperalgesia and inflammatory phenomona in the design of mild analgesic assays.

I. Terminology

Increased sensitivity to pain (hyperalgesia) has been induced in small laboratory animals by the subcutaneous and intradermal injection of a wide variety of irritants. All of these irritants elicit oedema formation but not by the same mechanism. Some irritants produce large oedemas within 30 min of injection. Upon microscopic examination of the irritated tissue, capillary damage is apparent, but few inflammatory cells are seen. Those irritants which act directly on capillaries, damaging them and thereby increasing their permeability, have been termed oedematous agents or "oedemagens" (VINEGAR et al., 1976c). Other irritants, called inflammatory agents or inflammagens elicit oedema formation slowly, over 1–4 h, and indirectly. Inflammagens mobilize inflammatory cells which, in the course of phagocytosing the irritant, release mediators of oedema formation. The distinction between oedemagen and inflammagen is of prime importance to the pharmacologist, as oedema resulting from the action of oedemagens (e.g. histamine, 5-hydroxytryptamine (5-HT) and bradykinin) is not affected by anti-inflammatory drugs, whereas the development of oedema by inflammagens is inhibited by this class of drug. Oedema produced by oedemagens is inhibited specifically by their respective antagonist (e.g. histamine-induced oedema by H_1 antihistaminic agents).

Although heat, redness, pain, and swelling are cited as the cardinal signs of inflammation, it is the microscopic signs of this process, presence of inflammatory cells and tissue oedema (WILHELM, 1971) which characterise the term inflammation as it is used in this chapter.

II. Historical Introduction to Analgesic Testing in Hyperalgesic Animals

Modern, quantitative, mild analgesic testing in laboratory animals began with the observations that the yeast-injected hind-limb of the rat was hyperalgesic to pressure and mild analgesic agents were able to reduce this increased sensitivity (Randall and Selitto, 1957). An analgesic assay was designed from these observations. In this assay, the subcutaneous injection of yeast rendered the rat hind-limb hyperalgesic to pressure. After the hyperalgesia developed, a mechanical force of increasing magnitude was applied to the hind-limb. The force (in mm Hg) at which the animals began to struggle was assumed to represent the pain threshold and served as the end point. Analgesia, produced by a test compound, resulted in an increase in the magnitude of the force needed to elicit a struggle. The anti-inflammatory drugs, sodium salicylate and phenylbutazone, as well as the narcotic analgesics morphine and codeine, produced dose-dependent increases in the pain threshold pressures (Randall and Selitto, 1957; Randall et al., 1957). Analgesia produced by the narcotic analgesics was believed to be due to a reduction in the central perception of the pain (Jaffe and Martin, 1975). Analgesia produced by the antiinflammatory drugs was assumed by Randall and Selitto (1957) to be the result of reduced oedema formation and a concomitant decrease in the degree of hyperalgesia. This suggested mechanism of drug action for aspirin was not consistent with data presented by Gilfoil et al., 1963, in which relatively low dose levels of aspirin (25 and 50 mg/kg p.o.) reduced the pain threshold in the Randall-Selitto assay without affecting the magnitude of the oedema. Before this difference was resolved, Winter and Flataker (1965a) reported that most of the force which made up the pain threshold pressure values published by previous authors was expended in overcoming the internal friction of the glass syringe plunger. This plunger transmitted the remaining force to the hind-limb. When Winter and Flataker (1965a) and van Arman et al. (1966) replaced the glass plunger with a teflon plunger, pain threshold pressures decreased appreciably. For example, the pain threshold pressures for the uninjected hindlimb were 155–175 mm Hg in the studies of Randall and Selitto (1957) and 120–135 mm Hg in those of Gilfoil et al. (1963). Using the teflon plunger, pain threshold pressures were 30–40 mm Hg (Winter and Flataker, 1965a). Importantly, the increased sensitivity resulting from the use of the teflon plunger made it possible for Winter and Flataker (1965a) to find that hypo-algesia developed immediately after the injection of yeast and persisted for 1 h. The degree of hyperalgesia returned to normal 1.5 h after the injection of yeast and then a strong, long-lasting hyperalgesia developed. These findings made it necessary for Winter and Flataker (1965a) to modify the protocol of the Randall-Selitto assay, for any drug effect measured at 1 h would take place during a period of hypo-algesia. There was no attempt made to explain the drug-induced analgesia which previous authors had reported at 1 h. In the Winter-Flataker modification, each test compound was administered 2 h after the hind-limb injection of 5 mg of yeast. The pain threshold was determined 1 h after the test compound was administered. Winter and Flataker (1965b) also changed the end point from the onset of the struggle reaction to vocalisation (a squeak) since the latter was found to yield more consistent results. Winter and Flataker (1965b) believed the new protocol made the assay insensitive to anti-inflammatory agents, since the test compounds were administered after the oedema, inflammation and high degree of hyperalgesia were established. In addition, only 1 h was allowed for the test compounds to act. This was considered to be too short an interval for an antiinflammatory agent to affect appreciably an established inflammation (WINTER, 1965). In spite of these considerations, WINTER and FLATAKER (1965b) found the anti-inflammatory drugs, aspirin and indomethacin, to be active in the modified test and ascribed local analgesic action to them. TAKESUE et al. (1969) observed the teflon plunger to stick after prolonged use and replaced it with a rubber diaphragm. Using this diaphragm and the protocol outlined by WINTER and FLATAKER (1965a), TAKE-SUE et al. (1969) found that orally administered aspirin, phenylbutazone and indomethacin produced dose-dependent increases in the pain threshold pressure. More recently, SWINGLE et al. (1971) modified the Randall-Selitto test so that quantal data was obtained and relative analgesic potency determined graphically using a probit plot. Cogent comments concerning the Randall-Selitto assay are included in reviews by WINTER (1965) and SWINGLE (1974).

In recent years, the concepts of mild analgesic testing introduced by RANDALL and SELITTO (1957) have been used in several animal models (VINEGAR et al., 1976b), as well as in a model utilizing humans (FERREIRA, 1972). To date, none have contributed as much as the original yeast-injected rat hind-limb model to the practical achievement of mild analgesic drug development. The choice of yeast as the irritant was based on the rapid production of a large oedematous response and the concomitant development of strong hyperalgesia. Cyproheptadine, an anti-5-HT-antihistamine agent (STONE et al., 1961), blocked the development of half of the acute oedematous response to yeast (Fig. 1). As histamine is not an irritant in the rat hind-limb

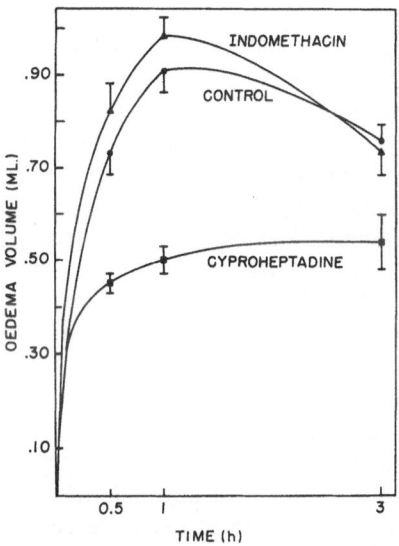

Fig. 1. Oedema volume produced as a function of time in the rat hind-limb by the subplantar injection of 0.10 ml of a 2.0% suspension of brewers yeast in pyrogen-free water 30 min after oral pretreatment with a 0.5% carboxymethylcellulose control (o), indomethacin (△), 4 mg/kg, and cyproheptadine (■), 10 mg/kg. Each point represents the mean of 16 animals

(VINEGAR et al., 1974), this finding indicated that half of the oedematous response to yeast resulted from 5-HT release and the direct capillary changes this amine produced (ROWLEY and BENDITT, 1956). Most of the yeast-induced oedema is produced in less than 30 min. In so short an interval there is little possibility that the actions of mobilized inflammatory cells are responsible for the oedema produced. It takes more than 60 min for carrageenin to mobilize 10–30 million neutrophils and subsequently to produce a significant oedema (greater than 0.2 ml) in the rat pleural cavity. The idea that the acute oedematous response to yeast was not due to a typical inflammation was supported by the failure of indomethacin to reduce the effect of yeast (Fig. 1) at a dose that inhibited the second phase of carrageenin hind-limb oedema by more than 60%. Indomethacin is a potent prostaglandin synthetase inhibitor (VANE, 1971) so this difference probably indicates the participation of prostaglandins in the carrageenin response, but not in that to yeast. One component of the acute rat hind-limb reaction to yeast (1–4 h) is the gradual development of a relatively small oedema volume which is associated with the mobilization of neutrophils and the development of inflammation. However, the large non-typical component of the total oedema predominates the early period of yeast-induced oedema and masks the small inflammatory component during the first few hours when the Randall-Selitto assay is carried out. Recently, rat hind-limb oedemas produced by enzymes and chemical irritants have been catagorised pharmacologically (VINEGAR et al., 1974). Utilising quantitative hind-limb volumetric techniques and various drugs as specific antagonists, oedema produced by a wide variety of irritants has been grouped into three pharmacological classes:

1. Highly sensitive to anti-inflammatory drugs and insensitive to anti-5-HT agents (e.g. the irritants carrageenin and kaolin)

2. Relatively insensitive to anti-inflammatory drugs and anti-5-HT agents (e.g. the irritants trypsin and elastase)

3. Highly sensitive to anti-5-HT agents and insensitive to anti-inflammatory drugs (e.g. the irritants dextran, hyaluronidase, acid phosphatase and 5-HT)

Yeast-induced rat hind-limb oedema represents a mixture of classes 2 and 3, since half of the immediate response can be blocked by cyproheptadine, whereas the remainder is insensitive to both anti-inflammatory and anti-5-HT drugs (Fig. 1). These unusual characteristics may be explained by the chemical heterogeneity of commercial yeast preparations. Enzymes as well as pyrogens are contained in these preparations. Due to this heterogeneity, a clear understanding of drug action on the yeast hyperalgesic assay of RANDALL and SELITTO (1957) is difficult to achieve (RANDALL, 1963). To avoid this problem, trypsin and carrageenin have been used to induce hyperalgesia in two new mild analgesic assays (VINEGAR et al., 1976a). Trypsin oedema (class 2) is unaffected by anti-5-HT and anti-inflammatory drugs and was used in the design of an assay in which these pharmacological agents are inactive. Carrageenin-induced oedema (class 1) is unaffected by anti-5-HT agents but can be severely inhibited by pretreatment with anti-inflammatory drugs. Advantage was taken of these characteristics in designing the carrageenin hyperalgesic assay to be sensitive to analgesic agents which have an anti-inflammatory component of action. The oedema-time curve and the hyperalgesia-time curve resulting from the subplantar injection of 500 µg of carrageenin were biphasic over the first 3 h (Fig. 2). The first phase of the hyperalgesia-time curve is due primarily to the trauma associated with

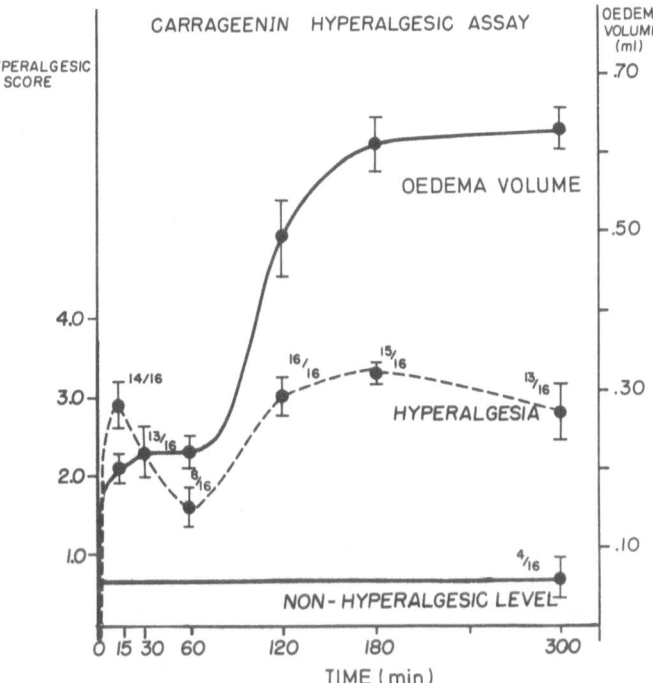

Fig. 2. Oedema volume-time curve produced by the subplantar injection of 500 μg of carrageenin and the hyperalgesia resulting from application of a 3.5 kg force to the inflamed hind-limb. Numerator of each fraction represents number of animals responding with a squeal or flight response in less than 2.3 sec. Each point represents the mean of 16 rats

the subplantar injection since much the same degree of hyperalgesia developed when the solvent was injected. The first phase of the hyperalgesia is short-lived. It peaks at 15 min and returns close to control level at 60 min. The second phase of the oedema-time curve and the hyperalgesia-time curve develops between 60 and 180 min. This is the period in which large numbers of neutrophils are free in the subplantar tissue, and tissue oedema and inflammation are evident histologically. By integrating the hyperalgesia-time data with the inhibitory effects of drugs on the first and second phase of carrageenin hind-limb oedema (VINEGAR et al., 1969) it was possible to design the carrageenin hyperalgesic assay to be sensitive to anti-inflammatory drugs. To achieve this sensitivity, the drugs were administered 1 h after the carrageenin and a 3.5 kg force applied 3 h after injection of the irritant. With this protocol, anti-inflammatory drugs inhibited the development of the second phase (60–180 min oedema, Fig. 2). This resulted in less inflammation and hyperalgesia at 3 h and "apparent" analgesic activity. Aspirin, phenacetin and acetaminophen (paracetamol) were active at relatively low dose levels in the carrageenin hyperalgesic assay (Table 1). Each of these drugs produced anti-inflammatory activity (VINEGAR et al., 1976 b).

The subplantar injection of trypsin in the rat resulted in the development of a hyperalgesia-time curve and an oedema-time curve which were both monophasic

Table 1. Activity of various drugs in the trypsin and carrageenin hyperalgesic assays

Drug	Trypsin hyperalgesic assay[a, b] ED$_{50}$ (mg/kg, p.o.)	Carrageenin hyperalgesic assay[a] ED$_{50}$ (mg/kg, p.o.)
Codeine phos.	42±9.4	34±10.9
Phenacetin	114±36.2	46±10.0
Acetaminophen	I[c] at 180	110±23.4
Aspirin	I at 360	56±19.6
Indomethacin	I at 5	1.7±0.37
Hydrocortisone	I at 25	20±4.3
Triprolidine	I at 1	I at 1
Cyproheptadine	I at 10	I at 10

[a] VINEGAR et al. 1976a.
[b] ED$_{50}$ represents the dose in mg/kg which reduced the average pain score of each drug-treated group 50% relative to solvent-fed control animals. The ED$_{50}$ was calculated graphically from dose-response curves. There were 6–8 animals at each dose-level. Every experiment contained a positive and negative control. The observer was blind to the drug treatment of each animal.
[c] I inactive.

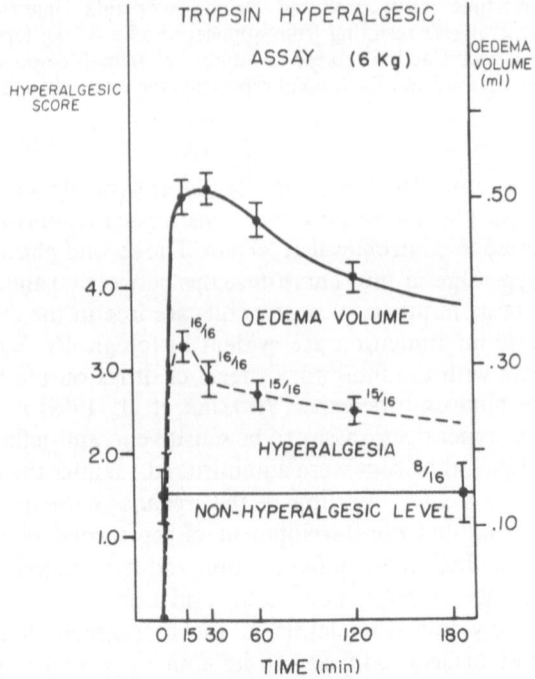

Fig. 3. Oedema volume-time curve produced by the subplantar injection of 100 µg of trypsin and the hyperalgesia resulting from application of a 6-kg force to the inflamed hind-limb. Numerator of each fraction represents number of animals responding with a squeal or flight response in less than 2.3 s. Each point represents the mean of 16 animals.

and parallel over the first 3 h (Fig. 3). Of the trypsin-injected animals 94% responded positively to a force of 6.0 kg applied at 1 h. This information was used in the design of the trypsin hyperalgesic assay. In this test, the drugs are administered 30 min after the subplantar injection of 100 µg of trypsin. After waiting 60 min for hyperalgesia to develop a 6.0 kg force is applied. With this protocol, the following three factors ensured that this hyperalgesic assay would not be affected by anti-inflammatory drugs:

1. Oedema development by the class 2 irritant trypsin is not affected by anti-inflammatory drugs.

2. The drugs are administered after most of the oedema and hyperalgesia have developed, in which case any anti-inflammatory effect would be minimal.

3. The drugs are allowed to act for only 30 min, a period too short for them to affect an established oedema and/or inflammation.

The effects of a wide variety of drugs were studied in the trypsin hyperalgesic assay (Table 1). Aspirin was inactive at 360 mg/kg, p.o. Acetaminophen produced less than 50% inhibition at 360 mg/kg; a dose which elicited profuse lacrimation and a large decrease in body temperature. At 180 mg/kg, a dose devoid of side-effects, acetaminophen was inactive. Interestingly, phenacetin was active in the trypsin hyperalgesic assay with an ED_{50} of 114 ± 36.2 mg/kg, p.o. These results indicate that a portion of the analgesia produced by phenacetin is independent of anti-inflammatory activity. Aspirin and acetaminophen lack this analgesic component. The mild analgesia they produce appears to result solely from anti-inflammatory activity, since they were active in the carrageenian hyperalgesic assay but inactive at dose levels devoid of obvious side-effects in the trypsin hyperalgesic assay. The strong, centrally acting analgesic codeine phosphate was active in both tests. Since these hyperalgesic tests were designed to detect mild analgesic compounds, inhibition by strong analgesic drugs was expected. Indomethacin and hydrocortisone were inactive in the trypsin test; the analgesia attributed to indomethacin in the clinic is thought to be the result of anti-inflammatory action (WOODBURY and FINGLE, 1975). The fact that indomethacin and hydrocortisone inhibited carrageenin-induced hyperalgesia confirms the rationale used in the experimental design of this test. In effect, the carrageenin hyperalgesic assay transforms anti-inflammatory activity to apparent analgesia. Similar reasoning can be used to explain the analgesia produced by aspirin, indomethacin and other anti-inflammatory drugs in the WINTER and FLATAKER (1965b) modification of the Randall-Selitto assay. In their protocol, the drugs are administered 2 h after the yeast is injected and the force applied 1 h later. Inflammation and strong hyperalgesia develop 1–3 h after the yeast is injected (see Fig. 1 in article by WINTER and FLATAKER, 1965b). Therefore, when the modified protocol is used, the development of inflammation and concomitant hyperalgesia that occurs between 2 and 3 h is liable to inhibition by anti-inflammatory drugs. Any decrease in hyperalgesia produced by these drugs will represent transformation of anti-inflammatory activity to apparent analgesia.

Two parameters determine the percentage of animals which perceive pain in hind-limb hyperalgesic assays: the magnitude of the applied force and the degree of hyperalgesia present at the time the force is applied. The magnitude of the force can be controlled quantitatively and the degree of hyperalgesia qualitatively. As the magnitude of the force is increased, the percentage of animals which perceive pain increases (Table 2). The relationship applies to normal as well as to carrageenin-,

Table 2. Pain score as a function of force in normal and irritant-injected rats

Force[a] (kg)	Normal rat hind-limb		Trypsin (100 µg)		Carrageenin (500 µg)		Yeast (2000 µg)	
	Average pain score (± S.E.)	% posi-tive	Average pain score (± S.E.)	% posi-tive	Average pain score (± S.S.)	% posi-tive	Average pain score (± S.E.)	% posi-tive
0.5	—	—	—	—	—	—	2.7±0.47	80
1.0	—	—	—	—	0.5±0.34	20	3.1±0.41	90
2.0	—	—	—	—	1.5±0.58	40	3.8±0.13	100
3.0	0.5±0.03	0	0.1±0.10	0	2.5±0.34	80	—	—
4.0	1.0±0.09	20	0.8±0.33	20	3.8±0.13	100	—	—
5.0	1.1±0.12	40	1.7±0.37	60	—	—	—	—
6.0	1.3±0.11	50	3.1±0.33	100	—	—	—	—
7.0	2.9±0.05	100	—	—	—	—	—	—

[a] The technique has been described in detail (VINEGAR et al., 1976a). Each force was applied for a maximum of 3.0 s. As soon as pain was perceived (flight response or vocalisation) the force was withdrawn. Arbitrary pain scoring was as follows:
  Score of 4—response in 0 –1.0 s
  Score of 3—response in 1.1–1.6 s
  Score of 2—response in 1.7–2.2 s
  Score of 1—response in 2.3–2.9 s
  Score of 0—response in 3.0 s
Positive responders perceived pain in less than 2.3 s. There were at least ten rats in each group.

trypsin- or yeast-injected animals. However, the irritant-injected animals are more sensitive. For example, there were no positive responders when a 3.0 kg force was applied for 3 s to the uninjected hind-limb of normal rats (Table 2). A force of 6.0 kg was required to cause 50% of the normal animals to respond and 7.0 kg to cause all to perceive pain. When these forces were applied 1 h after the injection of 100 µg of trypsin into the hind-limb, there was a moderate increase in sensitivity. The 3.0 kg force still was without effect, but all trypsin-injected animals responded to 6.0 kg. Three hours after the injection of 500 µg of carrageenin, there was severe inflamma-tion in the rat hind-limb. A 3.0 kg force applied to the carrageenin-injected animals resulted in 80% responding positively. A force of 4.0 kg was required to cause all of the carrageenin-injected animals to perceive pain. Yeast-injected animals developed strong hyperalgesia to pressure at 3 h. Only 2.0 kg was required in order to cause all yeast-injected animals to perceive pain (Table 2). These findings indicate that differ-ent degrees of hyperalgesia were produced by trypsin, carrageenin and yeast. One hour after the injection of trypsin, a mild degree of hyperalgesia was present which was a consequence of the oedema formed and the trauma of the hindlimb injection. Moderate hyperalgesia developed 3 h after the injection of carrageenin. This resulted from the combined effects of a weak oedemagenic reaction (1st phase) and a severe inflammation (2nd phase, Fig. 2). The strong hyperalgesic response to yeast at 3 h was due to a large mixed oedemagenic and inflammagenic reaction. These findings indicate that the degree of hyperalgesia present at any instant is the result of non-inflammatory as well as inflammatory processes. The exact mechanisms responsible

Table 3. Hyperalgesia produced in the rat hind-limb by handling and subplantar injection

Treatment	Average pain score[a] at 1 h	
	First test[b]	Retest[c]
Untouched prior to scoring procedure	0.3±0.12	1.3±0.90
Simulated subplantar injection[d]	0.9±0.20	1.4±0.25
Subplantar injection of pyrogen-free saline[e]	1.2±0.21	2.4±0.18
Subplantar injection of 0.1% trypsin[e]	2.8±0.25	3.0±0.21

[a] Each pain score represents the mean ± S.E. of 30 animals (three experiments containing 10 rats in each group). See Table 2 for explanation of scoring procedure.
[b] Average pain score obtained after application of a 6.0 kg force to the rat hind-limb.
[c] The reapplication of a 6.0 kg force within 15 s of the first test.
[d] Rats were removed from cage, placed in stainless steel cylinder with hind-limbs exposed and held for injection without introduction of needle.
[e] Injection volume was 0.10 ml.

for the hyperalgesia are unknown. Recent mechanistic studies indicate that prostaglandins may be responsible for the hyperalgesia which accompanies mild trauma by sensitizing pain receptors to mechanical or chemical stimuli (MONCADA et al., 1975).

In our experience, the general health and pretreatment of the animals is of overriding importance in experiments which utilise the development of hyperalgesia to mechanical force to measure mild analgesic activity. When rats are used, they must be free of both the acute and subacute pneumonias which pervade many commercial breeding colonies. Animals with infection will in general respond sluggishly to a mildly painful stimulus. In their stressed condition, the development of inflammation and concomitant hyperalgesia are reduced relative to healthy animals. Each manipulation of the animals prior to the application of mechanical force (injection of the irritant, administration of drug and pretest trial) may contribute significantly to the degree of hyperalgesia present at the time of test. For example, the successive application of a 6.0 kg force to one hind-limb of "untouched" animals (rats put in individual cages the night before the experiment and not manipulated until the force was applied) produced higher pain scores when the force was applied a second time (Table 3). Simulating a hind-limb injection by handling the animals or injecting pyrogen-free saline, which is not an irritant, in the rat hind-limb also resulted in high pain scores, indicating that hyperalgesia had developed. These results suggest that awareness, learning, as well as sensitization, may contribute importantly to the degree of hyperalgesia present in acute studies. Each parameter that contributes will have a specific time course of development and decay. A portion of the degree of hyperalgesia which results from the injection and/or handling of the animals appears to wear off rapidly (Fig. 2, note decrease in hyperalgesia which occurs between 15 and 60 min). This rapid decrease in hyperalgesia may represent the hypoalgesia reported by WINTER and FLATAKER (1965a) 1 h after the injection of trypsin. That is, their animals still were hyperalgesic relative to untouched animals. This relative change in the degree of hyperalgesia may explain the ability of RANDALL and SELITTO (1957), RANDALL et al. (1957) and GILFOIL et al. (1963) to measure drug-induced mild analgesia. For if hypo-algesia was indeed present at 1 h, it would not have been possible for them to measure these drug affects.

A crucial aspect in the design of hyperalgesic assays which will detect mild analgesic activity is the need to obtain the highest possible sensitivity to these agents. To achieve this degree of sensitivity in assays which depend on the development of hyeralgesia to mechanical stimulation the smallest force that will produce an adequate percentage of positive responders (e.g., greater than 90%) must be used. In addition, the most sensitive end point should be employed. WINTER and FLATAKER (1965 a) used vocalisation as the end point. They were convinced from their data that vocalisation was a more consistent end point than the flight reaction, as is doubtless true. However, as they indicated, vocalisation usually occurs after the flight reaction. Thus, although vocalisation is a more consistent end point than the flight reaction (struggle) it entails the use of a stronger or longer-lasting force and the concomitant loss of sensitivity to mild analgesic agents.

B. Non-Hyperalgesic Mild Analgesic Assays

I. Stretching Tests

Inhibition of stretching (writhing) in the mouse has been used as an index of analgesia ever since mild as well as strong analgesics were found to reduce the number of stretches produced by phenylquinone (SIEGMUND et al., 1957), acetic acid (KOSTER et al., 1959) and acetylcholine (COLLIER et al., 1968). Unfortunately, these assays lack pharmacological specificity (WHITTLE, 1964; CHERNOV et al., 1967). Non-steroid antiinflammatory drugs and antihistamine drugs as well as CNS depressants and stimulants, local anaesthetics and sympathomimetic drugs inhibit stretching. In spite of this shortcoming, stretching assays are widely used as no other simple test is available for assaying mild analgesia in the mouse.

The non-specificity of the mouse assay has made it difficult to uncover the mechanism(s) responsible for eliciting this complex syndrome. Recently, PGE_1 and PGE_2 were found to be among the most potent inducers of stretching (COLLIER and SCHNEIDER, 1972). PG-induced stretching was inhibited by morphine but not by aspirin. The inactivity of aspirin was related, in theory, to the concept that aspirin inhibits the biosynthesis of PGs but not their direct effects (VANE, 1971). The possibility that PGs mediated the stretching produced by acetic acid was investigated by comparing the activity of various drugs after local and subcutaneous administration. Aspirin and indomethacin were the only drugs active locally (intraperitoneal administration, Table 4) at low dose levels in the mouse and rat. Their high potency strongly suggested a specific pharmacological action. Interestingly, equivalent intraperitoneal (local) doses of aspirin and indomethacin inhibited arachidonic acid-induced diarrhoea in mice 50%. This assay is an in vivo measure of PG synthetase inhibition (BARUTH and RANDALL, 1974). The high potency and equivalent ED_{50}s of these anti-inflammatory drugs in both assays suggested identical mechanisms of inhibition. Presumably, aspirin and indomethacin act by irreversible inactivating the cyclo-oxygenase of PG synthetase (ROME and LANDS, 1975). This concept was reinforced, indirectly, by the inactivity of locally injected sodium salicylate, phenacetin, acetaminophen and hydrocortisone (Table 4). These anti-inflammatory drugs do not irreversibly inhibit PG synthetase.

Table 4. Activity of various drugs in the acetic acid stretching assay

Drug	Acetic acid stretching assay[a] ED_{50}[b], mg/kg		
	Mouse		Rat
	Local drug adm.[c] i.p.	Systemic drug adm.[d] s.c.	Local drug adm.[e] i.p.
Codeine phosphate	I[f] at 0.4	5	I at 1
Phenacetin	I at 15	94 ± 13.8	I at 1
Acetaminophen	I at 15	I at 240	I at 1
Sodium salicylate	I at 15	I at 150	I at 1
Aspirin	<4	145 ± 88.0	<0.2
Indomethacin	<0.4	I at 2	<0.2
Hydrocortisone	I at 4	I at 40	I at 1
Chlorpheniramine	I at 1	I at 10	I at 1
Methysergide	I at 0.4	I at 4	I at 1
Atropine sulphate	I at 2	I at 5	I at 1

[a] Stretching was induced in male ICR mice, 18–22 g, by the i.p. injection of 0.4 ml/20 g.b.wt. of a 0.6% solution of acetic acid in pyrogen-free water (KOSTER et al., 1959) and in Sprague-Dawley rats, 160–180 g, by the i.p. injection of 1.00 ml of a 0.6% solution of acetic acid. The average # of stretches produced by each drug-treated and carboxymethylcellulose solvent-fed control group in the 5–15-min-period following acetic acid injection was determined.
[b] ED_{50} represents the dose in mg/kg which reduced the average # of stretches in each drug-treated group 50% relative to solvent-fed control animals. The ED_{50} was calculated graphically from dose-response curves.
[c] 0.4 ml of drug/20 g.b.wt. was administered 5 min before the injection of acetic acid. A 0.8% solution of acetic acid was used to compensate for the dilution produced by local drug administration.
[d] 0.4 ml of drug/20 g.b.wt. was administered 20 min before the injection of acetic acid.
[e] 0.5 ml of drug/100 g.b.wt. was administered 5 min before the injection of acetic acid.
[f] I: inactive.

C. Assessment of Mild Analgesia in Humans

I. Clinical Evaluation of Mild Analgesic Agents

Since publication of an incisive review of mild analgesic drugs by BEAVER (1966), there has been renewed interest in the clinical testing of these agents. In a randomised double-blind crossover study of the pain of unresectable cancer (MOERTEL et al., 1972), aspirin (650 mg, approximately 10 mg/kg) was found to be superior to all the marketed analgesics tested, which included codeine (65 mg) and propoxyphene (65 mg). Analogous clinical findings were reported recently for alleviation of the pain resulting from dental surgery (COOPER and BEAVER, 1975). In one double-blind study, aspirin (650 mg) was superior to placebo (p<0.01), whereas codeine (30 mg) showed no difference. In another study, codeine (60 mg) was more efficacious than placebo for certain measures of effect. However, codeine at 60 mg produce a significant number of side-effects. In these clinical papers, no attempt was made to explain the superiority of aspirin over codeine. A logical explanation is that the pain from unresectable cancer and post-dental surgery is a result of the inflammation which accompanies them. Aspirin is able to reduce this inflammation and thus the accompanying pain, whereas codeine, which lacks anti-inflammatory activity, does not appreciably affect these painful conditions. This suggestion that the analgesia produced by aspirin is a consequence of its anti-inflammatory activity is not new (Randall, 1963; Beaver, 1966). It was reinforced by a comparison of the efficacy of aspirin and codeine in the carrageenin hyperalgesic assay and their clinically effective doses. A dose of aspirin of 70 mg/kg produced 50% inhibition in the carrageenin hyperalgesic assay. When species differences in body surface area and volume are taken into account, a dose of 70 mg/kg in rats is equivalent to 10 mg/kg (650 mg) in humans. That is, the dose of aspirin in rats which provided strong analgesia in the carrageenin hyperalgesic assay is equivalent to the effective analgesic dose in humans. This relationship did not apply to the results obtained with codeine. A dose of 35 mg/kg of this centrally acting analgesic was required to produce 50% inhibition in the carrageenin hyperalgesic assay (Table 1). In rats, 35 mg/kg is equivalent to 7 mg/kg in humans. This is a relatively high dose of codeine which cannot be administered clinically due to adverse reactions.

D. Conclusion

The pharmacological findings obtained from the new hyperalgesic assays in rodents, as well as the clinical considerations just presented, suggest that pain can be categorised into three pharmacological classes:

1. Pain of non-inflammatory aetiology defined by sensitivity to centrally acting analgesic agents and insensitivity to anti-inflammatory drugs.

2. Pain of inflammatory aetiology defined by sensitivity to anti-inflammatory drugs and relative insensitivity to centrally acting analgesics.

3. Pain of mixed aetiology defined by moderate sensitivity to both anti-inflammatory drugs and centrally acting analgesic agents.

In man, a pain syndrome that responds to codeine (65 mg) but not to aspirin (650 mg) would be a member of class 1. Conversely, pain which responded to aspirin and codeine elicited a measurable degree of pain relief would be placed in class 3.

For more than 50 years, combined chemotherapy of a centrally acting narcotic analgesic, usually codeine, and APC (aspirin, phenacetin and caffeine) was routinely prescribed for most patients with mild to moderate pain. The efficacy of this combination can be inferred from its popularity to this day. This long-lived success can readily be explained by the above classification, since patients with pain of all three classes would obtain some measure of relief. However, as progress is made in our understanding of the mechanisms of pain and inflammation and the important role of inflammatory processes in many pain syndromes becomes evident, this classification should lead to more rational and efficacious chemotherapeutic combinations. For example, the combination of an anti-inflammatory steroid with a non-steroid anti-inflammatory agent, each inhibiting inflammation by different mechanisms, may be more beneficial in pain of class 2 aetiology than the usual codeine-APC combination, since codeine is doing little to alleviate the pain of inflammatory aetiology.

Similarly, for the treatment of class 1 pain the combination of codeine and phenacetin may be more efficacious than codeine and aspirin since phenacetin, unlike aspirin, has a central component to its analgesic activity which differs from that of codeine. An important advantage of the prudent use of the above classification would be the elimination of the use of narcotic analgesics for the treatment of pain syndromes of class 2 in which they are of little value. It is now up to the clinical pharmacologist carefully to characterise each pain syndrome pharmacologically in order that the most beneficial chemotherapeutic treatment of each class may be determined.

Acknowledgements. The authors wish to thank Dr. Robert A. Maxwell, Dr. Donald H. Namm, and Dr. Helen L. White for their advice and constructive criticism in the preparation of this manuscript.

References

Baruth, H., Randall, L. O.: Anti-inflammatory activity of the carbazole, C-5720. Fed. Proc. **33**, 557 (1974)

Beaver, W. T.: Mild analgesics: a review of their clinical pharmacology. Amer. J. med. Sci. **251**, 576—599 (1966)

Chernov, H. I., Wilson, D. E., Fowler, F., Plummer, A. J.: Non-specificity of the mouse writhing test. Arch. int. Pharmacodyn. **167**, 171—178 (1967)

Collier, H. O. J., Dinneen, L. C., Johnson, C. A., Schneider, C.: The abdominal constriction response and its suppression by analgesic drugs in the mouse. Brit. J. Pharmacol. **32**, 295—310 (1968)

Collier, H. O. J., Schneider, C.: Nociceptive response to prostaglandins and analgesic actions of aspirin and morphine. Nature (New Biol.) **236**, 141—143 (1972)

Cooper, S. A., Beaver, W. T.: Evaluation of mild analgesics in outpatients. Clin. Pharmacol. Ther. **17**, 231 (1975)

Feldberg, W., Saxena, P. N.: Further studies on prostaglandin E_1 fever in cats. J. Physiol. (Lond.) **219**, 739—746 (1972)

Ferreira, S. H.: Prostaglandins, aspirin-like drugs and analgesia. Nature (New Biol.) **240**, 200—203 (1972)

Gilfoil, T. M., Klavins, K., Grumbach, L.: Effects of acetylsalicylic acid on the edema and hyperesthesia of the experimentally inflamed rat's paw. J. Pharmacol. exp. Ther. **142**, 1—5 (1963)

Jaffe, J. H., Martin, W. R.: Narcotic analgesics and antagonists. In: Goodman, L. S., Gilman, A. (Eds.): The Pharmacological Basis of Therapeutics, pp. 245—283, New York-Toronto-London: MacMillan 1975

Koster, R., Anderson, M., deBeer, E. J.: Acetic acid for analgesic screening. Fed. Proc. **18**, 412 (1959)

Moertel, C. G., Ahmann, D. L., Taylor, W. F., Schwartau, N.: A comparative evaluation of marketed analgesic drugs. New Engl. J. Med. **286**, 813—815 (1972)

Moncada, S., Ferreira, S. H., Vane, J. R.: Inhibition of prostaglandin biosynthesis as the mechanism of analgesia of aspirin-like drugs in the dog knee joint. Europ. J. Pharmacol. **31**, 250—260 (1975)

Randall, L. O.: Non-narcotic analgesics. In: Root, W. S., Hofmann, F. G. (Eds.): Physiological Pharmacology, Vol. I, pp. 313—416. New York-London: Academic Press 1963

Randall, L. O., Selitto, J.: A method for measurement of analgesic activity on inflamed tissue. Arch. int. Pharmacodyn. **111**, 209—219 (1957)

Randall, L. O., Selitto, J., Valdes, J.: Anti-inflammatory effects of xylopropamine. Arch. int. Pharmacodyn. **113**, 233—249 (1957)

Rome, L. H., Lands, W. E. M.: Inhibition of prostaglandin biosynthesis. Fed. Proc. **34**, 790 (1975)

Rowley, D. A., Benditt, E. P.: 5-Hydroxytryptamine and histamine as mediators of the vascular injury produced by agents which damage mast cells in rats. J. exp. Med. **103**, 399—411 (1956)

Siegmund, E., Cadmus, R., Lu, G.: A method for evaluating both non-narcotic and narcotic analgesics. Proc. Soc. exp. Biol. (N. Y.) **95**, 729—731 (1957)

Stone, C. A., Wenger, H. C., Ludden, C. T., Stavorski, H. M., Ross, C. A.: Antiserotonin-antihista-
  minic properties of cyproheptadine. J. Pharmacol. exp. Ther. **131**, 73—84 (1961)
Swingle, K. F.: Evaluation for anti-inflammatory activity. In: Scherrer, R. A., Whitehouse, M.
  (Eds.): Anti-inflammatory Agents: Chemistry and Pharmacology, pp. 33—122. New York:
  Academic Press 1974
Swingle, K. F., Grant, T. J., Kvam, D. C.: Quantal responses in the Randall-Selitto assay. Proc.
  Soc. exp. Biol. (N. Y.) **137**, 536—538 (1971)
Takesue, E. I., Schaeffer, W., Jukniewicz, E.: Modification of the Randall-Selitto analgesic appara-
  tus. J. Pharm. (Lond.) **21**, 788—789 (1969)
Van Arman, C. G., Nuss, G. W., Winter, C. A., Flataker, L.: Proteolytic enzymes as mediators of
  pain. In: Rocha e Silva, M. (Ed.): Pharmacology of pain. New York: Pergammon Press 1966,
  pp. 25—32
Vane, J. R.: Inhibition of prostaglandin synthesis as a mechanism of action for aspirin-like drugs.
  Nature (New Biol.) **231**, 232—235 (1971)
Vinegar, R., Macklin, A. W., Truax, J. R., Selph, J. L.: Pedal edema formation in normal and granu-
  locytopenic rats. In: White Cells in Inflammation. Van Arman, C. G. (Ed.). Springfield-Illi-
  nois: Charles C. Thomas 1974, pp. 111—138
Vinegar, R., Schreiber, W., Hugo, R.: Biphasic development of carrageenan edema in rats. J.
  Pharmacol. exp. Ther. **166**, 96—103 (1969)
Vinegar, R., Truax, J. F., Selph, J. L.: Quantitative comparison of the analgesic and anti-inflammatory activities of aspirin, phenacetin and acetaminophen in rodents. Europ. J. Pharmacol. **37**,
  23—30 (1976 b)
Vinegar, R., Truax, J. F., Selph, J. L.: Quantitative studies of the pathway to acute carrageenan
  inflammation. Fed. Proc. **35**, 2447—2456 (1976 c)
Vinegar, R., Truax, J. F., Selph, J. L., Welch, R. M., White, H. L.: Potentiation of the anti-inflamma-
  tory and analgesic activity of aspirin by caffeine in the rat. Proc. Soc. exp. Biol. (N. Y.) **151**,
  556—560 (1976 a)
Whittle, B. A.: The use of changes in capillary permeability in mice to distinguish between nar-
  cotic and non-narcotic analgesics. Brit. J. Pharmacol. **22**, 246—253 (1964)
Wilhelm, D. L.: Inflammation and healing. In: Anderson, W. A. D. (Ed.): Pathology, pp. 14—67.
  St. Louis: C. V. Mosby 1971
Winter, C. A.: The physiology and pharmacology of pain and its relief. In: DeStevens, G. (Ed.):
  Analgesics, pp. 10—61. New York: Academic Press 1965
Winter, C. A., Flataker, L.: Reaction thresholds to pressure in edematous hindpaws of rats and
  responses to analgesic drugs. J. Pharmacol. exp. Ther. **150**, 165—171 (1965 a)
Winter, C. A., Flataker, L.: Nociceptive thresholds as affected by parenteral administration of
  irritants and of various nociceptive drugs. J. Pharmacol. exp. Ther. **148**, 373—379 (1965 b)
Woodbury, D. M., Fingle, E.: Analgesic-antipyretics, anti-inflammatory agents, and drugs em-
  ployed in the therapy of gout. In: Goodman, L. S., Gilman, A. (Eds.): The Pharmacological
  Basis of Therapeutics, pp. 325—358. New York-Toronto-London: MacMillan 1975

CHAPTER 27

Inhibition of Cell Migration in vivo and Granuloma Formation

M. DI ROSA

A. General Introduction

I. Mechanisms of Cell Migration

Cell migration is a cardinal feature of the inflammatory response. This phenomenon is characterised by emigration of leucocytes from small blood vessels and their accumulation in inflamed or injured tissues. The early morphological event is the movement of leucocytes from the center to the periphery of the bloodstream, followed by the adhesion of the cells to the luminal surface of the vascular endothelium, especially of the postcapillary venules.

Although the mechanism of white cell adhesiveness is not clear, most evidence suggests that essential changes occur in the endothelial cells, and leucocyte sticking is secondary to the endothelial damage brought about by the injurious stimulus (GRANT, 1965). However, electron microscopic studies of inflamed venules have failed to detect any alteration in the endothelial surface (MARCHESI and FLOREY, 1960; FLOREY and GRANT, 1961; WILLIAMSON and GRISHAM, 1961).

These observations led SPECTOR and WILLOUGHBY (1963) to suggest that changes occurring at molecular level may involve the electrochemical forces operative at cell surfaces causing reduction in the energy of repulsion between two cells in close contact. It has also been suggested that both divalent cations and cationic proteins may act as ligands between negatively charged cell surfaces causing cell adhesiveness (BANGHAM, 1964; JANOFF and ZWEIFACH, 1964; THOMPSON et al., 1967).

Leucocyte adhesion to the endothelial surface is followed by the egress of these cells from the blood vessels. Detailed electron microscopic studies have established that leucocytes migrate between the endothelial cells and not through them (MARCHESI and FLOREY, 1960; MARCHESI, 1961; FLOREY and GRANT, 1961; WILLIAMSON and GRISHAM, 1961).

The leucocyte penetrates the endothelium of the vessel by thrusting out and inserting pseudopodia at interendothelial junctions. The white cell, assuming amoeboid movements, forces itself through a narrow gap by radically modifying its shape and reaches the external surface of the endothelium where it is arrested by the basement membrane. The vascular basement membrane, a barrier consisting of fibers and filaments arranged to form an unstructured network (LUFT, 1965), acts as a filter and arrests the leucocytes for a variable period. Finally, the leucocytes enter the surrounding connective tissue, either by moving parallel to the basement membrane until they find a suitable gap for exit (FLOREY and GRANT, 1961), or by secreting extracellularly proteolytic enzymes which break down the basement membrane (COCHRANE and AIKIN, 1966).

In the acute response, the accumulation of leucocytes at the inflammatory site may be explained by three different mechanisms: (1) chemotaxis, (2) increased leakiness of vessels, (3) proliferation of a small population of emigrated cells by mitotic division (WILKINSON, 1974).

This last mechanism may be disregarded, since acute responses are characterised by a large predominance of polymorphonuclear leucocytes which are short-lived (few days of life span) and unable to divide. However, cell division plays an important role in chronic inflammation and will be considered later in this chapter.

The second possibility implies that vasoactive substances which are known to increase vascular permeability should also possess chemotactic activity. Despite the differences in time courses for increased vascular permeability and leucocyte migration in several types of acute inflammation (WILHELM and MASON, 1960; HURLEY and SPECTOR, 1961), the problem has been extensively investigated. None of the vasoactive substances which play a role in the acute response—histamine, 5-hydroxytryptamine (5-HT), bradykinin, slow reacting substance in anaphylaxis (SRS-A), lymph node permeability factor or prostaglandins—is a strong chemotactic factor for leucocytes (WARD et al., 1965, 1966; BOREL, 1970; SORKIN et al., 1970; KAY and AUSTEN, 1971). The only exception seems to be prostaglandin E_1 which attracts neutrophils (KALEY and WEINER, 1971). This observation was recently confirmed by HIGGS et al. (1975) who also demonstrated that rabbit polymorphonuclear leucocytes release prostaglandin E_1 during phagocytosis. The release of a chemotactic factor by phagocytosing leucocytes has been proposed as an important control mechanism for local leucocyte migration which would continue as long as phagocytosis is occurring (HIGGS et al., 1975). However, a possible interaction of these vasoactive substances with other humoral or cellular factors to promote or enhance leucocyte migration cannot be excluded.

A large body of evidence suggests that chemotaxis is the most important mechanism for the accumulation of leucocytes into the inflamed area. Chemotaxis has been defined as "enhanced movement of cells in the presence of chemical substances and especially migration towards and away from such substances" (HERBERT and WILKINSON, 1971). These substances, named cytotaxins (KELLER and SORKIN, 1967a), are hydrosoluble, diffusible peptides and proteins with a molecular weight between 6000 and 300000 (WARD, 1967). Cytotactic activity, however, is also exhibited by low molecular weight non-protein substances such as the aforementioned prostaglandin E_1, hydroxy acids derived from arachidonic acid (TURNER et al., 1975b) and thromboxane B2 (BOOT et al., 1976). The evidence for a chemotactic activity of cAMP is rather confusing for the reported ability of this nucleotide to attract leucocytes (LEAHY et al., 1970; BECKER, 1971) has not been confirmed (KALEY and WEINER, 1971; WISSLER et al., 1972); furthermore, it was found to inhibit chemotactic migration of neutrophils (TSE et al., 1972). The role of these low molecular weight substances in chemotaxis is worth consideration, particularly in the light of evidence which suggests that highly chemotactic substances, casein (TURNER et al., 1975a) and complement fraction C5a (WISSLER et al., 1974) owe their activity to low molecular weight impurities. Cytotaxins have been isolated from inflammatory exudates as well as from the circulating blood (WARD et al., 1966; KELLER and SORKIN, 1968a). The chemotactic activity shown in vivo by several cytotaxins correlates with the activity they exhibit when tested in vitro (HURLEY, 1964; KELLER and SORKIN, 1968b).

The intimate mechanism by which cytotaxins stimulate the directional movement of leucocytes is not entirely understood. It is accepted that it implies a molecular recognition mechanism of the cytotaxin by the responding cell, probably by means of specific receptors (KELLER and SORKIN, 1967b). There is indirect evidence that two types of esterase are involved, which probably control the potassium pump (BEKER and WARD, 1967; WARD and BEKER, 1967).

II. The Sequence of Cell Migration

The population of white cells which emigrate into the damaged tissue is mainly composed of neutrophilic polymorphonuclear granulocytes (polymorphs, PMNs) and mononucleocytes (monocytes and lymphocytes). Other cells (plasma cells, fibroblasts, basophilic granulocytes) are poorly represented in the cellular infiltrate although eosinophilic granulocytes are prominent in allergic reactions or inflammation involving parasites.

All types of inflammation commence with an emigration of polymorphs; later, mononuclear cells become dominant in inflammatory exudates. The mechanism of the polymorphs' replacement by mononuclear cells has several interpretations (SPECTOR and WILLOUGHBY, 1963; SPECTOR, 1969). The most usual view has been that mononuclear emigration occurs after egress of polymorphs from injured vessels has virtually ceased. An alternative hypothesis suggests a concurrent emigration of both polymorphs and mononuclears, the polymorphs then moving away unimpaired or suffering destruction leaving mononuclear cells to predominate (PAZ and SPECTOR, 1962).

SPECTOR (1969) made a critical appraisal of both these hypotheses. He considered the possible existence of separate mechanisms controlling the escape of each type of cell (HURLEY et al., 1966), the suggestion that polymorphs had to be present in the inflamed area as a prerequisite for mononuclear migration (PAGE and GOOD, 1958), the quantitative measurement of both polymorphs' and mononuclear cells' migration into granulomata of various ages from 2 days to 3 months (SPECTOR et al., 1967) and the variability of the relative proportion of polymorphs and mononuclear cells emigrating at the inflammatory sites according to the animal strain (SULTZER, 1968), and in conclusion, he strongly supported the view that "polymorphs and mononuclears compete for the chance to emigrate".

III. Fate of Emigrated Cells

1. Polymorphs

Polymorphonuclear granulocytes emigrate into the inflamed area within a few hours of the application of the injurious stimulus.

Polymorphs have a variety of activities which are intimately connected with the pathogenesis of inflammatory reactions. They are highly phagocytic, contain efficient bactericidal mechanisms and possess a rich pattern of potential generators of inflammation mediators (hydrolytic enzymes), usually confined within intracytoplasmatic granules (lysosomes). These granules discharge their contents outside the cell by two different release processes (HENSON, 1974): active secretion (non-cytotoxic release) or following cell destruction (cytotoxic release).

These two processes are not mutually exclusive; indeed, they occur concomitantly, helping to generate and amplify the local inflammatory response.

Cytotoxic release is dominant when a large number of polymorphs are attracted into the damaged tissue, e.g. by bacterial cytotoxins, with massive cell destruction and pus or abscess formation. The polymorph is in fact an "end cell", unable to transform into other cell types, and is easily destroyed. This cell is, however, highly motile and thus has a chance to escape from the inflamed site into the bloodstream. Although the number of infiltrating polymorphs varies according to the nature and intensity of the stimulus, the number of these cells at the inflamed site in most types of inflammation progressively declines after 24 h either because of destruction or escape; the result is an increasing predominance of mononuclear cells.

2. Mononuclear Cells

Mononuclear cells infiltrating the inflamed area are mainly represented by monocytes and lymphocytes. Monocytes enter the inflamed tissues concurrently with polymorphs and by the same route. The slowness of their movement allows polymorphs to predominate in the early stages, although some cell-specific chemotactic mechanisms may possibly be implicated in controlling polymorph/monocyte emigration (WILKINSON, 1974).

The monocyte belongs to the mononuclear phagocyte system (VAN FURTH et al., 1972). After egress from the circulation to enter the inflamed area, the monocyte transforms into a macrophage, the basic unit of chronic inflammation. The macrophage is characterised by enlarged cytoplasm, numerous lysosomes and abundant endoplasmic reticulum. The cell is highly phagocytic with the cytoplasm containing prominent phagocytic vacuoles into which lysosomes discharge their enzymes. The nature of the inflammatory agent virtually controls the fate of macrophages in inflamed areas. If it is non-toxic and easily digestible, the cell degrades the ingested material and then tends to migrate elsewhere, possibly after only one division. Phagocytosis of toxic material causes the cell to die. If the macrophage ingests non-toxic but indigestible material, it may become a resting cell unable to divide but capable of survival for months or possibly years (SPECTOR and RYAN, 1969).

Lymphocytes probably migrate from the bloodstream and enter the inflamed areas by passing through the cytoplasm of the endothelial cells of postcapillary venules, whereas the egress of polymorphs and monocytes occurs between the endothelial cells (WILKINSON, 1974).

This process tends to exclude a chemotactic emigration; indeed, a chemotactic factor for lymphocytes has never been clearly demonstrated, although some investigations suggest that lymphocytes may actually be attracted by some chemotactic factors produced by sensitized lymphocytes (WARD et al., 1971).

Furthermore, it has been recently reported that large immunoblast-like lymphocytes from mouse and man migrate towards chemical attractants in Boyden chambers and that this migration is chemotactic (WILKINSON et al., 1976).

Lymphocyte infiltration is characteristic of inflammatory reactions involving cellular immunity. Although in inflammatory exudates lymphocytes may undergo morphological alterations (enlargement), the transformation of these cells into macrophages is generally excluded; lymphocyte and macrophage cell lines are clearly distinguished as separate (SPECTOR, 1969). However, at inflammatory sites a multiple, if ill-understood, interaction between lymphocytes and macrophages certainly occurs.

As a possible mechanism of this interaction, it has been proposed that the secretion of lymphokines by sensitized lymphocytes activates macrophages, a process which includes the release of prostaglandin E_1, which in turn is able to inhibit further lymphokines secretion (MORLEY, 1974).

This postulated homeostatic mechanism also provides the basis for a stimulating hypothesis on the pathogenesis of rheumatoid arthritis (RA) which could be due to a defective lymphocyte reactivity towards prostaglandin E_1(MORLEY, 1974).

IV. Granuloma Formation and Evolution

The granulomatous inflammatory exudate (granuloma) is the typical feature of established (chronic) inflammatory reactions. The granuloma is histologically characterised by the local accumulation of a variety of mononuclear cell types, commonly known as macrophages, histiocytes, epithelioid cells, giant cells, lymphocytes and fibroblasts (SPECTOR, 1969). Despite the large number of important diseases of animals and man characterised by granulomatous lesion (e.g. tuberculosis, leprosy), the pathogenesis of the granulomatous response is still poorly understood.

The crucial problem in chronic granulomatous inflammation concerns the mechanism sustaining the persistence, for months or even years, of mononuclear cell infiltration. The chronic mononuclear infiltrate may be considered as dependent on three different mechanisms: (1) longevity of exudate cells, (2) continual fresh recruitment from the circulation and (3) mitotic division of emigrated cells.

These three possibilities, which are not mutually exclusive, have been widely explored. Conflicting conclusions largely prevailed, mainly because of the basic variety of experimental approaches and the paucity of quantitation of the observed phenomena. SPECTOR and his associates were the first to attempt to quantitate the relevance of each mechanism in sustaining granulomatous lesions of different age induced by different stimuli (SPECTOR, 1969). They used a variety of cell labels, such as colloidal carbon, which is taken up by the cytoplasm of phagocytic cells, and/or tritiated thymidine, which is incorporated into the DNA of the nuclei of cells about to divide (SPECTOR et al., 1965; SPECTOR and COOTE, 1965; SPECTOR and LYKKE, 1966). They identified two main types of granuloma: high turnover granuloma and low turnover granuloma (SPECTOR, 1969). The granuloma induced by *Bordetella pertussis* vaccine is representative of the high turnover reaction with the fresh recruitment from the circulation of about 2.10^5 cells each day (SPECTOR et al., 1967). In low turnover lesions (carrageenin granuloma), the number of new emigrated cells was 10–20 times less (RYAN and SPECTOR, 1969).

Following whole body irradiation, which, by destroying bone marrow, deprives animals of the precursors of infiltrating cells, a rapid decline of cell number was observed in high turnover granulomata, while in low turnover granulomata cell counts were virtually unaffected (RYAN and SPECTOR, 1970). The rate of cell division is also different in the two types of granuloma. Thus, in high turnover granulomata, the number of cells undergoing mitotic activity is about 10 times higher than in low turnover granulomata (SPECTOR and RYAN, 1969).

The rates of both cell entrance and proliferation seem to depend on the nature of the injurious agent which is distributed into a quite different proportion of cells according to the type of granuloma. Thus, killed bacteria *(B. pertussis)* are detectable in a small percentage of macrophages (SPECTOR et al., 1968), while in carrageenin granuloma virtually all macrophages (about 80%) contain the irritant (MONIS et al., 1968). The unequal distribution of the injurious agent represents a further element of discrimination between the two types of granuloma and may also be correlated with the observed high or low turnover rate because of the relative infrequency of DNA synthesis in the cells that had ingested particles (SPECTOR et al., 1968).

Despite these sharp differences, high and low turnover granulomata are not considered to be two clear-cut types of lesion. Indeed, they are regarded as two extremes of the same chronic inflammatory process, with a large number of intermediate situations according to the maturity of the lesion and the intensity of the injurious stimulus (SPECTOR, 1969). Consistent with this view are a number of experiments demonstrating a gradual transformation of high turnover granulomata to low turnover responses (SPECTOR and HEESOM, 1969). This gradual transformation could be dependent on a natural selection of macrophages reacting to phagocytosed foreign indigestible material on the basis of the postulated existence of two populations of macrophages. One population, in an attempt to degrade the indigestible irritant, releases lysosomal enzymes thus stimulating continued emigration and proliferation of mononuclear cells (high turnover rate). The other population of macrophages tends to neutralize the indigestible irritant by long term sequestration within the cytoplasm (low turnover rate).

The first population of cells, suffers a high death rate because of the activation of digestive enzymes and is gradually replaced (natural selection) by long-lived macrophages which survive because of the paucity of their cytoplasmic enzymes. According to this hypothesis, "high turnover granuloma is merely a stage on the road to a low turnover reaction" (SPECTOR, 1969).

B. Models for Leucocyte Emigration in vivo

I. Generalities

The quantitative assessment of leucocyte emigration into inflamed areas has not received due attention, taking into account the dominant role played by white cell infiltration in the inflammatory process. This concept is supported by the relatively small number of experimental models specifically designed to evaluate leucocyte emigration, as compared with the plethora of tests developed to assess other aspects of the inflammatory reaction, such as increased vascular permeability or oedema formation. There has also been inadequate utilisation of available models for studying the effect of anti-inflammatory drugs on leucocyte emigration in vivo. This situation prevails, in our opinion, for two main reasons. Firstly, the study of leucocyte migration requires technical procedures more elaborate and usually less reproducible than those commonly employed to assess anti-inflammatory drugs. Secondly, the study of leucocyte migration is a subject that lies on the borderline between pathology, immunology and pharmacology.

Each investigator seems influenced by the specific background of his own discipline. Pathologists are generally interested in the static morphology of the cells, paying little attention to the quantitative aspects of cell migration. Pharmacologists are preferentially attracted by chemical mediators without considering that increased vascular permeability is only a transient phase of the inflammatory process. Finally, immunologists have for a long while virtually neglected immune phenomena which occur in non-immune inflammation. Thus, few people have worked on leucocyte migration and the effects on it of anti-inflammatory drugs. Because of this, attention has been preferentially given to methods which have actually been used to evaluate the effect of anti-inflammatory drugs on leucocyte emigration.

II. Histological Method

This method can be used in every type of inflammation at any site. However, the irritant is usually injected intradermally or subcutaneously; then, at different intervals, the inflamed tissue is excised and processed for histological section, or alternatively a "spread" can be made on slides (SPECTOR and WILLOUGHBY, 1964). However, the subsequent microscopic examination of these specimens takes a long time, is very tedious and allows only a semiquantitative evaluation of leucocyte emigration (KOLOUCH, 1939; PAGE et al., 1962; HURD and ZIFF, 1968; DI ROSA and WILLOUGHBY, 1971; DI ROSA et al., 1971).

III. Cell Collection From Cavities

1. Natural Cavities

a) Peritoneal Cavity

Since the classic experiments by METCHNIKOFF (1892), the peritoneal cavity has been a favourite site for the study of inflammatory reactions. Leucocytes emigrate into the peritoneal cavity after the intraperitoneal injection of an irritant. At different intervals, usually from 3 to 24–48 h, cells can be collected by peritoneal lavage and total and differential counts determined. Different animal species (rat, guinea pig, mice) and several irritants have been used, such as mineral oil (GEORGE and VAUGHAN, 1962), bacterial endotoxins, glycogen, compound 48/80 (FRUHMAN, 1962), formalin (WILHELMI, 1965), casein (HYMES et al., 1967) and new born calf serum (THOMPSON and VAN FURTH, 1970). The mouse peritoneal cavity has been extensively used for quantitative studies on the kinetics of mononuclear phagocytes during acute inflammation (VAN FURTH et al., 1973). Despite the simplicity of the technique, the peritoneal cavity has been poorly employed to assess the effect of anti-inflammatory drugs on cellular exudation.

b) Pleural Cavity

The basic procedure of this method is to induce an acute inflammatory exudate in the rat through intrapleural injection of an irritant. At the required time after the injection, the animal is killed, the chest wall opened and the exudate removed, possibly by washing the cavity with a known volume of fluid (saline, Hank's solution, etc.) to ensure a complete recovery of the exudate. Volume, protein content, total and differential leucocyte counts and possibly other evaluations may be carried out on the collected exudate.

A large variety of substance has been used to induce pleurisy: turpentine (SPECTOR, 1956; SPECTOR and WILLOUGHBY, 1957, 1959; HURLEY and SPECTOR, 1965), Evans blue (HOLTKAMP et al., 1958; WEISBACH et al., 1963; SANCILIO and RODRIGUEZ, 1966), arabic gum (GALBER and FOSDICK, 1965), a mixture of carrageenin and Evans blue (SANCILIO, 1968, 1969), glycogen, dextran, homologous serum, histamine, saline (HURLEY et al., 1966; DI ROSA et al., 1972; DI ROSA, 1974), kaolin (VINEGAR et al., 1973), carrageenin (DI ROSA, 1974; AMMENDOLA et al., 1975), calcium pyrophosphate (WILLOUGHBY et al., 1975). Despite the extensive use of this model, the evaluation of the inflammatory reaction is usually confined to the measurement of exudate volume.

However, some investigators have made quantitative measurements of cell migration (HURLEY et al., 1966; DI ROSA et al., 1972; VINEGAR et al., 1972, 1973; DI ROSA, 1974; AMMENDOLA et al., 1975). The use of dextran to induce pleurisy for evaluation of anti-inflammatory drugs on leucocyte emigration has been recommended because its mild irritating properties allow an easy differentiation of emigrated cells; it also induces approximately equal migration of polymorphs and mononuclears, although at different times (DI ROSA et al., 1972; DI ROSA, 1974).

c) Joints

α) Dog Knee Joint

A method to quantify the inflammatory reaction induced by the injection of microcrystalline sodium urate into canine knee joint was described by McCARTY et al. (1966). One hind leg of the anaesthetized dog is immobilised with the femur and tibia mantained at a 90° angle. The knee joint is catheterized and injected with 15 mg of monosodium urate crystals suspended in pyrogen-free physiological salt solution. At different times after the intra-articular injection, small aliquots of exudate are removed for determination of leucocyte counts (PHELPS and McCARTY, 1966).

β) Rabbit Knee Joint

The rabbit knee joint has been used to elicit an articular arthritis by DUMONDE and GLYNN (1962). Rabbits were sensitized with a suspension of heterologous fibrin in Freund's complete adjuvant and subsequently challenged with an intra-articular injection of fibrin. The method was later modified by replacing fibrin with ovalbumin, an antigen obtainable in a pure and soluble form (CONSDEN et al., 1971). Technical difficulties in recovering suitable samples of synovial fluid from the inflamed joint have discouraged the routine use of this method for the determination of leucocyte migration. However, leucocyte counts in the washouts of the rabbit knee joints have been recently reported (BLACKAM et al., 1974).

γ) Chicken Intertarsal Joint

The arthritis elicited by the injection of a suspension of urate crystals into the intertarsal joint of pigeons was first proposed as a model of acute inflammation (BRUNE et al., 1974a, 1974b). Subsequentely, the model has been used for chickens in order to obtain sufficient amounts of joint fluid for total and differential leucocyte counts as well as for biochemical investigations (BRUNE and GLATT, 1974a, 1974b). The cellular emigration, which has been evaluated for up to 8 h, is largely represented by polymorphonucleocytes.

2. Artificial Cavities

a) "Skin Window"

The "skin window" technique, first described by REBUCK and his co-workers (REBUCK et al., 1951; REBUCK and MELLINGER, 1953; REBUCK and YATES, 1954; REBUCK and CROWLEY, 1955), has become very popular because it represents a simple test to study leucocyte migration in human subjects as well as animals. An approximately 10–20 mm^2 area of skin is scraped with a blade and the resulting lesion is covered by a sterile circular cover slip. The cover slip, protected by a piece of cardboard, is fixed to the skin by tape. Scraping the skin serves as an inflammatory stimulus for leucocytes which migrate to the under surface of the cover slip. Cover slips are removed and replaced at different intervals, usually over 1 to 12 h. The cover slips are air dried and stained for microscopic qualitative and quantitative cell counts. The skin window technique is used mainly for the qualitative study of inflammatory exudates in man because total counts of emigrated leucocytes are difficult or even impossible, and usually only semiquantitative determinations are attainable.

b) "Skin Chamber"

To achieve a better quantification of total cell counts at any one stage of inflammation, several modifications of the original skin window technique have been proposed (PERILLIE and FINCH, 1964; GOWLAND, 1964; RIDDLE and BARNHART, 1965; SOUTHAM and LEVIN, 1966; BARNHART, 1968; SENN et al., 1969; HOLLAND et al., 1971).

All these methods are based on the use of plastic chambers instead of the cover slip to collect the inflammatory exudates. These plastic chambers (skin chambers), although differing in minor details in their shape, volume and technical arrangements, have all been designed to allow periodical drainage of the exudate without being removed from the skin lesion. The withdrawn fluid is used to obtain total leucocyte counts and to prepare smears for microscopic examination. In some experiments, chambers are filled with serum or with fluids in order to study their effect on leucocyte mobilisation.

All the methods of cell collection from both natural or artificial cavities have the great advantage of being easy technical procedures coupled with reproducible quantitative and qualitative measurements of leucocyte emigration. This situation has favoured the use of these experimental models which, however, are quite different from known pathological lesions. Leucocytes emigrating into a cavity come in contact mainly, if not only, with plasma substrates, while in the large majority of pathological lesions emigrated cells are surrounded by connective tissue. The interaction between leucocytes and connective tissue substrates, possibly altered by the injurious stimulus, represents an important modulating factor of the inflammatory process, e.g. through the generation of chemotactic factors or antigenic determinants (WILLOUGHBY and DI ROSA, 1971). This is at least one aspect of the inflammatory response which is missed when these methods are used. Nevertheless, the procedures are useful tools in the study of leucocyte migration in vivo, especially when the method is used critically.

IV. Cell Collection From Early Granulomata

The degree of cellular influx into a granuloma has been used as an assay method for leucocyte emigration. The assay should be limited to the early stages of the inflammatory reaction in order to quantitate the arrival of new cells. In the later stages, mitosis and/or longevity of the emigrated cells may interfere with the interpretation of the results. The cellular exudation into a carboxymethylcellulose pouch occurring in rats at $7^{1}/_{2}$ h has been assessed by ISHIKAWA et al. (1969). Leucocyte counts measured 5 days after inducing a croton oil granuloma pouch have also been reported (VARSA-HANDLER et al., 1967).

The implantation of a small round pellet of non-resorbable plastic sponge under the skin of the rat has been used as a technique to assess cellular emigration (SAXENA, 1960). At different intervals, not exceeding 24 h after the implant, the sponge is removed and the cells are recovered by centrifuging the sponge in a small test tube containing a balanced salt solution. An alternative procedure for recovering the cells has been recently proposed by FORD-HUTCHINSON et al. (1975) who squeezed the sponge using a plastic syringe containing saline.

A quantitative procedure for the study of cells in experimentally induced granulomata in mice has been proposed by PAUL et al. (1972). Granuloma formation was induced by subcutaneous injection of either antigenic (tetanus toxoid) or non-antigenic substances (aluminium phosphate). After intervals ranging from 1 to 28 days, granulomata were dissected and subjected to dispersion and digestion by incubation with collagenase and pronase. A complete dispersion of the cells was obtained. Samples of the incubation fluid were used for total and differential cell counts.

Methods described in this section have not been specifically designed to assay leucocyte emigration. The risk of interference due to cell proliferation and/or cell longevity has been already pointed out. However, they seem potentially useful to study cell kinetics also in the later stages of the granulomatous reaction. The problem is how to discern newly arrived cells from those already present or derived from recent divisions at the site of the lesion. Possibly, a combination of these methods with the cell labelling techniques (see next paragraph) would be an effective method to achieve this.

V. Cell Labelling

The basic principle of this method is to label leucocytes with a radioactive marker and to determine their accumulation at the inflamed area by radioactivity measurements. Radioactive diisopropylfluorophosphate has been proposed as a specific label for human granulocytes (ATHENS et al., 1959; MAUER et al., 1960). Although this technique was potentially suitable for studies on inflammation, it has been mainly used for investigations of granulocyte kinetics (ATHENS et al., 1961a, 1961b; BISHOP et al., 1968).

A method specifically designed for studying leucocyte chemotaxis in vivo has been recently described by PERPER et al. (1974a). Rat peritoneal cell suspensions, collected 1 or 3 days following intraperitoneal injection of sodium caseinate, are labelled in vitro with ^{51}Cr and then injected intravenously into isologous recipients in which an inflammatory reaction is induced. In recipient rats, labelled circulating leucocytes from 1 day peritoneal exudates were all identified as neutrophils, whereas after injecting cells from 3 day exudates, only labelled mononuclears were circulating.

The accumulation of both cell types into the hind paw following subplantar injection of carrageenin was determined by direct scintillation counting following amputation of the paw. The radioactivity in the controlateral paw, not injected with carrageenin, was used as a measure of non-inflammatory-related circulating radioactivity. The kinetics of cell emigration was cell type specific since a time-related accumulation of neutrophils (max. 1–5 h) and mononuclears (max. 5–18 h) was observed in accordance with histologic evaluation. In contrast, no time-related accumulation of either labelled erythrocytes or lymph node lymphocytes was seen. This observation excludes the possibility that radioactivity in the inflamed area was due to non-specific particle sequestration.

This method, although involving quite sophisticated procedures and calculations, allows an actual quantitative measurement of leucocyte migration and seems useful for studies on chemotaxis in vivo.

C. Models for Granuloma Formation in vivo

I. Cotton-Pellet Granuloma

This rather simple test in rats was introduced by MEIER et al. (1950) who observed that the formation of granuloma tissue following the subcutaneous implantation of a cotton-wool-pellet was inhibited by cortisone. In the original procedure, pellets weighing 40 mg prepared from cotton dental rolls were implanted along the flanks of the rat. Seven days later granuloma tissue, represented by a compact mass, was easily excised and the wet and dry weight determined. The net dry weight, i.e. after subtracting the weight of the cotton-pellet, was used as an index of granuloma tissue formation.

The cotton-pellet granuloma method has been widely employed, although several modifications have been proposed in order to improve the precision of the assay. An important source of variability arises from the initial size, i.e. the weight and particularly the surface of the cotton-pellet (ROBINSON and ROBSON, 1964; BENZI and FRIGO, 1964). Granuloma tissue growth has been reported to be enhanced by adding killed bacteria (GANLEY et al., 1958), turpentine (CHRISTIAN and WILLIAMSON, 1958) or carrageenin (BUSH and ALEXANDER, 1960) to the pellet prior to implantation. Septic inflammation, which may alter the granulomatous reaction, can be prevented by using sterilized pellets or by adding antibiotics to them (WINTER and PORTER, 1957).

The initial phase of the inflammatory reaction to subcutaneous implantation of cotton-pellets in rats is characterised by increased permeability of the vessels in the connective tissue surrounding the implant, with the pellet undergoing a rapid saturation ('soaking') by the fluid escaping from the vessels (MEYER et al., 1953). The presence in the pellet of pontamine sky blue dye injected intravenously can be demonstrated within the first 20 min after implantation (PENN and ASHFORD, 1963). Early permeability changes in the implant region are responsible for a transient transudative phase during the first three, which is followed by an exudative phase occurring between 3 and 72 h (SHWINGLE and SHIDEMAN, 1972). The fluid absorbed by the pellet greatly influences the wet weight of the granuloma, so that reproducible assessments are only achieved by determining the dry weight, which correlates well with the amount of granulomatous tissue formed.

The growth of the granulomatous tissue depends on the proliferation of fibroblasts and the new connective tissue synthesis, this latter occurring approximately 3–4 days after the implantation of the cotton-pellet (SWINGLE and SHIDEMAN, 1972). The duration of the implantation influences the granuloma formation, which is a time-related reaction. A continuous increase in the granuloma dry weight has been observed for up to 3 months (DI PASQUALE and MELI, 1965). However, the greatest rate of increase occurs during the first few weeks; thus, the majority of assessments have been confined to 7–14 days granulomata.

The inhibition exhibited by both steroid and non-steroid anti-inflammatory drugs on cotton-pellet granuloma formation is dose-related, the inhibition being characterised as a flat slope of the log dose-response curve (WINDER et al., 1962; WINTER, 1966). Drugs to be tested should always be administered by the oral route in order to avoid local irritation which may produce non-specific granuloma inhibition (CYGIELMAN and ROBSON, 1963). Food intake restriction or impairment in body growth by administered drugs may also produce false positives in the assay. These artifacts may be eliminated by expressing the dry weight of the granuloma in relation to the body weight (DI PASQUALE and MELI, 1965).

II. Granuloma Pouch

The granuloma pouch technique was introduced by SELYE (1953) and modified by ROBERT and NEZAMIS (1957). The basic procedure consists of making a pouch in the back of the rat by injecting sterile air (25 ml). Subsequently, dilute croton oil is introduced into the pouch to induce granulomatous tissue formation. One or 2 days later the pouch is deflated to stimulate exudate formation. Occasionally, the pouch is compressed manually in order to prevent the formation of adhesions. The response is evaluated 4–14 days later on the basis of the volume of the fluid collected from the pouch and the weight or thickness of the pouch wall.

Besides croton oil, several other irritants have been proposed, such as carrageenin (HIGHTON, 1963; BENITZ and HALL, 1963; GOLDSTEIN and SCHNALL, 1963; BORIS and STEVENSON, 1965; FUKUHARA and TSURUFUJI, 1969a, 1969b), mycobacterial adjuvant (BOBALIK and BASTIAN, 1967), D-α-tocopherol (GLENN et al., 1963), turpentine (TRNAVSKÝ et al., 1962; INNERFIELD et al., 1966; DELAUNAY and BAZIN, 1965).

Although seriously criticised by WHITEHOUSE (1965) as an effective assay method for granulomatous reaction, the granuloma pouch has been frequently used for the assay of steroid anti-inflammatory drugs because these drugs effectively inhibit both exudative and proliferative components of the response. Non-steroid anti-inflammatory drugs usually exhibit only a weak effect on the granuloma pouch.

III. Carrageenin Granuloma

Carrageenin, a sulphated polysaccharide extracted from the alga *Chondrus Chrispus* (DI ROSA, 1972), injected subcutaneously in the guinea pig induces the development of a granulomatous tissue containing large amounts of collagen (ROBERTSON and SCHWARTZ, 1953) which is initially accumulated at microsomal level (LOWTHER et al., 1961). The granuloma tissue formation is maximal at about 1 week and is completely resorbed at 46 weeks (JACKSON, 1957; SLACK, 1957).

The cellular evolution of carrageenin granuloma in the guinea pig has been described by WILLIAMS (1957). In the rat, the lesion is characterised by an intense histiocyte proliferation and macrophage differentiation providing a useful tool for the study of structure and function of macrophages (BENITZ and HALL, 1959; MONIS et al., 1968) in a typical low turnover granuloma (SPECTOR, 1969).

Carrageenin granuloma is not easily dissectable; thus technical difficulties discouraged an extensive use of this model to assess anti-inflammatory drugs. However, carrageenin granuloma has been widely employed to elucidate the role of ascorbic acid (ROBERTSON and HINDS, 1956; SLACK, 1958; ROBERTSON et al., 1959), as well as of hormonal factors (ROBERTSON and SANBORN, 1958; FISHER and PAAR, 1960) in collagen metabolism. Carrageenin granuloma is the favourite model for studies on biochemical aspects of connective tissue formation and the effects on it of anti-inflammatory drugs (TRNAVSKÝ, 1974).

IV. Plastic Ring Granuloma

A method for quantitative evaluation of granulomatous tissue formation has been proposed by RUDAS (1960). A circle of skin is removed from the back of the rat and a plastic (polyvinylchloride) ring is incorporated into the wound. By this procedure contractions of the wound edges are inhibited and the epithelization of the wound is prevented. The plastic ring also induces regular growth of the granulation tissue which covers the wound. After 7 days the granulation tissue is removed and weighed. Both steroid and non-steroid anti-inflammatory drugs have been reported to be effective in inhibiting the granulomatous response. The method is also recommended to test drugs which influence wound healing.

V. Filter Paper Granuloma

This method, described by D'ARCY and HOWARD (1967) is based on the observation that the presence of a filter paper disc on the chorio-allontoic membrane of an 8 day chick embryo, when incubated at 37° C for 4 days, produces an inflammatory reaction in the membrane. The granulation tissue, which contains fibroblasts and inflammatory cells, was found to be very constant in weight. Drugs, solubilised or suspended, were dropped onto the surface of each disc immediately prior to implantation. The inflammatory response was inhibited by several steroid or non-steroid anti-inflammatory drugs. The inhibition was graded according to the amount of drug used. By observing changes in chick embryos, this method also provides additional information on the toxic or other side-effects of the drug on an early stage of development of an animal.

D. Inhibition of Cell Migration in vivo

I. Steroids

1. Neutrophils

The number of neutrophils circulating in the blood is usually increased by steroid administration in the rat (FRUHMAN, 1962), rabbit (GERMUTH et al., 1951), mouse (THOMPSON and VAN FURTH, 1970) and man (BOGGS et al., 1964). Despite the larger number of circulating neutrophils, the majority of reports have shown a reduced accumulation of these cells in the inflamed areas.

Cellular exudation into the peritoneal cavity of mice injected with living *E. coli* or with bacterial extracts was inhibited by large doses (100–300 mg/kg) of hydrocortisone (MEIER and ECKLIN, 1960). However, in rats with experimental peritonitis only a slight decrease in cell migration was observed following prednisolone administration (WILHELMI, 1965), while treatment with cortisone failed to prevent polymorph migration (HORVÁTH et al., 1955).

These data are at variance with a recent report demonstrating a suppressive effect of betamethasone on neutrophil mobilisation into the peritoneal cavity of rats injected with *E. coli* endotoxin (WATNICK et al., 1974). A marked reduction of cellular migration after implantation of a non-resorbable plastic sponge in rats was observed with moderate doses (10 mg/kg) of hydrocortisone (SAXENA, 1960).

The role of adrenal glands in leucocyte migration, as well as the doses at which steroids are effective, has been examined by FRUHMAN (1962). He found that adrenalectomized rats were still able to mobilise large amounts of neutrophils into the peritoneal fluid in response to the local injection of bacterial polysaccharide. Treatment of intact animals with hydrocortisone by subcutaneous injection inhibited neutrophil mobilisation only when a massive dose (100 mg/kg) was used. In contrast, the drug was effective at smaller doses when locally administered. The great difference in dose requirements between local and general administration was interpreted as a direct effect by steroids, probably upon small blood vessels. This concept had been stressed by GERMUTH (1956) who also regarded the inhibition of leucocyte migration by steroids as a result of the suppressive effect of these drugs on the vascular response.

The inhibitory effect of steroids when locally applied was shown in experiments with the carboxymethylcellulose pouch method. Several steroids (hydrocortisone, prednisolone, betamethasone, fluoroformylone, triamcinolone, fluocinolone) have been tested by suspending them directly in the irritant solution (ISHIKAWA et al., 1969). The leucocyte emigration into the pouch fluid was markedly reduced by these steroids according to the dose applied and the relative anti-inflammatory potency as assayed with other methods such as granuloma test, thymus involution and liver glycogen deposition (LERNER et al., 1964). No significant changes in vascular permeability were observed for the pouch fluid volume and protein content; these were unaffected by steroids even at dose levels at which 70–80% of leucocyte migration was inhibited. Betamethasone (0.2 mg/kg i.p.) was found to decrease by more than 50% of the number of neutrophils which are mobilised in the pleural cavity of rats injected with kaolin (VINEGAR et al., 1972). These observations, suggesting a rather specific effect of steroids on leucocyte migration, are further supported by some experiments with ^{51}Cr labelled neutrophils (PERPER et al., 1974b). In rats treated orally with 1 mg/kg of paramethasone there was a substantial inhibition (61%) of neutrophil accumulation in the carrageenin inflamed paw.

It is interesting that ^{51}Cr labelled leucocytes previously incubated with 5×10^{-4} hydrocortisone when transferred to untreated recipients failed to accumulate at the inflammatory site.

Experiments carried out in human subjects with the skin window technique showed that treatment with hydrocortisone (200 mg) was associated with a striking reduction in the number of cells in the exudate (BOGGS et al., 1964). The qualitative character of the exudate was not modified by steroids, for differential leucocyte counts were similar before and after the treatment. Prednisolone and dexamethasone have been recently assayed in normal subjects with the skin chamber technique (PETERS et al., 1972). The normal mobilisation of granulocytes was slightly decreased by prednisolone, while a significant increase was observed following dexamethasone administration. A qualitative difference between the two steroids is suggested on the basis of their respective ability to increase the absolute granulocyte blood counts, much more pronounced for dexamethasone, and to decrease the mobility of these cells, which was exhibited only by prednisolone.

2. Mononuclear Cells

Anti-inflammatory steroids decrease the number of circulating lymphocytes and monocytes (HILLS et al., 1948; GERMUTH et al., 1951; QUITTNER et al., 1951; BOGGS et al., 1964; THOMPSON and VAN FURTH, 1970). Systemically administered or topically applied steroids decrease the number of lymphocytes in inflamed areas (CUMMINGS et al., 1952; REBUCK and MELLINGER, 1953). A similar decrease in the number of migrating mononuclear phagocytes represents a typical effect of anti-inflammatory steroids (DOUGHERTY and SCHNEEBELI, 1950; MICHAEL and WHORTON, 1951; CUMMINGS et al., 1952; CRADDOCK et al., 1967; THOMPSON and VAN FURTH, 1973; WATNICK et al., 1974). The reaction to old tuberculin in the skin of sensitized rats was depressed by cortisone (10 mg/kg), which was more effective in reducing the mononuclear component while polymorphs were less affected (GELL and HINDE, 1951). Cortisone seems more effective in preventing mononuclear cell infiltration than in inhibiting proliferation of indigenous histiocytes. Experiments with ^{51}Cr labelled monocytes have shown a marked inhibition in the ability of these cells to accumulate into the carrageenin-inflamed paw of rats treated with 1 mg/kg paramethasone (PERPER et al., 1974b).

Early experiments with the skin window technique in humans revealed that the inhibition exhibited by steroids on leucocyte migration was more pronounced on monocytes than on polymorphs which were only slightly affected (REBUCK et al., 1951; REBUCK and MELLINGER, 1953).

With the same technique, BOGGS et al. (1964) found with hydrocortisone a fourfold reduction in the leucocyte number in the exudate but were unable to detect any difference in the sensitivity of neutrophils and mononuclear cells, for the differential cell counts remained unchanged.

The mechanism underlying the reduced influx of monocytes at the inflammatory site following steroid administration has been extensively investigated in mice in relation to the kinetics of these cells and their precursor in bone marrow (THOMPSON and VAN FURTH, 1970, 1973). The prolonged monocytopenia induced by hydrocortisone is considered to be a consequence of reduced release of newly formed monocytes from the bone marrow, resulting in a prolonged sojourn of these cells in this compartment. During an inflammatory response, the reduced number of monocytes in the exudate is attributed to a diminished egress of these cells from the peripheral blood.

The above reported evidence quite unequivocally demonstrates that following steroid treatment a reduced number of leucocytes appears in the injured areas. There is, however, some doubt that steroids suppress cell migration by a specific effect on circulating leucocytes, for these agents can reduce the number of emigrated cells by several different ways, e.g. by reducing vascular permeability, by inhibiting release of cells from bone marrow and by reducing cell division. Possibly, each mechanism may play a major, if not exclusive, role according to the animal species, the type of inflammation, the individual steroid agent and the dose used.

II. Non-Steroid Anti-Inflammatory Drugs

The effect of non-steroid anti-inflammatory drugs on cell migration has not been extensively investigated. Furthermore, in the majority of reports only total leucocyte migration has been evaluated without differentiation of the cell type. This basic situation may explain, at least in part, some discrepancies that exist in the literature; the different experimental approaches may also be responsible. Phenylbutazone administered to the rat (200 mg/kg) reduces cellular exudation in the early granuloma following implantation of non-resorbable plastic sponge (SAXENA, 1960), as well as in the peritoneal cavity injected with formalin (WILHELMI, 1965). According to FORD-HUTCHINSON et al. (1975), leucocyte migration into plastic sponge exudate in rat is also depressed by a smaller dose of phenylbutazone (50 mg/kg), as well as by indomethacin (3 mg/kg) and aspirin (150 mg/kg). The inhibition of leucocyte migration by aspirin (VINEGAR et al., 1973) and by several classic non-steroid anti-inflammatory drugs in rat carrageenin pleurisy has been also observed (AMMENDOLA et al., 1975).

The cellular emigration in rat carrageenin foot oedema has been studied by DI ROSA et al. (1971) histologically following administration of several representative non-steroid anti-inflammatory drugs, i.e. aspirin (150 mg/kg), indomethacin (2 mg/kg) phenylbutazone (50 mg/kg) and mefenamic acid (50 mg/kg). The treatment with these drugs, administered orally 1 h prior to the carrageenin injection, caused a suppression of the total number of leucocytes emigrating at both 4 and 6 h; the effect was most marked on the mononuclear cells. In order to study more closely the observed inhibition on mononuclear cells, rats were used in which a depletion of circulating polymorphs was achieved by treatment with methotrexate (WILLOUGHBY and GIROUD, 1969). In these rats, the total number of leucocytes emigrating into the carrageenin-injected paw was almost unaffected, but emigrated cells were virtually all mononuclear (95%). A combination of polymorphonucleocyte depletion with non-steroid anti-inflammatory drug treatment produced an almost total suppression of the cellular exudate (DI ROSA et al., 1971).

The selective inhibition of mononuclear cell emigration by non-steroid anti-inflammatory drugs is also supported by experiments with dextran pleurisy in the rat; this is a quantitative method in contrast to microscopic examination which allows only semiquantitative evaluation (DI ROSA et al., 1972). In these experiments, polymorph emigration was only slightly prevented, while mononuclear cell emigration was substantially depressed. The calculated ED_{50} values (mg/kg) at 24 h were: indomethacin 7.5, phenylbutazone 60, aspirin and flufenamic acid 180.

The potency ratio exhibited by these drugs in suppressing mononucleocyte emigration closely agrees with their efficacy on various experimental models of inflammation, as well as with their clinically established antirheumatic activity. Furthermore, cellular exudation induced in the rat by intrapleural injection of homologous serum, which consists virtually of polymorphs, remains completely unaffected by non-steroid anti-inflammatory drugs (DI ROSA, 1974).

The poor susceptibility of polymorphs to non-steroid agents may explain the failure of indomethacin and similar drugs to prevent leucocyte emigration in synovitis of the dog knee joint induced by urate crystals, and in monoarticular arthritis in the rabbit, both of which are inflammatory responses characterised by cellular emigration mainly sustained by polymorphs (VAN ARMAN et al., 1970; BLACKHAM et al., 1974). These data, however, conflict with the inhibition by indomethacin of polymorph emigration in the dog knee joint synovitis (PHELPS and McCARTY, 1967), or in a different type of experimental inflammation such as carrageenin oedema, as well as in kaolin or carrageenin pleurisy (VAN ARMAN et al., 1971a, 1971b; VINEGAR et al., 1971, 1972, 1973). It must be also mentioned that sodium salicylate was found slightly to increase polymorph emigration occurring in urate crystal arthritis in chickens (BRUNE and GLATT, 1974b).

The view that non-steroid anti-inflammatory drugs selectively inhibit mononuclear cell chemotaxis in vivo recently received strong support from experiments with ^{51}Cr labelled leucocytes (PERPER et al., 1974b). Indomethacin (5 mg/kg), phenylbutazone (100 mg/kg) and mefenamic acid (300 mg/kg) reduced mononuclear cell emigration in rat carrageenin foot oedema while no significant inhibition was exhibited by these drugs on polymorph accumulation in the inflamed paw.

These data have been interpreted on the basis of a possible ability of these drugs to alter the integrity of the cell membrane. The external coat of the macrophage cell membrane is, in fact, characterised by the presence of heavy mucopolysaccharides (CARR, 1970). The cellular synthesis of such compounds is inhibited by indomethacin, phenylbutazone and mefenamic acid (WHITEHOUSE, 1965), as well as by corticosteroids which also decrease mononuclear cell emigration.

Other evidence of the action of these drugs on the surface activity of the cells derives from the inhibition of colloidal carbon phagocytosis exhibited in vivo by indomethacin and phenylbutazone, as well as from the ultrastructural alterations observed by electron microscopy in monocytes and macrophages adherent to the surface of strips of cellophane implanted in rats treated with indomethacin (DI ROSA et al., 1971). These agents also affect the central bone marrow stores of monocytes, as demonstrated by the development of carrageenin oedema in radiation chimaera experiments. Irradiated rats receiving bone marrow from normal donors reacted to injected carrageenin in a similar way to non-irradiated controls. In contrast, in irradiated rats receiving bone marrow from donors previously treated with indomethacin or with phenylbutazone, the oedema was greatly reduced and was virtually indistinguishable from that of irradiated rats which did not receive bone marrow

(Di Rosa et al., 1971). The hypothesis was advanced that the main mode of action of non-steroid anti-inflammatory drugs is primarily on the monocytes, and that their effect is possibly due to an impairment of an energy-supplying enzyme system which is reponsible for the movements of cell surface. This hypothesis received suggestive and stimulating support by the demonstration that anti-inflammatory agents are able to inhibit the adenosine triphosphate-induced contractile process in rat leucocytes (Görög and Kovàks, 1974).

III. Immunosuppressive Agents

This discussion of the effect of immunosuppressive agents on leucocyte emigration will be strictly confined to non-specific inflammatory responses. The drastic decrease induced by immunosuppressive agents in the number of circulating leucocytes and the remarkable general toxicity of these agents are the main factors responsible for the inadequate appraisal of the action of these drugs on cellular emigration. It is, in fact, rather difficult to judge whether the observed inhibition of white cell exudation is a specific effect or is merely a consequence of the induced general impairment of animal reactivity. The narrow margin between tolerable and toxic or even lethal doses is a source of additional problems.

The inflammatory response to subcutaneous injection of egg white in rabbits treated with nitrogen mustard (neutropenia) was characterised by a decreased neutrophil emigration and also by a marked delay in lymphocyte infiltration (Page and Good, 1958). With the same technique, it was later shown that 6-mercaptopurine, according to the dose and the period of treatment, virtually eliminates the participation of mononuclear cells in inflammation (Page et al., 1962). The inhibition of mononuclear cell emigration at the inflamed site exhibited by 6-mercaptopurine has been also demonstrated in guinea pigs (Phillips and Zweiman, 1970). Treatment with this drug greatly decreased the production and mobilisation of mononuclear phagocytic cells from the bone marrow (Hurd and Ziff, 1968).

Actinomycin D and puromycin specifically blocked mononuclear cell infiltration of rabbit subcutaneous areas injected with egg white, while aminopterin, 5-fluorouracil, cytoxan, 8-azaguanine and chloromycetin were ineffective (Page, 1964). Other immunosuppressive agents, such as methotrexate, cyclophosphamide and chlorambucil also prevented mononucleocyte emigration (Hersch and Freireich, 1968; Watnick et al., 1974). Furthermore, colchicine decreased polymorph emigration in urate crystal arthritis (Malawista and Seegmiller, 1965; Brune and Glatt, 1974 b).

However, these findings are at variance, at least in part, with other observations, although obtained in different experimental conditions. For example, cyclophosphamide failed to prevent the accumulation of either mononucleocytes or neutrophils in carrageenin inflamed rat paw in experiments carried out using ^{51}Cr labelled leucocytes (Perper et al., 1974 b). Furthermore, methotrexate did not influence the mononuclear cell response of the rat to intradermal injection of either fibrinogen or Freund's adjuvant (Willoughby and Giroud, 1969).

After a week methotrexate produced a selective agranulocytosis when given to rats by an intraperitoneal regimen (Willoughby and Spector, 1968; Willoughby and Giroud, 1969). Since these agranulocytic rats were able to react normally to inflammatory stimuli such as thermal injury, skin burn and intrapleural injection of turpentine, it was suggested that polymorphs were not an essential feature of the inflammatory response in the rat. This conclusion was in contrast to several other findings which demonstrated a close relation between the inhibition of the inflammatory response and the depletion of circulating polymorph populations (VAN ARMAN et al., 1971 b; VINEGAR et al., 1971; ARRIGONI-MARTELLI and RESTELLI, 1972).

The question was also reinvestigated by WILLOUGHBY's group by exploring in rat carrageenin oedema the effect of a variety of immunosuppressive agents, including methotrexate, cyclophosphamide, chlorambucil, busulphan, 6-mercaptopurine and azathiopurine. With the exception only of azathiopurine, all the agents exhibited an anti-inflammatory effect which appeared to be correlated with a reduction in the number of infiltrating polymorphonuclear cells (DUKES et al., 1973).

IV. Endogenous Substances

Leucocyte accumulation at the inflamed site is induced by cytotaxins which are formed through different pathways (WILKINSON, 1974). The existence of endogenous inactivators of cytotaxins is suggested by the short half-life (less than 20 min) of these factors in the circulating blood (WARD et al., 1966), whereas their activity presists in vitro for hours without any loss (KELLER, 1972). Furthermore, endogenous inhibitors of leucocyte chemotaxins have been discovered in sera of various patients showing impaired leucocyte responsiveness and reduced emigration of these cells (WARD and SCHLEGEL, 1969; PAGE et al., 1968). The considerable interest of these findings deserves further work to elucidate the endogenous regulatory mechanisms of leucocyte accumulation in vivo.

The key role of $3'5'$ c-AMP in controlling a variety of essential leucocyte properties is supported by a large number of observations. An increase of intracellular $3'5'$ cAMP level is associated with the inhibition of several leucocyte functions such as lysosomal enzyme release (WEISSMANN et al., 1971a, 1971b; ZURIER et al., 1973), migration and mobility (DIMITROV et al., 1969; JOHNSON et al., 1972; PICK, 1972), phagocytosis and microbicidal activity (BOURNE et al., 1971) and response to antigenic stimuli (BOURNE et al., 1974). These in vitro observations may explain the anti-inflammatory activity exhibited in vivo by $3'5'$ cAMP in several types of experimental inflammations (BERTELLI et al., 1966, 1973, 1974; ICHIKAWA et al., 1972a, 1972b).

Although in these experiments no attention was given to leucocyte migration, these data are at variance with the increased ^{51}Cr labelled polymorph migration observed in carrageenin injected paws of rats treated with dibutyryl-$3'5'$ cAMP (PERPER et al., 1974b). The same treatment was without effect on mononuclear cell emigration and did not reduce the paw swelling.

Normal human plasma contains a fraction showing experimental anti-inflammatory activity (MCARTHUR et al., 1972). The fraction has an apparent molecular weight below 1000 and is resistant to acidic, proteolytic and thermal degradation (FORD-HUTCHINSON et al., 1973). It has been recently reported that this plasma fraction inhibits the migration of polymorphonuclear and mononuclear leucocytes into inflammatory exudates produced by the intrapleural injection of carrageenin or turpentine, or by the subcutaneous implantation of polyvinyl sponges in the rat (FORD-HUTCHINSON et al., 1975). The mechanism of this effect is still under investigation; however, it does not involve complement depletion.

E. Inhibition of Granuloma Formation

I. Steroid Anti-Inflammatory Drugs

Granuloma inhibition by anti-inflammatory steroids has been shown by several experimental methods in which granuloma growth was induced by a large variety of stimuli (see Section C). Cotton-pellets granuloma provides a simple test to evaluate the activity of these steroids since their ability to reduce the amount of granulation tissue closely correlates with their effects on thymus involution and liver glycogen deposition (LERNER et al., 1964). Also, the granuloma pouch assay has been extensively used for the assay of anti-inflammatory steroids, although because of the difficult dissection of the pouch wall, the measure was sometimes restricted to exudate volume. Thus, the effect of the tested drug was measured on serous exudation and not on granuloma growth (WHITEHOUSE, 1965).

These methods, as well as those of less extended use, such as plastic ring granuloma or filter paper granuloma in chick embryos, are based on the weight assay of dissected granuloma, which is indeed a rough measure for a complicated process such as granulomatous tissue formation (RUDAS, 1960; D'ARCY and HOWARD, 1967). On the other hand, detailed biochemical studies have only been carried out in carrageenin granuloma, which has never become a routine assay test. Furthermore, no satisfactory information on cell composition and turnover in these granulomata under the influence of anti-inflammatory steroids has been achieved. This situation represents a typical example of the inadequate co-operation between scientific disciplines mentioned above.

Biochemical studies on the granulomatous tissue have been carried out in order to elucidate the mechanism of action of anti-inflammatory steroids. The majority of these investigations have been focussed on the evaluation of the collagen content of the granulation tissue, as measured by the concentration of hydroxyproline. Corticosteroids usually decrease the hydroxyproline content of granulation tissue (ROBERTSON and SANBORN, 1958; TRNAVSKÝ et al., 1962; ORONSKY and NOCENTI, 1967; FUKUHARA and TSURUFUJI, 1969a), although some negative results have been reported (JORGENSEN, 1962). Some studies with prednisolone, methylprednisolone and cortisone have shown that this effect seems related to an inhibition of synthesis rather than to an increased catabolism of collagen (KÜHN et al., 1964; NIMNI and BAVETTA, 1964; KIVIRIKKO et al., 1965). Betamethasone also strongly decreases the incorporation of ^{3}H-proline into the hydroxyproline of collagen from carrageenin granuloma (FUKUHARA and TSURUFUJI, 1969b). Possibly, the inhibition is not specific for collagen since it was concomitantly observed for non-collagen proteins and seems rather to be an aspect of the ability of steroids to inhibit general protein synthesis (FUKUHARA and TSURUFUJI, 1969a; EBERT and PROCKOP, 1967). This inhibition is probably due to a multiple intracellular action of steroids which may influence the activity of messenger ribonucleic acid, polyribosomal function or ribosomal aggregation (GOULD and MANNER, 1967). However, it must be mentioned that there is a considerable amount of evidence showing that collagen undergoes breakdown under the influence of anti-inflammatory steroids (DOUGHERTY et al., 1973). Collagenolytic enzymes are probably induced by hydrocortisone through the production of messenger RNA, with a subsequent synthesis of proteolytic enzymes (HOUCK et al., 1968).

It has also been shown that steroids inhibit the incorporation of ^{35}S into rat cartilage, this data suggesting a reduced synthesis of sulphated mucopolysaccharides (ANASTASSIADES and DZIEWIATKOWSKI, 1970). The decrease of both collagen and mucopolysaccharides in the granulomatous tissue under the influence of steroids may possibly depend on a unique mechanisms, i.e. a depression of the synthetic and metabolic activity produced by these agents in fibroblasts which may be considered as target cells (DOUGHERTY et al., 1973).

II. Non-Steroid Anti-Inflammatory Drugs

Non-steroid anti-inflammatory drugs usually exhibit a moderate inhibition of granulomatous tissue formation. An exception is indomethacin which is able to inhibit cotton-pellet granuloma at dose levels comparable to hydrocortisone (WINTER et al., 1963). A similar result has been observed by comparing, among other drugs, indomethacin and betamethasone in rat carrageenin granuloma pouch (FUKUHARA and TSURUFUJI, 1969a). It is interesting, however, that in these experiments betamethasone was able to reduce a pre-existing granuloma, while non-steroid anti-inflammatory drugs (indomethacin, phenylbutazone, aspirin) failed do so. Although there is a wide variability in results from different laboratories, there is general agreement that non-steroid anti-inflammatory drugs inhibit cotton-pellet granuloma formation exhibiting a potency ratio which correlates with their clinical efficacy (WINTER et al., 1963; WINDER et al., 1965). Other methods seem less precise in achieving such correlation (RUDAS, 1960; D'ARCY and HOWARD, 1967). The minor susceptibility of granulomatous tissue to be inhibited by non-steroid anti-inflammatory drugs is reflected, at a biochemical level, by the relative insensitivity of collagen synthesis to be reduced by these drugs when used at doses comparable with those exhibiting an effect on granulomatous tissue. Phenylbutazone and salicylates do not modify hydroxyproline concentration (DANIEL-MOUSSARD and QUESSON, 1961; JORGENSEN, 1962). However salicylate, in contrast to the inefficacy of phenylbutazone and indomethacin, has a specific inhibitory effect on collagen synthesis without modifying the synthesis of non-collagen proteins (FUKUHARA and TSURUFUJI, 1969b). These results are at variance with recent observations demonstrating a suppression of collagen synthesis by indomethacin and phenylbutazone, while salicylate was hardly effective (KULONEN and POTILA, 1975).

In chronic experiments in rats, sodium salicylate (300 mg/kg during 8 weeks) accelerated the metabolic turnover, maturation and degradation of collagen, as studied by the incorporation of ^{14}C-hydroxyproline (TRNAVSKÁ et al., 1968). In a similar experiment, phenylbutazone (100 mg/kg during 3 weeks) was found to inhibit collagen synthesis without affecting collagen maturation in normal rats (TRNAVSKÝ and TRNAVSKÁ, 1971) while in animals with adjuvant arthritis, collagen maturation was accelerated (TRNAVSKÝ, 1974). It is evident that the reports on the effect of non-steroid anti-inflammatory drugs are far from unequivocal, the discrepancies probably resulting from the differences in dose regimen and experimental conditions.

III. Immunosuppressive Agents

Immunosuppressive agents have not been frequently tested in non-immune inflammatory granulomata. One of the few investigations concerns the effect of several agents (6-mercaptopurine, cyclophosphamide, methotrexate) on cotton-pellet and

Freund's adjuvant granulomata (STEVENS and WILLOUGHBY, 1969). These chronic inflammatory reactions were little affected by the treatment, while some types of acute inflammation (thermal injury and turpentine pleurisy) were strongly inhibited. Thus, immunosuppressive agents seem to have a non-specific effect on the vascular changes of acute inflammation, whereas they exhibit only a modest effect on granulomatous inflammatory lesions. This is a rather surprising result, considering the immune mechanisms involved in chronic inflammation (SPECTOR, 1969; ALLISON and DAVIES, 1974).

IV. Endogenous Substances

The effect of 3'5' cAMP has been evaluated on carrageenin-induced granuloma pouch in the rat (ICHIKAWA et al., 1972b). Either local (intrapouch) or systemic (intraperitoneal) administration of 3'5' cAMP inhibited granuloma formation (pouch wall wet weight) as well as serous exudation (pouch fluid volume), according to the dose used. The simultaneous administration of theophylline resulted in a greater suppression of the inflammatory response. The inhibition of granuloma formation may possibly depend on the regulatory effect of 3'5' cAMP on the function of phagocytic cells in the injured region.

The role of histamine in the formation of granulomatous tissue has been poorly investigated. Futhermore, conflicting results have been reported. The idea that histamine, released from mast cells, may stimulate the proliferative stage of inflammation (RILEY, 1955) was supported by the marked inhibition of granuloma pouch or cotton-pellet granuloma observed in rats treated with the compound 48/80 (STERN et al., 1956; BHATT and SANYAL, 1964).

In contrast to these results, daily subcutaneous injections of histamine inhibited the growth of granulomatous tissue induced by implantation of formalin-soaked filter paper discs (SAEKI et al., 1975). The inhibition was removed by simultaneous administration of the H_2 receptor antagonist burimamide, whereas the H_1 receptor antagonist mepyramine was ineffective. It was suggested that histamine has a biphasic effect: low concentrations promote granuloma growth while higher concentrations induce inhibition. The suppressive effect of histamine may depend on an inhibition of fibroblast growth caused by an increased intracellular level of 3'5' cAMP, possibly induced by activation of H_2 receptors (OTTEN et al., 1972; LICHTENSTEIN and GILLESPIE, 1973).

F. Conclusions

It is virtually impossible to assemble all the data in a comprehensive picture. The paucity of knowledge on some basic mechanisms of cell migration and granuloma formation, as well as the heterogeneity of the models used to mimic the inflammatory response, represent serious obstacles to satisfactory rationalisation. Although most of the morphological events of cell migration have been identified, the biochemical aspects of the process are far from being clearly understood.

The granulomatous lesion suffers from the same inadequate approach. However, the quantification of cell kinetics in some types of granuloma represents a substantial achievement, although it cannot simply be extended to other similar types of lesion.

Results obtained in a definite experimental situation are, in fact, too often considered as representative of the entire process under investigation, this generalisation possibly accounting for most of the discrepant or conflicting interpretations. Nevertheless, most reports demonstrate a suppression of leucocyte migration by both steroid and non-steroid anti-inflammatory drugs. The effect of steroids in reducing mononuclear cell emigration is clear, while their inhibition of polymorph escape is more equivocal. Nonsteroid drugs have not been extensively evaluated in their ability to effect leucocyte emigration. These drugs, however, selectively inhibit mononuclear cell migration without modifying polymorph accumulation in the inflamed area. Immunosuppressive agents inhibit cell migration possibly by a non-specific mechanism, for their effect seems to be related to the general toxicity of these agents. Steroids are very effective in inhibiting granulomatous tissue formation in a large variety of experimental models, whereas chronic lesions appear to be less sensitive to both non-steroid drugs and immunosuppressive agents. Endogenous mechanisms involved in the regulation of leucocyte migration and granuloma growth are obscure, although they possibly represent the key to a basic understanding of the entire inflammatory process.

Inhibition of leucocyte migration, mainly of mononuclear cells, into the inflamed area, seems at present the only common mechanism shared by both steroid and non-steroid anti-inflammatory drugs. Although these drugs have a multiplicity of interfering mechanisms, their effect on cell migration appears a promising area which deserves further investigation.

Acknowledgement. The author wishes to thank Dr. Giuliana Ammendola for her helpful cooperation during the preparation of the manuscript.

References

Allison,A.C., Davies,P.: Mechanisms underlying chronic inflammation. In: Velo,G.P., Willoughby,D.A., Giroud,J.P. (Eds.): Future Trends in Inflammation, pp.449—480. Padua: Piccin Medical Books 1974

Ammendola,G., Di Rosa,M., Sorrentino,L.: Leucocyte migration and lysosomal enzymes release in rat carrageenin pleurisy. Agents Actions 5, 250—255 (1975)

Anastassiades,T., Dziewiatkowski,D.: The effect of cortisone on the metabolism of connective tissue in the rat. J. Lab. clin. Med. 75, 826—839 (1970)

Arrigoni-Martelli,E., Restelli,A.: Release of lysosomal enzymes in experimental inflammations: effect of anti-inflammatory drugs. Europ. J. Pharmacol. 19, 191—198 (1972)

Athens,J.W., Haab,O.P., Raab,S.O., Mauer,A.M., Ashenbruker,H., Cartwright,G.E., Wintrobe,M.M.: Leukokinetic studies. IV. The total blood, circulating and marginal granulocyte pool and the granulocyte turnover rate in normal subjects. J. clin. Invest. 40, 989—995 (1961b)

Athens,J.W., Mauer,A.M., Ashenbrucker,H., Cartwright,G.E., Wintrobe,M.M.: Leukokinetic studies. I. Method for labeling leukocytes with diisopropylfluorophosphate (DFP³²). Blood 14, 303—333 (1959)

Athens,J.W., Raab,S.O., Haab,O.P., Mauer,A.M., Ashenbrucker,H., Cartwright,G.E., Wintrobe,M.M.: Leukokinetic studies. III. The distribution of granulocytes in the blood of normal subjects. J. clin. Invest. 40, 159—164 (1961a)

Bangham,A.D.: The adhesiveness of leukocytes with special reference to zeta protentials. Ann. N.Y. Acad. Sci. 116, 945—949 (1964)

Barnhart,M.I.: Role of blood coagulation in acute inflammation. Biochem. Pharmacol. 17 suppl., 205—219 (1968)

Becker, E. L.: Biochemical aspects of the polymorphonuclear response to chemotactic factors. In: Biochemistry of the Acute Allergic Reactions, p. 243. Austen, K. F., Becker, E. L. (Eds.). Oxford-Edinburgh: Blackwell 1971

Beker, E. L., Ward, P. A.: Partial biochemical characterization of the activated esterase required in the complement-dependent chemotaxis of rabbit polymorphonuclear leucocytes. J. exp. Med. **125**, 1021—1030 (1967)

Benitz, K. F., Hall, L. M.: Local morphological response following a single subcutaneous injection of carrageenin in the rat. Proc. Soc. exp. Biol. (N.Y.) **102**, 442—445 (1959)

Benitz, K. F., Hall, L. M.: The carrageenin-induced abscess as a new test for anti-inflammatory activity of steroids and non steroids. Arch. int. Pharmacodyn. **144**, 185—195 (1963)

Benzi, G., Frigo, G. M.: Interferenza di alcuni fattori sul test del granuloma da cotton pellet. Farmaco, Ed. prat. **19**, 327—337 (1964)

Bertelli, A., Amato, G., Caciagli, F.: Inhibition of kinins formation by cyclic 3'5'-AMP in anaphylactic shock in the guinea pig. Pharm. Res. Commun. **5**, 29—36 (1973)

Bertelli, A., Breschi, M. C., Caciagli, F.: Effects of cyclic nucleotides on the inflammatory reaction. In: Velo, G. P., Willoughby, D. A., Giroud, J. P. (Eds.): Future Trends in Inflammation, pp. 267—276. Padua: Piccin Medical Books 1974

Bertelli, A., Cerrati, A., Perazzoli, A. G., Rossano, M. A.: Attività antiflogistica del 3'5' AMP ciclico. Atti Accad. med. lombarda **21**, 601—604 (1966)

Bhatt, K. G. S., Sanyal, R. K.: The role of histamine and 5-hydroxytryptamine in inflammatory process. J. Pharm. Pharmacol. **16**, 385—393 (1964)

Bishop, C. R., Athens, J. W., Boggs, D. R., Warner, H. R., Cartwright, G. E., Wintrobe, M. M.: Leukokinetic studies. XIII. A non-steady-state kinetic evaluation of the mechanism of cortisone-induced granulocytosis. J. clin. Invest. **47**, 249—260 (1968)

Blackam, A., Farmer, J. B., Radziwonik, H., Westwick, J.: The role of prostaglandins in rabbit monoarticular arthritis. Brit. J. Pharmacol. **51**, 35—44 (1974)

Bobalik, G. R., Bastian, J. W.: Effect of various antiphlogistic agents on adjuvant-induced exudate formation in rats. Arch. int. Pharmacodyn. **166**, 466—472 (1967)

Boggs, D. R., Athens, J. W., Cartwright, G. E., Wintrobe, M. M.: The effect of adrenal glucocorticosteroids upon the cellular composition of inflammatory exudates. Amer. J. Path. **44**, 763—773 (1964)

Boot, J. R., Dawson, W., Kitchen, E. A.: The chemotactic activity of thromboxane B_2: a possible role in inflammation. J. Physiol. **257**, 47—48 P (1976)

Borel, J. F.: Studies on chemotaxis. Effect of subcellular fractions on neutrophils and macrophages. Int. Arch. Allergy **39**, 247—271 (1970)

Boris, A., Stevenson, R. H.: The effects of some non-steroidal anti-inflammatory agents on carrageenin-induced exudate formation. Arch. int. Pharmacodyn. **153**, 205—210 (1965)

Bourne, H. R., Lehrer, R. I., Cline, M. J., Melmon, K. L.: Cyclic 3'5'-adenosine monophosphate in the human leukocyte: synthesis, degradation, and effects on neutrophils candidacidal activity. J. clin. Invest. **50**, 920—929 (1971)

Bourne, H. R., Lichtenstein, L. M., Melmon, K. L., Henney, C. S., Weinstein, Y., Shearer, G. M.: Modulation of inflammation and immunity by cyclic AMP. Science **184**, 19—27 (1974)

Brune, K., Bucher, K., Walz, D.: The avian microcrystal arthritis. II. Central versus peripheral effects of sodium salicylate, acetaminophen and colchicine. Agents Actions **4**, 27—33 (1974a)

Brune, K., Glatt, M.: The avian microcrystal arthritis. III. Invasion and enzyme-release from leukocytes at the site of inflammation. Agents Actions **4**, 95—100 (1974a)

Brune, K., Glatt, M.: The avian microcrystal arthritis. IV. The impact of sodium salicylate, acetaminophen and colchicine on leukocyte invasion and enzyme liberation in vivo. Agents Actions **4**, 101—107 (1974b)

Brune, K., Walz, D., Bucher, K.: The avian microcrystal arthritis. I. Simultaneous recording of nociception and temperature effect at the inflamed joint. Agents Actions **4**, 21—26 (1974b)

Bush, I. E., Alexander, R. W.: An improved method for the assay of anti-inflammatory substances in rats. Acta. endocr. (Kbh.) **35**, 268—276 (1960)

Carr, I.: The fine structure of the mammalian lymphoreticular system. Int. Rev. Cytol. **27**, 283—348 (1970)

Christian, J. J., Williamson, H. O.: Effect of crowding on experimental granuloma formation in mice. Proc. Soc. exp. Biol. (N.Y.) **99**, 385—387 (1958)

Cochrane, C. G., Aikin, B. S.: Polymorphonuclear leukocytes in immunologic reactions. The destruction of vascular basement membrane in vivo and in vitro. J. exp. Med. **124**, 733—752 (1966)

Consden, R., Doble, A., Glynn, L. E., Nind, A. P.: Production of a chronic arthritis with ovalbumin. Its retention in the rabbit knee joint. Ann. rheum. Dis. **30**, 307—315 (1971)

Craddock, C. G., Winkelstein, A., Matsuyuki, Y., Lawrence, J. S.: The immune response to foreign red blood cells and the participation of short-lived lymphocytes. J. exp. Med. **125**, 1149—1172 (1967)

Cummings, M. M., Drummond, M. C., Michael, M., Bloom, W. L.: The influence of cortisone on artificially induced peritoneal exudates. Bull. Johns Hopk. Hosp. **90**, 185—191 (1952)

Cygielman, S., Robson, J. M.: The effect of irritant substances on the deposition of granulation tissue in the cotton pellet test. J. Pharm. Pharmacol. **15**, 794—797 (1963)

Daniel-Moussard, H., Quesson, M.: Etude microchimique du granulome silicotique experimental chez le rat. IV. Action de certaines substances pharmacodynamiques sur les mucopolysaccharides et la vitesse d'echange du soufre. Bull. Soc. Chim. biol. (Paris) **43**, 215—226 (1961)

D'Arcy, F. P., Howard, E. M.: A new anti-inflammatory test, utilizing the chorio-allantoic membrane of the chick embryo. Brit. J. Pharmacol. **29**, 378—387 (1967)

Delaunay, A., Bazin, S.: Metabolic changes in connective tissue during an inflammatory process. In: Non-steroidal Anti-inflammatory Drugs, pp. 25—34. Garattini, S., Dukes, M. N. G. (Eds.). Amsterdam: Excerpta Medica 1965

Dimitrov, N. V., Miller, J., Ziegra, S. R.: The effect of caffeine on glucose metabolism of polymorphonuclear leukocytes. J. Pharmacol. (Kyoto) **168**, 240—243 (1969)

Di Pasquale, G., Meli, A.: Effect of body weight changes on the formation of cotton pellet-induced granuloma. J. Pharm. Pharmacol. **17**, 379—382 (1965)

Di Rosa, M.: Biological properties of carrageenan. J. Pharm. Pharmacol. **24**, 89—102 (1972)

Di Rosa, M.: Prostaglandins, leucocytes and non-steroidal anti-inflammatory drugs. Pol. J. Pharmacol. **26**, 25—36 (1974)

Di Rosa, M., Papadimitriou, J. M., Willoughby, D. A.: A histopathological and pharmacological analysis of the mode of action of non-steroidal anti-inflammatory drugs. J. Path. **105**, 239—256 (1971)

Di Rosa, M., Sorrentino, L., Parente, L.: Non-steroidal anti-inflammatory drugs and leucocyte emigration. J. Pharm. Pharmacol. **24**, 575—577 (1972)

Di Rosa, M., Willoughby, D. A.: Screens for anti-inflammatory drugs. J. Pharm. Pharmacol. **23**, 297—298 (1971)

Dougherty, T. F., Schneebeli, G. L.: Role of cortisone in regulation of inflammation. Proc. Soc. exp. Biol. (N.Y.) **75**, 854—859 (1950)

Dougherty, T. F., Stevens, W., Schneebeli, G. L.: Functional and morphological alterations produced in target cells by anti-inflammatory steroids. Recent Progr. Hormone Res. **29**, 287—328 (1973)

Dukes, M., Chan, W. C., Willoughby, D. A.: The effect of various immunosuppressive agents on the vascular and cellular response to carrageenan in the rat. J. Path. **109**, 151—161 (1973)

Dumonde, D. C., Glynn, L. E.: The production of arthritis in rabbits by an immunological reaction to fibrin. Brit. J. exp. Path. **43**, 373—383 (1962)

Ebert, P. S., Prockop, J. D.: Influence of cortisol on the synthesis of sulfated mucopolysaccharides and collagen in chick embryos. Biochim. biophys. Acta (Amst.) **136**, 45—55 (1967)

Fisher, E. R., Paar, J.: Carrageenin granuloma in the guinea pig and rat. Arch. Path. **70**, 565—575 (1960)

Florey, H. W., Grant, L. H.: Leucocyte migration from small blood vessels stimulated with ultraviolet light; an electron microscope study. J. Path. Bact. **82**, 13—17 (1961)

Ford-Hutchinson, A. W., Insley, M. Y., Elliott, P. N. C., Sturgess, E. A., Smith, M. J. H.: Anti-inflammatory activity in human plasma. J. Pharm. Pharmacol. **25**, 881—886 (1973)

Ford-Hutchinson, A. W., Smith, M. J. H., Elliott, P. N. C., Bolam, J. P., Walker, J. R., Lobo, A. A., Badcock, J. K., Colledge, A. J., Billimoria, F. J.: Effect of a human plasma fraction on leucocyte migration into inflammatory exudates. J. Pharm. Pharmacol. **27**, 106—112 (1975)

Fruhman, G. J.: Adrenal steroids and neutrophil mobilization. Blood **20**, 355—363 (1962)

Fukuhara, M., Tsurufuji, S.: The effect of locally injected anti-inflammatory drugs on the carrageenin granuloma in rats. Biochem. Pharmacol. **18**, 475—484 (1969a)

Fukuhara, M., Tsurufuji, S.: The effect of locally injected anti-inflammatory drugs on the synthesis of collagen and non collagen protein of carrageenin granuloma in rats. Biochem. Pharmacol. **18**, 2409—2414 (1969 b)

Galber, W. L., Fosdick, L. S.: A possible mechanism for the anti-inflammatory effects of proteolytic enzymes. Proc. Soc. exp. Biol. (N.Y.) **120**, 160—163 (1965)

Ganley, O. H., Graessle, O. E., Robinson, H. J.: Anti-inflammatory activity of compounds obtained from egg yolk, peanut oil, and soybean lecithin. J. Lab. clin. Med. **51**, 709—714 (1958)

Gell, P. G. H., Hinde, I. T.: Histology of tuberculin reaction and its modifications by cortisone. Brit. J. exp. Path. **32**, 516—529 (1951)

George, M., Vaughan, J. H.: In vitro cell migration as a model of delayed hypersensitivity. Proc. Soc. exp. Biol. (N.Y.) **111**, 514—521 (1962)

Germuth, F. G.: The role of adrenocortical steroids in infection, immunity and hypersensitivity. Pharmacol. Rev. **8**, 1—24 (1956)

Germuth, F. G., Nedzel, G. A., Ottinger, B., Oyama, J.: Anatomical and histological changes in rabbits with experimental hypersensitivity treated with compound E and ACTH. Proc. Soc. exp. Biol. (N.Y.) **76**, 177—182 (1951)

Glenn, E. M., Miller, W. L., Schlagel, C. A.: Metabolic effects of adrenocortical steroids in vivo and in vitro: relationship to anti-inflammatory effects. Recent Progr. Hormone Res. **19**, 107—191 (1963)

Goldstein, S., Schnall, M.: A three-stage sequential screening program for the detection of anti-inflammatory agents using a carrageenin-induced abscess. Arch. int. Pharmacodyn. **144**, 269—277 (1963)

Görög, P., Kovaks, I. B.: Adenosine triphosphate-induced contractile process in rat lymphocytes and its inhibition by anti-inflammatory drugs. Brit. J. Pharmacol. **50**, 316—318 (1974)

Gould, B. S., Manner, G.: The action of hydrocortisone on collagen formation with special reference to its action on ribosomal aggregation. Biochim. biophys. Acta (Amst.) **138**, 189—192 (1967)

Gowland, E.: Studies on the emigration of polymorphonuclear leucocytes from skin lesions in man. J. Path. Bact. **87**, 347—352 (1964)

Grant, L.: The sticking and emigration of white blood cells in inflammation. In: Zweifach, B. W., Grant, L., McCluskey, R. T. (Eds.): The Inflammatory Process, pp. 197—244. New York-London: Academic Press 1965

Henson, P. M.: Mechanisms of mediator release from inflammatory cells. In: Weissmann, G. (Ed.): Mediators of Inflammation, pp. 9—50. New York-London: Plenum Press 1974

Herbert, W. J., Wilkinson, P. C.: A Dictionary of Immunology. Oxford and Edinburgh: Blackwell 1971

Hersch, E. M., Freireich, E. J.: Host defence mechanisms and their modification by cancer chemotherapy. In: Busch, H. (Ed.): Methods in Cancer Research, Vol. IV, pp. 355—451. New York-London: Academic Press 1968

Higgs, G. A., McCall, E., Youlten, L. J. F.: A chemotactic role for prostaglandins released from polymorphonuclear leucocytes during phagocytosis. Brit. J. Pharmacol. **53**, 539—546 (1975)

Highton, T. C.: The effect of sera from patients with rheumatoid arthritis on carrageenin granuloma pouchs, skin wounds and weight gain in rats. Brit. J. exp. Path. **44**, 137—144 (1963)

Hills, A., Forsham, P. H., Finch, C. A.: Changes in circulating leucocytes induced by administration of pituitary adrenocorticotrophic hormone (ACTH) in man. Blood **3**, 755—786 (1948)

Holland, J. F., Senn, H., Banerjee, T.: Quantitative studies of localized leukocyte mobilization in acute leukemia. Blood **37**, 499—511 (1971)

Holtkamp, D. E., Wang, R., Doggett, M.: Rapid method for measurement of anti-inflammatory activity utilizing fluid volume of experimentally-inflamed pleural cavity of the rat. Fed. Proc. **17**, 379 (1958)

Horváth, G., Ludány, G., Vajda, G.: Die Wirkung von Cortison auf die Auswanderung der Leukozyten und ihre Bacterienphagozytose. Arch. int. Pharmacodyn. **100**, 357—360 (1955)

Houck, J. C., Sharma, V. K., Patel, Y. M., Gladner, J. A.: Induction of collagenolytic and proteolytic activities by anti-inflammatory drugs in the skin and fibroblast. Biochem. Pharmacol. **17**, 2081—2090 (1968)

Hurd, E. R., Ziff, M.: Studies on the anti-inflammatory action of 6-mercaptopurine. J. exp. Med. **128**, 785—800 (1968)

Hurley, J. V.: Substances promoting leucocyte emigration. Ann. N.Y. Acad. Sci. **116**, 918—935 (1964)

Hurley, J. V., Ryan, G. B., Friedman, A.: The mononuclear response to intrapleural injection in the rat. J. Path. Bact. **91**, 575—587 (1966)

Hurley, J. V., Spector, W. G.: Delayed leucocityc emigration after intradermal injection and thermal injury. J. Path. Bact. **82**, 421—429 (1961)

Hurley, J. V., Spector, W. G.: A topographical study of increased vascular permeability in acute turpentin-induced pleurisy. J. Path. Bact. **89**, 245—254 (1965)

Hymes, W. F., Gilbert, J. B., Mengoli, H. F., Watne, A. L.: Inhibition of migration of rat peritoneal exudate cells by ascites tumor fluid fractions. Nature (Lond.) **213**, 108—110 (1967)

Ichikawa, A., Hayashi, H., Minami, M., Tomita, K.: An acute inflammation induced by inorganic pyrophosphate and adenosine triphosphate, and its inhibition by cyclic 3′5′-adenosine monophosphate. Biochem. Pharmacol. **21**, 317—331 (1972a)

Ichikawa, A., Nagasaki, M., Umezu, K., Hayashi, H., Tomita, K.: Effect of cyclic 3′5′ monophosphate on edema and granuloma induced by carrageenin. Biochem. Pharmacol. **21**, 2615—2626 (1972b)

Innerfield, I., Cohen, H., Zweil, P.: Effect of orally administered proteolytic enzymes on carbon tetrachloride induced granuloma pouch. Proc. Soc. exp. Biol. (N.Y.) **123**, 871—874 (1966)

Ishikawa, H., Mori, Y., Tsurufuji, S.: The characteristic feature of glucocorticoids after local application with reference to leucocyte migration and protein exudation. Europ. J. Pharmacol. **7**, 201—205 (1969)

Jackson, D. S.: Connective tissue growth stimulated by carrageenin. I. The formation and removal collagen. Biochem. J. **65**, 277—284 (1957)

Janoff, A., Zweifach, B. W.: Production of inflammatory changes in the micro-circulation by cationic proteins extracted from lysosomes. J. exp. Med. **120**, 747—764 (1964)

Johnson, G. S., Morgan, W. D., Pastan, I.: Regulation of cell motility by cyclic AMP. Nature (Lond.) **235**, 54—56 (1972)

Jorgensen, O.: Influence of some antirheumatic compounds on formation of granulation tissue. Acta pharmacol. (Kbh.) **19**, 251—258 (1962)

Kaley, G., Weiner, R.: Effect of prostaglandin E$_1$ on leukocyte migration. Nature (New Biol.) **234**, 114—115 (1971)

Kay, A. B., Austen, K. F.: The IgE-mediated release of an eosinophil leukocyte chemotactic factor from human lung. J. Immunol. **107**, 899—902 (1971)

Keller, H. U.: Chemotaxis and its significance for leucocyte accumulation. Agents Actions **2**, 161—169 (1972)

Keller, H. U., Sorkin, E.: Studies on chemotaxis. V. On the chemotactic effect of bacteria. Int. Arch. Allergy **31**, 505—517 (1967a)

Keller, H. U., Sorkin, E.: Studies on chemotaxis. VI. Specific chemotaxis in rabbit polymorphonuclear leucocytes and mononuclear cells. Int. Arch. Allergy **31**, 575—586 (1967b)

Keller, H. U., Sorkin, E.: Studies on chemotaxis. X. Inhibition of chemotaxis of rabbit polymorphonuclear leucocytes. Int. Arch. Allergy **34**, 513—520 (1968a)

Keller, H. U., Sorkin, E.: Chemotaxis of leucocytes. Experientia (Basel) **24**, 641—652 (1968b)

Kivirikko, K. I., Laitinen, O., Aer, J., Halme, J.: Studies with ^{14}C-proline on the action of cortisone on the metabolism of collagen in the rat. Biochem. Pharmacol. **14**, 1445—1451 (1965)

Kolouch, F.: The lymphocyte in acute inflammation. Amer. J. Pathol. **15**, 413—428 (1939)

Kühn, K., Iwangoff, P., Hammerstein, F., Stecker, K., Durruti, M., Holzmann, H., Korting, G. W.: Untersuchungen über den Stoffwechsel des Kollagens. II. Der Einbau von (^{14}C) Glycin in Kollagen bei mit Prednison-behandelten Ratten. Z. physiol. Chem. **337**, 249—256 (1964)

Kulonen, E., Potila, M.: Effect of antirheumatic drugs on sponge-induced granulation tissue, rheumatoid synovial tissue, matrix-free tendon cells and fibroblasts plasma membranes in vitro. Biochem. Pharmacol. **24**, 1671—1678 (1975)

Leahy, D. R., McLean, E. R., Bonner, J. T.: Evidence for cyclic-3′,5′-adenosine monophosphate as chemotactic agent for polymorphonuclear leukocytes. Blood **36**, 52—54 (1970)

Lerner, L. J., Bianchi, A., Turkheimer, A. R.: Anti-inflammatory steroids: potency, duration and modification of activities. Ann. N.Y. Acad. Sci. **116**, 1071—1077 (1964)

Lichtenstein, L. M., Gillespie, E.: Inhibition of histamine release by histamine controlled by H$_2$ receptor. Nature (Lond.) **244**, 287—288 (1973)

Lowther, D. A., Green, N. M., Chapman, J. A.: Morphological and chemical studies of collagen formation. II. Metabolic activity of collagen associated with subcellular fractions of guinea pig granulomata. J. biophys. Biochem. Cytol. **10**, 373—388 (1961)

Luft, J. H.: The ultrastructural basis of capillary permeability. In: Zweifach, B. W., Grant, L., McCluskey, R. T. (Eds.): The Inflammatory Process, pp. 121—159. New York-London: Academic Press 1965

McArthur, J. N., Smith, M. J. H., Freeman, P. C.: Anti-inflammatory substances in human serum. J. Pharm. Pharmacol. **24**, 669—671 (1972)

McCarty, D. J. Jr., Phelps, P., Pyenson, J.: Crystal-induced inflammation in canine joints. I. An experimental model with quantification of the host response. J. exp. Med. **124**, 99—114 (1966)

Malawista, S. E., Seegmiller, J. E.: The effect of pretreatment with colchicine on the inflammatory response to microcrystalline urate. A model for gouty inflammation. Ann. intern. Med. **62**, 648—657 (1965)

Marchesi, V. T.: The site of leucocyte emigration during inflammation. Quart. J. exp. Physiol. **46**, 115—118 (1961)

Marchesi, V. T., Florey, H. W.: Electron micrographic observations on the emigration of leucocytes. Quart. J. exp. Physiol. **45**, 343—348 (1960)

Mauer, A. M., Athens, J. W., Ashenbrucker, H., Cartwright, G. E., Wintrobe, M. M.: Leukokinetic studies. II. A method for labeling granulocytes in vitro with radioactive diisopropyl-fluorophosphate (DFP^{32}). J. clin. Invest. **39**, 1481—1486 (1960)

Meier, R., Ecklin, B.: Die Wirkung des Hydrocortisons auf die infektionsbedingte lokale Leukozytenansammlung. Experientia (Basel) **16**, 204—205 (1960)

Meier, R., Schuler, W., Desaulles, P.: Zur Frage des Mechanismus der Hemmung des Bindegewebswachstums durch Cortisone. Experientia (Basel) **6**, 469—471 (1950)

Metchnikoff, E.: La patologie comparée de l'inflammation. Paris: Masson 1892

Meyer, R. K., Stucki, J. C., Aulsebrook, K. A.: Effect of pregnancy and lactation on granuloma tissue formation and joint permeability in rats. Proc. Soc. exp. Biol. (N.Y.) **84**, 624—628 (1953)

Michael, M., Whorton, C. M.: Delay of the early inflammatory response by cortisone. Proc. Soc. exp. Biol. (N.Y.) **76**, 754—759 (1951)

Monis, B., Weinberg, T., Spector, G. J.: The carrageenan granuloma in the rat. A model for the study of the structure and function of macrophages. Brit. J. exp. Path. **49**, 302—310 (1968)

Morley, J.: Prostaglandins and lymphokines in arthritis. Prostaglandins **8**, 315—326 (1974)

Nimni, M. E., Bavetta, L. A.: Collagen synthesis and turnover in the growing rat under the influence of methyl prednisolone. Proc. Soc. exp. Biol. (N.Y.) **117**, 618—623 (1964)

Oronsky, A. L., Nocenti, M. R.: Influence of hydrocortisone acetate on chemical composition of experimental granulomas. Proc. Soc. exp. Biol. (N.Y.) **125**, 1297—1301 (1967)

Otten, J., Johnson, G. S., Pastan, I.: Regulation of cell growth by cyclic adenosine 3'5'-monophosphate. Effect of cell density and agents which alter cell growth on cyclic adenosine 3'5'-monophosphate levels in fibroblasts. J. biol. Chem. **247**, 7082—7087 (1972)

Page, A. R.: Inhibition of the lymphocyte response to inflammation with antimetabolites. Amer. J. Path. **45**, 1029—1044 (1964)

Page, A. R., Condie, R. M., Good, R. A.: Effect of 6-mercaptopurine on inflammation. Amer. J. Path. **40**, 519—530 (1962)

Page, A. R., Gewurz, H., Pickering, R. J., Good, R. A.: The role of complement in the acute inflammatory response. In: Miescher, P. A., Grabar, P. (Eds.): Immunopathology, Vth International Symposium, pp. 221—230. Basel: B. Schwabe & Co. 1968

Page, A. R., Good, R. A.: A clinical and experimental study of the function of neutrophils in the inflammatory response. Amer. J. Path. **34**, 645—670 (1958)

Paul, S. D., Athanassiades, T. J., Speirs, R. S.: A quantitative procedure for the study of cells in experimentally induced granulomas. Proc. Soc. exp. Biol. (N.Y.) **139**, 1090—1095 (1972)

Paz, R. A., Spector, W. G.: The mononuclear cell response to injury. J. Path. Bact. **84**, 85—103 (1962)

Penn, G. B., Ashford, A.: The inflammatory response to implantation of cotton pellets in the rat. J. Pharm. Pharmacol. **15**, 798—803 (1963)

Perillie, P. E., Finch, S. C.: Quantitative studies of the local exudative cellular reaction in acute leukemia. J. clin. Invest. **43**, 425—430 (1964)

Perper, R. J., Sanda, M., Chinea, G., Oronsky, A. L.: Leukocyte chemotaxis in vivo. I. Description of a model of cell accumulation using adoptively transferred ^{51}Cr labeled cells. J. Lab. clin. Med. **84**, 378—393 (1974 a)

Perper, R. J., Sanda, M., Chinea, G., Oronsky, A. L.: Leukocyte chemotaxis in vivo. II. Analysis of the selective inhibition of neutrophil or mononuclear cell accumulation. J. Lab. clin. Med. **84**, 394—406 (1974 b)

Peters, W. P., Holland, J. F., Senn, H., Rhomberg, W., Banerjee, T.: Corticosteroid administration and localized leukocyte mobilization in man. New Engl. J. Med. **282**, 342—345 (1972)

Phelps, P., McCarty, D. J. Jr.: Crystal induced inflammation in canine joints. II. Importance of polymorphonuclear leukocytes. J. exp. Med. **124**, 115—126 (1966)

Phelps, P., McCarty, D. J. Jr.: Suppressive effect of indomethacin on crystal-induced inflammation in canine joints and on neutrophilic motility in vitro. J. Pharmacol. (Kyoto) **158**, 546—553 (1967)

Phillips, S. M., Zweiman, B.: Cellular mechanisms in the depression of delayed hypersensitivity by 6-mercaptopurine. Fed. Proc. **29**, 701 (1970)

Pick, E.: Cyclic AMP affects macrophage migration. Nature (New Biol.) **238**, 176—177 (1972)

Quittner, H., Wald, N., Sussman, L. N., Antopol, W.: The effect of massive doses of cortisone on the peripheral blood and the bone marrow of the mouse. Blood **6**, 513—521 (1951)

Rebuck, J. W., Crowley, J. H.: A method of studying leukocytic functions in vivo. Ann. N.Y. Acad. Sci. **59**, 757—794 (1955)

Rebuck, J. W., Mellinger, R. C.: Interruption by topical cortisone of leukocytic cycles in acute inflammation in man. Ann. N.Y. Acad. Sci. **56**, 715—732 (1953)

Rebuck, J. W., Smith, R. W., Margulis, R. R.: The modification of leukocytic functions in human windows by ACTH. Gastroenterology **19**, 644—657 (1951)

Rebuck, J. W., Yates, J. L.: The cytology of the tuberculin reaction in skin windows in man. Amer. Rev. Tuberc. **69**, 216—226 (1954)

Riddle, J. M., Barnhart, M. I.: The eosinophil as a source for profibrinolysin in acute inflammation. Blood **25**, 776—794 (1965)

Riley, J. F.: Pharmacology and functions of the mast cells. Pharmacol. Rev. **7**, 267—277 (1955)

Robert, A., Nezamis, J. E.: The granuloma pouch as a routine assay for antiphlogistic compounds. Acta endocr. (Kbh.) **25**, 105—112 (1957)

Robertson, W. van B., Hinds, H.: Polysaccharide formation in repair tissue during ascorbic acid deficiency. J. biol. Chem. **221**, 791—796 (1956)

Robertson, W. van B., Hiwett, J., Herman, C.: The relation of ascorbic acid to the conversion of proline to hydroxyproline in the synthesis of collagen in the carrageenan granuloma. J. biol. Chem. **234**, 105—108 (1959)

Robertson, W. van B., Sanborn, E. C.: Hormonal effects on collagen formation in granulomas. Endocrinology **63**, 250—252 (1958)

Robertson, W. van B., Schwartz, B.: Ascorbic acid and the formation of collagen. J. biol. Chem. **201**, 689—696 (1953)

Robinson, V., Robson, J. M.: Production of an anti-inflammatory substance at a site of inflammation. Brit. J. Pharmacol. **23**, 420—432 (1964)

Rudas, B.: Zur quantitativen Bestimmung von Granulationsgewebe in experimentell erzeugten Wunden. Arzneimittel-Forsch. **10**, 226—229 (1960)

Ryan, G. B., Spector, W. G.: Natural selection of long-lived macrophages in experimental granulomata. J. Path. **99**, 139—151 (1969)

Ryan, G. B., Spector, W. G.: Macrophage turnover in inflamed connective tissue. Proc. roy. Soc. B. **175**, 269—292 (1970)

Saeki, K., Yokoyama, J., Wake, K.: Inhibition of granulation tissue growth by histamine. J. Pharmacol. **193**, 910—917 (1975)

Sancilio, L. F.: Effect of acetylsalicylic acid and hydrocortisone on the pleural response to Evans Blue-carrageenin. Proc. Soc. exp. Biol. (N.Y.) **127**, 597—600 (1968)

Sancilio, L. F.: Evans Blue-carrageenan pleural effusion as a model for the assay of non steroidal antirheumatic drugs. J. Pharmacol. **168**, 199—204 (1969)

Sancilio, L. F., Rodriguez, R.: Effect of non-steroidal anti-inflammatory drugs in the Evans Blue pleural effusion. Proc. Soc. Exp. biol. (N.Y.) **123**, 707—710 (1966)

Saxena, P. N.: Effect of drugs on early inflammatory reaction. Arch. int. Pharmacodyn. **126**, 228—237 (1960)

Selye, H.: On the mechanism through which hydrocortisone affects the resistance of tissue to injury. J. Amer. med. Ass. **152**, 1207—1213 (1953)

Senn, H., Holland, J. F., Banerjee, T.: Kinetic and comparative studies on localized leukocyte mobilization in normal man. J. Lab. clin. Med. **74**, 742—756 (1969)

Slack, H. G. B.: Connective tissue growth stimulated by carrageenin. 2. The metabolism of sulphated polysaccharides. Biochem. J. **65**, 459—464 (1957)

Slack, H. G. B.: Connective tissue growth stimulated by carrageenin. 3. The nature and amount of polysaccharide produced in normal and scorbutic guinea pigs and the metabolism of a chondroitin sulphuric acid fraction. Biochem. J. **69**, 125—134 (1958)

Sorkin, E., Stecher, V. J., Borel, J. F.: Chemotaxis of leucocytes and inflammation. Ser. Haematol. **3**, 131—162 (1970)

Southam, C. M., Levin, A. G.: A quantitative Rebuck technic. Blood **27**, 734—738 (1966)

Spector, W. G.: The mediation of altered capillary permeability in acute inflammation. J. Path. Bact. **72**, 367—380 (1956)

Spector, W. G.: The granulomatous inflammatory exudate. Int. Rev. exp. Path. **8**, 1—55 (1969)

Spector, W. G., Coote, E.: Differentially labelled blood cells in the reaction to paraffin oil. J. Path. Bact. **90**, 589—598 (1965)

Spector, W. G., Heesom, N.: The production of granulomata by antigen-antibody complexes. J. Path. **98**, 31—39 (1969)

Spector, W. G., Heesom, N., Stevens, J. E.: Factors influencing chronicity in inflammation of rat skin. J. Path. Bact. **96**, 203—213 (1968)

Spector, W. G., Lykke, A. W. J.: The cellular evolution of inflammatory granulomata. J. Path. Bact. **92**, 163—177 (1966)

Spector, W. G., Likke, A. W. J., Willoughby, D. A.: A quantitative study of leucocyte emigration in chronic inflammatory granulomata. J. Path. Bact. **93**, 101—107 (1967)

Spector, W. G., Ryan, G. B.: New evidence for the existence of long living macrophages. Nature (Lond.) **221**, 860 (1969)

Spector, W. G., Walters, M. N. I., Willoughby, D. A.: The origin of the mononuclear cells in inflammatory exudates induced by fibrinogen. J. Path. Bact. **90**, 181—192 (1965)

Spector, W. G., Willoughby, D. A.: Histamine and 5-hydroxytryptamine in acute experimental pleurisy. J. Path. Bact. **74**, 57—65 (1957)

Spector, W. G., Willoughby, D. A.: The demonstration of the role of mediators in turpentine pleurisy in rats by experimental suppression of the inflammatory changes. J. Path. Bact. **77**, 1—17 (1959)

Spector, W. G., Willoughby, D. A.: The inflammatory response. Bact. Rev. **27**, 117—154 (1963)

Spector, W. G., Willoughby, D. A.: Anti-inflammatory agents. In: Laurence, D. R., Bacharach, A. L. (Eds.): Evaluation of Drugs Activities: Pharmacometrics, Vol. II, pp. 815—826. London-New York: Academic Press 1964

Stern, P., Niculin, A., Misirlija, A., Ciglar, M.: Histamin im Entzündungsprozeß. Naunyn-Schmiedebergs Arch. exp. Path. Pharmak. **227**, 522—527 (1956)

Stevens, J. E., Willoughby, D. A.: The antiinflammatory effect of some immunosuppressive agents. J. Path. **97**, 367—373 (1969)

Sultzer, B. M.: Genetic control of leucocyte responses to endotoxin. Nature (Lond.) **219**, 1253—1254 (1968)

Swingle, K. F., Shideman, F. E.: Phases of the inflammatory response to subcutaneous implantation of a cotton pellet and their modification by certain anti-inflammatory agents. J. Pharmacol. (Kyoto) **183**, 226—234 (1972)

Thompson, P. L., Papadimitriou, J. M., Walters, M. N. I.: Suppression of leucocytic stiking and emigration by chelation of calcium. J. Path. Bact. **94**, 389—396 (1967)

Thompson, J., van Furth, R.: The effect of glucocorticosteroids on the kinetics of mononuclear phagocytes. J. exp. Med. **131**, 429—442 (1970)

Thompson, J., van Furth, R.: The effect of glucocorticosteroids on the proliferation and kinetics of promonocytes and monocytes of the bone marrow. J. exp. Med. **137**, 10—21 (1973)

Trnavská, Z., Trnavský, K., Kühn, K.: The influence of sodium salicylate on the metabolism of collagen. Biochem. Pharmacol. **17**, 1493—1500 (1968)

Trnavský, K.: Some effects of anti-inflammatory drugs on connective tissue metabolism. In: Scherrer, R. A., Whitehouse, M. W. (Eds.): Anti-inflammatory Agents, Vol. II, pp. 303—326. New York-London: Academic Press 1974

Trnavský, K., Trnavská, Z.: The influence of phenylbutazone on collagen metabolism in vivo. Pharmacology 6, 9—16 (1971)

Trnavský, K., Trnavská, Z., Malinský, J.: A comparative study on the effects of salycilates and of the antiphlogistic corticoids on the inflammatory reactivity of connective tissue. Arch. int. Pharmacodyn. 137, 199—211 (1962)

Tse, R. L., Phelps, P., Urban, D.: Polymorphonuclear leukocyte motility in vitro. VI. Effect of purine and pyrimidine analogues: possible role of cyclic AMP. J. Lab. clin. Med. 80, 264—274 (1972)

Turner, S. R., Campbell, J., Lynn, W. S.: Arachidonic acid. A precursor of polymorphonuclear leukocyte (PMN) chemotaxis. Clin. Res. 23, 54 A (1975 a)

Turner, S. R., Tainer, J. A., Lynn, W. S.: Biogenesis of chemotactic molecules by the arachidonate lipoxygenase system of platelets. Nature (Lond.) 257, 680—681 (1975 b)

Van Arman, C. G., Bokelman, D. L., Risley, E. A., Nuss, G. W.: Changes in the rat's foot with carrageenan inflammation and indomethacin treatment. Fed. Proc. 30, 386 (1971 a)

Van Arman, C. G., Carlson, R. P., Risley, E. A., Thomas, R. H., Nuss, G. W.: Inhibitory effect of indomethacin, aspirin and certain other drugs on inflammation induced in rat and dog by carrageenan, sodium urate and ellagic acid. J. Pharmacol. 175, 459—468 (1970)

Van Arman, C. G., Risley, E. A., Kling, P. J.: Correlation between white-cell count and inflammatory swelling induced by carrageenan. Pharmacologist 13, 284 (1971 b)

Van Furth, R., Cohn, Z. A., Hirsch, J. G., Humphrey, J. H., Spector, W. G., Langevoort, H. L.: The mononuclear phagocyte system: a new classification of macrophages, monocytes, and their precursor cells. Bull. Wld. Hlth Org. 46, 845—852 (1972)

Van Furth, R., Diesselhoff-Den Dulk, M. M. C., Mattie, H.: Quantitative study on the production and kinetics of mononuclear phagocytes during an acute inflammatory reaction. J. exp. Med. 138, 1314—1330 (1973)

Varsa-Handler, E. E., Handler, E. S., Gordon, A. S.: Quantification of cellular influx into the croton oil-induced pouch. Effect of prednisolone. Proc. Soc. exp. Biol. (N.Y.) 124, 562—566 (1967)

Vinegar, R., Truax, J. F., Selph, J. L.: Pedal-edema formation in agranulocytic rats. Fed. Proc. 30, 385 (1971)

Vinegar, R., Truax, J. F., Selph, J. L.: Some characteristics of the pleural mobilization of neutrophils produced by kaolin. In: Abstracts of 5th International Congress of Pharmacology. San Francisco 1972, p. 242

Vinegar, R., Truax, J. F., Selph, J. L.: Some quantitative temporal characteristics of carrageenin-induced pleurisy in the rat. Proc. Soc. exp. Biol. (N.Y.) 143, 711—714 (1973)

Ward, P. A.: A plasmin-split fragment of C3 as a new chemotactic factor. J. exp. Med. 126, 189—206 (1967)

Ward, P. A., Beker, E. L.: Mechanism of the inhibition of chemotaxis by phosphonate esters. J. exp. Med. 125, 1001—1020 (1967)

Ward, P. A., Cochrane, C. G., Müller-Eberhard, H. J.: The role of serum complement on chemotaxis of leukocytes in vitro. J. exp. Med. 122, 327—346 (1965)

Ward, P. A., Cochrane, C. G., Müller-Eberhard, H. J.: Further studies on the chemotactic factor of complement and its formation in vitro. Immunology 11, 141—153 (1966)

Ward, P. A., Offen, C. D., Montgomery, J. R.: Chemoattractants of leucocytes, with special reference to lymphocytes. Fed. Proc. 30, 1721—1729 (1971)

Ward, P. A., Schlegel, R. J.: Impaired leucotactic responsiveness in a child with recurrent infection. Lancet 1969 II, 344—347

Watnick, A. S., Gilchrest, H., Kearney, S., Sabin, C.: The effect of clonixin, betamethasone and cyclophosphamide on endotoxin-induced cellular mobilization, pp. 235—247. In: Future Trends in Inflammation. Velo, G. P., Willoughby, D. A., Giroud, J. P. (Eds.). Padua: Piccin Medical Books 1974

Weisbach, J. A., Burns, C., Macko, E., Douglas, B.: Studies in the synthesis and pharmacology of aporphines. J. med. Chem. 6, 91—97 (1963)

Weissmann, G., Dukor, P., Sessa, G.: Studies on lysosomes: mechanisms of enzyme release from endocytic cells and a model for latency in vitro. In: Forscher, B.K., Houck, J.C. (Eds.): Immunopathology of Inflammation, pp. 107—117. Amsterdam: Excerpta Medica 1971a

Weissmann, G., Dukor, P., Zurier, R.B.: Effect of cyclic AMP on release of lysosomal enzymes from phagocytes. Nature (New Biol.) **231**, 131—135 (1971b)

Whitehouse, M.W.: Some biochemical and pharmacological properties of anti-inflammatory drugs. In: Progress in Drug Research, Vol. VIII, pp. 321—429. Basel-Stuttgart: Birkhäuser 1965

Wilhelm, D.L., Mason, B.: Vascular permeability changes in inflammation: the role of endogenous permeability factors in mild thermal injury. Brit. J. exp. Path. **41**, 487—506 (1960)

Wilhelmi, G.: Influence of non-steroidal anti-inflammatory drugs on experimental serositis. In: Garattini, S., Dukes, M.N.G. (Eds.): Non Steroidal Anti-inflammatory Drugs, pp. 174—179. Amsterdam: Excerpta Medica 1965

Wilkinson, P.C.: Chemotaxis and inflammation. Edinburgh-London: Churchill Livingstone 1974

Wilkinson, P.C., Russel, R.J., Pumphrey, R.S.H., Sless, R., Parrott, D.M.V.: Studies on chemotaxis of lymphocytes. In: Future Trends in Inflammation, Vol. II, pp. 243—247. Giroud, J.P., Willoughby, D.A., Velo, G.P. (Eds.). Basel: Birkhäuser 1976

Williams, G.: A histological study of the connective-tissue reaction to carrageenin. J. Path. Bact. **73**, 557—562 (1957)

Williamson, J.R., Grisham, J.W.: Electron microscopy of leukocytic margination and emigration in acute inflammation in dog pancreas. Amer. J. Path. **39**, 239—244 (1961)

Willoughby, D.A., Di Rosa, M.: A unifying concept for inflammation: a new appraisal of some old mediators. In: Immunopathology of Inflammation, pp. 28—38. Forscher, B.K., Houck, J.C. (Eds.). Amsterdam: Excerpta Medica 1971

Willoughby, D.A., Dunn, C.J., Yamamoto, S., Capasso, F., Deporter, D.A., Giroud, J.D.: Calcium pyrophosphate-induced pleurisy in rats: a new model of acute inflammation. Agents Actions **5**, 35—38 (1975)

Willoughby, D.A., Giroud, J.P.: The role of polymorphonuclear leucocyte in acute inflammation in agranulocytic rats. J. Path. **98**, 53—60 (1969)

Willoughby, D.A., Spector, W.G.: Inflammation in agranulocytic rats. Nature (Lond.) **219**, 1258 (1968)

Winder, C.V., Wax, J., Scotti, L., Scherrer, R.A., Jones, E.M., Short, F.W.: Anti-inflammatory, antipyretic and antinociceptive properties of N-(2,3-xylyl)anthranilic acid (mefenamic acid). J. Pharmacol. **138**, 405—413 (1962)

Winder, C.V., Wax, J., Welford, M.: Anti-inflammatory and antipyretic properties of N-(2,6-dichloro-m-tolyl) anthranilic acid (CI-583). J. Pharmacol. **148**, 422—429 (1965)

Winter, C.A.: Nonsteroid anti-inflammatory agents. In: Progress in Drug research, Vol. X, pp. 139—203. Basel-Stuttgart: Birkhäuser 1966

Winter, C.A., Porter, C.C.: Effect of alterations in side chain upon anti-inflammatory and liver glycogen activities of hydrocortisone esters. J. Amer. pharm. Ass., sci. Ed. **46**, 515—519 (1957)

Winter, C.A., Risley, E.A., Nuss, G.W.: Anti-inflammatory and antipyretic activities of indomethacin, 1-(p-chlorobenzoyl)-5-methoxy-2-methyl-indole-3-acetic acid. J. Pharmacol. **141**, 369—376 (1963)

Wissler, J.H., Sorkin, E., Stecker, V.J.: In: Antibiotics and Chemotherapy, Vol. XIX, pp. 442—463. Schonfeld, H., Brockman, R.W., Hahn, F.E. (Eds.). Basel: Karger 1974

Wissler, J.H., Stecker, V.J., Sorkin, E.: Biochemistry and biology of a leucotactic binary peptide system related to anaphylatoxin. Int. Arch. Allergy **42**, 722—749 (1972)

Zurier, R.B., Hoffstein, S., Weissmann, G.: Mechanism of lysosomal enzyme release from human leucocytes: I. Effects of cyclic nucleotides and colchicine. J. Cell Biol. **58**, 27—41 (1973)

CHAPTER 28

Inhibition of Fever

C. ROSENDORFF and C. J WOOLF

A. Introduction

Fever is a pathological alteration in the thermoregulatory performance of an animal resulting in an elevation in its deep body temperature to an abnormally high level. This disturbance in temperature regulation is produced by a variety of processes including infection, tissue damage, immunological disorders and some neoplasms.

The frequency of occurrence of the febrile response to disease among most mammals makes it tempting to ascribe a survival value to fever. Many claims have been made about its protective role (BENNET and NICOSTRI, 1960). In the lizard, fever is protective against bacterial infections (KLUGER et al., 1975), but in man a beneficial role for fever is controversial (KLASTERSKY and KASS, 1970). On the other hand, fever increases the lethality of endotoxin in rabbits, mice and rats (ATWOOD and KASS, 1964). Fever may, of course, be deleterious to the host but be of survival value to the infective agent.

In clinical practice, the indications for antipyretic drug therapy are not clear (CONE, 1969; DONE, 1959; HUNTER, 1973; SMITH, 1970). The alleviation of the discomfort of the patient and the risk of febrile convulsions in children must be balanced against the diagnostic value of fever and the toxic and allergic side effects of the antipyretic. However, antipyretic drugs are used extremely commonly and it is consequently important to understand their mechanism of action. Before discussing the antipyretic drugs in detail, we will briefly describe some features of the pathogenesis of fever which are pertinent to theories about the mechanism of action of antipyretic agents. The genesis of fever is described in detail in Chapter 18.

B. Pathogenesis of Fever

I. Exogenous and Endogenous Pyrogen

The pyrogenicity of lipopolysaccharide extracted from the cell walls of gram-negative bacteria, endotoxin or bacterial pyrogen (BP), has been recognised for some time. However, it was only in 1948 that BEESON provided the first evidence that BP and other exogenous pyrogens may act through the release of an endogenous pyrogen (EP) from body tissues. The interactions between BP and EP are now fairly well understood (ATKINS, 1960; ATKINS and BODEL, 1972; GANDER and GOODALE, 1975; RAWLINS and CRANSTON, 1973). The production of EP by a variety of cells, consequent on their interaction with a number of "activators," of which BP is one, is illustrated in Figure 1.

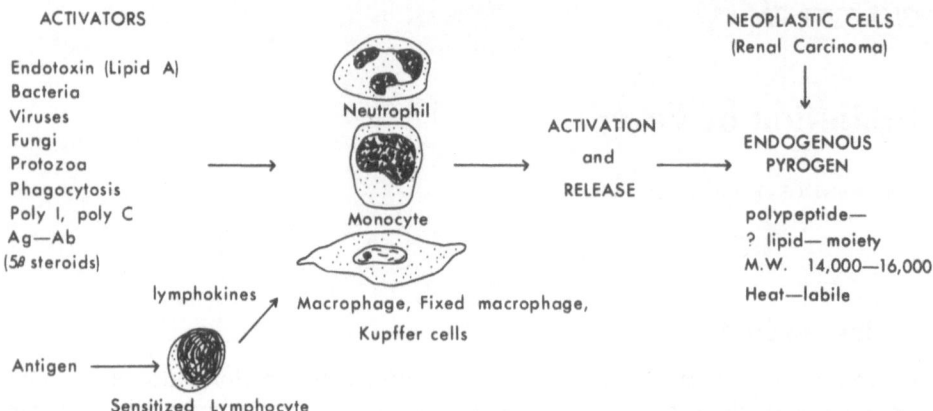

Fig. 1. Production of endogenous pyrogen (EP); a summary of experiments performed on rabbit and human systems. Not all cells illustrated have been found to produce EP in man. The 5-β-steroids activate only human leucocytes and require a longer incubation period than other activators. Actual mechanisms of activation and release are not clear but are presumed to involve protein synthesis of an enzyme which converts an inactive precursor to active EP. Cellular integrity is important for the production and release of EP. Whether EP is a single substance or whether different cells exposed to different activators produce different pyrogens is not known

There is much about EP that remains to be determined, particularly its exact chemical composition (Murphy et al., 1971), the nature of the feedback, if any, it exerts on the cells that produce it (Root et al., 1970), the kinetics of its clearance from plasma (Larber et al., 1971; Rawlins and Cranston, 1973) and, of great importance, its mode of entry into and action on the central nervous system (CNS) (Cooper and Veale, 1973).

II. Site of Action of Pyrogens

The hypothalamus is the major site of the neural control of temperature regulation, integrating information from peripheral and central temperature sensors and activating either heat loss or heat production pathways.

Microinjections of BP (Villablanca and Myers, 1965) and EP (Jackson, 1967) into the anterior hypothalamic/preoptic (AH/PO) regions of the cat produced fevers of shorter latency and requiring much lower doses of the pyrogen than did intravenous injections. Cooper et al. (1967) found that while both BP and EP produced fevers when microinjected into the AH/PO regions of the rabbit, the fever produced by BP had a longer latency of onset than EP-induced fever. Subsequent investigations into the site of action of pyrogens have indicated that the maximum sensitivity, with greatest amplitude of response and shortest latent period, does reside in the AH/PO regions of the rabbit (Rosendorff and Mooney, 1971), the rhesus monkey (Myers et al., 1974), the squirrel monkey (Lipton and Fossler, 1974) and the rat (Veale and Cooper, 1975). The doses of both BP and EP required centrally to produce a fever are at least two orders of magnitude less than that needed to produce a fever by intravenous administration.

Although MYERS et al. (1974) have proposed a direct action of BP on the neural elements of the hypothalamus, COOPER et al. (1967) suggest that direct microinjections of BP into the hypothalamus require the local production of EP to produce a fever, either by recruitment of leucocytes or possibly via glial cells. The whole problem of the passage of both bacterial and endogenous pyrogens into cerebral tissue and their subsequent actions to produce an alteration in the neural activity of appropriate neurones is poorly understood at present. Work by FELDBERG et al. (1971) and COOPER and VEALE (1972) has demonstrated that it is likely that leucocyte pyrogen enters the hypothalamus via the blood stream and that either the pyrogen or its pyrogenic mediators are removed via the CSF.

III. Mechanism of Action of Pyrogens

1. Change in Set-Point or Gain?

The traditional interpretation of fever has been that the rise in body temperature is the result of a change in a set-point signal within the hypothalamus. The level at which the body temperature is controlled is altered but the temperature control mechanisms are otherwise unchanged (COOPER, 1972). Theoretical aspects of an adjustable set-point have been discussed by HAMMEL et al. (1963). In 1970, MITCHELL et al. suggested that the results of neurophysiological investigations into the mechanisms of fever were more compatible with a change in the gain of the feedback control system than with a change in the set-point.

While EISENMAN (1974) has found a depression in central thermosensitivity in rabbits given pyrogen (a result compatible with a change in gain), STITT et al. (1974) failed to find any change in the central thermosensitivity of rabbits with prostaglandin E fever, and claim that the fever is a result of an upward displacement of a central reference point. CABANAC and MASSONNET (1974), using a behavioural technique in man, support the idea that fever is a result of an alteration in the body's thermostat, and that body temperature is then regulated normally about this higher level. The controversy has not yet been satisfactorily resolved.

2. Role of Prostaglandins

The mechanism of action of antipyretics will remain obscure until a detailed understanding of the pathogenesis of fever is attained. A major advance appeared to have been made with the suggestion that prostaglandins of the E series (PGE) mediate pyrogen fever.

PGE was first shown to be pyrogenic by MILTON and WENDLANDT (1971 b). This pyrogenic property is shared in a variety of animals (see FELDBERG and MILTON, 1973; and Chap.18; VEALE and COOPER, 1974) and the site of action is practically identical to that of pyrogen (i.e. AH/PO regions) (STITT, 1973; VEALE and COOPER, 1973; WOOLF et al., 1975b). These observations led to the idea that PGE mediated pyrogen fever. Supporting this idea, FELDBERG and GUPTA (1973) and PHILLIP-DORMSTON and SIEGERT (1974) showed that PGE levels in the CSF of cats and rabbits rose very significantly during pyrogen fever.

In 1971, VANE demonstrated that the aspirin-like drugs inhibited prostaglandin synthetase and suggested that this would help explain their antipyretic activity.

FELDBERG et al. (1973) and HARVEY et al. (1975) have since shown that the elevated PGE levels in the CSF of the cat and rabbit, present during fever, fall during antipyresis. These results seem strong if indirect evidence that PGE does have a role in the pathogenesis of fever. The fact that both BP and PGE_1 require an intact hypothalamic α-adrenoceptor system supports this model of fever (LABURN et al., 1975).

Despite the attractiveness of the theory, reports of a dissociation between pyrogen and prostaglandin fevers are now accumulating. Newborn lambs can respond to pyrogen even when they fail to react to PGE_1 (PITTMAN et al., 1975). Particular lesions in the AH/PO regions abolish the response to intracerebral injections of PGE_1 and EP, but not to intravenous EP in the rabbit (VEALE and COOPER, 1975). Further evidence against a role for PGE has come from CRANSTON et al. (1975b), who have found that the elevated PGE levels in the CSF of rabbits receiving intracerebral injections of EP were effectively prevented by pretreatment with an appropriate dose of salicylate, which did not, however, affect the fever. Moreover, they have found that PGE fever is attenuated by a prostaglandin antagonist, while EP fever is not (CRANSTON et al., 1976). The impact of these recent observations on the strong body of evidence for prostaglandin involvement in fever (FELDBERG and MILTON, 1973, and Chap. 18; VEALE and COOPER, 1974; LABURN et al., 1975; WOOLF et al., 1975b) has yet to be evaluated.

3. Role of Monoamines and Cyclic-AMP

The neural networks of the hypothalamus have numerous synaptic interconnections. A variety of putative transmitters, particularly monoamines, have been proposed as having specific functions in the activation of different temperature regulatory pathways (HELLON, 1972, 1974; HENSEL, 1973). Most of this work has involved the microinjection of different transmitters (e.g. COOPER et al., 1965) and observation of the effects on body temperature. Other experimental approaches have utilised the depletion of monoamines (e.g. WOOLF et al., 1975a) or the antagonism of the putative transmitters with blocking agents (e.g. DHAWAN and DUA, 1971). The results of these studies indicate that these putative transmitters have a role in temperature regulation but that this role differs in different species. Pyrogens and prostaglandins, by activating heat production and conservation pathways and inhibiting heat loss pathways, are likely to activate some synapses which utilise monoamines as transmitters. If so, interference with the production, release and receptor interaction of different transmitters will affect fever in different animals (see Sect. D).

In the rabbit, noradrenaline microinjections into the AH/PO regions produces a hyperthermia and an intact α-adrenoceptor mechanism is necessary for the development of both PGE_1 and BP'fevers (LABURN et al., 1975). It has been proposed that cAMP mediates this α-adrenoceptor mechanism (LABURN et al., 1974; WOOLF et al., 1975b). The dibutyryl derivative of cAMP is pyrogenic when injected into the AH/PO regions of the rabbit (WOOLF et al., 1975b) or when injected intracerebroventricularly (PHILLIP-DORMSTON and SIEGERT, 1975b). Both pyrogen and prostaglandin fevers are potentiated by theophylline, a nucleotide phosphodiesterase inhibitor (WOOLF et al., 1975b), and the levels of cAMP in the CSF of the rabbit are elevated during BP fever (PHILLIP-DORMSTON and SIEGERT, 1975a). An adenylate cyclase inhibitor has been found to attenuate both BP and PGE fever, but fails to

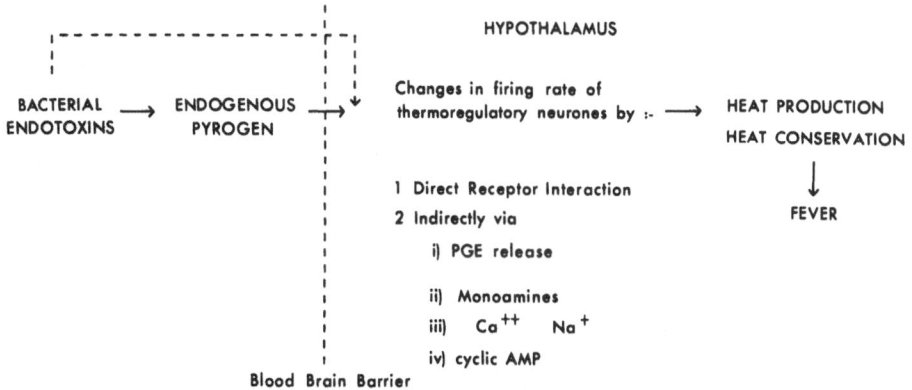

Fig. 2. Pathogenesis of fever; a summary of some salient features believed to occur during development of fever. Although bacterial pyrogens (BP) certainly stimulate EP production, it is not certain whether EP is essential for the pyrogenic properties of BP or whether BP has some inherent activity of its own. The mode of entry of pyrogens into the hypothalamus has yet to be elucidated. Both BP and EP alter firing rate and thermosensitivity of temperature-sensitive neurones, but it is not clear if this is a direct interaction with the specific neurones or whether some mediators which are themselves pyrogenic are produced. Prostaglandins have been provisionally assigned a role in fever by many workers but whether this is an essential "in series" function, is still not clear. Monoamines are unlikely to have a specific function in the pathogenesis of fever, but are more likely to act as transmitters in the hypothalamic temperature regulatory pathways. Although changes in the ionic content of the CSF alters body temperature, the significance of these findings to fever are still to be evaluated. Cyclic-AMP has been speculatively assigned a role in the pathogenesis of fever in the rabbit, but its role in other species is less certain

affect cAMP fever in the rabbit (WOOLF et al., 1976). A role for cAMP in the pathogenesis of fever in cats has also been suggested (CLARK et al., 1974), but more recent evidence (DASCOMBE and MILTON, 1975) fails to support the suggestion.

4. Ionic Mechanisms in Fever

Changes in the relative amounts of sodium and calcium in the CSF of a number of animals affect the body temperature (FELDBERG et al., 1970; MYERS, 1971, 1974). When the ratio of sodium to calcium is abnormally high, fever results. Excess calcium abolishes the sodium fever and the fever due to BP and PGE (DEY et al., 1974). Although MYERS and TYTELL (1972) have found changes in the relative amounts of sodium and calcium extruded into the CSF during fever, no changes in PGE levels were found in the cat during sodium fever (DEY et al., 1974).

Figure 2 summarises some of the CNS events postulated to occur during fever.

C. Antipyretics

The term antipyretics will be reserved for non-steroid anti-inflammatory, analgesic, antipyretic drugs: the aspirin-like drugs. Other drugs which modify fever but in a different fashion will be mentioned separately. Drugs which remove the primary cause of a particular fever, such as antibiotics, antimitotic agents and immunosuppressants, will not be discussed.

The antipyretic effects of extracts of Cinchona bark, containing quinine, have been recognised for many centuries. Following a shortage of Peruvian bark during the Seven Years War (1756–1763), a substitute was found by using extracts of willow bark which contains salicin, the glucoside of salicyl alcohol. In a letter to the President of the Royal Society, the Rev. Mr. Edmund Stone in 1763 described the efficacy of the bark of the willow in curing "agues and intermitting disorders;" since the willow "delights in a moist or wet soil, where agues chiefly abound," this follows the general maxim "that many natural maladies carry their cures along with them." Salicylate was first used as an antipyretic by BUSS in 1875, and acetylsalicylate in 1899 by DRESSER, although it had been synthesised by VON GERHARDT in 1853. The first para-aminophenol drug used as an antipyretic was acetanilid in 1886, but because of excessive toxicity it has been withdrawn from use. Phenacetin was introduced in 1887 and although acetaminophen (paracetamol) was recognised as an antipyretic in 1893, it has only fairly recently been reintroduced clinically. The pyrazolone derivatives, antipyrine and amidopyrine, were first used in 1884 but the danger of blood dyscrasias has severely limited their use. Phenylbutazone and oxyphenbutazone are too toxic for routine antipyretic usage and their indication is limited to their anti-inflammatory activities. Indomethacin, an indole derivative with potent antipyretic properties, is not usually used for the clinical reduction of fever. More recently, anthranilic acid derivatives, such as mefanamic acid, have been found to be potent antipyretic agents. Until the discovery by VANE and his colleagues that aspirin-like drugs inhibit prostaglandin synthesis (VANE, 1971; FERREIRA and VANE, 1974), there was no adequate explanation of the mechanism of the anti-inflammatory, analgesic and antipyretic properties of a chemically very disparate group of compounds.

I. Possible Sites of Action on Antipyretics

During the course of investigations into the mechanism of action of antipyretic agents, a variety of sites of action have been proposed. The following is a review of these sites. Figure 3 summarises the possible sites of action of antipyretics in the sequential processes involved in the development of fever.

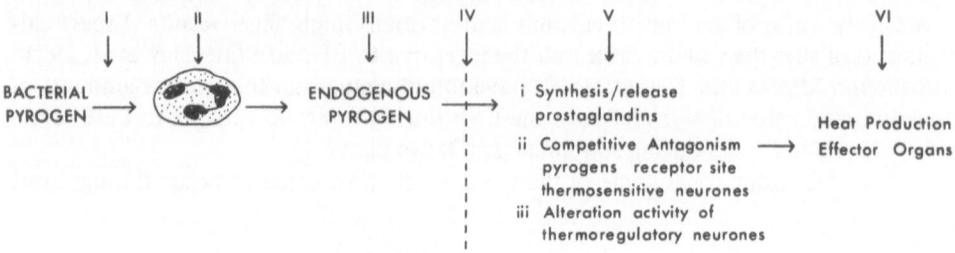

Fig. 3. Possible sites of action of antipyretics. I. Inactivation of BP. II. Inhibition of EP production or release. III. Inactivation of EP. IV. Prevention of access of EP to the central nervous thermoregulatory centres. V. Antagonism of the effects of EP on thermoregulatory centres of hypothalamus, either competitively, or by inhibiting production or release of indirect mediators. VI. Inhibition of heat production and conservation. Experimental evidence favours site V (see text)

1. Inactivation of Bacterial Pyrogen (Site I)

A reaction between antipyretics and exogenous pyrogens rendering the pyrogens inactive, and therefore unable to stimulate the EP-producing cells, could prevent the generation of fever. However, GANDER et al. (1967) showed that incubation of BP with salicylate failed to affect its pyrogenicity.

2. Inhibition of Endogenous Pyrogen Production or Release (Site II)

In the 1950s and 1960s in an impressive series of papers from Barry Wood's laboratory, the importance of EP in the production of fever was demonstrated (see ATKINS and BODEL, 1971). An interference in the production or release of EP would prevent the development of fever. GANDER et al. (1967) incubated leucocytes with salicylate and found that the amount of EP produced was markedly reduced. A number of workers have attempted to repeat this work using the same and different antipyretics and EP-producing systems. None have succeeded in duplicating the inhibiting effect of antipyretics on EP production found by GANDER et al. (see Table 1). VAN MIERT et al. (1971) showed that the amount of EP generated in vivo in rabbit plasma by BP injections was unaffected by pretreatment with salicylate, although the salicylate inhibited fever. CLARK and CUMBY (1975) have recently reported similar observations for indomethacin in cats. Furthermore, the efficacy of a variety of antipyretics, including salicylate, in reducing the fever produced by the administration of EP in a variety of animals (ADLER et al., 1969; CRANSTON et al., 1970b; LIN and CHAI, 1972; CLARK and ALDERDICE, 1972) is incompatible with the GANDER hypothesis of leucocyte inhibition as the sole mechanism of action of antipyretics. Nevertheless, there are still some discrepancies between the effects of salicylate pretreatment on BP fever in the rabbit (WOOLF et al., 1975b) where the antipyretic very significantly reduced the fever, and EP fever (CRANSTON et al., 1971b) where salicylate failed to affect the fever.

Table 1. Antipyretics and the production of endogenous pyrogen

Species	Antipyretic	Dose	Effect	Reference
1. Rabbit leucocytes	Salicylate	4 mM	Decreased EP	GANDER et al. (1967)
2. Rabbit leucocytes	Acetylsalicylate	—	No effect	LIN and CHAI (1972)
3. Rabbit leucocytes	Salicylate phenylbutazone	8 mM 0.5–1.0 mg/ml	No effect	VAN MIERT et al. (1971)
4. Rabbit leucocytes	Acetylsalicylate	2 –20 mM	No effect	HOO et al. (1972)
5. Cat leucocytes	Salicylate paracetamol	0.1–10 mM 0.1– 3 mM	No effect	CLARK and MOYER (1972)
6. Cats in vivo	Indomethacin	500 µg/kg	No effect	CLARK and CUMBY (1975)
7. Goat leucocytes	Salicylate phenylbutazone	8 mM 0.5–1.0 mg/ml	No effect	VAN MIERT et al. (1971)

3. Inhibition of Endogenous Pyrogen Activity (Site III)

Incubation of EP with acetylsalicylate (HOO et al., 1972; LIN and CHAI, 1972), with salicylate (GRUNDMAN, 1969) and with indomethacin (CLARK and CUMBY, 1975) has failed in any way to alter its pyrogenic activity. Antipyretics do not affect the generation of EP or its pyrogenic activity, and the amount and potency of EP is the same in animals rendered afebrile with antipyretics as in febrile animals not given antipyretics (VAN MIERT et al., 1971; CLARK and CUMBY, 1975).

4. Access of Endogenous Pyrogen to the Central Nervous System (Site IV)

In 1968 COOPER et al. found that whilst salicylate administered intraverebroventricularly failed to prevent a fever produced by intravenous EP, salicylate given systemically was effective in abolishing the fever. On the basis of these results, they proposed that salicylate attenuated pyrogen fever by limiting the passage of EP into the pyrogen sensitive areas of the hypothalamus. Subsequently, however, repeated investigations have not only shown that both intracerebral and intraventricular injections of salicylates are effective against BP and EP fevers, but that the doses required are far lower than those needed to produce antipyresis by intravenous administration (CRANSTON et al., 1971c; CRANSTON and RAWLINS, 1972; LIN and CHAI, 1972; CLARK and ALDERDICE, 1972; AVERY and PENN, 1974). Salicylates therefore exert their antipyretic activity in the same area that pyrogens exert their pyretic activity—that is the AH/PO region of the hypothalamus.

5. Hypothalamic Thermoregulatory Centres (Site V)

Microinjection investigations have repeatedly demonstrated that pyrogens act centrally, mainly on a small area of the hypothalamus (AH/PO), an area, moreover, that is recognised to be of great importance in thermoregulation. It is therefore most likely that, since the antipyretics leave the EP-producing system intact and fail to prevent EP entry into the CNS, they act in the AH/PO region. The microinjection work of CRANSTON et al. (1970b) has substantiated this concept by demonstrating that the major antipyretic action of salicylate resides in the anterior hypothalamus, and that in other sites it is relatively inactive. Furthermore, the dose of antipyretics required to attenuate a fever diminishes substantially when the antipyretics are administered directly in the AH/PO region of the hypothalamus (LIN and CHAI, 1972). The site of action of antipyretics having been established, what remains to be elucidated is their mode of action, a subject we will discuss in Section C.II.

6. Suppression of Heat Production (Site VI)

The prevention or attenuation of fever produced by antipyretics could be explained if they inhibited the generation of body heat, either by acting on the neural pathways of the hypothalamus or on peripheral heat production effector organs. If this were the case, then antipyretics would cause a hypothermia in afebrile animals, or in animals exposed to a cold stress that activates their heat production pathways. Table 2 demonstrates that with few exceptions the antipyretic drugs fail to affect the thermoregulatory performance of afebrile animals. Where there is a fall, it is usually not

Table 2. Effect of antipyretics on afebrile animals

Species	Antipyretic	Dose		Route	Ambient temps.	Effect on core temp.	Reference
1. Rabbit	Salicylate	300	mg/kg	i.v.	TN	Nil	Cranston et al. (1970a)
Rabbit	Salicylate	0.6	mg	intraventricularly	TN	Nil	Cranston and Rawlins (1972)
2. Rabbit	Salicylate	6–30	µg	intracerebrally	10° C	Nil	Pittman et al. (1974)
3. Rabbit	Salicylate	300	mg/kg	i.v.	TN but cooled	Nil	Cranston et al. (1970a)
4. Rabbit	Salicylate	360	mg	i.v.	AH/PO		
5. Rabbit	Amidopyrine	120	mg/kg	s.c.	TN	Decrease	Bruns et al. (1950)
6. Rabbit	Indomethacin	30	mg/kg	s.c.	TN	Nil	Kandasamy et al. (1975)
Rabbit	Ketoprofen	3	mg/kg	s.c.	TN	Nil	Kandasamy et al. (1975)
7. Cat	Salicylate	100	mg/kg	i.v.	TN	Nil	Clark (1970)
Cat	Paracetamol	50	mg/kg	i.v.	TN	Nil	Clark (1970)
8. Cat	Indomethacin	40	µg/kg	i.v.	TN	Non d.d. decrease	Clark and Cumby (1975)
9. Cat	Indomethacin	2–25	mg/kg	i.v.	TN	Decrease	Milton (1973)
10. Cat	Indomethacin	2	mg/kg	i.v.	6–9° C	Decrease	Cranston et al. (1975a)
Cat	Salicylate	120	mg/kg	i.v.	6–9° C	Nil	Cranston et al. (1975a)
	Paracetamol	50	mg/kg	i.v.	6–9° C	Nil	Cranston et al. (1975a)
11. Cat	Salicylate	1	mg	intraventricularly	TN	Decrease	Clark and Alderdice (1972)
Cat	Paracetamol	1	mg	intraventricularly	TN	Decrease	Clark and Alderdice (1972)
12. Rat	Salicylate	30–300	mg/kg	i.p.	5° C	Decrease	Satinoff (1972)
13. Rat	Salicylate	300	mg/kg	i.p.	4° C	Decrease	Francesconi and Mager (1975)
14. Rat	Indomethacin	10	mg/kg	i.v.	TN	Nil	Feldberg and Saxena (1975)
Rat	Acetylsalicylate	25	mg/kg	i.p.	TN	Nil	Feldberg and Saxena (1975)
15. Rat	Salicylate	5	µg	AH/PO	TN	Nil	Avery and Penn (1974)
16. Man	Salicylate	3.6	g	p.o.	TN	Nil	Rosendorff and Cranston (1968)

TN = Thermoneutral.
d.d. = dose-dependent.

dose dependent, e.g. indomethacin in the cat (CLARK and CUMBY, 1975). The fever produced in the rabbit by hypothalamic cooling is not abolished by salicylate (CRANSTON et al., 1970a).

Although intrahypothalamic microinjections of salicylate are without effect in the afebrile rat in a thermoneutral environment (AVERY and PENN, 1974), intraperitoneal injections of salicylate in rats exposed to a cold environment produce a marked hypothermia (SATINOFF, 1972; FRANCESCONI and MAGER, 1975). This appears to be a unique case, because exposure to a cold ambient temperature does not alter the effect of antipyretics in the cat (CRANSTON et al., 1975a) or of salicylate in the rabbit (PITTMAN et al., 1976).

Table 2 shows that the vast majority of authors who have investigated this problem have been unable to demonstrate a hypothermic effect of antipyretics in afebrile animals. It is therefore improbable that antipyretics act in any way other than to antagonise the cellular events initiated and maintained by EP; they have no intrinsic activity. Any hypothermic effect produced is probably non-specific and represents activation of systems other than those found during fever. Although the increased lipid solubility of those drugs which do produce a hypothermia (in particular amidopyrine) has been used to explain their antipyretic action by allowing for easier access to the AH/PO region (COOPER and VEALE, 1973), this property is unlikely to be relevant because direct microinjection of a variety of antipyretics into the hypothalamus of the afebrile animal is without effect on body temperature (see Table 2).

II. Possible Mechanisms of Antipyretic Action

In Section C, we have indicated that antipyretics appear to act on the anterior hypothalamic/preoptic regions of the brain and that they only act in the presence of pyrogens. The following are some of the more likely possible mechanisms of action.

1. Inhibition of Prostaglandin Synthesis/Release

Fever research is currently beset by the embarrassing situation that while an essential role for PGE is being increasingly challenged, the generally accepted explanation of the mechanism of action of antipyretic drugs is based on their ability to inhibit prostaglandin synthetase (VANE, 1971; FLOWER and VANE, 1972, 1974; FLOWER, 1974; FERREIRA and VANE, 1974). Inhibition of prostaglandin synthesis has been demonstrated in the brain tissue of dogs, rabbits, mice, gerbils, and cats (see FERREIRA and VANE, 1974). Paracetamol, which is an antipyretic but not an anti-inflammatory drug, selectively inhibits prostaglandin synthetase of brain tissue but not that of spleen (FLOWER and VANE, 1972).

The relative potencies of prostaglandin synthetase inhibitors differ in different tissues and also depend upon the method of assessment. Generally speaking, the order of potency of some antipyretics tested in comparable situations is: meclofenamic acid > niflumic acid > indomethacin > mefanamic acid > flufinamic acid > naproxen > phenylbutazone > ibuprofen > aspirin (FLOWER, 1974). Not all of these drugs have been tested for their antipyretic activity in a quantitative fashion; moreover, a comparison between the potency of a reaction determined in vitro and a biological effect in vivo is difficult because factors such as absorption, distribution, biotransformation and biological half-life influence the in vivo but not the in vitro potency. Another difficulty is that the antipyretics are tested against BP and EP, the potency of which differs from batch to batch.

In spite of these problems, Table 3 demonstrates that the order of antipyretic potency of these drugs is very similar to their potency in inhibiting prostaglandin synthetase. ZIEL and KRUPP (1975) in particular have found a very significant correlation between the antipyretic activity and prostaglandin synthetase inhibition of a number of drugs in the rat. If antipyretics do not act by inhibiting prostaglandin production then this correlation is a most remarkable coincidence.

Since the site of action of pyrogen is central, antipyretics injected intravenously must gain ready access to the brain. Thirty minutes after a 50 mg/kg i.v. injection of salicylate into the febrile rabbit, the brain level of salicylate is of the order of 12.8 µg/ ml brain water (RAWLINS et al., 1973). RAWLINS et al. derived from results of FLOWER and VANE (1972) that such a concentration of salicylate should inhibit prostaglandin synthetase by at least 50%.

Antipyretics do not abolish fever induced by injections of PGE in the rat (MILTON and WENDLANDT, 1971a), in the cat (MILTON, 1973; SCHOENER and WANG, 1974; and CLARK and CUMBY, 1975) and the rabbit (KANDASAMY et al., 1975; WOOLF et al., 1975b). Antipyretics therefore do not antagonise the effects of PGE once synthesized.

Antipyretics are effective in abolishing the non-specific fever which follows some hours after the intracisternal and intraventricular microinjections of saline and calcium-free artificial CSF and which have been shown to be associated with an elevated PGE in the CSF (DEY et al., 1974). Salicylate failed to affect the short-latency fever produced by dibutyryl cAMP (Db-cAMP) in the rabbit (WILLIES et al., 1975), whereas antipyretics reduced the Db-cAMP fever in the cat (CLARK et al., 1974), which is of long onset and therefore more likely to be non-specific (DASCOMBE and MILTON, 1975).

2. Competitive Antagonism Between Pyrogens and Antipyretics for a Receptor Site

Once pyrogen has entered the hypothalamus, it alters the activity and thermosensitivity of specific neurones. Hypothetically, pyrogen could either interact directly with neuronal membrane receptors, or it could act indirectly through mediators; for example, by increasing the production or release of prostaglandins. How these indirect mediators of pyrogen would then act to alter neuronal activity in a specific fashion is not understood.

If EP acts directly at neuronal receptor sites, then competition for the site with antipyretics might explain their antipyretic action (RAWLINS et al., 1971; RAWLINS, 1973). This idea was introduced to explain the finding that salicylate pretreatment in the rabbit was ineffective in preventing EP fever, while the same dose of salicylate given 4 h after the development of the fever was very effective (CRANSTON et al., 1971b). It was suggested that the relationship between the hypothalamic concentration of EP and temperature change was non-linear and that the high concentration of EP in the hypothalamus at the start of the fever would not be antagonised to the same extent as the lower concentration later in the fever (RAWLINS, 1973). Although VAN MIERT et al. (1971) and GANDER et al. (1967) have also found that salicylate pretreatment fails to prevent an EP fever in the rabbit, COOPER et al. (1968) found the opposite, namely that salicylate pretreatment was effective in inhibiting EP fever. Moreover, salicylate pretreatment is very effective against BP fevers in the rabbit (GANDER et al., 1967; WOOLF et al., 1975b), and pretreatment with other antipyretics, including acetylsalicylate is effective in the prevention of fever produced by both BP (BAKER et al., 1963; DASCOMBE and MILTON, 1972; KANDASAMY et al., 1975; HARVEY et al., 1975) and EP (VAN MIERT et al., 1972; LIN and CHAI, 1972). In other species also, pretreatment with salicylate and other antipyretics is effective in reducing BP and EP fevers (Table 3). The failure of salicylate pretreatment to affect EP fever in the rabbit therefore needs to be further investigated before it can be used convincingly to explain either the nature of the antagonism between pyrogen and antipyretics, or the role of PGE in fever (CRANSTON et al., 1975b).

CLARK and COLDWELL (1972) have shown a change in the log dose-response curve of EP in the cat with salicylate and paracetamol pretreatment, which could be compatible with a competive antagonism, but other explanations are possible.

It is difficult to imagine substances as different as salicylate, indomethacin and the anthranilic acid derivatives all competing with EP for the same receptor site. Further studies of the structure-activity relationships of the different antipyretics (e.g. CRANSTON et al., 1971a) must be made, and further dose-response curves studied, before any conclusions on the type of interaction—whether competitive, allosteric or indirect—between EP and antipyretic can be drawn.

3. Alteration in the Activity of Neurones in the Hypothalamus

Salicylate alters the ionic permeability of molluscan neurones (BARKER and LEVITAN, 1971), and also the potential across phospholipid bilayer membranes (McLAUGH-LIN, 1973). Salicylate could therefore have a direct effect on neural activity by altering membrane potentials. This is, however, unlikely to be the mechanism of action because antipyretics appear to be effective only in the presence of pyrogens (Table 2).

The effect of pyrogens on the single unit activity of hypothalamic neurones has been studied. Systemically administered BP depresses the spontaneous activity and sensitivity of warm sensitive neurones and increases both the spontaneous activity and thermosensitivity of cold sensitive neurones in rabbits (CABANAC et al., 1968), and cats (WIT and WANG, 1968; EISENMAN, 1969). EP when microinjected into the hypothalamus of the cat has a very similar effect within 2 min, before body temperature has changed (SCHOENER and WANG, 1975).

WIT and WANG (1968) found that acetylsalicylate administered systemically had no effect on hypothalamic neuronal activity in the absence of pyrogen, but that it produced a return in the responsiveness of neurones depressed by intravenous BP. Microinjections of acetylsalicylate into the hypothalamus antagonise the effect of locally microinjected EP on hypothalamic neurones, but are without effect when microinjected alone (SCHOENER and WANG, 1975).

Because of the technical difficulties of iontophoresing EP onto appropriate hypothalamic neurones, the changes it produces, whether direct or indirect, are difficult to assess. BECKMAN and ROSKOWSKA-RUTTIMANN (1974) have reported that salicylate iontophoresed onto rat hypothalamic neurones altered their neuronal activity. The warm sensitive neurones in particular increased their activity. Although this result

Table 3. Effect of antipyretics on pyrogen fever

Species	Antipyretic	Dose	Route	Pyrogen	Route	Effect	Reference
1. Rabbit	Acetylsalicylate	500 mg/kg	i.g. simultaneously with pyrogen	BP	i.v.	+++	BAKER et al. (1963)
	Salicylate	500 mg/kg				+	BAKER et al. (1963)
	Carsalam	500 mg/kg				++++	
	Paracetamol	500 mg/kg				++++	
2. Rabbit	Paracetamol	125 mg/kg	p.o. 30 min after pyrogen	BP	i.v.	++	CASHIN and HEADING (1968)
3. Rabbit	Acetylsalicylate	100 mg/kg	i.v. 15 min before pyrogen	BP	i.v.	+++	DASCOMBE and MILTON (1972)
4. Rabbit	Salicylate	120 mg fol. by .75 mg/min	i.v. 40 min before pyrogen	BP	i.v.	+++	WOOLF et al. (1975b)
5. Rabbit	Indomethacin	30 mg/kg	s.c. before pyrogen	BP	i.c.v.	++++	KANDASAMY et al. (1975)
6. Rabbit	Ketoprofen	3 mg/kg	i.p. 30–60 min before pyrogen	BP	i.v.	++++	HARVEY et al. (1975)
	Acetylsalicylate	75 mg/kg				++++	
	Paracetamol	150 mg/kg					
7. Rabbit	Indomethacin	5 mg/kg	i.p. 60 min before pyrogen	BP	i.v.	++++	GANDER et al. (1967)
	Salicylate	250 mg/kg		LP		+++	GANDER et al. (1967)
		250 mg/kg				Nil	
8. Rabbit	Salicylate	100 mg/kg	i.v. 60 min after pyrogen	BP	i.v.	+	VAN MIERT et al. (1971)
		100 mg/kg	i.v. 15 min after pyrogen	LP	i.v.	Nil	VAN MIERT et al. (1971)
	Acetylsalicylate	250 mg/kg	p.o. 60 min before pyrogen	BP/LP	i.v.	+++	VAN MIERT et al. (1971)
	Phenylbutazone	50 mg/kg	i.v. 15 min before pyrogen	BP/LP	i.v.	+++	VAN MIERT et al. (1971)
9. Rabbit	Salicylate	300 mg	i.v. before pyrogen	LP	i.v.	++	COOPER et al. (1968)
		300 mg	i.v. before pyrogen	LP	i.c.v.	Nil	COOPER et al. (1968)

Table 3 (continued)

Species	Antipyretic	Dose	Route	Pyrogen	Route	Effect	Reference
10. Rabbit	Salicylate	120–240 mg/kg followed by 0.75–1.5 mg/kg	i.v.	LP	i.v. infusion	d.d.++	Cranston et al. (1970b)
		.12, .6, 1.2 mg	i.c.v. 4 h after pyrogen	LP	i.v.	d.d.++	
11. Rabbit	Salicylate	1.2 mg followed by 360 mg followed by 2 mg/min	i.c.v. i.v. 3 h after pyrogen	LP	i.c.v.	+++	Cranston et al. (1970a)
12. Rabbit	Salicylate	240 mg fol. 1.5 mg/min	i.v. at 1, 2, 3, & 4 h after	LP	i.v. in-fusion	effective antipyresis only at 4 hrs	Cranston et al. (1971b)
13. Rabbit	Salicylate	6–30 µg	AH/PO midbrain	LP	i.v.	+++	Cranston and Rawlins (1972)
14. Rabbit	Salicylate	240 mg fol. by 1.5 mg/min	i.v. 60 min before pyrogen	LP	in-fusion	Nil	Cranston et al. (1975b)
15. Rabbit	Acetysalicylate	25–50 mg/kg	i.v. 3 h after pyrogen	LP	i.c.v.	d.d.++	Lin and Chai (1972)
		25, 50, 100 mg/kg	i.v. 5 min before pyrogen	LP	i.v.	d.d.+++	Lin and Chai (1972)
		2.5 mg	i.c.v.	LP	i.c.v.	+++	Lin and Chai (1972)
		2 mg	AH/PO	LP	i.c.v.	+++	Lin and Chai (1972)
16. Cat	Salicylate	25, 100 mg/kg	i.v. 4 h after pyrogen	BP	i.c.v.	d.d.++	Clark (1970)
	Paracetamol	10, 50 mg/kg	i.v. 4 h after pyrogen	BP	i.c.v.	d.d.+++	Clark (1970)
	Salicylate	10, 25, 50 mg/kg	i.v.	BP	i.v.	++	Clark (1970)
	Paracetamol	10, 25 mg/kg	i.v.	BP	i.v.	+++	Clark (1970)

	Drug	Dose	Pyrogen	Administration	Route	Effect	Reference
17. Cat	Salicylate	0, 25, 1.0 mg	LP	i.c.v. 30 min before pyrogen	i.v.	d.d. ++	CLARK and ALDERDICE (1972)
	Paracetamol	0.5, 1.0 mg	LP	i.c.v. 30 min before pyrogen	i.v.	d.d. ++	CLARK and ALDERDICE (1972)
18. Cat	Salicylate	20, 40 mg/kg	LP	i.v. 30 min before pyrogen	i.v.	+++	CLARK and MOYER (1972)
	Paracetamol	5, 10 mg/kg	LP	i.v. 30 min before pyrogen	i.v.	+++	CLARK and MOYER (1972)
19. Cat	Indomethacin	2 mg/kg	BP	i.v. before	i.c.v.	++++	MILTON (1973)
	Paracetamol	50 mg/kg		i.v. and during		++++	MILTON (1973)
	Acetylsalicylate	25 mg/kg		i.p. pyrogen		+++	MILTON (1973)
20. Cat	Acetylsalicylate	100 mg/kg	LP	i.v. 8 min before pyrogen	i.c.v.	+++	SCHOENER and WANG (1974)
21. Cat	Indomethacin	5–40 µg/kg	LP	i.v. 30 min before pyrogen	i.v.	d.d. ++++	CLARK and CUMBY (1975)
22. Monkey	Salicylate	300, 600, 1200 mg	BP	i.g.	AH/PO	d.d.	MYERS et al. (1974)
23. Rat	Indomethacin	2.5 mg/kg	BP	i.v.	i.c.v.	+++	FELDBERG and SAXENA (1975)
	Paracetamol	50 mg/kg	BP	i.v.	i.c.v.	++	FELDBERG and SAXENA (1975)
24. Rat	Salicylate	5 µg	BP	AH/PO	i.p.	+++ Antipyretic potency	AVERY and PENN (1974)
25. Rat	Diclofenac sodium	0.3, 1, 0, 3.0 mg/kg	Yeast suspension	p.o.	i.m.	0.54 mg/kg	ZIEL and KRUPP (1975)
	Indomethacin	1, 3, 10 mg/kg	Yeast susp.	p.o.	i.m.	1.2 mg/kg	ZIEL and KRUPP (1975)
	Flufenamic acid	10, 30, 100 mg/kg	Yeast susp.	p.o.	i.m.	14 mg/kg	ZIEL and KRUPP (1975)
	Mefanamic acid	10, 30, 100 mg/kg	Yeast susp.	p.o.	i.m.	16 mg/kg	ZIEL and KRUPP (1975)
	Phenylbutazone	10, 30, 100 mg/kg	Yeast susp.	p.o.	i.m.	35 mg/kg	ZIEL and KRUPP (1975)
	Oxyphen-butazone	30, 100, 300 mg/kg	Yeast susp.	p.o.	i.m.	150 mg/kg	ZIEL and KRUPP (1975)
	Acetylsalicylate	30, 100, 300 mg/kg	Yeast susp.	p.o.	i.m.	185 mg/kg	ZIEL and KRUPP (1975)

Table 3 (continued)

Species	Antipyretic	Dose	Route	Pyrogen	Route	Effect	Reference
26. Mice	4-Aminopyrine	3.125, 6.25, 12.5 mg/kg	p.o.	BP	i.c.v.	3.9 mg/kg	CASHIN and HEADING (1968)
	Mefanamic acid	3.125, 6.25, 12.5 mg/kg	p.o.	BP	i.c.v.	4.0 mg/kg	CASHIN and HEADING (1968)
	Flufenamic acid	3.125, 6.25, 12.5 mg/kg	p.o.	BP	i.c.v.	4.8 mg/kg	CASHIN and HEADING (1968)
	Indomethacin	3.125, 6.25, 12.5 mg/kg	p.o.	BP	i.vi.c.v.	6.3 mg/kg	CASHIN and HEADING (1968)
	Paracetamol	6, 25, 12.5, 25 mg/kg	p.o.	BP	i.c.v.	6.8 mg/kg	CASHIN and HEADING (1968)
	Phenylbutazone	6, 25, 12.5, 25 mg/kg	p.o.	BP	i.c.v.	8.9 mg/kg	CASHIN and HEADING (1968)
	Ibufenac	6, 25, 12.5, 25 mg/kg	p.o.	BP	i.c.v.	10.5 mg/kg	CASHIN and HEADING (1968)
	Acetylsalicylate	12.5, 25, 50 mg/kg	p.o.	BP	i.c.v.	15.8 mg/kg	CASHIN and HEADING (1968)
27. Man (adult)	Salicylate	2 g followed by 20 mg/min	i.v.	LP	i.v.	+++	ADLER et al. (1969)
28. Man (adult)	Salicylate	2 g followed by 15 mg/min	i.v.	Natural fevers	—	+++	ROSENDORFF and CRANSTON (1968)
29. Man (children)	Acetylsalicylate	5–12 mg/kg	p.o.	Natural fevers	—	+++	HUNTER (1973)
	Paracetamol	5–12 mg/kg	p.o.		—	No diff. in antipyretic activity	
30. Man (children)	Acetylsalicylate	75–300 mg	p.o.	Natural fevers	—	Combination greater antipyresis than drugs alone	STEELE et al. (1972)
	Paracetamol combination	80–240 mg					

The number of crosses is a relative indication of the attenuation of the fever by the antipyretic compared to control fevers. p.o. per os, i.c.v. intracerebroventricularly, s.c. subcutaneous, i.p. intraperitoneal, i.m. intramuscular, i.g. intragastrically.

was interpreted as a possible mechanism of salicylate antipyresis, this explanation is improbable because firstly the amount of salicylate iontophoresed is likely to have been higher than that usually found effective for antipyresis, and secondly intrahypothalamic microinjections of salicylate in the rat do not produce a hypothermia (AVERY and PENN, 1974).

III. Antipyresis

Although the mechanism of action of pyrogens is not certain, there is considerable information on the actual effect of antipyretics on fever. Table 3 summarises most recent quantitative investigations on the antipyretic activity of different compounds. This activity depends on the species tested, the type and dose of antipyretic used, the route of administration of the antipyretic and its relationship to the time of administration of pyrogen, whether BP or EP. A common method of testing antipyretic drugs is to use the pyrexic effect of injections of yeast suspension. Because the actual mode of fever in this situation is not clear and because comparison between fevers in different experiments is difficult, these investigations have not been included except for the careful and systematic work of ZIEL and KRUPP (1975).

Rabbits are used most often in fever investigations, followed in frequency by cats, rats, and monkeys. The relative efficacy of different antipyretics in natural fever in man is difficult to assess, and only one experimental investigation using an artificially induced EP fever in man has been carried out (ADLER et al., 1969).

What is clear from Table 3 is that, except for the pretreatment of rabbits with salicylate, all antipyretics are effective in preventing or reducing both BP and EP fevers whether given before, simultaneously with, or after the pyrogen. The dose of antipyretic required is lowest when injected directly into the hypothalamus; more is required for intracerebroventricular injections and up to a hundred fold more for intravenous injections. In all studies in which a number of different doses has been used, the antipyretic effect is dose-dependent. The relative potencies of the different antipyretics are much the same in different animals.

D. Inhibition of Fever by Other Means

Although the antipyretics are the agents most commonly used to reduce fever, other drugs have been found to affect fever, particularly in experimental situations. Theoretically, there are two methods of reducing fever. The first is to interfere with the pathogenesis of fever either peripherally or centrally, and the second is to increase heat loss and thereby overcome the thermoregulatory capacity of the body.

I. Increased Heat Loss

Tepid sponging is commonly used especially in children to increase heat loss during fever but is less effective than antipyretics (HUNTER, 1973). Tepid sponging together with antipyretics is more effective than either alone.

II. Monoamine Blockade and Depletion

The monoamines are thought to have a role in the thermoregulatory pathways of homeotherms. Attempts have been made to investigate pharmacologically the requirements for intact pathways involving catecholamines and 5-hydroxytryptamine (5-HT) as transmitters in a variety of animals during fever (see Table 4).

Unfortunately, much of the evidence is conflicting. Reserpine, which depletes all monoamines, was effective in reducing fever in rabbits when used by Desprez et al. (1966) and Metcalf and Thomson (1975), but not when used by Cooper et al. (1967) and Tangri et al. (1975). In the rabbit, noradrenaline microinjections produce a hyperthermia (Cooper et al., 1965), and both catecholamine depletion (Teddy, 1971; Metcalf and Thomson, 1975; Laburn et al., 1975) and α-adrenoceptor blockade attenuated fever (Laburn et al., 1975). In the cat, noradrenaline microinjections produce a hypothermia (Feldberg and Myers, 1964) and catecholamine depletion results in a potentiation of fever (Harvey and Milton, 1974).

Recent unpublished work from our laboratory has shown that 5-HT depletion or antagonism does not affect pyrogen fever in the rabbit, whereas it is reported to attenuate fever in the cat (Milton and Harvey, 1975), results which are again compatible with the different role of this monoamine in the different animals.

Prostaglandin fevers are inhibited by catecholamine depletion and α-adrenoceptor blockade in the same way as BP fevers in the rabbit (Laburn et al., 1975; Kandasamy et al., 1975); both may require an intact α-adrenoceptor system to produce their effects. In the cat, 5-HT depletion reduced low-dose PGE fevers (Milton and Harvey, 1975), but we have found no similar effects in the rabbit (unpublished observations).

III. Cholinergic Blockade

The cholinomimetic substance carbachol and the anticholinesterase eserine result in a hypothermia in the rabbit when injected intracerebroventricularly at a variety of ambient temperatures; microinjections of acetylcholine itself were, however, without effect (Bligh et al., 1971). Cooper et al. (1965) found no response to intrahypothalamic acetylcholine and eserine in the rabbit. Tangri et al. (1975) have shown that while nicotine blockers (d-tubocurarine and chlorisondamine) attenuate BP fever in the rabbit, atropine has no effect, indicating a possible nicotinic mechanism in the development of fever. Veale and Cooper (1975), however, found that atropine blocks both pyrogen and prostaglandin fever in the rabbit.

E. Conclusion

Antipyretic drugs do not affect the production of EP or its entry into the pyrogen-sensitive areas of the brain, and they act in the same area of the brain as pyrogen. Until the details are known of how pyrogen acts to alter the activity of different neurone populations in the hypothalamus, explanations of the mechanism of antipyretics must necessarily remain speculative. The antipyretics are generally without effect on the afebrile animal and only reduce body temperature in the presence of pyrogen, presumably by some kind of anatagonism. Whether they competively anta-

Table 4. The effect of monoamine blockade/depletion on fever

Species	Drug	Monoamine	Pyrogen	Effect	Reference
1. Rabbit	Cyproheptidine	5-HT blockade	BP	Decreased	CANAL and ORNESI (1961)
2. Rabbit	Reserpine	Monoamine depl.	BP	Decreased	DESPREZ et al. (1966)
3. Rabbit	Reserpine	Monoamine depl.	BP	Nil	COOPER et al. (1967)
4. Rabbit	PCPA	5-HT depl.	LP	Potentiated	GIARMAN et al. (1968)
5. Rabbit	α-Methyltyrosine	catecholamine depl.	LP	Decreased	GIARMAN et al. (1968)
6. Rabbit	PCPA	5-HT depletion	LP	Potentiated	TEDDY (1971)
7. Rabbit	α-Methyltyrosine	catecholamine depl.	LP	Decreased	TEDDY (1971)
	6-Hydroxydopamine	Catecholamine depl.	BP	Decreased	LABURN et al. (1975)
	Phenoxybenzamine	α-Adrenoceptor block.	BP	Decreased	LABURN et al. (1975)
	Propranolol	β-Adrenoceptor block.	BP	Nil	LABURN et al. (1975)
8. Rabbit	Reserpine	Monoamine depl.	BP	Decreased	METCALF and THOMSON (1975)
	α-Methyltyrosine	Catecholamine depl.	BP/LP	Decreased	METCALF and THOMSON (1975)
	PCPA	5-HT depl.	BP/LP	Nil	METCALF and THOMSON (1975)
	α-MT + PCPA	Monoamine depl.	BP/LP	Nil	METCALF and THOMSON (1975)
9. Rabbit	Reserpine	Monoamine depl.	BP	Nil	TANGRI et al. (1975)
	Phenoxybenzamine	α-Adrenoceptor blockade	BP	Nil	TANGRI et al. (1975)
	UML 491	5-HT blockade	BP	Nil	TANGRI et al. (1975)
	α-Methyltyrosine	Catecholamine depl.	BP	Nil	TANGRI et al. (1975)
10. Rabbit	Cyproheptidine	5-HT antagonism	BP	Decreased	KANDASAMY et al. (1975)
	Cinanaserine	5-HT antagonism	BP	Nil	KANDASAMY et al. (1975)
	Phenoxybenzamine	α-Adrenoceptor blockade	BP	Decreased	KANDASAMY et al. (1975)
11. Cat	Methysergide	5-HT blockade	BP	Decreased	MILTON and HARVEY (1975)
	PCPA	5-HT depletion	BP	Decreased	MILTON and HARVEY (1975)
	6-Hydroxydopamine	Catecholamine depl.	BP	Potentiated	MILTON and HARVEY (1975)
12. Cat	PCPA	5-HT depletion	LP	Nil	VEALE and COOPER (1975)

gonise the interaction of pyrogen with a receptor, or prevent the synthesis or release of an indirect mediator of fever such as prostaglandin and/or monoamines, is uncertain. The inhibitory activity of the antipyretics on prostaglandin synthetase correlates well with their antipyretic potency. Further work is required either to validate this interpretation of their antipyretic activity or to dismiss it as a coincidence.

The role of prostaglandins in the pathogenesis of fever is still not completely resolved. Recent investigations, including work in our laboratory, have however provided a possible explanation for the evidence challenging an essential role for prostaglandins in fever (Cranston et al., 1975 b; Cranston et al., 1976).

Ziel and Krupp (1976) have now shown that EP can activate a cerebral prostaglandin synthetase system, increasing the synthesis of PGE from its precursor arachidonic acid. Bacterial pyrogen did not have this effect, but antipyretic drugs were able to inhibit the increased synthesis of PGE induced by EP. Unfortunately the effect of EP on the other derivatives of arachidonic acid such as prostaglandin endoperoxide and the thromboxanes was not measured. Arachidonic acid itself produces a fever when injected centrally in the rat (Splawinski et al., 1974), in the cat (Clark and Cumby, 1976), and in the rabbit (Laburn et al., 1977). This fever is reduced by the simultaneous administration of the antipyretics aspirin and indomethacin (Splawinski et al., 1974; Laburn et al., 1977). In the rabbit, however, prostaglandin antagonists failed to modify significantly the arachidonic acid fever (Laburn et al., 1977). This implies that derivatives of arachidonic acid other than PGE, formed distal to prostaglandin synthetase, such as prostaglandin endoperoxide and the thromboxanes, may also be pyrogenic.

Therefore if bacterial pyrogen acts by causing the production and release of endogenous pyrogen from white blood cells and the reticuloendothelial system, and the EP acts on the hypothalamus to activate the prostaglandin synthetase system, this would explain both the elevated levels of PGE found in fever and the antipyretic activity of prostaglandin synthetase inhibitors. Moreover, if in addition to PGE, other derivatives of arachidonic acid are also pyrogenic, then the apparent dissociation between pyrogen and prostaglandin fevers can be reconciled with the accumulated evidence favouring a role for PGE in fever (Feldberg and Milton, 1974; Veale and Cooper, 1974).

References

Adler, R. D., Rawlins, M., Rosendorff, C., Cranston, W. I.: The effect of salicylate on pyrogen fever in man. Clin. Sci. **37**, 91—97 (1969)

Atkins, E.: Pathogenesis of fever. Physiol. Rev. **40**, 580—646 (1960)

Atkins, E., Bodel, P. T.: Role of leucocytes in fever. In: Wolstenholme, G. E. W., Birch, J. (Eds.): Pyrogen and Fever; a Ciba Foundation Symposium, pp. 81—97. London: Churchill Livingston 1971

Atkins, E., Bodel, P. T.: Fever. New Engl. J. Med. **228**, 27—34 (1972)

Atwood, P. R., Kass, E. H.: Relationship of body temperature to the lethal action of bacterial endotoxin. J. clin. Invest. **43**, 151—159 (1964)

Avery, D. D., Penn, P. E.: Blockade of pyrogen induced fever by intrahypothalamic injection of salicylate in the rat. Neuropharmacology **13**, 1179—1185 (1974)

Baker, J. A., Hayden, J., Marshall, P. G., Palmer, C. H. R., Whittet, T. D.: Some antipyretics related to aspirin and phenacetin. J. Pharm. (Lond.) **15**, 97—100 T (1963)

Barker, J. L., Levitan, H.: Salicylate effect on membrane permeability of molluscan neurones. Science **172**, 1245—1247 (1971)

Beckman, A. L., Roskowska-Ruttimann, E.: Hypothalamic and septal neuronal responses to iontophoretic application of salicylate in rats. Neuropharmacology **13**, 393—348 (1974)

Beeson, P. B.: Temperature elevating effect of a substance obtained from polymorphonuclear leucocytes. J. clin. Invest. **27**, 525—531 (1948)

Bennet, I. L., Nicostri, A.: Fever as a mechanism of resistance. Bact. Rev. **24**, 16—34 (1960)

Bligh, J., Cottle, W. H., Maskrey, M.: Influence of ambient temperature on the thermoregulatory responses to 5-hydroxytryptamine, noradrenaline, and acetylcholine injected into the lateral cerebral ventricles of sheep, goats, and rabbits. J. Physiol. (Lond.) **212**, 371—382 (1971)

Bruns, F., Hahn, F., Schild, W.: Über den Wirkungsmechanismus und die Angriffspunkte der Narkotika, Kramgifte und Antipyretika. Naunyn-Schmiedeberg's Arch. exp. Path. Pharmak. **209**, 104—129 (1950)

Cabanac, M., Massonnet, B.: Temperature regulation during fever: change of set-point or change of gain? A tentative answer from a behavioural study in man. J. Physiol. (Lond.) **238**, 561—568 (1974)

Cabanac, M., Stolwick, J. A. J., Hardy, J. D.: Effects of temperature and pyrogens on single unit activity in the rabbit brain stem. J. appl. Physiol. **24**, 645—652 (1968)

Canal, N. C., Ornesi, A.: Serotonina encefalica e ipertemia da vaccino. Atti Accad. med. lombarda. **16**, 69—73 (1961)

Cashin, C. H., Heading, C. E.: The assay of antipyretic drugs in mice using intracerebral injections of pyretogenins. Brit. J. Pharmacol. **34**, 148—158 (1968)

Clark, W. G.: The antipyretic effects of acetaminaphen and sodium salicylate on endotoxin-induced fever in cats. J. Pharmacol. exp. Ther. **175**, 469—475 (1970)

Clark, W. G., Alderdice, M. T.: Inhibition of leucocyte pyrogen induced fever by intracerebroventricular administration of salicylate and acetaminaphen in the cat. Proc. Soc. exp. Biol. (N.Y.) **140**, 399—403 (1972)

Clark, W. G., Coldwell, B. A.: Competitive antagonism of leucocyte pyrogen by sodium salicylate and acetaminaphen. Proc. Soc. exp. Biol. (N.Y.) **141**, 669—672 (1972)

Clark, W. G., Cumby, H. R.: The antipyretic effect of indomethacin. J. Physiol. (Lond.) **248**, 625—638 (1975)

Clark, W. G., Cumby, H. R.: Antagonism by antipyretics of the hyperthermic effect of a prostaglandin precursor, sodium arachidonate in the cat. J. Physiol. **257**, 581—595 (1976)

Clark, W. G., Cumby, H. R., Davis, H. E., IV: The hyperthermic effect of intracerebroventricular cholera enterotoxin in the unanaesthetized cat. J. Physiol. (Lond.) **240**, 493—504 (1974)

Clark, W. G., Moyer, S. G.: The effects of acetaminaphen and sodium salicylate on the release and activity of leucocyte pyrogen in the cat. J. Pharmacol. exp. Ther. **181**, 183—191 (1972)

Cone, T. E.: Diagnosis and treatment: children with fevers. Pediatrics **43**, 290—293 (1969)

Cooper, K. E.: The body temperature set-point during fever. In: Bligh, J., Moore, R. E. (Eds.): Essays on Temperature Regulation, pp. 141—162. Amsterdam: North Holland 1972

Cooper, K. E., Cranston, W. I., Honour, A. J.: Effects of intraventricular and intrahypothalamic injections of noradrenaline and 5-hydroxytryptamine on body temperature of conscious rabbits. J. Physiol. (Lond.) **181**, 852—864 (1965)

Cooper, K. E., Cranston, W. I., Honour, A. J.: Observations on the site and mode of action of pyrogens in the rabbit brain. J. Physiol. (Lond.) **191**, 325—337 (1967)

Cooper, K. E., Grundman, M. J., Honour, A. J.: Observations on sodium salicylate as an antipyretic. J. Physiol. (Lond.) **196**, 56—57 (1968)

Cooper, K. E., Veale, W. L.: The effect of injecting an inert oil into the cerebral ventricular system upon fever produced by intravenous leucocyte pyrogen. Canad. J. Physiol. Pharmacol. **50**, 1066—1071 (1972)

Cooper, K. E., Veale, W. L.: Exchange between blood-brain cerebrospinal fluid of substances which can induce or modify febrile responses. In: Schönbaum, E., Lomax, P. (Eds.): The Pharmacology of Thermoregulation, pp. 278—288. Basel: S. Karger 1973

Cranston, W. I., Duff, G. W., Hellon, R. F., Mitchell, D.: Effect of a prostaglandin antagonist on the pyrexia caused by PGE and leucocyte pyrogen in rabbits. J. Physiol. (Lond.) (1976) in press

Cranston, W. I., Hellon, R. F., Luff, R. H., Rawlins, M. D., Rosendorff, C.: Observations on the mechanism of salicylate induced antipyresis. J. Physiol. (Lond.) **210**, 593—600 (1970a)

Cranston, W. I., Hellon, R. F., Mitchell, D.: Is brain prostaglandin synthesis involved in response to cold. J. Physiol. (Lond.) **249**, 425—434 (1975a)

Cranston, W. I., Hellon, R. F., Mitchell, D.: A dissociation between fever and prostaglandin concentration in the cerebrospinal fluid. J. Physiol. (Lond.) **253**, 583—592 (1975b)

Cranston, W. I., Luff, R. H., Rawlins, M. D.: Antipyretic properties of some metabolic and structural analogues of sodium salicylate. J. Physiol. (Lond.) **216**, 81—82 P (1971a)

Cranston, W. I., Luff, R. H., Rawlins, M. D., Rosendorff, C.: The effects of salicylate on temperature regulation in the rabbit. J. Physiol. (Lond.) **208**, 251—259 (1970b)

Cranston, W. I., Luff, R. H., Rawlins, M. D., Wright, V. A.: Influence of the duration of experimental fever on salicylate antipyresis in the rabbit. Brit. J. Pharmacol. **41**, 344—351 (1971b)

Cranston, W. I., Rawlins, M. D.: Effects of intracerebral microinjections of sodium salicylate on temperature regulation in the rabbit. J. Physiol. (Lond.) **222**, 257—266 (1972)

Cranston, W. I., Rawlins, M. D., Luff, R. H., Duff, G. W.: Relevance of experimental observations to pyrexia in clinical situation. In: Wolstenholme, G. E. W., Birch, J. (Eds.): Pyrogens and Fever: a Ciba Foundation Symposium, pp. 155—164. London: Churchill Livingstone 1971c

Dascombe, M. J., Milton, A. S.: The effect of caffeine on the antipyretic action of aspirin administered during endotoxin induced fever. Brit. J. Pharmacol. **46**, 548—549 P (1972)

Dascombe, M. J., Milton, A. S.: The effects of cyclic adenosine 3'5'-monophosphate and other adenine nucleotides on body temperature. J. Physiol. (Lond.) **250**, 143—166 (1975)

Desprez, R., Helman, R., Oats, J. A.: Inhibition of endotoxin fever by reserpine. Proc. Soc. exp. Biol. (N.Y.) **122**, 746—749 (1966)

Dey, P. K., Feldberg, W., Gupta, K. P., Milton, A. S., Wendlandt, S.: Further studies on the role of prostaglandins in fever. J. Physiol. (Lond.) **241**, 629—646 (1974)

Dhawan, B. W., Dua, P. R.: Evidence for the presence of alpha-adrenergic receptors in the central thermoregulatory mechanisms of rabbits. Brit. J. Pharmacol. **43**, 497—503 (1971)

Done, A. K.: Uses and abuses of antipyretic therapy. Pediatrics **23**, 774—780 (1959)

Eisenman, J. S.: Pyrogen induced changes in the thermosensitivity of septal and preoptic neurones. Amer. J. Physiol. **216**, 330—334 (1969)

Eisenman, J. S.: Depression of preoptic thermosensitivity by bacterial pyrogen in rabbits. Amer. J. Physiol. **227**, 1067—1073 (1974)

Feldberg, W., Gupta, K. P.: Pyrogen fever and prostaglandin activity in cerebrospinal fluid. J. Physiol. (Lond.) **228**, 41—53 (1973)

Feldberg, W., Gupta, K. P., Milton, A. S., Wendlandt, S.: Effects of pyrogen and antipyretics on prostaglandin activity in cisternal CSF of unaneasthetized cats. J. Physiol. (Lond.) **234**, 279—303 (1973)

Feldberg, W., Milton, A. S.: Prostaglandin fever. In: Schönbaum, E., Lomax, P. (Eds.): The Pharmacology of Thermoregulation, pp. 302—310. Basel: S. Karger 1973

Feldberg, W., Myers, R. D.: Effects on temperature of amines injected into the cerebral ventricles. A new concept of temperature regulation. J. Physiol. (Lond.) **173**, 226—236 (1964)

Feldberg, W., Myers, R. D., Veale, W. L.: Perfusion from cerebral ventricle to cisterna magna in the unanaesthetized cat. Effect of calcium on body temperature. J. Physiol. (Lond.) **207**, 403—416 (1970)

Feldberg, W., Saxena, P. W.: Prostaglandins, endotoxin, and lipid A on body temperature in rats. J. Physiol. (Lond.) **249**, 601—615 (1975)

Feldberg, W., Veale, W. L., Cooper, K. E.: Does leucocyte pyrogen enter the hypothalamus via cerebrospinal fluid. Int. Union Physiol. Sci. **9**, 175 (1971)

Ferreira, S. H., Vane, J. R.: New aspects of the mode of action of non-steroid anti-inflammatory drugs. Ann. Rev. Pharmacol. **14**, 57—73 (1974)

Flower, R. J.: Drugs which inhibit prostaglandin synthesis. Pharmacol. Rev. **26**, 33—67 (1974)

Flower, R. J., Vane, J. R.: Inhibition of prostaglandin synthesis in brain extracts explains the antipyretic activity of paracetamol (4-acetaminaphenol). Nature (Lond.) **240**, 410—411 (1972)

Flower, R. J., Vane, J. R.: Inhibition of prostaglandin synthesis. Biochem. Pharmacol. **23**, 1439—1450 (1974)

Francesconi, R. P., Mager, M.: Salicylate, tryptophan, and tyrosine hypothermia. Amer. J. Physiol. **228**, 1431—1435 (1975)

Gander, G. W., Chaffee, J., Goddale, F.: Studies upon the antipyretic action of salicylates. Proc. Soc. exp. Biol. (N.Y.) **126**, 205—209 (1967)

Gander, G. W., Goodale, F.: The role of granulocytes and mononuclear leucocytes in fever. In: Lomax, J., Schönbaum, E., Jacob, J. (Eds.): Temperature regulation and Drug Action, pp. 51—58. Basel: S. Karger 1975

Giarman, N. J., Tanaka, C., Mooney, J., Atkins, E.: Serotonin, norepiniphrine and fever. Advanc. Pharmacol. **60**, 307—317 (1968)

Grundman, M. J.: D. Phil. Thesis. University of Oxford (1969)

Hammel, H. T., Jackson, D. C., Stolwick, J. A. J., Hardy, J. D., Stromme, S. B.: Temperature regulation by proportional control with an adjustable set-point. J. appl. Physiol. **18**, 1146—1154 (1963)

Harvey, C. A., Milton, A. S.: The effect of intraventricular 6-hydroxydopamine on the response of the conscious cat to pyrogen. Brit. J. Pharmacol. **50**, 135—136 P (1974)

Harvey, C. A., Milton, A. S., Straughan, D. W.: Prostaglandin E$_1$ levels in cerebral spinal fluid of rabbits and the effects of bacterial pyrogen and antipyretic drugs. J. Physiol. (Lond.) **248**, 26—27 P (1975)

Hellon, R. F.: Central transmitters and thermoregulation. In: Bligh, J., Moore, R. E. (Eds.): Essays of Temperature Regulation, pp. 71—86. Amsterdam: North Holland 1972

Hellon, R. F.: Monoamines, pyrogens, and cations; their actions on central control of body temperature. Pharmacol. Rev. **26**, 289—322 (1974)

Hensel, H.: Neural processes in thermoregulation. Physiol. Rev. **53**, 948—1017 (1973)

Hoo, S. L., Lin, M. T., Wei, R. D., Chai, C. V., Wong, S. C.: Effects of sodium acetylsalicylate on the release of pyrogen from leucocytes. Proc. Soc. exp. Biol. (N.Y.) **139**, 1155—1158 (1972)

Hunter, J.: Study of antipyretic therapy in current use. Arch. Dis. Childh. **48**, 313—315 (1973)

Jackson, D. L.: A hypothalamic region responsive to localised injections for pyrogens. J. Neurophysiol. **30**, 586—602 (1967)

Kandasamy, B., Giroult, J. M., Jacob, J.: Central effects of a purified bacterial pyrogen, prostaglandin E$_1$ and biogenic amines on the temperature in the awake rabbit. In: Lomax, J., Schönbaum, E., Jacob, J. (Eds.); Temperature Regulations and Drug Action, pp. 124—132. Basel: S. Karger 1975

Klastersky, J., Kass, E. H.: Is suppression of fever or hypothermia useful in experimental and clinical infectious diseases? J. infect. Dis. **121**, 81—86 (1970)

Kluger, M. J., Ringler, D. H., Anver, M. R.: Fever and survival. Science **188**, 166—168 (1975)

Laburn, H. P., Mitchell, D., Rosendorff, C.: Effects of prostaglandin antagonism on sodium arachidonate fever in rabbits. J. Physiol. (Lond.) in press (1977)

Laburn, H., Rosendorff, C., Willies, G., Woolf, C.: A role for noradrenaline and cyclic AMP in prostaglandin E$_1$ fever. J. Physiol. (Lond.) **240**, 49—50 P (1974)

Laburn, H., Woolf, C. J., Willies, G. H., Rosendorff, C.: Pyrogen and prostaglandin fever in the rabbit. II. Effects of noradrenaline depletion and adrenergic receptor blockade. Neuropharmacology **14**, 405—411 (1975)

Larber, D., Tenebaum, M., Thurstan, S., Gander, G. W., Goodale, F.: The fate of circulating leucocyte pyrogen in the rabbit. Proc. Soc. exp. Biol. (N.Y.) **137**, 896—910 (1971)

Lin, M. T., Chai, C. V.: The antipyretic effect of sodium salicylate on pyrogen induced fever in the rabbit. J. Pharmacol. exp. Ther. **180**, 603—609 (1972)

Lipton, J. M., Fossler, D. E.: Fever produced in the squirrel monkey by intravenous and intracerebral endotoxin. Amer. J. Physiol. **226**, 1022—1027 (1974)

McLaughlin, S.: Salicylate and phospholipid bilayer membranes. Nature (Lond.) **243**, 234—236 (1973)

Metcalf, G., Thomson, J. W.: The effect of various amine-depleting drugs on the fever response exhibited by rabbits to bacterial or leucocyte pyrogen. Brit. J. Pharmacol. **53**, 21—27 (1975)

Milton, A. S.: Prostaglandin E$_1$ and endotoxin fever, and the effect of aspirin, indomethacin, and 4-acetaminophenol. Advanc. Biosci. **9**, 495—500 (1973)

Milton, A. S., Harvey, C. A.: Prostaglandins and monoamines in fever. In: Lomax, P., Schönbaum, E., Jacob, J. (Eds.): Temperature Regulation and Drug Action, pp. 133—142. Basel: S. Karger 1975

Milton, A. S., Wendlandt, S.: The effects of 4-acetaminophenol on the temperature response of the conscious rat to the intracerebral injection of prostaglandin E$_1$, adrenaline and pyrogen. J. Physiol. (Lond.) **217**, 33—34 P (1971 a)

Milton, A.S., Wendlandt, S.: Effects on body temperature of prostaglandins of the A, E, and F series injected into the third ventricle of unanaesthetized cats and rabbits. J. Physiol. (Lond.) **218**, 325—336 (1971 b)

Mitchell, D., Snellen, J. W., Atkins, A. R.: Thermoregulation during fever: change of set-point or change of gain. Pflügers Arch. ges. Physiol. **321**, 293—302 (1970)

Murphy, P. A., Chesney, P. J., Wood, W. B.: Purification of an endogenous pyrogen with an appendix on assay methods. In: Wolstenholme, G. E. W., Birch, J. (Eds.): Pyrogens and Fever: a Ciba Foundation Symposium, pp. 59—72. London: Churchill Livingstone 1971

Myers, R. D.: Hypothalamic mechanisms of pyrogen action in the cat and monkey. In: Wolstenholme, G. E. W., Birch, J. (Eds.): Pyrogens and Fever, a Ciba Foundation Symposium, pp. 131—153. London: Churchill Livingstone 1971

Myers, R. D.: Ionic concepts of the set-point for body temperature. In: Lederis, K., Cooper, K. E. (Eds.): Recent Studies of Hypothalamic Function, pp. 371—390. Basel: S. Karger 1974

Myers, R. D., Rudy, T. A., Yaksh, T. L.: Effect in the rhesus monkey of salicylate on centrally induced endotoxin fever. Neuropharmacology **10**, 775—778 (1971)

Myers, R. D., Rudy, T. A., Yaksh, T. L.: Fever produced by endotoxin injected into the hypothalamus of the monkey and its antagonism by salicylate. J. Physiol. (Lond.) **243**, 167—193 (1974)

Myers, R. D., Tytell, M.: Fever: reciprocal shift in brain sodium to calcium ratio as the set-point temperature rises. Science **178**, 765—777 (1972)

Phillip-Dormston, W. K., Siegert, R.: Prostaglandins of the E and F series in rabbit cerebrospinal fluid during fever induced by Newcastle disease virus, E Coli-endotoxin or endogenous pyrogens. Med. Microbiol. Immunol. **159**, 279—284 (1974)

Phillip-Dormston, W. K., Siegert, R.: Adenosine $3',5'$cyclic monophosphate in rabbit cerebrospinal fluid during fever induced by E coli-endotoxin. Med. Microbiol. Immunol. **161**, 11—13 (1975 a)

Phillip-Dormston, W. K., Siegert, R.: Fever produced in rabbits by N^6O^2-dibutyryl adenosine $3',5'$cyclic monophosphate. Experientia (Basel) **31**, 471—472 (1975 b)

Pittman, Q. J., Veale, W. L., Cooper, K. E.: Temperature responses of lambs after centrally injected prostaglandins and pyrogens. Amer. J. Physiol. **228**, 1034—1038 (1975)

Pittman, Q. J., Veale, W. L., Cooper, K. E.: Observations on the effect of salicylate on fever and the regulation of body temperature against cold. Canad. J. Physiol. Pharmacol. **54**, 101—106 (1976)

Rawlins, M. D.: Mechanism of salicylate induced antipyresis. In: Schönbaum, E., Lomax, P. (Eds.): The Pharmacology of Thermoregulation, pp. 311—324. Basel: S. Karger 1973

Rawlins, M. D., Cranston, W. I.: Clinical studies on the pathogenesis of fever. In: Schönbaum, E., Lomax, P. (Eds.): The Pharmacology of Thermoregulation, pp. 264—277. Basel: S. Karger 1973

Rawlins, M. D., Luff, R. H., Cranston, W. I.: Regional brain salicylate concentrations in afebrile and febrile rabbits. Biochem. Pharmacol. **22**, 2639—2642 (1973)

Rawlins, M. D., Rosendorff, C., Cranston, W. I.: The mechanism of action of antipyretics. In: Wolstenholme, G. E. W., Birch, J. (Eds.): Pyrogens and Fever: a Ciba Foundation Symposium, pp. 175—187. London: Churchill Livingstone 1971

Root, R. K., Nordlund, J. J., Woolf, S. M.: Factors affecting the quantitative production and assay of human leucocyte pyrogen. J. Lab. clin. Med. **75**, 679—693 (1970)

Rosendorff, C., Cranston, W. I.: Effects of salicylate on human temperature regulation. Clin. Sci. **35**, 81—91 (1968)

Rosendorff, C., Mooney, J. J.: Central nervous system sites of action of a purified leucocyte pyrogen. Amer. J. Physiol. **220**, 597—603 (1971)

Satinoff, E.: Salicylate: action on normal body temperature in rats. Science **176**, 532—533 (1972)

Schoener, E. P., Wang, S. C.: Sodium acetylsalicylate effectiveness against fever induced by leucocyte pyrogen and prostaglandin E1 in the cat. Experientia (Basel) **30**, 383—384 (1974)

Schoener, E. P., Wang, S. C.: Leucocyte pyrogen and sodium acetylsalicylate on hypothalamic neurones in the cat. Amer. J. Physiol. **229**, 185—190 (1975)

Smith, D. S.: Fever and the paediatrician. J. Pediat. **77**, 935—936 (1970)

Splawinski, J. A., Reichenberg, K., Vetulani, J., Marchaj, J., Kalvza, J.: Hyperthermic effect of intraventricular injects of arachidonic acid and prostaglandin E2 in the rat. Pol. J. Pharmacol. Pharm. **26**, 101—107 (1974)

Steele, R. W., Franklin, S. H., Bass, J. W., Shirkey, H. C.: Oral antipyretic therapy: evaluation of aspirin acetaminophen combination. Amer. J. Dis. Child. **123**, 204—206 (1972)

Stitt, J. T.: Prostaglandin E_1 fever induced in rabbits. J. Physiol. (Lond.) **232**, 163—179 (1973)

Stitt, J. T., Hardy, J. D., Stolwijk, J. A. J.: PGE_1 fever: its effect on thermoregulation at different low ambient temperatures. Amer. J. Physiol. **227**, 622—629 (1974)

Tangri, K. K., Bhargava, A. K., Bhargava, K. P.: Significance of central cholinergic mechanisms in pyrexia induced by bacterial pyrogen in rabbits. In: Schönbaum, E., Lomax, P., Jacob, J. (Eds.): Temperature Regulation and Drug Action, pp. 65—74. Basel: S. Karger 1975

Teddy, P. J.: Discussion contribution. In: Wolstenholme, G. E. W., Birch, J. (Eds.): Pyrogen and Fever, a Ciba Foundation Symposium, pp. 124—127. London: Churchill Livingstone 1971

Van Miert, A. S. J. A. M., Van Essen, J. A., Tromp, G. A.: The antipyretic effect of pyrozalone derivative and salicylates on fever induced with leucocytes or bacterial pyrogen. Arch. int. Pharmacodyn. **197**, 288—391 (1971)

Vane, J. R.: Inhibition of prostaglandin synthesis as a mechanism of action of aspirin-like drugs. Nature (New Biol.) **231**, 232—235 (1971)

Veale, W. L., Cooper, K. E.: Species differences in the pharmacology of thermoregulation. In: Schönbaum, E., Lomax, P. (Eds.): The Pharmacology of Thermoregulation, pp. 282—301. Basel: S. Karger 1973

Veale, W. L., Cooper, K. E.: Evidence for the involvement of prostaglandins in fever. In: Lederis, K., Cooper, K. E. (Eds.): Recent Studies of Hypothalamic Function, pp. 359—370. Basel: S. Karger 1974

Veale, W. L., Cooper, K. E.: Comparison of sites of action of prostaglandin E_1 leucocyte pyrogen in brain. In: Schönbaum, E., Lomax, P., Jacob, J. (Eds.): Temperature Regulation and Drug Action, pp. 218—226. Basel: S. Karger 1975

Villablanca, J., Myers, R. D.: Fever produced by microinjections of typhoid vaccine into the hypothalamus of cats. Amer. J. Physiol. **208**, 703—707 (1965)

Willies, G. H., Woolf, C. J., Rosendorff, C.: The effect of sodium salicylate on dibutyryl cyclic AMP fever in the conscious rabbit. Neuropharmacology **15**, 9—10 (1975)

Wit, A., Wang, S. C.: Temperature sensitive neurones in preoptic/anterior hypothalamic regions: actions of pyrogens and acetylsalicylate. Amer. J. Physiol. **215**, 1160—1169 (1968)

Woolf, C. J., Laburn, H. R., Willies, G. H., Rosendorff, C.: Hypothalamic heating and cooling in monoamine depleted rabbits. Amer. J. Physiol. **228**, 569—574 (1975a)

Woolf, C. J., Willies, G. H., Laburn, H. P., Rosendorff, C.: Pyrogen and prostaglandin fever in the rabbit. I. Effects of salicylate and the role of cyclic AMP. Neuropharmacology **14**, 397—403 (1975b)

Woolf, C. J., Willies, G. H., Rosendorff, C.: Does cyclic AMP have a role in the pathogenesis of fever in the rabbit? Naturwissenschaften **63**, 94 (1976)

Ziel, R., Krupp, P.: Effect on prostaglandin synthesis and antipyretic activity of non steroid anti-inflammatory drugs. In: Schönbaum, E., Lomax, P., Jacob, J. (Eds.): Temperature Regulation and Drug Action, pp. 233—241. Basel: S. Karger 1975

Ziel, R., Krupp, P.: Influence of endogenous pyrogen on the cerebral prostaglandin-synthetase system. Experientia (Basel) **32**, 1451—1453 (1976)

CHAPTER 29

Evaluation of the Toxicity
of Anti-Inflammatory Drugs

P. W. DODGE, D. A. BRODIE, and B. D. MITCHELL

A. Introduction

I. Historical Overview

The importance of the problem of anti-inflammatory drug toxicity comes into perspective when it is recognised that there are approximately 40 million people in the United States suffering from arthritis (EMMITT, 1975). About half of this population is under medical care and the other half is self-treated; of those under medical care, one-third require chronic drug administration, and the remainder, intermittent administration. Arthritis is a prevalent disease worldwide: if there were a 10% incidence of drug-related side-effects (a conservative estimate), there would be the possibility of drug-induced toxicity in 5 million patients per year of those under medical treatment, and at least twice this number for those patients who would self-administer an anti-inflammatory drug such as aspirin.

The complexity and variability of rheumatic disease can be appreciated from the classification of the disease by the American Rheumatoid Association into 13 major classes with 73 subclasses (DECKER et al., 1964). The number of drugs available for the therapy of rheumatic conditions has rapidly increased in the last decade with the promise of an even wider choice in the decade to come. Pharmacological treatment of rheumatic disease has been a mixed blessing, and the initial clinical enthusiasm for each new drug has abated as the incidence of clinical toxicity increases with wider usage. Identification of potential clinical toxicity is the responsibility of the pharmacologist and toxicologist, and this review will examine the animal models available for prediction of clinical toxicity and indicate the relative value of current methodology. Since it is axiomatic that all drugs produce toxicity at some dose, the major toxicity produced by anti-inflammatory drugs will be considered in detail, rather than all reported toxic effects which include the allergic or idiosyncratic reactions that can be anticipated with any class of drugs.

The prediction of clinical toxicity from animal data of anti-inflammatory drugs ranges from excellent to impossible (LEVY, 1974). It is complicated by several factors: antirheumatic therapy is usually chronic; drug therapy is palliative; the drugs do not alter the degenerative course of the disease; and patient susceptibility to side effects is extremely variable. While lethality and organ toxicity can be determined in several animal species by administering high dose levels acutely or chronically, this is expensive and time-consuming and is related to the toxic dose. The current problem is to devise animal models that will predict toxicity from acute studies and provide a therapeutic index based on activity to side effects rather than on activity to lethality. Research for the development of new anti-inflammatory agents has expanded greatly so that accurate toxicity assessment and prediction from preclinical data would reduce the number of drugs taken to clinical trial and indicate their advantage over established therapy. Retrospectively, it has been possible to identify several toxic or unwanted effects produced by anti-inflammatory drugs. New animal models for toxicity will be judged by prospective clinical comparison of new agents with drugs in current use.

The development of therapy for rheumatoid arthritis (RA) began in folk medicine when extracts of willow bark were used for treatment over a hundred years ago (RODNAN and BENEDEK, 1970). The bitter glycoside salicin was discovered in the early 1800s; salicylic acid was made from salicin and its sodium salt was later used in rheumatic fever. When large doses were prescribed, salicylate toxicity was identified and one of the major problems turned out to be gastric intolerance. Acetylsalicylic acid (aspirin) was said to be synthesized in the search for a substitute which had fewer gastric problems (RODNAN and BENEDEK, 1970). In the late 1920s, the use of gold for RA was suggested (FORESTIER, 1929), but it was not until the late 1930s to mid-1940s that sufficient clinical trials had been carried out to consider gold as important therapy in the disease (FORESTIER, 1935; SNYDER et al., 1939; ELLMAN et al., 1940). Salicylates remained the major drug for treatment, and during this time several congeners were prepared in order to reduce toxicity. While this was success-ful in the case of antipyrine, since the compound was effective and did not produce gastric distress, its use and that of a close analogue, aminopyrine, caused serious blood dyscrasias (RODNAN and BENEDEK, 1970). The results of this early attempt to improve anti-inflammatory drugs appear to characterise the class; as one side effect is removed, other equally limiting toxicity has appeared.

A congener of these agents, phenylbutazone, was introduced into therapy in the early 1950s (BURNS et al., 1952), and this agent along with its hydroxy analogue, oxyphenylbutazone, was used in patients refractive to other anti-inflammatory agents, but the problem of gastrointestinal toxicity remained. At the same time, the clinical trial of steroid anti-inflammatory agents (HENCH et al., 1949) marked the beginning of a new era and radical departure in drug therapy for the treatment of arthritis. However, these agents, while apparently innocuous in short-term therapy, proved to have severe and life-threatening adverse reaction when given over a long term (BERLINGER, 1974). In the early 1960s, another major change in therapy oc-curred with the discovery of a non-steroid anti-inflammatory drug, indomethacin (WINTER et al., 1963; MICHOTTE and WAUTERS, 1964), which is chemically unrelated to the salicylates, the steroids, or phenylbutazone. However, there was still no great separation of therapeutic activity and adverse reactions. Two classes of compounds, the antimalarial drugs and D-penicillamine (JAFFE, 1963; DAY et al., 1974), have been used with increasing frequency from the early 1960s as alternative therapy. In the 1970s, successors to indomethacin such as alclofenac, ibuprofen, and ketoprofen appeared in clinical trial and therapy in Europe. These drugs are less potent than indomethacin, share many of its side effects, but offer alternatives to this drug.

B. Evaluation of Toxicity in Man

The major toxicities of anti-inflammatory drugs occur in several organ systems: the gastrointestinal tract, CNS, haematopoetic process, kidney, skin, liver, and eye. The currently marketed anti-arthritic drugs present both the physician and patient with side-effects which often are severe enough to interrupt therapy. These drugs differ in

Table 1. Adverse reactions of anti-inflammatory drugs (Bach, 1973; Cuthbert, 1974; Physician's desk reference, 1975)

Drug class	Average daily dose, Gm	GI	CNS	Skin	Blood	Renal	He-patic	Ocular
Salicylates (acetylsalicylic acid)	1.8–5.0 p.o.	+ +	+ +	+	+	+	+	
Gold (sodium aurothioglycate)	0.01–0.05 s.c.	+	+	+ +	+ +	+		
Steroids (prednisolone)	0.005–0.030 p.o.	+ +	+	+	+	+		
Phenylbutazone	0.4–0.6 p.o.	+ +	+	+	+ +	+	+	
Indomethacin	0.05–0.2 p.o.	+ +	+ +	+	+	+	+	+
Antimalarials (hydroxy-chloroquine)	0.2–0.6 p.o.	+	+	+	+ +			+ +
D-penicillamine	0.3–0.6 p.o.	+		+	+	+ +	+	+
Arylalkanoic acids (ibuprofen)	0.9–1.6 p.o.	+	+	+	+	+	+	

+ + Major reaction   p.o. Per os
+   Minor reaction   s.o. Subcutaneous

the incidence of side reaction with different organ systems and certain of the agents have specific organ toxicity, such as: ocular toxicity produced by antimalarials (Hen-kind, 1965; Carr, 1968), taste loss produced by D-penicillamine (Day et al., 1974), or headache with indomethacin (Cuthbert, 1974). Generally, as the potency of the medication increases, so do the side effects and this necessitates careful evaluation by the physician of the benefit-to-risk ratio. The major adverse reactions of anti-inflammatory drugs are listed in Table 1; each group of drugs has side effects which range from annoying to life-threatening. The problem of producing an anti-inflammatory agent without the restricting side effects has not been solved. This is due in part to the lack of appropriate animal models, particularly in the area of CNS side-effects which cannot be quantitatively determined in animals (Keeney, 1974).

I. Gastrointestinal Tract

Gastrointestinal side effects, while usually not life-threatening, are often responsible for eliminating the drug from the therapeutic regime. All of the available anti-inflammatory drugs affect the gastrointestinal system and most of them have ulcero-genic potential (Hart, 1970). Nausea, vomiting and gastric distress occur in about 10% of the patients taking large doses of salicylate and occult bleeding occurs in about 70% (A.M.A., 1973). While the amount of blood lost per day is small (about 4 ml/day, Prescott, 1972), gastric distress and the threat of massive bleeding can limit the utility of the drug in many patients. Protection of the stomach by antacids or giving medication with milk offers little help (CROFT et al., 1972), and the blood loss can be severe enough to produce iron deficiency anaemia (PRESCOTT, 1972).

Gastrointestinal disturbances such as nausea, gastrointestinal distress, indigestion, vomiting, stomatitis, and diarrhoea have been reported in 15–25% of patients taking indomethacin or phenylbutazone (PRESCOTT, 1972; KAMMERER, 1974), and peptic ulceration has also been reported with indomethacin (FISCHER and RINKOFF, 1969; LEVY and GASPAR, 1975; TAYLOR et al., 1968). Gastrointestinal disturbances are found with antimalarials and gold (KAMMERER, 1974), but since these drugs are known to have other toxicities, the patients are generally watched more closely and drug therapy can be stopped before major damage occurs. The incidence of peptic ulcer in rheumatic patients appears to be increasing and there is evidence that anti-inflammatory drugs exacerbate pre-existing ulcers and should be contra-indicated in the presence of an active ulcer (A.M.A., 1973). One major difference in the gastrointestinal toxicity of steroids is that they produce "silent ulcers" which occur relatively rapidly and painlessly while there is usually some warning of gastrointestinal irritation with the non-steroid anti-inflammatory drugs (GARB et al., 1965; CUSHMAN, 1970).

II. Central Nervous System

CNS disturbances connected with anti-inflammatory therapy include tremors, weakness, ataxia, headache, vertigo, blurring of vision, diplopia, confusion, and agitation (KAMMERER, 1974). The classic symptom of salicylism is tinnitus and hearing loss (KAMMERER, 1974; A.M.A., 1973; PEREZ and HAYDEN, 1968); the ototoxic effects are reversible and are used to determine the maximum tolerated daily dose (A.M.A., 1973). Headache, giddiness and depression are encountered with phenylbutazone therapy (PRESCOTT, 1972). Indomethacin headache is usually frontal (HEALEY, 1967) and occurs in 20–60% of patients (O'BRIEN, 1968). It is of a severe throbbing nature especially in the morning and may be associated with dizziness, vomiting, and confusion (HODGKINSON and WOOLF, 1973; CUTHBERT, 1974). Antimalarial therapy and high doses of steroids have been reported to produce changes in mental attitude or psychosis (BROOKES, 1966; BOSTON U., 1972).

III. Dermatological Disorders

Urticaria is a common complication of anti-inflammatory therapy (ALMEYDA and BAKER, 1970; FARR, 1970) and is seen with aspirin (MATHEWS and STAGE, 1974; DE WECK, 1974), phenylbutazone, indomethacin (PRESCOTT, 1972) and gold therapy. Gold-induced dermatitis is the most serious dermatological problem (WALZER and FEINSTEIN, 1971; QUE, 1968; MYERS, 1971). Exfoliative dermatitis has been reported with chloroquine therapy and prolonged administration may cause bluish pigmentation of the skin (A.M.A., 1973). Systemic corticosteroid therapy has been known to cause skin trauma (DAVID, 1972).

IV. Haematopoietic System

Salicylate prolongation of bleeding time (QUICK, 1970) is usually considered a side effect in therapy of RA; however, this effect may have therapeutic application in the reduction of mortality and frequency of myocardial infarction (ELWOOD et al., 1974).

Bone marrow depression is a serious adverse effect which has been reported with phenylbutazone (A.M.A., 1973; WOODLIFF and DOUGAN, 1964; BRUMETT, 1972) and steroid therapy (STREETEN, 1975); this is manifested by leucopenia, pancytopenia, agranulocytosis, and aplastic anemia (PRESCOTT, 1972). Also the tolerance of plasma to heparin is raised while fibrinolytic activity falls. Blood dyscrasias are frequent with antimalarial therapy (MANSON-BAHR, 1972) and gold therapy (CANADA, 1973; KAY, 1973; ENGLAND and SMITH, 1972; ROSA and KRA, 1974).

V. Ocular Disturbances

Serious eye complications associated with the use of chloroquine and hydroxychloroquine are frequent (CARR et al., 1968; HILL, 1963; HENKIND, 1965; PERCIVAL and MEANOCK, 1968; RUBIN, 1968). Diplopia is reversible, but blurred vision due to corneal opacities and chorioretinitis may signal an irreversible damage. Progressive impairment of vision after discontinuation of the drug may lead to blindness (MANSON-BAHR, 1972). Retinal sensitivity has been a complaint with indomethacin therapy (BURNS, 1968), but is reversible when the drug is discontinued.

VI. Renal Side Effects

Renal toxicity has been reported as a side effect of salicylate therapy but a recent study suggests that aspirin, per se, is not the cause of kidney damage, but rather an additive effect with other analgesics (CAUGHEY et al., 1974). Toxic nephritis has been reported with gold therapy (STEELE, 1975; SILVERBERG et al., 1970; MYERS, 1971), but it is not a common side effect as it is with D-penicillamine therapy (HIRSCHMAN and ISSELBACHER, 1965); use of both drugs would be contra-indicated in patients with impaired renal function. Changes in kidney function are also noted with steroid therapy and phenylbutazone treatment.

VII. Miscellaneous Side Effects

Allergy to salicylates can produce asthma severe enough to necessitate discontinuation of the medication (ANON, 1969). Hepatic damage has been reported with both salicylates (ANON, 1973; WOLFE et al., 1974; ATHREYA et al., 1973) and phenylbutazone (PRESCOTT, 1972), while steroids cause a wide range of side effects ranging from necrotizing arteritis (DE LANGE and DORENBOS, 1972) to osteoporosis with pathological fracture (BUCHANAN et al., 1970). Antimalarials have been shown to cross the placental barrier and cause injury to the fetus (MANSON-BAHR, 1972) and there is also risk of cochlear damage (HART and NAUNTON, 1964) with these agents.

C. Methods Used to Evaluate Toxicity in Animals

The World Health Organization (1966), GOLDENTHAL (1968), and ZBINDEN (1964) have published guidelines for preclinical evaluation of drug safety. It is obvious, because of the high cost of manpower, space, and animals, that acute tests to predict potential toxicity would be preferable to chronic drug administration. Unfortunately, only gastrointestinal damage, photosensitivity, and chloroquine-induced eye damage can be predicted by acute drug administration. Anti-inflammatory drugs offer a unique challenge to toxicological assessment because of the diverse types of chemical structures associated with this pharmacological activity (WHITEHOUSE, 1965); LEVY (1974) has recently reviewed the toxicological methodology for evaluating this class of drugs. It is too large a task to discuss all of the potential clinical side effects of anti-inflammatory drugs, but there are certain recurring organ toxicities that are characteristic of this class of drugs. This part of the review will be confined to a discussion of the availability of animal models to predict clinical toxicity in the following systems: gastrointestinal, haematopoietic, hepatic, renal, ocular, CNS, and skin.

I. Gastrointestinal

Gastrointestinal ulceration is a well-known side effect following the administration of steroid as well as non-steroid anti-inflammatory drugs to man. Extensive preclinical experimentation has been carried out to develop suitable animal models for estimating potential gastrointestinal damage from new anti-inflammatory drugs. Non-steroid anti-inflammatory drugs produce gastric lesions in a variety of common laboratory animals. These gastric lesions may be observed grossly or following fixation and staining for histological examination.

The gastric mucosa of the mouse is damaged by aspirin (HINGSON and ITO, 1971). Although this species would be very inexpensive to use, the small size of the animals requires the inconvenience of fixation and histological examination to visualise properly the gastric damage. Steroid as well as non-steroid anti-inflammatory drugs produce gastric damage in the dog (DAVISON et al., 1966; HURLEY and CRANDALL, 1964; MAX and MENGUY, 1970), but the size and expense of this animal limits its use in routine screening for potential gastrointestinal damage.

The rat and guinea pig have been employed extensively to evaluate visually acute gastric damage produced by anti-inflammatory drugs (WILHELMI, 1961; ANDERSON, 1964a, 1964b; DOMENJOZ, 1960; BRODIE and CHASE, 1969; HITCHENS et al., 1967; JOHANSSON and LINDQUIST, 1971). For non-steroid anti-inflammatory drugs, these methods vary slightly in design, but generally the animals are fasted overnight and then receive a single dose of the compound to be evaluated; they are killed within 4 h following that dose. The stomach is removed and mucosal damage is visually determined using various scoring systems. Experiments in rats of different ages have shown that juvenile animals are less sensitive than adults to the gastric damage produced by non-steroid anti-inflammatory drugs (WILHELMI, 1972; BONFILS, 1959; KOHUT and NICAK, 1969). Chronic drug administration for the demonstration of gastric lesions is not warranted since gastric lesions occur less frequently in non-fasted animals or in animals that have ingested faeces (ANDERSON, 1964a, 1964b; BRODIE et al., 1971a). The lesions are not chronic in nature and there is virtually no evidence of damage 24 h after the last dose.

Gastric damage may be manifested as blood loss without ulceration. Chromium-51 (^{51}Cr) labelled erythrocytes are employed in humans to measure gastrointestinal blood loss (EBAUGH et al., 1958). EDELSON and DOUGLAS (1973) have adapted this method to the rat using pooled (homologous) ^{51}Cr labelled red cells from rats. This procedure was suggested to be superior to using labelled red cells from the same animal (autologous), as performed by Owen et al. (1954) in the dog and Cohen (1965) in the rat. Phillips (1973) has described a method to assess gastrointestinal microbleeding in the dog using ^{59}Fe.

Assessment of gastric damage induced by steroid anti-inflammatory drugs requires somewhat different methodology than non-steroid anti-inflammatory agents. It seems clear that in steroid-treated patients, the relative incidence of duodenal vs. gastric ulcers is much less than that encountered with non-steroid anti-inflammatory drugs (Cushman, 1970). Robert and Nezamis (1958) have described a method where multiple gastric ulcers were produced with steroid anti-inflammatory drugs. The test steroid was administered subcutaneously once a day for 4 days to fasted rats. The test can be used quantitatively since it is expressed as an ulcer index. An important characteristic of the steroid-induced ulcer is its location. It is always found in the glandular (pyloric) portion of the stomach where the mucosa is similar to that of the human stomach. Ingle et al. (1951) showed that some non-fasted rats receiving high doses of cortisone acetate developed gastric ulcers in 3 weeks. Kahn et al. (1963) and Skoryna et al. (1958) studied the effects of chronic intermittent cortisone administration on healing of cautery-induced gastric ulcers in the rat. Steroid treatment resulted in far more persistent and extensive lesions than were seen in the control groups.

Although the most prominent pathological finding with non-steroid anti-inflammatory drugs has been in the stomach, intestinal lesions have been reported as well (Kirsner and Ford, 1955; Hucker et al., 1966; Levrat and Lambert, 1960). These lesions, as in the case of gastric lesions, can be demonstrated following single oral doses of the drug, primarily in the rat. Wax et al. (1975) have described a method for visualising both gastric and intestinal lesions 24 h following a single dose of a number of non-steroid anti-inflammatory drugs. Following the administration of indomethacin in the rat, Brodie et al. (1970, 1971a) and Wax et al. (1970) demonstrated that food deprivation or bile duct ligation inhibited or significantly reduced the incidence of intestinal ulcers induced with indomethacin, aspirin, and the fenamates. The use of a marker dye, pontamine sky blue, facilitated the detection of aspirin-induced intestinal lesions in the rat.

II. Kidney

The majority of compounds used for anti-inflammatory purposes are not particularly toxic to the human kidney (Levy, 1974). Gold, penicillamine, and salicylates have been implicated in kidney disease (Burry, 1973). Leblanc and Vernet (1973) have stated that phenylbutazone has a direct toxic action on the kidney tubules.

There are a large number of kidney function tests described in the literature which are based on the ability of the kidneys to excrete solutes or to concentrate urine. Doubts have been raised as to whether any one or a combination of several of these tests is adequate to detect early renal damage without resorting to histological inspection of renal tissue. Foulkes and Hammond (1975) have discussed the pros and cons of the "routine" tests. Tests commonly employed to predict kidney damage are: simple urinalysis for glucose, amino acids, epithelial cells, protein, etc.; PAH clearance; creatinine excretion as a measure of glomerular filtration rate; glutamic oxaloacetic transaminase and phenol red excretion to predict tubular damage.

Although studies are very limited, anti-inflammatory drugs do not appear to share a common mechanism for producing kidney toxicity in laboratory animals. In a comparative study using rats, oxyphenbutazone and phenylbutazone decreased the renal excretion of sodium and water, whereas indomethacin was without effect. Also, in contrast to indomethacin, oxyphenbutazone produced a rise in the corticomedullary sodium concentration gradient (BARTELHEIMER and SENFT, 1968).

Gold is toxic to the kidney and experimental animals given high doses usually die of renal insufficiency (HARVEY, 1970). JASMIN (1957) demonstrated nephrocalcinosis in rats following massive doses of sodium aurothiomalate for 6 days. This toxicity was demonstrated only in adrenalectomized animals receiving deoxycorticosterone acetate. BOKELMAN et al. (1971) demonstrated a strain-specific renal toxicity with a non-steroid anti-inflammatory drug; 1-p-chlorobenzylidine-5-methoxy-2-methyl-3-indene acetic acid produced a strain and sex-related haematuria in rats. The animals were treated with drug up to 25 weeks and histological examination revealed lesions of the renal papilla.

In contrast to gastrointestinal toxicity, there does not appear to be any simple acute methods available to predict renal toxicity. The evaluation of a new chemical entity would require chronic drug administration with periodic kidney function tests and histological examination of the kidney.

III. Haematopoietic System

Steroid and non-steroid anti-inflammatory drugs have been implicated in a variety of clinical toxicities concerning the formed elements of the blood. Leucocytosis has been described in children during therapy with prednisone, prednisolone, and triamcinolone (JOHN, 1966). Agranulocytosis and thrombocytopenia have been attributed to treatment with phenylbutazone and its metabolite, oxyphenbutazone (HUGULEY, 1964; ARMSTRONG and SCHERBEL, 1961). Sodium aurothiomalate has been implicated in deaths due to agranulocytosis, aplastic anaemia, pancytopaenia, and thrombocytopenia (ANON, 1971). Although haematological toxicity has been a clinical problem with anti-inflammatory drugs, little published data on investigations of this toxicity in laboratory animals is available. Administration of indomethacin to mice for 6 days produced a severe anaemia, but this finding does not appear to reflect the clinical findings with this drug (KEICHLINE, 1971). The anaemia may have been secondary to blood loss from the gastrointestinal tract. HOWELL et al. (1973) have developed an in vitro bone marrow culture procedure (human and rodent) which may find application in drug toxicity studies. Unfortunately, the effect of anti-inflammatory drugs in this system has not been reported to date. WEINER and PILIERO (1970) have stated that no satisfactory preclinical model exists for a variety of disturbing blood effects including agranulocytosis and thrombocytopenia. It is apparent that, currently, drug toxicity to the formed elements of the blood in laboratory animals is best determined by chronic drug administration, with periodic evaluation of haematological parameters at selected intervals during the study (ZBINDEN, 1964).

IV. Liver

The liver is affected adversely by many types of drugs including non-steroid anti-inflammatory drugs. There are a variety of ways of classifying hepatic lesions induced by various chemical substances. PLAA (1975) discusses three basic types of injury produced by drugs.

The first is acute hepatic necrosis, which is associated with exposure to carbon tetrachloride, chloroform, benzene etc., and which has been extensively described in the literature. This type of hepatic injury is easily reproducible in laboratory animals, but is seldom caused by compounds employed therapeutically.

A second type of injury is intrahepatic cholestasis with a diminution in bile flow and a retention of bilirubin, leading to jaundice. This condition has been seen in a series of unrelated drugs such as anabolic steroids, phenothiazines, certain antimicrobials and oral hypoglycaemics. The reproduction of this lesion with these agents has not proven successful in laboratory animals. Ibufenac, a non-steroid anti-inflammatory drug, produced evidence of disturbances of liver function in 14 out of 36 patients in a study reported by THOMPSON et al. (1964). There were elevations in serum glutamic oxaloacetic transaminase (SGOT) and serum glutamic pyruvic transaminase (SGPT) levels. Two of the patients developed jaundice, indicating the possibility of cholestasis, but this was not substantiated by laboratory findings. The occurrence of this hepatotoxicity with ibufenac could not have been anticipated from chronic drug administration to dogs (26 weeks) and rats (27 weeks) prior to the clinical studies.

A third type of hepatic lesion produced by drugs is a condition resembling viral hepatitis. Examples of compounds producing this toxicity are iproniazid, cinchophen, and zoxazolamine. Phenylbutazone and indomethacin have also been associated with this condition in the human in rare instances (SMETANA, 1963; SCHAFF-NER and RAISFELD, 1969). Salicylates also have been implicated in producing liver damage (ATHREYA et al., 1973) and hepatitis (WOLFE et al., 1974) in clinical studies. As in the case of cholestatic lesions, this type of hepatic toxicity is not reproducible in laboratory animals.

Ibufenac and phenylbutazone have been shown to reduce bilirubin and o-aminophenol conjugation in rat liver slices and rabbit liver homogenates (HARGREAVES, 1965), as well as producing jaundice in humans. Further work is needed before the feasibility of using this type of in vitro system to predict cholestatic hepatotoxicity can be determined. To date, it is apparent that there is little predictability of hepatotoxicity induced by anti-inflammatory agents from animals to the human. Chronic toxicity studies in a variety of animal species, with liver function tests and histological examination, are essential in preclinical drug evaluation, but appear to have minimal predictive value.

V. Skin

Cutaneous reactions to anti-inflammatory agents in humans have been a common clinical problem. Miscellaneous skin reactions have been described for phenylbutazone, oxyphenbutazone, indomethacin, gold (ALMEYDA and BAKER, 1970), salicylates (BAKER and MOORE-ROBINSON, 1970), and steroids (ASHTON et al., 1970); many types, including urticaria, angio-oedema, pruritus, toxic epidermal necrolysis, discoid eczema, and photosensitivity, have been cited. With the exception of drug-induced photosensitivity, there is no suitable animal model available for predicting the development of these reactions in the clinical situation. Photosensitivity reactions in albino mice, following parenteral administration of drugs such as tetracycline and chlorpromazine, have been observed using long-wave fluorescent light (ISON and DAVIS, 1969; ROTHE and JACOBUS, 1968). SAMS (1966) and SAMS and EPSTEIN (1967) produced a photosensitivity response in guinea pigs with chlorpromazine, demethyl-chlortetracycline and chlorthiazide using both artificial light and sunlight. A method for the production of drug-induced phototoxicity in swine has also been described (BAY et al., 1970). A large number of drugs known to produce phototoxicity in animals are active in the previously described animal models. Unfortunately, no anti-inflammatory drugs have been evaluated in these laboratory procedures to see whether they are predictive for photosensitivity reactions in humans for this class of drugs.

VI. Eye

Certain anti-inflammatory drugs (chloroquine, steroids, indomethacin) have been reported to affect the eye adversely (POTTS and GONASUN, 1975). Experimentally-induced chloroquine retinopathy was first produced in the cat after 4–8 weeks oral administration (MEIER-RUGE, 1965). BERNSTEIN et al. (1963) showed that following intravenous administration of chloroquine to pigmented rabbits, the drug appears in the choroid and iris tissues of the eye 6–12 h later. They have demonstrated in the rat as well as in the rabbit, that the drug is concentrated far more in eye tissue than in other tissues of the body. DALE et al. (1965) confirmed the pigmentary deposits of chloroquine in pigmented rabbits with an 11-month feeding study. It is thought that the drug localises in the melanin-containing parts of the eye. FRANCOIS and MAUD-GAL (1965) produced chloroquine keratopathy in albino rats which could be seen after 6 weeks of drug administration. GLEISER et al. (1968) produced degenerative dose-dependent changes in the retina of pigs following chronic oral dosing with chloroquine for 17–106 days.

Experimentally, steroid cataracts can be produced in rabbits by 2 mg of betamethasone applied subconjunctively for 41 weeks. However, no eye pathology in animals has been reported with indomethacin.

VII. Central Nervous System

Certain classes of anti-inflammatory drugs have produced clinical toxicity related to the CNS (BACH, 1973). Steroids and chloroquine have produced toxic psychoses, nervousness, and insomnia. Severe frontal headaches and vertigo are often experienced during treatment with indomethacin. High doses of salicylates have been associated with tinnitis. These subjective side-effects cannot be detected in laboratory animals and usually require clinical studies in hundreds of patients before their relative frequency of occurrence can be elucidated.

D. Correlation of Experimental Models With Clinical Toxicity

I. Non-Steroid Anti-Inflammatory Drugs

1. Salicylates

Gastrointestinal irritation is the most common side-effect of salicylate administration. Salicylates in various forms were used in therapy of arthritis since the early 1800s and gastrointestinal irritation was well-recognised as a problem in their use.

Although scattered reports appeared on the production of gastrointestinal bleeding by salicylates from 1916 to 1950 (SMITH and SMITH, 1966), little attention was paid to them and negative reports (SMITH and SMITH, 1966) made it a controversial subject. In the mid-1950s, several clinical reports appeared which confirmed the observation that salicylates did damage the gastrointestinal mucosa and increased faecal blood loss (LANGE, 1957; STUBBÉ, 1958; ALVAREZ and SUMMERSKILL, 1958; SCOTT et al., 1961; MODELL and PATTERSON, 1951; KELLY, 1956; MUIR and COSSAR, 1955). Animal correlation of gastric damage was published in the late 1930s (BARBOUR and DICKERSON, 1938), but as with the clinical data more complete studies and investigation of mechanism of action did not appear until more than 2 decades later (LEVRAT and LAMBERT, 1960; ANDERSON, 1964a, 1964b; DAVENPORT, 1967; BRODIE and CHASE, 1969; VANE, 1971). Interest has continued since the problem of aspirin-induced gastric bleeding as a source of gastric ulceration has been documented both retrospectively (CHAPMAN and DUGGAN, 1969) and prospectively (DUGGAN, 1972), and research papers on toxicity associated with chronic administration are beginning to appear (ST. JOHN et al., 1973). Clinical and experimental interest in the problem of gastrointestinal toxicity of salicylates was stimulated by the introduction of other non-steroid anti-inflammatory drugs and spurred the development of test procedures which could compare the potential toxicity of these agents.

In rats, the acute toxicity of salicylates is in the range of 3000–5000 mg/kg p.o., and its therapeutic dose for reduction of inflammation is about 100–300 mg/kg, which gives a good margin of safety. The problem of the clinical significance of gastrointestinal bleeding with the salicylates has been debated extensively (LANGMAN, 1974; INGELFINGER, 1974; SPIRO, 1974; SMITH and SMITH, 1966). In the United States alone it is estimated that over 600–1000 metric tons of salicylates are used annually (INGELFINGER, 1974; MENGUY, 1969) and if gastrointestinal bleeding were a major problem, it would occur much more frequently than has been reported with the widespread self-administration. The incidence rate has been reported to be about 15/1 000 000 hospital admissions/year (INGELFINGER, 1974).

Experimentally, salicylates produce intestinal as well as gastric damage (BRODIE et al., 1970) and it is also clear that there is a local irritation effect as well (ROTH and VALDES-DAPENA, 1963). This had led to a continuing discussion of whether gastrointestinal damage produced by salicylates is caused by their local action on the gastric mucosa or whether the effects are due to changes produced by circulating drugs. Animal data have shown that gastric damage can be produced when aspirin is given by any route of administration (BARBOUR and DICKERSON, 1938; ANDERSON, 1964b; PFEIFFER and LEWANDOWSKI, 1971; BRODIE and HOOKE, 1971), while sodium salicylate has been shown to produce gastric bleeding in rats only when given by the oral route (BRODIE and HOOKE, 1971). These data suggest that toxicity of salicylates may depend on the pharmaceutical formulation. At first, this question may appear to be academic since it is extremely rare that arthritic patients use salicylates in any other form than by oral administration. However, the question assumes practical importance when enteric coated or special pharmaceutical formulations are prepared which are designed to bypass the stomach and to be released and absorbed in the intestine (LEONARDS and LEVY, 1967). If gastrointestinal damage is due to a local effect, these preparations should reduce the potential for gastric haemorrhage; however, if the damage is due to circulating levels of salicylates, then the danger to the patient remains regardless of the dosage form. At the present time this question remains unresolved; however, studies on the mechanism of action of aspirin-induced gastric bleeding have indicated that the presence of acid in the stomach is a causal factor (BRODIE and CHASE, 1969), due to acid back diffusion through damage to a break in the gastric mucosal acid barrier (DAVENPORT, 1967; IVEY, 1973; COOKE, 1973).

Salicylates produce gastrointestinal damage in many species of animals (TAYLOR and CRAWFORD, 1968; ANDERSON, 1964a; EDER, 1964). However, availability, size, cost, and sensitivity have made the rat the species of choice for comparitive tests. Also, analytical procedures have been developed which will detect aspirin-induced gastric damage and bleeding in rats and dogs at doses equivalent to those used in the clinical treatment of arthritis (EDELSON and DOUGLAS, 1973; PHILLIPS, 1973). This provides a means both for studying new pharmaceutical formulations of salicylates and for the evaluation of experimental models of arthritis where activity and toxicity can be assessed in the same animal to provide a therapeutic index.

Gastrointestinal damage is not the only clinical toxicity of salicylates which can be detected in animals. Clinical changes in blood clotting, acid base balance and liver function have been reported (ATHREYA et al., 1973; SMITH and SMITH, 1966; BACH, 1973). Nephrotoxicity has been difficult to detect in animals by administration of the salicylates (CLAUSEN and HARVALD, 1961) and at the present time there is no method to detect idiosyncratic reactions or allergy reactions (SMITH, 1971) to salicylates in animals. Folklore that aspirin damages the heart is not substantiated in animals or in clinical reports of toxicity.

It has been suggested that the mechanism of action of anti-inflammatory agents may be due to their effect on prostaglandin synthetase (VANE, 1971). It has also been postulated that the gastrointestinal damage due to anti-inflammatory agents is due to this same mechanism (NEZAMIS et al., 1971; PAULUS and WHITEHOUSE, 1973), which would indicate that gastric irritation is an intrinsic part of anti-inflammatory activity and that it is not possible to separate the two functions (CUTHBERT, 1974) produced by a drug such as indomethacin. A comparison of anti-inflammatory activity, gastrointestinal toxicity and prostaglandin synthetase inhibition suggests that there is a relationship between the three actions (PAULUS and WHITEHOUSE, 1973). However, recent evidence has come to light that it is possible to separate the activity on prostaglandin synthetase from that of anti-inflammatory activity, and while the anti-inflammatory effect may not be related to the reduction of prostaglandin synthetase, the production of gastrointestinal damage is directly related to this effect (DODGE et al., 1974). Although it is not yet confirmed, it appears possible that new drugs could be tested in vitro for their effect on prostaglandin synthetase and those compounds which do not have this effect, but still retain anti-inflammatory activity, would be interesting candidate drugs. This would provide a biochemical means for the evaluation of potential anti-inflammatory drugs.

The teratogenic effect of salicylates in animals has been clearly demonstrated (WALKER, 1971), but whether this finding has clinical implications is still controversial (WARKANY, 1966). The wide self-administration of aspirin and aspirin-containing preparations make this an extremely complex problem. It is clear that aspirin can cross the placental barrier and alter the newborn blood-clotting mechanism (BLEYER and BRECKENRIDGE, 1970).

The CNS toxicity produced by salicylates has not been studied extensively in animals. The tinnitis, which is a major side effect in salicylate therapy, conceivably could be detected by the same methods that are used to show hearing loss with aminoglycoside antibiotics. However, to date, a search of the literature has not revealed studies of this toxicity in animals.

2. Indomethacin

There is a high incidence of side-effects associated with the use of indomethacin. A survey of clinical trials (O'Brien, 1968) stated that few patients can tolerate more than 100 mg/day of indomethacin without some type of untoward effect. At doses of 150–200 mg/day, over 50% of the patients taking the drug have some toxic reaction; the most frequently encountered are associated with the CNS and the gastrointestinal tract. Of 210 patients in 6 controlled studies, 47.1% had headache and 18.6% severe abdominal pain, while of 1663 patients in 18 uncontrolled studies, 20.9% had headache and only 7.7% had abdominal pain. In the controlled studies, 0.47% of the patients developed ulcers while in the uncontrolled studies 2.1% developed such ulcers. Presumably in the double-blind studies, the patients were seen at regular intervals, and carefully and specifically questioned about signs of intoxication. As a result, the drug may have been discontinued more promptly and fewer peptic ulcers developed. As with aspirin, gastric ulceration is a more common toxicity than is ulceration of the small intestine, although specific reports of indomethacin-induced intestinal damage have been cited in the literature (Thompson and Rowe, 1965; Sturges and Krone, 1973). In the absence of frank ulceration, gastrointestinal bleeding has been reported with clinical administration of indomethacin (Wanka et al., 1964; Winship, 1970).

There appears to be good correlation between indomethacin-induced gastrointestinal damage in human and laboratory animals. The rat appears to be the animal of choice because of cost and ease of ulcer production. Administration of a single dose of indomethacin can lead to gastric and intestinal ulceration and gastrointestinal haemorrhage (Brodie et al., 1970; Wilhelmi and Menassé-Gdynia, 1972; Menassé-Gdynia and Krupp, 1974; Wax et al., 1975; Di Pasquale and Welaj, 1973).

The side-effects involving the CNS described with indomethacin therapy are headache, vertigo, depression, mental confusion, and other psychological reactions such as detachment and depersonalisation (Calabro, 1971; Honing, 1973). The frontal headaches associated with indomethacin therapy constitute a unique side-effect amongst the non-steroid anti-inflammatory drugs. As yet, there is no suitable animal model for predicting these CNS side-effects in man.

Indomethacin has also been associated with side-effects involving the eye, liver, kidney, and skin. As is the case with the CNS effects, these toxicities are not predictable from animal experiments. Burns (1968) described reduced retinal sensitivity and corneal deposits associated with indomethacin therapy. This is in contrast to a statement by Daviddorf (1973) indicating no toxic ocular effects with the drug. There have been isolated cases of hepatitis with biliverdinemia reported in association with indomethacin therapy (Fenech et al., 1967; Kelsey et al., 1967). Marsh et al. (1971) described a proliferative glomerulonephritis which developed in two patients shortly after indomethacin therapy. Allergic reactions have also been reported during indomethacin therapy. MATHEWS and STAGE (1974) have recommended that indomethacin be administered with caution to patients with a prior history of aspirin sensitivity whether the previous reaction has been asthmatic or urticarial in nature.

3. Phenylbutazone

Phenylbutazone is poorly tolerated by many patients. Some type of side-effect was noted in 10–45% of patients and medication may have to be discontinued in 10–15%. A survey of adverse reactions to non-steroid anti-inflammatory drugs was published by CUTHBERT (1974); in the case of phenylbutazone, the profile shows that adverse reactions involving the blood predominate, with gastrointestinal effects in second place, in terms of fatal reactions. A total of 1276 reports were received in the period June 1964 to January 1973: 398 (204 fatal) were blood disorders, which included 163 reports of aplastic anaemia (121 fatal); 59 were reports of thrombocytopenia (18 fatal); 95 were reports of agranulocytosis, leucopenia or pancytopenia (44 fatal), and haemorrhage from the gastrointestinal tract was recorded in 104 cases (27 fatal). Comparison with prescribing statistics showed that approximately 40 reports and 9 deaths are associated with each million prescriptions for phenylbutazone. Oxyphenbutazone, a known metabolite of phenylbutazone, showed an almost identical profile.

As has been discussed with the salicylates and indomethacin, gastrointestinal toxicity is easily predictable using the animal models previously described in this chapter. In contrast, changes in the peripheral blood and bone marrow in animal toxicity studies are usually only secondary to the gastrointestinal pathology produced by non-steroid anti-inflammatory drugs and rarely, if ever, can a direct depressant effect on the bone marrow be demonstrated.

A less serious clinical side-effect associated with phenylbutazone therapy is water and electrolyte retention and oedema formation. BARTELHEIMER and SENFT (1968) demonstrated, in rats, that phenylbutazone and oxyphenbutazone decreased the renal excretion of sodium and water in the rat. This finding therefore represents another relatively rare instance of predictability of clinical side effects from laboratory animal studies.

Phenylbutazone, like indomethacin, is responsible for other less prevalent clinical adverse reactions which cannot be predicted from animal models, including: CNS effects (insomnia, euphoria, and nervousness), hepatitis and cutaneous reactions.

4. Arylalkanoic Acids

Several arylalkanoic acid derivatives are in clinical use throughout the world. The more prominent of these include ibuprofen, alclofenac, naproxen, and ketoprofen. These compounds share, to varying degrees, the adverse reactions of the previously mentioned non-steroid anti-inflammatory drugs (CUTHBERT, 1974). This similarity extends to the prediction of clinical side effects from animal models. The majority of clinical toxicities associated with these drugs is similar to that of indomethacin and phenylbutazone, but a few unique characteristics can be mentioned.

Ibuprofen is very closely related to a hepatotoxic drug, ibufenac, although ibuprofen is not hepatotoxic itself. The occurrence of hepatotoxicity with ibufenac could not have been anticipated on the basis of the results of animal studies conducted before the drug was made available for clinical trial (THOMPSON et al., 1964). The profile of adverse reactions of ibuprofen are similar to indomethacin (CUTHBERT, 1974).

Alclofenac has been associated with a high proportion of reports of skin reaction (CHAMBERLAIN and WRIGHT, 1975). They are generally assumed to be allergic, appearing 8–12 days after treatment and subsiding upon withdrawal of the drug.

Naproxen was marketed in the United Kingdom in 1973 with the suggestion that the gastrointestinal tolerance might be better than with some other non-steroid anti-inflammatory drugs. However, the use of the drug has been associated with a significant incidence of gastrointestinal bleeding (CUTHBERT, 1974).

Much additional clinical experience is needed to assess the possible advantages of the arylalkanoic acids with regard to clinical adverse reactions.

5. Gold

The use of gold as an anti-inflammatory agent has been hampered by a number of problems. While there appear to be adequate clinical studies indicating that gold is the only agent available to date which will retard the progress of the disease (SIGLER et al., 1972), its use requires care and special knowledge. Gold therapy has usually been reserved as a last resort treatment, but its proponents indicate that the general concern for its toxicity by the medical community is not warranted and that these compounds deserve earlier use (KAMMERER, 1974). A major problem in gold therapy is the fact that the drug must be given by injection, the patient carefully monitored and the dose adjusted to each patient by the physician. However, the results produced by gold therapy indicate that there is a great benefit-to-risk ratio.

One of the goals in this area has been the development of an orally active gold compound, and it appears that this has been achieved in animals (WALZ et al., 1974). Clinically, the major side effects of gold therapy has been dermatological (KAMMERER, 1974), but it has not been possible to reproduce this routinely in animals (FENNEL, 1969). However, chronic administration of gold can reproduce some of the allergic responses seen in man by examination of peripheral blood in rabbits (NINEHAM, 1963). The effect on the haematopoietic system is serious but not common. Clinically, parenteral administration of gold in rats produces kidney damage and toxicity to other organs (WALZ et al., 1974) and it also can produce teratogenic effects (KIDSTON et al., 1970). Gastric toxicity has been uncommon with parenteral gold (KAMMERER, 1974); however, an incidence of 10% of gastrointestinal haemorrhage was reported in adverse drug reaction reports (CUTHBERT, 1974). Experimentally, both oral and parenteral gold produced gastric erosions in rats (WALZ et al., 1974; SHRIVER et al., 1975). As indicated by WALZ et al. (1974), assessment of toxicity in gold compounds requires chronic administration since acute studies do not give an accurate picture of the toxicity of these agents. Current research in this area indicates that animal tests of potentially useful new gold formulations are available to assess the potential clinical toxicity.

II. Steroids

Although the effectiveness of corticosteroids in the treatment of inflammation has been known for almost 20 years, their use is often questioned due to the frequency and severity of side-effects. Major synthetic efforts have been conducted in order to separate the anti-inflammatory activity from the other steroid actions and although some success has been achieved in separating the adverse effects on the electrolytic balance and glucose metabolism, the same was not true in the case of the more serious problems of osteoporosis and the decreased resistance to infection. The lack of success could be due to either a direct relationship between the side-effects and the anti-inflammatory activity or to the inadequacy of the animal models used. The attempts to reduce the side-effects though have resulted in the development of locally active compounds and in the use of longer-acting systemic compounds (POPPER and WATNICK, 1974).

The exact relationship of glucocorticoid therapy to peptic ulceration of the stomach is still not clear, although the clinical impression is that the incidence is increased after glucocorticoid therapy. In animals, short-term administration produced no change in acid secretion. Longer term administration in the dog showed that acid secretion usually rose, unlike in the rat where no changes were observed. In animals, adrenalectomy seems to reduce gastric secretion significantly, which is restored after administration of glucocorticoids. It has also been shown that the viscosity and quantity of mucous secreted appears to fall after ACTH or cortisone in dogs (CUSHMAN, 1970). The absorptive functions of the small intestine appear to be directly affected by the glucocorticoids. In the adrenalectomized animal, for example, a reduced rate of glucose absorption is observed (CUSHMAN, 1970).

Corticosteroids in usual clinical doses impair cellular immune responses, such as delayed-type skin reactions to tuberculin. In massive doses, they may have some effect on antibody formation in animals, although this has not been clearly demonstrated (STREETEN, 1975). Their effects on protein and carbohydrate metabolism have been demonstrated in both man and animals. The glucocorticoids inhibit the transport of amino acids into the muscle and reduce new protein synthesis. Enhancement of gluconeogenesis contributes to the aggravation of diabetes in patients. All of the corticosteroids increase urinary losses of potassium and therefore cause hypokalemia. Glucocorticoids increase the excitability of the brain cortex in man and large doses in animals have resulted in a lowering of the threshold to electric shock.

E. Summary

In the development of new anti-inflammatory agents or the assessment of formulations of existing drugs experimentally, major emphasis has been placed on drugs which are free of gastrointestinal damage since this is one of the most common side-effects and can be easily detected in animals. It is conceivable that anti-inflammatory agents can be developed which do not produce the major side effect of gastrointestinal damage, but this does not make such an agent automatically superior to those available at present. It requires adequate clinical trial to determine whether other side-effects will appear which may not be as life-threatening, but which are as detrimental to the quality of life. It should also be emphasised that toxicity related to the CNS such as headache, psychosis, and peripheral neuritis may be difficult or impossible to assess in animals so that, regardless of excellent therapeutic ratios in acute and chronic tests, the completion of acceptable Phase I clinical trials and efficacy in early Phase II studies, the final assessment of a new anti-inflammatory agent will depend on several years of evaluation in thousands of arthritic patients.

The incidence of the side effects of anti-inflammatory drugs suggests that the treatment of arthritis with these agents must be closely monitored, particularly if more than one agent is used for therapy. The primary use of these drugs, even with the possibility of severe adverse reactions, is undertaken with the hope of the physician to improve the quality of life for these patients and the physician must use appropriate therapy for the individual patient based on a benefit-to-risk consideration. Assessment of toxicity in animals will aid in the development of agents which permit the best possible ratio.

References

Almeyda, J., Baker, H.: Drug reactions. XII. Cutaneous reactions to anti-rheumatic drugs. Brit. J. Derm. **83**, 707—711 (1970)

Alvarez, A. S., Summerskill, W. H. J.: Gastrointestinal haemorrhage and salicylates. Lancet **1958 II**, 920—925

A.M.A. Department of Drugs: Anti-rheumatic agents. In: A.M.A. Drug Evaluations, 2nd Ed. Acton, Massachusetts: Publishing Sciences Group, Inc. 1973

Anderson, K. W.: A study of the gastric lesions induced by aspirin in laboratory animals. Arch. int. Pharmacodyn. **152**, 379—391 (1964 a)

Anderson, K. W.: A study of the gastric lesions induced in laboratory animals by soluble and buffered aspirin. Arch. int. Pharmacodyn. **152**, 392 (1964 b)

Anon: Asthma from aspirin. Brit. med. J. **1**, 6 (1969)

Anon: Gold for rheumatoid arthritis. Brit. med. J. **1**, 471—472 (1971)

Anon: Liver injury by salicylates. Brit. med. J. **2**, 732 (1973)

Armstrong, F. B., Scherbel, A. L.: Review of toxicity of oxyphenylbutazone: report of a case of thrombocytopenic purpura. J. Amer. med. Ass. **175**, 614—615 (1961)

Ashton, H., Beveridge, G. W., Stevenson, C. J.: Therapeutics: XI. Immuno-suppressive drugs. Brit. J. Derm. **83**, 326 (1970)

Athreya, B. H., Gorske, A. L., Myers, A. R.: Aspirin-induced abnormalities of liver function. Amer. J. Dis. Child. **126**, 638—641 (1973)

Bach, G. L.: Adverse reactions of anti-rheumatic drugs. Int. J. clin. Pharmacol. **7**, 198—205 (1973)

Baker, H., Moore-Robinson, M.: Drug reactions. IX. Cutaneous responses to aspirin and its derivatives. Brit. J. Derm. **82**, 319 (1970)

Barbour, H. G., Dickerson, V. C.: Gastric ulceration produced in rats by oral and subcutaneous aspirin. Arch. int. Pharmacodyn. **58**, 78—87 (1938)

Bartelheimer, V. H. K., Senft, G.: Zur Lokalisation der tubulären Wirkung einiger antirheuma-tisch wirkender Substanzen. Arzneimittel-Forsch. **18**, 567—570 (1968)

Bay, W. W., Gliser, C. A., Dukes, T. W., Brown, R. S.: The experimental production of drug-in-duced phototoxicity in swine. Toxicol. appl. Pharmacol. **17**, 538—547 (1970)

Berlinger, F. G.: Use and misuse of steroids. Postgrad. Med. **55**, 153—157 (1974)

Bernstein, H., Zvaifler, N., Rubin, M., Mansour, A. M.: The ocular deposition of chloroquin. In-vest. Ophthal. **2**, 384—392 (1963)

Bleyer, W. A., Breckenridge, R. T.: Studies on the detection of adverse drug reactions in the new-born. II. The effects of prenatal aspirin on newborn hemostasis. J. Amer. med. Ass. **213**, 2049—2053 (1970)

Bokelman, D. L., Bagdon, W. J., Mattis, P. A., Stonier, P. F.: Strain dependent renal toxicity of a nonsteroid anti-inflammatory agent. Toxicol. appl. Pharmacol. **19**, 111—124 (1971)

Bonfils, S.: La diminution du pouvoir pathogene, generale et gastrique de la phenylbutazone chez le rat impubere. 6e Congr. Int. de Therapeutique, Strasbourg 1959

The Boston U. Med. Center: Acute adverse reactions to prednisone in relation to dosage. Clin. Pharmacol. Ther. **13**, 694—698 (1972)

Brodie, D. A., Chase, B. J.: Evaluation of gastric acid as a factor in drug-induced gastric hemor-rhage in the rat. Gastroenterology **56**, 206—213 (1969)

Brodie, D. A., Cook, P. G., Bauer, B. J., Dagle, G. E.: Indomethacin-induced intestinal lesions in the rat. Toxicol. appl. Pharmacol. 17, 615—624 (1970)

Brodie, D. A., Hooke, K. F.: Effects of route of administration on the production of gastric hemorrhage in the rat by aspirin and sodium salicylate. Amer. J. dig. Dis. 16, 985—989 (1971a)

Brodie, D. A., Tate, C. L., Hooke, K. F.: Aspirin: intestinal damage in rats. Science 170, 183—185 (1971b)

Brookes, D. B.: Chloroquine psychosis. Brit. med. J. 1, 983 (1966)

Brumett, R. E.: Antipyretic anti-inflammatory drugs. Pharm. Index 14, 4—8 (1972)

Buchanan, W. W., Samuels, B. M., Jasani, M. K., Anderson, W. M., O'Brien, J. A., Boyle, G. N., Boyle, I. T.: Do oral corticosteroids cause osteoporosis in rheumatoid arthritis? Ann. rheum. Dis. 29, 560—561 (1970)

Burns, C. A.: Indomethacin, reduced retinal sensitivity and corneal deposits. Amer. J. Ophthal. 66, 825—835 (1968)

Burns, J. J., Schulert, A., Chenkin, T., Goldman, A., Brodie, B. B.: The physiological disposition of phenylbutazone (Butazolidin), a new anti-rheumatic agent. J. Pharmacol. exp. Ther. 106, 375—376 (1952)

Burry, H. C.: Drug-induced nephropathies. Proc. roy. Soc. Med. 66, 897—900 (1973)

Calabro, J. J.: Indomethacin: a current view of its use in rheumatic disorders. Drug. Ther. 1, 34—38, 43—44 (1971)

Canada, A. T.: Gold-induced thrombocytopenia. Amer. J. Hosp. Pharm. 30, 340—342 (1973)

Carr, R. E., Henkind, P., Rothfield, N., Siegel, I. M.: Ocular toxicity of antimalarial drugs. Long-term follow-up. Amer. J. Ophthal. 66, 738—744 (1968)

Caughey, D. E., Isdale, I. C., Tweed, J. M., Treadwell, B. L. J., Laing, J. K., Kirk, J., Highton, T. C., Palmer, D. G., Wigley, R. D., Morrison, R. B., Couchman, K., Reay, B., Fowles, M., Caughey, E.: Aspirin and the kidney. New Zealand Rheumatism Association Study. Brit. med. J. 1, 593—596 (1974)

Chamberlain, M. A., Wright, V.: A double-blind trial to assess the value of alclofenac compared with phenylbutazone in the management of rheumatoid arthritis. Ann. rheum. Dis. 34, 186—189 (1975)

Chapman, B. L., Duggan, J. M.: Aspirin and uncomplicated peptic ulcer. Gut 10, 443—450 (1969)

Clausen, E., Harvald, B.: Nephrotoxicity of different analgesics. Acta med. scand. 170, 469—474 (1961)

Cohen, Y.: Aspirin induced digestive bleeding studied by Cr^{51}-labeled red cells in the rat. In: Isotopes in Experimental Pharmacology. Chicago: University of Chicago Press 1965

Cooke, A. R.: The role of acid in the pathogenesis of aspirin-induced gastrointestinal erosions and hemorrhage. Amer. J. dig. Dis. 18, 225—237 (1973)

Croft, D. N., Cuddigan, J. H. P., Sweetland, C.: Gastric bleeding and benorylate, a new aspirin. Brit. med. J. 3, 545 (1972)

Cushman, P. Jr.: Glucocorticoids and the gastrointestinal tract: current status. Gut 11, 534—539 (1970)

Cuthbert, M. F.: Adverse reactions to non-steroidal anti-rheumatic drugs. Curr. med. Res. Opin. 2, 600—610 (1974)

Dale, A., Parkhill, E., Layton, D.: Studies on chloroquine retinopathy in rabbits. J. Amer. med. Ass. 193, 141—143 (1965)

Davenport, H. W.: Salicylate damage to the gastric mucosal barrier. New Engl. J. Med. 276, 1307—1312 (1967)

David, D. J.: Skin trauma in patients receiving systemic corticosteroid therapy. Brit. med. J. 2, 614—616 (1972)

Daviddorf, F. H.: Ocular toxicity of systemic drugs. A review of the effects of seven commonly used agents. Ohio St. med. J. 68, 1022—1026 (1973)

Davison, C., Hertig, D. H., Devine, R.: Gastric hemorrhage induced by non-narcotic analgesic agents in dogs. Clin. Pharmacol. Ther. 7, 239—249 (1966)

Day, A. T., Golding, J. R., Lee, P. N., Butterworth, D.: Penicillamine in rheumatoid disease: a long-term study. Brit. med. J. 1, 180—183 (1974)

Decker, J. L., Bollet, A. J., Duff, I. F., Shulman, M. D., Stollerman, G. H.: Primer on the rheumatic diseases. Part I. J. Amer. med. Ass. 190, 127—140 (1964)

Di Pasquale, G., Welaj, P.: Ulcerogenic potential of indomethacin in arthritic and non-arthritic rats. J. Pharm. (Lond.) **25**, 831—832 (1973)

Dodge, P. W., Brodie, D. A., Young, P. R., Krause, R. A., Tekeli, S.: Prevention of anti-inflammatory drug-induced gastric lesions in rats by ABBOTT-29590. Amer. J. dig. Dis. **19**, 449—457 (1974)

Domenjoz, R.: The pharmacology of phenylbutazone analogues. Ann. N.Y. Acad. Sci. **86**, 263 (1960)

Duggan, J. M.: Aspirin ingestion and perforated peptic ulcer. Gut **13**, 631—633 (1972)

Ebaugh, F. G., Clemens, T. Jr., Rodnan, G., Peterson, R. E.: Quantitative measurement of gastrointestinal blood loss. Amer. J. Med. **25**, 169—181 (1958)

Edelson, J., Douglas, J. F.: Measurement of gastrointestinal blood loss in the rat: the effect of aspirin, phenylbutazone, and seclazone. J. Pharmacol. exp. Ther. **184**, 449—452 (1973)

Eder, H.: Chronic toxicity studies on phenacetin. N-acetyl-p-amino-phenol (NAPA) and acetylsalicylic acid on cats. Acta Pharmacol. (Kbh.) **21**, 197—204 (1964)

Ellman, P., Lawrence, J. S., Thorold, G. P.: Gold therapy in rheumatoid arthritis. Brit. med. J. **2**, 314—316 (1940)

Elwood, P. C., Cochrane, A. L., Burr, M. L., Sweetnam, P. M., Williams, G., Welsby, E., Hughes, S. J., Renton, R.: A randomized controlled trial of acetylsalicylic acid in the secondary prevention of mortality from myocardial infarction. Brit. med. J. **1**, 436—440 (1974)

Emmitt, R. B.: Arthritis and drug therapy. In: Cyrus J. Lawrence Reports. New York: Cyrus J. Lawrence, Inc. 1975

England, J. M., Smith, D. S.: Gold-induced thrombocytopenia and response to dimercaprol. Brit. med. J. **2**, 748—749 (1972)

Farr, R. S.: Presidential message. The need to re-evaluate acetylsalicylic acid (aspirin). J. Allergy **45**, 321—328 (1970)

Fenech, F. F., Bannister, W. H., Grech, J. L.: Hepatitis with biliverdinemia in association with indomethacin therapy. Brit. med. J. **3**, 155—156 (1967)

Fennel, C.: The use of "Myocrisin." Vet. Rec. **84**, 259 (1969)

Fischer, I., Rinkoff, S.: Gastrointestinal hemorrhage caused by indomethacin. Amer. J. Gastroent. **51**, 42—47 (1969)

Forestier, J.: La chrysotherapie dans les rhumatismes chromigues. Bull. Soc. Méd. Paris **44**, 323 (1929)

Forestier, J.: Rheumatoid arthritis and its treatment by gold salts. The results of six years' experience. J. Lab. clin. Med. **20**, 827—840 (1934—1935)

Foulkes, E. C., Hammond, P. B.: Toxicology of the kidney. In: Toxicology: The Basic Science of Poisons. New York: MacMillan 1975

Francois, J., Maudgal, M.: Experimental chloroquine keratopathy. Amer. J. Ophthal. **60**, 459—464 (1965)

Garb, A. E., Soule, E. H., Bartholomew, L. G., Cain, J. C.: Steroid-induced gastric ulcer. A clinicopathologic study. Arch. intern. Med. **116**, 899—906 (1965)

Gleiser, C., Bay, W., Dukes, T., Brown, R., Read, W., Pierce, K.: Study of chloroquine toxicology and a drug-induced cerebrospinal lipodystrophy in swine. Amer. J. Path. **53**, 24—45 (1968)

Goldenthal, E. J.: Current views on safety evaluation of drugs. F.D.A. Papers **2**, 13—18 (1968)

Hargreaves, T.: Inhibition of conjugation by anti-inflammatory drugs. Nature (Lond.) **208**, 1101—1102 (1965)

Hart, C. W., Naunton, R. F.: The ototoxicity of chloroquine sulphate. Arch. Otolaryng. (Chicago) **80**, 407—411 (1964)

Hart, F. D.: Anti-inflammatory drugs in the treatment of rheumatic diseases. Practitioner **205**, 597—603 (1970)

Harvey, S. C.: Heavy metals and heavy-metal antagonists. In: The Pharmacological Basis of Therapeutics, 4th. Ed. New York: MacMillan 1970

Healey, L. A. Jr.: Hazards of drugs for rheumatoid arthritis. Gen. Practit. **36**, 110—114 (1967)

Hench, P. S., Kendall, E. C., Slocumb, C. H., Polley, H. F.: The effect of a hormone of the adrenal cortex (17-hydroxy-11-dehydrocorticosterone: compound E) and of pituitary adrenocorticotropic hormone on rheumatoid arthritis. Proc. Mayo Clin. **24**, 181—197 (1949)

Henkind, P.: Iatrogenic eye manifestations in rheumatic disease. Geriatrics **20**, 12—19 (1965)

Hill, K.: Ocular complications of drug therapy. J. Maine med. Ass. **54**, 35—39 (1963)

Hingson, D. J., Ito, S.: Effect of aspirin and related compounds on the fine structure of mouse gastric mucosa. Gastroenterology **61**, 156 (1971)

Hirschman, S. Z., Isselbacher, K. J.: The nephrotic syndrome as a complication of penicillamine therapy. Ann. intern. Med. **62**, 1297—1300 (1965)

Hitchens, J. T., Goldstein, S., Sambuca, A., Shemano, I.: Ulcerogenic effects of non-steroidal anti-inflammatory agents in rats. Pharmacologist **9**, 242 (1967)

Hodgkinson, R., Woolf, D.: A five-year clinical trial of indomethacin in osteoarthritis of the hip. Practitioner **210**, 392—396 (1973)

Honing, W. J.: The use of indomethacin after meniscectomy. A double-blind trial against placebo. J. int. Med. Res. **1**, 231—239 (1973)

Howell, T., Andrews, T. M., Watts, R. W. E.: Toxic effects of drugs on bone marrow cultures. Brit. med. J. **7**, 48 (1973)

Hucker, H. B., Zacchei, A. G., Cox, S. V., Brodie, D. A., Cantwell, N. H. R.: Studies on the absorption, distribution, and excretion of indomethacin in various species. J. Pharmacol. exp. Ther. **153**, 237—249 (1966)

Huguley, C. M.: Drug-induced blood dyscrasias II. Agranulocytosis. J. Amer. med. Ass. **188**, 817—818 (1964)

Hurley, J. W., Crandall, L. A.: The effect of salicylates upon the stomachs of dogs. Gastroenterology **46**, 36—43 (1964)

Ingelfinger, F. J.: The side effects of aspirin. New Engl. J. Med. **290**, 1196—1197 (1974)

Ingle, D. J., Prestrud, M. C., Nezamis, J. E.: Effects of administering large doses of cortisone acetate to normal rats. Amer. J. Physiol. **166**, 171 (1951)

Ison, A. E., Davis, C. M.: Phototoxicity of quinoline methanols and other drugs in mice and yeast. J. invest. Derm. **52**, 193—198 (1969)

Ivey, K. J.: Gastric mucosal barrier—recent advances. Acta hepatogastroent. **20**, 517—524 (1973)

Jaffe, I. A.: Comparison of the effect of plasmapheresis and penicillamine on the level of circulating rheumatoid factor. Ann. rheum. Dis. **22**, 71—76 (1963)

Jasmin, G.: Prevention of experimental polyarthritis with sodium aurothiomalate. J. Pharmacol. exp. Ther. **120**, 349—353 (1957)

Johansson, H., Lindquist, B.: Anti-inflammatory drugs and gastric mucus. Scand. J. Gastroent. **6**, 49—54 (1971)

John, T. J.: Leukocytosis during steroid therapy. Amer. J. Dis. Child. **111**, 68—70 (1966)

Kahn, D. S., Phillips, M. J., Skoryna, S. C.: Chronic experimental gastric ulcer in the rat receiving intermittent cortisone administration. Exp. molec. Path. **2**, 481—490 (1963)

Kammerer, W. H.: Drugs for arthritis and rheumatic disease. In: Drugs of Choice 1975. St. Louis: The C. V. Mosby Co. 1974

Kay, A.: Depression of bone marrow and thrombocytopenia associated with chrysotherapy. Ann. rheum. Dis. **32**, 277—278 (1973)

Keeney, J. P.: Update on new drugs for the treatment of arthritis and rheumatism. Lehman Brothers' Health Care Trends **2**, 15 (1974)

Keichline, L. D.: Indomethacin-induced hemolytic anemia in mice. Fed. Proc. **30**, 386, abstract 1083 (1971)

Kelly, J. J. Jr.: Salicylate ingestion: a frequent cause of gastric hemorrhage. Amer. J. med. Sci. **232**, 119—128 (1956)

Kelsey, W. M., Scharyj, M.: Fatal hepatitis probably due to indomethacin. J. Amer. med. Ass. **199**, 586—587 (1967)

Kidston, M. E., Beck, F., Lloyd, J. B.: The teratogenic effect of myocrisin injection in rats. Proc. anat. Soc. Great Britain Ireland **108**, 590 (1970)

Kirsner, J. B., Ford, H.: Phenylbutazone-effect on basal gastric secretion and the production of gastroduodenal ulcerations in the dog. Gastroenterology **29**, 18—23 (1955)

Kohut, A., Nicak, A.: Effect of epinephrine, epinephrectomy, and adrenodemedullation on phenylbutazone gastric ulceration in the young and adult rat. In: 4th Int. Congr. Pharmacology, abstracts 106, 107 (1969)

Lange, H. F.: Salicylates and gastric hemorrhage. I. Occult bleeding. Gastroenterology **33**, 770—777 (1957)

Lange, W. E. de, Dorenbos, H.: Corticotrophins and corticosteroids. In: Side Effects of Drugs, Vol. VII. Amsterdam: Excerpta Medica 1972

Langman, M. J. S.: Aspirin is not a major cause of acute gastrointestinal bleeding. In: Controversy in Internal Medicine. Philadelphia: W. B. Saunders 1974

Leblanc, A., Vernet, A.: The nephrotoxicity of drugs. Praxis **62**, 31—37 (1973)

Leonards, J. R., Levy, G.: The role of dosage form in aspirin-induced gastrointestinal bleeding. Clin. Pharmacol. Ther. **8**, 400—408 (1967)

Levrat, M., Lambert, R.: Ulceres medicamenteux chez le rat. 3. L'acide acetyl-salicyliyide. Gastroenterologia (Basel) **94**, 273—289, 337—350 (1960)

Levy, L.: Assessment of the toxicity of anti-inflammatory drugs. In: Anti-Inflammatory Agents: Chemistry and Pharmacology, Vol. II. London: Academic Press 1974

Levy, N., Gaspar, E.: Rectal bleeding and indomethacin suppositories. Lancet **1975 I**, 577

Manson-Bahr, P. E. C.: Antiprotozoal drugs. In: Side Effects of Drugs, Vol. VII. Amsterdam: Excerpta Medica 1972

Marsh, F. P., Almeyda, J. R., Levy, L. S.: Non-thrombocytopenic purpura and acute glomerulonephritis after indomethacin therapy. Ann. rheum. Dis. **30**, 501—505 (1971)

Mathews, J. I., Stage, M. H.: Indomethacin, aspirin, and urticaria. Ann. intern. Med. **80**, 771 (1974)

Max, M., Menguy, R.: Influence of adrenocorticotropin cortisone, aspirin, and phenylbutazone on the rate of exfoliation and the rate of renewal of gastric mucosal cells. Gastroenterology **58**, 329—336 (1970)

Meier-Ruge, W.: Experimental investigation of the morphogenesis of chloroquine retinopathy. Arch. Ophthal. (Chicago) **73**, 540—544 (1965)

Menassé-Gdynia, R., Krupp, P.: Quantitative measurement of gastrointestinal bleeding in rats: the effect of non-steroidal anti-inflammatory drugs. Toxicol. appl. Pharmacol. **29**, 389—396 (1974)

Menguy, R.: Gastric mucosal injury by aspirin. Gastroenterology **51**, 430—432 (1969)

Michotte, L. J., Wauters, M.: Clinical test of indomethacin. Acta rheum. scand. **10**, 273—280 (1964)

Modell, W., Patterson, R.: Intestinal bleeding associated with acetylsalicylic acid. J. Amer. med. Ass. **147**, 124—126 (1951)

Muir, A., Cossar, I. A.: Aspirin and ulcer. Brit. med. J. **1**, 1—12 (1955)

Myers, A. R.: Chrysotherapy in rheumatoid arthritis. Mod. Treatm. **8**, 761—768 (1971)

Nezamis, J. E., Robert, A., Stowe, D. F.: Inhibition by prostaglandin-E_1 of gastric secretion in the dog. J. Physiol. (Lond.) **218**, 369—383 (1971)

Nineham, A. W.: Gold compounds—their chemistry, pharmacology, and pharmacy. A. I. R. Arch. interamer. Rheum. (Rio de J.) **6**, 113—140 (1963)

O'Brien, W. M.: Indomethacin: a survey of clinical trials. Clin. Pharmacol. Therap. **9**, 94—107 (1968)

Owen, C. A., Bollman, J. L., Grindlay, J. H.: Radiochromecin labeled erythrocytes for the detection of gastrointestinal hemorrhage. J. Lab. clin. Med. **44**, 238—245 (1954)

Paulus, H. E., Whitehouse, M. W.: Nonsteroid anti-inflammatory agents. Ann. Rev. Pharmacol. **13**, 107—119 (1973)

Peck, H. M.: An appraisal of drug safety evaluation in animals and the extrapolation of results to man. In: Importance of Fundamental Principles in Drug Evaluation. New York: Raven Press 1968

Percival, S. P. B., Meanock, I.: Chloroquine: ophthalmological safety and clinical assessment in rheumatoid arthritis. Brit. med. J. **3**, 579—584 (1968)

Perez, L. F., Hayden, R. C.: Salicylate ototoxicity: a human temporal bone report. Arch. Otolaryng. (Chicago) **87**, 368—372 (1968)

Pfeiffer, C. J., Lewandowski, L. G.: Comparison of gastric toxicity of acetylsalicylic acid with route of administration in the rat. Arch. int. Pharmacodyn. **190**, 5—13 (1971)

Phillips, B. M.: Aspirin-induced gastrointestinal microbleeding in dogs. Toxicol. appl. Pharmacol. **24**, 182—189 (1973)

Plaa, G.: Toxicology of the liver. In: Toxicology: The Basic Science of Poisons. New York: MacMillan 1975

Popper, T. L., Watnick, A. S.: Anti-inflammatory steroids. In: Anti-inflammatory Agents: Chemistry and Pharmacology, Vol. II. London: Academic Press 1974

Potts, A. M., Gonasun, L. M.: Toxicology of the eye. In: Toxicology: The Basic Science of Poisons. New York: MacMillan 1975

Prescott, L. F.: Antipyretic analgesics and drugs used in rheumatic diseases and gout. In: Side Effects of Drugs, Vol. VII. Amsterdam: Excerpta Medica 1972

Que, G. S.: Metals. In: Side Effects of Drugs, Vol. VI. Baltimore, Maryland-Amsterdam: Williams & Wilkins & Excerpta Medica 1968

Quick, A. J.: Salicylates and bleeding. J. Amer. med. Ass. **212**, 1524 (1970)

Robert, A., Nezamis, J. E.: Ulcerogenic property of steroids. Proc. Soc. exp. Biol. (N.Y.) **99**, 443—447 (1958)

Rodnan, G. P., Benedek, T. G.: The early history of anti-rheumatic drugs. Arthr. Rheum. **13**, 145—165 (1970)

Rosa, R. M., Kra, S. J.: Gold-induced thrombocytopenic purpura. Conn. Med. **38**, 592—594 (1974)

Roth, J. L. A., Valdes-Dapena, A.: Mechanisms of salicylate gastrointestinal erosion and hemorrhage. In: Pathophysiology of Peptic Ulcer. Montreal: McGill University Press 1963

Rothe, W. E., Jacobus, D. P.: Laboratory evaluation of the phototoxic potency of quinoline methanols. J. med. Chem. **11**, 366—368 (1968)

Rubin, M.: Prolonged pharmacotherapy and the eye. A symposium. The antimalarials and the tranquilizers. Dis. nerv. Syst. **29** (Suppl.), 67—76 (1968)

St. John, D. J. B., Yeomans, N. D., de Boer, W. G. R. M., Path, M. R. C.: Chronic gastric ulcer induced by aspirin: an experimental model. Gastroenterology **65**, 634—641 (1973)

Sams, W. M.: The experimental production of drug phototoxicity in guinea pigs using artificial light sources. Arch. Derm. **94**, 773—777 (1966)

Sams, W. M., Epstein, J. H.: The experimental production of drug phototoxicity in guinea pigs using sunlight. J. invest. Derm. **48**, 89—94 (1967)

Schaffner, F., Raisfeld, I. H.: Drugs and the liver: a review of metabolism and adverse reactions. Adv. intern. Med. **15**, 221—251 (1969)

Scott, J. T., Porter, I. H., Lewis, S. M., Dixon, A. St. J.: Studies of gastrointestinal bleeding caused by corticosteroids, salicylates, and other analgesics. Quart. J. Med. **30**, 167—188 (1961)

Shriver, D. A., White, C. B., Snador, A., Rosenthale, M. E.: A profile of the rat gastrointestinal toxicity of drugs used to treat inflammatory diseases. Toxicol. appl. Pharmacol. **32**, 73—83 (1975)

Sigler, J. W., Bluhm, G. B., Duncan, H., Sharp, J. T., Ensign, D. C., McCrum, W. R.: A double-blind study on the effects of gold salts in the treatment of rheumatoid arthritis (RA). Arthr. Rheum. **15**, 125—126 (1972)

Silverberg, D. S., Kidd, E. G., Shnitka, T. K., Ulan, R. A.: Gold nephropathy. A clinical and pathologic study. Arthr. Rheum. **13**, 812—825 (1970)

Skoryna, S. C., Webster, D. R., Kahn, D. S.: A new method of production of experimental gastric ulcer: the effects of hormonal factors on healing. Gastroenterology **34**, 1—11 (1958)

Smetana, H. F.: The histopathology of drug-induced liver disease. Ann. N.Y. Acad. Sci. **104**, 821—846 (1963)

Smith, A. P.: Response of aspirin-allergic patients to challenge by some analgesics in common use. Brit. med. J. **2**, 494—496 (1971)

Smith, M. J. H., Smith, P. K.: The salicylates—a critical bibliographic review. New York: Interscience Publishers 1966

Snyder, R. G., Traeger, C., Kelly, L.: Gold therapy in arthritis; observations on 100 cases treated with gold sodium thiosulphate and Aurocein. Ann. intern. Med. **12**, 1672—1681 (1939)

Spiro, H. M.: Aspirin is dangerous for the peptic ulcer patient. In: Controversy in Internal Medicine, Vol. II. Philadelphia, Pennsylvania: W. B. Saunders 1974

Steele, A. D.: Rheumatoid arthritis. In: Current Therapy. Philadelphia, Pennsylvania: W. B. Saunders 1975

Streeten, D. H. P.: Corticosteroid therapy. J. Amer. med. Ass. **232**, 944—947 (1975)

Stubbé, L. Th. F. L.: Occult blood in faeces after administration of aspirin. Brit. med. J. **2**, 1062—1066 (1958)

Sturges, H. F., Krone, C. L.: Ulceration and structure of the jejunum in a patient on long-term indomethacin therapy. Amer. J. Gastroent. **59**, 162—169 (1973)

Taylor, L. A., Crawford, L. M.: Aspirin-induced gastrointestinal lesions in dogs. J. Amer. vet. med. Ass. **152**, 617—619 (1968)

Taylor, R. T., Huskisson, E. C., Whitehouse, G. H., Dudley Hart, F., Trapnell, D. H.: Gastric ulceration occurring during indomethacin therapy. Brit. med. J. **1968** IV, 734

Thompson, H. E., Rowe, H. J.: Evaluation of indomethacin, a non-steroid agent, in rheumatic diseases. Ariz. Med. **22**, 289—290 (1965)

Thompson, M., Stephenson, P., Percy, J. S.: Ibufenac in the treatment of arthritis. Ann. rheum. Dis. **23**, 397—404 (1964)

Vane, J. R.: Inhibition of prostaglandin synthesis as a mechanism of action for aspirin-like drugs. Nature (New Biol.) **231**, 232—235 (1971)

Walker, B. E.: Induction of cleft palate in rats with anti-inflammatory drugs. Teratology **4**, 39—42 (1971)

Walz, D. T., Dimartino, M. J., Sutton, B. M.: Design and laboratory evaluation of gold compounds as anti-inflammatory agents. In: Anti-inflammatory Agents: Chemistry and Pharmacology, Vol. I. London: Academic Press 1974

Walzer, R., Feinstein, R.: Gold dermatitis. Arch. Derm. **104**, 107—109 (1971)

Wanka, J., Jones, L. I., Wood, P. H. N., Dixon, A. S. J.: Indomethacin in rheumatic disease. A controlled clinical trial. Ann. rheum. Dis. **23**, 218—225 (1964)

Warkany, J.: Are salicylates teratogenic? In: Proceedings of the Conference on Effects of Chronic Salicylate Administration. June 13—14, 1966. National Inst. of Arthritis & Metabolic Diseases. Bethesda, Maryland: U.S.D.H.E.W. 1966

Wax, J., Clinger, W. A., Varner, P., Bass, P., Winder, C. V.: Relationship of the enterohepatic cycle to ulcerogenesis in the rat small bowel with flufenamic acid. Gastroenterology **58**, 772—780 (1970)

Wax, J., Winder, C. V., Tessman, D. K., Stephens, M. D.: Comparative activities, tolerances and safety of non-steroidal anti-inflammatory agents in rats. J. Pharmacol. exp. Ther. **192**, 172 (1975)

Weck, A. L. de.: Immunological and non-immunological mechanisms of intolerance reactions to aspirin. Int. J. clin. Pharmacol. Toxicol. Suppl. **6**, 31—35 (1974)

Weiner, M., Piliero, S. J.: Non-steroid anti-inflammatory agents. Ann. Rev. Pharmacol. **10**, 171—198 (1970)

Whitehouse, M. W.: Some biochemical and pharmacological properties of anti-inflammatory drugs. Fortschr. Arzneimittel-Forsch. **8**, 323—429 (1965)

Wilhelmi, G.: Pharmacological properties of butazolidin and of its calcium and sodium salts. Indian J. Physiol. Pharmacol. **5**, 113—124 (1961)

Wilhelmi, G., Menassé-Gdynia, R.: Gastric mucosal damage by non-steroid anti-inflammatory agents in rats of different ages. Pharmacology **8**, 321—328 (1972)

Winship, D. H.: Basal and histamine stimulated human gastric acid secretion. Lack of effect of indomethacin in therapeutic doses. Gastroenterology **58**, 762—765 (1970)

Winter, C. A., Risley, E. A., Nuss, G. W.: Anti-inflammatory and antipyretic activities of indomethacin, 1-(p-chlorobenzoyl)-5-methoxy-2-methylindole-3-acetic acid. J. Pharmacol. exp. Ther. **141**, 369—376 (1963)

Wolfe, J. D., Metzger, A. L., Goldstein, R. C.: Aspirin hepatitis. Ann. intern. Med. **80**, 74—76 (1974)

Woodliff, H. J., Dougan, L.: Acute leukaemia associated with phenylbutazone treatment. Brit. med. J. **1964** I, 744—746

World Health Organization Scientific Group: Principles for the testing of drugs for teratogenicity. WHO Techn. Rep. Ser. 341. Geneva: WHO 1966

Zbinden, G.: The problem of the toxicologic examination of drugs in animals and their safety in man. Clin. Pharmacol. Ther. **5**, 537—545 (1964)

Pharmacology
of the Anti-Inflammatory Agents

CHAPTER 30

Prostaglandin Synthetase Inhibitors I

T. Y. SHEN

A. Introduction

The prostaglandins (PGs) are a group of lipid-soluble C_{20}-carboxylic acids containing an oxygenated five-membered ring and two parallel aliphatic side-chains. Chemically they are named as substituted prostenoic (1) or prostadienoic (2) acids.

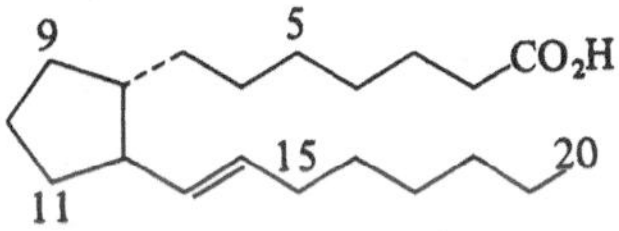

Five primary series of PGs (A, B, D, E, and F) are classified by the substitutions in the cyclopentyl moiety:

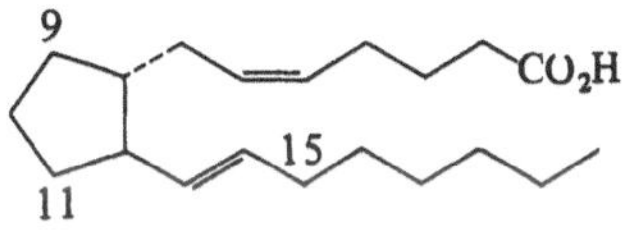

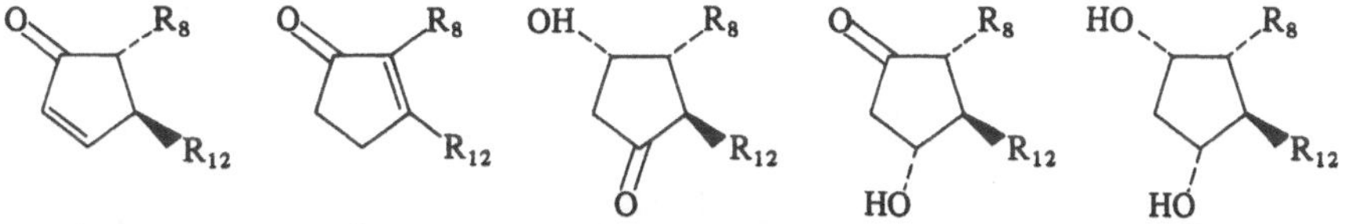

| A | B | D | E | F |

For example:
PGE$_1$ (-)-11α,15(S)-dihydroxy-9-oxo-13-*trans*-prostenoic acid

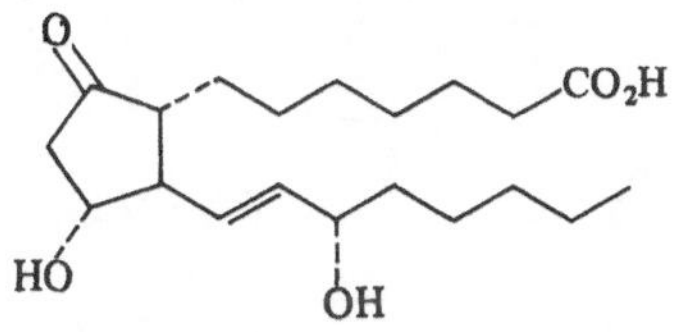

PGF$_{2\alpha}$(-)-9α,11α,15(S)-trihydroxy-5-*cis*-13-*trans*-prostadienoic acid

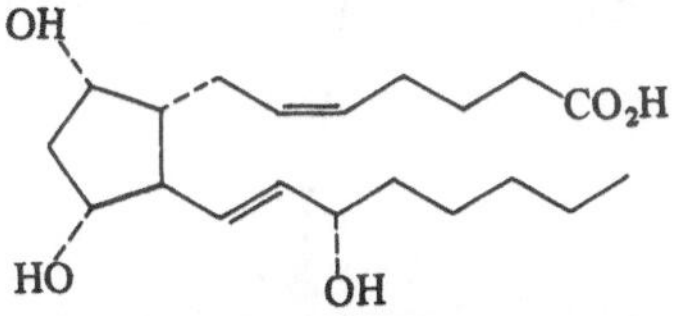

The biosynthesis of PGs from their unsaturated fatty acid precursors has been discussed in detail in Chapter 11. Reactions carried out by the multi-enzyme complex, commonly termed PG synthetase, are still being elucidated. Several excellent reviews on the biosynthetic pathways and their inhibitors have been published. As background for the discussion of synthetase inhibitors, a schematic description of our current understanding is depicted below:

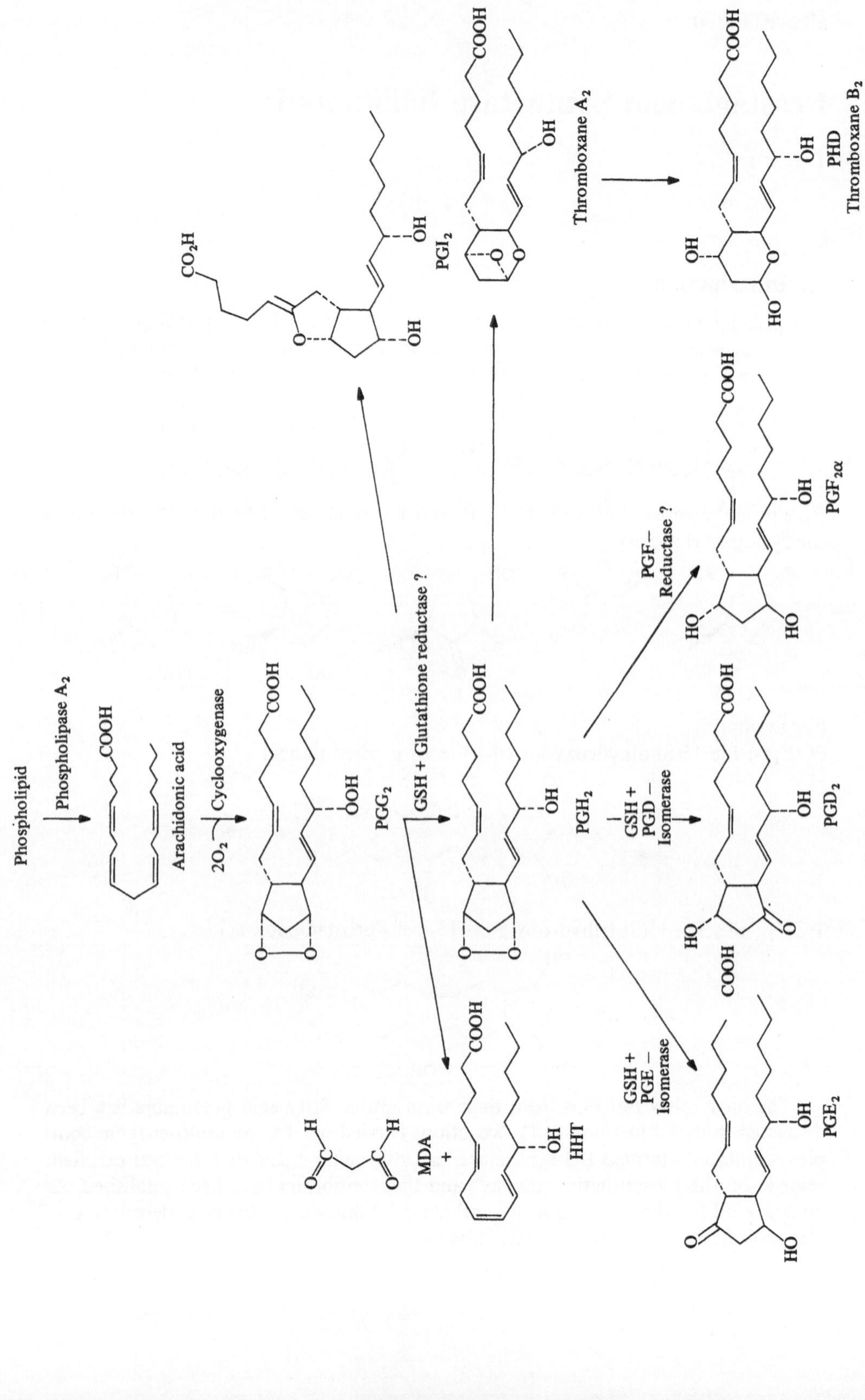
Phospholipid
Phospholipase A_2
COOH
Arachidonic acid
$2O_2$
Cyclooxygenase
COOH
OOH
PGG_2
GSH + Glutathione reductase ?
COOH
OH
PGH_2
MDA
+
COOH
OH
HHT
CO_2H
OH
OH
PGI_2
COOH
OH
Thromboxane A_2
COOH
OH
HO
OH
PHD
Thromboxane B_2
PGF–
Reductase ?
COOH
HO
HO
OH
$PGF_{2\alpha}$
GSH +
PGD –
Isomerase
COOH
HO
OH
PGD_2
GSH +
PGE –
Isomerase
COOH
HO
OH
PGE_2

The PG synthetase pathway may also be considered as an integral part of the emerging arachidonic acid cascade, which includes the lipoxygenase pathway as shown below:

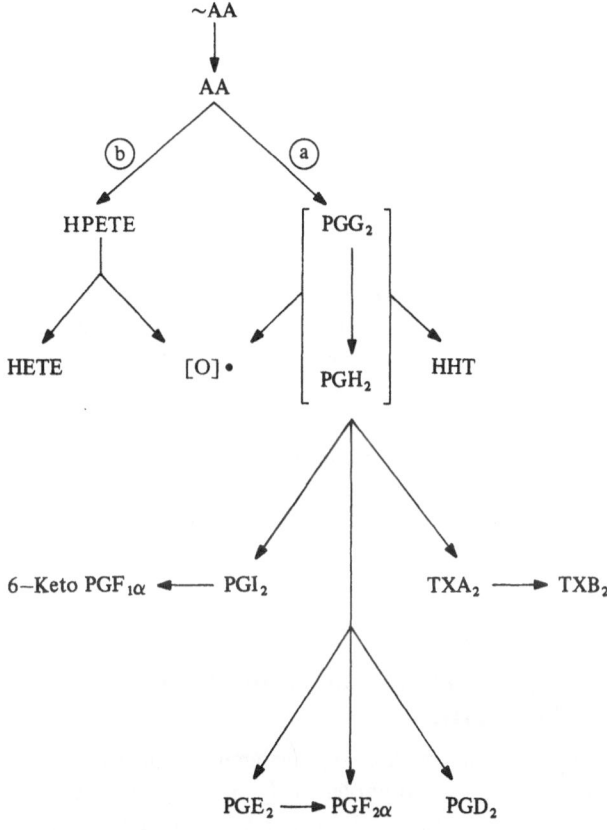

The arachidonic acid (AA) cascade

(a) PG synthetase pathway

(b) Lipoxygenase pathway

Interest in PG synthetase inhibitors in the past few years has been greatly stimulated by the discovery that aspirin-like drugs block PG biosynthesis (VANE, 1971). In the search for non-steroid anti-inflammatory agents, this finding provided a new mechanistic concept as well as a biochemical approach. Perhaps more importantly, medically useful inhibitors such as aspirin and indomethacin soon became valuable research tools in discerning the possible involvement of PGs—which are extremely potent, often present in nanogram quantities and metabolically unstable—in numerous physiological systems. The elucidation of new roles of PGs and other metabolites, such as thromboxanes (HAMBERG et al., 1975), in the synthetase pathway in turn stimulated a wider interest in the search for better or more selective inhibitors as new therapeutic agents. As a result, a variety of chemical structures, acidic and non-acidic, synthetic and naturally occurring, as well as many known pharmacological agents, have been identified as PG synthetase inhibitors. Most of these inhibitors were evaluated in crude "synthetase" preparations from various tissues. In addition, isolated cells, such as the human platelets (SMITH and WILLIS, 1971) and epidermal cells (FORSTRÖM et al., 1974), dog spleens (FERREIRA et al., 1971), isolated gastrointestinal tissues (VAN NUETEN, 1976), human rheumatoid synovium (ROBINSON et al., 1975) and various in vivo models, have been used recently to measure the systemic effect of some inhibitors. The synthetase complex carries out multi-step conversions involving several co-factors. Its sensitivity to drug inhibition is much influenced by the concentrations of substrates, co-factors, Cu^{++}, etc. It has also shown tissue specificity in many instances. Consequently, the observed overall activities of these inhibitors in more than 40 different systems can be best compared in a semiquantitative manner only. Other characteristics of the inhibitors such as competitiveness or non-competitiveness with substrates, the site of enzymic inhibition, selective inhibition of PGE vs. PGF, PG antagonism, etc., also influence their pharmacological effects.

For the sake of convenience and clarity, only selected literature reports up to the beginning of 1976 were reviewed. Numerous patents on potential non-steroid anti-inflammatory drugs, most of them undoubtedly PG synthetase inhibitors, have purposely been left out. A diversity of inhibitors are classified according to their primary pharmacological properties and/or chemical structure types and are discussed below.

B. Inhibition of Synthetase by Substrate Analogues and Fatty Acid Derivatives

The biosynthetic precursors of PGs are endogenous unsaturated fatty acids, which are released from glycerides and cholesterol esters by the action of acylhydrolases. Arachidonic acid (5) (all-cis-5,8,11,14-eicosatetraenoic acid) is the precursor for the E_2 and F_2 series, whereas di-homo-γ-linolenic acid (6) (all-cis-8,11,14-eicosatrienoic acid) is the precursor for the E_1 and F_1 series.

(5)   (6)

I. Unsaturated Fatty Acids

Not unexpectedly, a number of unsaturated fatty acids, particularly those containing acetylenic linkages, are inhibitors of the synthetase. The acetylenic analogue of arachidonic acid, eicosa-3,8,11,14-tetraynoic acid (7), is a non-substrate, irreversible inhibitor of E_2 synthesis at $1.0–5.0$ μM. The 8,11,14-triynoic analog (8) is also active.

$$C_5H_9C\overset{14}{\equiv}\overset{}{C}-CH_2-C\overset{11}{\equiv}\overset{}{C}-CH_2-C\overset{8}{\equiv}\overset{}{C}-CH_2-C\overset{5}{\equiv}\overset{}{C}-(CH_2)_3CO_2H \qquad (7)$$

$$C_5H_9C\equiv C-CH_2-C\equiv C-CH_2-C\equiv C-(CH_2)_6CO_2H \qquad (8)$$

Table 1

Fatty acid		Unsaturation						Ki μM
Arachidonic	20:4		5c	8c	11c	14c		1.7
	20:6	2c	5c	8c	11c	14c	17c	2.5
	20:5		5c	8c	11c	14c	17c	
	20:4		5c	8c	12t	14c		
Eicosatrienoic	20:3			8c	12t	14c		0.12
Linolenic	18:3				9c	12c	15c	15
Linoleic	18:2				9c	12c		
Oleic	18:1				9c			22
	18:1				10a			10

c = *cis* olefin; t = *trans* olefin; a = acetylene.

Changing the number, position, and/or geometry of the all-*cis* olefinic bonds in eicosatetra or trienoic acids yielded additional inhibitors. Examples of some fatty acid inhibitors in the sheep seminal vescicle (SSV) system are given in Table 1 (FLOWER, 1974).

Several C_{18} fatty acids have shown modest inhibitor activity only. The presence of an acetylenic linkage either at 9 or 12 is preferred, whereas no significant difference was found with the remaining *cis* or *trans* double bonds. The inhibitory activity of (7) was shown to be biphasic: an instantaneous concentration dependent effect and a time dependent irreversible destruction of the catalytic site. The latter action requires oxygen uptake and the formation of the lipid peroxide intermediate, an interesting phenomenon also observed with aspirin and indomethacin discussed below. The biosynthesis of PGE_2 by the microsomal fraction from human epidermis was also inhibited by linoleic, linolenic, and eicosatrienoic acids at 1–2 mM concentrations (ZIBOH et al., 1973).

Some substituted acetylenic compounds have been found to be potent irreversible enzyme inhibitors of the k_{cat} type. Following the abstraction of an α-proton, the acetylene (9) isomerizes to a highly electrophilic allene species (10) which could react with a nucleophile of the active-site to form a stable adduct.

(9)   (10)

(DOWNING et al., 1972). Conceivably similar mechanisms may be involved in the irreversible inhibition of cyclo-oxygenase by the acetylenic fatty acids.

These fatty acid derivatives are conformationally flexible. The biphasic inhibition found with some examples indicate that further analysis of parameters, such as binding with the active site, possible formation of an active intermediate at the catalytic site and chemical inactivation of the enzyme, may lead to the design of better inhibitors.

II. Bicyclic Analogues

A variety of analogues of PGs have been synthesized as PG agonists or antagonists. An oxaprostaglandin analogue, 5-oxaprost-13-*trans*-enoate (11), and related structures were reported to be competitive inhibitors of bovine seminal vesicle (BSV) PG synthetase with a K_i of 32 μM (MCDONALD-GIBSON et al., 1973) for (11).

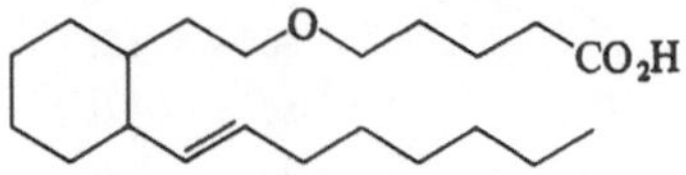

(11)

Bicyclic analogues of endoperoxide PGH_2 (12) such as (13)–(16) have shown highly potent PG-like activities (BUNDY, 1975; COREY et al., 1975, 1976; MALMSTEN, 1976).

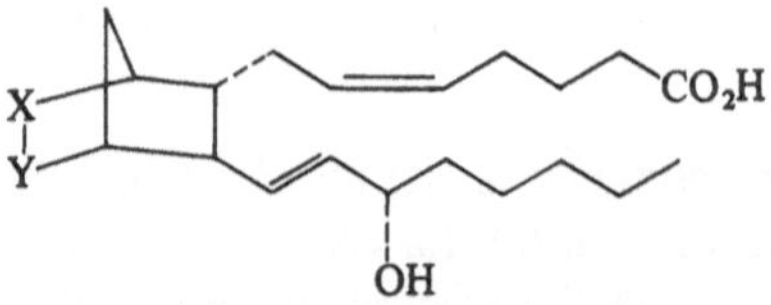

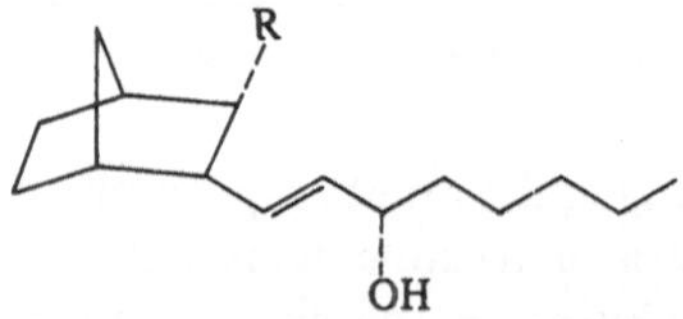

X – Y		
O – O	PGH_2	(12)
O – CH_2		(13)
CH_2 – O		(14)
N = N		(15)
CH = CH		(16)
CH_2 – CH_2		(17) 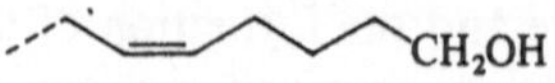

R

$(CH_2)_6CO_2H$ (18)

CH_2OH (19)

Compound (18) competitively inhibits the formation of PGE, but not PGFα from 8,11,14-eicosatrienoic acid at ca. 1 mM (WLODAWER et al., 1971). The corresponding Δ^5 ("2" series) analogues (16), (17), and (19) were recently found to be more potent inhibitors of PGE_2 synthesis at <0.5 mM (LEENEY et al., 1976). The selective synthetase inhibitory activity of these PGH analogues, even though modest, suggests that other analogues of fatty acids and PG intermediates may exert multiple effects on the synthesis and action of prostaglandins. The pharmacological actions of these inhibitors in vivo need to be thoroughly investigated.

C. Regulation of Enzymic Factors: Co-Factors, Stimulation, and Catabolism

Several co-factors are required in the stepwise biosynthesis of PGs. Therefore, the overall production of PGs by the synthetase system is subject to regulation by co-factor inhibitors or other enzymic stimulators. The level of PGs may also be manipulated by altering the activity of the catabolic enzyme, 15-hydroxy-PG dehydrogenase

I. Regulation of Biosynthesis

The fatty acid oxygenase is a phenol-activated enzyme which requires an activity factor for optimal activity (LANDS et al., 1976). It is stimulated by haemoglobin or haem compounds and inhibited by haem enzyme inhibitors such as azide ion and 3-amino-1,2,4-triazole (PANGANAMALA et al., 1974). It is also inhibited by copper complexing agents such as diethyldithiocarbamate. Nevertheless, the question of whether the oxygenase is a metalloenzyme remains unsolved.

The mechanism of the initial oxygenation steps is still under investigation. The possible involvement of superoxide anion (O_2-) is not clear, but the requirement of a singlet oxygen ($^1O_2$) and a free hydroxyl radical ($\cdot OH$) have been proposed (PANGANAMALA et al., 1976). A recent report showed that a hydroxyl radical scavenger, chlorpromazine (20) inhibits the oxygenation of arachidonic acid in both microsomal and platelet systems whereas a singlet oxygen scavenger, 1,4-diazabicyclo[2,2,2]octane (21), does not. The requirement for H_2O_2 in PG biosynthesis has not

(20)   (21)

been unequivocally established, but a scheme involving an Fe^{++}-enzyme complex was postulated (PANGANAMALA et al., 1974, 1976).

$$H_2O_2 + Fe^{++}\text{-enzyme} \rightarrow \cdot OH^- + Fe^{+++}\text{-enzyme}$$

The observed stimulating effect of phenolic compounds such as hydroquinone, eugenol (22), p-aminophenol, 5-hydroxyindole acetic acid (23), etc., may be attributed to their ability to generate H_2O_2 through a quinone-hydroquinone cycle.

(22)   (23)

Other phenolic compounds, such as 2,7-dihydroxynaphthalene, were found to be potent inhibitors at 2 μM (TAKEGUCHI and SIH, 1972). Vitamin E, α-tocopherol (24), is weakly inhibitory. Other antioxidants, e.g., butylated hydroxyanisole, α-naphthol and ethoxyquin (25), are non-competitive inhibitors at 10^{-6} M (VANDERHOEK and LANDS, 1973).

(24)   (25)

The cyclo-oxygenase-stimulating effect of phenolic compounds counteracts the inhibitory action of some anti-inflammatory drugs, such as indomethacin (26), flurbiprofen (27), and ibuprofen (28). In the case of fenamates (29) and (30), an enhancement of inhibition with a reduced ID_{50} value was observed (EGAN et al., 1976).

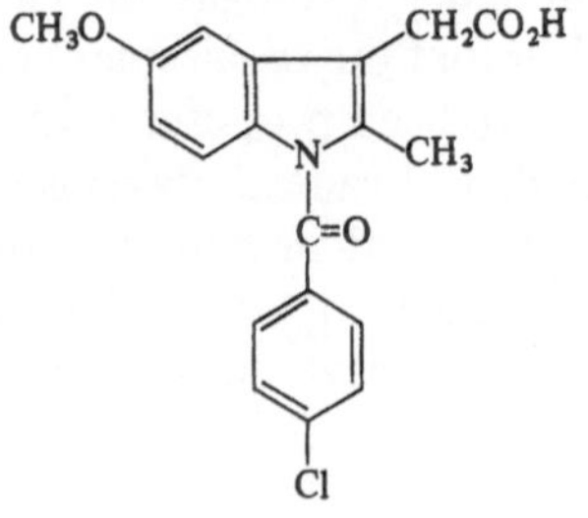

(26) 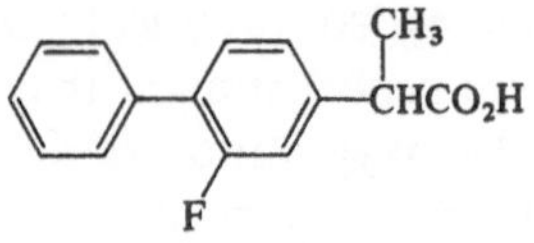   (27) 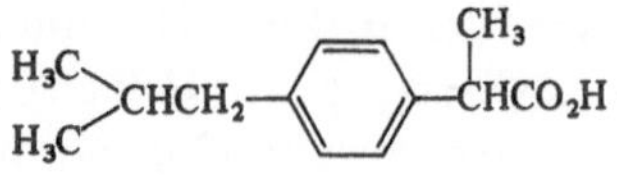   (28)

The flavonoid rutin, quercetin-3-rutinoside (31), is another polyphenolic substance. Interestingly, the 7-hydroxyethylated derivative stimulates PG synthesis in the microsomal fraction of human skin homogenate at 60 µg/ml, whereas the tri (7,3′,4′) and tetra (5,7,3′,4′) substituted derivatives are inhibitors at 20 µg/ml. These properties have been related to their effects on inflammatory and microvascular permeability (ARTURSON and JONSSON, 1975).

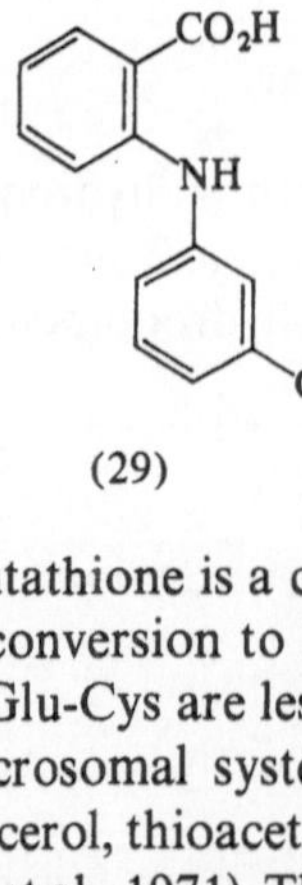

(29) 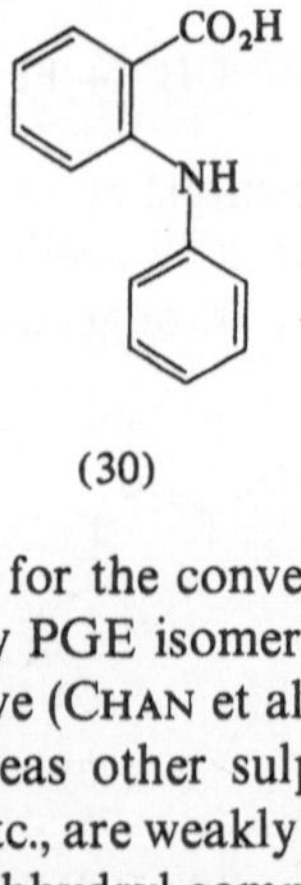   (30) 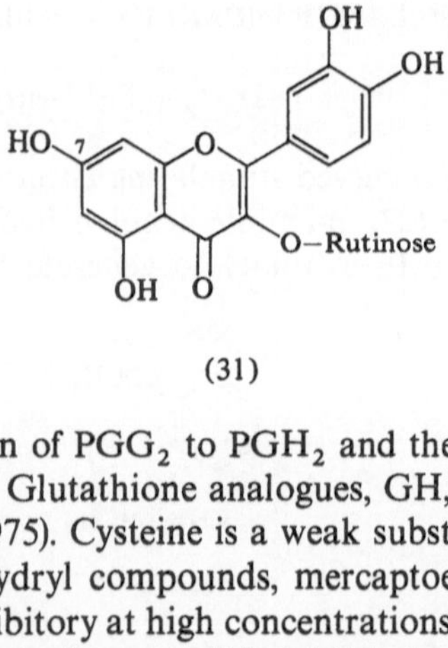   (31)

Glutathione is a co-factor for the conversion of PGG_2 to PGH_2 and the subsequent conversion to PGE_2 by PGE isomerase. Glutathione analogues, GH, GSAc, and γ-Glu-Cys are less effective (CHAN et al., 1975). Cysteine is a weak substitute in the microsomal system whereas other sulphhydryl compounds, mercaptoethanol, thioglycerol, thioacetamide, etc., are weakly inhibitory at high concentrations (TAKEGUCHI et al., 1971). These sulphhydryl compounds also reversibly inhibit the platelet system in vitro and in vivo (VARGAFTIG et al., 1974). The inhibitory effect is reversed by Cu^{++}, although there seems to be no direct relationship between Cu^{++} chelation and antagonism of arachidonic acid effect on platelets. In our laboratory, chelating agents D-penicillamine (32) and 5-amino-1-phenyltetrazole (33) are inactive at 100 µg/ml in the SSV system (SHEN et al., 1974).

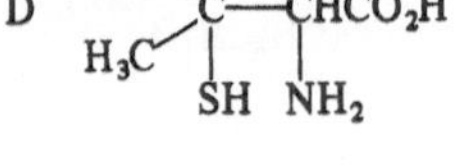

(32) 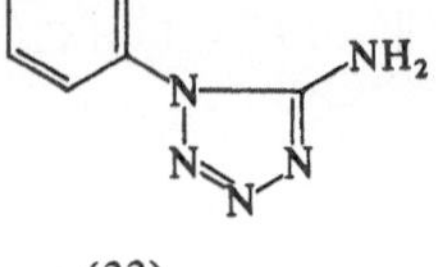   (33)

An interesting stimulation of PG synthesis by the rat renal papilla in vitro was observed after incubation with angiotensin II (10 ng/ml), possibly by activation of acyl hydrolase and increase of the substrate levels (DAMON et al., 1975).

PGF is formed from PGE by PGE 9-keto-reductase. It is not yet certain whether the conversion of PGH_2 into $PGF_{2\alpha}$ is enzyme catalyzed. Cupric ions and Cu^{++}-dithiothreitol complex enhanced the formation of PGF at the expense of other PGs, possibly by non-enzymic reduction of PG endoperoxides (CHAN et al., 1975). On the other hand, the Zn^{++}-dithiothreitol complex stimulated the formation of PGE_2. These findings clearly indicate the feasibility of regulating both the level and type of PGs.

II. Catabolic Enzymes

Most PGs are metabolically inactivated by oxidation of the 15-hydroxyl group, saturation of the Δ^{13} double bond, and oxidation of the two side-chains. The PG 15-hydroxy dehydrogenase (PGDH), an NAD^+-dependent enzyme, is most significant in the inactivation of PGE and PGF. A number of moderately potent inhibitors have been reported. Among these are PG and fatty acid analogues, NAD^+ antagonists, purine and pyrimidine nucleosides, sulphhydryl inhibitors and Ca^{++} ions. Poly-phosphoretin phosphate and diphloretin phosphate inhibit the pulmonary inactivation of PGE_2, $F_{2\alpha}$ and $F_{2\beta}$ at 10^{-7} M. Several anti-inflammatory agents, e.g., indomethacin (26), niflumic acid (34) and meclofenamic acid (35), inhibit PGDH at 10^{-4} M concentrations. The indomethacin inhibition is non-competitive with re-

(34)   (35)

spect to PGE_1. The inhibitory activity of these PG synthetase inhibitors has also shown tissue specificity. The concentrations required are generally higher for PGDH than for synthetase inhibition. Further investigations are needed to ascertain the in vivo effects of these multi-action inhibitors on various physiological responses (HANSEN, 1974).

D. Inhibition by Non-Steroid Anti-Inflammatory Agents

I. An Overview of Structure-Activity Relationship

1. Correlation of PG Synthetase Inhibition With Anti-Inflammatory Action

The mechanisms of action of non-steroid anti-inflammatory drugs (NSAID) have been investigated extensively, especially after the introduction of indomethacin and other aryl acids in recent years. In biochemical or cellular biological terms, many possible mechanisms have been considered (SHEN, 1972; BRUNE et al., 1976). Among these, the suggestion of PG synthetase inhibition was particularly noteworthy on account of the following observations:

1. The biosynthesis of PGs is significantly inhibited by NSAID at concentrations (0.1–10 µg/ml) comparable to their therapeutic levels in man and in animal models. In contrast, much higher (10^{-5}–10^{-3} M) concentrations of these drugs are required to regulate other proposed mechanisms.

2. The PG synthetase is readily inhibited by a number of α-methyl aryl acetic acids with the S($+$) absolute configuration, but not by their R($-$) enantiomers. It is noteworthy that this very high degree of stereospecificity is the same as observed in in vivo anti-inflammatory assays but not shared by any other in vitro systems. For example, the uncoupling of oxidative phosphorylation and the stabilization of erythrocyte membrane are equally responsive to both S and R isomers.

3. A remarkable parellelism has been observed between the structure-activity relationships for in vivo anti-inflammatory actions and in vitro PG synthetase inhibition for several series of NSAID. The correlation is particularly good for more potent aryl acids which may have similar pharmacodynamic characteristics.

The correlation between anti-inflammatory action and PG synthetase inhibition has been discussed widely. Bearing in mind that differential metabolisms, distribution barriers, albumin-binding and other systemic factors often exert a profound influence on the overall in vivo efficacy of any enzyme inhibitors, the observed general correlation, e.g., with indomethacin analogues described below, is truly remarkable. Nevertheless, one would not expect similar correlations for NSAID in all cases. The relative potency of PG synthetase inhibitors is profoundly influenced by in vitro experimental conditions, e.g., source of enzyme preparations, concentration of substrates, co-factors, Cu^{++}, phenolic, and sulphhydryl reagents, etc. The effect of substrate concentration on ID_{50} of several typical synthetase inhibitors are illustrated in Table 2 (CUSHMAN and CHEUNG, 1976).

Many NSAID may well have different or multiple mechanisms of action to inhibit the dynamic and complex inflammatory process in vivo. Fenamates (see Sect. D.V.) have shown both synthetase inhibition and PG antagonism. Others may interfere with PG metabolism through actions on PG catabolic enzymes, cyclonu-

Table 2. Effect of substrate concentrations on inhibitory potency of anti-inflammatory agents

	ID_{50} (µM) (1 mM arachidonate)			ID_{50} (µM) (1µM arachidonate)
	$F_{2\alpha}$	E_2	D_2	E_2
Meclofenamic acid (35)	14	7	14	0.6
Indomethacin (26)	31	40	31	0.6
Niflumic acid (34)	150	100	250	0.3
Naproxen (59)	480	370	480	0.8
Ibuprofen (28)	500	650	600	6
Phenylbutazone (77)	370	430	—	37
Aspirin	>10000	9000	>10000	1100
Benzydamine (101)	1100	(stimulation)	1500	160

cleotide pathways, etc. Still others may exert their anti-arthritic action primarily at some immunological mechanisms which are partially or indirectly regulated by PGs. Thus, the simple question of correlating in vitro PG synthetase inhibition with in vivo anti-inflammatory action becomes academic if not kept in perspective. From the application viewpoint, the synthetic inhibitory activity of a compound may be a good indicator of its intrinsic or local anti-inflammatory potency. The possible use of a combination of synthetase inhibition assay and protein binding assay to improve the correlation with in vivo anti-inflammatory activity has been suggested (GRY-GLEWSKI et al., 1976). Naturally, a reasonable correlation in a given chemical series would facilitate the synthetic modifications. On the other hand, any unsatisfactory correlation should not discourage investigators from studying the anti-arthritic potential of a new lead in animal models. In the case of non-acidic agents, it is highly probable that both the pharmacokinetics and the modes of PG inhibition will vary according to their structure differences. If PG inhibition is not necessary for anti-inflammatory action, neither is it sufficient. As PGs are involved in many physiological processes, it is not surprising that various pharmacological agents should also inhibit the synthetase system. Further understanding of PG biochemistry will not only improve the selectivity of inhibitors but also provide a rational basis for combining several desirable pharmacological properties in a more effective therapeutic agent.

2. General Structure-Activity Relationship

Among PG synthetase inhibitors the acidic NSAID, particularly the aryl acids, represent a predominant group. Chemically they may be divided into several subclasses: salicylates, indomethacin analogues, phenyl acetic acids, fenamic acids and enolic compounds. Most of them inhibit the cyclo-oxygenase by competing with the substrate arachidonic acid at the active site. The aromatic moieties in these compounds are sterically and electronically similar to the polyene system in arachidonic acid, possibly interacting with a common binding site. Attempts have been made to refine the geometry of this hypothetical binding site, originally postulated from in vivo anti-inflammatory data, by more sophisticated calculations and model building (see Sect. G.V.). In general, these NSAID possess two non-coplanar hydrophobic or aromatic moieties and an acidic group. The in vitro enzyme inhibition and in vivo anti-inflammatory activities are often enhanced significantly by electronegative substituents such as fluorine and chlorine, at a specific position of the molecule. Interestingly, the more potent halogen-containing flurbiprofen (27) and meclofenamic acid (35) are time-dependent, irreversible inhibitors, whereas their less potent halogen-free congeners are only reversible inhibitors (ROME and LANDS, 1975). The mechanism of action of aspirin has been attributed to its ability to acetylate the cyclo-oxygenase (ROTH et al., 1975; ROME et al., 1976). Sodium salicylate has less than one-tenth of the enzyme inhibitory activity (SMITH et al., 1975). The molecular mechanisms of other irreversible inhibitors are still under investigation. Not unexpectedly, there are notable differences in optimal structural features and substituents among subclasses of aryl acids. These differences may reflect alternative modes of binding and changes in their physicochemical requirements. Similar spatial arrangements of hydrophobic or aromatic moieties are also found in the non-acidic PG synthetase inhibitors. However, since the site of action (e.g., cyclo-oxygenase) and kinetics of only a few inhibitors have been determined, the relationship between acidic and non-acidic inhibitors remains to be elucidated.

II. Salicylates

Since the original observation by Vane (1971), the inhibition of PG synthetase by aspirin and other salicylates has been studied extensively in many systems. The biological effects resulting by this inhibition are described elsewhere in this mono-graph. Following the isolation of cyclo-oxygenase, it was reported (Roth et al., 1975; Rome et al., 1976) that aspirin quantitatively and selectively acetylated the oxygenase at its functional stage. Serum proteins and, denatured oxygenase were not acetylated nearly as rapidly. Optimal acetylation also seemed dependent upon the presence of haemprotein activators that give optimal enzymic activity of the oxygenase. The acylation was partially, but not completely, blocked by pre-incubation of the enzyme with indomethacin which presumably changed the configuration of the active site.

$$\text{(36)}$$

The tissue specificity of aspirin was demonstrated by its inhibitory potencies on the release of $PGF_{2\alpha}$ from human platelets and synovium, a sixfold difference in ID_{50} (29 vs. 172 μM, respectively) was observed. As both systems were equally sensitive to indomethacin (ID_{50} 1.33 and 1.08 μM, respectively), this may explain the profound effect of aspirin on platelet function at its anti-arthritic therapeutic doses (Patrono et al., 1976).

The in vitro inhibition by aspirin is about four times more potent than salicylic acid. In the SSV system used in our laboratory, replacement of the phenolic OH by SH or OCH_3 completely abolishes the activity. The methyl ester of aspirin is also much less active. Gentisic acid, the 5-hydroxy metabolite without any 0-acetyl group, is almost as effective as aspirin. However, it may be noted that gentisic acid also has the hydroquinone structure, which may inhibit the enzyme by a different mechanism. The 6-hydroxy isomer, γ-resorcyclic acid, is as active as gentisic acid against rabbit kidney synthetase (Blackwell et al., 1975).

The structure specificity of salicylates was demonstrated in our laboratory by the examination of a large number of substituted salicylates with substituents at 3, 4, and 5 positions, e.g., 3-methoxy, 3-chloro, 4-phenyl, 5-phenoxy, 5-t-butyl, and 5-bromo, etc. All of them are inactive as PG-synthetase inhibitors in the SSV system and are also inactive in anti-inflammatory assays in vivo.

The real exceptions are analogues with 5-fluorinated phenyl and certain 5-het-eroaryl substituents, such as diflunisal (36), and the 5-(1-pyrryl) derivative (37) of salicylic acid. In these cases, both the anti-inflammatory and PG synthetase inhibi-tion appeared to be not significantly affected by the presence or absence of an 0-acetyl group. In view of the importance of trans-acetylation in the inactivation of cyclooxygenase by aspirin, the mode of enzyme inhibition by diflunisal and its 0-acetyl derivative are being compared. The non-acetylating salicylate, diflunisal, ex-erts its anti-inflammatory and analgesic effects in man with a concomitant decrease of the excretion of 7α-hydroxy-5,11,diketotetranorprostane-1,16-dioic acid (38), the major urinary metabolite of PGE$_1$ and PGE$_2$. On the other hand, unlike aspirin it did not produce any significant effect on platelet aggregation, bleeding time, etc., at its therapeutic doses (STEELMAN et al., 1976). Apparently, a partial separation of PG-related pharmacological effects has been achieved.

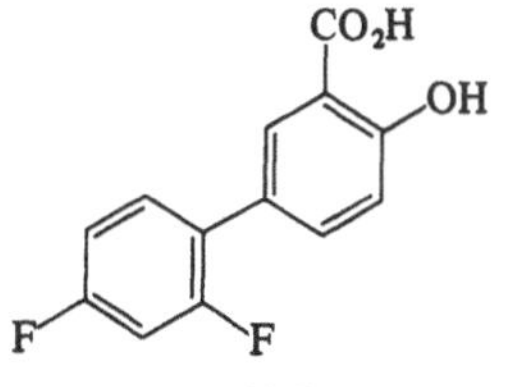

(36)

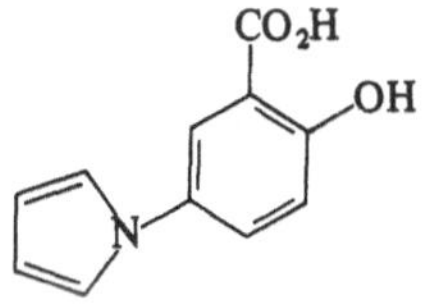

(37)

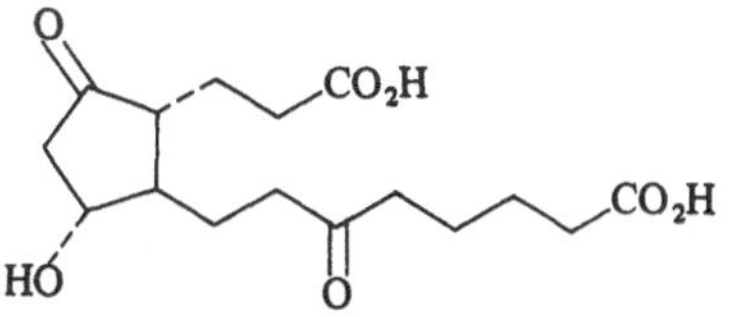

(38)

III. Indomethacin, Sulindac, and Congeners

Since the original observation by VANE (1971) that indomethacin (26) is a potent inhibitor of PG synthetase, it has been widely used as a reference compound in numerous PG synthetase systems. Some recent examples are shown in Table 3. Indomethacin is a time-dependent, concentration-dependent, substrate-competitive, irreversible inhibitor (SMITH and LANDS, 1971; ROME and LANDS, 1975; KU and WASVARY, 1975). Its site of inhibition is the formation of PGG from precursor fatty acids by cyclo-oxygenase (MIYAMOTO et al., 1976), thereby blocking the subsequent formation of prostaglandins E, F, and thromboxanes. The p-chlorobenzoyl group in indomethacin is chemically labile with a half-life of 1 h at pH 10. However, unlike aspirin no transacylation of cyclo-oxygenase has been observed.

The in vivo PG synthetase inhibition by indomethacin was demonstrated by a 77–98% reduction of the urinary metabolite 15-keto-13,14-dihydro PG in patients treated with 200 mg of indomethacin (HAMBERG and SAMUELSSON, 1972). At higher concentrations (10^{-4}–10^{-5} M), indomethacin was also reported to be a non-competitive inhibitor of PGDH in vitro (HANSEN, 1974). The possible role of indomethacin on the PG turnover in different tissues and species remains to be elucidated.

Regarding the structure-activity relationship of indomethacin and its congeners, a highly specific pattern is readily discernible from the evaluation of many analogues in our laboratory. The correlation of in vitro PG synthetase inhibition with the in vivo anti-inflammatory activity, as measured by the carrageenin-foot oedema assays, is remarkably good for this series. Three notable characteristics of these inhibitors, namely, significant activity at therapeutic levels of drug concentration (μg/ml), requirement for well-defined stereochemical configuration and a preference for certain types of chemical substituents, are equally well observed in both in vitro and in vivo systems. The relative activities of a group of selected indomethacin analogues are shown in Table 4.

Table 3. Inhibition of PG synthesis by indomethacin in various in vitro systems

Enzyme source	ID_{50} (μM)	References
Bovine seminal vesicles (BSV)	0.07	DEMBINSKA-KIEĆ et al. (1976)
	0.6	CUSHMAN and CHEUNG (1976)
	0.63	VIGDAHL and TUKEY (1975)
	1	YANAGI and KOMATSU (1976)
	1.4	HORODNIAK et al. (1974)
	2.8	HORODNIAK et al. (1975)
	6	ZIEL and KRUPP (1975)
	6.5	KU and WASVARY (1975)
	7.5	CARMINATI and LERNER (1975)
	15	ADAMS et al. (1975)
	20	DEBY et al. (1975)
Sheep seminal vesicles (SSV)	0.45	HAM et al. (1972)
	0.5	GAUT et al. (1976)
Goat seminal vesicles	5.6	WISEMAN et al. (1975)
Guinea pig lung	0.6	TOLMAN et al. (1976)
Dog spleen	0.17	FLOWER et al. (1973)
Rabbit brain	0.6	DEMBINSKA-KIEĆ et al. (1976)
	3.6	FLOWER et al. (1973)
Rabbit kidney	3.7	BLACKWELL et al. (1975)
	0.15	DEMBINSKA-KIEĆ et al. (1976)
Rat platelets	2.2	PATRONO et al. (1975)
Human platelets	1.3	PATRONO et al. (1976)
Human synovium	0.003	KANTROWITZ et al. (1975)
	0.5	CROOK and COLLINS (1975)
	2.2	PATRONO et al. (1976)
Human epidermal cells	3	FÖRSTRÖM et al. (1974)

Table 4. Indomethacin and Sulindac analogues Anti-inflammatory activity

Indole series	Man daily dose	Rat carrageenin oedema ED_{50} mg/kg	PG synthetase inhibition (SSV)[a] ID_{50} μM
(26) (Indomethacin)	75–100 mg	2.4	0.4
(39) (MK-825)	200 mg	4	0.6
(40)		ca. 1.1	0.6
(41) (Metabolite)		ca. 50	1.5
(42) (MK-555)	2–3 g	25	10
(43) (MK-410)	1–1.5 g	15	2.2
Indene Series			
(50) (MK-715)	200–400 mg	4	2
(52) (Sulindac)	300–400 mg	4.9	—
(51) (Sulphide metabolite)		2	2.2
Others			
(45)		Inactive	Inactive
(47)			ca. 3
(48)		≥50	30
(49)		9	3

[a] The PG synthetase inhibition assay of these compounds and others in the following tables, marked by (SSV)*, were carried out by HAM, HUMES and associates in our laboratories using the procedure described in HAM et al., 1972.

In comparing the relative potency of various analogues, it may be pointed out that the dimethylamino analogue (MK-825) (39) was equally as efficacious as indomethacin in man at approximately twice the dosage. The benzyl analogues, MK-555 (42) and MK-410 (43), also showed clinical efficacy respectively at 2 g/day and 1 g/day levels. The p-fluoro analogue (40) is at least as active as indomethacin in several animal models. A general parallelism between in vitro and in vivo activities is discernible.

The requirement for a sinister absolute configuration at the asymmetric center in MK-555 (42), MK-410 (43), and their p-methoxy analogue (44), is consistently shown by the dominant, if not exclusive, activity of the three S(+) enantiomers. As described below, this stereospecificity was also demonstrated by several α-methylarylacetic acids. Two major metabolites of indomethacin, the desbenzoyl (45) and desbenzoyldesmethyl derivatives (46), are completely inactive. Modest activity in vitro and in vivo were shown by the desmethyl metabolite (41). The effects of various substituents on the indole ring and the acetic acid side-chain on the in vivo and in vitro activities are exemplified by analogues (47) to (49).

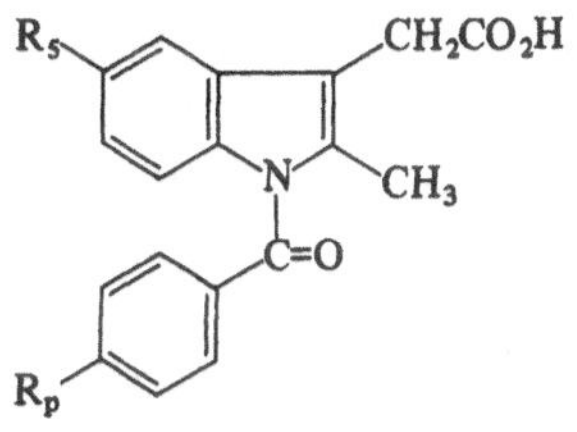

	R_s	R_p
(26)	CH_3O	Cl
(39)	$(CH_3)_2N$	Cl
(40)	CH_3O	F
(41)	OH	Cl

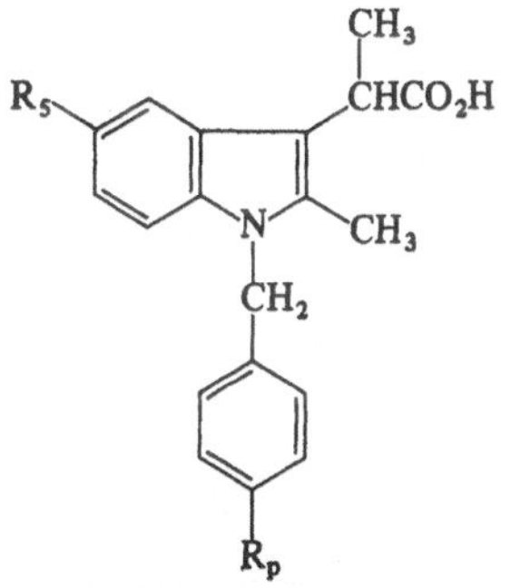

	R_s	R_p
(42)	CH_3O	Cl
(43)	CH_3O	SCH_3
(44)	CH_3O	CH_3O

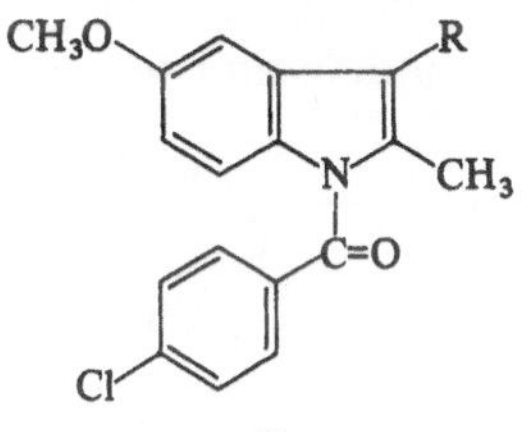

	R
(47)	CH_2CH_2OH
(48)	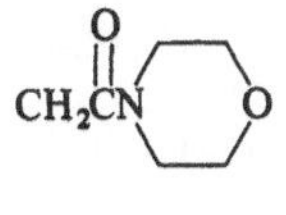 $CH_2CN\text{(morpholine)}$

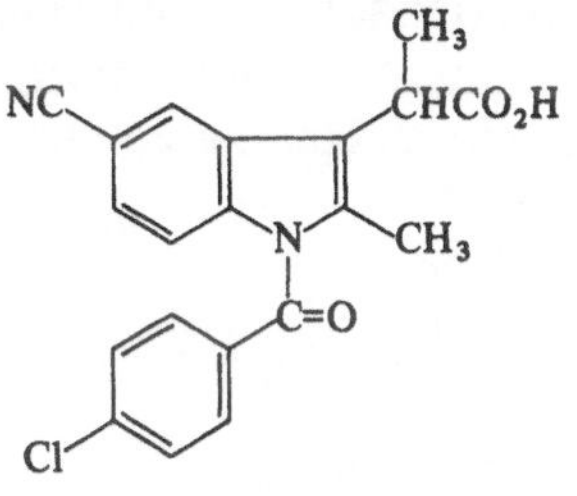

(49)

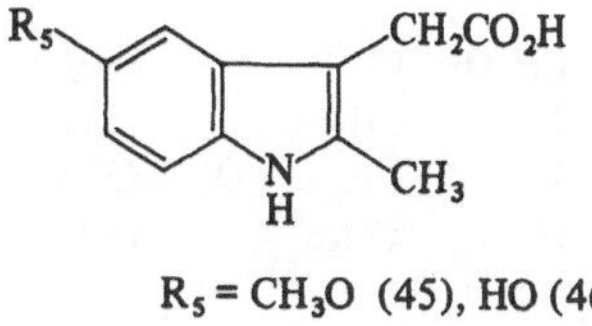

$R_s = CH_3O$ (45), HO (46)

Electronically and stereochemically 1-benzylidenyl indene is isosteric with N-benzoyl indole. A semi-quantitative parallelism between the indene and indole series in terms of anti-inflammatory and PG synthetase inhibition has been observed. For example, the indene isotere of indomethacin, MK-715 (50), is pharmacologically very similar to indomethacin and comparably active in vitro.

Sulindac (52) (MK-231, Clinoril) is a new anti-arthritic agent with clinical efficacy comparable to that of indomethacin but with an improved patient tolerance (SHEN et al., 1972; VAN ARMAN et al., 1972). Interestingly, sulindac is not an inhibitor of PG synthetase in vitro, whereas the corresponding sulphide analogue is a very potent one. The metabolism of sulphoxide is known to form sulphide and sulphone in the following manner:

$$CH_3S \rightleftharpoons \quad \underset{\underset{O}{\downarrow}}{CH_3S} \longrightarrow CH_3SO_2$$

sulphide   suphoxide   sulphone

In man, as well as in animals, the sulphide metabolite (51) of sulindac has a long serum half life of 18 h and is considered the active species of sulindac. The sulphone metabolite (53) is inactive both in vivo and in vitro. Thus, the pharmacodynamics of sulindac rationalises the use of sulindac as a pro-drug of a potent and long-acting PG synthetase inhibitor (the sulphide) for anti-arthritic therapy:

Absorption   Sulindac (pro-drug) minimal local gastrointestinal irritation
                                              ↓
Circulation   sulphone ← Sulindac ↔ sulphide   systemic PG synthesis inhibition
                                              ↓
Excretion   sulphone   Sulindac   (inactive urinary metabolite)

The marked reduction of synthetase inhibition, accompanying the change of the oxidation stage of the 4′-substituent in these indene acetic acids from sulphide to sulphoxide or sulphone, further indicates the high degree of structure specificity for this series of inhibitors (see Table 4). X-ray crystallographic studies have shown that the configuration of the *cis* isomer of indene isotere (50) is almost identical to that of indomethacin (HOOGSTEEN and TRENNER, 1970; KISTENMACHER and MARSH, 1972). The *cis* isomer is also 5 times more active than the *trans* geometrical isomer (54) in vivo and in vitro. Again, a common active site for indole and indene isoteres is

cis   trans

	R_s	R_p		
	CH$_3$O	Cl	(50)	
	F	CH$_3$S	(51)	
	F	CH$_3$S→O	(52)	
	F	CH$_3$SO$_2$	(53)	
			(54)	

indicated. A hypothetical receptor site for these compounds was initally proposed on the basis of anti-inflammatory data in vivo (SHEN, 1964). Recently, taking into consideration the mechanism of cyclo-oxygenase, a refined model was suggested (GUND and SHEN, 1977; see Sect. G.V.) on the basis of quantum mechanical (complete neglect of differential overlap, CNDO) and chemical mechanical calculations. This model also accommodates a number of arylacetic acids which are potent anti-inflammatory agents.

IV. Substituted Aryl Aliphatic Acids

Aryl aliphatic acid is a generic name for a large group of substituted phenyl or heterocyclic aliphatic acids which have been found to possess moderate to potent anti-inflammatory, analgesic, and antipyretic activities. Since 1971, a number of these have been reported to be PG synthetase inhibitors (see Table 5). Many others not yet evaluated in this enzyme system are expected to be inhibitors also. The spatial arrangement of the aryl moiety is frequently in accordance with the contour of the hypothetical "receptor site," derived from the study of indomethacin analogues (SHEN, 1964). However, a number of others, e.g., prodolic acid (75), are distinctly different stereochemically (GREENBERG, 1975). The preferred substituents for

Table 5. Inhibition of PG synthetase by aryl aliphatic acids

	ID_{50} (μM)	Enzyme source	References
Ibuprofen (28)	1.5	(SSV)*	HAM et al. (1972)
	6	(BSV)	CUSHMAN and CHEUNG (1976)
	1	(Human synovium)	KANTROWITZ et al. (1975)
MK-830 (55)	0.2	(SSV)*	
Fenclorac (56)	0.05	(BSV)	PROCACCINI et al. (1976)
	0.01	(Human synovium)	CROOKS and COLLINS (1975)
			NUSS et al. (1976)
Flurbiprofen (27)	0.01	(Human synovium)	KANTROWITZ et al. (1975)
	0.7	(SSV)*	
	7	(BSV)	ADAMS et al. (1975)
Ketoprofen (57)	0.12	(SSV)*	
Fenoprofen (58)	2	(Human synovium)	PATRONO et al. (1976)
	4	(Rat platelets)	PATRONO et al. (1974)
			HO and ESTERMAN (1974)
Naproxen (59)	0.8	(BSV)	CUSHMAN and CHEUNG (1976)
	1.8	(BSV)	KU and WASVARY (1975)
	6.1	(SSV)*	
Pirprofen (d) (60)	1.2	(BSV)	KU and WASVARY (1975)
(l)	8.3	(BSV)	KU and WASVARY (1975)
	3.5	(SSV)*	
Diclofenac (61)	1.7	(BSV)	ZIEL and KRUPP (1975)
	0.3	(SSV)*	
C 8012 (71)	31	(SSV)	GAUT et al. (1976)
	0.1	(SSV)	
(70)	0.03	(SSV)*	
Suprofen (65)			DECLERCK et al. (1975)

higher potency vary according to the nature of aryl moieties in each series, although a preponderance of Cl or fluoro substituents are frequently incorporated (ROME and LANDS, 1975).

A notable feature among several more potent families is the α-methylacetic acid side-chain with the sinister (S) absolute configuration as found with some indomethacin analogues discussed above. The rectus (R) enantiomers are usually, though not always, much less active (SHEN, 1972; GAUT et al., 1976). For example, compound 70 is 2.5 times more potent than indomethacin in the carrageenin foot oedema assay and more than 5 times in the SSV PG synthetase system, whereas its laeveorotatary enantiomer is practically inactive.

Most of these acids are chemically stable, substrate-competitive inhibitors of cyclo-oxygenase. A few metabolites, e.g., the 4′-hydroxy metabolite of flurbiprofen (ADAMS et al., 1975), were found to have moderate activity also. Interestingly, the activity of the carbonyl propionic acid derivative, fenbufen (67), was attributable to the corresponding acetic acid (72) formed as a metabolite in vivo (TOLMAN et al., 1976).

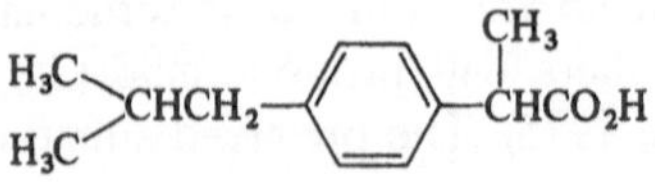

Ibuprofen (28)

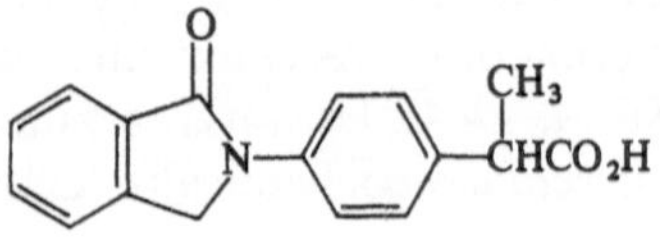

Indoprofen (66)

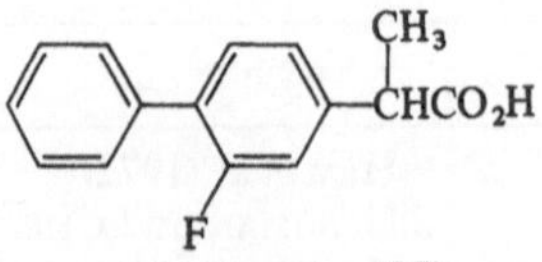

Flurbiprofen (27)

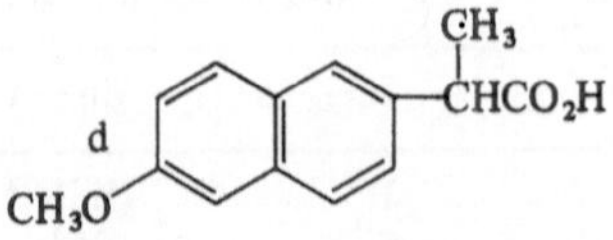

Naproxen (59)

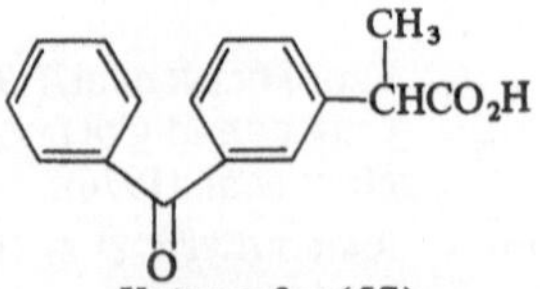

Ketoprofen (57)

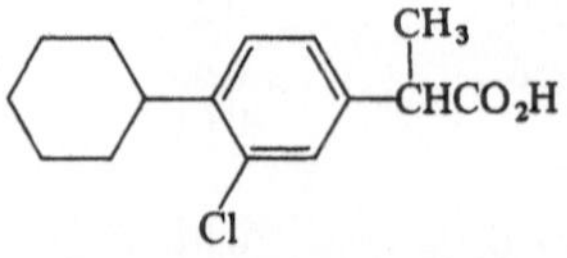

MK–830 (55)

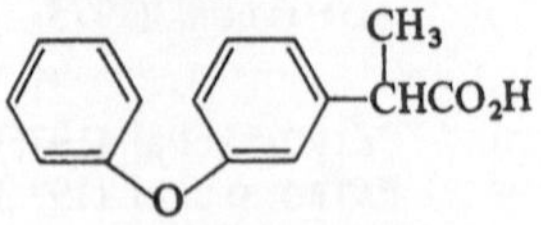

Fenoprofen (58)

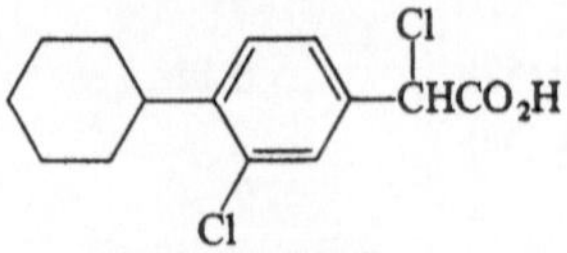

Fenclorac (56)

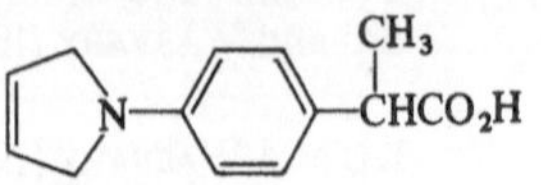

Piroprofen (60)

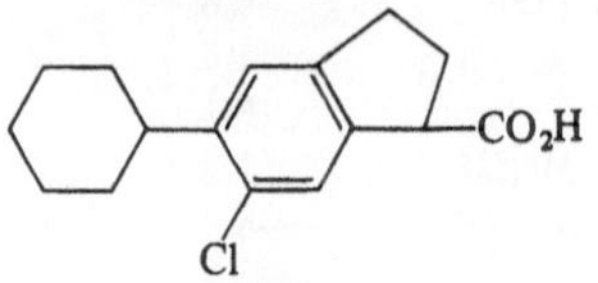

(64)

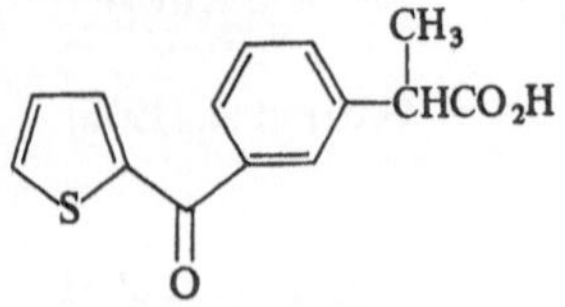

Suprofen (65)

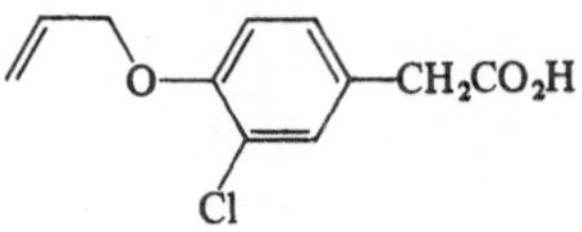

Alclofenac (63)

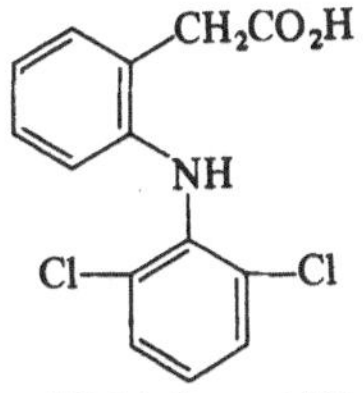

Dichlofenac (61)

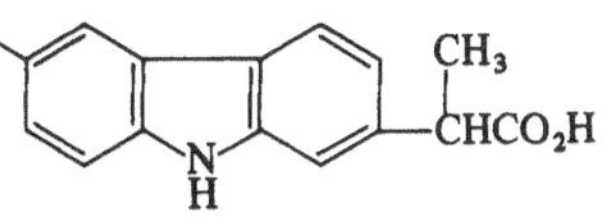

C-8012 (71)

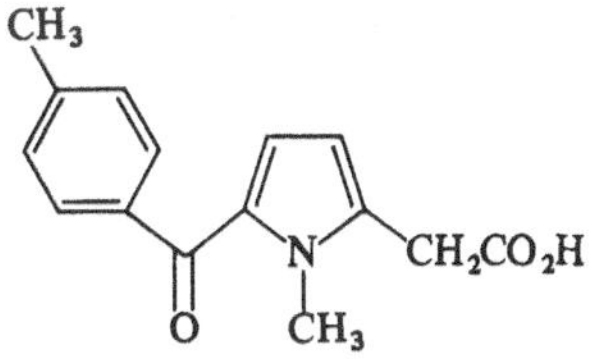

Tolmetin (62)

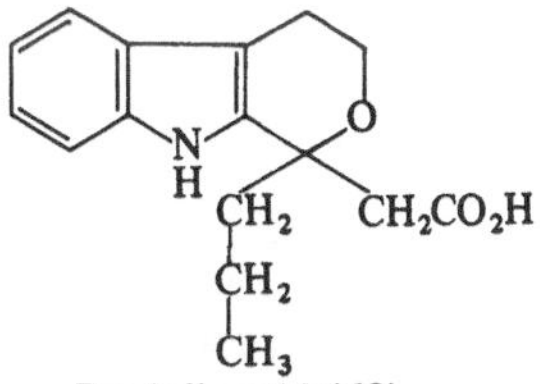

Prodolic acid (69)

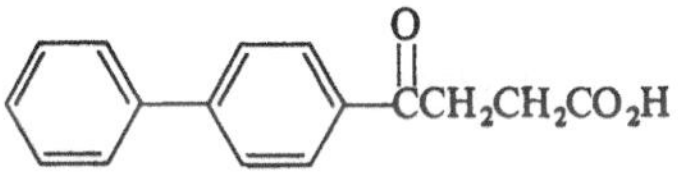

Fenbufen (67)

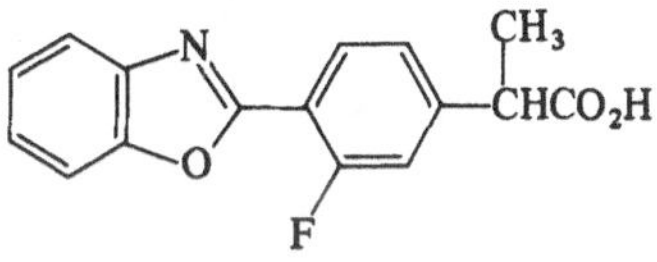

(70)

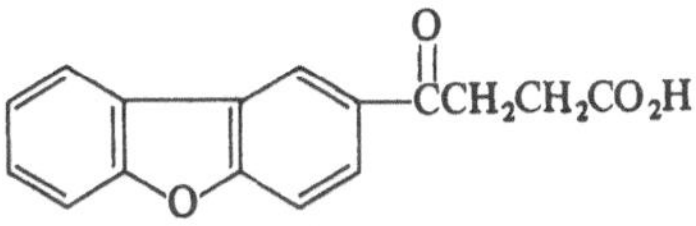

Furoprofen (68)

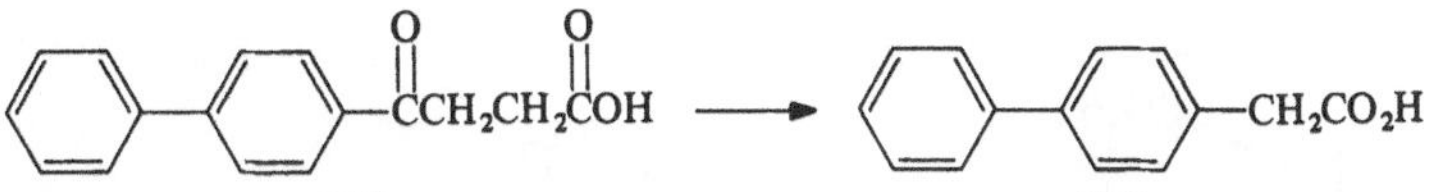

(67) → (72)

An acidic function on the aliphatic side-chain, e.g., CO_2H or tetrazole, is optimal for high potency. Moderate activities have been found with alcohol derivatives. It should be recognized that some of these derivatives, e.g., CH_2CHO and $CH_2CH_2NH_2$, may be oxidized in vivo to the corresponding acetic acid.

Most of these anti-inflammatory aliphatic acids were developed by the standard carrageenin induced foot oedema assay in rats. In spite of their similar PG synthetase inhibition in vitro, variations of their tissue distribution and metabolism in man may account for, at least in part, differences in their anti-arthritic efficacies.

V. Fenamates

Fenamates are a group of N-aryl anthranilic acid which possess significant anti-inflammatory and antinociceptive activities. They are potent inhibitors of PG synthetase (Table 6) as well as PG antagonists. The relatively poor correlation of their PG synthetase inhibition and in vivo anti-inflammatory potency may partly be attributable to their dual mechanisms of action. A cyclized analogue (73) and two aza analogues, niflumic acid (34) and clonixin (74), are comparably active as enzyme inhibitors. Clonixin is less anti-inflammatory but possesses a higher degree of analgesia involving both central and peripheral actions.

For synthetase inhibition the optimal stereochemistry and the position of substituents (e.g., CF_3 and CO_2H) are well defined by a comparison of a group of cyclized analogues with their acyclic congers. A comparison of various analogues and partial structures of fenamic acids (CUSHMAN and CHEUNG, 1976) showed that the diphenylamine moiety is the minimal structure that can serve as a moderately potent competitive inhibitor of PG synthetase. The 0-carboxyl group and a *m*-alkyl substituent greatly enhance the potency further. Like aspirin and indomethacin, fenamates inhibit all PG products equally, presumably by blocking the cyclo-oxygenase. On the other hand, the PG antagonistic property of fenamates and their analogues have not been compared. Such a study should shed further light on the stereochemical and physicochemical requirements for PG antagonists.

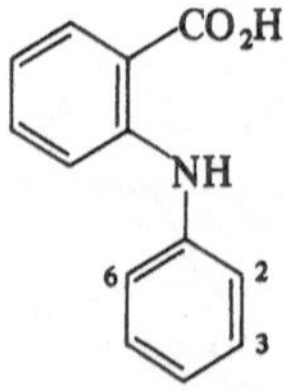

2,3 di Me	Mefanamic acid (73)
3–CF_3	Flufenamic acid (29)
2,6–diCl–3–Me	Meclofenamic acid (35)

| 3–CF_3 | Niflumic acid (34) |
| 3–Cl–2–Me | Clonixin (74) |

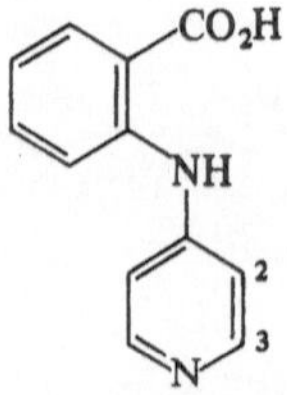

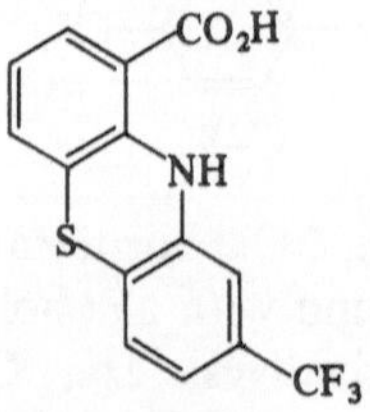

SKF 22908
(73)

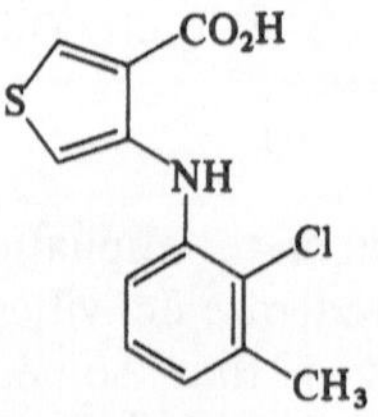

HOE 895
(75)

A series of substituted anthranilic acids, e.g. (76), was found to inhibit the BSV microsomal PG synthetase. A regressional analysis using the de novo model of FREE-WILSON was applied successfully in estimating the structure-activity relationship. The in vitro potency of (76), about one tenth that of indomethacin, correlated well with its local anti-inflammatory action. Its systemic activity was reduced to the level of aspirin on account of strong binding to serum albumin (GRYGLEWSKI et al., 1976).

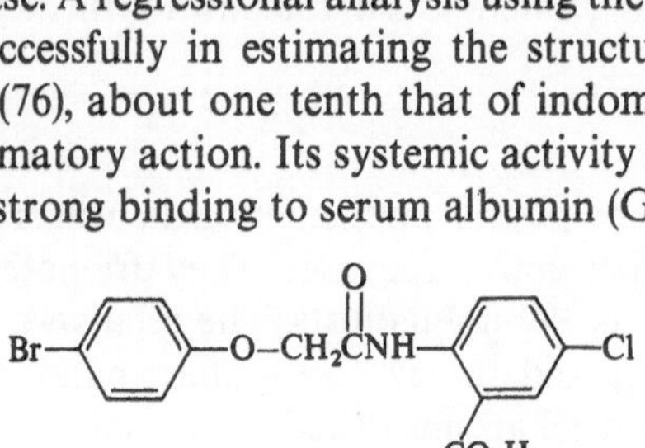

(76)

Table 6. Inhibition of PG synthetase by fenamates

	ID_{50} µM	Enzyme source	References
Mefenamic acid (73)	0.046	(g.p.l.)	TOLMAN et al. (1976)
	0.7	(BSV)	CUSHMAN and CHEUNG (1976)
	3.2	(BSV)	KU and WASVARY (1975)
	1.9	(Rabbit kidney)	BLACKWELL et al. (1975)
	2	(SSV)*	
Flufenamic acid (29)	0.8	(BSV)	CUSHMAN and CHEUNG (1976)
	3	(BSV)	ZIEL and KRUPP (1975)
	30	(BSV)	HORODNIAK et al. (1975)
	0.2	(Human synovium)	KANTROWITZ et al. (1975)
Meclofenamic acid (35)	0.6	(BSV)	CUSHMAN and CHEUNG (1976)
	2.6	(BSV)	KU and WASVARY (1975)
	1.4	(Rabbit kidney)	BLACKWELL et al. (1975)
	0.1	(Dog spleen)	FLOWER and VANE (1974)
Niflumic acid (34)	0.3	(BSV)	CUSHMAN and CHEUNG (1976)
	0.11	(Dog spleen)	FLOWER and VANE (1974)
	1.2	(SSV)*	
Clonixin (74)	0.3	(BSV)	CUSHMAN and CHEUNG (1976)
SKF 22908 (73)	33	(BSV)	HORODNIAK et al. (1975)
	2	(SSV)*	

VI. Other Acidic Anti-Inflammatory Agents

The importance of the carboxylic acid function in salicylates and aryl aliphatic acids as PG synthetase inhibitors has been well recognized. Several classes of aromatic structures bearing an acidic function such as enolic hydroxyl or a tetrazole group are also anti-inflammatory agents (see Table 7).

Table 7. Inhibition of PG synthetase by other acidic anti-inflammatory agents

	ID_{50} µM	Enzyme source	References
Phenylbutazone (77)	4.88	(g.p.l.)	TOLMAN et al. (1976)
	12.6	(SSV)*	HAM et al. (1972)
	7.25	(Dog spleen)	FLOWER and VANE (1974)
	15	(Rabbit kidney)	BLACKWELL et al. (1975)
	20	(BSV)	VIGDAHL and TUKEY (1975)
	37	(BSV)	CUSHMAN and CHEUNG (1976)
	98	(BSV)	KU and WASVARY (1975)
	500	(BSV)	ZIEL and KRUPP (1975)
	875	(BSV)	HORODNIAK et al. (1975)
Oxyphenbutazone (78)	540	(BSV)	ZIEL and KRUPP (1975)
	730	(BSV)	KU and WASVARY (1975)
Sudoxicam (81)	7	(SSV)*	
Azapropazone (82)	3	(SSV)*	
R-807	5	(BSV)	VIGDAHL and TUKEY (1975)

In a BSV system, phenylbutazone (77) inhibits the formation of both PGE_2 and $PGF_{2\alpha}$ but has no effect on malondialdehyde (FLOWER et al., 1973). Its activity, like that of other anti-inflammatory acids, is more pronounced at low substrate concentrations (CUSHMAN and CHEUNG, 1976). When Cu^{++} was added to a SSV system to increase the production of $PGF_{2\alpha}$ vs. PGE_2, an apparent selective inhibition of PGF_2 by phenylbutazone at 80 μM was observed (STONE et al., 1975).

Sulphinpyrazone (79), originally developed as an uricosuric drug, was recently applied as an antithrombotic agent by virtue of its inhibition of platelet aggregation. Interestingly, in both in vitro platelet aggregation and PG synthetase assays, the sulphide metabolite (80) is more potent. This is analogous to the findings with Sulindac and its sulphide metabolite mentioned above.

Sudoxicam (81) was the forerunner of a group of long-acting and potent anti-inflammatory agents including its close analogue W 8495 (84). Azapropazone (82) is active in man at 800 mg/day. R 807 (83) is a newer member of the acidic sulphonamides. The relatively low in vitro potency of these compounds, such as compared with many carboxylic acids described above, probably reflects some differences in pharmacological profiles and pharmacokinetics.

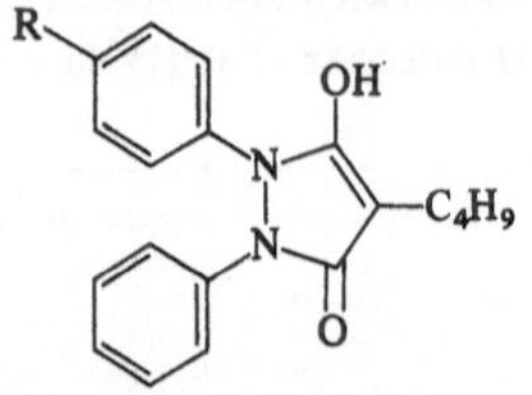

R = H   Phenylbutazone (77)

OH   Oxyphenbutazone (78)

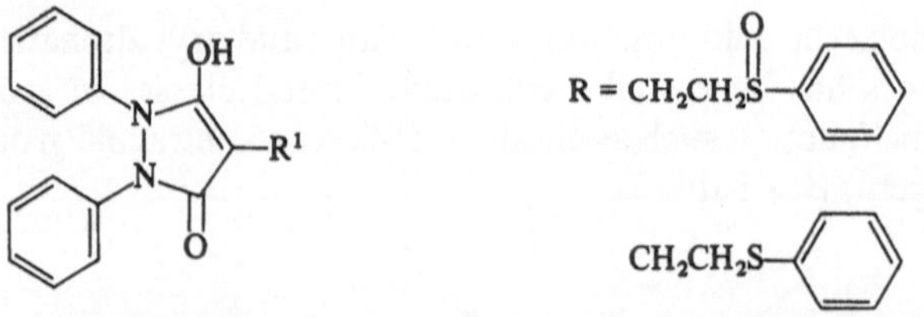

$R = CH_2CH_2\overset{\overset{O}{\|}}{S}-\bigcirc$ Sulphinpyrazone (79)

$CH_2CH_2S-\bigcirc$ (80)

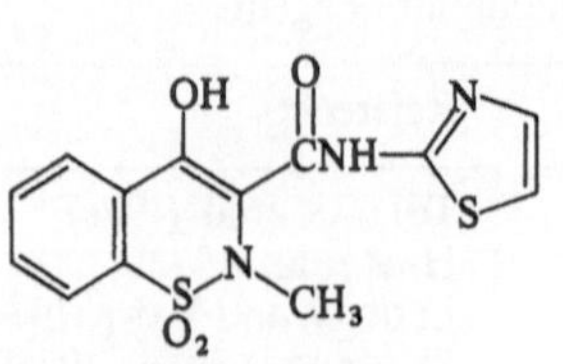

Sudoxicam (81)

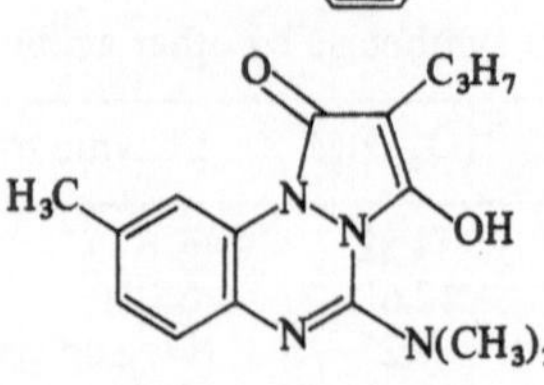

Azapropazone (82)

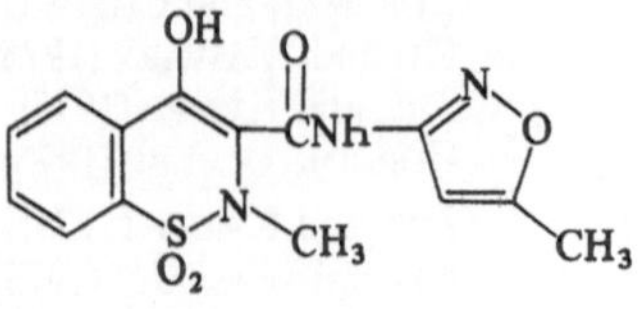

W 8495 (84)

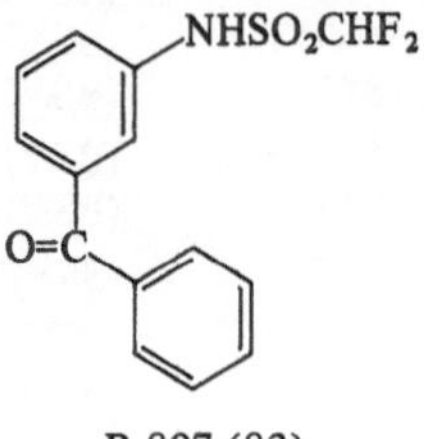

R 807 (83)

VII. Non-Acidic Anti-Inflammatory Agents

After the initial evaluation of various acidic anti-inflammatory agents as PG synthetase inhibitors, it was soon discovered that several non-acidic anti-inflammatory agents also displayed enzyme inhibitory activities. In particular, they possess a five-membered heteroaryl group substituted with two or three phenyl groups, either fused or in angular fashion:

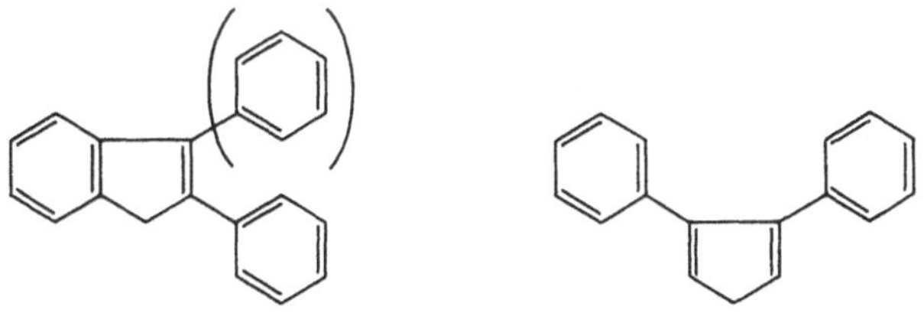

The preference for activity-enhancing substituents, such as methoxy, halogen or hydrophobic groups, further distinguishes them from acidic enols discussed in Section D.VI. above.

In our laboratory, an old experimental anti-inflammatory drug, indoxole, (85) was found to be a good inhibitor of the SSV synthetase system with an ID_{50} 0.5 µg/ml. Similar structures, such as (86) and bimetopyrol (87) were also active. The most potent compound of this type appears to be flumizole (88), in accordance with the reported anti-inflammatory activities of these compounds. Other inhibitors with similar structures are L-8027 (89) and ditazol (90). SL 573 (91) is a member of the anti-inflammatory quinazolinon family. Diftalone (92) and the moderate immuno-suppressive flazalone (93) are both weak PG synthetase inhibitors.

Table 8. Inhibition of PG synthetase by non-acidic anti-inflammatory agents

	ID_{50} µM	Enzyme source	References
Indoxole (85)	1.5	(SSV)*	HAM et al. (1972)
(86)	1.0	(SSV)*	
Bimetopyrol (87)		(SSV)*	
Flumizole (88)	0.2	(SSV)*	
	0.7	(Goat SV)	WISEMAN et al. (1975)
L-8027 (89)	22	(BSV)	DUVIVIER et al. (1975)
Ditazol	6.4	(Rat platelet)	PATRONO et al. (1975)
SL 573 (91)	5	(BSV)	YANAGI and KOMATZU (1976)
Diftalone (92)	170	(BSV)	CARMINATI and LERNER (1975)
Flazalone (93)	350	(BSV)	CUSHMAN and CHEUNG (1976)
(94)	50	(SSV)*	
(95)	5	(SSV)*	
(96)	2.5	(SSV)*	

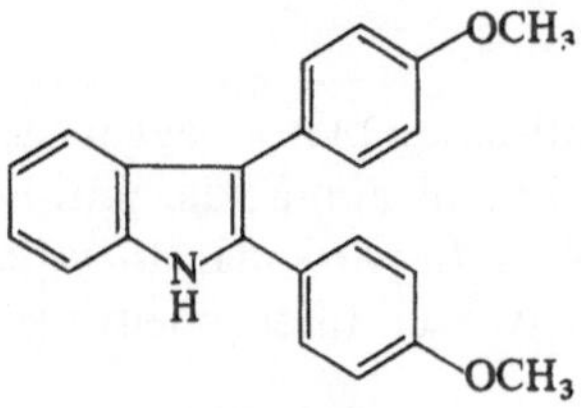

Indoxole (85)

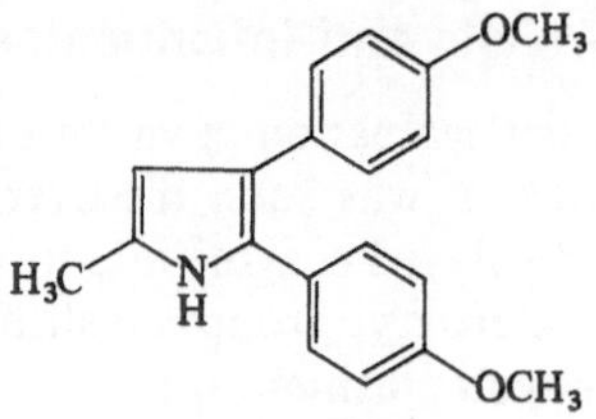

Bimetopyrol (87)

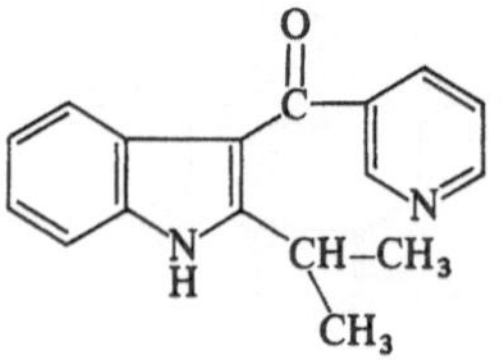

L 8027 (89)

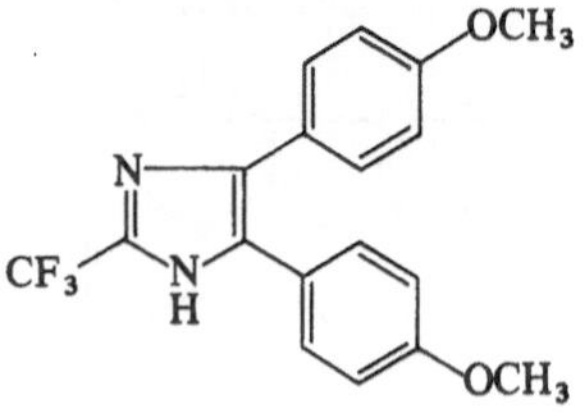

Flumizole (88)

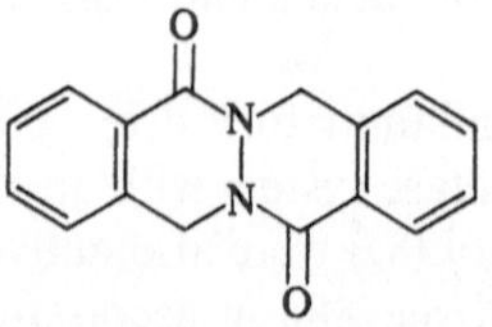

Diftalone (92)

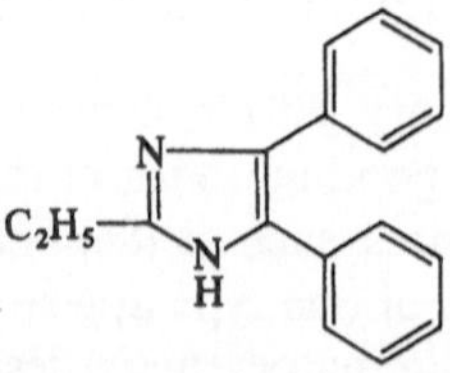

(86)

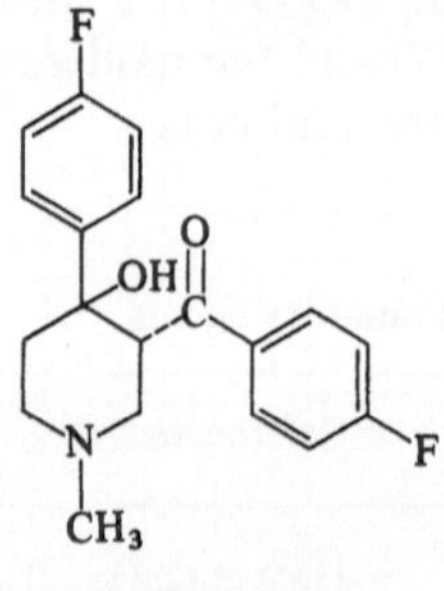

Flazalone (93)

In another series, the modest activity of 2-phenylbenzoxazole (94) was greatly surpassed by its aza analogues, the [4,5-b] and [5,4-b] oxazolopyridines. The in vitro activity of the highly potent members, e.g. (95) and (96), are in the same range of the better known aryl aliphatic acids. The site of action of these non-acidic inhibitors has not been elucidated. The poor systemic anti-inflammatory activity and the lack of toxicity of some of the potent enzyme inhibitors may be attributed to their rapid metabolic inactivation.

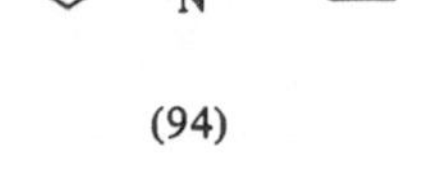

(94) 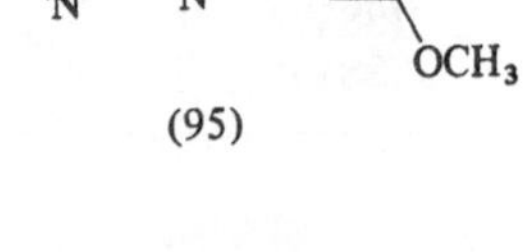   (95) 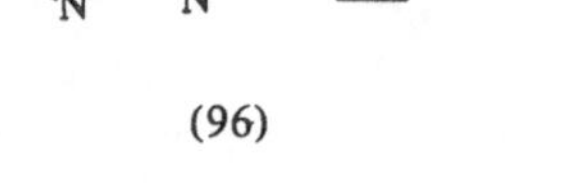   (96)

E. Effects of Corticosteroids

Corticosteroids are potent anti-inflammatory agents. In many in vitro and in vivo systems, however, they have not been shown to be inhibitors of the PG synthetase. In our laboratory, cortisone, hydrocortisone, prednisolone, and dexamethasone are all inactive at 50 μg/ml in the SSV system. The topical anti-inflammatory triamcinolone acetonide and dexamethasone are also ineffective in human epiderm microsomes (HSIA et al., 1974). On the basis of indirect data, the possible inhibition of the release of arachidonic acids and not the synthesis of PG, by anti-inflammatory steroids was suggested (LEWIS and PIPER, 1975; HONG and LEVINE, 1976). Very recently, hydrocortisone and dexamethasone were shown to inhibit PGE_2 production in culture media from explants of human rheumatoid synovia at 10^{-5} M and 10^{-6} M, respectively. The suppression of levels of PGE_2 and PGF_2 was not due to increased PG degradation (KANTROWITZ et al., 1975). In a follow-up experiment (ROBINSON et al., 1976), the synthetase of PGE_2 and $PGF_{2\alpha}$ by rheumatoid synovial cultures was reduced to <10% of controls by dexamethasone at 10^{-9} M and hydrocortisone at 10^{-8} M. The inhibitory effect is not due to a direct interaction of corticosteroids with the synthetase. In another related study, a reversible inhibition of PG synthesis by hydrocortisone at 5×10^{-6} M was demonstrated with $HSDM_1C_1$ strain of mouse fibrosarcoma cells. As the ratio of PGE_2 to PGF_2 was unaltered, the locus of inhibition was probably at a stage prior to endoperoxide formation (TASHJIAN et al., 1975). These independent observations are in accordance with the conclusion that corticosteroids inhibit the production of prostaglandins at the phospholipase level.

F. Inhibition and Stimulation by Other Pharmacological Agents

I. Anti-Arthritic and Related Compounds

Benzydamine (97), an analgesic agent, and flazalone (93), an experimental immunoregulant, are weakly or non-competitive with arachidonic acid in the BSV microsomal system. They inhibit the conversion of arachidonate (1 μM) to PGE_2 with I_{50} 160 and 350 μM respectively. At high concentrations of arachidonic acid (1 mM) they augment the synthesis of PGE_2 while inhibiting the production of $PGF_{2\alpha}$ and PGD_2. This marked change of inhibitory pattern, as a function of substrate concentration, is not found with other acidic NSAID like indomethacin and phenylbutazone (CUSHMAN and CHEUNG, 1976).

Ditazol (90)   SL 573 (91)   (97)

Thiabendazole [2-(4-thiazolyl)-benzimidazole] (98) is a broad spectrum anthelmintic antifungal agent with a modest analgesic property. It inhibits SSV synthetase at 5–10 γ/ml. There is no correlation between its anti-infective and synthetase inhibitory activities. A more potent anthelmintic analogue, cambendazole, (99), is devoid of synthetase inhibition. On the other hand, some 5-substituted derivatives of (98), e.g., the 5-CF$_3$O (100) and 5-(p-fluorophenyl) (101) analogues, are synthetase inhibitors. The chemical structure resemblance between these analogues and 2-phenyloxzolopyridines described in Section D.VII. is noted.

R = H   Thiabendazole   (98)

(CH$_3$)$_2$CHOCNH   Cambendazole   (99)

CF$_3$O   (100)

F—⟨ ⟩—   (101)

Sulphasalazine, (102), useful in ulcerative colitis, is an inhibitor of PG synthesis with a potency comparable to that of aspirin. Chemically, sulphasalazine may be considered as a 5-substituted salicylic acid in the general category of some active salicylates discussed in Section D.V.

The reduced metabolites of sulphasalazine, sulphapyridine, and 5-aminosalicylic acid, are not active. It was suggested that the bacteriostatic activity of sulphapyridine may protect sulphasalazine from microbial reduction and thus preserve its anti-inflammatory activity (COLLIER et al., 1976).

(102)

Sodium aurothiomalate inhibits SSV dioxygenase at 50 μM in a time-dependent manner (PENNEYS et al., 1974; DEBY et al., 1973).

In a BSV system, sodium aurothiomalate and aurothioglucose inhibit the PGF$_{2\alpha}$ synthesis and stimulate PGE$_2$ synthesis at high concentrations (0.4–2 mM) (STONE et al., 1975).

Chloroquinine (103) and hydroxychloroquine (104) were also reported to inhibit PGF$_{2\alpha}$ synthesis while stimulating PGE$_2$ synthesis (GREAVER and McDONALD-GIBSON, 1972; STONE et al., 1975).

Dimethyl sulphoxide (DMSO) in concentrations of from 10–50% inhibits the synthesis of PGF$_{1\alpha}$ but stimulates the synthesis of PGE$_1$ to as high as 15-fold of BSV microsomes (LA HANN and HORITA, 1975). At higher concentrations, DMSO inhibits the formation of both PGE and PGF. This effect was attributed to its ability to trap·OH involved in the biosynthesis (PANGANAMALA et al., 1976).

Tomatin, a naturally occurring anti-inflammatory substance, is moderately active at 10 µM. Maleopimaric acid (105), a modestly active inhibitor of the complement system is also a weak PG synthetase inhibitor at 30 µM.

Retinoic acid (106) activates skin phospholipase A_2 to liberate arachidonic acid but inhibits the formation of PGE_2 at higher concentrations (160 µM in vitro). As a consequence, topical application of retinoic acid on guinea pig skin resulted an initial erythema with an elevation of skin PGE_2 but a reduction of PGE_2 levels after chronic treatment (ZIBOH, 1975).

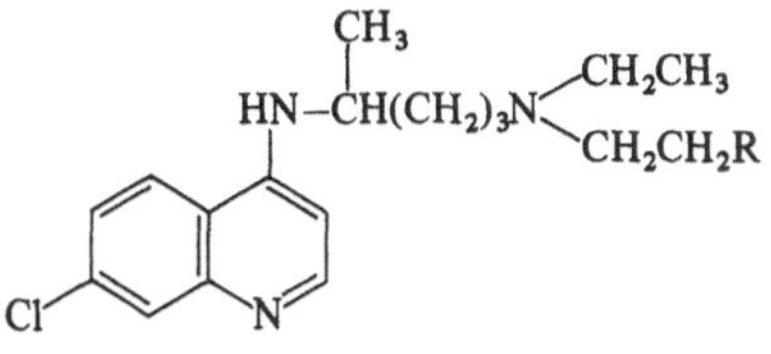

R = H   Chloroquine (103)

= OH   Hydroxychloroquine (104)

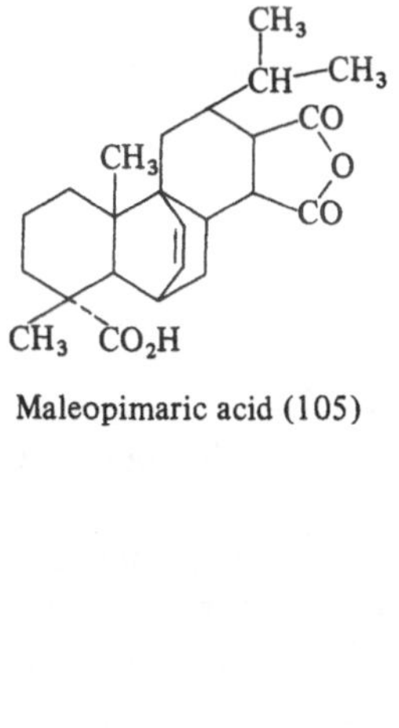

Maleopimaric acid (105)

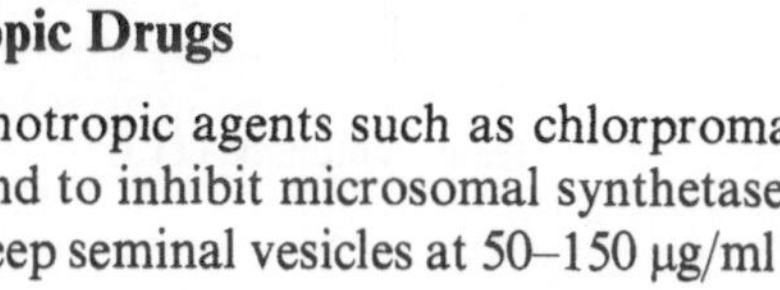

Retinoic acid (106)

II. Psychotropic Drugs

Tricyclic psychotropic agents such as chlorpromazine (20), amitriptyline (107), etc., have been found to inhibit microsomal synthetase from guinea pig lung (LEE, 1974), bovine and sheep seminal vesicles at 50–150 µg/ml (KRUPP and WEST, 1975).

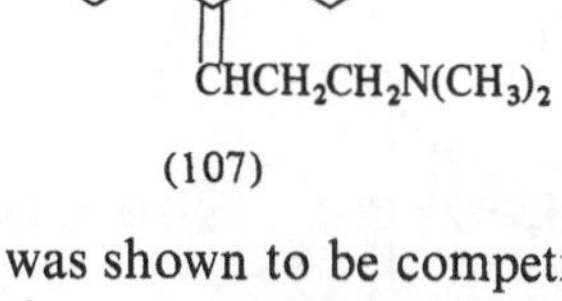

(107)

The inhibition of metrotiline was shown to be competitive to the substrate. The synthetase inhibitory activity of these compounds may be partially related to their anti-depressant activity and modest anti-inflammatory activity in a few cases, but no significant correlation is apparent. The chemical nature of the tricyclic ring system, whether phenothiazine, as in (20), or dibenzocycloheptatriene, as in (107), is not critical, neither is the structure of the aliphatic amino side-chain in these compounds. Indeed, other tricyclic ring systems, such as dibenzothiophene (108), xanthone (109), fluorenone (110) and an uncyclized benzophenone (111), even without a basic amino alkyl side-chain, are inhibitory at ≤ 10 μg/ml in the SSV system. Their activities are further enhanced by an amino substitution in the ring. It is of interest to note that structures (108)–(110) are the same type of aryl moieties commonly found in aryl acids discussed in Section D.IV. above. The mechanistic implications of this similarity at the enzyme level remain to be ascertained.

(108)   (109)   (110)   (111)

Monoamine oxidase inhibitors such as phenelzine (112) (at 10^{-7} M), tranylcypromine (113) (at 10^{-6} M), and pargyline (114) (at 10^{-4} M) are also inhibitors of the guinea pig lung synthetase (LEE, 1974). The potency of the latter two are comparable to that of indomethacin and aspirin in the same system, respectively.

III. Sulphhydryl Reagents and Derivatives

Ethacrynic acid (115) is a potent diuretic agent containing an SH-binding α,β-unsaturated ketone moiety. Its renal vasodilation effect may be mediated by an increase of synthesis and release of PGs. It is not an inhibitor of the SSV PG synthetase up to 50 μg/ml. N-ethyl maleimide (116) is also inactive at 50 μg/ml. Interestingly, other hydrophobic α,β-unsaturated compounds such as (117) (121) inhibit the SSV PG synthetase at 10 μg/ml in our laboratory. Vulpinic acid (121) is also a potent inhibitor at 30 μM. The therapeutic potential of many inhibitors of this type is severely limited by their non-specific toxicities.

Phenelzine (112)   Tranylcypromine (113)

Pargyline (114)

(115)   (116)

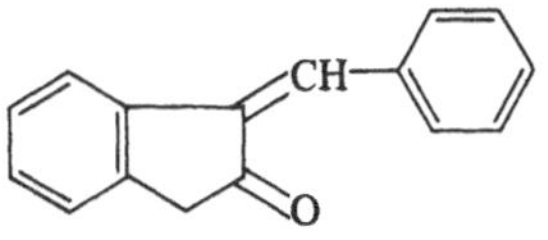

(117)

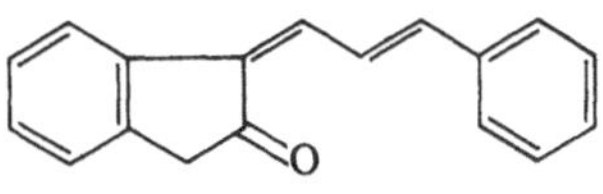

(118)

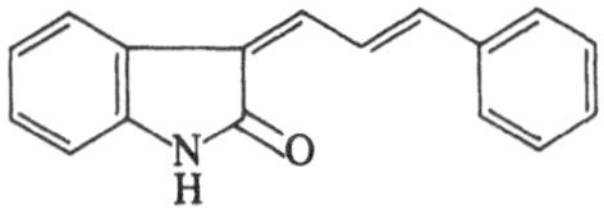

(120)

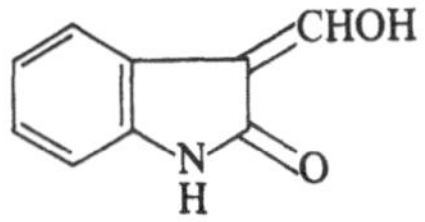

(119)

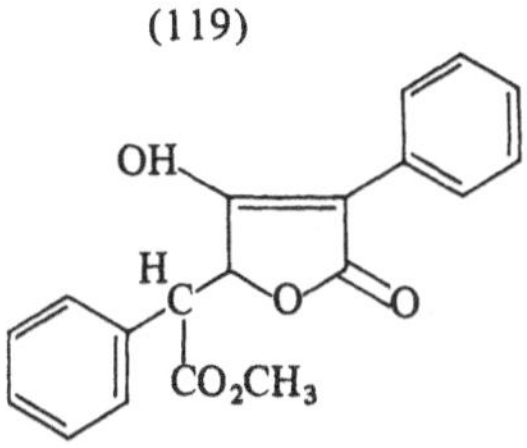

(121)

Sodium diethyldithio carbamate inhibits PG synthetase at ~ 10 µg/ml. The site of action is not at the fatty acid substrate site. It is a copper chelating agent and probably prevents the interaction of oxygen with the enzyme. Free SH compounds such as cysteamine, cysteine, and D-penicillamine (32), are not effective inhibitors. In some cases, the introduction of a heteroaryl hydrophobic moiety, e.g. (122), (123), and (124), enhances the potency and reduces the inhibitory concentration to the 10–50 µg/ml range in the SSV system.

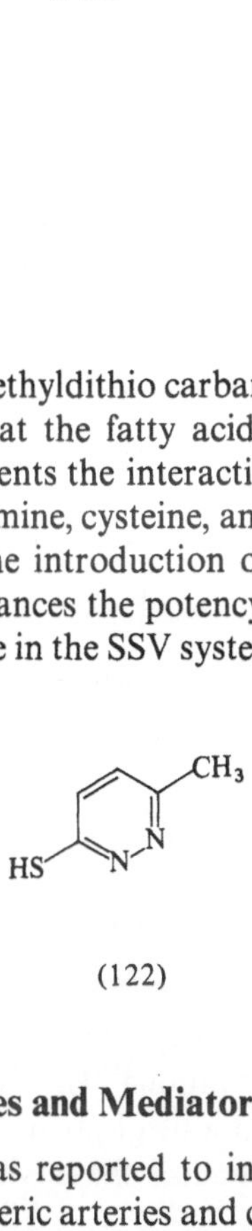

(122)

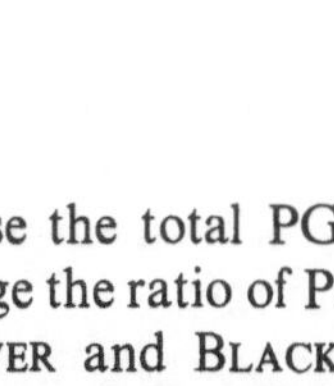

(123)

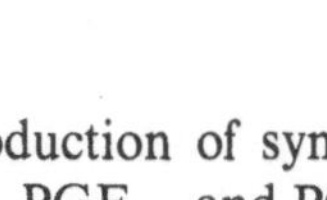

(124)

IV. Hormones and Mediators

Bradykinin was reported to increase the total PG production of synthetase from bovine mesenteric arteries and change the ratio of PGE_2, $PGF_{2\alpha}$, and PGD_2 slightly. It stimulates phospholipase (FLOWER and BLACKWELL, 1976). It also stimulates PGE-9 keto reductase which, in the presence of $NADP^+$, converts PGE_2 to $PGF_{2\alpha}$. Both bradykinin and cGMP increased the Vm without affecting the Km of the enzyme (WONG et al., 1975).

The effects of insulin and glucagon on PG synthesis and on membrane phospholipase activity in rat liver were studied. Both PGF_2 and PGE_2 synthesis was significantly depressed in insulin-treated (1 U intravenously or intraportally) rat liver homogenate. Glucagon produced a slight inhibition. Both insulin and glucagon in-

Table 9. Relative activities of hormonal agents

	Hormonal	Anti-inflammatory	PG synthetase inhibitors
Indomethacin		High	1
Clomiphene (125)	Potent oestrogen	Weak	1
Diethylstilboestrol (DES)	Potent oestrogen	Moderate	0.18
MER-25	Anti-oestrogen		0.02
MER-29 (126)	Weak anti-oestrogen		0.01

creased phospholipase activity in vivo but inhibited phospholipase in vitro (POLON-OVSKI et al., 1975).

Several non-steroid oestrogens and anti-oestrogens have also been found to be PG synthetase inhibitors in vitro (LERNER, 1975). There is no apparent correlation between their hormonal, anti-inflammatory or synthetase inhibitory activities. Clomiphene (125), a weak oestrogen is equipotent with indomethacin in the BSV microsomal preparation. MER-29 (126) is a non-oestrogenic inhibitor of cholesterol synthesis.

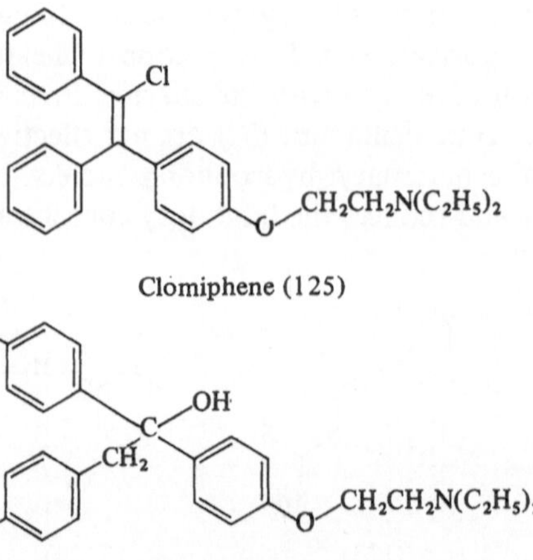

Clomiphene (125)

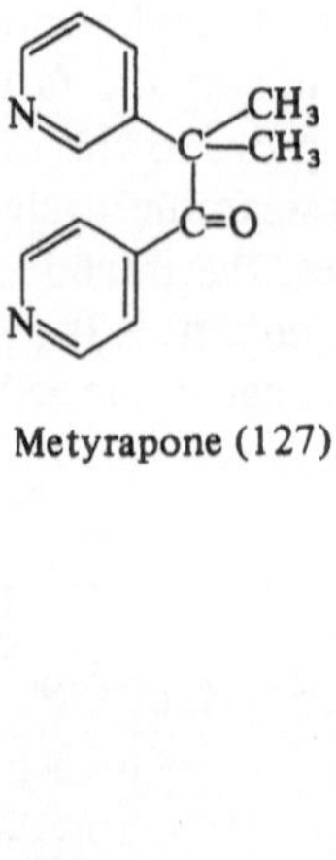

Metyrapone (127)

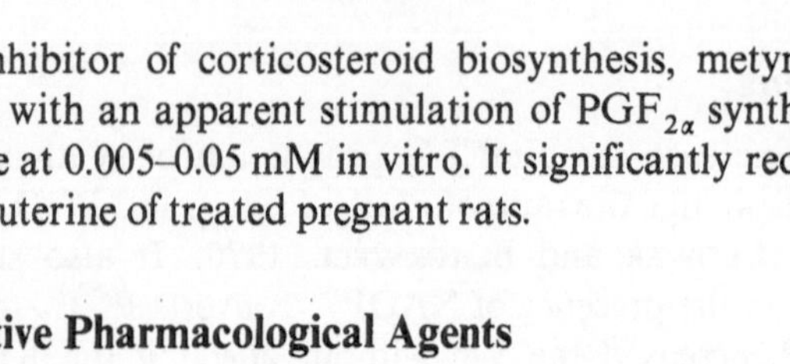

MER−29 (126)

An inhibitor of corticosteroid biosynthesis, metyrapone (127), inhibits PGE_2 synthesis with an apparent stimulation of $PGF_{2\alpha}$ synthesis of pregnant uterine homogenate at 0.005–0.05 mM in vitro. It significantly reduces the in vitro PG release from the uterine of treated pregnant rats.

V. Inactive Pharmacological Agents

The above discussions have illustrated the sensitivity of the PG synthetase system to a large variety of chemical structures. Thus, it is of interest to note that many pharmacological agents whose activities may be related to membrane action or peripheral to those of anti-inflammatory-analgesic drugs, are devoid of significant effects on the synthetase system. For example, potent narcotic analgesics, such as morphine, codeine, 5,9-diethyl-2-OH-6,7-benzomorphane and D-propoxyphene are not synthetase inhibitors. Morphine and apomorphine have been reported to be stimulators (COLLIER and McDONALD-BIBSON, 1975).

Colchicine, the mitotic inhibitor for the treatment of gout, was reported to be a synthetase stimulator (ROBINSON et al., 1975). Colchicine also stimulates collagenase production by synovial cells. Whether these activities are directly or indirectly related to the inhibition of microtubule assembly by colchicine is not clear.

Other examples of inactive pharmacological agents, including the anti-rheumatic D-penicillamine and 5-mercaptopyridoxine (JAFFE, 1974), are shown in the following table.

Table 10. Inactive pharmacological agents

Agent	Pharmacological action
Benemid	Uricosuric
Quinine	Antimalarial
D-Penicillamine	Anti-rheumatic
N-Acetyl cysteine	Mucolytic
N-Mercaptopropionyl glycine	Sulphydryl
MK-290	Anti-arthritic (rat)
5-Mercaptopyridoxine	Anti-rheumatic
6-Mercaptopurine	Anti-metabolite
Curcumin	Anti-inflammatory
Tilorone	Interferon inducer, immunosuppressive
Capsacin	Counter-irritant
Cytochalasin B	Microfilament inhibitor

G. The Search for New Inhibitors

I. Current Research Trend

With a better understanding of the biosynthesis and physiological roles of PGs and related mediators, the search for new synthetase inhibitors has put increasing emphasis on selectivity and efficacy. The therapeutic value of synthetase inhibitors in the treatment of arthritis has been well established. New inhibitors with less gastrointestinal irritation and other potential side-effects are obviously of interest. Application of synthetase inhibitors to other inflammatory conditions, e.g. dermatological, ocular, and periodontal diseases, would require inhibitors with different physicochemical and metabolic characteristics.

PGs are involved in many other physiological processes; the potential application of synthetase inhibitors in these areas would prefer compounds devoid of antiinflammatory activity and associated side-effects. Narrow spectrum agents affecting individual intermediates in the synthetic pathway or with much more pronounced tissue or organ specificity would be desirable. In this regard, knowledge about the physiological distribution of substrates, co-factors and their regulatory mechanisms may suggest possible new approaches.

Several recent findings have demonstrated another level of complexity of the PG synthetase system. Notable examples are the fractionation of the cyclooxygenase (MIYAMOTO et al., 1976), the elucidation of the thromboxane pathway (HAMBERG et al., 1975), the discovery of PGI_2 (MONCADA et al., 1976) which counteracts some actions of thromboxanes, and the growing appreciation of the roles of lipoxygenase metabolites. The self-destruction of cyclo-oxygenase has been attributed to an oxygen-centered radical species which is produced during the enzymic conversion of the hydroperoxide PGG_2 (EGAN et al., 1976). Similar radicals are formed in the transformation of hydroperoxide metabolites in the arachidonic acid cascade and may contribute significantly to the inflammatory process (KUEHL et al., 1977). These related pathways are sensitive to inhibition by a variety of chemical structures.

From these, prototypes of inhibitors with multiple or specific sites of action in the synthetase system are gradually emerging. On the other hand, because of the complexity, the overall efficacy and selectivity of new inhibitors will have to be defined in vivo in pertinent animal models. As with other PG studies, the successful development of a clinically useful biosynthesis regulator depends much upon the quantitative determination of its pharmacological profile in vivo.

II. Biochemical and Physiological Specificity

The specific of PG synthetase inhibitors may be considered at two different levels: enzymic specificity and tissue specificity. The complex synthetase pathways described above offer multiple sites of inhibition. Inhibitors of phospholipase-A_2, e.g., mepacrine (quinacrine), would block metabolites of both lipoxygenase and cyclo-oxygenase pathways. As inhibitors of cyclo-oxygenase, aspirin and indomethacin block the synthesis of PGG, PGH, thromboxanes, as well as PGE and PGF. Agents inhibiting the conversions of PGG and PGH should spare thromboxane. It also seems feasible to maintain, or even stimulate, the activity of PGI_2 synthetase, either by prevention of its destruction by oxygen-centered radicals or by selective synthetase stimulators. The net result would be a more favourable ratio of the local concentrations of PGI_2 and thromboxanes at the target site to achieve some beneficial effects. After the formation and interconversions of PGE, PGF, and other metabolites are clarified, presumably one may find even more specific inhibitors. In practice, the identification of specificity is complicated by the sensitivity of the synthetase system to minor changes of substrate concentration, co-factors, stimulators, and possible feedback mechanisms.

Superimposed upon the biochemical specificity is the well recognised tissue specificity. Following the demonstration that PG synthetase from rabbit brain is more sensitive to inhibition by 4-acetamidophenol than synthetase from dog spleen (FLOWER and VANE, 1972), differential inhibition of synthetase from various tissues by anti-inflammatory drugs have been reported (FERREIRA and VANE, 1974; BHATTACHERJEE and EAKINS, 1975; PATRONO et al., 1976). For example, aspirin is 31-fold more potent in acetylating and inhibiting cyclo-oxygenase in human platelets compared with enzyme from sheep seminal vesicles (MAJERUS and STANFORD, 1977). Thus, the relative potency of synthetase inhibitors should ideally be determined with enzyme preparations from target tissues in man. The synthetase from human rheumatoid synovial tissue was found to be similar to the enzyme system from other sources in terms of pH profile and sensitivity to drug inhibition (CROOK and COLLINS, 1975). In a recent comparison, the blood platelets and synovial tissue from the same patients were superfused in vitro with anti-inflammatory drugs, and the inhibitory effects on $PG_{1\alpha}$ and $PGF_{2\alpha}$ production were evaluated (PATRONO et al., 1976).

Indomethacin and fenoprofen inhibited both systems approximately to the same extent. On the other hand, aspirin was about six times more potent in inhibiting $PGF_{2\alpha}$ production by platelets than by synovium from the same patient.

In addition to tissue origin, many other factors also contribute to differences in drug sensitivity. The inhibition of PG synthetase from the microsomal fractions of the anterior uvea and conjunctiva by indomethacin is 25–100 times less than that by a neutral compound indoxole. However, indomethacin becomes 2–4 times as potent as indoxole when these drugs are instilled into the conjunctival sac. In addition to pharmacodynamic parameters, e.g., drug penetration, protein-binding and metabolism, other factors such as substrate concentration, temperature, co-factors and pH used in the in vitro experiment may also contribute to the observed differences. Similarly, aspirin has little inhibitory activity against the ocular synthetase in vitro, but results in marked inhibition following systemic administration (BHATTACHERJEE and EAKINS, 1975). In spite of the complexity, these observations, nevertheless, illustrate the feasibility in seeking more specific inhibitors as therapeutic agents.

III. Pharmacodynamic and Metabolic Control

The general influence of pharmacokinetics on drug efficacy has been emphasized in previous discussions. While poor absorption and rapid metabolism are detrimental to systemic effects, the same properties may be advantageously exploited in the development of topical synthetase inhibitors for dermatological, ocular, and periodontal diseases. One may use compounds of this type to exert anti-inflammatory action topically and locally, with a minimal degree of systemic actions and side effects only.

Another approach which minimizes undesirable side effects of PG synthetase inhibitors is the use of a pro-drug. As described above, sulindac is an inactive synthetase inhibitor and presumably does not produce local gastrointestinal irritation during its absorption. It is readily converted into a long-acting sulphide metabolite to produce its anti-arthritic actions. Although our knowledge about factors controlling the tissue distribution of chemical agents is still insufficient, conceivably some pro-drugs may yield active metabolites with higher affinity for the target tissue. Alternatively, one may use elevated enzyme activities in the disease state, e.g., higher concentration of lysosomal enzymes in the inflamed tissue, to liberate active drugs from their precursors or conjugates. The N-acetyl-D-glucosaminide of prednisolone (128) (HIRSCHMANN et al., 1964) may be considered as a prototype in this kind of selective drug delivery. The protein binding and tissue distribution of acidic and

(128)

(129)

basic molecules are influenced oppositely by any change of tissue pH; the neutral compounds are generally less affected (BRUNE et al., 1976). The correlation of in vitro and in vivo activities, therefore, is often less satisfactory when a group of analogues with basic, acidic, and neutral substituents, even with very similar ring structures, are compared. As anti-inflammatory aryl acids (DEBY et al., 1975) are noted for their exaggerated activity in the adjuvant arthritis assays, and since other cellular and immunological events play more prominent roles in this chronic inflammatory model, the relationship between in vivo potency and PG synthetase activity is further distorted. Statistically significant correlation has been found with antipyretic activity, but the relationship with antinociceptive activity is also less distinct (ZIEL and KRUPP, 1975).

IV. Multiple-Action Inhibitors

To achieve higher efficacy, a PG synthetase inhibitor with PG antagonistic properties would be desirable. Such an agent would block both the formation and the action of PG(s). Considering the similarity in stereochemistry of several intermediates and metabolites in the PG synthetase pathway, it is reasonable that some substrate-competitive inhibitors of the synthetic enzymes may block the PG receptor as well. The synthetase inhibitor, flufenamic acid (29) is reported to.be a moderately potent antagonist of PGF. Indomethacin (26) and mefanamic acid (73) also reversibly interfere with PGE_1 induced smooth muscle contractions. Fenbufen and phenylbutazone (77) are less effective, and aspirin is not active (TOLMAN and PARTRIDGE, 1975). Interestingly, the PG antagonist SC 19220 (129) (BENNETT and POSNER, 1971) has a tricyclic structure not too different from some nonacidic PG synthetase inhibitors described in Section D.VII. A more thorough evaluation of other synthetase inhibitors in the PG receptor assays may clarify the structure-activity relationship and facilitate the design of more effective dual action inhibitors.

Some synthetase inhibitors are also moderate inhibitors of other enzymes involved in the metabolism of PG and cyclonucleotides. For example, indomethacin inhibits 15-hydroxyprostaglandin dehydrogenase at 10^{-5} M (HANSEN, 1974) and cAMP phosphodiesterase at 10^{-4} M (CIOSEK et al., 1974; NEWCOMBE et al., 1974). These concentrations are higher than the inhibitory concentration for cyclo-oxygenase; therefore the physiological significance of these properties of indomethacin remains in question (BEATTY et al., 1976). On the other hand, as the biological roles of individual prostaglandins, cyclonucleotides, and their metabolizing enzymes are progressively elucidated, it may be attractive to use a multiple action synthetase inhibitor with an optimal activity profile for maximum efficacy.

Another approach to enhance the anti-arthritic potency of PG synthetase inhibitors is to increase their antiproteolytic and/or immunoregulatory activities. Again, the characteristics of some anti-inflammatory compounds have indicated the possible combination of these properties in one molecule. Indeed, in view of the broad biochemical profiles of many NSAID and the structural diversity of many new PG synthetase inhibitors, the development of multiple-action inhibitors as more effective anti-arthritic agents is only waiting for dedicated chemical and biological commitments.

V. Synthetic and Physicochemical Approaches

The extensive structure-activity relationship of PG synthetase inhibitors outlined above has provided medicinal chemists with many potential leads for synthetic explorations. For safety enhancement and novel pharmacological profiles, the non-acidic types may offer greater opportunities. More detailed mechanistic studies of various non-acidic inhibitors, particularly their relationship to acidic inhibitors, are still awaited.

With aryl acids, a prominent stereochemical feature is readily discernible. Previously, hypothetical "receptor contours" were proposed for indomethacin analogues (SHEN, 1964) and fenamates (SCHERRER, 1974) on the basis of their anti-inflammatory activities in vivo. Following the identification of cyclo-oxygenase as the site of action of indomethacin and related compounds, a conformational study of these inhibitors and arachidonic acid has resulted in a refined model (GUND and SHEN, 1977). The receptor model explains the stereospecific transformation of arachidonic acid into the cyclic *endo*-diperoxide (PGG) and rationalizes the structure-activity relationship for cyclo-oxygenase substrates and inhibitors (Fig. 1).

The molecular conformation of PGs has been investigated by physicochemical methods such as X-ray crystallography, circular dichroism and nuclear magnetic resonance (LEOVEY and ANDERSEN, 1975; ANDERSEN et al., 1976). The binding of prostaglandins and analogues to the lipocyte PGE was shown to exhibit a high

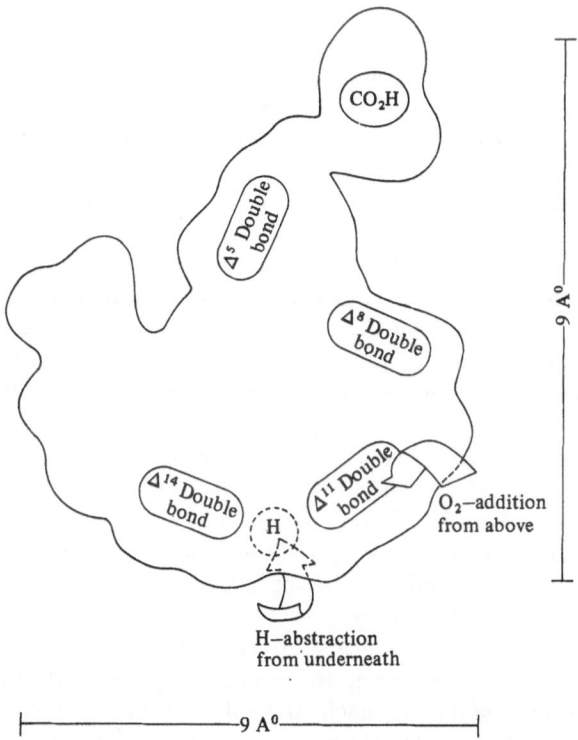

Fig. 1. The binding site of fatty acid substrate and inhibitors of prostaglandin synthetase

degree of structural specificity, particularly at the 9-keto or 15-hydroxy position (OIEN et al., 1975). The activity enhancing effect of chemical substituents in anti-inflammatory drugs, such as Cl and F in aryl acetic acids, has also been demonstrated in in vitro cyclo-oxygenase inhibition (ROME and LANDS, 1975).

These analyses are essentially retrospective and by no means exclusive. Nevertheless, they provide a rationale for observed structure-activity relationship and a guide to further refinement of PG synthetase inhibitors. Interesting activities have been found with several bicyclic analogues of PGH and a variety of PGE and PGF modifications. Synthetic analogues of thromboxanes will undoubtedly emerge very soon. The chemical diversity of these synthetic analogues of PGs should increase the probability of finding more selective regulators of PG metabolism.

H. Pharmacokinetics of Prostaglandin Synthetase Inhibitors

The importance of pharmacokinetics to drug actions is well appreciated. The in vivo manifestation of an intrinsic in vitro property of any chemical agent is subject to variations in the extent and rate of absorption, tissue distribution, metabolic disposition and pattern of excretion. Physiological distribution barriers, e.g., the so-called "blood-brain barrier" and the selective localisation of drugs, often change both the efficacy and side-effects. With PG synthetase inhibitors, the observed in vitro potency seems to correlate well with in vivo anti-inflammatory action of most acidic agents but less so with moderately active or non-acidic agents. It was also noted that, in spite of their broad anti-inflammatory-analgesic and antipyretic actions, on the whole, non-steroid anti-arthritic agents appear to be relatively well tolerated in man even after chronic administration. The severity of their side-effects is much less than that one might expect from non-specific systemic inhibitors of the biosynthesis of PGs. Indeed, even the well-known gastrointestinal irritation has been partially dissociated from the anti-inflammatory action of some newer drugs in animals and in man.

These apparently selective actions are at least partly attributable to their pharmacokinetic properties. The tissue distributions of indomethacin in rats was shown by YESAIR et al. (1970) to favour the extracellular fluid by radio autography. Similar concentration of indomethacin and phenylbutazone, but not antipyrine, in inflamed tissue, the stomach, small intestine and kidney, was shown by BRUNE et al. (1976). In chickens, acidic drugs like indomethacin and phenylbutazone accumulate in the fluid of inflamed joints to a level occur of three times higher than in the non-inflamed joint. On the other hand, this does not occur with the non-acidic compounds antipyrine and indoxole. This distribution pattern may be explained as follows:

1. Acidic NSAID have a very high affinity for serum proteins (>90% bound). Their distribution into the inflamed tissue is facilitated by extravasation of plasma proteins through damaged capillary.

2. Only non-ionized organic acids are permeable to cell membranes. The local acidity (lower pH) of inflamed tissue and stomach suppresses the ionization of drugs like phenylbutazone and indomethacin and enhances their penetration into intracellular space. A similar concentrating process may take place in H^+ secreting cells in the renal tubules.

Microenvironment   Cell   Intracellular space
low pH   membrane   higher pH

$$RCO_2^- + H^+ \rightleftharpoons RCO_2H \rightleftharpoons RCO_2H \rightleftharpoons RCO_2^- + H^+$$

This is in accordance with the observation that a better correlation of in vitro PG synthetase inhibition and in vivo activity for certain compounds is obtained if their relative affinity for serum protein is also taken into consideration (GRYGLEWSKI et al., 1976).

There is a parallel kinetic relationship between the concentration of indomethacin in the synovial fluid and its plasma level. The drug level in the two compartments are apparently in equilibrium. The plasma half-life of aryl carboxylic acids varies from 2 to 18 h. Acidic enolic compounds like phenylbutazone and sudoxicam have half-life values in man of 72 and 24–96 h respectively. For non-acidic agents, the half-life as well as their tissue distribution patterns depend on their diverse chemical structural features. As the in vivo efficacy of anti-inflammatory acids may be generally related to the area under the curve of plasma level ($\approx$ synovial level) vs. time, the pharmacokinetics of these compounds will naturally further influence the relationship of their in vitro and in vivo activities. As discussed above, the overall efficacy, duration of action and tolerance of sulindac are the consequences of multiple pharmacokinetic factors.

Many anti-inflammatory acids undergo enterohepatic recirculation. Their conjugated metabolites, e.g., acyl glucuronide, are secreted through the bile duct. Some of the metabolites are cleaved in the gut regenerating the free acid which is then reabsorbed in the lower intestine. The repeated exposure of this part of the gastrointestinal tract to the PG synthetase inhibitor leads to local damage of mucosal barrier, etc.

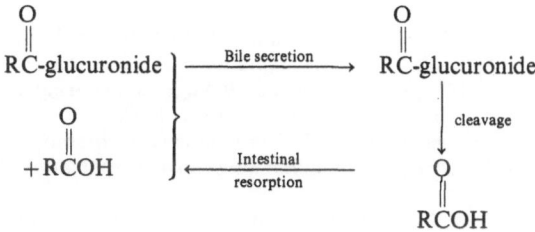

These studies indicate that one may improve the clinical efficacy as well as the safety of PG synthetase inhibitors through the elucidation and optimization of their pharmacokinetic parameters.

I. Conclusion

It is remarkable that, within a short span of five years since the first observation with aspirin and indomethacin, such a variety of chemical structures have been identified as inhibitors of the PG synthetase system. Their importance to the control of inflammatory process, regardless of the degree of quantitative correlation, is well established. Further characterization of these inhibitors in terms of their enzymatic, pharmacological, and pharmacokinetic properties undoubtedly will provide medicinal chemists with needed insight to synthesize more selective and efficacious inhibitors for arthritis and other related inflammatory disorders. The major questions in this field in the next five to ten years may also change from "What?" to "When?" and "How?" to use this newly defined major class of pharmacological agents.

References

Adams, S. S., Bresloff, P., Risdall, P. C.: The contribution of metabolism to the anti-inflammatory activity of flurbiprofen. Scand. J. Rheum. 4 Suppl. 8, S 11—S 19 (1975)

Anderson, N. H., Ramwell, P. W., Leovey, E. M. K., Hohnson, M.: Biological consequences of prostaglandin molecular conformations. In: Samuelsson, B., Paoletti, R. (Eds.): Advances in Prostaglandin and Thromboxane Research, Vol. I, pp. 271—289. New York: Raven Press 1976

Arturson, G., Jonsson, C. E.: Stimulation and inhibition of biosynthesis of prostaglandins in human skin by some hydroxyethylated rutosides. Prostaglandins 10, 941—948 (1975)

Beatty, C. H., Bocek, R. M., Young, M. K., Novy, M. J.: Effect of indomethacin on cyclic AMP phosphodiesterase activity in myometrium from pregnant rhesus monkeys. Prostaglandins 11, 713—725 (1976)

Bennett, A., Posner, J.: Studies on prostaglandin antagonists. Brit. J. Pharmacol. 42, 584—594 (1971)

Bhattacherjee, P., Eakins, K. E.: Inhibition of the ocular effects of sodium arachidonate by antiinflammatory compounds. Prostaglandins 9, 175—182 (1975)

Blackwell, G. J., Flower, R. J., Vane, J. R.: Some characteristics of the prostaglandin synthesizing system in rabbit kidney microsomes. Biochim. biophys. Açta 398, 178—190 (1975)

Brune, K., Glatt, M., Graf, P.: Mechanisms of action of anti-inflammatory drugs. Gen. Pharmacol. 7, 27—33 (1976)

Brune, K., Graf, P., Glatt, M.: Inhibition of prostaglandin synthesis in vivo by non-steroid antiinflammatory drugs: evidence for the omportance of pharmacokinetics. Agents Actions 6, 159—164 (1976)

Bundy, G. L.: The synthesis of prostaglandin endoperoxide analogs. Tetrahedron Lett. 1975—1960 (1975)

Carminati, P., Lerner, L. J.: Effect of diftalone and other nonsteroidal anti-inflammatory agents on synthesis of prostaglandins. Proc. Soc. exp. Biol. (N.Y.) 148, 455—458 (1975)

Chan, J. A., Nagasawa, M., Takeguchi, C., Sih, C. J.: On agents favouring prostaglandin F formation during biosynthesis. Biochemistry 14, 2987—2991 (1975)

Ciosek, C. P. Jr., Ortel, R. W., Thanassi, N. M., Newcombe, D. S.: Indomethacin potentiates PGE, stimulated cyclic AMP accumulation in human synovidcytes. Nature (Lond.) 251, 148—150 (1974)

Collier, H. O. J., Francis, A. A., McDonald-Gibson, W. J., Saeed, S. A.: Inhibition of prostaglandin biosynthesis by sulphasalazine and its metabolites. Prostaglandins 11, 219—225 (1976)

Collier, H. O. J., McDonald-Bibson, W. J.: Inhibition by drugs on the stimulation of prostaglandin biosynthesis induced by apomorphine. International Conference on Prostaglandins, Florence, 1975, pp. 27, Abs. 1975

Corey, E. T., Nicolaou, K. C., Machida, C. Y., Malmsten, C. L., Samuelsson, B.: Synthesis and biological properties of 9, 11-920-prostanoid: highly active biochemical mimic of prostaglandin endoperoxides. Proc. nat. Acad. Sci. (Wash.) 72, 3355—3358 (1975)

Corey, E. J., Shibasaki, M., Nicolaou, K. C., Malmsten, C. L., Samuelson, B.: Simple stereocontrolled total synthesis of a biologically active analog of the prostaglandin endoperoxides (PGH$_2$, PGG$_2$). Tetrahedron Lett. 737—740 (1976)

Crook, D., Collins, A. J.: Prostaglandin synthetase activity from human rheumatoid synovial tissue and its inhibition by nonsteroidal anti-inflammatory drugs. Prostaglandins 9, 857—865 (1975)

Cushman, D. W., Cheung, H. S.: Effect of substrate concentration on inhibition of prostaglandin synthetase of bull seminal vesicles by anti-inflammatory drugs and fenamic acid analogs. Biochim. biophys. Acta **424**, 449—459 (1976)

Damon, A., Heimberg, M., Oates, J. A.: Enrichment of rat tissue lipid with fatty acids that are prostaglandin precursors. Biochim. biophys. Acta **388**, 318—330 (1975)

Deby, C., Bacq, Z. M., Simon, D.: In vitro inhibition of the biosynthesis of a prostaglandin by gold and silver. Biochem. Pharmacol. **22**, 3141—3243 (1973)

Deby, C., Descamps, M., Binon, F., Bacq, Z. M.: Correlation between anti-inflammatory properties and inhibition of prostaglandin biosynthesis in vitro. Biochem. Pharmacol. **24**, 1089—1092 (1975)

De Clerck, F., Vermylen, J., Reneman, R.: Effects of suprofen, an inhibitor of prostaglandin biosynthesis, on platelet function, plasma coagulation and fibrinolysis. II. In vivo experiments. Arch. int. Pharmacodyn. **217**, 68—79 (1975)

Dembinska-Kiec, A., Zmuda, A., Krupinska, J.: Inhibition of prostaglandin synthetase by aspirin-like drugs in different microsomal preparations. In: Samuelsson, B., Paoletti, R. (Eds.): Advances in Prostaglandin and Thromboxane Research, Vol. I, pp. 99—103. New York: Raven Press 1976

Downing, D. T., Barve, J. A., Gunstone, F. D., Jacobsberg, M., Lie, K. J.: Structural requirements of acetylenic fatty acids for inhibition of soybean lipoxygenase and prostaglandin synthetase. Biochem. biophys. Acta. **280**, 343—347 (1972)

Duvivier, J., Wolf, D., Heusghem, C.: Enzymatic properties of prostaglandin synthetase for bovine seminal vesicles. Biochimie **57**, 521—528 (1975)

Egan, R. W., Eckert, C. A., Galavage, M., Humes, J. L., Kuehl, Jr., F. A.: The influence of phenols and related compounds on inhibition of prostaglandin biosynthesis by nonsteroidal anti-inflammatory agents. Fed. Proc. **35**, 1652 (1976)

Egan, R. W., Paxton, J., Kuehl, F. A., Jr.: Mechanism for irreversible self-deactivation of prostaglandin synthetase. J. biol. Chem., **251**, 7329—7335 (1976)

Ferreira, S. H., Moncada, S., Vane, J. R.: Indomethacin and aspirin abolish prostaglandin release from the spleen. Nature (New Biol.) **231**, 237—239 (1971)

Ferreira, S. H., Vane, J. R.: New aspects of the made of action of non-steroidal anti-inflammatory drugs. Ann. Rev. Pharmacol. **14**, 57—73 (1974)

Flower, R. J.: Drugs which inhibit prostaglandin biosynthesis. Pharmacol. Rev. **26**, 33—67 (1964)

Flower, R. J., Blackwell, G. J.: The importance of phospholipase-A$_2$ in prostaglandin biosynthesis. Biochem. Pharmacol. **25**, 285—291 (1976)

Flower, R. J., Cheung, H. S., Cushman, D. W.: Quantitative determination of prostaglandins and malondialdehyde formed by the arachidonate oxygenase (prostaglandin synthetase) system of bovine seminal vesicle. Prostaglandins **4**, 325—341 (1973)

Flower, R. J., Vane, J. R.: Inhibition of prostaglandin synthetase in brain explains the anti-pyretic activity of paracetamol. Nature (New Biol.) **240**, 410—411 (1972)

Flower, R. J., Vane, J. R.: Inhibition of prostaglandin biosynthesis. Biochem. Pharmacol. **23**, 1439—1450 (1974)

Förström, Goldyne, M. E., Winkelmann, R. K.: Prostaglandin production by human epidermal cells in vitro: a model for studying pharmacologic inhibition of prostaglandin synthesis. Prostaglandins **8**, 107—115 (1974)

Gaut, Z. N., Baruth, H., Randall, L. O., Ashley, C., Paulstrud, J. R.: Stereoisometric relationships among anti-inflammatory activity, inhibition of platelet aggregation, and inhibition of prostaglandin synthetase. Prostaglandins **10**, 59—66 (1976)

Greaves, M. W., McDonald-Gibson, M. J.: Anti-inflammatory agents and prostaglandin biosynthesis. Brit. med. J. **5825**, 527 (1972)

Greenberg, R.: Some pharmacological effects of prodolic acid, a new anti-inflammatory compound, indicative of inhibition of prostaglandin synthesis. Canad. J. Physiol. Pharmacol. **53**, 186—189 (1975)

Gryglewski, R. J., Ryznerski, Z., Gorczyca, M., Krupinska, J.: Design of new prostaglandin synthetase inhibitors in a group of N-(2-carboxy-phenyl) phenoxy acetomides and their anti-inflammatory activity. In: Samuelson, B., Paoletti, R. (Eds.): Advances in Prostaglandin and Thromoxane Research, Vol. I, pp. 117—120. New York: Raven Press 1976

Gund, P., Shen, T. Y.: A model for the prostaglandin synthetase cyclooxygenation site and its inhibition by antiinflammatory arylacetic acids. J. med. Chem. **20**, 1146—1152 (1977)

Ham, E. A., Studies on the mode of action of non-steroidal anti-inflammatory agents. In: Ramwell, P. W., Pharriss, B. B. (Eds.): Prostaglandins in Cellular Biology, pp. 345—352. New York: Plenum Press 1972

Hamberg, M., Samuelson, B.: On the metabolism of prostaglandin E_1 and E_2 in the guinea pig. J. biol. Chem. **247**, 3495 (1972)

Hamberg, M., Svensson, J., Samuelson, B.: Thromboxanes: a new group of biologically active compounds derived from prostaglandin endoperoxides. Proc. nat. Acad. Sci. (Wash.) **72**, 2994—2998 (1975)

Hansen, H. S.: Inhibition by indomethacin and aspirin of 15-hydroxyprostaglandin dehydrogenase in vitro. Prostaglandin **8**, 95—111 (1974)

Hirschmann, R., Strachan, R. G., Buchschacher, P., Sarett, L. H., Steelman, S. L., Silber, R.: An approach to an improved anti-inflammatory steroid, the synthesis of 11β, 17-dihydroxy-3,20-dione-1,4-pregnadien-21-yl 2-acetamido-2-deoxy-β-D-glucopyrandoside. J. Amer. chem. Soc. **86**, 3903 (1964)

Ho, P. P. K., Esterman, M. A.: Fenoprofen: inhibitor of prostaglandin synthesis. Prostaglandins **6**, 107—113 (1974)

Hong, S. C. L., Levine, L.: Inhibition of arachidonic acid release from cells as the biochemical action of anti-inflammatory corticosteroids. Proc. nat. Acad. Sci. (Wash.) **73**, 1730—1734 (1976)

Hoogsteen, K., Trenner, N. R.: Structure and conformation of cis and trans isomers of 1-(p-chlorobenzylindene)-2-methyl-5-methoxy-3-indenyl acetic acid. J. org. Chem. **35**, 521 (1970)

Horodniak, J. W., Julius, M., Zarembo, J. E., Bender, A. D.: Inhibitory effects of aspirin and indomethacin on the biosynthesis of PGE_2 and $PGF_{2\alpha}$. Biochem. biophys. Res. Commun. **57**, 539—545 (1974)

Horodniak, J. W., Matz, E. D., Walz, D. T., Sutton, B. M., Berkoff, C. E., Zarembo, J. E., Bender, D. A.: Inhibition of prostaglandin synthetase and carageenan-induced edema by tricyclic analogs of flufenamic acid. Res. Commun. chem. Path. Pharmacol. **11**, 533—542 (1975)

Hsia, S. L., Ziboh, V. A., Snyder, D. S.: Naturally occurring and synthetic inhibitors of prostaglandin synthetase of the skin. In: Vane, J. R., Robinson, H. R. (Eds.): Prostaglandin Synthetase Inhibitors, pp. 353—361. New York: Raven Press 1974

Jaffe, I.: U.S. Patent, No. 3, 852, 454 (1974)

Kantrowitz, F., Robinson, D. R., McCuire, M. B., Levine, L.: Corticosteroids inhibit prostaglandin production by rheumatoid synovia. Nature (Lond.) **258**, 737—739 (1975)

Kistenmacher, T. J., Marsh, R. E.: Crystal and molecular structure of an anti-inflammatory agent, indomethacin, 1-(p-chlorobenzoyl)-5-methoxy-2-methyl-indole-3-acetic acid. J. Amer. chem. Soc. **94**, 1340—1345 (1972)

Krupp, P., West, M.: Inhibition of prostaglandin synthetase by psychotropic drugs. Experientia (Basel) **31**, 330—331 (1975)

Ku, E. C., Wasvary, J. M.: Inhibition of prostaglandin synthetase by pirprofen studies with sheep seminal vesicle enzyme. Biochim. biophys. Acta **384**, 360—368 (1975)

Kuehl, F. A., Jr., Humes, J. L., Beveridge, G. C., Van Arman, C. G., Egan, R. W.: Biologically active derivatives of fatty acids, prostaglandins, thromboxanes and endoperoxides. Inflammation **2**, 285—294 (1977)

La Hann, T. R., Horita, A.: Effects of dimethyl sulfoxide (DMSO) on prostaglandin synthetase. Proc. West. pharmacol. Soc. **18**, 81—82 (1975)

Lands, W. E. M., Cook, H. W., Rome, L. H.: Prostaglandin biosynthesis: consequences of oxygenase mechanism upon in vitro assays of drug effectiveness. In: Samuelsson, B., Paoletti, R. (Eds.): Advances in Prostaglandin and Thromboxane Research, Vol. I, pp. 7—17. New York: Raven Press 1976

Lee, R. E.: The influence of psychotropic drugs and prostaglandin biosynthesis. Prostaglandins **5**, 63—72 (1974)

Leeney, T. J., Marsham, P. R., Ritchie, G. A. F., Senior, M. W.: Inhibitors of prostaglandin biosynthesis: a bicyclo-(2,2,1)-peptene analogue of "2" series prostaglandins and related derivatives. Prostaglandins **11**, 953—960 (1976)

Leovey, E. M. K., Anderson, N. H.: Molecular basis of prostaglandin potency. II. Proton NMR studies of the conformation of prostaglandin $F_{2\alpha}$. Prostaglandins 10, 789—794 (1975)

Lerner, L. J., Carminati, P., Schiatti, P.: Correlation of anti-inflammatory activity with inhibition of prostaglandin synthesis activity of nonsteroidal anti-estrogens and estrogens. Proc. Soc. exp. Biol. (N.Y.) 148, 329—332 (1975)

Lewis, G. P., Piper, P. J.: Inhibition of release of prostaglandins as an explanation of some of the actions of anti-inflammatory cortico-steroids. Nature (Lond.) 254, 308—311 (1975)

Majerus, P. W., Stanford, N.: Comparative effects of aspirin and diflunisal on prostaglandin synthetase from human platelets and sheep seminal vesicles. Brit. J. clin. Pharmac. 4, 15S—18S (1977)

Malmsten, C.: Some biological effects of prostaglandin endoperoxide analogs. Life Sci. 18, 169—176 (1976)

McDonald-Gibson, R. G., Flack, J. D., Ramwell, P. W.: Inhibition of prostaglandin biosynthesis by 7-oxa and 5-oxa-prostaglandin analogues. Biochem. J. 132, 117—120 (1973)

Miyamoto, T., Ogino, N., Yamamoto, S., Hayaishi, O.: Purification of prostaglandin endoperoxide synthetase from bovine vesicular gland microsomes. J. biol. Chem. 251, 2629—2636 (1976)

Moncada, S., Gryglewski, R., Bunting, S., Vane, J. R.: An enzyme isolated from arteries transforms prostaglandin endoperoxides to an unstable substance that inhibits platelet aggregation. Nature 263, 663—665 (1976)

Newcombe, D. S., Thanassi, N. M., Ciosek, C. P. Jr.: Cartilage cyclic nucleotide phosphodiesterase inhibition by anti-inflammatory agents. Life Sci. 14, 505—519 (1974)

Nuss, G. W., Smyth, R. D., Dreder, C. H., Hitchings, M. J., Mir, G. N., Reavey-Cartwell, N. H.: Fencloras, a new nonsteroidal anti-inflammatory agent. Fed. Proc. 35, 774 (1976)

Oien, H. G., Mandel, L. R., Humes, J. L., Taub, D., Hoffsommer, R. D., Kuehl, F. A. Jr.: Structural requirements for the binding of prostaglandins. Prostaglandins 9, 985—995 (1975)

Panganamala, R. V., Sharma, H. M., Geer, J. G., Cornwell, D. G.: A suggested role for hydrogen peroxide in the biosynthesis of prostaglandins. Prostaglandins 8, 3—11 (1974)

Panganamala, R. V., Sharma, H. M., Heikila, R. E., Geer, J. C., Cornwell, D. G.: Role of hydroxyl radical scavengers dimethyl sulfoxide, alcohols, and methional in the inhibition of prostaglandin biosynthesis. Prostaglandins 11, 599—607 (1976)

Patrono, C., Ciabattoni, G., Greco, F., Grossi-Belloni, D.: Comparative evaluation of the inhibitory effects of aspirin-like drugs on prostaglandin production by human platelets and synovial tissue. In: Samuelsson, B., Paoletti, R. (Eds.): Advances in Prostaglandins and Thromboxane Research, Vol. I, pp. 125—131. New York: Raven Press 1976

Patrono, C., Ciabattoni, G., Grossi-Belloni, D.: In vitro and in vivo inhibition of prostaglandin synthesis by fenoprofen, a nonsteroid anti-inflammatory drug. Pharmacol. Res. Commun. 6, 509—518 (1974)

Patrono, C., Ciabattoni, G., Grossi-Belloni, D.: Release of prostaglandin $F_{1\alpha}$ and $F_{2\alpha}$ from superfused platelets: quantitative evaluation of the inhibitory effects of some aspirin-like drugs. Prostaglandins 9, 557—568 (1975)

Penneys, N. S., Ziboh, Gottlieb, N. L., Katz, S.: Inhibition of prostaglandin synthesis and human epiderman enzymes by aurothiomalate in vitro: possible actions of gold in pemphigus. J. invest. Derm. 63, 356—361 (1974)

Polonovski, J., Bard, D., Bereziat, G., Colard, O.: Modifications de la synthese des prostaglandines dans le foie de rat sous l'influence de l'insuline et du glucagon. C.R. Soc. Biol. (Paris) 168, 1208—1215 (1975)

Pong, S. S., Levine, L.: Prostaglandin synthetase systems of rabbit tissues and their inhibition by nonsteroidal anti-inflammatory drugs. J. Pharmacol. exp. Ther. 196, 226—230 (1976)

Procaccini, R. L., Smyth, R. D., Rush, K., Reavey-Cantwell, N. H.: Studies on the inhibition of prostaglandin synthetase by fenclorac, a new nonsteroidal anti-inflammatory agent. Fed. Proc. 35, 774 (1976)

Robinson, D. R., McCuire, M. B., Bastian, D. E.: Corticosteroid inhibition of prostaglandin synthesis by rheumatoid synovia. Fed. Proc. 35, Abstract 735 (1976)

Robinson, D. R., Smith, H., McGuire, M. B., Levine, L.: Prostaglandin synthesis by rheumatoid synovium and its stimulation by colchicine. Prostaglandins 10, 67—85 (1975)

Rome, L. H., Lands, W. E. M.: Structural requirements for time-dependent inhibition of prostaglandin biosynthesis by anti-inflammatory drugs. Proc. nat. Acad. Sci. (Wash.) **72**, 4863—
4865 (1975)

Rome, L. H., Lands, W. E. M., Roth, G. J., Majerus, P. W.: Aspirin as a quantitative acetylating
reagent for the fatty acid oxygenase that forms prostaglandins. Prostaglandins **11**, 23—29
(1976)

Roth, G. J., Stanford, N., Majerus, P. W.: Acetylation of prostaglandin synthase by aspirin. Proc.
nat. Acad. Sci. (Wash.) **72**, 3073—3076 (1975)

Scherrer, R. A.: Introduction to the chemistry of anti-inflammatory and anti-arthritic agents. In:
Scherrer, R. A., Whitehouse, M. W. (Eds.): Anti-inflammatory Agents, Vol. I, pp. 29—43. New
York: Academic Press 1974

Shen, T. Y.: Synthesis and biological activity of some indomethacin analogs. In: Proceedings
International Symposium on Nonsteroidal Anti-inflammatory Drugs, pp. 13—20, 1964

Shen, T. Y.: Perspectives in non-steroidal anti-inflammatory agents. Angew. Chemie **11**, 460—472
(1972)

Shen, T. Y., Ham, E. A., Cirillo, V. J., Zanetti, M.: Structure-activity relationship of certain prostaglandin synthetase inhibitors. In: Vane, J. R., Robinson, H. R. (Eds.): Prostaglandin Synthetase Inhibitors, pp. 19—31. New York: Raven Press 1974

Shen, T. Y., Witzel, B. E., Jones, H., Linn, B. O., McPherson, J., Greenwald, R., Fordice, M., Ja-
cobs, A.: Synthesis of a new anti-inflammatory agent, cis-5-fluoro-2-methyl-1-(p-methylsulfinyl) benzylidenyl) indene-3-acetic acid. Fed. Proc. **31**, 577 (1972)

Smith, J. B., Willis, A. L.: Aspirin selectively inhibits prostaglandin production in human platelets.
Nature (New Biol.) **231**, 235—237 (1971)

Smith, M. J. H., Ford-Hutchinson, A. W., Elliott, P. N. C.: Prostaglandins and the anti-inflammatory activities of aspirin and sodium salicylate. J. Pharm. (Lond.) **27**, 473—478 (1975)

Smith, W. L., Lands, W. E. M.: Stimulation and blockade of prostaglandin biosynthesis. J. biol.
Chem. **246**, 6700—6702 (1971)

Steelman, S. L., Smit Sibinga, C. T., Schulz, P., Van den Heuvel, W. J. H., Tempero, K. F.: The effect
of diflunisal on urinary prostaglandin excretion, bleeding time and platelet aggregation in
normal human subjects. In: Proceedings XIII International Congress of Internal Medicine,
p. 215, 1976

Stone, K. J., Mathes, S. J., Gibson, P. P.: Selective inhibition of prostaglandin biosynthesis by gold
salts and phenylbutazone. Prostaglandins **10**, 241—251 (1975)

Takeguchi, C., Kohno, K., Sih, S. J.: Mechanism of prostaglandin biosynthesis. I. Characterisation
and assay of bovine prostaglandin synthetase. Biochemistry **10**, 2372—2376 (1971)

Takeguchi, C., Sih, S. J.: A rapid spectrophotometric assay for prostaglandin synthetase: application to the study of non-steroidal anti-inflammatory agents. Prostaglandins **2**, 169—184
(1972)

Tashjian, A. H. Jr., Voelkel, E. F., McDonough, J., Levine, L.: Hydrocortisone inhibits prostaglandin production by mouse fibrosarcoma cells. Nature (Lond.) **258**, 739—741 (1975)

Tolman, E. L., Birnbaum, J. E., Chiccarelli, F. S., Panagides, J., Sloboda, A. E.: Inhibition of prostaglandin activity and synthesis by fenbufen (a new non-steroidal anti-inflammatory agent) and
one of its metabolites. In: Samuelsson, B., Paoletti, R. (Eds.): Advances in Prostaglandin and
Thromboxane Research, Vol. I, pp. 133—138. New York: Raven Press 1976

Tolman, E. L., Partridge, R.: Multiple sites of interaction between prostaglandins and nonsteroidal anti-inflammatory agents. Prostaglandins **9**, 349—359 (1975)

Van Arman, C. G., Risley, E. A., Nuss, G. W.: Pharmacologic properties of an anti-inflammatory
agent 5-fluoro-2-methyl-1-(p-methylsulfinyl benzylidene)-inden-3-yl-acetic acid. Fed. Proc.
31, 577 (1972)

Vanderhoek, J. Y., Lands, W. E. M.: Acetylenic inhibitors of sheep vesicular gland oxygenase.
Biochim. biophys. Acta **296**, 374—381 (1973)

Vane, J. R.: Inhibition of prostaglandin synthesis as a mechanism of action for aspirin-like drugs.
Nature (New Biol.) **231**, 232 (1971)

Van Nueten, J. M.: Antagonism of arachidonic acid hydroperoxide on isolated gastro-intestinal
tissues as a measure of the inhibition of prostaglandin biosynthesis. In: Samuelsson, B.,
Paoletti, R. (Eds.): Advances in Prostaglandin and Thromboxane Research, Vol. I, pp. 139—
145. New York: Raven Press 1976

Vargaftig, B. B., Tranier, Y., Chignard, M.: Inhibition by sulfhydryl agents of arachidonic acid-induced platelet aggregation and release of potential inflammatory substances. Prostaglandins **8**, 133—147 (1974)

Vigdahl, R. L., Tukey, R. H.: Inhibition of prostaglandin synthetase by anti-inflammatory agents R-805 and R-807. Pharmacologist **17**, 226 (1975)

Wiseman, E. H., McIlhenny, H. M., Bettis, J. W.: Flumizole, a new nonsteroidal anti-inflammatory agent. J. pharm. Sci. **64**, 1469—1475 (1975)

Wlodawer, P., Samuelsson, B., Albonico, S. M., Corey, E. J.: Selective inhibition of prostaglandin synthetase by a bicyclo (2,2,1,) heptane derivative. J. Amer. chem. Soc. **93**, 2815—2816 (1971)

Yanagi, Y., Komatsu, T.: Inhibition of prostaglandin biosynthesis by SL-573. Biochem. Pharmacol. **25**, 937—941 (1976)

Yesair, D. W., Callahan, M., Remington, L., Kenster, C. J.: Role of the enterohepatic cycle of indomethacin on its metabolism, distribution in tissues, and its excretion by rats, dogs, and monkeys. Biochem. Pharmacol. **19**, 1579—1590 (1970)

Ziboh, V. A.: Regulation of prostaglandin E_2 biosynthesis in guinea pig skin by retinoic acid. Acta derm.-venereol (Stockh.) **74** Suppl., 56—60 (1975)

Ziboh, V. A., McElligott, T., Hsia, S. L.: Prostaglandin E_2 biosynthesis in human skin: subcellular localisation and inhibition by unsaturated fatty acids and anti-inflammatory drugs. Advanc. Biosci. **9**, 457—460 (1973)

Ziel, R., Krupp, P.: The significance of inhibition of prostaglandin synthesis in the selection on nonsteroidal anti-inflammatory agents. Advanc. Biosci. **9**, 457—460 (1973)

Ziel, R., Krupp, P.: The significance of inhibition of prostaglandin synthesis in the selection of non-steroidal anti-inflammatory agents. Int. J. clin. Pharmacol. **12**, 186—191 (1975)

CHAPTER 31

Mode of Action of Anti-Inflammatory Agents Which are Prostaglandin Synthetase Inhibitors

S. H. FERREIRA and J. R. VANE

This review is mainly concerned with the mechanism of action of those non-steroid anti-inflammatory drugs used to ameliorate the signs and symptoms of human acute and chronic inflammation which have the common property of inhibiting fatty acid oxidative cyclization, in particular the formation of prostaglandins (PGs) and thromboxanes. We have retained for this group of substances the term PG synthetase inhibitors because thromboxane synthetase can be selectively inhibited by substances which do not affect PG synthesis and do not show anti-inflammatory activity (MONCADA et al., 1976). Other types of non-steroid anti-inflammatory agents are reviewed in subsequent chapters.

A. Mediators and Inflammatory Responses

It is recognised that inflammation differs from species to species, in the same species from one tissue to another and also in the same tissue according to the type of traumas; yet the early inflammatory events induced by various trauma in different species and tissues have much in common, as far as signs and symptoms are concerned.

Several highly active substances are liberated locally in tissues during inflammatory reactions. Amongst these are histamine, 5-hydroxytryptamine (5-HT), slow reacting substance of anaphylaxis (SRS-A), various chemotactic factors, bradykinin (Bk), rabbit aorta contracting substance (RCS), which is now equated mainly with thromboxane A_2 (HAMBERG et al., 1976), and PGs of the E and F series. The involvement of these substances in inflammation has been proposed or demonstrated (see Chapters 5–16).

In different types of inflammation, some mediators may have more prominent roles than others; this is shown by the actions of antagonists. The sequence of mediator release may also be important. For instance, in anaphylactic shock there is an explosive and simultaneous release of histamine, SRS-A, PGE_2 and $PGF_{2\alpha}$ and RCS (see PIPER and VANE, 1971). However, in the inflammatory response to subcutaneous injection of carrageenin in the rat, there is a sequential release as shown by testing the exudate for pharmacological activity (WILLIS, 1969a, 1969b). At first, there was an output of histamine, which then tended to decline perhaps because the preformed stores in mast cells had been exhausted. WILLIS then detected Bk. There was little PG activity (< 5 ng/ml) until 3 h after the carrageenin injection but then the concentration gradually rose to an average plateau of 80 ng/ml between 18 and 24 h.

The lack of activity in the first 3 h may not reflect lack of PG formation; the presence of PGs in biological fluids depends on the balance between generation and removal and little is known about inactivation within the interstitial spaces. Furthermore, with such highly potent substances, a local vascular effect may be exerted before the amounts overflowing into the exudate reach detectable levels.

As the concentration of PGs in the exudate rose, so did that of histamine, reaching more than 1 μg/ml at 24 h. This secondary release of histamine may be associated with fresh synthesis, for in many situations "nascent histamine" formation has been described (SCHAYER, 1960), due to increased activity of histidine decarboxylase.

The results of WILLIS (1969a, 1969b) were reinforced by those of DI ROSA et al. (1971a, 1971b), who used depleting agents or antagonists to study the role of different mediators in rat paw oedema induced by carrageenin. In order to abolish the first phase of the response, they had to use a combination of antagonists of histamine and 5-HT or had to deplete both agents with compound 48/80. A kininogen-depleting agent (cellulose sulphate), presumably preventing formation of Bk, depressed the $1^1/_2-2^1/_2$ h oedema. Recently, using a Bk potentiating peptide, FERREIRA et al. (1974b, 1974c) concluded that Bk release began immediately after carrageenin injection and persisted for up to 6 h. PGs were detected after Bk release and DI ROSA et al. (1971b) noted that it was the "prostaglandin phase" of the oedema which was most susceptible to aspirin-like drugs. It was this phase also which coincided with the arrival of polymorphonuclear leucocytes (PMN cells) in large numbers. Other results by DI ROSA et al. (1971a) suggested that the early phase of turpentine-induced pleurisy in the rat was mainly histamine mediated and that 5-HT and kinins were much less important in this type of inflammation.

The invasion of the inflamed area by PMN cells may also be important for the maintenance of PG generation (and thereby of the inflammation). HIGGS and YOULTEN (1972) and HIGGS et al. (1975) showed that phagocytosis was accompanied by PG release and suggested that this could constitute a control mechanism for further influx of phagocytes, since PGE_1 is leucotactic (KALEY and WEINER, 1971a, 1971b). Phagocytosis (and therefore leucotaxis) would continue for as long as the injurious agent or tissue debris was present.

There is another enzyme involved in arachidonic acid transformation which is not inhibited by aspirin-like drugs. This is a lipoxygenase, isolated from human platelets and guinea pig lung by HAMBERG and SAMUELSSON (1974a, 1974b), HAMBERG et al. (1974) and NUGTEREN (1975). This enzyme generates a 12-hydroperoxide derivative of arachidonic acid (HPETE) and 12-L-hydroxy-5,8,10,14-eicosatetraenoic acid (HETE) (see Chap. 12). The importance of HETE in inflammatory processes may well lie in the fact that it exhibits chemotaxis for polymorphonuclear leucocytes (TURNER et al., 1975).

Phagocytosis also leads to the release of lysosomal enzymes which can damage the tissue further. Acid phosphatase and β-glucuronidase appear at the same time as PGE_2 in the carrageenin-induced exudate (ANDERSON et al., 1971; WILLIS et al., 1972). This finding led to the suggestion that phospholipases liberated from the lysosomes release arachidonic acid from phospholipids, which in turn is converted to PGs by tissue enzymes (ANDERSON et al., 1971).

It is little realized, however, that the major increase in vascular permeability following carrageenin injection in the rat paw occurs within 2 h, at a time when the oedema is still developing (GARCIA LEME et al., 1973a). This observation has been questioned by DOHERTY and ROBINSON (1975), but their results may reflect an in-

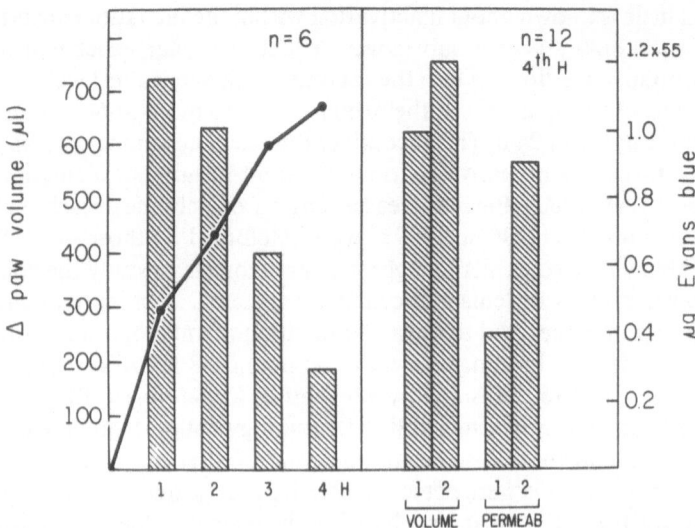

Fig. 1. Relationship between oedema and increased vascular permeability induced by injection of carrageenin in the paw. Left panel shows a comparison between rat paw volume *(black line)* and increase in permeability *(bars)*. Right panel shows the effect of a second injection (2) of carrageenin (100 μg) 3 h after the first injection (*1*). Measurements were made 4 h after the first injection. Values are the mean of 6 paws, in each time interval (Zanin et al., 1976)

crease in blood flow rather than permeability increase. In fact, Zanin et al. (1976) using a different method, confirmed Garcia Leme's observations (Fig. 1). This may well be the reason why aspirin-like drugs have little effect upon oedema formation when given after carrageenin challenge. The second panel of Figure 1 shows that a second injection of carrageenin produces a further increase in permeability. This indicates that the reduction in the permeability increase observed after the second hour results from a cessation of the trauma rather than from a loss of responsiveness of the vessels. This interpretation questions the importance of migrating cells as well as the idea of sequential liberation of mediators in acute inflammation, especially the existence of a pure "prostaglandin phase" in carrageenin oedema (Di Rosa et al., 1971a, 1971b). On the other hand, it implies that during the period in which the trauma is effective (2 h) there is a concomitant release of 5-HT, Bk, and PGs (see discussion later). It must be pointed out, however, that there is no way in which to settle the problem until the role of migrating cells in the development of acute inflammatory reaction is defined: some authors correlate the intensity of the inflammation with the white cell counts (Van Arman and Carlson, 1974) while others find no correlation (Brune et al., 1974; Brune and Glatt, 1974). Glatt et al. (1974) injected urate crystals into the intertarsal joints of chickens. At 1 h, concentrations of PGE_2 and $PGF_{2\alpha}$ were at a peak but there were no detectable PMN cells present. In animals treated with colchicine, which further delayed PMN cell migration, the prostaglandin concentration peaked at 2 h again, before invasion by PMN cells.

So far, we have mainly considered the inflammatory response induced by carrageenin. The importance of this acute model resides in its sensitivity to the anti-inflammatory drugs of proven value in acute as well as in human chronic inflammation—perhaps a reflection of the involvement of the same repertoire of mediators in both situations. Chronic inflammation differs from acute by the increased activity of cellular components such as fibroblasts and macrophages and by the presence of destructive lesions. Aspirin-like drugs only diminish the symptomatology without affecting the progression of chronic diseases, such as arthritis.

As far as the signs and symptoms are concerned, the arrival of new cells and the consequent change from acute to chronic inflammation, does not seem to involve new mediators, but only increased amounts of the existing ones. Each inflammatory sign or symptom is caused by the co-ordinated action of several inflammatory mediators and this must also depend on the sensitivity of the responding cells. This interplay is very important and the absence of any one factor can substantially change the final response. Generally speaking, even though the inflammatory response has an abundance of mediators each one has importance; otherwise it would be difficult to reduce preferentially, some of the signs or symptoms. Although we cannot prevent the outcome of most chronic inflammatory diseases, because we do not know how to prevent the ongoing tissue injury, we can at least ameliorate the situation and sometimes even recover impaired functions.

We shall now analyse the possible sites of anti-inflammatory action of aspirin-like drugs. The term "aspirin-like" drugs is a pharmacological rather than a chemical definition and includes compounds of diverse nature (although the majority are organic acids) which qualitatively show the same spectrum of antipyretic, analgesic and anti-inflammatory actions as does aspirin. The term anti-inflammatory is used in the loose clinical connotation; that is to describe agents which lessen or prevent inflammatory signs or symptoms.

B. Mechanism of Anti-Inflammatory Action

It has been suggested that aspirin-like drugs act in vivo by releasing an endogenous anti-inflammatory substance rather than by blocking the action or release of an inflammatory mediator. MAICKEL et al. (1965) and BRODIE (1965) some time ago suggested that they could be acting by releasing adrenocortical steroids from their binding with plasma proteins. Although adrenalectomy sometimes reduces the anti-inflammatory action of salicylates, COLLIER (1969) has summarized the reasons for not attributing the effect of adrenalectomy to a block of glucocorticoid release. These are: (a) adrenalectomy does not reduce the effects of phenylbutazone and fenamates on granulation, although granulation is very sensitive to glucocorticoids; (b) therapeutic doses of salicylates do not stimulate adrenocorticoid secretion in animals or man; (c) the antiphlogistic activity of glucocorticoids markedly differs from that of salicylates in ultraviolet (UV) erythema and in the tuberculin reaction. It should be added that in most experimental situations, aspirin-like drugs inhibit the synthesis and release of PGs whilst corticoids are usually without effect (see later).

Recently MCARTHUR et al. (1971) suggested that aspirin-like drugs act by releasing an endogenous anti-inflammatory peptide from plasma protein. However, no peptide which could be related to the anti-inflammatory properties of aspirin-like drugs has been isolated (see Chap. 15).

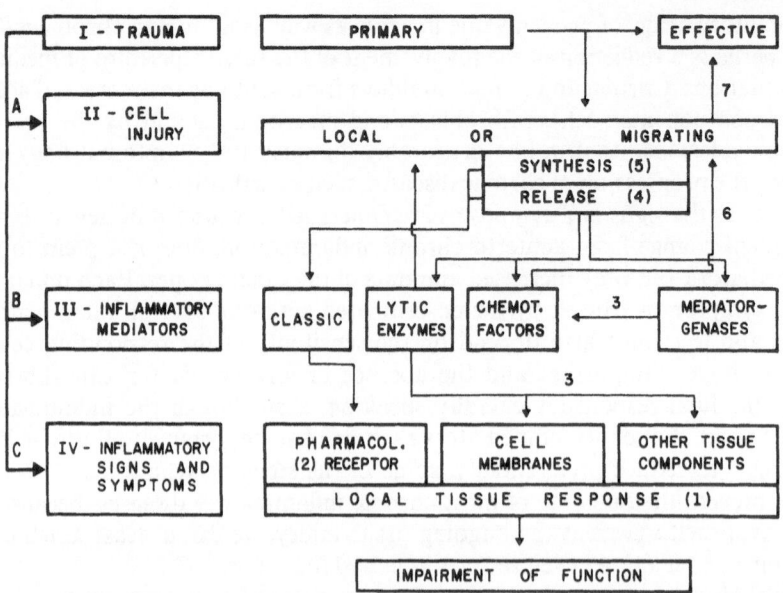

Fig. 2. Pathways leading to inflammation. Four components of inflammation can usually be recognized. Trauma (*I*) causes injury (*II*) to local or migrating cells. This leads to appearance of local inflammatory mediators (*III*) which induce tissue response (*IV*) that are the basis of inflammatory signs or symptoms *(arrow A)*. In some instances, a trauma can induce formation of inflammatory mediators, acting directly on plasma systems *(arrow B)*. A trauma can produce a sign or a symptom directly *(arrow C;* burning, for example) but in such instances anti-inflammatory drugs are of little or no use

Discussion of the mechanism of action of aspirin-like drugs is facilitated by describing the main steps of an inflammatory reaction sensitive to such agents (see Fig. 2).

Inflammatory mediators can be classified into three groups: (a) the direct-acting, classic ones such as histamine, Bk, PGs, etc., which act via pharmacological receptors (receptor-mediators); (b) lytic enzymes of cellular or plasma origin which directly damage the integrity of local or migrating cells; (c) chemotactic factors which regulate migration of cells to the site of inflammation. A mediator-genase is an enzyme or a cascade of enzymes which, when activated, generates a particular inflammatory mediator.

I. Actions on Step 1: Diminution of the Capability of Tissue Cells to Respond to Inflammatory Mediators

Vessels are mainly involved in causing the classical acute inflammatory signs and symptoms. These are vasodilatation (or erythema) and increased vascular permeability (or oedema; see Chap. 16). Sensory nerves subserve pruritus, hyperalgesia and overt pain whereas migrating cells, together with leaking vessels, contribute to the sign referred to as "tumor."

1. Increased Dilatation and Vascular Permeability

As amply discussed in this book, reduction in vasodilatation and increased vascular permeability are used to assess anti-inflammatory drugs. Stabilization of the walls of small vessels may prevent vascular dilatation and the increase of vascular permeability brought about by injurious stimuli. This seems to occur in diabetic rats, in which the effects of histamine, 5-HT, Bk or phlogogenic materials like dextran, ovomucoid, carrageenin or cellulose sulphate, were unspecifically reduced (GOTH et al., 1957; GARCIA LEME et al., 1973 b).

Corticosterone reduces vasodilatation (resulting in decreased blood flow) and vascular exudation (ASHTON and COOK, 1952; SPAIN et al., 1952; MOON and TER-SHAKOVIC, 1952, 1954; WYMAN et al., 1954). Recently, GARCIA LEME and WILHELM (1975) re-stated the importance of corticosteroids as regulators of direct vascular responsiveness to mediators such as histamine and 5-HT. In this context, MUNCK (1971) suggested that corticosteroids decrease the utilization of glucose by peripheral tissues by blocking its transport into the cell, possibly by preventing phosphorylation. SCHAYER (1964) proposed that the anti-inflammatory action of corticosteroids was caused by the passive attachment of the steroid to the microvascular smooth muscle cells, thus interfering with dilatation.

Salicylates uncouple oxidative phosphorylation (BRODY, 1956) and this has led to the suggestion that the reduction in ATP synthesis would interfere with glycogen and protein synthesis or with cell membrane permeability (for review, see WHITEHOUSE, 1965). Such an action during therapy with aspirin-like drugs would cause a general reduction in responsiveness of the vessels to all stimuli causing permeability increases. This does not happen, as we shall discuss later. Furthermore, a substance well known as an uncoupler of oxidative phosphorylation such as 2,4-dinitrophenol, does not exhibit anti-inflammatory activity (see WINTER, 1965).

Some of the putative inflammatory mediators, especially Bk, cause a contraction of isolated strips of vascular tissue, an effect which is antagonized by aspirin-like drugs. However, there is doubt whether this effect is selective (COLLIER, 1969). It probably reflects an inhibition of a background or stimulated production of prostaglandins which sensitizes the isolated smooth muscle preparations to the agonists (VANE and FERREIRA, 1975). For example, addition of Bk to slices of bovine mesenteric vessels stimulated PG synthesis (TERRAGNO et al., 1975).

When an injected substance causes mediator release, it is difficult to assess in vivo whether an anti-inflammatory agent is directly inhibiting the activity of the released substance(s) or blocking the formation or release of the substance(s). Certainly, many unspecific trauma and specific stimuli, like Bk induce a quick local formation and release of PGs (PIPER and VANE, 1971; VANE and FERREIRA, 1975). A recent example comes from MESSINA et al. (1975) who studied the vasodilator effect of Bk in the cremaster muscle. They concluded that the effect of Bk was at least in part mediated by a local release of PGs, since they found that vascular effects of Bk, but not of PGs, were reduced by PG synthetase inhibitors.

When the direct vascular effects of several inflammatory mediators have been studied in vivo, no general pattern of action of aspirin-like drugs has emerged. Phenylbutazone or aspirin were not effective in reducing the oedema produced by intra-plantar injections of mediators such as histamine or 5-HT or phlogogenic stimuli like chicken egg white, 48/80, polyvinylpyrrolidone or dextran (BONTA, 1965; GARCIA LEME et al., 1973a). Furthermore, the increased vascular permeability induced by Bk or peptides prepared from fibrin, was unaffected by local administration of salicylate in rats (SPECTOR and WILLOUGHBY, 1963). However, STARR and WEST (1967) found that calcium aspirin and antipyretics inhibited the wealing induced by intradermal injection of Bk, histamine or 5-HT in the rat. ARRIGONI-MARTELLI (1967) also found that aspirin, flufenamic acid, phenylbutazone, or sodium salicylate (in decreasing order of potency) inhibited the increased vascular permeability induced by Bk. In guinea pig, aspirin or sodium salicylate did not reduce the increase of permeability induced by Bk (COLLIER and SHORLEY, 1960; LEWIS, 1963). In the rabbit, LISH and MacKINNEY (1963) found that aspirin-like drugs diminished the permeability increase caused by Bk (but not that induced by histamine), although NORTHOVER and SUBRAMANIAN (1962) found no effect on the Bk response. It is possible that all these discrepancies between species or investigators depend on whether or not there is a release of PG caused by the trauma of injection in that particular species or experiment.

In short, if we accept that a drug is acting on some general mechanism which subserves the responsiveness of the tissues, it should reduce the direct effects of all inflammatory mediators and phlogogenic stimuli. It is difficult to conclude that this is a relevant mechanism for the anti-inflammatory action of aspirin-like drugs.

2. Pain and Hyperalgesia

The same argument can be applied for pain and hyperalgesia. If aspirin-like drugs were unspecifically depressing the responsiveness of nerve cells or pain receptors, they should show a pattern of pharmacological effects similar to that of a local anaesthetic. For this reason, it is difficult to reconcile the experimental observations with the suggested mechanism of analgesia of aspirin-like drugs via an inhibition of oxidative phosphorylation (LIM, 1966), or through a direct action upon membrane permeability (LEVITON and BARKER, 1972). Although aspirin-like drugs can reduce the algesic action of some inflammatory mediators, such as Bk (GUZMAN et al., 1962, 1964), they do not affect incapacitation induced in dogs by intra-articular injection of PGs. On the other hand, indomethacin has no analgesic effect on the pain-producing activity of Bk injected into a knee joint already sensitized with PGs. The problem is discussed in more detail in Chapter 17 but we must stress that aspirin-like drugs are analgesic only when there is an inflammatory process or a local synthesis and release of PGs. They do not affect the normal functions of pain receptors but restore to normal the lowered threshold to pain caused by inflammation. This contrasts with morphine which by a central action reduces the threshold to stimuli applied on normal as well as on inflamed regions.

3. Increased Fibroblast Proliferation and Secretion

A prolonged trauma usually stimulates fibroblast proliferation and secretion. This effect is probably through the formation of mediators such as the endogenous peptide described by CASTOR (1972). This peptide, which can be obtained from leucocytes, stimulates the production of hyaluronate by cultures of synovial fibroblasts and may account in part for proliferation of connective tissue in vivo. If so, fibroblast proliferation and secretion may be generally similar to other inflammatory events, i.e. the result of stimulation of an "effector cell" (fibroblast) by one or more of the locally released inflammatory mediators.

How can reduction of the increased fibroblast proliferation and secretion be beneficial to ameliorate the inflammatory process? In vitro and in vivo, depending on dose, sodium salicylate, phenylbutazone or indomethacin inhibit collagen biosynthesis (see TRNAVSKY, 1974 and Chapters 3 and 19). Abolition of PG synthesis by aspirin-like drugs may explain the fact that they impair scar formation, for PGs are known to stimulate biosynthesis of collagen (BLUMENKRANTZ and SONDERGAARD, 1972). However, non-steroid anti-inflammatory drugs are much less effective in causing changes in collagen fractions than steroids and their effect on granulomas does not seem to depend on an effect on collagen synthesis.

The effects of aspirin-like drugs on the maturation of collagen into the insoluble form seem to be of interest. Adjuvant arthritis in rats is thought to be a good model of many facets of human arthritis (GLENN and KOOYERS, 1966; Chap. 23). It is an autoimmune disease in which the conversion of soluble into insoluble collagen is unspecifically retarded. Acceleration of conversion of soluble to insoluble collagen may cause reduction of inflammatory signs and symptoms by reducing the possible activation of enzymes which generate kinin or complement. Sodium salicylate and phenylbutazone stimulate the conversion of soluble into insoluble collagen, in contrast to the increased degradation of soluble collagen that these agents can cause in normal animals (TRNAVSKÁ et al., 1972).

Formation of granulation tissue depends also on the synthesis of mucopolysaccharide by fibroblasts which is sometimes considerably increased in chronic inflammation. This constitutes the amorphous ground substance and its synthesis normally precedes that of collagen. Non-steroid anti-inflammatory drugs may affect mucopolysaccharide synthesis (a) by inhibiting glucosamine-6-phosphate synthetase (SCHÖNHÖFER, 1966, 1967); (b) by blocking incorporation of glucosamine into the polysaccharide chain (KALBHEN et al., 1967a, b); (c) by interfering with the production of glucuronic acid (LEE and SPENCER, 1969; MORETTI et al., 1966); and (d) by interfering with polysaccharide sulphation (BRÖHR and KALBHEN, 1968; ROGER and KALBHEN, 1968). Increased synthesis of glucosamine-6-phosphate correlates with the swelling of inflamed hind paws of adjuvant arthritic rats (FUJIHIRA et al., 1971) but there is no indication that the reduction of swelling by non-steroid anti-inflammatory drugs results from an inhibition of this enzyme. Aspirin-like drugs affect many facets of connective tissue metabolism but, as TRNAVSKY (1974) points out, their action in the overall metabolism "still does not satisfactorily explain their beneficial effects on rheumatic diseases."

At present, it is difficult to evaluate the contribution of a possible inhibition of mucopolysaccharide formation to the amelioration of signs and symptoms in chronic inflammation. Even if aspirin-like drugs have such an action, they still have dramatic effects in acute experimental models in which proliferation and fibroblast secretion does not play an important role.

II. Action on Step 2: Pharmacological Receptor Antagonism

One dogma of contemporary pharmacology is that the effect induced by an endogenous mediator results from its interaction with a specific site on the cell membrane referred to as a pharmacological receptor. The identification of possible specific antagonists of such receptors was, in the last two decades, ever present in the minds of those trying to understand the anti-inflammatory actions of aspirin-like drugs. COLLIER (1969) pointed out that the blockade by aspirin-like drugs of the broncho-constriction induced by Bk in guinea pigs, showed several features of receptor inhibition: (a) it occurs in the absence of CNS or of adrenal glands; (b) it is surmountable by higher doses of Bk, which can in turn be overcome by higher doses of aspirin; (c) its onset is rapid and (d) aspirin does not antagonise bronchoconstriction induced by acetylcholine, histamine or 5-HT. However, antagonism of the bronchocon-striction induced by other very dissimilar molecules, such as arachidonic acid and ATP, clearly spoke against a typical receptor antagonism. Moreover, in the isolated guinea pig ileum, aspirin antagonized contractions induced by arachidonic acid peroxide but not those induced by Bk (JAQUES, 1959) and there was no receptor antagonist action against other inflammatory mediators (GARCIA LEME and ROCHA E SILVA, 1965). In general, a receptor antagonism demonstrated on smooth muscle preparations should also be demonstrable on vascular permeability, as with antago-nists of adrenaline, 5-HT and histamine. On the present experimental evidence, it must be concluded that there is little ground to think that aspirin-like drugs act as anti-inflammatory or analgesic substances through a direct antagonism of a known mediator at its receptor site.

III. Action on Step 3: Inhibition of Extracellular Enzymic Activities Which Generate Inflammatory Mediators or Cause Injury to Cell Membranes and/or Tissue Components

A trauma can by itself activate a plasma enzyme system which directly (activation of alternate pathway of complement) or indirectly (activation of Hageman factor caus-ing Bk formation) generates substances responsible for inflammatory signs and symptoms (arrow B, Fig. 2). Carrageenin is one such trauma, because it releases kinin when incubated with plasma (ROTHSCHILD, 1967) and also activates the complement system (WARD and COCHRANE, 1965). Activation of plasma enzymes can also be indirectly induced by the trauma, i.e. secondary to the release of enzymes extruded by injured cells (see Chapters 9 and 14). In addition to the activation of plasma enzymes, other lytic enzymes (lysosomal enzymes or other hydrolases, for example) can be released into the inflammatory exudate either from injured local cells or during phagocytic activity of migrating cells (HIRSCH and COHN, 1960; WEISSMANN et al., 1971 a, 1971 b).

Binding of non-steroid anti-inflammatory agents to plasma proteins is well estab-lished and in recent years there have been many attempts to correlate such in vitro findings with clinical efficacy. The association with protein is reflected in some properties of the aspirin-like drugs such as inhibition of denaturation of plasma protein (MIZUSHIMA, 1964, 1965; MIZUSHIMA and KOBAYASHI, 1968), inhibition of binding to bovine albumin of urate (BLUESTONE et al., 1969), 2,4,6-trinitrobenz-aldehyde or 5-dimethylaminonaphthalene-sulphonamide (DNSA) (SKIDMORE and WHITEHOUSE, 1966; GRANT et al., 1971 a), and acceleration of sulphydryl-disulphide interchange (GERBER et al., 1967). Relevance of these binding properties to a reduc-tion of inflammatory signs and symptoms is obscure.

Aspirin-like drugs partially block the hypotension induced by kallikrein (NORTH-OVER and SUBRAMANIAN, 1961) as well as the release of kinin during oedema induced by kaolin (BONTA and DE VOS, 1965) or thermic oedema (ARRIGONI-MARTELLI et al., 1969). An explanation for these findings could be the inhibition of kininogenases similar to that observed with soya bean trypsin inhibitor (WEBSTER and PIERCE, 1960) or Trasylol (KRAUT et al., 1963). NORTHOVER and SUBRAMANIAN (1961) found that aspirin and phenylbutazone inhibited kinin formation by guinea pig serum kinino-genase or human salivary kininogenase. However, using purified bovine substrate, DAVIES et al. (1966) were unable to confirm this inhibition by several aspirin-like compounds.

Inhibition of enzymes responsible for the formation of Bk is not accepted as a relevant effect of aspirin-like drugs (see Chap. 14). Furthermore, those in vivo experiments in which a reduced release of Bk was observed, may reflect the fact that formation of Bk was inhibited consequent upon a diminution of the inflammatory response. Another possibility is that the substance being bioassayed as Bk was in part composed of PGs, which would accompany Bk in the usual process of ethanol extraction and resemble its activity on isolated smooth muscles such as the rat uterus. It is clear that the criteria for identification of Bk need to be made more stringent, especially by using more specific assay tissues. The rat uterus responds to many substances, including the PGs and effects of the PGs would survive the usual pharmacological antagonists. Strips of cat terminal ileum (FERREIRA and VANE, 1967) provide a more selective bioassay for Bk.

Besides formation of kinin there are at least two other enzymic activities in inflammatory exudates the blockade of which could partially explain the anti-inflammatory action of aspirin-like drugs; these are lysosomal enzymes and complement components. As discussed in Chapters 8 and 9, lysosomal enzymes and related hydrolytic enzymes can break down many tissue components and degradation of tissue is one of the basic features of chronic inflammation. Repeated intra-articular injection of lysosomal enzymes can induce several signs and symptoms of chronic inflammation (see WEISSMANN, 1972). Inflammatory exudates contain a large variety of enzymic activities. They originate from various sources. Collagenase, for instance, is present in polymorphonuclear leucocytes (LAZARUS et al., 1968), in skin (FULLMER et al., 1966) and rheumatoid synovium (EVANSON et al., 1967). A specific inhibitor of any lysosomal enzyme certainly would be of value in controlling inflammation. Flufenamic acid and aspirin, but not phenylbutazone and ibufenac, inhibit collagenase activity of a lysosomal preparation in vitro (ANDERSON, 1969). To our knowledge, there is no lysosomal enzyme that is selectively inhibited in vivo by aspirin-like drugs.

There have also been reports that aspirin-like drugs have anti-complementary action. Cobra venom and zymosan deplete C^3 and diminish inflammatory responses. FICHEL et al. (1958) found that salicylate and cortisone had an anti-complement effect through an anti-esterase activity. Recently, DI PERRY and AUTERY (1974) showed that aspirin, flufenamic acid, indomethacin and phenylbutazone inhibited in vitro the activation of several components of complement. However, the relevance of this observation to an anti-inflammatory effect is unclear for they were shown to be effective on the complement system in vivo only in very high doses (100 mg/kg, i.v. for indomethacin).

Finally, we should comment about the fibrinolytic activity of aspirin-like drugs. There is a parallelism between anti-inflammatory activity and fibrinolytic activity for salicylic acid derivatives, butazone, fenamates, and indomethacin (VON KAULLA, 1963; GRYGLEWSKI, 1966; GRYGLEWSKI and GRYGLEWSKA, 1966; ROUBAL and NEMECK, 1966a, 1966b). The fibrinolytic activity of these compounds is thought to be due to an inhibition of the actions of certain endogenous inhibitors of the fibrin-dissolving system of plasma (VON KAULLA, 1968). Activation of fibrinolytic activity of plasma may be important to minimise inflammatory reactions in which formation of thrombi is a usual component, as occurs in the Arthus reaction. But it is difficult to accept that, even in those models, activation of fibrinolysis plays a relevant role in the anti-inflammatory action of aspirin-like drugs, because of the very high concentration (30–100 mM) necessary to demonstrate this activity in vitro.

IV. Action on Step 4: Inhibition of the Release of Intracellular Lytic Enzymes or Mediator-Genases or Stored Receptor-Mediators

Injury of local or migrating cells can cause the release of pre-formed mediators or the release of lytic enzymes by mediator-genases. The enzymes may be dispersed in the cell cytoplasm or stored within organelles such as lysosomes.

Histamine and SRS-A can be released from mastocytes by an immediate type of hypersensitivity, passive cutaneous anaphylaxis (PCA), and this release can be suppressed in vivo by disodium cromoglycate (ORANGE and AUSTEN, 1968, and Chap. 34). However, aspirin-like drugs have no consistent effects in this model (UBATUBA et al., 1975) and are ineffective in blocking histamine release during anaphylaxis in isolated guinea pig lung (PIPER and VANE, 1969a, 1969b).

Unspecific binding of aspirin-like drugs to cell membrane proteins could help to stabilize lysosomal membranes and inhibit platelet aggregation or red cell lysis. Some of these effects could be relevant to the amelioration of inflammatory signs and symptoms because they would ultimately block the release either of inflammatory mediators or of lytic enzymes. But how relevant are the actions of aspirin-like drugs on lysosomal membranes to their anti-inflammatory action? The effect of aspirin-like drugs on lysosome membranes in vitro have been inconsistent. Some investigators report labilization and others stabilization. These discrepancies possibly reflect differences in methodology (HYTTEL and JORGENSSEN, 1970; HICHENS, 1974). Glucocorticoids, as shown by WEISSMANN and THOMAS (1964), have a direct stabilizing action on lysosome membranes against disrupting trauma such as hypoxia, bacterial, and chemical toxins or UV light. Although very much depending on the preparation of the lysosome, buffer conditions and disrupting stimuli, several aspirin-like drugs stabilize lysosomes in vitro (MILLER and SMITH, 1966; TANAKA and IZUKA, 1968; BROWN and SCHWARTZ, 1969; IGNARRO, 1971). Recently, IGNARRO renewed interest in lysosomal membrane stabilization as a possible mechanism of action of aspirin-like drugs (IGNARRO, 1971; IGNARRO and COLOMBO, 1972). However, the rank order of potency of the drugs tested was inverted when inhibition of oedema was compared with inhibition of extrusion of lysosome enzymes, i.e. aspirin > phenylbutazone > indomethacin (see FERREIRA and VANE, 1974a).

The experiments of CHAYEN are possibly relevant to the discussion because they show that in a more complex system (a very thin fragment of human skin), aspirin-like drugs are effective stabilizing agents (CHAYEN et al., 1970, 1971; CHAYEN and BITENSKY, 1971). ANDERSON (1970) found that phenylbutazone reduced the increased lysosomal enzyme activity in the paws of rats with adjuvant arthritis. HICHENS (1974) interpreted these effects, as well as those described by COPPI and BONARDI (1968) and IGNARRO and SLYWKA (1972), as secondary to the reduction of cellular infiltration. The interference of aspirin-like drugs in the migration of cells into tissues is still a matter of controversy, but they have little or no effect on the cell content of acute inflammatory exudates (VAN ARMAN and CARLSON, 1974; BRUNE et al., 1974; HIGGS et al., 1976; see Table 1).

Most of the lysosomal enzymes in inflammatory exudates are thought to be derived from leucocytes, especially from PMN cells, released during phagocytosis. Inhibition of phagocytosis, lysosomal degranulation or fusions of lysosomes with vacuoles (MALAWISTA and BODEL, 1967), may ameliorate inflammatory reaction by avoiding extrusion of the enzymes. Colchicine affects PMN cell functions by disrupting microtubules and consequently blocking the fusion of phagocytic vacuoles with lysosomes (see Chapters 8 and 9). In vivo, it does not seem that aspirin-like drugs interfere with the phagocytic function of PMN cells, for there was no change in the content of lysosome enzymes in inflammatory exudates (WILLIS et al., 1972).

Incidentally, GLATT et al. (1974) recorded an increase in PG production in the colchicine-treated animals and HIGGS et al. (1975) have noted a similar increase in carrageenin-induced formation of PGs in rats treated with colchicine. These observations are in accord with those of ROBINSON and LEVINE (1974) who found that colchicine stimulated PG production by rheumatoid synovial membrane preparations maintained in vitro in organ culture, but they pose the problem of the basis for the anti-inflammatory actions of colchicine. DENKO (1975) has provided evidence that colchicine directly antagonises the activity of PGE_1 in inflammation.

Even disregarding the fact that aspirin-like drugs may have a labilizing effect on lysosomal membranes (GRANT et al., 1971 b), it is difficult to accept that this stabilization of the membrane is relevant as a mechanism of anti-inflammatory and analgesic effect of aspirin-like drugs. This conclusion had already been reached by WINTER in 1966.

Other cells, as well as leucocytes, may release preformed mediators. Mastocytes, when stimulated by chemical or immunological stimuli, release histamine and SRS-A (see Chapters 11, 33, and 34).

The involvement of platelets in inflammation has been proposed by many authors (O'BRIEN, 1968a, 1968b; ROBERTSON and KHAIRALLAH, 1974; VARGAFTIG, 1974; REDEI and KELEMEN, 1969; GOROG and KOVACS, 1969; SILVER et al., 1974). Their role in causing increased endothelial permeability was linked to a focal release of 5-HT, histamine, PGs and/or other vasoactive substances by the local aggregation of circulating platelets. This aggregation was thought to be induced by basement membrane collagen exposed during endothelial contraction or damage caused by released inflammatory mediators (ROBERTSON and KHAIRALLAH, 1974) or by the initial trauma. Aspirin-like drugs inhibit the second phase of platelet aggregation induced by several types of trauma through an inhibition of the cyclo-oxygenase of PG synthetase, which in turn reduces the formation of thromboxane A_2 (HAMBERG et al., 1976). Thus, inhibitors of PG synthesis may derive their anti-inflammatory activity, at least in part, by reducing the release of inflammatory mediators from platelets.

In experiments designed to elucidate whether platelets participate in acute inflammation, UBATUBA et al. (1975) showed that the oedema in response to carrageenin, anti-platelet serum or passive cutaneous anaphylaxis was similar both in controls and thrombocytopenic rats. Thus, there was no evidence that the release of mediators from platelets contributes to the acute inflammatory response. Platelets, however, may be important in models such as the Arthus reaction, since thrombocytopenic rats exhibit a reduced Arthus reaction (MARGARETTEN and McKAY, 1971).

PGs may, in some instances, attenuate the inflammatory process by reducing receptor mediator release. WALKER (1973) showed that PGs, especially PGE_1 and PGE_2, inhibited the anaphylactic release in vitro of histamine from passively sensitized human lung tissue. However, they were considerably less potent than isoprenaline. E-type PGs also reduce the anaphylactic release of mediators from leucocytes taken from allergic patients (LICHTENSTEIN and BOURNE, 1971) and from rat mast cells (KOOPMAN et al., 1971). However, TAUBER et al. (1973) found that low concentrations of PGs increased mediator release; they suggested that the effects of PGs on mediator release depended on whether they increased or decreased cAMP in the cell.

When PG synthesis in lung tissue was suppressed by indomethacin, the release of SRS-A was markedly enhanced but that of histamine was inhibited. From these results, WALKER (1973) suggested that PGs may regulate the release of SRS-A or may be formed from the same precursor as SRS-A. The fact that SRS-A release increases in the presence of indomethacin, may contribute to the general lack of effect of aspirin-like drugs in asthma. GRYGLEWSKI et al. (1975) found histamine release in shocked guinea pig lungs was increased by indomethacin.

DAWSON and TOMLINSON (1974) investigated whether SRS-A is a derivative of arachidonic acid. They loaded isolated lungs from sensitized guinea pigs with labelled arachidonic acid and then challenged them. In the presence of cromoglycate, SRS-A release was suppressed but that of PGs was not. When the lungs were treated with a PG synthetase inhibitor, release of radioactivity was suppressed but SRS-A release continued. They concluded that SRS-A was unlikely to be formed from arachidonic acid. The fact that cromoglycate reduced the release of SRS-A but did not modify PG release, also counts against a major involvement of PG in those asthmatics who respond to cromoglycate. In summary, although PGs may modulate the release of other inflammatory mediators, the fact that PG synthetase inhibitors do not usually exacerbate inflammation suggests that this is not an important mechanism.

V. Action on Step 5: Inhibition of the Synthesis of Inflammatory Mediators

Aspirin-like drugs in vitro at high concentrations inhibit the synthesis of histamine and this has been suggested as one of the multiple ways by which these agents could block inflammation (SKIDMORE and WHITEHOUSE, 1966). In contrast to aspirin-like drugs, anti-histamine drugs are anti-inflammatory only in some special types of inflammation such as urticaria, hay fever and certain manifestations of anaphylaxis. Passive cutaneous anaphylaxis in the rat, for example, is inhibited by anti-histamines but not consistently by aspirin-like drugs. Moreover, there is no indication that aspirin-like drugs are effective in inflammatory reactions in which histamine release plays a relevant role.

The first clear demonstration of an inhibitory action of aspirin-like drugs at low concentrations on the release of a substance by a traumatic stimulus, was made by PIPER and VANE (1969a, 1969b) who showed that a previously unidentified biologically active material, which they named rabbit aorta contracting substance (RCS), was released from guinea pig lung during anaphylaxis, along with histamine, SRS-A, and PGs. The RCS release was blocked by aspirin. Owing to methodological problems, they failed to notice that there was also inhibition of PG synthesis. Evidence to link RCS into the biosynthetic pathway came from VARGAFTIG and DAO HAI (1971) who showed that the PG precursor, arachidonic acid, also generated RCS when infused into guinea pig lungs. Very recently, the main component of RCS activity has been re-named thromboxane A_2 by HAMBERG et al. (1976).

In 1971, it was shown in three different systems and species that the generation or release of PGs was inhibited by aspirin-like drugs. These were a cell-free preparation of PG synthetase (VANE, 1971), a suspension of human platelets (SMITH and WILLIS, 1971) and the dog perfused spleen stimulated by catecholamine (FERREIRA et al., 1971). At that time, release of PGs was already equated with synthesis (PIPER and VANE, 1971), because it was known that cells do not store PGs. These findings have been confirmed in a large number of species using a wide range of analytical techniques, including thin-layer and gas chromatography, radiometric, and polarographic assays, as well as radioimmunoassays.

VANE's (1971) suggestion that inhibition of PG synthesis explained the anti-inflammatory activity of aspirin-like drugs, enormously stimulated research in the field of inflammation. In contrast to all other hypotheses about the mechanism of anti-inflammatory, analgesic, and antipyretic activity of aspirin-like drugs, inhibition of PG synthesis encompasses observations made by biochemists, physiologists, pharmacologists, and pathologists, and forms the only unified view until now presented (see discussion later). Many points that we shall briefly discuss in this section on PGs have already been discussed in this book and have been the subject of several recent reviews (FERREIRA and VANE, 1974a, 1974b, 1974c; FLOWER, 1974).

1. Prostaglandin Synthesis and Release

In different types of inflammation, some mediators may have a more prominent role than others and this, as we have already pointed out, is shown by the actions of antagonists. But what determines which mediators are released by an inflammatory trauma? Looking at so many diverse types of inflammatory response and taking into account the restricted repertoire of inflammatory mediators, we are led to conclude that it is the chemical nature of the trauma, as well as its intensity and duration, that finally determine the cellular elements involved. In addition, the activation of one or several plasma enzyme systems will depend on its chemical nature. In order to interfere rationally in the final common pathway of inflammation, i.e. in the genesis of signs and symptoms, it is necessary to define the relative participation of each mediator in each specific inflammatory process and to understand their mechanism of synthesis and release.

Early in our involvement with the PGs, we put forward the hypothesis that "distortion of cell membranes could trigger the synthesis and release of prostaglandins" (FERREIRA and VANE, 1967; PIPER and VANE, 1971). The concentration of substrate, arachidonic acid or dihomo-γ-linolenic acid, is probably the rate-limiting step in the synthesis of PGs and activation of membrane phospholipase should play a key role. Chemical or mechanical stimulation probably activates this or another lipase and inhibition of PG release in some systems (mepacrine in the lungs; VARGAFTIG and DAO HAI, 1972) is considered to be due to an inhibitory effect on phospholipase. Aspirin-like drugs generally lack activity on lipases (FLOWER and BLACKWELL, 1976).

Integrity of the cell membrane depends on synthesis of phospholipids, and arachidonic acid is utilised in this process. Phospholipid biosynthesis is an energy-dependent process, whereas PG biosynthesis is not. What happens when both processes proceed simultaneously in the same environment? The synthesis of PGs would certainly jeopardize the synthesis of phospholipids, putting at risk the membrane integrity. Thus, it is necessary to postulate that PG synthetase is compartmentalized within the cells so that arachidonic acid normally favours the enzymic systems involved in the synthesis of phospholipids. The breaking of this barrier may be as relevant as the increased phospholipase activity for the generation of PGs. The stabilizing effect of corticoids upon membranes (thus protecting the compartmentalization of the PG synthetase enzymes) has been suggested as a mechanism for these agents to block the release of PGs in some in vivo or in vitro systems (GRYGLEWSKI, 1975). This idea is supported by two pieces of evidence: (a) although there is free arachidonic acid within cells, generation of PGs only occurs in the presence of a traumatic stimulus (FLOWER and BLACKWELL, 1976), and (b) arachidonic acid injected into rat paws induces oedema only when it is accompanied by a phlogogenic stimulus such as carrageenin (VAN ARMAN, 1972; LEWIS et al., 1975; SMITH et al., 1975). An alternative view is that cyclo-oxygenase, like phospholipase, is activated by cell trauma.

It is important to stress that generation of PGs is normally accompanied by the formation of several other biologically active substances from the same substrate by a complex system of aspirin-sensitive enzymes. For example, arachidonic acid is metabolized by platelets in two main pathways of oxidation, one via lipoxygenase forming HPETE and HETE, and the other via cyclo-oxygenase into the endoperoxides (PGG_2 and PGH_2), which instead of yielding PGs are mainly converted into C_{17}-hydroxy acid (HTT) and a hemiacetal derivative named thromboxane B_2 via the unstable intermediate thromboxane A_2 (SAMUELSSON et al., 1975; see also Chap. 12). The endoperoxides as well as the thromboxanes may be important for the induction of inflammatory signs or symptoms, for fatty acid hydroperoxides have been shown to cause erythema and overt pain (FERREIRA, 1972).

It should not be overlooked that PGG_2, the intermediate in the synthesis of PGs and thromboxanes, is a lipid peroxide and such substances can damage membrane protein (LEWIS and WILLS, 1962; DESAI and TAPPEL, 1963; HUNTER et al., 1964). Other linear lipoperoxides which are concomitantly synthesized, may also be active. The importance of lipoperoxides in maintaining and amplifying the cell injury caused by a trauma, is not known. If this role of lipoperoxides is shown to be important, it will indicate that aspirin-like drugs can affect more than just the symptoms of the disease. In this respect, it is worth mentioning that PGs can cause erosion of bone by releasing calcium (TASHJIAN et al., 1975). Aspirin-like drugs prevent this effect.

PGs have been detected in many forms of damage in both animals and man, including carrageenin and endotoxin inflammation (WILLIS, 1969a; DI ROSA et al., 1971a; MONCADA et al., 1975; HERMAN and MONCADA, 1975; ARTURSON et al., 1973), anaphylaxis (PIPER and VANE, 1969a), monoarticular arthritis (BLACKHAM et al., 1974), experimental uveitis (EAKINS et al., 1972b), allergic contact eczema (GREAVES et al., 1971), UV-induced inflammation (GREAVES and SØNDERGAARD, 1970), burn injury (JONSSON, 1971) and rheumatoid arthritis (HIGGS et al., 1974). However, in some situations, especially in those models which are insensitive to aspirin-like drugs, PG generation may not take place, or if it does it is unimportant for the maintenance of the inflammation. In this respect, UBATUBA et al. (1975) were unable to show an effect of PG synthetase inhibitors on passive cutaneous anaphylaxis in the rat. In this model, the release of amines due to the involvement of mastocytes plays a more relevant role than does the release of PGs.

The origin of PGs present in an inflammatory exudate is still a matter of debate. The importance of PMN cells to the local concentration of PGs is supported by the findings that: (a) up to 150 ng/ml of PGE_1 can be detected in aqueous humour when it contains many PMN cells in experimental immunogenic uveitis in rabbits, whereas the rabbit iris or ciliary body only generates PGE_2 (EAKINS et al., 1972b); (b) the appearance of PGs in the carrageenin oedema parallels the migration of leucocytes (WILLIS et al., 1972; DI ROSA et al., 1971a); (c) certain immunosuppressive agents affect the "prostaglandin phase" of carrageenin oedema, possibly by diminishing migration of PMN cells and monocytes. However, production of PGs by the local cells may also be important since the inflammatory reaction, though diminished, progresses in the absence of PMN cells (WILLOUGHBY and GIROUD, 1969; DI ROSA et al., 1971b). Furthermore, the content of PGs in sponge exudates induced by carrageenin did not correlate with the presence of migrating cells, for colchicine reduced white cell count by 80%, but increased PG concentrations in the exudate (HIGGS et al., 1975).

Finally, it is possible that the PG which is relevant for the development of an inflammatory sign and symptom is not present in the exudate but is produced by the effector cells themselves; this will be discussed in the following sections.

2. Prostaglandins and Inflammatory Signs and Symptoms

The strength of the hypothesis which considers inhibition of PG synthesis as the mechanism of the anti-inflammatory, analgesic and antipyretic action of non-steroid anti-inflammatory drugs, lies not only in the fact that they inhibit the generation of PGs in vitro and in vivo in a multitude of preparations but also in the growing evidence that PGs play a part in the genesis of inflammatory erythema, oedema, pain, and fever. Description and discussion about the participation of the several putative mediators of inflammation in the genesis of inflammatory signs and symptoms can be found in Chapters 11, 14, and 16–18. We intend to discuss only a few aspects in which PGs diverge from other mediators.

PGE$_1$, PGE$_2$, PGF$_{2\alpha}$, and PGD$_2$ show different pharmacological action in many biological systems, but similar effects on cutaneous vessels (erythema and oedema), sensitization of sensory nerves (hyperalgesia) and fever when injected into the CNS. Generally, PGE$_1$ is more potent than PGE$_2$ which is the most frequent PG in inflammatory exudates. PGF$_{2\alpha}$ is the weaker and in a few instances, as for example in the skin of rats, may inhibit the increase of vascular permeability induced by other substances (WILLOUGHBY, 1968).

a) Vasodilatation and Increased Vascular Permeability

There are two features of the vascular effects of PGs not shared by other putative mediators of inflammation: a sustained action and the ability to counteract the vasoconstriction caused by substances such as noradrenaline and angiotensin. The erythema induced by intradermal injection or subdermal infusions (FERREIRA, 1972) well illustrates the long-lasting action of PGs (sometimes up to 10 h). All PGs cause erythema, and PGE$_1$ is effective at doses as low as 1 ng; for F$_{1\alpha}$ 1 µg is needed (SOLOMON et al., 1968; JUHLIN and MICHAELSSON, 1969). This long-lasting action confers a very important property upon the PGs, in that the appearance and the magnitude of their effects not only depend on the actual concentration but also upon the duration of their release or infusion (FERREIRA, 1972).

In contrast to the long-lasting effects upon cutaneous vessels and superficial veins, the vasodilator action of PGs on other vascular beds is over within a few minutes. However, in some cases, there then remains a long-lasting reduction in response to vasoconstrictor substances (HOLMES et al., 1963; SIGGINS, 1972). It may well be that the long duration of PG erythema in man is partially due to a reduced local reactivity to the sympathetic mediator. In addition to this direct effect on the skin vessels, PGs may also be causing vasodilatation by blockade of the sympathetic control mechanism since they inhibit release of the adrenergic mediator in vitro (HEDQVIST, 1971). CHAPNICK et al. (1976) have now shown that in cat kidney in vivo, PGE$_2$ or PGA$_2$ attenuate the action of sympathetic nerve stimulation, presumably through reducing mediator release.

Although most active substances exhibit a general relationship between ability to increase vascular permeability and erythema formation, these effects result from actions on different components of the vessel. Erythema represents a local pooling of blood due to a relaxation of the smooth muscles of the walls of arterioles and venules, whereas increased vascular permeability results from the contraction of the venular endothelial cells (MAJNO et al., 1972). PGs, like Bk, histamine, and 5-HT, cause increased vascular permeability by inducing vascular leakage at the post-capillary and collecting venules (KALEY and WEINER, 1971 b).

PGs seem to be more effective in producing vasodilatation than oedema. PGE$_1$ when compared with histamine in guinea pig skin, produces an equivalent and much longer-lasting erythema but a smaller weal (SOLOMON et al., 1968). Similarly, in man histamine, Bk, and PGE$_1$ each cause erythema and oedema when injected intradermally. However, PGE$_1$ induces a long-lasting erythema and a much less pronounced oedema (FERREIRA, 1972). No difference has been found in the duration of the increased vascular permeability induced by histamine or PG (CRUNKHORN and WILLIS, 1971).

The long-lasting erythema induced by PGE_1 (measured by increase in temperature) is also seen in rat paw (ABERG, 1973). As in pain and oedema, aspirin-like drugs did not modify the direct effects of PGs but attenuated the local increase in temperature produced by carrageenin. Histamine and Bk also produce erythema; however, to our knowledge there has been no systematic study of their potency or possible synergism on cutaneous vasculature.

Most of the inflammatory mediators cause cutaneous vasodilatation and only when the effects of one mediator really predominate can blockade of its synthesis or its action be fully expressed. The joint participation of several mediators may be the reason why the development of UV erythema on albino guinea pig skin can be delayed but not abolished by aspirin-like drugs (WILHELMI and DOMENJOZ, 1951), and it may well be why erythema is the first symptom to appear and usually the last to disappear during the inflammatory process.

PGE_1, PGE_2, and PGA_2, but not $PGF_{2\alpha}$, cause oedema when injected into the hind paws of rats (GLENN et al., 1972). PGE_1 was as effective (on a weight basis) as Bk, although higher doses (40–80 µg) instead of causing increased effects as did Bk, produced erythema without oedema. When PGE_1 was given together with histamine or 5-HT, it elicited an additive effect rather than a synergistic one. We investigated this interaction further and found that in the rat paw there was no addition of effect between Bk and histamine in doses producing maximal effects but the effects of both agents were magnified by PGE_1 (MONCADA et al., 1973).

Similar potentiating activity of PGE_1 on Bk-induced rat paw oedema has been described by LEWIS et al. (1975).

If PG is indeed sensitizing blood vessels to the permeability effects of other mediators (as has been demonstrated for pain receptors, see Chap. 17), then the action of the anti-inflammatory drugs on oedema can be explained as a removal of this sensitisation. This reasoning implies that the contribution of PGs to the oedema of inflammation is by increasing the effects of the other known mediators, such as histamine and Bk, rather than through a direct action of their own. This idea, first propounded by FERREIRA (1972) studying pain, was tested on paw swelling induced by carrageenin in rats in which endogenous PG release had been abolished by indomethacin. In another group of similarly treated rats, we added low concentrations (100 or 500 ng) of PGE_1 to the carrageenin injection (MONCADA et al., 1973). The addition of PGE_1 to the carrageenin in the indomethacin-treated rats strikingly increased the oedema formation. PGE_2, but not $PGF_{2\alpha}$ or Bk, had a similar effect. This potentiation was seen even when PGE_1 was given 90 or 180 min after the carrageenin injection (FERREIRA et al., 1974b). The treatment of animals with indomethacin was important in order to reveal the potentiating effects of PGs in the later stages; otherwise the oedema was already sufficiently developed (presumably because of endogenous PG release) to mask any further potentiation. No potentiation of oedema was observed when PGE_1 was given 15 min before the injection of carrageenin. We conclude that PGs of the E series can sensitize the vessels to the permeability-increasing effects of the other mediators locally released by carrageenin. Furthermore, our results indicate that when a continuous generation of PG occurs, it can increase the development of oedema throughout the inflammatory reaction.

Histamine, 5-HT, and Bk have all been implicated in carrageenin oedema because the oedema is partially reduced by treatment of the rats with antagonists of histamine or 5-HT. Bk, for which no direct antagonist is known, could still be responsible for the oedema in these rats (Van Arman et al., 1966). Ferreira et al. (1974b, 1974c) found that the initial as well as the late phase of carrageenin oedema was potentiated by a specific Bk potentiator (BPP$_{9a}$; Ferreira, 1965; Greene et al., 1972). This potentiation was blocked by soya bean trypsin inhibitor, which blocks kinin generating enzymes. The early enhancement of the oedema indicates that generation of Bk commences just after the injection of carrageenin. This has also been observed by Bonta et al. (1976).

In the guinea pig, PGE$_1$ and PGE$_2$ also potentiate the increase of vascular permeability induced by histamine, Bk as well as passive cutaneous analphylaxis, reverse passive Arthus and delayed hypersensitivity reactions (Williams and Morley, 1973).

Thomas and West (1973) studied the effects of PGs on the permeability increase in rat skin induced by Bk or histamine. They found that small doses of PGE$_1$ selectively potentiated Bk; PGE$_2$ had no effect and PGF$_{2\alpha}$ inhibited the effects of other mediators, as previously shown by Willoughby (1968). PGE$_1$ had no effect upon the increase of vascular permeability induced by dextran.

Eakins et al. (1975) showed that inhibitors of PG biosynthesis markedly reduced the effects of Bk on contraction of pupil and on the increase of protein caused by intracorneal injection of Bk. Simultaneous injection of PGE$_2$ restored the responses induced by Bk.

The degree of potentiation of the other inflammatory mediators by PGs of the E series might depend on the vascular bed being studied. The intriguing finding that PGF$_{2\alpha}$ inhibits the increase in permeability caused by histamine or 5-HT in rat paw (Willoughby, 1968), may be explained by a venular constriction induced by PGF$_{2\alpha}$ which counteracts the effects of contraction of the venular endothelial cells ultimately responsible for the permeability increase. This effect of PGF$_{2\alpha}$ may be peculiar to rat skin, since Bk oedema in the rabbit was not inhibited. In the rabbit, PGF$_{2\alpha}$ also enhanced the increased permeability induced by Bk (Harrison, 1973). We found, however, that PGF$_{2\alpha}$ in equal amounts was ineffective in reducing the potentiation induced by PGs on the oedema caused by carrageenin in the rat paw. Brune et al. (1974) made similar observations in urate inflammation induced in the pigeon.

All these results support the idea that oedema is the result of the simultaneous action of several mediators, the concentration of which may vary during the development of the process. The relative contribution of each mediator depends on the nature of the traumatizing stimulus. When aspirin-like drugs are ineffective in reducing the oedema induced by a phlogogenic agent, the involvement of PGs in that particular type of inflammation is probably minimal.

b) Pain and Hyperalgesia

Although "it seems inescapable that small and subtle anti-nociceptive effects of aspirin can be demonstrated in the laboratory with brief noxious stimulation not obviously related with inflammation" (Winder, 1959), the noxious stimulation used in experiments which seem to support a central component for the action of aspirin-like drugs is probably due to PGs release. This would happen with radiant heat or electrical stimulation by implanted electrodes (WINDER, 1959; DUBAS and PARKER, 1971; BONNYCASTLE et al., 1953).

Aspirin-like drugs are capable of acting on the CNS, as shown by their antipyretic effects, and it is possible that pain threshold may be lowered during fever due to the release of PGs in the nervous tissue. But the main site of action of aspirin-like drugs is peripheral (see Chap. 17).

The hyperalgesic effects of PGs were described by SOLOMON et al. (1968). However, PGs were disregarded as mediators of pain because of their ineffectiveness as pain-producing substances on the blister base (HORTON, 1963). It was the demonstration in man that PGs sensitized pain receptors not only to mechanical but also to chemical stimulation, and moreover that pain-producing substances like Bk or histamine lack this sensitizing activity (FERREIRA, 1972), which paved the way to understanding the relationship between inhibition of PG synthesis and the analgesic effect of aspirin-like drugs.

The contribution of PGs to the development of inflammatory pain or hyperalgesia is discussed in length in Chapter 17. In summary, PGs unlike other inflammatory mediators, produce a long-lasting sensitization of the pain receptors to mechanical and chemical stimulation. Due to this long-lasting effect, minute amounts of PG released during the development of inflammation will slowly sensitize the pain receptors. Thus, abolition of the synthesis of PGs by aspirin-like drugs removes the background necessary for pain-triggering substances such as Bk to produce overt pain (see Fig.4, Chap.17). In a tissue sensitized by PGs, histamine causes itching before inducing pain. Aspirin-like drugs do not block the effect of PGs, which rules out the possibility of an effect upon the responsiveness of the receptors themselves.

Fatty acid hydroperoxides can also cause pain in man (FERREIRA, 1972). The intensity of the pain produced by intradermal injections of hydroperoxides of arachidonic, linoleic, and linolenic acids was greater than that induced by either the parent fatty acids or acetylcholine, Bk, histamine or PGE_1. Thus, lipoperoxides formed during arachidonic acid metabolism may also be important as pain-producing substances. It should also be remembered that thromboxane A_2 (RCS) has strong pharmacological activity in that it contracts rabbit aorta and many other arterial muscle strips (PIPER and VANE, 1969a, 1969b; PALMER et al., 1973; NEEDLEMAN et al., 1976), as do the lipid peroxides mentioned above (FERREIRA, 1972; GRYGLEWSKI and VANE, 1972a, 1972b; FERREIRA and VARGAFTIG, 1974). These observations take on a new importance now that it is known that lipid peroxides can be generated enzymically in platelets and lung (HAMBERG et al., 1974). This pathway, together with the formation of thromboxane A_2 accounts for the major part of the metabolism of arachidonic acid in these tissues. These observations, together with the high activity of the endoperoxides and of thromboxane A_2, all add force to the suggestion (VANE, 1972) that each intermediate generated in the cascade of arachidonic acid metabolism has its own contribution to make to the inflammatory process. With a vigorous activation of the PG-generating system by a trauma, the formation of intermediates could exceed their conversion to PG or thromboxane, thus leading to acute pain. It is not yet known whether the thromboxanes are also pain-producing substances.

The main problem in our explanation about the analgesic effects of aspirin-like drugs through inhibition of PG biosynthesis, derives from the existence of drugs such as paracetamol (acetaminophen) which display analgesic effects without substantial anti-inflammatory action. Small doses of aspirin also have such an effect. We shall discuss the problem in Section D, but it is necessary to stress the lack of precision of statements which imply that a drug is analgesic because it is "anti-inflammatory." Is hyperalgesia or pain present because there is erythema, oedema, migrating cells or fibroblast stimulation? It is well known that one symptom may occur in the absence of another. For example, dextran or a passive cutaneous anaphylaxis causes oedema without hyperalgesia (VAN ARMAN et al., 1966; HIGGS et al., 1976). We suggest that hyperalgesia occurs only when a trauma releases pain mediators, and the PGs are among such substances.

c) Fever

Fever is often associated with inflammation and occurs when the trauma induces the formation of endogenous pyrogen. PGE_1 is the most powerful pyretic agent known, when injected either into the cerebral ventricles or directly into the anterior hypothalamus (MILTON and WENDLANDT, 1971; FELDBERG and SAXENA, 1971 a, b; see Chapters 18 and 28 for reviews). The hyperthermic effect is dose-dependent, almost immediate and lasts for about 3 h. PGE_1 causes fever by an action on the same region as that on which monoamines and pyrogens act to affect temperature.

As in peripheral inflammatory responses, there is a generation of PGE-like substance in the CNS during fever (FELDBERG and GUPTA, 1973), and the concentrations in CSF rise several-fold after intravenous pyrogen, sometimes to as much as 35 ng/ml.

Aspirin-like drugs do not abolish either the formation of endogenous pyrogen by leucocytes (CLARK and MOYER, 1972) or the pyretic action of PGs injected into the third ventricle of cats. However, they inhibit both the generation of PGs in the CNS and the fever caused by pyrogens or 5-HT given into the cerebral ventricles. The five to tenfold increase in PG release into the CSF observed at the height of endotoxin-induced fever in dogs was suppressed by the administration of indomethacin (MILTON, 1973).

There have recently been a few observations (see Chapters 18 and 28) which apparently contradict the PG theory. The most significant was that pyrogen injected intraventricularly causes a fever which is only partially reduced by salicylates. FELDBERG and MILTON (Chap. 18) have discussed the problem in length but there is an alternative explanation for such observations. At high concentrations, pyrogens might cause fever by a direct effect, which cannot be blocked by aspirin-like drugs. In such a situation, it is possible that any PG which is released will potentiate this direct action, as happens with the pain-producing activity of Bk in the dog spleen (FERREIRA et al., 1973 a).

3. Correlation Between in vitro Inhibition of Prostaglandin Synthesis and Anti-Inflammatory Activity

Inhibition of PG biosynthesis is a general feature of aspirin-like drugs and has already been demonstrated in more than forty different biological systems. It has also been used as a tool for investigating the participation of PGs in many physiological or pathological events, such as tonus of isolated intestinal and bronchial preparations (FERREIRA et al., 1972; BENNETT and POSNER, 1971; ECKENFELS and VANE,

1972; FARMER et al., 1972), uterine contractions (VANE and WILLIAMS, 1973; AIKEN, 1972; POYSER et al., 1970; CHESTER et al., 1972; AIKEN, 1974; WILLIAMS and VANE, 1975); ovary function (ORCYZK and BEHRMAN, 1972; O'GRADY et al., 1972; ARMSTRONG and GRINWICH, 1972; LINDNER et al., 1974); control of lipolysis (ILLIANO and CUATRECASAS, 1971), control of the release of the sympathetic mediator (HEDQVIST, 1971; FERREIRA et al., 1973b; HEDQVIST, 1974) and local regulation of blood flow in kidney (HERBACYZNSKA-CEDRO and VANE, 1973; McGIFF et al., 1974; ANGGARD and LARSSON, 1974), adipose tissue (BOWERY and LEWIS, 1973) and haemodynamic shock (CULP et al., 1971; COLLIER et al., 1973). For a review of these fields, see FERREIRA and VANE (1974a).

Inhibition of PG biosynthesis, therefore, is not restricted to any one species or tissue and has been seen in vitro on preparations of subcellular fractions, homogenates or isolated organs and tissue slices, and in many organs in vivo. Thus all the evidence points to the effect being a general one depending only on the drug reaching the enzyme.

The absolute potency of the non-steroid anti-inflammatory drugs against PG synthetase varies not only with the source of the enzyme preparations but also with experimental conditions and the way in which the enzyme is prepared. However, the general trend of potency is independent of the enzyme preparation, although the rank order may change (see Chapters 12 and 30).

During this last 5 years it has been observed that the absolute potency, as well as the relative potencies, of these drugs varies considerably from one enzyme preparation to another. This is at least due to the differences in assay conditions, but the much more important question of whether enzymes from different sources are differentially sensitive to the inhibitory action of these drugs constitutes a fascinating problem in itself. There is already some evidence for this. On rabbit brain synthetase, for instance, the ratio of activity between indomethacin and aspirin is 17:1 (FLOWER et al., 1972), whereas on bovine seminal vesicles it is 2140:1 (HAM et al., 1972). This important observation, which may reflect a series of "isoenzymes," can explain the variations in activity within the group of compounds. For instance, the antipyretic, analgesic drug 4-acetamidophenol (acetaminophen or paracetamol), which is ten times less effective than aspirin on the dog spleen synthetase, has almost the same potency as aspirin on rabbit brain (FLOWER and VANE, 1972). Thus, the fact that paracetamol has antipyretic and analgesic without anti-inflammatory activity, can be explained by the differential sensitivity of the PG synthetase from different tissues. Just as the anti-inflammatory activity of aspirin-like drugs correlates well with their action against spleen enzyme, so also the antipyretic activity correlates with their action against the brain enzyme (FLOWER and VANE, 1972).

Other examples of differential enzyme sensitivity are also available. There is a thousand-fold variation of the ID_{50} of indomethacin against PG synthetase from different tissue of the rabbit (BHATTACHERJEE and EAKINS, 1973). On the spleen enzyme, the ID_{50} was 0.05 µg/ml, in close agreement with FLOWER and VANE (1972). However, on kidney enzyme, the ID_{50} was 5.0 µg/ml, on the iris ciliary body, 18.5 µg/ml and on the retina 50 µg/ml.

However, the diverse susceptibility of PG synthetase enzymes from different tissue to aspirin-like drugs and especially to indomethacin, should be interpreted cautiously as pointed out by GRYGLEWSKI (1975), since these preparations from different tissues may be unequally influenced by co-factors, substrate concentration and the pH. Examining 12 anti-inflammatory drugs for inhibition of microsomal preparation of PG synthetase in three tissues from four species, Dembinska-Kieĉ et al. (1976) found no organ or species specificity. But they found that a weak anti-inflammatory drug which possesses good analgesic and antipyretic activity, selectively inhibited PG synthetase in brain microsomes. This result points to what may be a very important physiopathological aspect of PGs. During a mild trauma it is not the PGs deriving from local or migrating cells which really matter for the sensitization of pain receptors, but that generated within the nerve endings themselves.

Pong and Levine (1976) have also studied PG synthetase systems from different tissues. When co-factors, substrate concentration etc. were all carefully controlled, the aspirin-like drugs had similar potencies on each enzyme. However, this may not represent the situation in vivo, where co-factors and substrate concentration may vary from tissue to tissue.

Perhaps the most striking correlation between inhibition of PG synthetase and anti-inflammatory activity was described for a pair of naproxen enantiomers and indomethacin analogues. In each instance, the one of each pair with anti-inflammatory activity also strongly inhibited PG synthetase, whereas the one with weak anti-inflammatory activity was also weak against the synthetase (Tomlinson et al., 1972; Ham et al., 1972). PG synthetase is the only in vitro system that responds to aryl acetic acids in the same sterospecific manner as in vivo animal models (Shen et al., 1974).

4. Inhibition of Prostaglandin Synthesis in vivo and Inflammatory Signs and Symptoms

For inhibition of PG biosynthesis to account for the anti-inflammatory action of aspirin-like drugs, it is important to show that normal therapeutic doses lead to effective plasma concentrations. Free plasma concentrations, during therapy with several aspirin-like drugs, often exceed those needed to inhibit PG synthesis from dog spleen, (Flower et al., 1972). Taking indomethacin as an example, the plasma concentration in man reaches $2 \mu g/ml$. Because of protein binding, the free plasma concentration would be $0.2 \mu g/ml$. However, the ID_{50} for indomethacin on dog spleen synthetase is only $0.05 \mu g/ml$. Thus, the free plasma concentrations can be more than sufficient to explain the anti-inflammatory activity of PG synthetase inhibitors and this has now been shown in man and several animal species.

Over the last few years, several drugs which are not anti-inflammatory in vivo have been described as inhibitors of preparations of PG synthetase in vitro. When one takes into account the many hazards that an orally-administered drug undergoes before reaching a peripheral microsomal enzyme, it is surprising that any relationship exists between in vitro inhibition of PG synthetase and the anti-inflammatory activity of the aspirin-like drugs. Yet for drugs where the activities have been compared, in carrageenin rat paw oedema as against PG synthetase, the group that is highly active on the enzyme showed stronger anti-inflammatory activity than the weakly active ones. However, the crucial test is their ability to block PG synthetase activity in vivo.

Therapeutic doses of aspirin or indomethacin inhibit PG production by human platelets (SMITH and WILLIS, 1971) and reduce the PG content of human semen (COLLIER and FLOWER, 1971; HORTON et al., 1973). The most persuasive evidence, however, comes from the work of HAMBERG (1972) who monitored the concentrations of the major metabolite of E_1 and E_2 in the urine of male and female subjects before and after treatment with therapeutic doses of indomethacin, aspirin, and salicylate. In female subjects, almost maximum inhibition (63–92%) was obtained after 1 day's treatment. In male subjects (who generally excreted more metabolite than females), the initial reduction was less, but reached similar low levels over a 3 day treatment period. Two days after the treatment was discontinued, the metabolite excretion had almost returned to control levels, although there was some variation. Indomethacin was the most potent, aspirin, and salicylate being some 15 times less active on a weight basis.

HIGGS et al. (1974) studied PGE levels in synovial fluid from arthritic patients. The mean concentration in patients not receiving aspirin-like drugs was 19 ng/ml. In those who were treated with aspirin-like drugs, the concentration was only 3 ng/ml.

WILLIS et al. (1972) showed that doses of aspirin-like drugs which are effective on the rat paw oedema induced by carrageenin were also effective in reducing the amount of PGs in the exudate from carrageenin air bleb in rats. They found that in this assay, sodium salicylate was as equally effective as aspirin. Sodium salicylate has only weak activity against PG synthetase in vitro (VANE, 1971), whereas it is as strong as aspirin in anti-inflammatory tests in vivo (COLLIER, 1969). WILLIS et al. (1972) suggested that salicylate may be inactive, but converted to an active metabolite in vivo—an interesting variation of one current view that aspirin is rapidly metabolised to salicylate in vivo! FLOWER and VANE (1974) studied the effects of some salicylic acid metabolites on PG synthetase. Gentisic acid was 32 times more potent than salicylic acid. HAMBERG (1972) has also shown salicylate to be as effective as aspirin against PG synthesis in man, so that the activity of salicylate against synthetase in vivo, in contrast to its ineffectiveness in vitro, seems to hold in at least two species.

There are several observations correlating appearance or disappearance of an inflammatory sign or symptom with an increased or decreased release or effectiveness of PGs. For instance, the oedema caused by carrageenin injected into the rat paw was less in animals immunized against PGs than in controls (FERREIRA et al., 1974a). Similarly, the carrageenin-induced hind paw inflammation was less in rats made deficient in essential fatty acids and indomethacin had no effect in the late phase of the oedema (BONTA et al., 1976). These results support both the involvement of PGs in the carrageenin oedema and our theory on the mechanism of aspirin-like drugs. BONTA et al., (1976), however, considered the effectiveness of indomethacin in the early phase of the oedema as supporting an alternative explanation for the mechanism of action of aspirin-like drugs. We have already pointed out that, in carrageenin oedema, although there is mild increase in permeability after the second hour, the main effect occurs within the first 2 h and this permeability increase is blocked by indomethacin (GARCIA LEME et al., 1973a; ZANIN et al., 1976). Thus, PGs are being released at an early stage of inflammation. In favour of this assertion is the fact that eicosatetraynoic acid (ETA, a specific inhibitor of PG formation) or SC-

Table 1. Comparison of the effects of different drugs on PG synthetase in vitro with inhibition of carrageenin oedema and PG production in vivo

	PG synthetase in vitro IC_{50} (µM)	Ref.	(a) Dose (mg/kg) given 3 times	% Inhibition of oedema (No. of rats)	% Reduction of PGs in sponge (No. of rats)
Indomethacin	0.17	(b)	4.0	55 (10)	>95 (13)
Phenylbutazone	7.25	(b)	100.0	50 (5)	>95 (6)
Aspirin	37.0	(b)	150.0	30 (5)	85 (10)
Sodium salicylate	800.0	(c)	150.0	30 (5)	80 (10)
Paracetamol	660.0	(b)	150.0	30 (5)	40 (5)
Dexamethasone	Inactive	(b)	0.1	45 (5)	30 (7)
Prednisolone	Inactive	(d)	5.0	45 (5)	0 (6)
Hydrocortisone	Inactive	(b)	20.0	45 (5)	0 (5)
Indomethacin	3.60	(e)	4.0	55 (10)	>95 (13)
Aspirin	150.0	(e)	150.0	30 (5)	85 (10)
Phenelzine	0.37	(e)	20.0	0 (5)	0 (5)
Desipramine	123.0	(e)	20.0	0 (5)	0 (5)
Chlorpromazine	170.0	(e)	20.0	0 (5)	0 (5)
Sodium aurothiomalate (gold) (i.m.)	10–100	(b)	1.0	20 (10)	35 (5)
Mepacrine	Inactive	(c)	150.0	20 (5)	0 (5)
Penicillamine	Inactive	(g)	30.0	0 (5)	0 (5)
Colchicine (s.c.)	Potentiates	(h)	1.5	85 (5)	+40 (6)

a Each drug was given orally, unless otherwise stated, to groups of 5–10 rats. Three doses were given; the first at the time of sponge implantation, the second 8 h later and the third after a further 13 h.
b from Flower et al. (1972).
c from Flower (1974).
d Blackwell and Parsons: personal communication (1975).
e from Lee (1974).
f from Deby et al. (1973).
g from Maddox (1973).
h from Robinson and Levine (1974).
Data from Higgs et al. (1976).

19 220 (a dibenzoxazepine hydrazide, a PG receptor antagonist) reduce carrageenin oedema commencing at a very early stage (Smith et al., 1974).

Recently, the effect of several anti-inflammatory drugs was tested on the generation of PGs induced by subcutaneous implantation of sterile polyester sponges impregnated with carrageenin (Higgs et al., 1976). Table 1 shows the result of the effects of several drugs on the content of PG in the exudates. Anti-inflammatory doses of hydrocortisone (20 mg/kg) and prednisolone (5 mg/kg) did not reduce PG concentrations in vivo. Phenelzine (20 mg/kg), chlorpromazine (20 mg/kg) or desipramine (20 mg/kg), which inhibit PG synthetase in vitro (Lee, 1974), did not significantly reduce the PG concentration in the exudates, or affect carrageenin-induced oedema (Table 1). This test provides a means of correlating in vivo anti-inflammatory activity with inhibition of PG biosynthesis. In fact, no drug is known which blocks PG synthesis in vivo without showing anti-inflammatory or analgesic-anti-pyretic activity.

SMITH et al. (1975) showed that acetylsalicylic acid and sodium salicylate, which are equally effective on carrageenin inflammation, had different effects on the arachidonic acid potentiation of carrageenin swelling of the rat paw. The authors favour the interpretation that the mechanism of action of non-steroid anti-inflammatory drugs results from an effect on cell migration, since both agents showed similar effect on their in vivo test. However, the main hindrance to accepting their correlation is that arachidonic acid potentiation of carrageenin occurs maximally within 1.5 h of the administration of carrageenin and cell migration is measured 9 h after implantation of a sponge. We have pointed out that salicylate has no effect in vitro but blocks the production of PGs in vivo (WILLIS et al., 1972; HIGGS et al., 1976). Since aspirin is metabolized to salicylate, the effect of aspirin upon PG synthesis is double, one rapid (possibly due to acetylation) and another later one due to active metabolites. In the experiments of SMITH et al. (1975), salicylate would be expected to fail to block arachidonic acid potentiation of carrageenin oedema because the oedema occurs so rapidly that it does not allow time for formation of the active metabolite of salicylate. An alternative explanation would be that in vivo the access to PG synthetase is slower for salicylates, so that they are effective only in slowly occurring processes, such as carrageenin oedema or cell migration into sponges implanted subcutaneously (see next section for cell migration).

PGs have been found in inflammatory exudates during the development of monoarticular arthritis in rabbits. Indomethacin reduced the concentration of PGs below detectable levels and caused partial reduction of the joint swelling and temperature (BLACKHAM et al., 1974). Endotoxin or carrageenin injected into the knee joint of the dog causes incapacitation which is closely related to the appearance of PGs in the joint fluid. There were no symptoms or PG release in joints locally treated with indomethacin (HERMAN and MONCADA, 1975). Indomethacin does not reduce the direct sensitizing action of exogenous PGs on the pain-producing effects of Bk (MONCADA et al., 1975; see Chap. 17).

In rheumatic diseases, PGs are present in synovial fluid and their concentration decreases during treatment with aspirin-like drugs (HIGGS et al., 1974; ROBINSON and LEVINE, 1974). A general relationship between intensity of the symptoms and content of PGs was observed. There was no correlation between total leucocyte count and PG content of synovial fluid (PATRONO et al., 1975). At the moment it is difficult to evaluate the importance of these clinical observations. We still do not know: (a) the origin of the PGs (from synovial membranes or from migrating cells?); (b) the significance of the actual concentration of PG in the exudate (PGs are quickly removed from joint cavities and we do not know if in an inflamed joint there is increased, normal or reduced clearance and destruction of PGs); (c) the importance of the PGs in the exudate rather than the tissues and nerve endings for the induction of the symptoms.

Rabbit eye responds to trauma in a very characteristic fashion—with miosis, local ocular vasodilatation and increased permeability of the blood-aqueous barrier, which is normally associated with raised levels of protein in the aqueous humour. PGs locally applied are able to reproduce such effects (for review see EAKINS, 1974). PGE_2-like activity is found in the secondary aqueous humour 1.5 h after paracentesis. Treatment of the animals with aspirin caused a marked fall in the appearance of PG and partially inhibited increased protein content in the secondary aqueous humour (Miller et al., 1973). In man, systemic administration of aspirin lowered the protein rise in aqueous humour due to anterior chamber paracentesis (Zimmerman et al., 1975).

Thus, there is an increasing number of observations indicative of parallelism between the appearance of an inflammatory sign or symptom and release of PGs. As pointed out in the beginning of this chapter, if the intensity of a trauma is less than that capable of causing a direct injury of the tissue, the development of inflammatory signs or symptoms results from a fine balance between tissue responsiveness and inflammatory mediators. The abolition of the synthesis or release of one mediator which normally synergises with other inflammatory mediators, has a profound effect on the symptomatology of the disease and this seems to hold true for drugs which inhibit the synthesis of PGs in vivo.

VI. Action on Step 6: Inhibition of Cell Migration

As leucocytes play an important role in the development of acute and chronic inflammation, inhibition of their migration might account for part of the anti-inflammatory effect of some drugs, such as corticoids and immunosuppressants. Nonsteroid anti-inflammatory drugs in doses which block increased permeability, seem: (a) to interfere with migration of cells in some models, such as pleurisy induced by carrageenin (Blackham and Owen, 1975), (b) not to interfere in others (Van Arman and Carlson, 1974), and (c) to have different effects depending on the type and intensity of the stimulus, such as in the migration of leucocytes into subcutaneous implanted sponges (Smith et al., 1975; Higgs et al., 1976).

At least three processes linked with cell migration can be influenced by drugs: (a) formation and activity of chemotactic factors, (b) marginalization of cells, and (c) the response of the migrating cells. The several chemotactic factors possibly act synergistically and their release by plasma systems depends on the intensity and type of trauma. Agents which strongly interfere with vascular permeability should reduce cell migration by reducing the chemotactic factors which originate from degradation of plasma proteins in the tissue spaces. Transudation of plasma protein per se is not a condition for generation of chemotactic factors, as illustrated by the fact that pleurisy exudates induced by turpentine are very poor in cells when compared with carrageenin exudates (Blackham and Owen, 1975). This observation stresses that a trauma, besides causing increased permeability, can also have the separate capability of inducing formation of chemotactic factors. Carrageenin induces formation of chemotactic factors directly via activation of complement or indirectly by releasing permeability factors from cells. Aspirin-like drugs, by blocking PG synthesis, may interfere with cell migration by a double mechanism: suppressing one of the chemotactic factors (PGs) and, indirectly, by reducing the contribution of PGs to the permeability increase, thus minimizing the formation of chemotactic factors generated from plasma exudate.

Inhibition of migration of PMN cells (Ford-Hutchinson et al., 1975) or monocytes (Di Rosa et al., 1971 b) has been suggested as a mode of action of non-steroid anti-inflammatory drugs. But how do these drugs affect leucocytes—by an action similar to immunosuppressant agents or corticoids? In fact, drugs which effectively reduce the cell number at the site of inflammation, have a profound effect on the resistance of animals to acute or chronic infection. That is not the case with aspirin-like drugs (ROBINSON et al., 1974). Arthritic patients under non-steroid therapy do not show reduced resistance to infection. This fact should be taken into account when proposing inhibition of leucocyte migration as an important mechanism of the anti-inflammatory action of non-steroid drugs.

Chemotactic factors seem to be a multifactorial system in most inflammations and this multiplicity of factors may be regarded as having survival value when one accepts the importance of leucocytes in dealing with a great number of inflammatory trauma, especially infections.

PGs show in vitro chemotactic effects for leucocytes (KALEY and WEINER, 1971a; HIGGS et al., 1975) at concentrations much higher than found in inflammatory exudates. The role of PGs as a leucotactic factor have been questioned by WARD (1974) on the basis of their low potency. Other products of arachidonic acid metabolism have also been shown to be highly chemotactic for leucocytes. These include HETE which is generated by a lipoxygenase (TURNER et al., 1975) and thromboxane B_2 (BOOT et al., 1976), as well as other oxidised unsaturated lipids (TURNER et al., 1975).

It is well established that PGs act synergistically with other mediators to increase permeability during inflammation. Thus, PGs contribute indirectly to cell migration when the inflammatory stimulus can induce generation of chemotactic factors from exuded plasma. PGs also increase the adhesiveness of circulating PMN cells to blood vessels (ATHERTON and BORN, 1973). Thus, continuous release of PGs during inflammation may facilitate cell migration. Inhibition of PG synthesis by non-steroid anti-inflammatory drugs may, therefore, be of importance in controlling cell migration in some inflammatory models. In other models, these effects of PGs may be overshadowed by more powerful chemotactic factors, so that aspirin-like drugs have little effect on cell migration.

VII. Action on Step 7: Inhibition of the Generation of the Effective Inflammatory Trauma

Immunocomplexes have been implicated in the pathogenesis of several human diseases. Although the primary cause of the diseases is frequently difficult to establish, the effective trauma has been related to an autoimmune disease. There are several immunological reactions in which aspirin-like drugs do have effects, such as systemic anaphylaxis induced by egg-white challenge in rabbit, Shwartzman reaction, reverse passive Arthus reaction, serum sickness, allergic encephalomyelitis in guinea pig, serum sickness in man and adjuvant arthritis (SHWARTZMAN and SCHNEIERSON, 1953; LEPPER et al., 1950; KANTOR, 1968; ROSENTHAL, 1974; VAN ARMAN et al., 1970; MOORE et al., 1952). Cytostatic effects (Chap. 35) could affect antibody formation but this response is not significantly impaired by non-steroid anti-inflammatory drugs (PERRY, 1941; MARMONT et al., 1965). In contrast to immunosuppressants, these drugs are effective in those immunopathological events subsequent to the interaction of an antigen and an established antibody. Antigen-antibody reactions in vitro were inhibited by non-steroid anti-inflammatory drugs but only at a toxic dosage (Kantor, 1968). Complement-reactive proteins decrease after salicylate therapy (Hill, 1952), but these reactions have not been causally related to the rheumatic process (Randall, 1963).

In rheumatoid diseases there are reduced sulphydryl levels, which led Lorber et al. (1964) to suggest that this change may contribute to the formation of autoantigen. Similarly, inhibition of autoantigen production due to inhibition of denaturation of proteins was proposed as a possible mode of action of aspirin-like drugs (Mizushima and Suzuki, 1965). Hichens (1974) remarks that "to speak of inhibiting in vivo production of an autoantigen is to overestimate the value of aspirin-like drugs, especially because it overlooks the fact that they exhibit most dramatic effects in experimental conditions not related to autoimmune phenomena."

The anti-inflammatory activity of PG synthetase inhibitors could in some diseases derive from minimizing a non-immunological trauma such as infections. In vitro, aspirin-like drugs inhibit bacterial growth (Wagner-Jauregg and Fischer, 1968; Schwartz and Mondel, 1972) but have no beneficial effect in vivo (Robinson et al., 1974).

In conclusion, there is no experimental evidence to support the idea that the general effects of non-steroid anti-inflammatory drugs result from a reduction of the intensity of the effectiveness of an immunological or chemical trauma, which is illustrated by the fact that they do not interfere in a large number of immunological reactions or in the progression of inflammatory lesions in chronic diseases. Inhibition of the release of PG seems to be the common denominator in those immunological reactions in which non-steroid anti-inflammatory agents ameliorate some inflammatory symptoms (for review see Vane, 1975; Ferreira, 1976).

Early in this review we suggested that lipoperoxides generated during activation of PG synthesis, play a role in amplifying the trauma by a direct association with membranal proteins, but this has yet to be demonstrated.

C. Side-Effects of Anti-Inflammatory Drugs Which are Prostaglandin Synthetase Inhibitors

When side-effects are shared by a group of compounds of diverse chemical structure but with the same therapeutic action, it suggests that the same mechanism of action underlies both processes. Several side-effects common to the non-steroid anti-inflammatory compounds have been described and we shall briefly discuss the possibility that they depend upon inhibition of PG biosynthesis.

The main side-effect observed with non-steroid anti-inflammatory drugs is gastric mucosal lesions although multiple lesions of the small intestine have been described for the more potent drugs (Brodie et al., 1970; Wax et al., 1975). There are four major factors which are generally taken into consideration in the analysis of the genesis of gastric lesions: (a) chemical composition of the drug or pharmaceutical formulations; (b) effect on acid secretion; (c) action on mucous membrane, and (d) vascular effect. There is a recent review about the pathology of aspirin-induced gastric damage by RAINSFORD (1975) with a thorough discussion of the factors involved in the induction of gastric lesions (see also Chap. 29).

The chemical composition of the drug, as well as the pharmaceutical formulation (with or without an antacid), is thought to be important because it can influence the amount of drug absorbed through the mucosa. An acid environment favours absorption as well as the accumulation of the drug inside mucosal cells (MARTIN, 1963), creating conditions for these drugs to interfere with a multitude of enzymes. Aspirin-like drugs can inhibit several mucosal enzymes and in fact inhibition of cytochrome oxidases (GANTER and GUYONNET, 1966) could lead to injury of the cells. However, against this idea is the fact that aspirin-like drugs cause gastric lesions even when given intravenously (see Chap. 29).

The effects of aspirin-like drugs on the mucosa may be by a direct sloughing of the protective mucous layer (RAINSFORD et al., 1968) or indirectly by inhibiting mucous production (JOHANSSON and LINDQUIST, 1970; RAINSFORD, 1970; NARUMI and KANNO, 1972) thus creating a condition for the back-diffusion of acid (DAVENPORT, 1967). This back-diffusion of acid has been related to the development of the damage and has been suggested as an explanation for the lowered acid secretion during non-steroid therapy. However, lowered acid output was recently suggested to be a direct action on the production of acid by these drugs (GLARBORG et al., 1974).

It is generally accepted that acid is necessary for the development of gastric lesions, but increased acid secretion does not seem to be the key factor on the lesions induced by aspirin-like drugs. However, in the rat indomethacin increased acid secretion (MAIN and WHITTLE, 1972) and as PGs inhibit acid secretion (SHAW and RAMWELL, 1968a), a continuous release in the stomach mucosa may act as a natural brake mechanism. Furthermore, PGE_2 in the rat causes vasodilatation as shown by the ratio of gastric mucosal blood flow to acid ouput which either remains unchanged or increases after administration of PGs (JACOBSON, 1970; MAIN and WHITTLE, 1974). BENNETT et al. (1973), suggested that PG vasodilatation possibly protects the integrity of the tissue against back-diffusion of acid or proteolytic enzymes. A factor that might be important for the maintenance of a "normal" concentration of PGs in the gastric mucosa is its very intense cell turnover. In favour of the importance of PG participation, DODGE et al. (1974) presented a correlation between gastro-intestinal damage and reduction of PG synthetase activity.

PGs, and especially their long-lasting synthetic derivatives, inhibit gastric lesions induced by many different stimuli. However, no specific effect on mucous, acid secretion or on the vascular bed could be implicated in the anti-ulcerogenic action. This led ROBERT (1975) to postulate a cytoprotective action for PGs. There is some structure-activity relationship here. PGs of the E series protect better than those of the A series, which are themselves better than those of the F series.

At the moment it is difficult to assess the relative importance of inhibition of PG synthetase or other enzymes in the genesis of the gastric lesions induced by aspirin-like drugs. The main reason is our ignorance of the trigger events or the sequence of physiopathological events which cause gastric lesions. What comes first, the breakdown of the mucosal barrier or the vascular lesions?

When one considers the variety of stimuli which can cause gastric lesions in the rat, it seems evident that the integrity of the gastric mucosa depends on a fine balance of influences and that interference in one component may cause an acute lesion. However, it was not possible to cause chronic lesions with aspirin-like drugs in rats (see Chap. 29) although gastro-intestinal blood loss was demonstrable (EDELSON and DOUGLAS, 1973).

Aspirin-like drugs can cause anything from a small to a massive blood loss. They can also increase bleeding time (QUICK and CLESCERI, 1960) and increase blood loss during parturition (LEWIS and SCHULMAN, 1973). It is not known how aspirin-like drugs cause vascular fragility (FRICK, 1956) but inhibition of platelet aggregation may be one of the components responsible for the increased bleeding time. Thromboxane A_2 (RCS), which is a strong vasoconstrictor, is released when platelets aggregate and this may also influence the bleeding time. Another factor in causing bleeding is the increased prothrombin time (QUICK and CLESCERI, 1960) but this may only be relevant in the presence of a bleeding tendency (SMITH, 1966).

Aspirin-like drugs after long-term administration to rats cause renal papillary necrosis, although they are relatively non-toxic in the human kidney (for review, see WISEMAN and REINERT, 1975, and Chap. 29). The kidney is another organ in which an acid environment at the inner medullary region will favour an increased intracellular concentration of non-steroid anti-inflammatory drugs. This could cause a toxic effect with consequent vascular necrosis. Inhibition of PG synthetase is probably a relevant factor since endogenous PGs contribute to auto-regulation (HERBACZYNSKA-CEDRO and VANE, 1973) as well as maintenance of resting blood flow and regulation of blood distribution between cortex and medulla. Aspirin-like drugs decrease blood flow to the inner cortex (for review see McGIFF et al., 1974), and reduction of synthesis of PGs may be the trigger mechanism for the renal papillary necrosis. The importance of a vascular component is shown by the occurence of similar lesions in patients with diabetes and vascular disease (BEESON, 1971). There is no agreement as to whether "analgesic nephropathy" induced by aspirin-phenacetin mixtures is due to phenacetin or to aspirin (see WISEMAN and REINERT, 1975). In this context it is interesting to note that phenacetin itself has no action against PG synthetase prepared from kidney (FLOWER and VANE, 1974) whereas paracetamol, which is its main metabolite, was four times as active as aspirin.

An antiproteinuric effect of aspirin-like drugs is easily demonstrable when there is a disturbed renal function. In such instances, indomethacin for example, decreases glomerular filtration rate and effective renal plasma flow, possibly via inhibition of PG synthesis (DONKER et al., 1975; ARISZ et al., 1975). In experimental models of nephritis, indomethacin affects protein excretion in autologous complex glomerulopathy but not in toxic nephropathy induced by puromycin (GRIBNAU, 1975).

As reviewed by AIKEN (1974) and WILLIAMS and VANE (1975), the prolongation and delay in parturition caused by aspirin-like drugs is almost certainly due to inhibition of PG biosynthesis. Such a conclusion implicates PG production in the parturition process, and this is most likely through the contractile action of PGs on uterine smooth muscle. A recent retrospective survey (LEWIS and SCHULMAN, 1973) showed that women taking aspirin had an average gestational period a week longer than the control group as well as significantly longer labour, with more blood loss. PGs may also play a part in the expulsion of uterine contents induced by abortifacients. For instance, WALTMAN et al. (1973) induced abortion by the intra-amniotic instillation of hypertonic saline. The time to abortion for 50 control women was 36.3 ± 2.75 h (mean $\pm$ s.e.m). In women treated with indomethacin this time was prolonged to 68.5 ± 4.8 h. In mice also, indomethacin prevented abortion induced by endotoxin (HARPER and SKARNES, 1972a, 1972b). VANE (1971) suggested that aspirin-like drugs should be tested as a treatment of premature labour. This has now been done with indomethacin and WIQVIST et al. (1976) conclude that indomethacin is a potent and useful drug in the treatment of premature labour.

We have discussed the side-effects which occur with high dosage or prolonged administration of aspirin-like drugs. There are two ideas underlying our comments: (a) the side-effects may derive from interference with intracellular enzymic systems which are important for the integrity of the cells or tissues: in this circumstance an acid environment may determine increased intracellular concentration (BRUNE, 1974), or (b) one of these enzyme systems is likely to be PG synthetase, especially in those organs in which PGs modulate normal physiological functions.

If the second possibility is demonstrated, PG synthetase inhibitors will continue to exhibit the same common side-effects unless new ones can be found with differential effects on the enzymes from different tissues.

The experimental evidence is sparse to support the suggestion (BRUNE, 1974) that aspirin-like drugs accumulate intracellularly at sites in which the lesions related to the side-effects occur. We favour the idea that unspecific inhibition of intracellular enzymes due to a high concentration of non-steroid anti-inflammatory agents, occurs only in toxic states caused by overdosage (for review see SMITH and DAWKINS, 1971).

D. Theories and Theories

Inhibition of an enzymic reaction is only pharmacologically meaningful when its participation can be demonstrated in the physiopathological process which the drug is able to modify. This obvious statement is frequently disregarded because inflammation is still poorly understood, so that any and every replicable effect of aspirin-like drugs can be proposed as a possible mechanism of action.

Non-steroid anti-inflammatory drugs have a high chemical reactivity towards proteins and it is not surprising that a great number of enzymic systems are inhibited in vitro. This fact paved the way to the conception that their mechanism of action derived from interference in various molecular or cellular events (WHITEHOUSE, 1974), i.e. that these drugs are polycompetent. In contrast with this "multiple effect theory," the PG theory relates the analgesic, antipyretic and anti-inflammatory action of aspirin-like drugs directly to inhibition of PG synthesis. The suggestion that this is the basic mechanism does not preclude other actions which may be important as explanations of differences in therapeutic usefulness, specific toxicity and effects not related to inflammation. For example, indomethacin—but not aspirin or phenylbutazone—inhibits the release of lysosomal enzymes from macrophages (FINLAY et al., 1975). In full therapeutic doses, salicylates affect respiration, possibly by a central stimulant effect. Phenylbutazone has many toxic effects not shared by other non-steroid anti-inflammatory drugs (MAUER, 1955).

As with all new theories, the PG theory has its dissenters and various criticisms were recently summarized by SMITH in an editorial (1975). The majority of his criticisms have already been answered in this review but his most pertinent query refers to analgesia. It has been suggested that the differential sensitivity of PG synthetase from various tissues could explain why agents without anti-inflammatory effect display analgesic and antipyretic activity (FLOWER et al., 1972, see Chap. 12). This idea may well explain the antipyretic effect but is still unsatisfactory with respect to analgesia. Low doses of aspirin-like drugs may act similarly to paracetamol because in arthritic patients they cause analgesia without a great effect on inflammatory oedema. The reason why the explanation is unsatisfactory derives from the idea that it is the concentration of a mediator in an inflammatory exudate that contributes to the development of a sign or symptom. If so, for the explanation to be correct, the threshold concentration of PGs for producing oedema should be smaller than that for causing hyperalgesia. There is no comparative study to support this assumption. In fact, indirect evidence indicates that for causing hyperalgesia, less PG is needed than for oedema, especially because the effects of PG on nerves are long-lasting, thus allowing small amounts generated over a long period of time to induce hyperalgesia. An alternative explanation is that the effective PG is generated by the injured effector cells and the PG synthetases of these cells present a differential sensitivity to aspirin-like drugs. One important factor which may account for the differential sensitivity of the enzymes is the access of the inflammatory drug to the enzymes. The structure of sensory nerves is so different from an endothelial cell that it is reasonable to suppose that the factors governing the access to the enzymes might also be different, favouring the inhibition of the PG synthetase of the nerves.

Recently, based on a pharmacokinetic interpretation, BRUNE (1974) suggested that aspirin-like drugs should specifically accumulate at the inflamed site and then exert their effects by acting unspecifically on any enzymic system. This suggested accumulation would favour sensory nerve endings, causing a more pronounced inhibition of the synthetase localized in these structures.

These speculations were made to stress our ignorance about a few aspects of the problem which might well be crucial for finding a satsifactory explanation. However, there are two positive findings which support the idea. Aspirin and paracetamol show similar potencies when tested on brain enzymes (FLOWER and VANE, 1972) and treatment of animals with paracetamol (and presumably aspirin) abolishes the release of PGs into CSF induced by pyrogen (see Chap. 18). There is no reason to think that the peripheral nervous system will behave differently towards a drug (although the opposite may be true, due to the blood-brain barrier). If hyperalgesia is caused by generation of PGs in the pain receptors themselves, then the dose necessary to produce analgesia would be the same as to block hyperthermia. This is what occurs with both aspirin and paracetamol. A pharmacokinetic factor or different sensitivity to the PGs from vessels may explain why increasing doses of paracetamol are not very effective in reducing inflammatory oedema. However, an explanation of the analgesic effect of aspirin-like drugs will only be satisfactory when the knowledge of the physiopathology of pain reaches a higher degree of maturity. Clearly, the demonstration that overt pain in inflammation results from the action of a mechanical or a chemical stimulation on a hyperalgesic background caused by PGs (FERREIRA, 1972; see Chap. 17) constitutes a step forward in support of the PG theory.

A theory is built on the basis of what is known and in this sense the PG theory has brought together a great number of observations which were present in the literature without an apparent link. An example is the inhibitory effect of aspirin-like drugs on the release of RCS from lungs or on platelet aggregation by collagen (see Chap. 5). This example also illustrates how the theory is evolving to encompass new observations. RCS activity was first thought to be due to a PG intermediate, perhaps the cyclic endoperoxide. It is now equated with a mixture of the cyclic endoperoxide and thromboxane A_2 (which accounts for most of the activity). Thromboxane A_2 aggregates platelets and its generation is also prevented by aspirin-like drugs. The actions of thromboxane A_2 upon vasculature and sensory nerves have not yet been established.

There is an apparent anomaly in the PG theory, for PGs can be anti-inflammatory in acute and chronic models (ASPINAL and CAMMARATA, 1969; ZURIER and QUAGLIATA, 1971; GLENN and ROHLOFF, 1972; ZURIER et al., 1973). These effects have only been shown with very large amounts of PGs which make it improbable that endogenously released PGs would display an important role as anti-inflammatory substances. Two mechanisms could account for these pharmacological effects of PGs, especially of PGE_1. They could act through a release of an endogenous anti-inflammatory factor and/or by inhibiting the release of inflammatory mediators. PGs given in such high doses (up to 1 mg a day) undoubtedly cause an increased vascular permeability and could be acting similarly to an irritant (see Chap. 15). It has been shown, however, that concentrations of PGE_1 or PGE_2 higher than those found in inflammatory exudates, block the release in vitro: (a) of histamine and SRS-A from lung fragments and basophils (LICHTENSTEIN and DE BERNARDO, 1971; TAUBER et al., 1973); (b) of lysosomal enzymes from human leucocytes (WEISSMANN et al., 1971a; ZURIER et al., 1973); (c) of lymphokine from macrophages (MORLEY, 1974). Furthermore, they prevent lymphocyte-mediated cytoxicity (HENNEY et al., 1972). These effects in vitro correlate with an increase in intracellular cAMP and may explain why administration of cAMP suppresses acute and chronic inflammation in several experimental models (ICHIKAWA et al., 1972a, b). The inhibitory effect of pharmacological doses of PGs has also been shown in vivo for cartilage destruction and lysosomal enzyme release (ASPINAL and CAMMARATA, 1969; ZURIER and BALLAS, 1973). If endogenous PGs were depressing cartilage destruction or lysosomal enzyme release in any type of inflammation, treatment with a PG synthetase inhibitor should accelerate the evolution of the physiopathological lesions; this does not happen. Thus, it is likely that endogenous PGs play a pro-inflammatory rather than an anti-inflammatory role and the anti-inflammatory effect of exogenous PGs is pharmacological, by either releasing endogenous anti-inflammatory substances or blocking the release of inflammatory mediators.

Initially, there seemed little evidence that the mechanism of action of the anti-inflammatory steroids was connected with the PG system, but evidence is now beginning to emerge. VANE (1971) could not demonstrate a direct inhibitory effect of steroids on a cell-free preparation of PG synthetase and in perfused spleens there was also no effect (FERREIRA et al., 1971). However, GREAVES and McDONALD-GIBSON (1972) reported inhibition of PG biosynthesis in unseparated homogenates of skin, using albeit high doses of fluocinolone or hydrocortisone. Later, they found that corticoids were ineffective upon purified preparations of skin enzyme. LEWIS and

Piper (1975) suggested that steroids inhibit not the synthesis of PG but its release from the fat pad during lipolysis. There is some experimental evidence to substantiate this concept (Chang et al., 1976), but Tashjian et al. (1975) found that corticoids inhibit PG production by mouse fibrosarcoma rather than its release from the cells. Gryglewski et al. (1975) found that either indomethacin or dexamethasone inhibited PG release induced by noradrenaline in the rabbit mesenteric bed. However, the dexamethasone inhibition was easily reversed by infusions of arachidonic acid, whereas that of indomethacin was not. They concluded that steroids may work by impairing the availability of the substrate for the enzyme. Kantrowitz et al. (1975) also found that steroids reduce PG production by isolated synovial membrane cells in culture. Thus, steroids could be affecting the PG synthetase system by limiting the substrate availability, possibly through "membrane stabilization" or by inhibition of phospholipase A_2. Such an activity would also reduce substrate availability for other enzymes which metabolize arachidonic acid, such as the lipoxygenase (which is not inhibited by aspirin). If this were so, it might be the basis of the improved performance of the steroids over the non-steroids against inflammation, especially in allergic conditions.

Another possibility is that the action of corticoids on PG content of inflammatory exudates is partly indirect. In aqueous humour from patients with untreated uveitis, Eakins et al. (1972a, 1972b) found a substantial amount of PGs which contrasts with that of patients treated with corticoids, in which little or none was detected. As corticoids have no effect on the PG synthetase enzymes of the eye, the inhibition was thought to derive from diminution in the numbers of migrating cells. However, corticoids must also have another basic mechanism of action since they are very effective in many clinical situations, such as asthma or haemodynamic shock, in which aspirin-like drugs have little or no clinical effect. Furthermore, even in vivo, only high doses of corticoids reduce the content of PGs from inflammatory exudates (see Table 1).

It is well known that topically applied steroids alleviate some of the allergic skin conditions. Much less is known about the effects of topical non-steroid anti-inflammatory agents, although one PG synthetase inhibitor (bufexamac) is marketed as a cream for topical use. Recently, Hsia et al. (1974) have studied the effects of indomethacin cream on the inflammation induced by sunburn. They showed that the reddening was completely abolished on the patch of skin to which the indomethacin was applied. It is likely, therefore, that in the next few years, PG synthetase inhibitors specifically designed for application to the skin will be tested against various inflammatory conditions, including those initiated by the allergic reaction.

In summary, the following observations support the "prostaglandin theory:"

1. All cells are capable of generating PGs and increased PG concentrations have been detected in most inflammatory exudates.

2. PGs of the E series mimic inflammatory symptoms. They have the special effect of enhancing the pro-inflammatory effect of other mediators: vasodilatation, increased vascular permeability and sensitization of pain receptors. They also induce fever. These effects are observed in concentrations likely to occur in inflammatory exudates but there is the possibility that the PGs generated by the traumatized effector cells are the most important for the genesis of the inflammatory signs or

symptoms. Intermediates in PG synthesis may also play a part in the inflammatory responses.

3. In vivo, aspirin-like drugs do not change the direct effect of PGs.

4. Aspirin-like drugs inhibit PG and thromboxane biosynthesis in concentrations attained in body fluids during therapy.

5. There is a general correlation between inhibition of PG synthesis in vitro and inflammatory activity. A few PG synthetase inhibitors do not show anti-inflammatory activity. However, drugs which inhibit PG synthesis in vivo display anti-inflammatory and antipyretic activity.

6. PG synthetase prepared from different tissues shows different sensitivities to aspirin-like drugs. This property may reflect a series of isoenzymes and can explain the variations in activity within the group of compounds capable of inhibiting PG synthesis in vivo. Paracetamol, which is antipyretic and analgesic without being anti-inflammatory, has equivalent activity to aspirin upon brain enzyme but much less on spleen enzyme. One factor that may govern in vivo the potency of a PG synthetase inhibitor, is its access to the enzyme within the cells.

7. Steroid anti-inflammatory drugs may also affect the PG system, but not by a direct inhibition of PG synthetase.

8. The fact that aspirin is a relatively non-toxic drug, consumed in enormous quantities throughout the world, suggests that PG synthetase is not an enzyme vital for the existence of the organism. This fits with the concept that PGs are modulators of the activity of the body, perhaps mainly involved in local communication between cells especially in defensive reactions induced by local damage.

9. Potent PG synthetase inhibitors are useful tools for defining the role that PGs play in the body. The evidence so far shows that PGs, as well as being important mediators of inflammation, fever and pain, also maintain the tone of some preparations of isolated smooth muscles, contribute to the expulsion of the foetus, modulate lipolysis and modulate catecholamine release from nerves. They also contribute to autoregulation of renal blood flow and to functional dilatation in adipose tissue.

10. It is not yet well understood how inhibition of PG synthesis relates to the side-effect of aspirin-like drugs, but there is likely to be a connection.

Considering that inhibition of PG synthesis is in vivo a common action of the group of anti-inflammatory agents referred to as aspirin-like drugs, we suggest that this group should collectively be referred to as "anti-inflammatory cyclo-oxygenase inhibitors" (ACI), in order to differentiate them from other types of anti-inflammatory agents such as corticoids, colchicine and immunosuppressive agents.

References

Aberg, G.: Interactions between salicylates and prostaglandins on the temperature of inflammatory rat paws. Int. Res. Commun. Syst. **9**, 3 (1973)

Aiken, J. W.: Aspirin and indomethacin prolong parturition in rats: evidence that prostaglandins contribute to expulsion of fetus. Nature (Lond.) **240**, 21—25 (1972)

Aiken, J. W.: Prostaglandins and prostaglandin synthetase inhibitors: studies on uterine motility and function. In: Robinson, H. J., Vane, J. R. (Eds.): Prostaglandin Synthetase Inhibitors, pp. 289—301. New York: Raven Press 1974

Anderson, A. J.: Effects of lysosomal collagenolytic enzymes, anti-inflammatory drugs and other substances on some properties of insoluble collagen. Biochem. J. 113, 457—463 (1969)

Anderson, A. J.: Lysosomal enzyme activity in rats with adjuvant-induced arthritis. Ann. rheum. Dis. 29, 307—313 (1970)

Anderson, A. J., Brocklehurst, W. E., Willis, A. L.: Evidence for the role of lysosomes in the formation of prostaglandins during carrageenin induced inflammation in the rat. Pharmacol. Res. Commun. 3, 13—19 (1971)

Änggård, E., Larsson, C.: Stimulation and inhibition of prostaglandin biosynthesis: opposite effects on blood pressure and intrarenal blood flow distribution. In: Robinson, H. J., Vane, J. R. (Eds.): Prostaglandin Synthetase Inhibitors, pp. 311—316. New York: Raven Press 1974

Arisz, L., Donker, A. J. M., Brentjens, J. R. H., Hemm, G. K. van der: Het effect van indometacine i op de proteinuri bij het nefrotisch syndroom. Ned. T. Geneesk. 119, 815 (1975)

Armstrong, D. T., Grinwich, D. L.: Blockade of spontaneous LH-induced ovulation in rats by indomethacin, an inhibitor of prostaglandin biosynthesis. Prostaglandins 1, 21—28 (1972)

Arrigoni-Martelli, E.: Antagonism of anti-inflammatory drugs on bradykinin-induced increase of capillary permeability. J. Pharm. (Lond.) 19, 617—620 (1967)

Arrigoni-Martelli, E., Corsico, N., Fognoloe, E.: Significance of the release of bradykinin in local inflammatory reactions and related effect of antiphlogistic drugs. In: Bertelli, A., Houck, J. C. (Eds.): Inflammation, Biochemistry, and Drug Interaction, Proceedings of an International Symposium, Italy 1968, pp. 185—188. Amsterdam: Excerpta Medica Foundation 1969

Arturson, G., Hamberg, M., Jonsson, C. E.: Prostaglandins in human burn blister fluid. Acta physiol. scand. 87, 270—276 (1973)

Ashton, N., Cook, C.: In vivo observations of the effects of cortisone upon the blood vessels in rabbit ear chambers. Brit. J. exp. Path. 33, 445—450 (1952)

Aspinall, R. L., Cammarata, P. S.: Effect of prostaglandin E_2 on adjuvant arthritis. Nature (Lond.) 224, 1320—1321 (1969)

Atherton, A., Born, G. V. R.: In vivo measurement of the adhesiveness of granulocytes to blood vessel walls. Bibl. anat. (Basel) 12, 138—145 (1973)

Beeson, P. B.: Pyelonephritis. In: Beeson, P. B., McDermott, W. (Eds.): Cecil-Loeb Textbook of Medicine, 13th Ed., pp. 1201—1205. Philadelphia-London-Toronto: W. B. Saunders Company 1971

Bennett, A., Posner, J.: Studies on prostaglandin antagonists. Brit. J. Pharmacol. 42, 584—594 (1971)

Bennett, A., Stamford, I. F., Unger, W. G.: Prostaglandin E_2 and gastric acid secretion in man. J. Physiol. (Lond.) 229, 349—360 (1973)

Bhattacherjee, P., Eakins, K. E.: Inhibition of the PG synthetase system in ocular tissue by indomethacin. Pharmacologist 15, 209 (1973)

Blackham, A., Farmer, J. B., Radziwonik, H., Westwick, J.: The role of prostaglandins in rabbit monoarticular arthritis. Brit. J. Pharmacol. 51, 35—44 (1974)

Blackham, A., Owen, R. T.: Prostaglandin synthetase inhibitors and leucocytic emigration. J. Pharm. (Lond.) 27, 201—203 (1975)

Blackwell, G. J., Parsons, M.: Personal communication (1975)

Bluestone, R., Kippen, I., Klinenberg, J. R.: Effect of drugs on urate binding to plasma protein. Brit. med. J. 1969 IV, 590—593

Blumenkrantz, N., Sondergaard, J.: Effect of prostaglandins E_1 and $F_{1\alpha}$ on the biosynthesis of collagen. Nature (New Biol.) 239, 246 (1972)

Bonnycastle, D. D., Cook, L., Ipsen, J.: Action of some analgesic drugs in intact and chronic spinal rats. Acta pharmacol. (Kbh.) 9, 332—336 (1953)

Bonta, I. L.: Time-effect course and drug antagonism pattern of various kinds of rat paw oedemas. In: Garattini, S., Dukes, M. N. G. (Eds.): Non-Steroidal Anti-Inflammatory Drugs, International Symposium, Milan 1964, p. 236. Amsterdam-London: Excerpta Medica Foundation 1965

Bonta,I.L., Bult,H., Ven,L.L.M. v. d., Noordhoek,J.: Essential fatty acid deficiency: a condition to discriminate prostaglandin and non-prostaglandin mediated components of inflammation. In: Giroud,J.P., Willoughby,D.A., Velo,G.P. (Eds.): Future Trends in Inflammation II, pp. 151—158. Basel: Birkhäuser Verlag 1976

Bonta,I.L., De Vos,C.J.: Presence of a slow-contraction inducing material in fluid collected from the rat paw oedema induced by serotonin. Experientia (Basel) 21, 34—35 (1965)

Boot,J.R., Dawson,W., Kitchen,E.A.: The chemotactic activity of thromboxane B₂, a possible role in inflammation. J. Physiol. (Lond.) 257, 47—48 P (1976)

Bowery,B., Lewis,G.P.: Inhibition of functional vasodilation and prostaglandin formation in rabbit adipose tissue by indomethacin and aspirin. Brit. J. Pharmacol. 47, 305—314 (1973)

Brodie,B.B.: Displacement of one drug by another from carrier or receptor site. Proc. roy. Soc. Med. 58 (Suppl.), 946—955 (1965)

Brodie,D.A., Tate,C.L., Hooke,K.F.: Aspirin: intestinal damage in rats. Science 170, 183—185 (1970)

Brody,T.M.: Action of sodium salicylate and related compounds on tissue metabolism in vitro. J. Pharmacol. exp. Ther. 117, 39—51 (1956)

Bröhr,H.J., Kalbhen,D.A.: Wirkung verschiedener Antirheumatica an die Sulfomucopolysac-charid-Synthese im Knorpel. Arch. int. Pharmacodyn. 176, 380—394 (1968)

Brown,J.H., Schwartz,N.L.: Interaction of lysosomes and anti-inflammatory drugs. Proc. Soc. exp. Biol. (N.Y.) 131, 614—620 (1969)

Brune,K.: How aspirin might work: a pharmacokinetic approach. Agents Actions 4, 230—232 (1974)

Brune,K., Glatt,M.: The avian microcristal arthritis. III. Invasion and enzyme-release from leukocytes at the site of inflammation. Agents Actions 2, 95—99 (1974)

Brune,K., Minder,B., Glatt,M., Schmid,L.: Do polymorphonuclear leucocytes function as me-diators in acute inflammation? In: Velo,G.P., Willoughby,D.A., Giroud,J.P. (Eds.): Future Trends in Inflammation, pp. 289—300. Padua-London: Piccin Medical Books 1974

Castor,C.W.: Connective tissue activation. IV. Regulatory effects of antirheumatic drugs. Arthr. Rheum. 15, 504—514 (1972)

Chang,J., Lewis,G.P., Piper,P.J.: The effects of anti-inflammatory steroids on levels of prosta-glandin in adipose tissue in vitro. Brit. J. Pharmacol. 56, 342—343 (1976)

Chapnick,B.M., Paustian,P.W., Klainer,E., Joiner,P.D., Hyman,A.L., Kadowitz,P.J.: Influence of prostaglandins E, A, and F on vasoconstrictor responses to norepinephrine, renal nerve stimulation and angiotensin in the feline kidney. J. Pharmacol. exp. Ther. 196, 44—52 (1976)

Chayen,J., Bitensky,L.: Lysosomal enzymes and inflammation with particular reference to rheu-matoid diseases. Ann. rheum. Dis. 30, 522—536 (1971)

Chayen,J., Bitensky,L., Butcher,R.G., Cashman,B.: Evidence for altered lysosomal membrane in synovial lining cells from human rheumatoid joints. Beitr. path. Anat. 142, 137—149 (1971)

Chayen,J., Bitensky,L., Butcher,R.G., Poulter,L.W., Ubhi,G.S.: Methods for direct measure-ment of anti-inflammatory action on human tissue maintained in vitro. Brit. J. Derm. 82, suppl. 6, 62 (1970)

Chester,R., Dukes,M., Slater,S.R., Walpole,A.L.: Delay of parturition in the rat by anti-inflam-matory agents which inhibit the biosynthesis of prostaglandins. Nature (Lond.) 240, 37—38 (1972)

Clark,W.C., Moyer,S.G.: The effects of acetaminophen and sodium salicylate on the release and activity of leukocytic pyrogen in the cat. J. Pharmacol. exp. Ther. 181, 183—191 (1972)

Collier,H.O.J.: A pharmacological analysis of aspirin. Advanc. Pharmacol. Chemother. 7, 333—405 (1969)

Collier,H.O.J., Shorley,P.G.: Analgesic antipyretic drugs as antagonists of bradykinin. Brit. J. Pharmacol. 15, 601—610 (1960)

Collier,J.G., Flower,R.J.: Effect of aspirin on human seminal prostaglandins. Lancet 1971 II, 852—853

Collier,J.G., Herman,A.G., Vane,J.R.: Appearance of prostaglandins in the renal venous blood of dogs in response to acute systemic hypotension produced by bleeding or endotoxin. J. Physiol. (Lond.) 230, 19 P—20 P (1973)

Coppi,G., Bonardi,G.: Effect of two non-steroidal anti-inflammatory agents on alkaline and acid phosphatases of inflamed tissues. J. Pharm. (Lond.) 20, 661—662 (1968)

Crunkhorn, P., Willis, A. L.: Cutaneous reactions to intradermal prostaglandins. Brit. J. Pharmacol. **41**, 49—56 (1971)

Culp, J. R., Erdös, E. G., Hinshaw, I. B., Holme, D. D.: Effects of anti-inflammatory drugs in shock caused by injection of living *E. coli* cells. Proc. Soc. exp. Biol. (N.Y.) **137**, 219—223 (1971)

Davenport, H. W.: Salicylate damage to the gastric mucosal barrier. New Engl. J. Med. **276**, 1307—1312 (1967)

Davies, G. E., Holman, G., Johnston, T. P., Lowe, J. S.: Studies on kallikrein: failure of some anti-inflammatory drugs to affect release of kinin. Brit. J. Pharmacol. **28**, 212—217 (1966)

Dawson, W., Tomlinson, R.: Effect of cromoglycate and eicosatetraynoic acid on the release of prostaglandins and SRS-A from immunologically challenged guinea pig lungs. Brit. J. Pharmacol. **52**, 107 P (1974)

Deby, C., Bacq, Z. M., Simon, D.: In vitro inhibition of the biosynthesis of a prostaglandin by gold and silver. Biochem. Pharmacol. **22**, 3141—3143 (1973)

Dembinska-Kieć, A., Zmuda, A. K., Krupinska, J.: Inhibition of prostaglandin synthetase by aspirin-like drugs in different microsomal preparations. In: Samuelsson, B., Paoletti, R. (Eds.): Advances in Prostaglandins and Thromboxane Research, pp. 99—103. New York: Raven Press 1976

Denko, W. C.: Anti-prostaglandin action of colchicine. Pharmacology (Basel) **13**, 219—227 (1975)

Desai, I. D., Tappel, A. L.: Damage to proteins by peroxidized lipids. J. Lipid Res. **4**, 204—207 (1963)

Di Perri, T., Auteri, A.: On the anticomplementary action of some non-steroidal anti-inflammatory drugs. In: Velo, G. P., Willoughby, D. A., Giroud, J. P. (Eds.): Future Trends in Inflammation, pp. 215—225. Padua-London: Piccin Medical Books 1974

Di Rosa, M., Giroud, J. P., Willoughby, D. A.: Studies of the mediators of the acute inflammatory response induced in rats in different sites by carrageenin and turpentine. J. Path. **104**, 15—29 (1971 a)

Di Rosa, M., Papadimitriou, J. M., Willoughby, D. A.: A histopathological and pharmacological analysis of the mode of action of non-steroidal anti-inflammatory drugs. J. Path. **105**, 239—256 (1971 b)

Dodge, P. W., Brodie, D. A., Young, P. R., Krause, R. A., Tekeli, S.: Prevention of antiinflammatory drug-induced gastric lesions in rats by ABBOTT-29 590. Amer. J. dig. Dis. **19**, 449—457 (1974)

Doherty, N. S., Robinson, B. V.: The inflammatory response to carrageenan. J. Pharm. (Lond.) **27**, 701—703 (1975)

Donker, A. J. M., Arisz, L., Brentjens, J. R. H., Hem, G. K. van der: Het effect van indomethacine i op de glomerulaire filtatie. Ned. T. Geneesk. **119**, 815 (1975)

Dubas, T. C., Parker, J. M.: A central component in the analgesic action of sodium salicylate. Arch. int. Pharmacodyn. **194**, 117—122 (1971)

Eakins, K. E.: Prostaglandins and prostaglandin synthetase inhibitors: actions in ocular disease. In: Robinson, H. J., Vane, J. R. (Eds.): Prostaglandin Synthetase Inhibitors, pp. 343—352. New York: Raven Press 1974

Eakins, K. E., Stier, C., Bhattacherjee, P., Greenbaum, L. M.: Actions and interactions of bradykinin, prostaglandin, and nonsteroidal antiinflammatory agents on the eye. Inflammation **1**, 117—125 (1975)

Eakins, K. E., Whitelock, R. A. F., Bennett, A., Martenet, A. C.: Prostaglandin-like activity in ocular inflammation. Brit. med. J. **1972 b** III, 452—453

Eakins, K. E., Whitelock, R. A. F., Perkins, E. S., Bennett, A., Ungar, W. G.: Release of prostaglandins in ocular inflammation in the rabbit. Nature (New Biol.) **239**, 248—249 (1972 a)

Eckenfels, A., Vane, J. R.: Prostaglandins, oxygen tension, and smooth muscle tone. Brit. J. Pharmacol. **45**, 451—462 (1972)

Edelson, J., Douglas, J. F.: Measurement of gastrointestinal blood loss in the rat: the effect of aspirin, phenylbutazone, and seclazone. J. Pharmacol. exp. Ther. **184**, 449—452 (1973)

Evanson, J. M., Jeffrey, J. J., Krane, S. M.: Human collagenase: identification and characterization of an enzyme from rheumatoid synovium in culture. Science **158**, 499—502 (1967)

Farmer, J. B., Farrar, D. G., Wilson, J.: The effect of indomethacin on the tracheal smooth muscle of the guinea pig. Brit. J. Pharmacol. **46**, 536 P—537 P (1972)

Feldberg, W., Gupta, K. P.: Pyrogen fever and prostaglandin-like activity in cerebrospinal fluid. J. Physiol. (Lond.) **228**, 41—53 (1973)

Feldberg, W., Saxena, P. N.: Fever produced by prostaglandin E₁. J. Physiol. (Lond.) **217**, 546—556 (1971a)

Feldberg, W., Saxena, P. N.: Further studies on prostaglandin E₁. Fever in cats. J. Physiol. (Lond.) **219**, 739—745 (1971b)

Ferreira, S. H.: A bradykinin potentiating factor (BPF) present in the venom of *Bothrops jararaca*. Brit. J. Pharmacol. **24**, 163—169 (1965)

Ferreira, S. H.: Prostaglandins, aspirin-like drugs and analgesia. Nature (New Biol.) **240**, 200—203 (1972)

Ferreira, S. H.: Prostaglandins and the immunological trauma. In: Lewis, G. P. (Ed.): The role of prostglandins in inflammation, pp. 75—83. Vienna: Hans Huber Publisher 1976

Ferreira, S. H., Flower, R. J., Parsons, M. F., Vane, J. R.: Reduction of the inflammatory response in rats immunized against prostaglandins. Prostaglandins **8**, 433—437 (1974a)

Ferreira, S. H., Harvey, E. A., Vane, J. R.: Hyperalgesia, inflammatory oedema and prostaglandins. In: Abstracts Sixth International Congress on Pharmacology, Helsinki 1974, Abstract 1001, 1975

Ferreira, S. H., Herman, A., Vane, J. R.: Prostaglandin generation maintains the smooth muscle tone of the rabbit isolated jejunum. Brit. J. Pharmacol. **44**, 328P—330P (1972)

Ferreira, S. H., Moncada, S., Parsons, M., Vane, J. R.: The concomitant release of bradykinin and prostaglandin in the inflammatory response to carrageenin. Brit. J. Pharmacol. **52**, 108P (1974b)

Ferreira, S. H., Moncada, S., Vane, J. R.: Indomethacin and aspirin abolish prostaglandin release from the spleen. Nature (New Biol.) **231**, 237—239 (1971)

Ferreira, S. H., Moncada, S., Vane, J. R.: Prostaglandin and the mechanism of analgesia produced by aspirin-like drugs. Brit. J. Pharmacol. **49**, 86—97 (1973a)

Ferreira, S. H., Moncada, S., Vane, J. R.: Some effects of inhibiting endogenous prostaglandin formation on the response of the cat spleen. Brit. J. Pharmacol. **47**, 48—58 (1973b)

Ferreira, S. H., Moncada, S., Vane, J. R.: Prostaglandins and the signs and symptoms of inflammation. In: Robinson, H. J., Vane, J. R. (Eds.): Prostaglandin Synthetase Inhibitors, pp. 175—187. New York: Raven Press 1974c

Ferreira, S. H., Vane, J. R.: Prostaglandins: their disappearance from and release into the circulation. Nature (Lond.) **216**, 868—873 (1967)

Ferreira, S. H., Vane, J. R.: Aspirin and prostaglandins. In: Ramwell, P. W. (Ed.): The Prostaglandins II, pp. 1—47. New York-London: Plenum Press 1974a

Ferreira, S. H., Vane, J. R.: New aspects of the mode of action of non-steroid anti-inflammatory drugs. Ann. Rev. Pharmacol. **14**, 57—73 (1974b)

Ferreira, S. H., Vane, J. R.: Inhibition of prostaglandin biosynthesis and the mechanism of action of non-steroidal anti-inflammatory agents. In: Velo, G. P., Willoughby, D. A., Giroud, J. P. (Eds.): Future Trends in Inflammation, pp. 171—185. Padua-London: Piccin Medical Books 1974c

Ferreira, S. H., Vargaftig, B. B.: Inhibition by non-steroid anti-inflammatory agents of rabbit aorta contracting activity generated in blood by slow reacting substance C. Brit. J. Pharmacol. **50**, 543—551 (1974)

Fichel, E. E., Frank, C. W., Boltax, A. J., Arcasoy, M.: Observations on the treatment of rheumatic fever with salicylate, ACTH, and cortisone. II. Combined salicylate corticoid therapy and attempts at rebound-suppression. Arthr. Rheum. **1**, 351—366 (1958)

Finlay, C., Davies, P., Allison, A. C.: Changes in cellular enzyme levels and the inhibition of selective release of lysosomal hydrolases from macrophages by indomethacin. Agents Actions **5**, 345—353 (1975)

Flower, R. J.: Drugs which inhibit prostaglandin biosynthesis. Pharmacol. Rev. **26**, 33—67 (1974)

Flower, R. J., Blackwell, G. J.: The importance of phospholipase in prostaglandin biosynthesis. Biochem. Pharmacol. **25**, 285—291 (1976)

Flower, R. J., Gryglewski, R., Herbaczynska-Cedro, K., Vane, J. R.: Effects of anti-inflammatory drugs on prostaglandin biosynthesis. Nature (New Biol.) **238**, 104—106 (1972)

Flower, R. J., Vane, J. R.: Inhibition of prostaglandin synthetase in brain explains the anti-pyretic activity of paracetamol (4-acetamido-phenol). Nature (Lond.) **240**, 410—411 (1972)

Flower, R. J., Vane, J. R.: Some pharmacologic and biochemical aspects of prostaglandin biosynthesis and its inhibition. In: Robinson, H. J., Vane, J. R. (Eds.): Prostaglandin Synthetase Inhibitors: Their Effects on Physiological Functions and Pathological States, pp. 9—18. New York: Raven Press 1974

Ford-Hutchinson, A. W., Smith, M. J. M., Elliott, P. N., Bolam, J. G., Walker, J. R., Lobo, A. A., Badcock, J. K., Colledge, A. J., Billimoria, F. J.: Effects of a human plasma fraction on leucocyte migration into inflammatory exudates. J. Pharm. (Lond.) 27, 106—112 (1975)

Frick, P. G.: Hemorrhagic diathesis with increased capillary fragility caused by salicylate therapy. Amer. J. med. Sci. 231, 402—406 (1956)

Fullmer, H. M., Gibson, W. A., Lazarus, G., Stamm, A. C.: Collagenolytic activity of the skin associated with neuromuscular diseases including ammyotrophic lateral sclerosis. Lancet 1966 I, 1007—1009

Fujihira, E., Tsubota, N., Nakazawa, M.: Effect of anti-inflammatory drugs on glucosamine-6-phosphate synthetase from inflamed tissue of rats. Chem. pharm. Bull. 19, 190—195 (1971)

Ganter, L. J., Guyonnet, J. C.: Histochemical study on experimental gastric lesions induced by acetylsalicyclic acid and other drugs in rats. Laval med. 37, 416—434 (1966)

Garcia Leme, J., Hamamura, L., Leite, M. P., Rocha e Silva, M.: Pharmacological analysis of the acute inflammatory process induced in the rat's paw by local injection of carrageenin and by heating. Brit. J. Pharmacol. 48, 88—96 (1973a)

Garcia Leme, J., Hamamura, L., Migliorini, R. H., Leite, M. P.: Influence of diabetes upon the inflammatory response of the rat. A Pharmacological analysis. Europ. J. Pharmacol. 23, 74—81 (1973b)

Garcia Leme, J., Rocha e Silva, M.: Competitive and non-competitive inhibition of bradykinin on the guinea-pig ileum. Brit. J. Pharmacol. 25, 50—58 (1965)

Garcia Leme, J., Wilhelm, D. L.: The effects of adrenalectomy and corticosterone on vascular permeability responses in the skin of the rat. Brit. J. exp. Path. 56, 402—407 (1975)

Gerber, D. A., Cohen, N., Giustra, R.: The ability of non-steroid anti-inflammatory compounds to accelerate a disulfide interchange reaction of serum sulphhydryl groups and 5,5'-dithiobis (2-nitrobenzoic acid). Biochem. Pharmacol. 16, 115—123 (1967)

Glaborg, J., Kaplan, E. L., Peskin, G. W.: Salicylate effects on gastric acid secretion. Scand. J. clin. Lab. Invest. 33, 31—38 (1974)

Glatt, M., Peskar, B., Brune, K.: Leukocytes and prostaglandins in acute inflammation. Experientia (Basel) 30, 1257—1259 (1974)

Glenn, E. M., Bowman, B. J., Rohloff, N. A.: Pro-inflammatory effects of certain prostaglandins. In: Ramwell, P. W., Pharriss, B. B. (Eds.): Prostaglandins in Cellular Biology, Vol. I, pp. 329—343. New York-London: Plenum Press 1972

Glenn, E. M., Kooyers, W. M.: Plasma inflammation units; an objective method for investigating effects of drugs on experimental inflammation. Life Sci. 5, 519—628 (1966)

Glenn, E. M., Rohloff, N. A.: Antiarthritic and anti-inflammatory effects of certain prostaglandins. Proc. Soc. exp. Biol. (N.Y.) 139, 290—294 (1972)

Gorög, P., Kovacs, I. B.: The alteration of platelet behaviour during various conditions and the effect of anti-inflammatory agents on the platelet aggregation and thrombus formation. In: Bertelli, A. B., Houch, J. C. (Eds.): Inflammation Biochemistry and Drug Interaction, pp. 197—203. Amsterdam: Excerpta Medica Foundation 1969

Goth, A., Nash, W. L., Nagler, M., Holman, J.: Inhibition of histamine release in experimental diabetes. Amer. J. Physiol. 191, 25—28 (1957)

Grant, N. H., Alburn, H. E., Singer, A. C.: Correlation between in vitro and in vivo models in anti-inflammatory drug studies. Biochem. Pharmacol. 20, 2137—2140 (1971a)

Grant, N. H., Rosenthale, M. E., Alburn, H. E., Singer, A. C.: Slowed lysosomal enzyme release and its normalization by drugs in adjuvant-induced polyarthritis. Biochem. Pharmacol. 20, 2821—2824 (1971b)

Greaves, M. W., McDonald-Gibson, W.: Inhibition of prostaglandin biosynthesis by corticosteroids. Brit. med. J. 1972 II, 83—84

Greaves, M. W., Søndergaard, J.: Pharmacological agents released in ultraviolet inflammation studied by continuous skin perfusion. J. invest. Derm. 54, 365—367 (1970)

Greaves, M. W., Søndergaard, J., McDonald-Gibson, W.: Recovery of prostaglandins in human cutaneous inflammation. Brit. med. J. 1971 II, 258—260

Greene, J. J., Camargo, A. C., Krieg, E., Stewart, J. M., Ferreira, S. H.: Inhibition of the conversion of angiotensin I to II and potentiation of bradykinin by small peptides present in *Bothrops jararaca* venom. Circulat. Res. **XXXI** Suppl. II, 62—71 (1972)

Gribnau, F. W. J.: Studies in Heymann-type nephritis and in puromycin aminonucleoside nephropathy. In: Gribnau, F. W. J. (Ed.): Indomethacin in Experimental Nephritis. Netherlands: 1975

Gryglewski, R.: The fibrinolytic activity of anti-inflammatory drugs. J. Pharm. (Lond.) **18**, 474 (1966)

Gryglewski, R. J.: Prostaglandins and prostaglandin synthesis inhibitors in etiology and treatment of inflammation. In: Proceedings Sixth International Congress of Pharmacology, Helsinki 1974, Vol. 5, pp. 151—160 (1975)

Gryglewski, R. J., Gryglewska, T. A.: The fibrinolytic activity of N-arylanthranilates. Biochem. Pharmacol. **15**, 1171—1175 (1966)

Gryglewski, R. J., Panczeko, B., Korbut, R., Grodzinska, L., Ocetkiewics, A.: Corticosteroids inhibit prostaglandin release from perfused mesenteric blood vessels of rabbit and from perfused lungs of sensitized guinea pig. Prostaglandins **10**, 343—355 (1975)

Gryglewski, R. J., Vane, J. R.: The release of prostaglandins and rabbit aorta contracting substance (RCS) from rabbit spleen and its antagonism by anti-inflammatory drugs. Brit. J. Pharmacol. **45**, 37—47 (1972a)

Gryglewski, R. J., Vane, J. R.: The generation from arachidonic acid of rabbit aorta contracting substance (RCS) by a microsomal enzyme preparation which also generates PGs. Brit. J. Pharmacol. **46**, 449—457 (1972b)

Guzman, F., Braun, C., Lim, R. K. S.: Visceral pain and the pseudo-affective response to intra-arterial injection of bradykinin and other algesic agents. Arch. int. Pharmacodyn. **136**, 353—384 (1962)

Guzman, F., Braun, C., Lim, R. K. S., Potter, G. D., Rodgers, D. W.: Narcotic and non-narcotic analgesics which block visceral pain evoked by intra-arterial injection of bradykinin and other algesic agents. Arch. int. Pharmacodyn. **149**, 571—588 (1964)

Ham, E. A., Cirillo, V. J., Zanetti, M., Shen, T. Y., Kuehl, F. A. Jr.: Studies on the mode of action of non-steroidal anti-inflammatory agents. In: Ramwell, P. W., Pharriss, B. B. (Eds.): Prostaglandins in Cellular Biology, pp. 343—352. New York: Plenum Press 1972

Hamberg, M.: Inhibition of prostaglandin synthesis in man. Biochem. biophys. Res. Commun. **49**, 720—726 (1972)

Hamberg, M., Samuelsson, B.: Prostaglandin endoperoxide. Novel transformation of arachidonic acid in human platelets. Proc. nat. Acad. Sci. (Wash.) **75**, 3400—3404 (1974a)

Hamberg, M., Samuelsson, B.: Prostaglandin endoperoxides. VII. Novel transformations of arachidonic acid in guinea pig lungs. Biochem. biophys. Res. Commun. **61**, 942—949 (1974b)

Hamberg, M., Svensson, J., Samuelsson, B.: Prostaglandin endoperoxides. A new concept concerning the mode of action and release of prostaglandins. Proc. nat. Acad. Sci. (Wash.) **71**, 3824—3828 (1974)

Hamberg, M., Svensson, J., Samuelsson, B.: Novel transformations of prostaglandin endoperoxides: formation of thromboxanes. In: Samuelsson, B., Paoletti, R. (Eds.): Advances in Prostaglandin and Thromboxane Research, Vol. I, pp. 19—27. New York: Raven Press 1976

Harper, M. J. K., Skarnes, R. C.: Inhibition of abortion and fetal death produced by endotoxin or prostaglandin $F_{2\alpha}$. Prostaglandins **2**, 295—309 (1972a)

Harper, M. J. K., Skarnes, R. C.: The role of prostaglandin in endotoxin-induced abortion and fetal death. In: Bergström, S., Raspe, G., Bernhard, S. (Eds.): Advances in the Biosciences, pp. 789—793. Vieweg: Pergamon Press 1972b

Harrison, R. G.: Prostaglandins, kinins, and amines synergistic effects on skin vascular permeability. Int. Res. Commun. Syst. (8.11.2) (1973)

Hedqvist, P.: Prostaglandin E compounds and sympathetic neuromuscular transmission. Ann. N.Y. Acad. Sci. **180**, 410—415 (1971)

Hedqvist, P.: Effect of prostaglandins and prostaglandin synthesis inhibitors on norepinephrine release from vascular tissue. In: Robinson, H. J., Vane, J. R. (Eds.): Prostaglandin Synthetase Inhibitors, pp. 303—309. New York: Raven Press 1974

Henney, C. S., Bourne, H. R., Lichtenstein, L. M.: The role of cyclic 3',5'-adenosine monophosphate in the specific cytolytic activity of lymphocytes. J. Immunol. **108**, 1526—1534 (1972)

Herbaczynska-Cedro, K., Vane, J. R.: Contribution of intra-renal generation of prostaglandin to autoregulation of renal blood flow in the dog. Circulat. Res. **33**, 428—436 (1973)

Herman, A. G., Moncada, S.: Release of prostaglandins and incapacitation after injection of endotoxin in the knee joint of the dog. Brit. J. Pharmacol. **53**, 465 P (1975)

Hichens, M.: Molecular and cellular pharmacology of the anti-inflammatory drugs: some in vitro properties to their possible modes of action. In: Scherrer, R. A., Whitehouse, M. W. (Eds.): Antiinflammatory Agents, Chemistry, and Pharmacology, Vol. 2, pp. 264—297. New York-San Francisco-London: Academic Press 1974

Higgs, G. A., Harvey, E. A., Ferreira, S. H., Vane, J. R.: The effect of anti-inflammatory drugs on the production of prostaglandins in vivo. In: Samuelsson, B., Paoletti, R. (Eds.): Advances in Prostaglandin and Thromboxane Research, Vol. 1, pp. 105—110. New York: Raven Press 1976

Higgs, G. A., McCall, E., Youlten, L. J. F.: A chemotactic role for prostaglandins released from polymorphonuclear leucocytes during phagocytosis. Brit. J. Pharmacol. **53**, 539—546 (1975)

Higgs, G. A., Vane, J. R., Hart, F. D., Wojtulewski, J. A.: Effects of anti-inflammatory drugs on prostaglandins in rheumatoid arthritis. In: Robinson, H. J., Vane, J. R. (Eds.): Prostaglandin Synthetase Inhibitors, pp. 165—173. New York: Raven Press 1974

Higgs, G. A., Youlten, L. J. F.: Prostaglandin production by rabbit peritoneal polymorphonuclear leukocytes in vitro. Brit. J. Pharmacol. **44**, 330 P (1972)

Hill, A. G. S.: C-reactive protein in rheumatic fever. Lancet **1952** II, 558—560

Hirsch, J. G., Cohn, Z. A.: Degranulation of polymorphonuclear leukocytes following phagocytosis of microorganisms. J. exp. Med. **112**, 1005—1040 (1960)

Holmes, S. W., Horton, E. W., Main, I. H. M.: The effect of prostaglandin E_1 on responses of smooth muscle to catecholamines, angiotensin, and vasopressin. Brit. J. Pharmacol. **21**, 538—543 (1963)

Horton, E. W., Jones, R. L., Marr, C. G.: Effects of aspirin on prostaglandin and fructose levels in human semen. J. Reprod. Fertil. **33**, 385—392 (1973)

Hsia, L. S., Ziboh, A., Snyder, D.: Naturally occurring and synthetic inhibitors of prostaglandin synthetase of the skin. In: Robinson, H. J., Vane, J. R. (Eds.): Prostaglandin Synthetase Inhibitors, pp. 353—361. New York: Raven Press 1974

Hunter, F. E., Scott, A., Hoffsten, P. E., Gebicki, J. M., Weinstein, J., Schneider, A.: Studies on the mechanism of swelling, lysis, and disintegration of isolated liver mitochondria, exposed to mixtures of oxidized and reduced glutathione. J. biol. Chem. **239**, 614—621 (1964)

Hyttel, J., Jorgensen, A.: Studies on lysosome stabilization by antirheumatic drugs. Europ. J. Pharmacol. **11**, 383—387 (1970)

Ichikawa, A., Hayashi, H., Minami, M., Tomita, K.: An acute inflammation induced by inorganic pyrophosphate and adenosine triphosphate, and its inhibition by cyclic 3'5'-adenosine monophosphate. Biochem. Pharmacol. **21**, 317—331 (1972 a)

Ichikawa, A., Nagasaki, M., Umezu, K., Hayashi, H., Tomita, K.: Effect of cyclic 3'5'-adenosine monophosphate on oedema and granuloma induced by carrageenin. Biochem. Pharmacol. **21**, 2615—2626 (1972 b)

Ignarro, L. J.: Effects of anti-inflammatory drugs on the stability of rat liver lysosomes in vitro. Biochem. Pharmacol. **20**, 2847—2860 (1971)

Ignarro, L. J., Colombo, C.: Enzyme release from guinea-pig polymorphonuclear leucocyte lysosomes inhibited in vitro by anti-inflammatory drugs. Nature (New Biol.) **239**, 155—157 (1972)

Ignarro, L. J., Slywka, J.: Changes in liver lysosomes fragility, erythrocyte membrane stability, and local and systematic lysosomal enzyme levels in adjuvant-induced polyarthritis. Biochem. Pharmacol. **21**, 875—886 (1972)

Illiano, G., Cuatrecasas, P.: Endogenous prostaglandins modulate lipolytic processes in adipose tissue. Nature (New Biol.) **234**, 72—74 (1971)

Jacobson, E. D.: Comparison of prostaglandin E_1 and norepinephrine on the gastric mucosal circulation. Proc. Soc. exp. Biol. (N.Y.) **133**, 516—519 (1970)

Jaques, R.: Arachidonic acid, an unsaturated fatty acid which produces slow contractions of smooth muscle and causes pain. Pharmacological and biochemical characterization of its mode of action. Helv. physiol. pharmacol. Acta **17**, 255—267 (1959)

Johansson, H., Lindquist, B.: The effect of calcium acetylsalicylate on the content and distribution of mucus in the rat stomach. Acta Soc. Med. upsalien. **75**, 85—89 (1970)

Jonsson, C. E.: Smooth muscle stimulating lipids in peripheral lymph after experimental burn injury. Scand. J. plast. reconstr. Surg. **5**, 1—5 (1971)

Juhlin, S., Michaelsson, G.: Cutaneous vascular reactions to prostaglandins in healthy subjects and in patients with urticaria and atopic dermatitis. Acta derm.-venereol. (Stockh.) **49**, 251—261 (1969)

Kalbhen, D. A., Domenjoz, R., Ehlers, K.: The effect of sodium salicylate on the ATP-level in normal and inflamed tissues. Life Sci. **6**, 1883—1886 (1967 a)

Kalbhen, D. A., Karzel, K., Domenjoz, R.: The inhibitory effects of some antiphlogistic drugs on the glucosamine incorporation into mucopolysaccharides synthesised by fibroblast cultures. Med. pharmacol. exp. (Basel) **16**, 185—189 (1967 b)

Kaley, G., Weiner, R.: Effect of prostaglandin E$_1$ on leucocyte migration. Nature (New Biol.) **234**, 114—115 (1971 a)

Kaley, G., Weiner, R.: Prostaglandin E$_1$: a potential mediator of the inflammatory response. Ann. N.Y. Acad. Sci. **180**, 338—350 (1971 b)

Kantor, T. G.: Anti-inflammatory drugs. In: Miescher, P. A., Müller-Eberhard, H. J. (Eds.): Textbook of Immunopathology, pp. 217—226. London: Grune 1968

Kantrowitz, F., Robinson, D., McGuire, M., Levine, L.: Corticosteroids inhibit prostaglandins production by rheumatoid synovia. Nature (Lond.) **258**, 737—739 (1975)

Kaulla, K. N. von: Chemistry of Thrombolysis: Human Fibrinolytic Enzymes. Springfield Ill.: Charles C. Thomas 1963

Kaulla, K. N. von: Structure-dependent fibrinolytic (clot-dissolving) activity of anti-inflammatory drugs and related compounds. Arzneimittel-Forsch. **18**, 407—412 (1968)

Koopman, W. J., Orange, R. P., Austen, K. F.: Immunochemical and biologic properties of rat IgE. III. Modulation of the IgE-mediated release of slow-reacting substance of anaphylaxis by agents influencing the level of 3′,5′-adenosine monophosphate[1]. J. Immunol. **105**, 1096—1102 (1971)

Kraut, H., Bhargava, N., Schultz, F., Zimmermann, H.: Isolierung des Kallikrein-Inaktivators. IV. Kristallisation und Aminosäurezusammensetzung. Vergleich mit dem Trypsin-Inhibitor von Kunitz und Northrop. Hoppe-Seylers Z. physiol. Chem. **334**, 230—235 (1963)

Lazarus, G. S., Brown, R. S., Daniels, J. R., Fullmer, H. M.: Human granulocyte collagenase. Science **159**, 1483—1485 (1968)

Lee, K. H., Spencer, M. R.: Studies on mechanisms of action of salicylates. V. Effect of salicylic acid on enzymes involved in mucopolysaccharides synthesis. J. pharm. Sci. **58**, 464—468 (1969)

Lee, R. E.: The influence of psychotropic drugs on prostaglandin biosynthesis. Prostaglandins **5**, 63—68 (1974)

Lepper, M. H., Candwell, E. R., Jr., Smith, P. K., Miller, B. F.: Effects of anaphylactic shock of salicylates, aminopyrine, and other chemically and pharmacologically related compounds. Proc. Soc. exp. Biol. (N.Y.) **74**, 254—258 (1950)

Levitan, H., Barker, J. L.: Effect of non-narcotic analgesics on membrane permeability of molluscan neurones. Nature (New Biol.) **239**, 55—57 (1972)

Lewis, A. J., Nelson, D. J., Sugrue, M. F.: On the ability of prostaglandin E$_1$ and arachidonic acid to modulate experimentally induced oedema in the rat paw. Brit. J. Pharmacol. **55**, 51—56 (1975)

Lewis, G. P.: Pharmacological actions of bradykinin and its role in physiological and pathological reactions. Ann. N.Y. Acad. Sci. **104**, 236—249 (1963)

Lewis, G. P., Piper, P. J.: Inhibition of release of prostaglandins as an explanation of some of the actions of anti-inflammatory corticosteroids. Nature (Lond.) **254**, 308—311 (1975)

Lewis, R. B., Schulman, J. D.: Influence of acetylsalicylic acid, an inhibitor of prostaglandin synthesis, on the duration of human gestation and labour. Lancet **1973 II**, 1159—1161

Lewis, S. E., Wills, E. D.: The destruction of -SH groups of proteins and amino acids by peroxides of unsaturated fatty acids. Biochem. Pharmacol. **11**, 901—912 (1962)

Lichtenstein, L. M., Bourne, H. R.: Inhibition of allergic histamine release by histamine and other agents which stimulate adenyl cyclase. In: Austen, K. F., Becker, E. L. (Eds.): Biochemistry of the Acute Allergic Reactions, pp. 161—174. London: Blackwell 1971

Lichtenstein, L. M., De Bernardo, R.: The immediate allergic response: in vitro action of cyclic AMP-active and other drugs on the two stages of histamine release. J. Immunol. **107**, 1131—1136 (1971)

Lim, R. K. S.: Salicylate analgesia. In: Smith, M. K., Smith, P. K. (Eds.): The Salicylates, pp. 151—202. New York-London-Sydney: Interscience Publishers 1966

Lindner, H. R., Zor, U., Bauminger, S., Tsafriri, A., Lamprecht, S. A., Koch, Y., Antebi, S., Schwartz, A.: Use of prostaglandin synthetase inhibitors in analyzing the role of prostaglandins in reproductive physiology. In: Robinson, H. J., Vane, J. R. (Eds.): Prostaglandin Synthetase Inhibitors, pp. 271—287. New York: Raven Press 1974

Lish, P. M., McKinney, G. R.: Pharmacology of methdilazine. II. Some determinants and limits of action on vascular permeability and inflammation in model systems. J. Lab. clin. Med. **61**, 1015—1028 (1963)

Lorber, A., Pearson, C. M., Meredith, W. L., Gantz-Mandell, L. E.: Serum Sulfhydryl determinations and significance in connective tissue diseases. Ann. intern. Med. **61**, 423—434 (1964)

Maddox, I. S.: Copper in prostaglandin biosynthesis. Biochim. biophys. Acta **306**, 74—81 (1973)

Maickel, R. P., Miller, F. P., Brodie, B. B.: Interaction of non-steroidal anti-inflammatory agents with corticosteroid binding to plasma proteins. Pharmacologist **7**, 182 (1965)

Main, I. H. M., Whittle, B. J. R.: Effects of prostaglandin E_2 on rat gastric mucosal blood flow, as determined by ^{14}C-aniline clearance. Brit. J. Pharmacol. **44**, 331 P—332 P (1972)

Main, I. H. M., Whittle, B. J. R.: Prostaglandins and prostaglandin synthetase inhibitors in gastrointestinal function and disease. In: Robinson, H. J., Vane, J. R. (Eds.): Prostaglandin Synthetase Inhibitors, pp. 363—372. New York: Raven Press 1974

Majno, G., Ryan, G. B., Gabbiani, G., Hirschel, B. J., Irlé, C., Joris, I.: Contractile events in inflammation and repair. In: Lepow, I. H., Ward, P. A. (Eds.): Inflammation, Mechanisms, and Control, pp. 13—27. New York-London: Academic Press 1972

Malawista, S. E., Bodel, P. T.: The dissociation by colchicine of phagocytosis from increased oxygen consumption in human leukocytes. J. clin. Invest. **46**, 786—789 (1967)

Margaretten, W., McKay, D. G.: The requirement for platelets in the active Arthus reaction. Amer. J. Path. **64**, 257—270 (1971)

Marmont, A. M., Rossi, F., Damasio, E.: Indomethacin in the treatment of rheumatic and non-rheumatic diseases, with special reference to systemic lupus erythematosus. In: Garattini, S., Dukes, M. M. G. (Eds.): International Symposium on Non-Steroid Anti-Inflammatory Drugs, International Congress Series 82, pp. 363—372. New York: Excerpta Medica Foundation 1965

Martin, B. K.: Accumulation of drug anions in gastric mucosal cells. Nature (Lond.) **198**, 896—897 (1963)

Mauer, E. F.: The toxic effects of phenylbutazone (Butazolidin): review of the literature and report of the twenty-third death following its use. New Engl. J. Med. **253**, 404—410 (1955)

McArthur, J. M., Smith, M. J. H., Hamilton, E. D.: Protein-bound peptides in human serum. Brit. med. J. **1971 IV**, 230

McGiff, J. C., Terragno, N. A., Itskovitz, H. D.: Role of renal prostaglandins as revealed by inhibitors of prostaglandin synthetase. In: Robinson, H. J., Vane, J. R. (Eds.): Prostaglandin Synthetase Inhibitors, pp. 259—269. New York: Raven Press 1974

Messina, E. J., Weiner, R., Kaley, G.: Inhibition of bradykinin vasodilation and potentiation of norepinephrine and angiotensin vasoconstriction by inhibitors of prostaglandin synthesis in skeletal muscle of the rat. Circulat. Res. **37**, 430—437 (1975)

Miller, J. D., Eakins, K. E., Atwal, M.: The release of PGE_2-like activity into aqueous humour after paracentesis and its prevention by aspirin. Invest. Opthal. **12**, 939—942 (1973)

Miller, W. S., Smith, J. G.: Effect of acetylsalicylic acid on lysosomes. Proc. Soc. exp. Biol. (N.Y.) **122**, 634—636 (1966)

Milton, A. S.: Prostaglandin E_1 and endotoxin fever, and the effects of aspirin, indomethacin, and 4-acetamidophenol. In: Bergström, S., Bwenhard, S. (Eds.): Advances in the Biosciences. International Conference on Prostaglandins, Vienna 1972, Vol. IX, pp. 495—500. Braunschweig: Pergamon Press-Vieweg 1973

Milton, A. S., Wendlandt, S.: Effects on body temperature of prostaglandins of the A, E, and F series on injection into the third ventricle of unanaesthetized cats and rabbits. J. Physiol. (Lond.) **218**, 325—336 (1971)

Mizushima, Y.: Inhibition of protein denaturation by antirheumatic or antiphlogistic agents. Arch. int. Pharmacodyn. **149**, 1—7 (1964)

Mizushima, Y.: Simple screening test for antirheumatic drugs. Lancet **1965 I**, 169—170

Mizushima, Y., Kobayashi, M.: Interaction of anti-inflammatory drugs with serum proteins, especially with some biologically active proteins. J. Pharm. (Lond.) **20**, 169—173 (1968)

Mizushima, Y., Suzuki, H.: Interaction between plasma proteins and antirheumatic or new antiphlogistic drugs. Arch. int. Pharmacodyn. **157**, 115—124 (1965)

Moncada, S., Ferreira, S. H., Vane, J. R.: Prostaglandins, aspirin-like drugs and the oedema of inflammation. Nature (Lond.) **246**, 217—219 (1973)

Moncada, S., Ferreira, S. H., Vane, J. R.: Inhibition of prostaglandin biosynthesis as the mechanism of analgesia of aspirin-like drugs in the dog knee joint. Europ. J. Pharmacol. **31**, 250—260 (1975)

Moncada, S., Needleman, S., Bunting, S., Vane, J. R.: Prostaglandin endoperoxide and thromboxane generating system and their selective inhibition. Prostaglandins **12**, 323—336 (1976)

Moon, V. H., Tershakovec, G. A.: Influence of cortisone upon acute inflammation. Proc. Soc. exp. Biol. (N.Y.) **79**, 63—65 (1952)

Moon, V. H., Tershakovec, G. A.: Effect of cortisone upon local capillary permeability. Proc. Soc. exp. Biol. (N.Y.) **85**, 600—603 (1954)

Moore, D. F., Lowenthal, J., Fuller, M., Jacques, L. B.: Inhibition of experimental arthritis by cortisone, salicylate, and related compounds. Amer. J. clin. Path. **22**, 936—943 (1952)

Moretti, A., Penati, M. R., Zambotii, V.: Effect of prednisolone and indomethacin on UDPG: NAD oxido-reductase in granulomatous tissue. Arq. Port. Bioquim. **9**, 259—260 (1966): (see Chem. Abs. **67**, 4753, 1967)

Morley, J.: Prostaglandins and lymphokines in arthritis. Prostaglandins **8**, 315—326 (1974)

Munck, A.: Glucocorticoid inhibition of glucose uptake by peripheral tissues; old and new evidence, molecular mechanisms, and physiological significance. Perspect. Biol. Med. **14**, 265—269 (1971)

Narumi, S., Kanno, M.: Effects of the non-steroidal antiphlogistics on the gastric mucosal barrier and hexosamine content in rats. Jap. J. Pharmacol. **22**, 675—684 (1972)

Needleman, P., Moncada, S., Bunting, S., Vane, J. R., Hamberg, M., Samuelsson, B.: Identification of an enzyme in platelet microsomes which generates thromboxane A_2 from prostaglandin endoperoxides. Nature (Lond.) **261**, 559—560 (1976)

Northover, B. J., Subramanian, G.: Analgesic-antipyretic drugs as inhibitors of kallikrein. Brit. J. Pharmacol. **17**, 107—115 (1961)

Northover, B. J., Subramanian, G.: Analgesic-antipyretic drugs as antagonists of endotoxin shock in dogs. J. Path. Bact. **83**, 463—468 (1962)

Nugteren, D. H.: Arachidonate lipoxygenase in blood platelets. Biochim. biophys. Acta (Amst.) **380**, 299—307 (1975)

O'Brien, J. R.: Effect of anti-inflammatory agents on platelets. Lancet **1968 a I**, 894—895

O'Brien, J. R.: Effects of salicylates on human platelets. Lancet **1968 b I**, 779—783

O'Grady, J. P., Caldwell, B. V., Auletta, F. J., Speroff, L.: The effects of an inhibitor of prostaglandin synthesis (indomethacin) on ovulation, pregnancy, and pseudopregnancy in the rabbit. Prostaglandins **1**, 97—106 (1972)

Orange, R. P., Austen, K. F.: Pharmacologic dissociation of immunologic release of histamine and slow reacting substance of anaphylaxis in rats. Proc. Soc. exp. Biol. (N.Y.) **129**, 836—841 (1968)

Orszyk, G. P., Behrman, H. R.: Ovulation blockade by aspirin or indomethacin: in vivo evidence for a role of prostaglandin in gonadotrophin secretion. Prostaglandins **1**, 3—20 (1972)

Palmer, M. A., Piper, P. J., Vane, J. R.: Release of rabbit aorta contracting substance (RCS) and prostaglandin induced by chemical or mechanical stimulation of guinea-pig lungs. Brit. J. Pharmacol. **49**, 226—242 (1973)

Patrono, C., Ciabattoni, G., Di Munno, O., Bombardieri, S., Greco, F., Grossi, D.: Evidence for in vivo and in vitro inhibition of prostaglandin synthesis in human synovial membrane by aspirin-like drugs. In: Proceedings of the Sixth International Congress of Pharmacology, Helsinki, Abstract 1447, 1975

Perry, C. E.: The action of salicylates on the development of anti-bodies following anti-typhoid inoculation. J. Path. Bact. **53**, 291—297 (1941)

Piper, P. J., Vane, J. R.: The release of prostaglandins during anaphylaxis in guinea-pig isolated lungs. In: Mantegazza, P., Horton, E. W. (Eds.): Prostaglandins, Peptides, and Amines, pp. 15—19. London-New York: Academic Press 1969 a

Piper, P. J., Vane, J. R.: Release of additional factors in anaphylaxis and its antagonism by anti-inflammatory drugs. Nature (Lond.) **223**, 29—35 (1969 b)

Piper, P. J., Vane, J. R.: The release of prostaglandin from lung and other tissues. Ann. N.Y. Acad. Sci. **180**, 363—385 (1971)

Pong, S. S., Levine, L.: Prostaglandin synthetase systems of rabbit tissues and their inhibition by non-steroidal anti-inflammatory drugs. J. Pharmacol. exp. Ther. **196**, 226—230 (1976)

Poyser, N. L., Horton, E. W., Thompson, C. J., Los, M.: Identification of prostaglandin $F_{2\alpha}$ released by distension of the guinea-pig uterus in vitro. Nature (Lond.) **230**, 526—528 (1970)

Quick, A. J., Clesceri, L.: Influence of acetylsalicylic acid and salicylamide on the coagulation of blood. J. Pharmacol. exp. Ther. **128**, 95—98 (1960)

Rainsford, K. D.: The effects of salicylates on gastric tissues. Ph. D. Thesis, University of London 1970

Rainsford, K. D.: The biochemical pathology of aspirin-induced gastric damage. Agents Actions **5**, 326—344 (1975)

Rainsford, K. D., Watkins, J., Smith, M. J. H.: Aspirin and mucus. J. Pharm. (Lond.) **20**, 941—943 (1968)

Randall, L. O.: Non narcotic analgesic. In: Rodt, W. S., Hofmann, F. G. (Eds.): Physiological Pharmacology: a Comprehensive Treatise, pp. 214—416. New York-London: Academic Press 1963

Redei, A., Kelemen, E.: Presence of platelets in acute experimental inflammatory oedema inhibited by salicylate or cortisone. In: Bertelli, A., Houck, J. C. (Eds.): Inflammation Biochemistry and Drug Interaction, Proceedings of an International Symposium, Italy 1968, pp. 261—265. Amsterdam: Excerpta Medica Foundation 1969

Robert, A.: The role of prostaglandins in the etiology and treatment of gastrointestinal diseases. In: Proceedings Sixth International Congress of Pharmacology, Helsinki **5**, 161—173 (1975)

Robertson, A. L., Khairallah, P. A.: Effects of angiotensin II on the permeability of the vascular wall. In: Page, I. H., Bumpus, F. M. (Eds.): Angiotensin, pp. 500—510. Berlin-Heidelberg-New York: Springer 1974

Robinson, D. R., Levine, L.: Prostaglandin concentrations in synovial fluid in rheumatic diseases: action of indomethacin and aspirin. In: Robinson, H. J., Vane, J. R. (Eds.): Prostaglandin Synthetase Inhibitors, pp. 327—343. New York: Raven Press 1974

Robinson, H. J., Phares, H. F., Graessle, O. E.: Prostaglandin synthetase inhibitors and infection. In: Robinson, H. J., Vane, J. R. (Eds.): Prostaglandin Synthetase Inhibitors, pp. 327—342. New York: Raven Press 1974

Roger, J., Kalbhen, D. A.: Der Adenosintriphosphat-Gehalt des Knorpels unter dem Einfluß verschiedener Antirheumatica in vitro. Arzneimittel-Forsch. **18**, 1512—1516 (1968)

Rosenthale, M. E.: Evaluation for immunosuppressive and anti-allergic activity. In: Scherrer, R. A., Whitehouse, M. W. (Eds.): Antiinflammatory Agents, Chemistry and Pharmacology, Vol. 2, pp. 123—192. New York-San Francisco-London: Academic Press 1974

Rothschild, A. M.: Pharmacodynamic properties of cellulose sulfate and related polysaccharides—a group of bradykinin-releasing compounds. In: Rocha e Silva, M., Rothschild, H. A. (Eds.): International Symposium on Vaso-Active Polypeptides: Bradykinin and Related Kinins, pp. 197—203. São Paulo: SBFTE 1967

Roubal, Z., Němeček, O.: Anti-inflammatory compounds exhibiting fibrinolytic activity. J. med. Chem. **9**, 840—842 (1966 a)

Roubal, Z., Němeček, O.: Activation of fibrinolysis by derivatives of diphenyldioxopyrazolidine. Nature (Lond.) **212**, 861 (1966 b)

Samuelsson, B., Hamberg, M., Malmsten, C., Svensson, J.: Physiological role of prostaglandin endoperoxides and thromboxanes in human platelets. In: Proceedings Sixth International Congress of Pharmacology, Helsinki, pp. 131—138, 1975

Schayer, R. W.: Relationship of induced histamine decarboxylase activity and (histamine) synthesis to shock from stress and from endotoxin. Amer. J. Physiol. **198**, 1187—1192 (1960)

Schayer, R. W.: A unified theory of glucocorticoid action. Perspect. Biol. Med. **8**, 71—84 (1964)

Schönhöfer, P.: Die Wirkung von entzündungshemmenden Pharmaka auf die Glucosamin-6-phosphat Synthese in Rattenleberhomogenaten. Med. pharmacol. exp. (Basel) **15**, 491—499 (1966)

Schönhöfer, P.: Eine kritische Bemerkung zur Vergleichbarkeit der Wirkung entzündungshemmender Pharmaka auf die Glucosamin-6-phosphat-Synthese in vitro und am Rattenpfotenödem in vivo. Med. pharmacol. exp. (Basel) **16**, 66—74 (1967)

Schwartz, C. S., Mandel, H. G.: The selective inhibition of microbial RNA synthesis by salicylate. Biochem. Pharmacol. **21**, 771—785 (1972)

Shaw, J. E., Ramwell, P. W.: Inhibition of gastric secretion in rats by prostaglandin E_1. In: Ramwell, P. W., Shaw, J. E. (Eds.): Prostaglandins, pp. 55—56. New York: Wiley 1968

Shen, T. Y., Ham, E. A., Cirillo, V. J., Zanetti, M.: Structure-activity relationship of certain prostaglandin synthetase inhibitors. In: Robinson, H. J., Vane, J. R. (Eds.): Prostaglandin Synthetase Inhibitors, pp. 19—31. New York: Raven Press 1974

Shwartzman, G., Schneierson, S. S.: Inhibition of the phenomenon of local tissue reactivity by corticosteroids, salicylates and compounds related to salicylate. Ann. N.Y. Acad. Sci. **56**, 733 (1953)

Siggins, G. R.: Prostaglandins and the microvascular system: physiological and histochemical correlations. In: Ramwell, P. W., Pharris, B. P. (Eds.): Prostaglandins in Cellular Biology, pp. 451—476. New York-London: Plenum Press 1972

Silver, M. J., Smith, J. B., Ingerman, C. M.: Blood platelets and the inflammatory process. Agents Actions **4**, 233—240 (1974)

Skidmore, I. F., Whitehouse, M. W.: Biochemical properties of anti-inflammatory drugs. VIII. Inhibition of histamine formation catalysed by substrate specific mammalian histidine decarboxylases. Drug antagonism of aldehyde binding to protein amino groups. Biochem. Pharmacol. **15**, 1965—1983 (1966)

Smith, J. B., Willis, A. L.: Aspirin selectively inhibits prostaglandin production in human platelets. Nature (New Biol.) **231**, 235—237 (1971)

Smith, M. J. H.: Toxicology. In: Smith, M. J. H., Smith, P. K. (Eds.): The Salicylates, pp. 233—306. New York-London: Interscience Publ. 1966

Smith, M. J. H.: Prostaglandins and aspirin: an alternative view. Agents Actions **5**, 315—317 (1975)

Smith, M. J. H., Dawkins, P. D.: Salicylate and enzymes. J. Pharm. (Lond.) **23**, 729—744 (1971)

Smith, M. J. H., Ford-Hutchinson, A. W., Elliott, P. N. C.: Prostaglandins and the anti-inflammatory activities of aspirin and sodium salicylate. J. Pharm. (Lond.) **27**, 473—478 (1975)

Smith, M. J. H., Ford-Hutchinson, A. W., Elliot, P. N. C., Bolam, J. P.: Prostaglandins and the anti-inflammatory activity of a human plasma fraction in carrageenin-induced paw oedema in the rat. J. Pharm. (Lond.) **26**, 692—698 (1974)

Solomon, L. M., Juhlin, L., Kirschenbaum, M. B.: Prostaglandin on cutaneous vasculature. J. invest. Derm. **51**, 280—282 (1968)

Spain, D. M., Molomut, N., Harber, A.: Studies of cortisone effects on the inflammatory response; alterations of histopathology of chemically induced inflammation. J. Lab. clin. Med. **39**, 383—389 (1952)

Spector, W. G., Willoughby, D. A.: Anti-inflammatory effects of salicylate in the rat. In: Dixon, A. St. J., Martin, B. K., Smith, M. J. H., Wood, P. H. N. (Eds.): Salicylates, an International Symposium, London 1962, pp. 141—147. London: J. and A. Churchill Ltd. 1963

Starr, M. S., West, G. B.: Bradykinin and oedema formation in heated paws of rats. Brit. J. Pharmacol. **31**, 178—187 (1967)

Tanaka, K., Iizuka, Y.: Suppression of enzyme release from isolated rat liver lysosomes by nonsteroidal anti-inflammatory drugs. Biochem. Pharmacol. **17**, 2023—2032 (1968)

Tashjian, A. H., Voelkel, E. F., McDonough, J., Levine, L.: Hydrocortisone inhibits prostaglandin production by mouse fibrosarcoma cells. Nature (Lond.) **258**, 739—741 (1975)

Tauber, A. I., Kaliner, M., Stechschulter, K. J., Austen, K. F.: Immunologic release of histamine and slow reacting substance of anaphylaxis from human lung. V. Effects of prostaglandins on release of histamine. J. Immunol. **111**, 27—32 (1973)

Terragno, D. A., Crowshaw, K., Terragno, N. A., McGiff, J. C.: Prostaglandin synthesis by bovine mesenteric arteries and veins. Circulat. Res. **36**, 176—180 (1975)

Thomas, G., West, G. B.: Prostaglandins as regulators of bradykinin responses. J. Pharm. (Lond.) **25**, 747—748 (1973)

Tomlinson, R. V., Ringold, H. J., Qureshi, M. C., Forchielli, E.: Relationship between inhibitors of prostaglandin synthesis and drug efficacy: support for the current theory on mode of action of aspirin-like drugs. Biochem. biophys. Res. Commun. **46**, 552—559 (1972)

Trnavská, Z., Grimová, J., Trnavský, K.: Collagen metabolism in adjuvant-induced arthritis in the rat. Ann. rheum. Dis. **31**, 334—338 (1972)

Trnavský, K.: Some effects of anti-inflammatory drugs on connective tissue metabolism. In: Scherrer, R. A., Whitehouse, M. W. (Eds.): Anti-inflammatory Agents: Chemistry and Pharmacology, Vol. 2, pp. 264—297. New York-San Francisco-London: Academic Press 1974

Turner, S. R., Campbell, J. A., Lynn, W. S.: Polymorphonuclear leukocyte chemotaxis toward oxidised lipid components of cell membranes. J. exp. Med. **141**, 1437—1441 (1975)

Ubatuba, F. B., Harvey, E. A., Ferreira, S. H.: Are platelets important in inflammation? Agents Actions **5**, 31—34 (1975)

Van Arman, C. G.: Personal communication (1972)

Van Arman, C. G., Carlson, R. P.: Anti-inflammatory drugs and the behaviour of leucocytes. In: Velo, G. P., Willoughby, D. A., Giroud, J. A. (Eds.): Future Trends in Inflammation, pp. 159—169. Padua-London: Piccin Medical Books 1974

Van Arman, C. G., Carlson, R. P., Risley, E. A., Thomas, R. H., Nuss, G. W.: Inhibitory effects of indomethacin, aspirin, and certain drugs on inflammation induced in rat and dog by carrageenin, sodium urate and ellagic acid. J. Pharmacol. exp. Ther. **175**, 459—468 (1970)

Van Arman, C. G., Nuss, G. W., Winter, C. A., Flataker, L.: Proteolytic enzymes as mediators of pain. In: Lim, R. K. S., Armstrong, D., Pardo, E. G. (Eds.): Pharmacology of Pain, Third International Pharmacological Meeting, Vol. 9, pp. 25—32. London-New York: Pergamon Press 1966

Vane, J. R.: Inhibition of prostaglandin synthesis as a mechanism of action for aspirin-like drugs. Nature (New Biol.) **231**, 232—235 (1971)

Vane, J. R.: Prostaglandins and the aspirin-like drugs. Hosp. Pract. **7**, 61—71 (1972)

Vane, J. R.: Aspirin. Proceedings of a Conference held at the Royal College of Physicians of London, 1974. In: Breckenridge, A. M. (Ed.): Advanced Medicine, Topics in Therapeutics, pp. 64—72. London: Pitman Medical Co. 1975

Vane, J. R., Ferreira, S. H.: Interactions between bradykinin and prostaglandins. International Symposium on the Chemistry and Biology of the Kallikrein-kinin System in Health and Disease. Fogarty International Center Proceedings 27. Life Sci. **16**, 804—805 (1975)

Vane, J. R., Williams, K. I.: The contribution of prostaglandin production to contractions of the isolated uterus of the rat. Brit. J. Pharmacol. **48**, 629—639 (1973)

Vargaftig, B. B.: Search for common mechanisms underlying the various effects of putative inflammatory mediators. In: Ramwell, P. W. (Ed.): The Prostaglandins II, pp. 205—276. New York-London: Plenum Press 1974

Vargaftig, B. B., Dao Hai, N.: Release of vaso-active substance from guinea-pig lungs by slow reacting substance C and arachidonic acid. Pharmacology (Basel) **6**, 99—108 (1971)

Vargaftig, B. B., Dao Hai, N.: Selective inhibition by mepacrine of the release of rabbit aorta contracting substance evoked by the administration of bradykinin. J. Pharm. (Lond.) **24**, 159—161 (1972)

Wagner-Jauregg, T., Fisher, J.: Über die Hemmung des Wachstums von *Lactobacillus casei* durch einige Antiphlogistica. Experientia (Basel) **24**, 1029—1031 (1968)

Walker, J. L.: The regulatory function of prostaglandins in the release of histamine and SRS-A from passively sensitized human lung tissue. In: Bergström, S., Bernhard, S. (Eds.): Advances in the Biosciences, International Conference on Prostaglandins, Vol. IX, pp. 235—240. Braunschweig: Pergamon Press-Vieweg 1973

Waltman, R., Tricomi, V., Palav, A. B.: Aspirin and indomethacin: effect on instillation abortion time of mid-trimester hypertonic saline-induced abortion. Prostaglandins **3**, 47—58 (1973)

Ward, P. A.: The inflammatory mediators. Ann. N.Y. Acad. Sci. **221**, 290—298 (1974)

Ward, P. A., Cochrane, C. G.: Bound complement and immunologic injury of blood vessels. J. exp. Med. **121**, 215—234 (1965)

Wax, J., Winder, C. V., Tessman, D. K., Stephens, M. D.: Comparative activities, tolerances and safety of non-steroidal anti-inflammatory agents in rats. J. Pharmacol. exp. Ther. **192**, 172—175 (1975)

Webster, M. E., Pierce, J. V.: Studies on plasma kallikrein and its relationship to plasmin. J. Pharmacol. exp. Ther. **130**, 484 (1960)

Weissmann, G.: Lysosomal mechanisms of tissue injury in arthritis. New Engl. J. Med. **286**, 141—147 (1972)

Weissmann, G., Dukor, P., Zurier, R. B.: Effect of cyclic AMP on release of lysosomal enzymes from phagocytes. Nature (New Biol.) **231**, 131—135 (1971a)

Weissmann, G., Thomas, L.: The effects of corticosteroids upon connective tissue and lysosomes. Recent Progr. Hormone Res. **20**, 215—245 (1964)

Weissmann, G., Zurier, R. B., Spieler, P. J., Goldstein, I. M.: Mechanisms of lysosomal enzyme release from leukocytes exposed to immune complexes and other particles. J. exp. Med. **134**, Suppl., 149—165 (1971b)

Whitehouse, M. W.: Some biochemical and pharmacological properties of anti-inflammatory drugs. Fortschr. Arzneimittel.-Forsch. **8**, 321—429 (1965)

Whitehouse, M. W.: Introduction and background to the regulation of inflammation and immune response. In: Scherrer, R. A., Whitehouse, M. W. (Eds.): Anti-inflammatory Agents, Vol. II, pp. 1—31. New York: Academic Press 1974

Wilhelmi, G., Domenjoz, R.: Vergleichende Untersuchungen über die Wirkung von Pyrazolen und Antihistaminen bei verschiedenen Arten der experimentellen Entzündung. Arch. int. Pharmacodyn. **85**, 129—143 (1951)

Williams, K. I., Vane, J. R.: Inhibition of uterine motility: the possible role of the prostaglandins and aspirin-like drugs. Pharmacol. Ther. B. **1**, 89—113 (1975)

Williams, T. J., Morley, J.: Prostaglandins as potentiators of increased vascular permeability in inflammation. Nature (Lond.) **246**, 215—217 (1973)

Willis, A. L.: Parallel assay of prostaglandin-like activity in rat inflammatory exudate by means of cascade superfusion. J. Pharm. (Lond.) **21**, 126—128 (1969a)

Willis, A. L.: Release of histamine, kinin, and prostaglandin during carrageenin-induced inflammation in the rat. In: Mantegazza, P., Horton, E. W. (Eds.): Prostaglandins, Peptides, and Amines, pp. 33—38. London-New York: Academic Press 1969b

Willis, A. L., Davidson, P., Ramwell, P. W., Brocklehurst, W. B., Smith, B.: Release and actions of prostaglandins in inflammation and fever: inhibition by anti-inflammatory and anti-pyretic drugs. In: Ramwell, P. W., Pharris, B. B. (Eds.): Prostaglandins in Cellular Biology, pp. 227—259. New York-London: Plenum Press 1972

Willoughby, D. A.: Effects of prostaglandins $PGF_{2\alpha}$ and PGE_1 on vascular permeability. J. Path. Bact. **96**, 381—387 (1968)

Willoughby, D. A., Giroud, J. P.: The role of polymorphonuclear leucocytes in acute inflammation in agranulocytic rats. J. Path. **98**, 53—60 (1969)

Winder, C. V.: Aspirin and algesimetry. Nature (Lond.) **184**, 494—497 (1959)

Winter, C. A.: Anti-inflammatory testing methods: comparative evaluation of indomethacin and other agents. In: Garattini, S., Dukes, M. N. G. (Eds.): Nonsteroidal Anti-Inflammatory Drugs, pp. 190—202. Amsterdam: Excerpta Medica Foundation 1965

Winter, C. A.: Non-steroid anti-inflammatory agents. Ann. Rev. Pharmacol. **6**, 157—174 (1966)

Wiseman, E. H., Reinert, H.: Anti-inflammatory drugs and renal papillary necrosis. Agents Actions **5**, 322—325 (1975)

Wiqvist, N., Lundström, V., Gréen, K.: Indomethacin and premature labour. In: Samuelsson, B., Paoletti, B. (Eds.): Advances in Prostaglandin and Thromboxane Research, Vol. II, p. 998. New York: Raven Press 1976

Wyman, L. C., Fulton, G. P., Schulman, M. H., Smith, L. L.: Vasoconstriction in the cheek pouch of the hamster following treatment with cortisone. Amer. J. Physiol. **176**, 335—340 (1954)

Zanin, T., Garcia Leme, J., Ferreira, S. H.: Edema e aumento de permeabilidade induzido pela carragenina. In: The Proceedings of 28th Meeting of S.B.P.C., Brazil, 1976

Zimmerman, T. J., Gravenstein, N., Sugar, A., Kaufman, H.: Aspirin stabilization of the blood-aqueous barrier in human eye. Amer. J. Opthal. **79**, 817—819 (1975)

Zurier, R. B., Ballas, M.: Prostaglandin E_1 (PGE_1) suppression of adjuvant arthritis. Histophatology. Arthr. Rheum. **16**, 251—257 (1973)

Zurier, R. B., Hoffstein, S., Weissmann, G.: Cytochalasin B: effect on lysosomal enzyme release from human leucocytes. Proc. nat. Acad. Sci. (Wash.) **70**, 844—848 (1973)

Zurier, R. B., Quagliata, F.: Effect of prostaglandin E_1 on adjuvant arthritis. Nature (Lond.) **234**, 304—305 (1971)

CHAPTER 32

Penicillamine and Drugs With a Specific Action in Rheumatoid Arthritis

E. C. HUSKISSON

For many years, the objective of much research into the drug treatment of rheumatic disease has been the development of better ways of suppressing inflammation. This approach has made little impact in rheumatoid arthritis (RA), a disease which appears to be more appropriately treated with specific drugs like D-penicillamine. Drugs of this type are not only more effective than anti-inflammatory drugs in RA but, with long-term therapy, they may alter the eventual outcome of the disease.

A. Classification of Antirheumatic Drugs

Antirheumatic drugs may be classified as shown in Table 1 (HUSKISSON, 1974). The first four classes should be regarded as nonspecific or symptomatic therapy. Analgesics only relieve pain. The nonsteroidal analgesic anti-inflammatory drugs in groups 2 and 3 relieve pain in the same way as simple analgesics but also reduce swelling and stiffness, which are regarded as manifestations of inflammation. The pure anti-inflammatory drugs, including steroids, suppress inflammation without having any direct analgesic effect. There is no evidence that any of these groups of drugs alters the course of RA, no matter how complete the suppression of inflammation achieved.

This chapter is concerned with drugs of group 5, those which have a specific action in RA. These compounds should not be regarded as anti-inflammatory drugs; the properties of the two classes of drugs are contrasted in Table 2. Both types of drug will produce relief of pain and reduction of swelling and stiffness in RA; whereas anti-inflammatory drugs will achieve this effect within a few days, specific drugs will take a few months. In many inflammatory arthropathies other than RA, penicillamine is not effective, but the anti-inflammatory drugs will be just as effective whatever the nature of the condition treated. Claims have been made that some of the specific drugs are effective in other diseases, for example gold in psoriatic arthropathy (WRIGHT, 1959), but very few formal trials have been carried out. These drugs

Table 1. Classification of drugs used for rheumatic diseases

Group 1	Simple analgesics e.g., paracetamol
Group 2	Analgesics with minor anti-inflammatory properties e.g., ibuprofen
Group 3	Analgesics with major anti-inflammatory properties e.g., indomethacin
Group 4	Pure anti-inflammatory drugs e.g., steroids
Group 5	Drugs with a specific action in RA e.g., D-penicillamine
Group 6	Drugs with a specific action in other diseases e.g., allopurinol

Table 2. Comparison of the properties of anti-inflammatory drugs and drugs with a specific action in RA

	Anti-inflammatory drugs	Drugs specific for RA
Relief of pain	Yes	Yes
Speed of action	Days	Months
Reduction in inflammation (swelling, stiffness)	Yes	Yes
Improvement in extra-articular disease e.g., nodules	No	Yes
Reduction in ESR	Slight or absent	Yes
Reduction in RF titre	No	Yes
Outcome of RA	Unchanged	Improved prognosis
Effectiveness in other arthropathies	Yes	Less or none
Effectiveness in animal models of inflammation	Yes	Usually none

Table 3. Compounds which may have a specific action in RA[a]

Definite	D-penicillamine; Gold salts; Chloroquine; Immunosuppressives; Levamisole
Possible	Clotrimazole; Alclofenac

[a] This list is probably incomplete and for some of the possible compounds, evidence is very limited.

are certainly not effective except in occasional arthropathies despite the presence of inflammation. In addition to their effect on pain and inflammation in RA, specific drugs lead to improvement in extra-articular features of the disease such as nodules, reduction in erythrocyte sedimentation rate (ESR) and rheumatoid factor (RF) titre, and may improve the prognosis of the disease.

Although gold has been available since the 1920s, it was D-penicillamine which awakened the interest of rheumatologists in this class of drugs and stimulated much work directed at finding the mode of action of similar drugs. Compounds which may have this type of action are listed in Table 3. It is convenient to consider D-penicillamine first and to compare its properties with other drugs of the same type.

B. Penicillamine

I. Actions in Man

Penicillamine ($\beta\beta$-dimethylcysteine; Fig. 1) is a degradation product of penicillin, prepared by hydrolysis. It was first used in RA because it was known to dissociate macroglobulins and it was believed that removal of RF might be useful. Jaffe (1962)

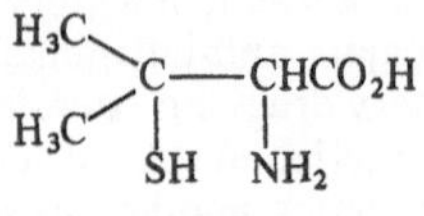

$$
\begin{array}{c}
H_3C \\
\diagdown \\
C\text{——}CHCO_2H \\
H_3C\diagup \mid \mid \\
SH NH_2
\end{array}
$$

Fig. 1. Penicillamine

showed that in vitro, or in the knee joint of a patient with RA, penicillamine produced prompt dissociation of RF. It was, however, clear that when the drug was given by mouth to patients, the effects were quite different (JAFFE, 1965); penicillamine had no immediate effect on circulating RF but there was a gradual reduction in titre, taking months to produce a maximum fall. The level of RF did not immediately rise when penicillamine was stopped, though the drug is cleared from the circulation within days. By contrast, plasmaphoresis produced an immediate but transient effect on RF titre (JAFFE, 1963). This suggests that penicillamine interferes with the production of RF. HUSKISSON et al. (1974) showed that there was no relationship between changes in RF titre and clinical response, and there is little evidence to suggest that RF plays any part in the pathogenesis of the disease; one recalls that RF is found in the blood in many chronic inflammatory conditions including infections. It seems, therefore, that the discovery of the beneficial effects of penicillamine was an example of the use of the right drug for the wrong reason. The right reason is still not apparent.

There are so many interesting aspects to penicillamine, including exotic side effects and unusual biochemical activities, that it is easy to fail to describe the type of response which patients can achieve. Such a patient is illustrated in Figure 2; she had suffered severe active RA for many years, which had persisted and progressed despite

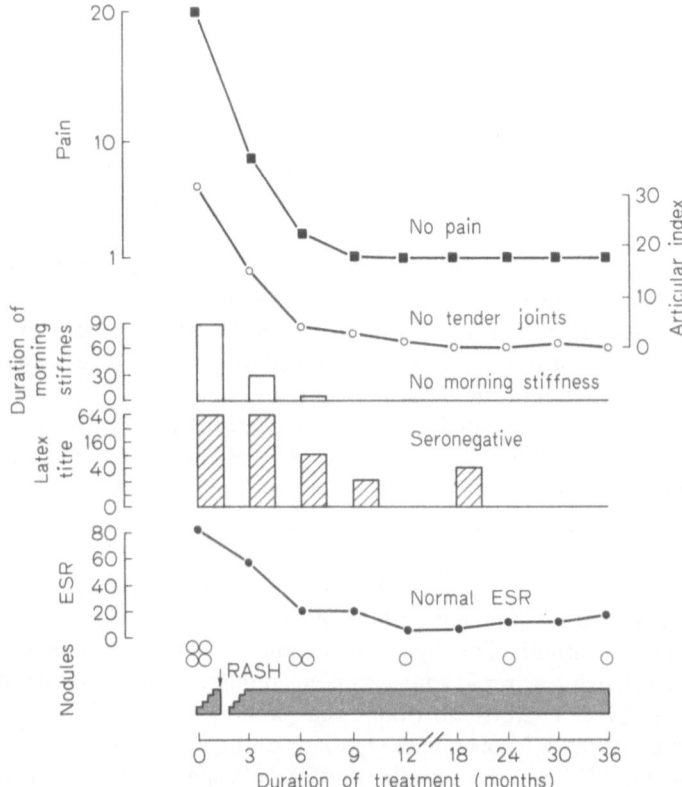

Fig. 2. The effects of penicillamine in a patient with RA

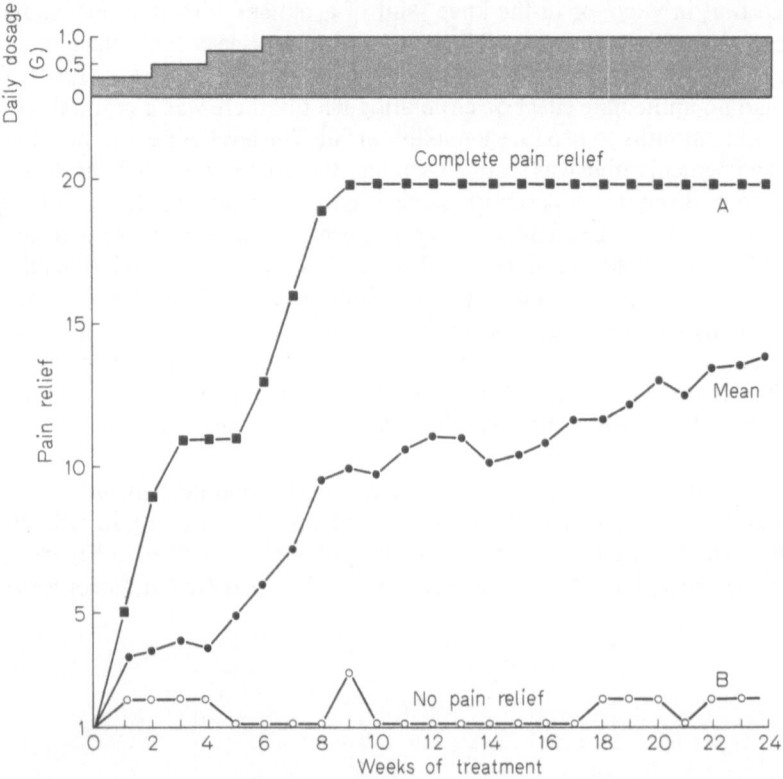

Fig. 3. Time course of the response to penicillamine showing the mean and extremes

treatment with many different anti-inflammatory drugs. The gradual response of her disease to penicillamine and the outcome after 3 years of treatment are illustrated; at this time she has no pain or morning stiffness, no tender joints or other evidence of active joint disease, a normal ESR, is seronegative and with just one rheumatoid nodule to remind her of the disease she once had.

The effectiveness of penicillamine has been demonstrated by the *Multicentre Trial Group* (1973) in a double-blind controlled trial involving 108 patients with severe RA. Penicillamine was superior to placebo in terms of reducing pain and the duration of morning stiffness, and increasing grip strength, articular index and functional capacity. The usual maintenance dose is between 500 mg and 1 g daily.

The rate of response to penicillamine is shown in Figure 3; the maximum improvement is produced after 4–6 months of treatment and the greatest mean change occurs in the 2nd month. This figure also shows the extreme responses that occur, one patient achieving a rapid and complete remission and another obtaining no benefit whatsoever. There is no doubt that some patients fail to respond—JAFFE (1970) estimated that 80% of courses were successful, GOLDING et al. (1970) obtained improvement in 75% and most authors give similar figures. Since penicillamine acts mainly on active joint disease, it is plain that patients with severe destructive changes (so-called burnt-out RA) may not benefit and various authors have noted this

(GOLDING et al., 1970; CAMUS et al., 1974). No other factors which affect the response can be identified. HUSKISSON et al. (1974) found that seronegative patients did as well as seropositive, and that there was no relationship between age, sex or duration of disease and response.

As well as influencing active joint disease, penicillamine may benefit nonarticular features, for example reducing the number of subcutaneous nodules (JAFFE, 1970), healing leg ulcers (GOLDING et al., 1970) and improving tenosynovitis, extensor tendon sheath swelling of the wrist and lymphadenopathy (*Multicentre Trial Group*, 1973). Some authors have obtained beneficial results in cases of rheumatoid vasculitis with peripheral gangrene (JAFFE, 1970; GOLDING et al., 1970). There is also a reduction in the requirement for other drugs including steroids.

Penicillamine has been compared with gold and found to be almost identical in its action (HUSKISSON et al., 1974). BERRY et al. (1975) found no significant difference in the clinical effects of penicillamine and azathioprine although there was a trend in favour of penicillamine. OTT and SCHMIDT (1974) found penicillamine more effective than steroids (prednisolone 15 mg daily).

The action of penicillamine on joints can also be demonstrated by reduction in technetium index and it has been suggested that this is a marker of the action of drugs of this type (HUSKISSON et al., 1976 b). That penicillamine reduces the technetium index while anti-inflammatory drugs do not, may be either because penicillamine is more effective or because it produces structural alterations such as a reduction in the amount of synovial tissue present.

Laboratory changes reported with penicillamine include gradual reductions in ESR and Latex test (JAFFE, 1970), increased urinary copper excretion (HUSKISSON and HART, 1972), decreased caeruloplasmin levels (ZUCKNER et al., 1970) and reduction in immunoglobulins and complement (BLUESTONE and GOLDBERG, 1973; HUSKISSON and BERRY, 1974). None of these changes has been shown to correlate with changes in the disease.

Penicillamine has many side effects. The most interesting are those which may have an immunological basis including rashes, thrombocytopaenia, proteinuria due to immune complex nephritis, drug-induced systemic lupus erythematosus (SLE), myasthenia gravis and Goodpasture syndrome. The side effects have been reviewed in detail elsewhere (HUSKISSON, 1976; MOWAT and HUSKISSON, 1975). Proteinuria occurs in about 15% of patients after between 4 and 18 months of treatment—about one in three of these patients will become nephrotic. In most cases, renal biopsy shows the presence of immune complexes, demonstrable by electron microscopy or immunofluorescent staining (JAFFE, 1968). If the drug is stopped when proteinuria develops, there is gradual recovery over a period of about 1 year (HUSKISSON and HART, 1972). However, some cases with modest proteinuria have continued to take the drug despite biopsy-proven immune complex nephritis, and the time course of the disappearance of the proteinuria was very similar (HUSKISSON, 1976). This suggests that the lesion is essentially benign and self-limiting, and is not associated with impairment of renal function probably because the immune complexes do not initiate cell proliferation and fibrosis in the glomerulus. Myasthenia gravis, SLE and Goodpasture syndrome are rare side effects. It is of considerable interest that the incidence of some of these problems appears to be much higher in RA than in two other diseases for which penicillamine is used, Wilson's disease and cystinuria.

Many patients are unable to continue penicillamine therapy, either because they do not respond, or because of some side effects. After 2 years of treatment about half of an initial group of patients will be well controlled and able to continue treatment.

Penicillamine is effective in about 50% of cases of Still's disease (Stocker and Schairer, 1974)—the lower incidence of success probably reflects the heterogeneity of Still's disease. Some cases are not juvenile RA but such diseases as ankylosing spondylitis, and are not therefore likely to respond. There is no good evidence that penicillamine is effective in other varieties of chronic polyarthritis such as psoriatic arthropathy, but it must be said that formal trials have not been carried out and a definite statement is therefore not possible.

II. Possible Mode of Action and Effects in Animal Models

The view that penicillamine is not an anti-inflammatory drug is supported by its lack of effect in conventional models. Liyanage and Currey (1972) showed no suppression of adjuvant arthritis. Arrigoni-Martelli and Bramm (1975) found no effect on the primary lesions of adjuvant arthritis, but an enhancement of the secondary lesions. Secondary lesions of adjuvant arthritis are usually regarded as a manifestation of cell-mediated immunity and their enhancement suggests that penicillamine might be an immunostimulant. This is supported by its effects in models of delayed hypersensitivity using pertussis vaccine as antigen (Arrigoni-Martelli et al., 1976; Dieppe et al., 1976). In these models, the inflammatory reaction to pertussis vaccine in sensitized animals is enhanced by penicillamine and suppressed by conventional anti-inflammatory drugs such as indomethacin. Also in support are enhancement of skin responsiveness to tuberculin in patients with RA after treatment with penicillamine (Berry and Huskisson, 1976) and the similarity of the effects of penicillamine and levamisole, a known immunostimulant, both in animal models and in RA. Levamisole is discussed in greater detail below.

There is some evidence that cell-mediated immune responses are depressed in patients with RA (Yu and Peter, 1974) and it has been postulated that the chronicity of inflammation in RA may be maintained by the persistence of a foreign antigen. In these circumstances, it is as logical to stimulate the appropriate cells to remove or conceal the antigen as it is to suppress the immunological reaction which represents the efferent loop of the pathway.

There is little support for the view that penicillamine is immunosuppressive. There is a fall in immunoglobulin levels (Bluestone and Goldberg, 1973) but this can be interpreted as normalisation rather than depression. Inhibition of lymphocyte stimulation has been described in mice (Schumacher et al., 1975) and inhibition of lymphocyte transformation in cultures (Roath and Willis, 1974).

A virus is perhaps the most popular candidate at present as the foreign antigen which initiates RA. Penicillamine inhibits polio virus replication by an effect on RNA synthesis (Jaffe et al., 1974), but there is no reason to believe that this is important in RA. Penicillamine is able to cleave the labile crosslinks of newly formed collagen (Herbert et al., 1974), but whereas this might be beneficial in inhibiting fibrosis in joints, it is unlikely to explain the fundamental effects which the drug displays on so many different aspects of the disease. The giving of copper supplements does not affect clinical response (*Multicentre Trial Group*, 1973) which does not correlate with changes in caeruloplasmin levels, suggesting that depletion of copper is not essential—penicillamine chelates many other metals which might be important. Pyridoxine supplements do not affect the response, suggesting that pyridoxine deficiency is not the answer.

C. Gold Salts

Gold therapy was introduced during the 1920s in the mistaken belief that RA had something to do with tuberculosis, and the equally mistaken belief that tuberculosis should be treated with gold. Its effectiveness was not satisfactorily confirmed until controlled clinical trials were reported by the *Empire Rheumatism Council* (1961). In this study, a course of injections of sodium aurothiomalate (Fig. 4) amounting to a total dose of 1 g, was shown to be superior to a course of injections of minute quantities of gold, in effect a placebo group. As well as improvement in clinical manifestations of arthritis, there was a fall in ESR and RF titre. There was no difference in radiological progression in the two groups, and X-ray changes did not parallel clinical progress. The advantage in the gold-treated group was apparent up to 18 months after the start of treatment, but thereafter there was a deterioration.

$$CO_2H \cdot CH(S \cdot Au) \cdot CH_2 \cdot CO_2H$$

Fig. 4. Sodium aurothiomalate ("gold")

Perhaps the most important reason why gold therapy has only recently been placed in proper perspective is the long-held view that it should be given as a "course." There is no good reason to believe that a brief spell of treatment would banish the disease forever, as antibiotics banish bacterial infection. Two studies have shown that the effects of gold can be maintained with continued therapy (VOREN-KAMP and DE BLECOURT, 1971; ROTHERMICH et al., 1973) and it is now usual to continue treatment indefinitely.

The effects of gold on RA are very similar to those of D-penicillamine (HUSKIS-SON et al., 1974). Both drugs promote the disappearance of nodules and improvement in other extra-articular features, as well as causing improvement in active synovitis. Side effects are less common with gold, but those which do occur are more likely to lead to withdrawal of treatment. After 2 years' treatment, there are twice as many patients well controlled and still receiving penicillamine as there are receiving gold.

In contrast to the *Empire Rheumatism Council* (1961), SIGLER et al. (1974) showed significantly slower radiological progression in patients receiving gold for 2 years compared with patients receiving placebo.

Two different gold salts have been used, sodium aurothiomalate and thioglucose. Both are effective, but thioglucose is better tolerated (ROTHERMICH et al., 1973).

Gold salts are not anti-inflammatory in man, having no immediate effect. Suppression of adjuvant arthritis has been reported by some but not all authors (WALZ et al., 1971). Gold is concentrated in synovium and remains in significant concentration for many years after a course of injections (GRAHAME et al., 1974). There is also evidence that gold is taken up by the reticuloendothelial system, is particularly concentrated in lymph nodes and accumulates in synovial macrophages (PERSELLIN and ZIFF, 1966). JESSOP et al. (1973) and VERNON-ROBERTS et al. (1973) showed suppression of cell migration and phagocytosis using a skin window technique both in man and animals. Compared with prednisolone, the effects of gold were delayed and prolonged.

It is tempting to think that gold and penicillamine act in the same way because their effects are so similar and because response to one correlates well with response to the other. It seems more likely, however, that gold acts by suppressing phagocytic cells, probably macrophages, perhaps by simply sitting in them and preventing them from taking up other particles. Again assuming that the chronicity of RA is maintained by the presence of a persistent antigen, it might be beneficial to prevent this antigen being taken up by macrophages.

Gold is not immunosuppressive, although it produces a slight fall in the levels of immunoglobulins (HUSKISSON and BERRY, 1974). STRONG et al. (1973) were able to show changes in lymphocyte transformation with cyclophosphamide, but not with gold. There is no evidence that gold is immunostimulant.

D. Chloroquine and Other Antimalarials

Chloroquine is a 4-amino quinolone compound (Fig. 5) used in the treatment of malaria. In RA it produces a useful suppression of disease activity in two-thirds of patients treated. This effect is achieved slowly, accompanied by reduction in ESR and RF titre. No changes in radiological manifestations of the disease have been demonstrated.

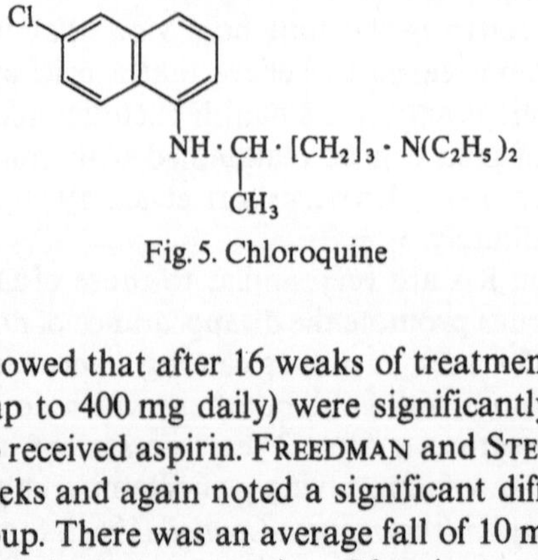

$$Cl \qquad NH \cdot CH \cdot [CH_2]_3 \cdot N(C_2H_5)_2$$
$$CH_3$$

Fig. 5. Chloroquine

FREEDMAN (1956) showed that after 16 weaks of treatment, patients treated with chloroquine sulphate (up to 400 mg daily) were significantly better than a control group. Both groups also received aspirin. FREEDMAN and STEINBERG (1960) extended this experience to 52 weeks and again noted a significant difference in favour of the chloroquine-treated group. There was an average fall of 10 mm/h in the ESR but no advantage in terms of radiological progression. Of patients treated with chloroquine, 90% felt that they had improved, 80% showed objective improvement, 15% had a complete remission and 5% deteriorated. These figures correspond closely to those for penicillamine and it is a feature of all these drugs that only about 80% of patients respond.

POPERT et al. (1961) compared chloroquine diphosphate (250 mg daily) with placebo for up to 2 years and showed similar clinical results but again with no significant difference in the rate of radiological progression in the two groups. There was a fall in the titre of RF in patients on chloroquine and it is of considerable interest that there was a significant correlation between changes in RF and change in clinical state; such a correlation has not been found with other drugs of this type. Chloroquine had no effect on RF in vitro in concentrations similar to those achieved in plasma of treated patients.

The usefulness of chloroquine has been limited by its effects on the eye: both corneal and retinal changes have been reported, the latter not always reversible when the drug is stopped (HOBBS et al., 1959). These side-effects can probably be avoided by giving only short courses of chloroquine, but the whole purpose of this type of treatment is to control the disease and this obviously requires that the drug be continued indefinitely. Apart from ocular toxicity, side-effects are not a problem; there are occasional gastro-intestinal disturbances and rashes. Chloroquine may exacerbate psoriasis and should not be used in psoriatic arthropathy. It is often useful in mild cases of SLE but not in other types of arthritis.

Mepacrine has also been found to be effective in an uncontrolled clinical trial (FREEDMAN and BACH, 1952).

Chloroquine is neither analgesic nor anti-inflammatory in animal models, and its mode of action is unknown. It accumulates in lymphocytes and reduces the responsiveness of lymphocytes from patients with RA to phytohaemagglutinin (PANAYI et al., 1973).

E. Levamisole

Levamisole is an imidazole anthelmintic, L-2,3,5,6-tetrahydro-6-phenylimidazo-[2,1-b]thiazole hydrochloride (Fig. 6). Its interest as a potential treatment for RA arises because it is known to be immunostimulant.

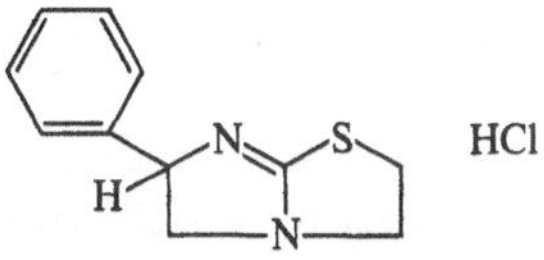

Fig. 6. Levamisole

The beneficial effects of levamisole in RA were first noted by SCHUERMANS (1975) who reported the results of 6 months' treatment in six patients. Striking objective and subjective improvement occurred within the 1st month of treatment, accompanied by reduction in ESR and conversion to negative of tests for RF in three patients. HUSKISSON et al. (1976b) compared levamisole, penicillamine and placebo. Comparison of levamisole and placebo-treated groups confirmed the effectiveness of levamisole under controlled conditions. Comparison of levamisole and penicillamine showed little difference between the effects of the two drugs. Levamisole-treated patients had significant relief of pain, reduction in the duration of morning stiffness, number of tender joints and joint swelling, accompanied by changes in ESR and RF titre. These effects were achieved slowly, reaching a peak after about 4 months of treatment, similar to the time course of penicillamine (Fig. 7). There was also a

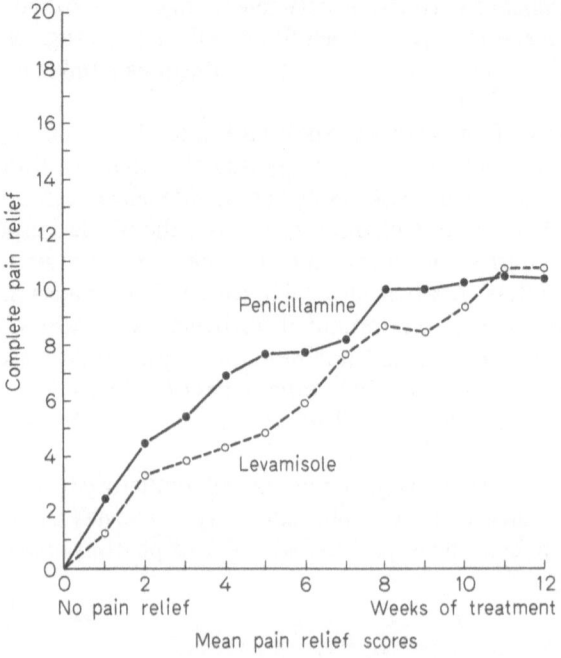

Fig. 7. Time course of the effects of levamisole and penicillamine to show delayed effects

significant reduction in technetium index, total white cell count and IgG level and a significant rise in haemoglobin. The treatment was not free of side effects—nausea, rashes, mouth ulcers, and disturbance of taste were mentioned; all these side effects occur with penicillamine.

Drugs may have many different actions which are not necessarily related to their effect in a particular disease. The effect of penicillamine in Wilson's disease is due to chelation of copper and its many other actions are presumably irrelevant to this disease. Thus, it should not be assumed that levamisole is active in RA because it is immunostimulant, although there is some evidence to support this view. Firstly, Huskisson et al. (1976b) showed a correlation between changes in skin responsiveness to tuberculin and pain relief, and also between enhancement of leucocyte migration inhibition to purified protein derivative (PPD) and pain relief. It is unusual to find such correlations and it is striking that with penicillamine, correlations have not been found between clinical and laboratory measurements. Secondly, levamisole and penicillamine appear to have in common a specific activity in RA and the ability to stimulate cell-mediated immune responses. The many other properties of penicillamine which have been suggested as a possible mode of action are not shown with levamisole—levamisole has not, for example, been shown to chelate copper or interfere with pyridoxine metabolism whilst penicillamine has not been shown to kill worms.

Levamisole is not an anti-inflammatory drug and this is confirmed by the absence of suppression of carrageenin pleurisy or the primary lesions of adjuvant arthritis (HUSKISSON et al., 1976a). However, secondary lesions of adjuvant arthritis were more severe in levamisole-treated animals. Penicillamine and levamisole had the same effect in pertussis vaccine oedema (ARRIGONI-MARTELLI et al., 1976) and in pertussis vaccine pleurisy (DIEPPE et al., 1976). Whereas anti-inflammatory drugs suppressed the inflammatory response in sensitized animals, penicillamine and levamisole enhanced it. This effect was greatest when the drugs were given around the time of challenge. These effects were interpreted as due to stimulation of cell-mediated immune responses. Support for this comes from the restoration of delayed hypersensitivity skin reactions by levamisole in old age and in patients with malignant disease (HIRSHAUT et al., 1973; TRIPODI et al., 1973).

The stimulation, or more properly restoration, of cell-mediated immune responsiveness could be related to increased phagocytosis. In RA, increased phagocytosis could enable a foreign antigen to be taken up by macrophages and subsequently processed. There is good evidence that levamisole increases phagocytosis. HOEBEKE and FRANCHI (1973) showed enhanced clearance of colloidal carbon in mice in vivo and LIMA et al. (1974) showed enhanced phagocytosis of sensitized sheep erythrocytes by mouse macrophages in vitro. This may explain the effects of levamisole in protecting against infection and malignancy in experimental animals (RENOUX and RENOUX, 1971, 1972a). It should be noted that increased phagocytosis of foreign material could aggravate some conditions and this may be reflected in the side effects of the drug.

Levamisole also has effects on lymphocytes, restoring responsiveness to agents such as phytohaemagglutinin in various diseases associated with poor response (DE CREE et al., 1974).

It has been suggested that levamisole may act on intracellular cAMP levels (LIMA et al., 1974) and in support of this, RENOUX and RENOUX (1972b) showed that the immunostimulant effect could be blocked by theophylline.

It is probable that levamisole has no direct effect on humoral immunity, although some authors have found increased antibody responses, for example, following influenza vaccination (BRUGMANS et al., 1973). This could be explained by increased phagocytosis or other cellular effects.

At this time, it is reasonable to suggest that penicillamine and levamisole are active in RA because of their immunostimulant effect and this may provide useful clues to the pathogenesis of the disease as well as to the development of a new class of compounds with which to treat the disease. It remains to be seen whether other compounds with a specific action will be shown to be immunostimulant; some like gold may act in a different way and it must be remembered that immunosuppressants produce similar clinical effects.

F. Other Imidazole Derivatives

There are many other imidazole derivatives which have attracted attention as anthelmintic or antifungal agents. One of these is clotrimazole (bis-phenyl (2 chlorphenyl-imidazolyl) methane), for which striking effects in RA have been claimed in an uncontrolled trial (WYBURN-MASON, 1974). This requires confirmation under controlled conditions.

G. Immunosuppressives

Immunosuppressives achieve similar results in RA as do penicillamine and gold. Their effect is slow and associated with changes in ESR and RF. There is radiological evidence for an improvement in outcome (*Cooperating Clinics Committee of the American Rheumatism Association*, 1970; Currey et al., 1974). Drugs of this type are certainly effective in a wider range of diseases than penicillamine; they are used for example, in psoriatic arthropathy, SLE and polymyositis, although they are more specific than the anti-inflammatory drugs.

The pharmacological properties of these drugs are discussed in Chapter 35.

Some explanation is needed of the apparent suppression of RA by both immunostimulant and immunosuppressive drugs. One must postulate that immunostimulants act on the afferent limb of the pathway, leading to improved processing of antigen, whereas immunosuppressives act on the efferent limb, blocking the organisms' capacity to respond.

H. Alclofenac

Alclofenac (4-allyloxy-3 chlorophenylacetic acid, Fig. 8) is an anti-inflammatory drug for which an additional specific action has been claimed. In animal models, such as the abdominal stretching test and carrageenin oedema, it demonstrates analgesic and anti-inflammatory activity (Wiggins, 1975). Short-term studies in man confirm the

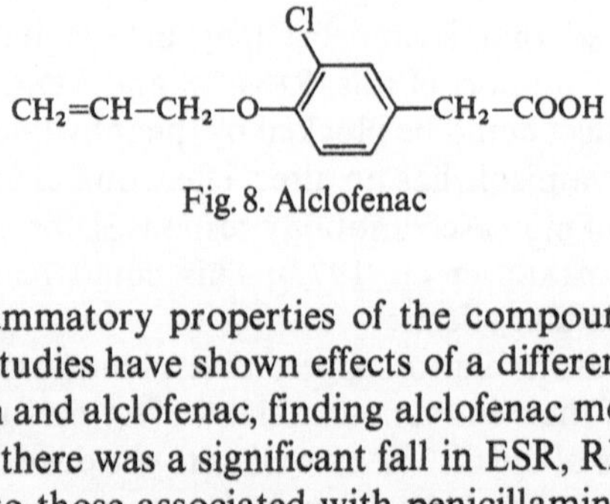

$$CH_2=CH-CH_2-O-\underset{Cl}{\overbrace{\hspace{2cm}}}-CH_2-COOH$$

Fig. 8. Alclofenac

analgesic and anti-inflammatory properties of the compound (Aylward and Davies, 1972). Long-term studies have shown effects of a different kind. Aylward et al. (1974) compared aspirin and alclofenac, finding alclofenac more effective. In patients treated with alclofenac, there was a significant fall in ESR, RF and levels of IgG and IgM—changes similar to those associated with penicillamine therapy. Unlike penicillamine, however, the reduction in ESR correlated with clinical changes. In a later study, Maddock et al. (1975) compared alclofenac and penicillamine. In the first few weeks of the trial, alclofenac was more effective, presumably because of its immediate anti-inflammatory effect. Apart from this, the effect of the drugs was similar, although alclofenac was better tolerated. In another long-term comparison of alclofenac and indomethacin, Aylward (1975) showed that there was significantly less radiological deterioration in patients treated with alclofenac. Aylward (1975) himself admitted that it was surprising to find an apparently straightforward anti-inflammatory drug having, in addition, the properties of another type of antirheumatic drug. His results require confirmation and it will be interesting to discover whether related acetic acid derivatives already undergoing clinical trials will show similar effects.

I. Steroids

At first sight, steroids appear to have more in common with anti-inflammatory drugs than with specific drugs. Their effect is common to all inflammatory arthropathies and is similar in its time course to that of nonsteroidal anti-inflammatories. Reduction in ESR is no greater than that produced by aspirin (*Empire Rheumatism Council*, 1957), and neither of these drugs reduces the titre of RF (*Joint Committee of the Medical Research Council and Nuffield Foundation*, 1960). These two studies produced different results in terms of radiological progression. The *Empire Rheumatism Council* (1957) compared cortisone (75 mg daily) and aspirin and showed no difference between the groups, except with respect to spread of radiological change to new joints which was significantly more frequent in patients on aspirin. Other radiological measurements showed no significant difference. The *Joint Committee of the Medical Research Council and Nuffield Foundation* (1960) compared prednisolone in mean doses of 10–20 mg daily with aspirin or other analgesics. There was significantly less radiological deterioration in the steroid-treated group. Such doses are, of course, associated with unacceptable manifestations of Cushing's disease. Thus, although steroids may be capable of preventing radiological progression, their action cannot be regarded as specific for RA.

J. Summary

Penicillamine is not just an anti-inflammatory drug. Although it relieves pain and suppresses manifestations of inflammation such as swelling, this action is accompanied by improvement in extra-articular features of RA such as nodules and by the disappearance of circulating RF. In contrast to the anti-inflammatory drugs, this action is achieved slowly, and whereas anti-inflammatory drugs are beneficial in any inflammatory arthropathy, the action of penicillamine depends upon the nature of the disease. For this reason, it is called "specific" to distinguish it from "non-specific" or symptomatic remedies like analgesic and anti-inflammatory drugs.

A number of drugs have this type of action in RA, including levamisole, gold salts, chloroquine, and immunosuppressives. It is unlikely that a common mode of action exists for these widely differing drugs and further subdivision of the group is likely when mechanisms of action are better understood.

There is no animal model which can be used to demonstrate this type of action in the way that experimental models of inflammation can be used to screen anti-inflammatory drugs. Most specific drugs are ineffective in relieving inflammation induced experimentally in animals. Some of these drugs are capable of enhancing cell-mediated immune responses, and this may be relevant to their action and useful in searching for further compounds.

Drugs of this type are capable of arresting the progress of RA and are, at the present time, the most promising new approach to the treatment of RA. Study of the mode of action of these drugs may shed light on the nature of the disease itself, as well as providing a therapeutic advance.

References

Arrigoni-Martelli, E., Bramm, E.: Investigations in the influence of cyclophosphamide, gold sodium thiomalate, and D-penicillamine on nystatin oedema and adjuvant arthritis. Agents Actions 5, 264—267 (1975)

Arrigoni-Martelli, E., Bramm, E., Huskisson, E. C., Willoughby, D. A., Dieppe, P. A.: Pertussis vaccine oedema: an experimental model for the action of penicillamine-like drugs. Agents Actions 6, 613—617 (1976)

Aylward, M.: Clinical studies on alclofenac in the treatment of rheumatic diseases: a drug in question. Curr. med. Res. Opin. 3, 274—285 (1975)

Aylward, M., Davies, D. B. S.: A double-blind crossover trial comparing a new antirheumatic agent alclofenac with phenylbutazone in chronic rheumatic disorders. Brit. J. clin. Pract. 26, 517—521 (1972)

Aylward, M., Parker, R. J., Maddock, J.: Studies on 4-alloxy-3 chlorophenylacetic acid (Alclofenac). Ann. rheum. Dis. 33, 268—272 (1974)

Berry, H., Huskisson, E. C. (1976) unpublished.

Berry, H., Liyanage, S. P., Durance, R. A.: A controlled trial of penicillamine and azathioprine in the treatment of rheumatoid arthritis. Scand. J. Rheum. Suppl. 8, 21—26 (1975)

Bluestone, R., Goldberg, L. S.: Effects of D-penicillamine on serum immunoglobulins and rheumatoid factor. Ann. rheum. Dis. 32, 50—52 (1973)

Brugmans, J., Schuermans, Y., de Cock, W., Thienpont, D., Janssen, P., Verhaegen, H., Van Nimmen, L., Louwagie, A. C., Stevens, E.: Restoration of host defense mechanisms in man by Levamisole. Life Sci. 13, 1499—1504 (1973)

Camus, J.-P., Crouzet, J., Guillien, P., Benichou, C., Lievre, J.-A.: Cent cas de polyarthrite rhumatoide commune traités par la D-pénicillamine. Ann. Med. interne (Paris) 125, 9—28 (1974)

Cooperating Clinics Committee of the American Rheumatism Association: A controlled trial of cyclophosphamide in rheumatoid arthritis. New Engl. J. Med. 283, 883—889 (1970)

Currey, H. L. F., Harris, J., Mason, R. M., Woodland, J., Beveridge, T., Roberts, C. J., Vere, D. W., Dixon, A. St. J., Davies, J., Owen-Smith, B.: Comparison of azathioprine, cyclophosphamide and gold in the treatment of rheumatoid arthritis. Brit. med. J. III, 764—766 (1974)

De Cree, J., Verhaegen, H., de Cook, H., Vanheule, R., Brugmans, J., Schuermans, V.: Impaired neutrophil phagocytosis. Lancet II, 294—295 (1974)

Dieppe, P. A., Willoughby, D. A., Huskisson, E. C., Arrigoni-Martelli, E.: Pertussis vaccine pleurisy: a model of delayed hypersensitivity. Agents Actions 6, 618—621 (1976)

Empire Rheumatism Council: Multicentre controlled trial comparing cortisone acetate and acetyl salicylic acid in the long-term treatment of rheumatoid arthritis. Ann. rheum. Dis. 16, 277—289 (1957)

Empire Rheumatism Council: Gold therapy in rheumatoid arthritis. Ann. rheum. Dis. 20, 315—340 (1961)

Freedman, A.: Chloroquine and rheumatoid arthritis. Ann. rheum. Dis. 15, 251—257 (1956)

Freedman, A., Bach, F.: Mepacrine and rheumatoid arthritis. Lancet II, 321 (1952)

Freedman, A., Steinberg, V. L.: Chloroquine in rheumatoid arthritis. Ann. rheum. Dis. 19, 243—256 (1960)

Golding, J. R., Wilson, J. V., Day, A. T.: Observations on the treatment of rheumatoid arthritis with penicillamine. Postgrad. med. J. 46, 599—605 (1970)

Grahame, R., Billings, R., Laurence, M., Marks, V., Wood, P. J.: Tissue gold levels after chrysotherapy. Ann. rheum. Dis. 33, 536—539 (1974)

Herbert, C. M., Lindberg, K. A., Jackson, M. I. V., Bailey, A. J.: Biosynthesis and maturation of skin collagen in scleroderma and effect of D-penicillamine. Lancet I, 187—192 (1974)

Hirshaut, Y., Pinsky, C., Marquardt, H., Oettgen, H. F.: Effects of levamisole on delayed hypersensitivity reactions in cancer patients. 64th meeting of the American Association for Cancer Research 14, 109 (1973)

Hobbs, H. E., Sorsby, A., Freedman, A.: Retinopathy following chloroquine therapy. Lancet II, 478—480 (1959)

Hoebeke, J., Franchi, G.: Influence of tetramisole and its optical isomers on the mononuclear phagocytic system. J. reticuloendoth. Soc. 14, 317—323 (1973)

Huskisson, E. C.: Recent drugs and the rheumatic diseases. Reports on Rheumatic Diseases 52, Arthritis and Rheumatism Council 1974

Huskisson, E. C.: Penicillamine and the rheumatologist: a review. Pharmatherapeutica 1, 24—39 (1976)

Huskisson, E. C., Berry, H.: Some immunological changes in rheumatoid arthritis among patients receiving penicillamine and gold. Postgrad. med. J. August suppl. 59—61 (1974)

Huskisson, E. C., Dieppe, P. A., Scott, P. J., Trapnell, J. C., Balme, H. W., Willoughby, D. A.: Immuno-stimulant therapy for rheumatoid arthritis. Lancet I, 393—395 (1976a)

Huskisson, E. C., Gibson, T. J., Balme, H. W., Berry, H., Burry, H. C., Grahame, R., Hart, F. D., Wojtulewski, J. A.: Trial comparing D-penicillamine and gold in rheumatoid arthritis. Ann. rheum. Dis. 33, 532—535 (1974)

Huskisson, E. C., Hart, F. D.: Penicillamine in the treatment of rheumatoid arthritis. Ann. rheum. Dis. 31, 402—404 (1972)

Huskisson, E. C., Scott, P. J., Balme, H. W.: Objective measurement of rheumatoid arthritis using the technetium index. Ann. rheum. Dis. 35, 81—82 (1976b)

Jaffe, I. A.: Intra-articular dissociation of the rheumatoid factor. J. Lab. clin. Med. 60, 409—421 (1962)

Jaffe, I. A.: Comparisons of the effects of plasmapheresis and penicillamine on the level of circulating rheumatoid factor. Ann. rheum. Dis. 22, 71—76 (1963)

Jaffe, I. A.: The effects of penicillamine on the laboratory parameters in rheumatoid arthritis. Arthr. Rheum. 8, 1064—1079 (1965)

Jaffe, I. A.: Effects of penicillamine on the kidney and on taste. Postgrad. med. J. October suppl. 15—18 (1968)

Jaffe, I. A.: The treatment of rheumatoid arthritis and necrotizing vasculitis with penicillamine. Arthr. Rheum. 13, 435—443 (1970)

Jaffe, I. A., Merryman, P., Ehrenfeld, E.: Further studies of the anti-viral effect of D-penicillamine. Postgrad. med. J. August suppl. 50—55 (1974)

Jessop, J. D., Vernon-Roberts, B., Harris, J.: Effects of gold salts and prednisolone on inflammatory cells. I. Phagocytic activity of macrophages and polymorphs in inflammatory exudates studied by a "skin-window" technique in rheumatoid and control patients. Ann. rheum. Dis. 32, 294—300 (1973)

Joint Committee of the Medical Research Council and Nuffield Foundation: A comparison of prednisolone with aspirin or other analgesics in the treatment of rheumatoid arthritis. Ann. rheum. Dis. 19, 331—337 (1960)

Lima, A. O., Javierre, M. Q., da Silva, W. D., Camara, D. S.: Immunological phagocytosis: effects of drugs in phosphodiesterase activity. Experientia (Basel) 30, 945—946 (1974)

Liyanage, S. P., Currey, H. L. F.: Failure of oral D-penicillamine to modify adjuvant arthritis or immune response in the rat. Ann. rheum. Dis. 31, 521 (1972)

Maddock, J., Rees, P., Holly, F., Aylward, M.: The influence of alclofenac treatment on acute-phase proteins, plasma tryptophan, and erythrocyte sedimentation rate in patients with rheumatoid arthritis. Curr. med. Res. Opin. 3, 286—297 (1975)

Mowat, A., Huskisson, E. C.: D-Penicillamine in rheumatoid arthritis. Clin. rheum. Dis. 1, 319—333 (1975)

Multicentre Trial Group: Controlled trial of D-penicillamine in severe rheumatoid arthritis. Lancet I, 275—280 (1973)

Ott, V. R., Schmidt, K. L.: Treatment of rheumatoid arthritis with D-penicillamine. Preliminary results of a controlled clinical trial. International Symposium on Penicillamine, 1974.

Panayi, G. S., Neill, W. A., Duthie, J. J. R., McCormick, J. N.: Action of chloroquine phosphate in rheumatoid arthritis. I. Immunosuppressive effect. Ann. rheum. Dis. 32, 316—318 (1973)

Persellin, R. H., Ziff, M.: The effect of gold salt on lysosomal enzymes of the peritoneal macrophage. Arthr. Rheum. 9, 57—65 (1966)

Popert, A. J., Meifers, K. A. E., Sharp, J., Bier, F.: Chloroquine diphosphate in rheumatoid arthritis. Ann. rheum. Dis. 20, 18—35 (1961)

Renoux, G., Renoux, M.: Effet immunostimulant d'un imidothiazol dans l'immunisation des souris contre l'infection par Brucella Abortus. C.R. Acad. Sci. (Paris) 272, 349—350 (1971)

Renoux, G., Renoux, M.: Levamisole inhibits and cures a solid malignant tumour and its pulmonary metastases in mice. Nature (New Biol.) **240**, 217—218 (1972a)

Renoux, G., Renoux, M.: Inhibition par la theophylline de la stimulation immunologique induite par le phenylimidothiazole. C.R. Acad. Sci. (Paris) **274**, 3149—3151 (1972b)

Roath, S., Willis, R.: The effects of penicillamine on lymphocytes in culture. Postgrad. med. J., August suppl. 56—67 (1974)

Rothermich, N. D., Philips, V. K., Bergen, W., Thomas, M. H.: Excerpta Med. int. Congr. Ser. **299**, 144 (1973)

Schuermans, Y.: Levamisole in rheumatoid arthritis. Lancet **I**, 111 (1975)

Schumacher, K., Maerker Alzer, G., Preuss, R.: Effect of D-penicillamine on lymphocyte function. Arzneimittel-Forsch. **25**, 603—606 (1975)

Sigler, J. W., Bluhm, G. B., Duncan, H., Sharp, J. T., Gusign, D. C., McCrum, W. R.: Gold salts in the treatment of rheumatoid arthritis. A double-blind study. Ann. intern. Med. **80**, 21—26 (1974)

Stocker, E., Schairer, H.: D-penicillamine in juvenile rheumatoid arthritis. International Symposium on Penicillamine, 1974.

Strong, J. S., Bartholomew, B. A., Smith, C. J.: Immunoresponsiveness of patients with rheumatoid arthritis receiving cyclophosphamide or gold salts. Ann. rheum. Dis. **32**, 233—237 (1973)

Tripodi, D., Parks, L. C., Brugmans, J.: Drug-induced restoration of cutaneous delayed hypersensitivity in anergic patients with cancer. New Engl. J. Med. **289**, 354—357 (1973)

Vernon-Roberts, B., Jessop, J. D., Dore, J.: Effects of gold salts and prednisolone on inflammatory cells. 2. Suppression of inflammation in the rat. Ann. rheum. Dis. **32**, 301—307 (1973)

Vorenkamp, E. O., de Blecourt, J. J.: Gold treatment in rheumatoid arthritis. Abstr. VII Europ. Rheumat. Congr. **10**, 1 (1971)

Walz, D. T., Di Martino, M. J., Misher, A.: Suppression of adjuvant-induced arthritis in the rat by gold sodium. Ann. rheum. Dis. **30**, 303—306 (1971)

Wiggins, L. F.: The chemical and biological background to alclofenac. Curr. med. Res. Opin. **3**, 241—248 (1975)

Wright, V.: Rheumatism and psoriasis. Amer. J. Med. **27**, 454—462 (1959)

Wyburn-Mason, R.: The significance of the effect of Clotrimazole on active rheumatoid disease. In: Abstracts of the 9th International Congress of Chemotherapy 1974

Yü, D. T. Y., Peter, J. B.: Cellular immunological aspects of "rheumatoid arthritis". Semin. Arthr. Rheum. **4**, 25—51 (1974)

Zuckner, J., Ramsey, R. H., Dorner, R. W., Gantner, G. E.: D-penicillamine in rheumatoid arthritis. Arthr. Rheum. **13**, 131—144 (1970)

CHAPTER 33

Antagonists of Histamine, 5-Hydroxytryptamine and SRS-A

A. F. GREEN, L. G. GARLAND, and H. F. HODSON

A. Classification of Antihistamines

Antihistamines that powerfully and selectively inhibit certain effects of histamine have been known° for over 25 years. The effects of histamine that they inhibit are contractile actions on the smooth muscle of the gut, uterus and bronchioles and capillary permeability responses. Some other effects of histamine are highly resistant to these antihistamines and they include stimulation of gastric secretion, relaxation of rat uterus and positive inotropic effects on isolated atria (LOEW, 1947; ASHFORD et al., 1949; DUTTA, 1949; TRENDELENBERG, 1960). Indeed, it has been demonstrated that gastric secretion induced by histamine is enhanced rather than diminished by antihistamines, including mepyramine (WOOD, 1948) and triprolidine (GREEN, 1953), perhaps in consequence of histamine release (Chap. 34, Sect. C.II.). Compounds that selectively inhibit histamine-induced gastric secretion and other effects of histamine resistant to the earlier antihistamines were first reported only in 1972 by BLACK and colleagues. They are referred to as antagonists at H_2 receptors, in distinction from the earlier antihistamines whose inhibitory effects at low concentrations character-ised a histamine receptor for which ASH and SCHILD in 1966 had suggested the symbol H_1. The distinction between H_1 and H_2 receptors is already well character-ised by studies both of selective agonists (ASH and SCHILD, 1966; BLACK et al., 1972) and antagonists (BLACK et al., 1972, 1973, 1975).

H_1 receptors are of particular significance in relation to anaphylactic broncho-constriction and local inflammatory responses of skin (Sect. H.). H_2 receptors are apparently activated by released histamine and play some part in moderating subse-quent histamine release (Chap. 34, Sect. C.II.). Both types of receptor are concerned in vasodilator and depressor responses to injected histamine (Sect. E.) and their relative contributions to vascular reactions associated with inflammation and allergy have yet to be worked out in detail.

B. Histamine H_1 Antagonists: Structure-Activity Relationships

As long ago as 1933, FOURNEAU and BOVET showed that the benzodioxan derivative (1) could protect experimental animals against histamine-induced bronchospasm. Many compounds related to (1) were subsequently prepared, but a clinically useful antihistamine drug did not emerge until 10 years later. In 1942, HALPERN reported the antihistaminic activity of a number of ethylenediamine derivatives of which the compound (2), later to be named phenbenzamine (Antergan), was outstanding. Con-current work along similar lines in the USA led to a series of aminoethyl ethers typified by diphenhydramine (3) (RIEVESCHL, 1947), which still enjoys extensive usage as an antihistamine drug.

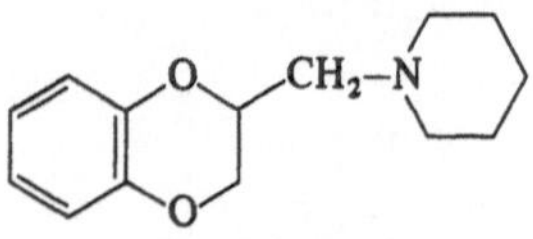

(1) 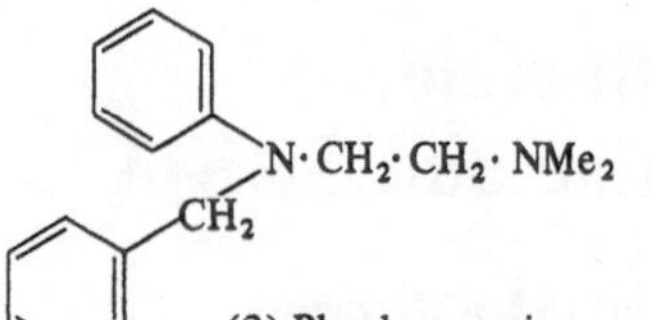   (2) Phenbenzamine 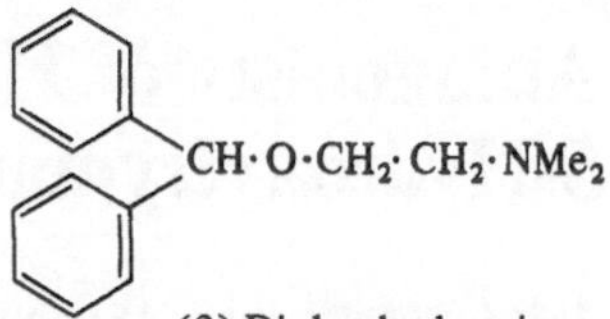   (3) Diphenhydramine

Following the introduction of diphenhydramine and phenbenzamine, work in many laboratories led to the synthesis of thousands of compounds with potent antihistaminic activity; all are more or less closely related to (2) and (3) and no fewer than 50 are currently in clinical use. Most of these compounds are either represented by the general structure (4) or can readily be derived from such a structure in a formal sense. In structure (4):

1. Ar^1 and Ar^2 are phenyl, substituted phenyl or heteroaryl (thienyl, pyridyl, etc.) groups

2. $X=N$, CH or CH-O-

3. $n=0$ or 1; i.e., a methylene group may optionally be present between the X function and one of the aryl groups

4. A is usually an ethylene group or a two-carbon fragment of a nitrogen hetero-cyclic system.

5. R^1 and R^2 are usually methyl groups, but can together form a small hetero-cyclic group, e.g. pyrrolidinyl in triprolidine (5).

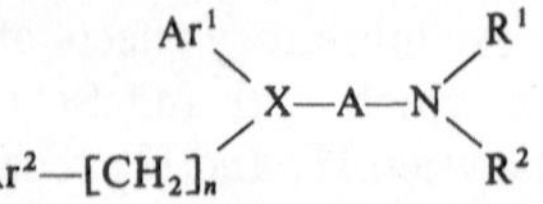

(4)

The detailed relationships between chemical structure and antihistaminic activity are complex and very few studies have been concerned with the systematic variation of one or more structural features. However, it is possible to consider the broad structural requirements for antagonist activity in the light of the general structure (4); the examples given illustrate most of the usual variants.

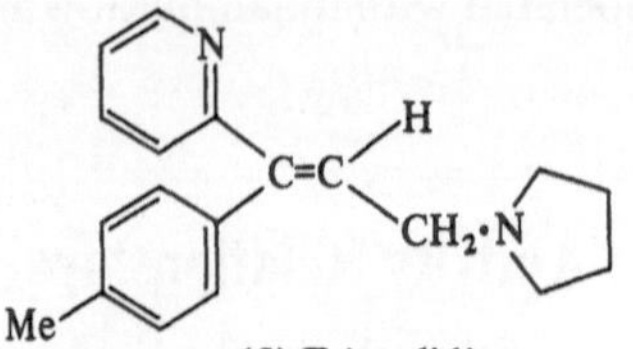

(5) Triprolidine 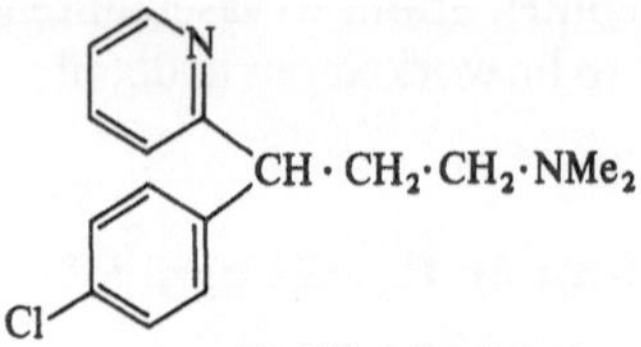   (6) Chlorpheniramine

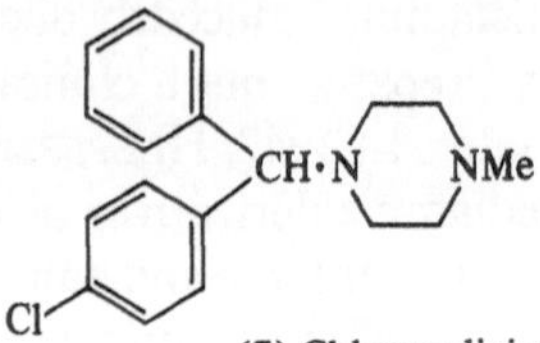

(7) Chlorcyclizine 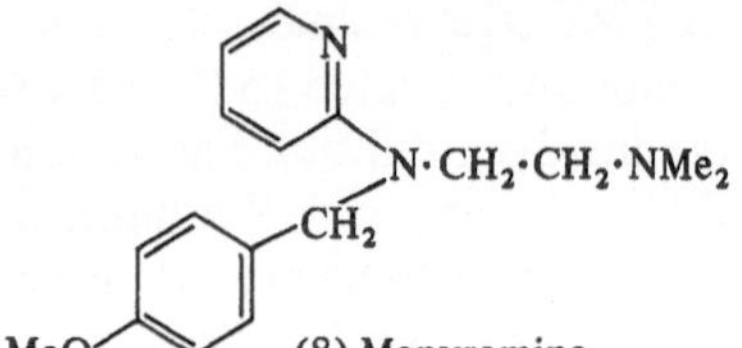   (8) Mepyramine

Two aromatic rings are present in nearly all potent antihistaminics. In triprolidine (5), chlorpheniramine (6), chlorcyclizine (7), and mepyramine (8) a phenyl ring is substituted in the *p*-position by a chloro, methyl or methoxy group, all small groups with some electron-releasing character.

The effect of aryl substitution is apparent from two independent studies, one on in vivo (ENSOR et al., 1954) the other on in vitro (HARMS and NAUTA, 1960) antihistaminic activity of a large number of diphenhydramine derivatives substituted in one or both of the phenyl nuclei. Together these studies covered a wide range of substituent types and position and the results have been incorporated into two quantitative parameter-activity studies (KUTTER and HANSCH, 1969; REKKER et al., 1975). Only those compounds with one *p*-substituent which was methyl, ethyl or a halogroup were better than diphenhydramine itself; *o*- and *m*-substituted compounds were inactive or less active than the parent and *p*-substitution of both phenyl rings led to a decrease in activity.

There are a number of cases where replacement of one phenyl group by a heteroaryl group leads to higher activity. Many of the potent antihistamines in clinical use were developed in this way; triprolidine (5), chlorpheniramine (6), mepyramine (8), and tripelennamine (9), for example have 2-pyridyl groups, while thenaldine (10) has a 2-thienyl group. Tricyclic antihistamines such as promethazine (11) and cyproheptadine (12) can be considered as diaryl compounds with a linking group (S, and CH=CH respectively).

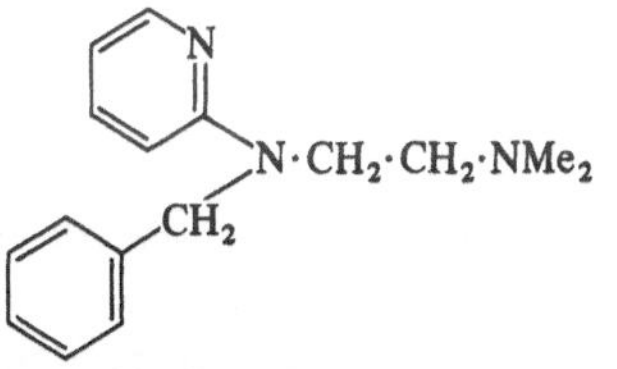

(9) Tripelennamine

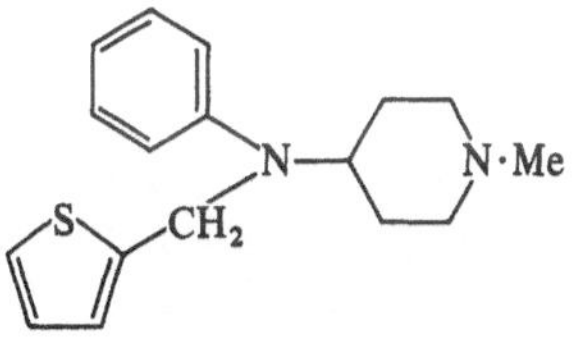

(10) Thenaldine

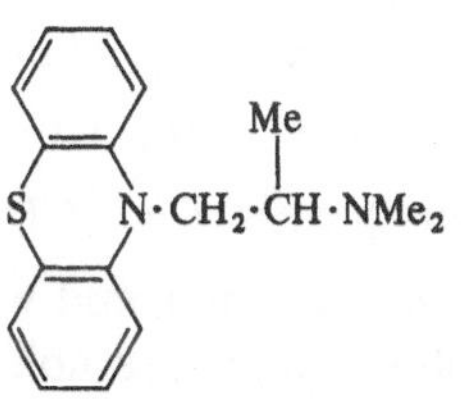

(11) Promethazine

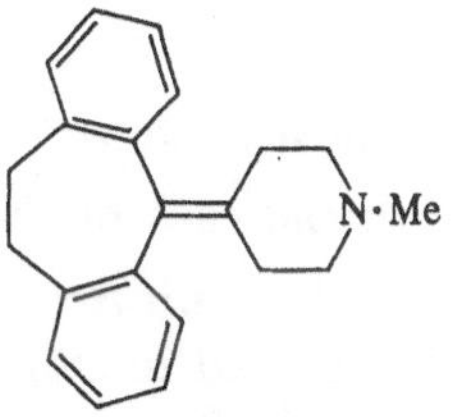

(12) Cyproheptadine

The basic terminus in nearly all cases is a tertiary amine. Often this is a dimethylamino group, but the basic nitrogen can be incorporated into a small saturated heterocyclic ring system; triprolidine (5), chlorcyclizine (7), thenaldine (10), and antazoline (13) exemplify different ways in which this can occur, but in every case the structural requirements of the general formula (4) are preserved and the nitrogen is tertiary and sufficiently strongly basic to be protonated at physiological pH. This tertiary nitrogen is more strongly basic than the primary amino group of histamine and if both compete for the same binding site, and if the interaction is purely electrostatic, the antihistamines will have a greater affinity at this site. Increased bulk around this basic centre leads to lower activity; for example, *N,N*-diethylamino compounds are invariably less active than the N,N-dimethylamino analogues. On the other hand, NAUTA et al. (1973) have recently shown that replacement of the dimethylamino group by the compact azetidine (14) group gave a 250-fold increase in activity in some compounds of the diphenhydramine series.

(13) Antazoline   (14)   (15) Pyrrobutamine

The broad similarity between these antihistaminic compounds suggests that they are all similarly bound at the same receptor site and there has been much speculation on the possible structural and conformational requirements of the ideal histamine H^1 receptor antagonist. It has been known for a long time that in the triprolidine series, the compounds in which the 2-pyridyl group is *trans* to the pyrrolidinomethyl group (cf 5) are more active than their *cis* isomers (ADAMSON et al., 1951). ISON and CASY (1971) recently confirmed these observations and showed that in the pyrrobutamine (15) series the more active of the geometrical isomers are those in which the phenyl group is *trans* to the pyrrolidinomethyl group (as depicted in 15) (CASY and ISON, 1970; ISON et al., 1973). Thus, it appears that for high activity in both series it is necessary to have a *trans* Ar^1—C$=$CH.CH$_2$.N$\diagup$ arrangement; the preferred conformation (CASY and ISON, 1970) is that in which Ar^1 (pyridyl or phenyl) is more or less coplanar with the double bond as illustrated in formula (16) while the plane of the Ar^2 or $Ar^2 \cdot CH_2$ group lies nearly at right angles. For the other antihistaminic drugs of general structure (4), it is possible for the molecules to adopt conformations similar to (16) with the two aromatic groups nearly at right angles and with the components of the $Ar^1 \cdot X$—C—C—N$\diagup$ system in a common plane and in some cases there is evidence that these are indeed the preferred conformations in solution (HAM, 1971). In the case of the dephenhydramines, with $X = $$\diagup$CH—O, a likely conformation is (17) with Ar^1 and the amino group coplanar and with an Ar^1-N distance similar to that in (16). The tricyclic antihistamines are able to achieve a conformation in which one of the aromatic rings is in the same plane as the 2-aminoalkyl side-chain, but the angle between the two aryl groups depends on the particular tricyclic systems. It is notable that the highly active (18) and cyproheptadine (12), for example, have almost the same geometry as the conformer (17) of diphenhydramine (CASY and ISON, 1970).

(16)   (17)

Most histamine H_1 antagonists then, are able to adopt conformations similar to those of (16) in which the $Ar^1 \ldots N{<}^{R^1}_{R^2}$ distance is close to the imidazole $\ldots NH_2$ distance in histamine. In these conformations the Ar^1-A-N moiety has similar shape and dimensions to those of the histamine molecule and could, therefore, be expected to occupy the same receptor site as the agonist; the Ar^2 group of the antagonist would then occupy a binding site not implicated in the agonist-receptor interaction (CASY and ISON, 1970).

(18)   (19)   (20)

Recent work by HANNA and AHMED (1973) supports these ideas on conformational requirements for antagonist activity. These workers prepared the *cis* and *trans* isomers of (20) both of which can formally a regarded as cyclic and more conformationally rigid forms of phenbenzamine; the *trans*-isomer prevented histamine-induced contractions of guinea pig ileum at concentrations as low as 2×10^{-9} M and the antagonistic effect could not readily be reversed, while the *cis*-isomer was active at concentrations of about 1×10^{-7} M, but was less persistent after washing.

Finally, it should be noted that stereoselectivity of action has been demonstrated in several antihistamines which have an asymmetric centre and which can, therefore, be resolved; one stereoisomer is usually much more active than the other. This is true, for example, of chlorpheniramine (6) and related compounds (BRITTAIN et al., 1959; SHAFI'EE and HITE, 1969; JAMES and WILLIAMS, 1974); other examples are quoted by WITIAK (1970) and in all these cases the asymmetric centre is adjacent to the aromatic rings. In contrast, promethazine (11) has an asymmetric centre α to the dimethylamino group and the *d*- and *l*-isomers have the same activity and toxicity (TOLDY et al., 1959); the asymmetry in the receptor must, then, be closely associated with the region which binds to the aromatic nuclei.

C. Histamine H_1 Antagonists: Inhibition of Responses to Histamine Involved in Inflammatory and Anaphylactic Reactions

Many descriptive reviews of the effects of H_1 antagonists on a variety of responses to histamine are already available (LOEW, 1947; FEINBERG et al., 1950; SCHACHTER, 1973; ROCHA E SILVA, 1977). It is therefore appropriate to confine this brief review to antihistaminic properties that are directly relevant to the interpretation of the studies of the anti-inflammatory and anti-anaphylactic effects of these substances that are described in Section H. As in that Section, the information is presented separately for each species because there are major differences in the sensitivity of different species to histamine and its antagonists. The differential effects of histamine and 5-hydroxytryptamine (5-HT) also vary in different species. This is illustrated by comparisons of the sensitivities of the skin to the permeability inducing effect of intradermal injections of these substances. The response is usually measured as the area of skin showing extravasation of an albumin-bound blue dye (usually Evans or Pontamine blue) that has been previously injected intravenously (i.v.) (this and alternative procedures are described more fully in Chap. 34, Sect. B.I.). Some comparisons of sensitivities to histamine and 5-HT and to the amine releasing substances compound 48/80 and polymyxin (see Sect. H.II.4.) are presented in Table 1 and the inhibitory effects of antihistamines in different species are compared in Table 2.

Table 1. PF Potency (EBD/mg) of histamine, 5-hydroxytryptamine and their liberators in different species of animal

Permeability factor	EBD[a]/mg when tested in			
	Guinea-pig[b]	Rat[b]	Rabbit[b]	Man[c]
Histamine	32 200	1 400	37 000	62 500
Compound 48/80	3 500	6 800	30	nt
Polymyxin B	1 120	14 900	< 20	nt
5-Hydroxytryptamine	60	16 200	< 20	nt

[a] Here the effective blueing dose (EBD) is defined as the amount of substance which in an injection volume of 0.1 ml on average induces, in the skin of a blued animal, a lesion that at the maximum development of the area of increased permeability is 6 mm in diameter. Permeability factor (PF) potency is defined as the number of EBD's per mg of substance.
[b] Except for polymyxin, figures from SPARROW and WILHELM (1957).
[c] Estimated from the data of STEWART and BLISS (1957), assuming the dosage-response line has a slope of 6.0.
nt = not tested.
(From: MILES and WILHELM, 1960).

Table 2. Inhibition of PF potency of histamine and compound 48/80 by various antihistamines given intravenously in guinea pigs (0.1 mg/kg), rats (0.5 mg/kg) and rabbits (0.1 mg/kg)—doses as base

	Factor of inhibition of PF[a]				
	Guinea pig		Rat		Rabbit
Antihistamine	Histamine	48/80	Histamine	48/80	Histamine
Triprolidine	1750	4	40	1.3	11
Chlorpheniramine	530	5	13	1.8	2
Mepyramine	47	3	37	1.1	9
Promethazine	12	2	100	3.0	4
Tripelennamine	6	7	10	1.5	3
Chlorcyclizine	1.6	1.7	19	2.0	2
Diphenhydramine	1.4	1.5	8	3.0	2
Antazoline	1.1	3	3	2.0	3
Thenalidine	0.8	1.0	5	1.7	1.0

[a] The ratio of the permeability factor potency of histamine in control and treated animals.
(From: WILHELM, 1973.)

I. Guinea Pig

The useful comparison of the effects of antihistamines on the permeability increasing effect of histamine in skin, presented in Table 2, is based partly on results published by WILHELM and MASON (1960), MILES and WILHELM (1960) and LOGAN and WIL-HELM (1966), and partly on unpublished results (MASON and WILHELM, cited in WILHELM, 1973). Of several antihistamines, triprolidine was the most potent. The duration of effect of i.v. doses of 0.1 mg/kg of triprolidine, chlorpheniramine (chlorprophenpyridamine), mepyramine and promethazine have also been compared; all but promethazine show a rapid fall off of effect between 1 and 3 h (LOGAN and WILHELM, 1966).

These same substances are also powerful inhibitors of other effects of histamine at H_1 receptors. Pertinent in relation to protection against anaphylaxis in guinea pigs, these compounds are highly effective in protecting guinea pigs against the bronchoconstrictor effects of an histamine aerosol. For example, in a study reported by GREEN (1953), the relative potencies of triprolidine:chlorpheniramine:mepyramine were related as 8.6:1.8:1.5, the ED_{50} of triprolidine being approximately 0.01 mg/kg i.p. These compounds are less active by the oral route than when given systematically in guinea pigs, though in comparisons of oral potency chlorpheniramine and triprolidine were more active than other antihistamines tested (MARGOLIN and TISLOW, 1950; GREEN, 1953).

II. Rat

The amounts of histamine required to produce a cutaneous permeability reaction are much larger than in guinea pigs (MILES and WILHELM, 1960, and Table 1) and larger doses of antihistamines are needed to inhibit these reactions than in guinea pigs (WILHELM, 1973, and Table 2). The relative potencies of the compounds tested are different from those in the guinea pig, but triprolidine and mepyramine are again among the preferred compounds from the viewpoints of both potency and specificity. BROCKLEHURST et al. (1960) found a 60–200-fold decrease in sensitivity to histamine 45 min after 50 mg/kg mepyramine i.p., an amount which is near to the maximum tolerated dose.

Oedema can be measured in rat hind feet following subcutaneous injection of histamine (approximately 9.1–0.2 mg) into the plantar area. This response can also be suppressed by mepyramine (PARRATT and WEST, 1958; STARR and WEST, 1967) and many other H_1 antagonists (MALING et al., 1974). The doses of antihistamines required are high. For example, the subcutaneous doses reducing oedema by 50% were approximately 15 mg/kg for triprolidine and 8 mg/kg for mepyramine. Some antihistamines were almost as active in antagonising 5-HT as histamine—e.g. promethazine and tripelennamine; cyproheptadine was more active in antagonising 5-HT.

Despite these low sensitivities to histamine, this amine—being present at high concentrations in rat tissues—plays some part as an inflammatory mediator but not as a mediator of respiratory anaphylaxis, the sensitivity of rat bronchial muscle to histamine being particularly low (Sect. H). In the rat, 5-HT appears to be more important a mediator than histamine and in consequence more attention has been given to antagonism of that amine (Sect. G).

III. Rabbit

Intradermal (i.d.) tests using the local blueing reaction at the site of i.d. injection of histamine in animals previously injected with an albumin-bound blue dye, show that the sensitivity of rabbits to histamine is comparable with that of guinea pigs and very much greater than that of rats (Table 1). The sensitivity of the histamine response to inhibition by triprolidine, mepyramine, and chlorpheniramine is substantially less than in guinea pigs (Table 2).

IV. Mouse

The threshold dose of histamine (base) which, when administered i.d. caused extravasation of an albumin-bound dye at the injection site, is about $0.12 \, \mu g$ (HALPERN et al., 1963; CASEY and TOKUDA, 1973). The permeability factor (PF) for comparison with those for other species (Table 1) is therefore about 10000 indicating a sensitivity to histamine between that of guinea pig and rat. Estimates of the threshold value for 5-HT vary—e.g. $0.0012 \, \mu g$ base (HALPERN et al., 1963) and $0.05 \, \mu g$ (CASEY and TOKUDA, 1973)—suggesting differences between strains. However, these values show that mouse skin is much less sensitive to histamine than to 5-HT and that its sensitivity to 5-HT is as great or greater than that of the rat.

A dose of mepyramine of 6 mg/kg subcutaneously (s.c.) reduced the sensitivity of skin to histamine by a factor of about 50 and whereas even 25 mg/kg did not appreciably change the sensitivity to 5-HT (HALPERN et al., 1963), a slight inhibitory effect on 5-HT has been observed with 50 mg/kg intraperitoneally (i.p.) (CASEY and TOKUDA, 1973). Promethazine at 1.56 mg/kg reduced the sensitivity to histamine by a factor of approximately 150 and at 12 mg/kg reduced the sensitivity to 5-HT. Both substances have been used to investigate antihistamine action in other inflammatory situations.

Similarly, antihistamines suppress the blueing response at the site of pricking histamine (1 mg/ml) into the pinna of mice injected i.v. with an albumin-bound dye, the ID_{50}s of mepyramine, diphenhydramine, and cyproheptadine administered s.c. 20 min previously being 1.34, 2.51, and 0.024 mg/kg (CHURCH and MILLER, 1975).

Antihistamines, also protect against the lethal effects of histamine. For example, in mice sensitized to histamine (and 5-HT) by prior treatment with *Bordetella pertussis* organisms, the lethality of histamine at 25 mg/kg i.p. was significantly reduced by chlorpheniramine (MED approximately 1 mg/kg i.p.) and by cyproheptadine (MED approximately 0.01 mg/kg i.p.) and was virtually abolished by larger amounts (GANLEY, 1962).

V. Man

The sensitivity of the human skin to i.d. injected histamine, exhibited as a weal and flare response, exceeds that of the skin of laboratory animals (Table 1). The weal response can be used as a quantitative measure of histamine and antihistamines action (BAIN, 1949, 1951). The most active antihistamines in man include chlorpheniramine (BAIN, 1951) and triprolidine (BAIN cited in GREEN, 1953; FOWLE et al., 1971; PECK et al., 1975). Clinically used doses are a good guide to relative potencies of antihistamines in man. Their dosage is limited by the drowsiness and impairment of concentration that they produce. Separation of peripheral antihistaminic reaction from central depressant effects have been claimed for some compounds but not substantiated (PECK et al., 1975).

D. Histamine H_2 Antagonists: Chemical Considerations

Soon after ASH and SCHILD (1966) had defined two distinct types of histamine receptor in pharmacological terms, KIER (1968a) proposed that the two agonist-receptor interactions of histamine involve two distinct conformations of the histamine monocation; this amino-protonated form represents >96% of the population at physiological pH. This proposal was based on molecular orbital calculations which suggested two preferred conformations for histamine: the *trans*-conformation (21), with an inter-nitrogen distance of 4.55 A, was assumed to be complementary to the H_1 receptor, and the *gauche*-conformation (22), with an inter-nitrogen distance of 3.60 A, complementary to the H_2 receptor. However, recent work (GANELLIN et al., 1973) on the conformational and biological properties of a series of methyl-substituted histamines suggests that the side-chain conformational preference of these compounds is not related to their ability to distinguish between H_1 and H_2 receptors. Thus, α-methyl, β-methyl, and N,N-dimethylhistamine (cf. 23) are agonists, but show no selectivity of action towards the different receptor types, despite the fact that the *trans/gauche* conformational ratios are predicted to be 0.1, 0.02, and 4 respectively. In contrast, 2-methyl and 4-methylhistamine (cf. 23) have very similar side-chain conformational preferences and yet 4-methylhistamine is a highly selective H_2 receptor agonist ($H_1:H_2=1:170$) while 2-methylhistamine is a more potent stimulant of H_1 than H_2 receptors ($H_1:H_2=8:1$).

(21)   (22)   (23)

Recently, DURANT et al. (1975) suggested a possible chemical differentiation of histamine H_1 and H_2 receptor agonists. Because 2-pyridyl and 2-thiazolylethylamine are potent selective H_1 agonists the imidazole tautomeric system is not essential for H_1 receptor agonist activity. On the other hand, all known potent H_2 receptor agonists are compounds which are capable of undergoing a 1,3-prototropic tautomerism, and the functional requirements of such agonists could then be defined by formula (24a⇌24b).

(24a)   (24b)

In the light of this suggested structural requirement for H_2 receptor stimulant activity, it is interesting to note that the only potent H_2 receptor antagonists described to date have an imidazole ring system. The first such compound to be described, burimamide (25) (BLACK et al., 1972), is a specific competitive histamine H_2-receptor antagonist with an ED_{50} of 6.1×10^{-6} M as an inhibitor of histamine-stimulated gastric secretion in the rat. Burimamide is orally ineffective in experimental animals, but a closely related and intrinsically equipotent compound, metiamide (26), was later reported to have good oral bioavailability and low toxicity in laboratory animals (BLACK et al., 1973; WYLLIE et al., 1972). A third compound of the same series, cimetidine (27), is slightly more potent than metiamide and is devoid of toxic effects noted with the first two compounds (BRIMBLECOMBE et al., 1975); cimetidine has a cyanoguanidine function in place of the thiourea function in (25) and (26). It is interesting to note that the latter two compounds, (26) and (27), possess the 4-methyl group which is present in the potent H_2 agonist 4-methylhistamine.

(25) Burimamide   (26) Metiamide

(27) Cimetidine

E. Inhibition of Cardiovascular Responses to Histamine by H_1 and H_2 Antagonists

The depressor effects of histamine in anaesthetised cats and dogs are reduced by antihistamines (LOEW, 1947; FEINBERG et al., 1950), the more active compounds, triprolidine and cyproheptadine, being effective at doses as low as 10 µg/kg i.v. (GREEN, 1953; STONE et al., 1961). However, these antihistamines do not suppress responses to elevated doses of histamine and this can now be explained in terms of histamine activating both H_1 and H_2 receptors (BLACK et al., 1972, 1975).

In the studies of BLACK et al. (1975), the dose-response curves for histamine in cats and dogs were shifted to the right by mepyramine (as by other H_1 antagonists) but the maximal decrease in sensitivity was less than tenfold. Metiamide (up to 2×10^{-6} mol/kg/min i.v.) alone had no appreciable effect on the histamine dose-response curve, but when administered in the presence of mepyramine, it caused dose-dependent displacements to the right greater than could be achieved with mepyramine alone. Similar results to these were obtained by FLYNN and OWEN (1975) in studies of the vasodilator response of both the mesentery and the hind limb

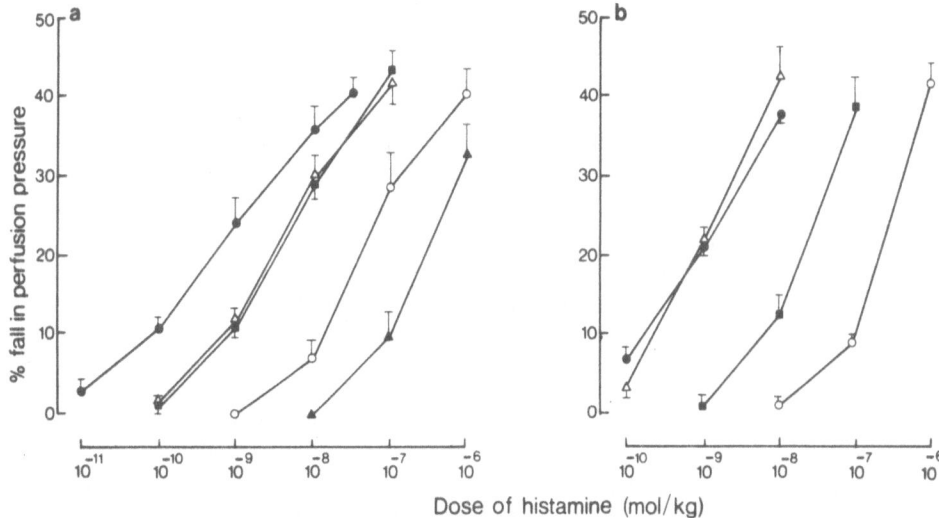

Fig. 1a and b. Anaesthetised cats. Vasodilator response to histamine in the hind limb perfused with blood at constant flow rates. Effects of mepyramine and metiamide on the responses to histamine. (a) Dose response curve to histamine in untreated cats (●); (△) after mepyramine 2.5×10^{-5} mol/kg; (■) after mepyramine 5×10^{-5} mol/kg; (○) after mepyramine 5×10^{-5} mol/kg plus metiamide 4×10^{-7} mol/kg/min; (▲) after mepyramine 5×10^{-5} mol/kg plus metiamide 2×10^{-6} mol/kg/min. (b) Dose response curve to histamine in untreated cats (●); (△) after metiamide 2×10^{-6} mol/kg/min; (■) after metiamide 2×10^{-6} mol/kg/min plus mepyramine 2.5×10^{-6} mol/kg; (○) after metiamide 2×10^{-6} mol/kg/min plus mepyramine 2.5×10^{-5} mol/kg. Vertical bars indicate s.e. mean. (From: FLYNN and OWEN, 1975).

in anaesthetised cats; the results in the latter preparation are illustrated in Figure 1. A synergistic effect between tripelennamine and the H_2 receptor antagonists has also been demonstrated in studies of vasodilator responses to histamine in canine paws (KRAFT and ZIMMERMAN, 1975).

In contrast with these results are those found by EYRE and WELLS (1973) in studies of the depressor actions of histamine and anaphylaxis in calves. These depressor responses were incompletely blocked by mepyramine and were increased by burimamide. Also, depressor responses that had been enhanced by burimamide were inhibited by mepyramine. Hence in this species, in contrast with cat and dog, activation of H_2 receptors appears to oppose the depressor action associated with activation of H_1 receptors.

These observations again emphasize the considerable variation between mammalian species in their response to physiologically occurring mediators and drugs. Another variation is exemplified by the positive chronotropic effect of histamine. This response of isolated guinea pig atria is mediated by activation of H_2 receptors and is blocked by burimamide (BLACK et al., 1972; LEVI and LEE, 1974), but the increased rate of beat caused by histamine in chicken hearts was reported to be resistant to burimamide and blocked by H_1 antagonists (EL-ACKAD et al., 1974).

F. Chemical and Pharmacological Classes
of 5-Hydroxytryptamine Antagonists

I. Chemical Classes

Antagonism of one or more of the effects of 5-HT is observed in compounds of widely diverse structural types. The following broad chemical classes can be distinguished: (a) lysergic acid derivatives; (b) aryloxyalkylamidines such as xylamidine and BW 501 C67 (Mawson and Whittington, 1970); (c) β-haloalkylamines; (d) tricyclic alkylamines, including many antihistamines such as cyproheptadine and the phenothiazine derivatives chlorpromazine and promethazine; (e) a wide variety of indole derivatives of which the only common feature is the indole nucleus. These include indole alkylamines such as tryptamine itself and benzyl-anti-serotonin, derivatives of carbazole, gramine, and harmine, indole acetamides, quaternary ammonium salts of N,N-dialkyltryptamines, and miscellaneous derivatives such as medmain: (f) arylguanidines and biguanides.

Many compounds of classes (a), (c), and (d) are also α-adrenoceptor blocking agents and, although the properties of antagonism of 5-HT and of noradrenaline do not run in parallel with structural changes, there is sufficient overlap of these properties to suggest that the receptors of the two amines are similar. Both amines powerfully stimulate adenyl cyclase. The tricyclic alkylamines of class (d) include compounds which possess antihistaminic and a variety of other properties.

II. "M" and "D" Receptors

The concept of "M" and "D" receptors for 5-HT was put forward by Gaddum and Picarelli (1957) to explain their observations in a study of the effect of antagonists in guinea pig ileum. "M" receptors are those blocked by morphine. They appeared to be associated with the nerve plexus. They are blocked also by other morphine-like analgesic narcotics. The response is apparently mediated by a cholinergic pathway, being abolished by atropine and by nerve blockade with cocaine. "D" receptors are those blocked by dibenzyline (phenoxybenzamine, dibenyline). They were considered to be probably associated directly with the smooth muscle fibres and were shown also to be blocked by lysergic acid diethylamide (LSD) and 5-benzoyloxygramine.

Several studies, reviewed by Gyermek (1966), add some support to this general concept. However, the mechanisms in the ileum preparation were found to be more complex than originally supposed and analysis of results led Day and Vane (1963) to conclude as follows. 5-HT contracts the longitudinal muscle of the guinea pig ileum mainly through receptors in nervous tissue and some of this action is sensitive to morphine. Smooth muscle receptors are of negligible importance in this tissue unless the neuronal mechanisms have been inactivated. Dibenzyline blocks smooth muscle receptors but also antagonises some of the effects of 5-HT on nerves whereas methysergide is a more specific antagonist of the muscle receptors. Since the responses to 5-HT of the stomachs of guinea pig, rat, and kitten are unaffected by morphine or hyoscine, the proportion of nerve receptors to muscle receptors probably varies not only from species to species but from one part of the alimentary tract to another. Their final conclusion was that the terms "M" and "D" receptors should be used only in the sense of the original definitions and should not be equated quantitatively with nerve and smooth muscle receptors.

III. "Musculotropic" and "Neurotropic" Receptors

An alternative classification of 5-HT antagonists has been suggested by GYERMEK (1966).

Type A, Typical musculotropic antagonists: These are effective in preparations in which the action of 5-HT is not dependent upon a nervous mechanism—e.g. the rat stomach strip and rat uterus. Notably specific compounds of this type are the lysergic acid derivatives LSD (lysergic acid diethylamide) (28), bromo-LSD (the 2-bromo derivative of (28), and methysergide (29), belonging to chemical class (a). These compounds contain the indole ethylamine residue of 5-HT embedded in a tetracyclic structure; in this situation the geometry of this residue corresponds closely to that which has been calculated (KIER, 1968b), using molecular orbital theory, for the single preferred conformation of 5-HT (30), as the protonated form, which is the predominant species at physiological pH. The more recently discovered peripheral antagonists exemplified by xylamidine (31) and BW 501 C67 (32) (COPP et al., 1967; MAWSON and WHITTINGTON, 1970) of chemical class (b), provide further examples, although these amidines apparently have no structural affinities with (28), (29) or (30). However, a possible conformation of xylamidine is represented by (33) in which form it could be expected to occupy the same receptor site as (30).

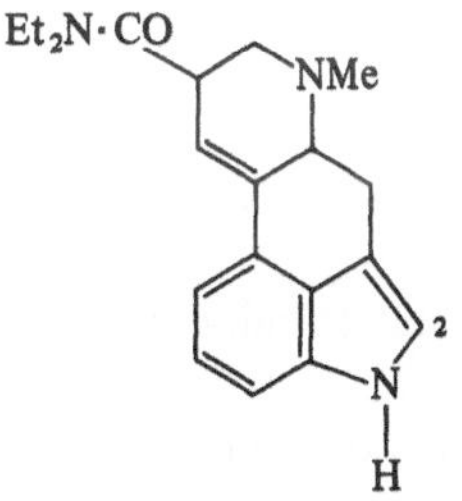

(28) LSD

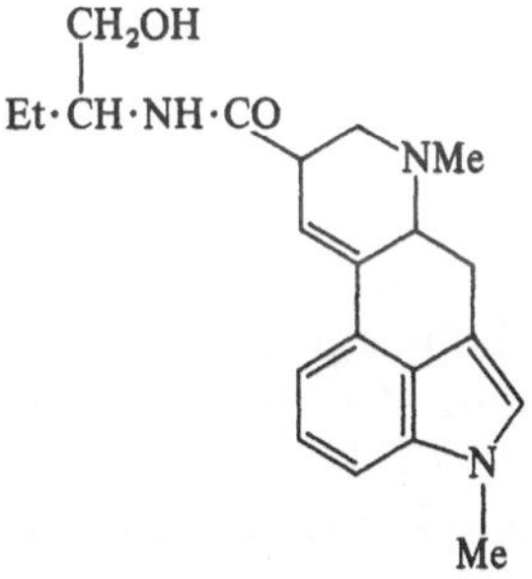

(29) Methysergide

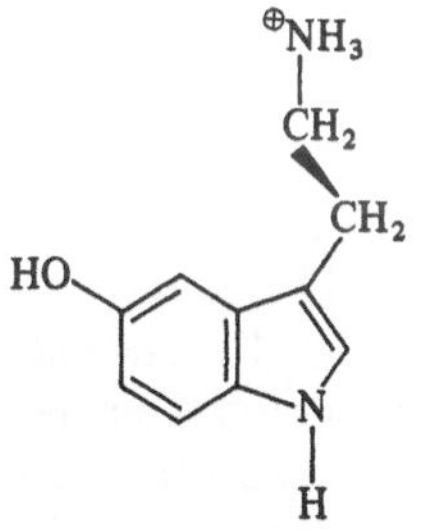

(30)

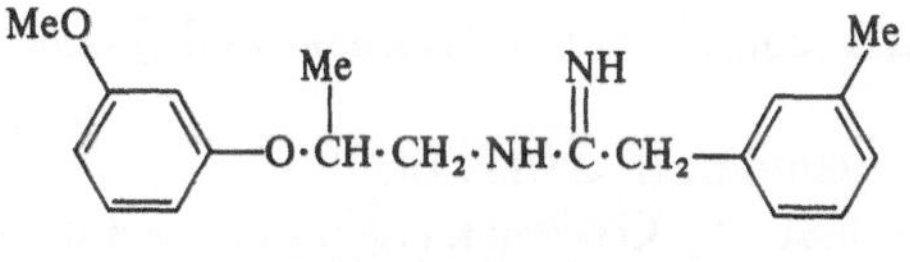

(31) Xylamidine

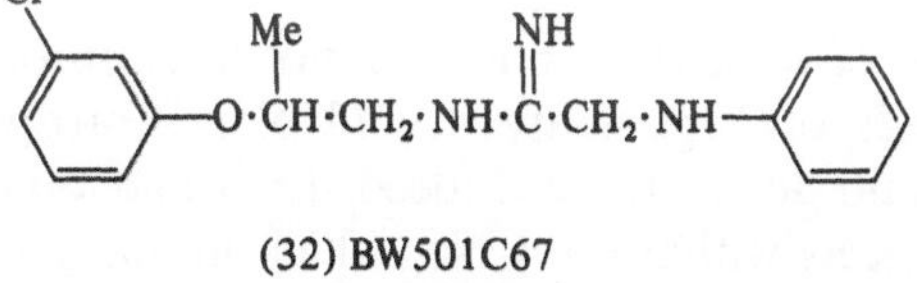

(32) BW501C67

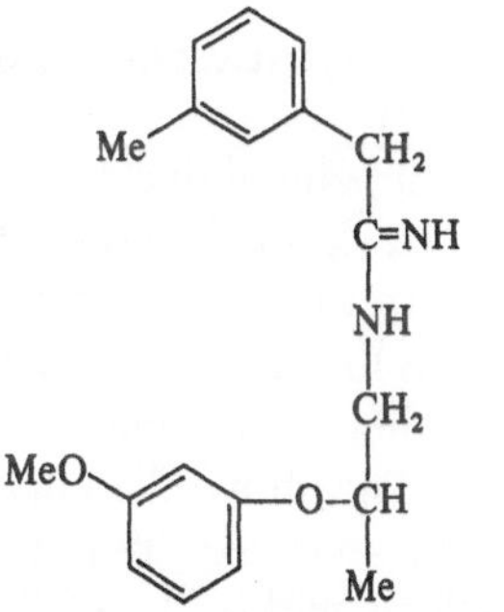

(33)

Non-specific antagonists of type A which are also α-adrenoceptor blocking agents include such lysergic acid derivatives as ergotamine and ergotoxine and also β-haloalkylamines, class (c), such as dibenzyline (34) in which it is difficult to visualise a structural resemblance to 5-HT. A number of potent antihistamines of the ethylenediamine class, in particular cyproheptadine (35) are also non-specific type A antagonists as are certain phenothiazines, among the best known of which are promethazine (36) and chlorpromazine (37). No clear relationship between structure and anti-5-HT activity has been discerned for these compounds of class (d).

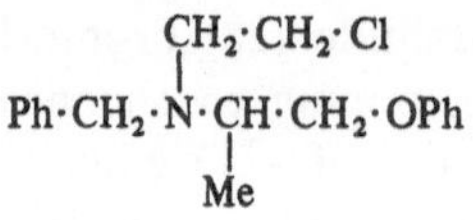

$CH_2 \cdot CH_2 \cdot Cl$

$Ph \cdot CH_2 \cdot N \cdot CH \cdot CH_2 \cdot OPh$

Me

(34) Dibenzyline

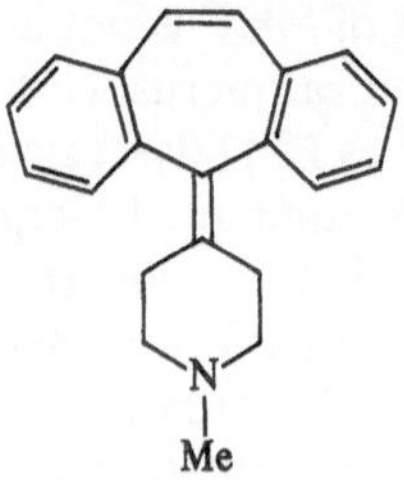

Me

(35) Cyproheptadine

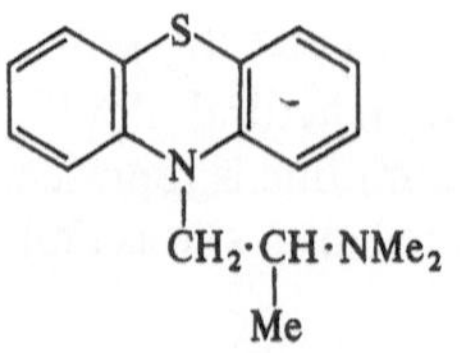

$CH_2 \cdot CH \cdot NMe_2$

Me

(36) Promethazine

Cl

$CH_2 \cdot CH_2 \cdot CH_2 \cdot NMe_2$

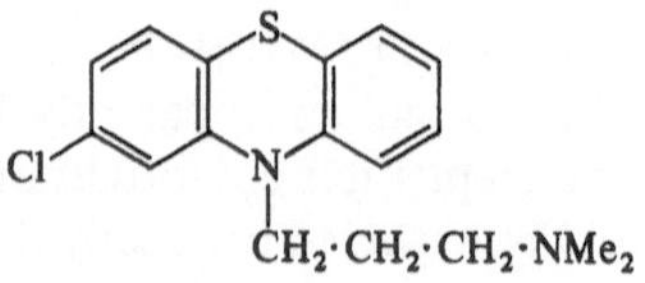

(37) Chlorpromazine

Type B, neurotropic antagonists: They have the following characteristics:

1. High potency in antagonising response to stimulation of nervous receptors by 5-HT and relatively low anti-cholinergic potency

2. Produce stimulant actions of various degress at autonomic ganglia prior to blocking their responsiveness to 5-HT.

Apart from cocaine and morphine-like agents they consist of three main groups, from chemical classes (e) and (f):

1. Indole acetamides—e.g. 5-hydroxyindole-3-acetamide (WOOLLEY and SHAW, 1957)

2. Quarternary indole alkylammonium compounds (GYERMEK and NADOR, 1957)

3. Guanidine derivatives, e.g. 2-anthrylguanidine (FASTIER, 1962).

It should be noted, however, that as discussed by GYERMEK (1966), the usefulness for research and any possible therapeutic purposes of compounds in groups (1) and (3) is limited by their cardiovascular side effects, and that of compounds in group (2) by their poor penetration into the CNS.

The above classification of GYERMEK is of value though it must not be supposed that so-called "musculotropic" compounds of Type A are devoid of neurotropic effects within the CNS, providing they gain access there. Indeed, LSD and other lysergic acid derivatives have profound effects within the CNS, which in many instances can be related to their effect on 5-HT receptors.

The present review is concerned only with the pharmacological properties of 5-HT antagonists (Type A), for it is only they which are known to have powerful and informative effects on the inflammatory reactions. No further consideration is given to the so-called neurotropic antagonists of Type B.

G. Antagonists of 5-Hydroxytryptamine: Inhibition of Responses to 5-HT Involved in Inflammatory and Anaphylactic Reactions

This review, in contrast to the comprehensive review on 5-HT antagonists prepared by GYERMEK (1966), is concerned only with the effects of the principal 5-HT antagonists on those responses to 5-HT that are involved in inflammatory and anaphylactic reactions.

Two main chemical types of selective 5-HT antagonists are available for anti-inflammatory studies. The first group consists of lysergic acid derivatives. Notable among these are LSD and methysergide which powerfully inhibit peripheral and central actions of 5-HT, and 2-bromolysergic acid diethylamide (brom-LSD, also known as BOL-148) which has a more selectively peripheral effect (DOEPFNER and CERLETTI, 1958; GYERMEK, 1966). The second group consists of powerful peripheral antagonists devoid of central actions of low toxicity and exemplified by xylamidine (COPP et al., 1967; MAWSON and WHITTINGTON, 1970) and BW 501 C 67 (MAWSON and WHITTINGTON, 1970). They are potentially useful tools but by comparison with the lysergic acid derivatives they have been little used. Cyproheptadine, which antagonises both 5-HT and histamine (STONE et al., 1961), is also frequently employed in inflammatory studies.

Information is presented separately for each species as these differ greatly in their sensitivity to 5-HT and its antagonists and different species are suitable for different kinds of experimentation.

I. Guinea Pig

By comparison with histamine, 5-HT appears to be a relatively unimportant mediator of inflammatory responses in the guinea pig. Nevertheless, studies of the cutaneous reaction to intradermal 5-HT show that this amine at relatively high concentrations increases capillary permeability in guinea pig skin (Table 1).

Bronchospasm is, however, caused in guinea pigs by intravenous injection of 5-HT at i.v. doses of 10–30 µg/kg. These responses are blocked by a variety of 5-HT antagonists (GYERMEK, 1966), and notably by methysergide (ED$_{50}$ 1 µg/kg i.v., BERETTA et al., 1965), methergoline (ED$_{50}$ ≃ 1.5 µg/kg i.v., BERETTA et al., 1965) and xylamidine (ED$_{100}$ 0.15 mg/kg i.v., COPP et al., 1967). Bronchospasm is caused also by inhalation of 5-HT in guinea pigs and this action too is well suppressed by LSD (ca. 0.02 mg/kg i.m., HERXHEIMER, 1955).

II. Rat

5-HT appears to play a more important role in the rat than in most other species. Tissue levels are generally fairly high (Sect. H) and measurements of the permeability response of the skin shows a much greater sensitivity to 5-HT than to histamine (Table 1). A commonly used method for evaluating the potency of 5-HT antagonists is to determine inhibition of the local oedema formation caused by injecting 5-HT into the feet of rats. The threshold dose of this amine for producing such an effect is

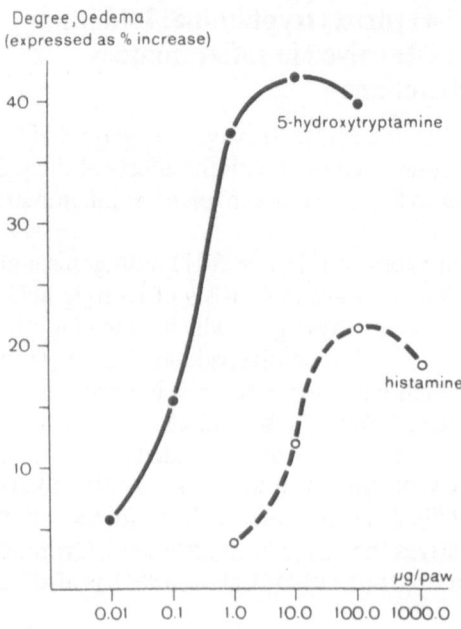

Fig. 2. Comparison of 5-HT and histamine in regard to their potency as oedema provoking agents in the rat's paw. (From: DOEPFNER and CERLETTI (1958) with permission of S. Karger AG, Basel, Switzerland)

about 0.01 µg, the sensitivity being about 200 times that to histamine (DOEPFNER and CERLETTI, 1958). Dose-response curves for the two amines are shown in Figure 2, and the time course of the oedema response in animals given a series of doses of methysergide in Figure 3. In this study, methysergide was administered s.c. 30 min before the 5-HT. This is a fairly common practice but it has been observed that the potent peripheral 5-HT antagonists, xylamidine and BW 501 C 67, are effective at lower oral dosage if given 5 h rather than 1 h before 5-HT injection (COPP et al., 1967; MAWSON and WHITTINGTON, 1970).

The following provides a guide to approximate ED_{50} values in the rat paw test:

Methysergide	s.c.	0.015 mg/kg	(MALING et al., 1974; BERETTA et al., 1965; DOEPFNER and CERLETTI, 1958)
	oral	0.2 mg/kg	(COPP et al., 1967)
LSD	s.c.	0.057 mg/kg	(DOEPFNER and CERLETTI, 1958)
Brom-LSD	s.c.	0.2 mg/kg	(DOEPFNER and CERLETTI, 1958)
Methergoline	s.c.	0.015 mg/kg	(BERETTA et al., 1965)
	oral	0.16 mg/kg	(MAWSON and WHITTINGTON, 1970)
Xylamidine	s.c.	0.04 mg/kg	(COPP et al., 1967)
	oral	0.4 mg/kg	
BW 501C67	oral	0.05 mg/kg	(MAWSON and WHITTINGTON, 1970)
Cyproheptadine	s.c.	0.03 mg/kg	(STONE et al., 1961)
	s.c.	0.1 mg/kg	(MALING et al., 1974)

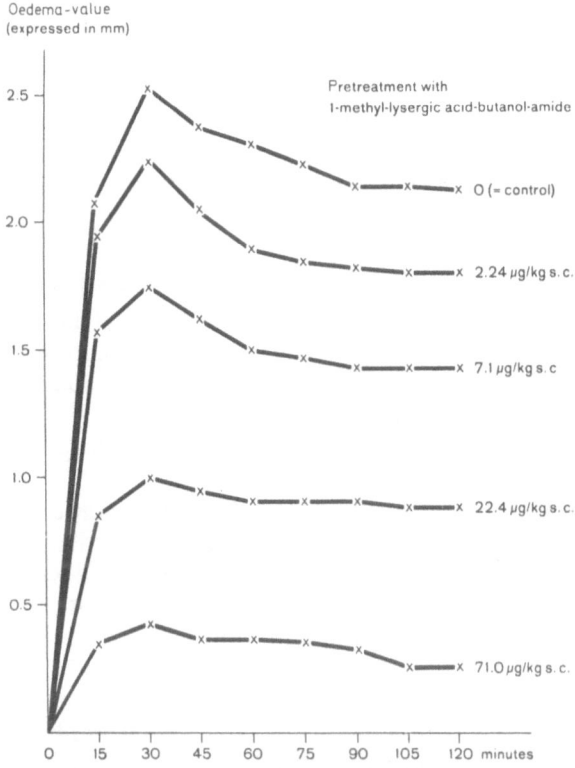

Fig. 3. Oedema values (difference of thickness in mm between the NaCl and 5-HT treated paw) obtained during the 2-h observation period in a control experiment and in four experiments with successively increasing doses of methysergide (1-methyl-lysergic acid butanolamide). Each curve represents the average values obtained from at least ten animals. (From: DOEPFNER and CERLETTI (1958) with permission of S. Karger AG, Basel, Switzerland)

Less information is available on antagonism of the increase in capillary permeability at the site of i.d. injection of 5-HT, but published data (HALPERN et al., 1959; WILHELM and MASON, 1960; JULOU et al., 1966) and our own unpublished information concerning BW 501 C 67 suggests that 5-HT antagonists are effective in skin tests at doses of similar magnitude to those effective in the paw test.

These compounds are also powerful antagonists of the pressor (GYERMEK, 1966; COPP et al., 1967) and bronchoconstrictor (CHURCH, 1975) effects of 5-HT in the rat as in other species (WOOLLEY and SHAW, 1957; STONE et al., 1961; BERETTA et al., 1965; FANCHAMPS et al., 1960; GYERMEK, 1966).

Cellular Response. The effect of s.c. injections of 5-HT on the reaction to implanted Ivalon sponges was studied by SCHERBEL et al. (1960). Daily administration of 1–30 mg 5-HT increased the inflammatory reaction but did not alter the fibroplasia, in contrast to histamine which increased the fibroplasia but not the inflammation. The effect of 5-HT was greatly potentiated when animals were pretreated with monoamine oxidase inhibitors and completely blocked following pretreatment with methysergide.

III. Rabbit

Tests using the local blueing reactions of skin show a low sensitivity to 5-HT (Table 1). Because of this it has been supposed that 5-HT plays little, if any, part in the mediation of responses to local tissue reaction in this species and the effect of antagonists has not been investigated. Where tests have been made, for example tests of inhibition of cutaneous anaphylaxis, 5-HT antagonists were ineffective.

IV. Mouse

Mouse skin is highly sensitive to 5-HT, the reported threshold for increasing capillary permeability to i.d. doses varying between $0.0012\,\mu g$ (HALPERN et al., 1963) and $0.05\,\mu g$ (CASEY and TOKUDA, 1973). These responses are abolished by 5-HT antagonists. For example, LSD at s.c. doses of 3 and 6 mg/kg, reduced 5-HT sensitivity by factors of 170 and 3000 times, respectively (HALPERN et al., 1963). Brom-LSD, at 4 mg/kg i.v., abolished the effect of a large i.d. dose $(0.5\,\mu g)$ of 5-HT (CASEY and TOKUDA, 1973).

Similarly, 5-HT antagonists suppress the blueing response at the site of pricking 5-HT (0.2 mg/ml) into the pinna of mice injected i.v. with an albumin-bound dye, the $ID_{50}s$ of methysergide and cyproheptadine, administered s.c. 20 min previously being 0.008 and 0.16 mg/kg, respectively (CHURCH and MILLER, 1975). In this test, cyproheptadine was more effective in antagonising histamine than 5-HT, whereas the converse was found in the rat paw test (MALING et al., 1974).

Oedema can be measured in the hind feet of mice following local injections of 5-HT and is reduced by LSD (0.1 mg/kg i.p., WEIS, 1963) and by other 5-HT antagonists (NORTHOVER and SUBRAMANIAN, 1962).

Large doses of 5-HT are lethal to mice $(LD_{50}\simeq 870\,mg/kg\ i.p.)$ and protection is afforded by 5-HT antagonists (e.g. methysergide, GELFAND and WEST, 1961). The lethal dose of 5-HT can be reduced to about 10 mg/kg i.v. by prior treatment of the animals with *B. pertussis* organisms and then the minimal protective doses of LSD and cyproheptadine were approximately 0.001 and 0.01 mg/kg i.p., respectively (GANLEY, 1962).

V. Man

The findings of KALZ and FEKETE (1961) in subjects injected i.v. with Coomassie blue are described in a subsequent section (H.V.2). They show low skin sensitivity to locally applied 5-HT and support the conclusion that this amine does not have an important role in cutaneous inflammatory responses in man. However, cyproheptadine did antagonise cutaneous reactions to 5-HT (KALZ and FEKETE, 1961). An observation of interest in relation to the use of methysergide in migraine and the release of 5-HT by 48/80, is that this 5-HT antagonist inhibited elevation of CSF pressure associated with injection of both 5-HT and 48/80 (SICUTERI, 1959).

H. Effects of Antagonists of Histamine (H_1 Receptors) and 5-HT in Various Types of Inflammation

The effects of antagonists of histamine at H_1 receptors and of 5-HT antagonists are referred to in several reviews dealing with inflammation (MILES and WILHELM, 1960; WILHELM, 1962, 1963; SPECTOR and WILLOUGHBY, 1963; WILLOUGHBY, 1973) and

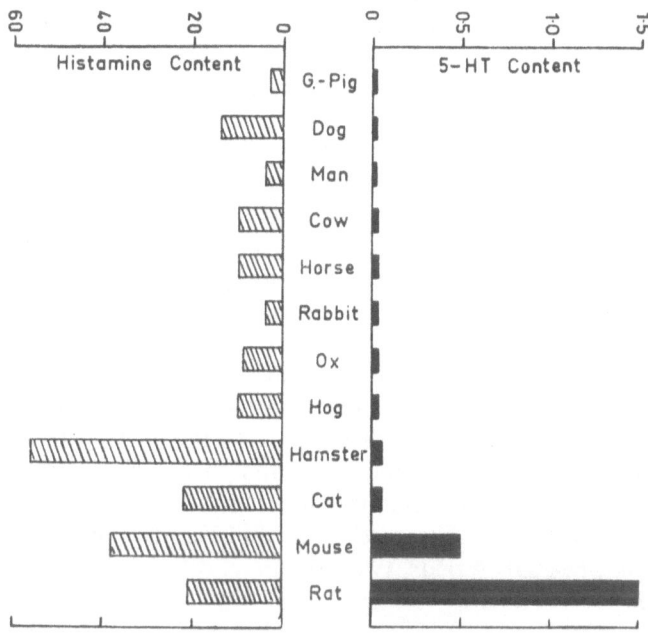

Fig. 4. Comparison of the 5-HT content (μg/g) of the ventral abdominal skin of different species with the histamine content (μg/g). (From: WEST (1957) with permission of S. Karger AG, Basel, Switzerland)

anaphylaxis (AUSTEN and HUMPHREY, 1963; STECHSCHULTE and AUSTEN, 1974). Reviews dealing with histamine and H_1 antihistamines (LOEW, 1947; SCHACHTER, 1973; ROCHA E SILVA, 1966, 1977) and with 5-HT and its antagonists (GARATTINI and VALZELLI, 1965; ERSPAMER, 1966) refer among many topics to inflammatory processes. This current review is much narrower in scope and concentrates on the effects of antagonists of histamine and 5-HT on inflammation in the common laboratory species, briefly mentioning comparative studies in man and bovine anaphylaxis. Information concerning the synthesis, distribution, storage, metabolism, and release of histamine and 5-HT is reviewed by LICHTENSTEIN and PLAUT in Chapter 11 and the role of these amines in vascular phenomena of inflammation are considered by YOULTEN in Chapter 16.

In considering the available information, it is appropriate to deal with each species separately. Species vary greatly in their sensitivity to histamine and 5-HT and their antagonists (Sect. C. and G.) and also in their tissue contents of these amines. For detailed results on tissue levels, the reviews referred to above should be consulted, but Figure 4 exemplifies the order of magnitude of the differences in skin amine contents. The amount of each mediator released by an inflammatory insult, together with the sensitivity to each mediator will in large measure influence the magnitude of the response and govern the change produced by appropriate antagonists. It should also be borne in mind when comparing results from different sources that the levels of amines varies in skin taken from different regions in the same animal (FELDBERG and MILES, 1953; WEST, 1957).

Other special difficulties in the interpretation of anti-inflammatory studies are as follows. One group of problems arises from the multiplicity of mediating substances, their interaction (e.g. prostaglandins sensitize to bradykinin and 5-HT; see MON-CADA et al., Chap. 17) and the progressive sequence of events, including enhanced synthesis and release. In consequence it may happen, for example, that an early contribution by one mediator (say histamine) is not revealed by an antagonist because the inflammation is measured at a time when the contribution of another mediator (say bradykinin) has become overwhelming. Interactions can extend to one mediator releasing another, a particularly relevant example in the present context being the release of histamine by 5-HT (FELDBERG and SMITH, 1953; SPARROW and WILHELM, 1957). Other problems arise because adequate information is not always available concerning the effectiveness, specificity of action and persistence of the antagonist used in the species in which an anti-inflammatory effect has been sought. Histamine or 5-HT antagonists which have other prominent effects (e.g. chlorpromazine, promethazine, diphenhydramine, LSD, and phenoxybenzamine) are poor tools for investigating the role of these amines in inflammatory processes by comparison with specific antihistamines like triprolidine and chlorpheniramine and specific 5-HT antagonists like methysergide, xylamidine, and BW 501 C 67.

I. Guinea Pig

1. Thermal and Ultraviolet Injury

WILHELM and MASON (1958, 1960) provided valuable information on the response of the guinea pig skin to mild thermal injury. It is gratifying that the heat applied, contact with a copper disk at 54° C for up to 30 s, does not produce an overt pain reaction in guinea pigs (or man). The reaction was assessed from the intensity of the

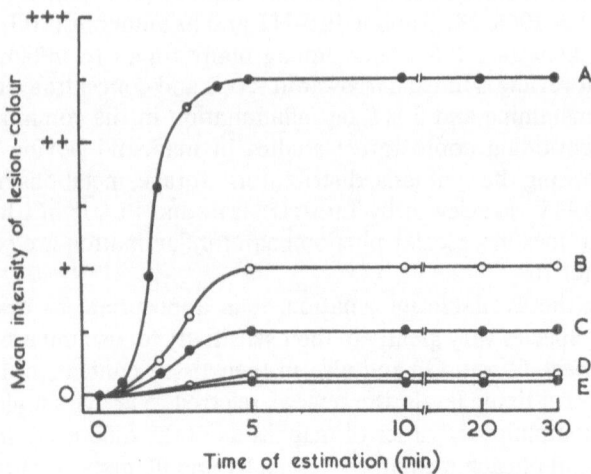

Fig. 5. Maturation of the immediate permeability effect in the blued guinea pig during the 30 min following a mild heat stimulus to the skin (A); and the influence of prior treatment with the antihistamine triprolidine, 0.02 µg. (B) and 2 µg. (D) intracutaneously, and 10 µg/kg (C) and 100 µg/kg (E) intravenously. (From: WILHELM and MASON, 1958)

blueing reaction at the exposed site, Pontamine blue having been injected i.v. Skin heated for 5 s became erythematous in 30–40 s and blueing was maximal in 5 min. This immediate response was readily inhibited by triprolidine either by injecting 0.02 μg in 0.1 ml of saline into the test site or by injecting 10 μg/kg i.v. (Fig. 5). Other antihistamines (0.1 mg/kg i.v.) inhibited the reaction and in order of decreasing effectiveness they rank roughly in the order of their relative potencies in suppressing the cutaneous reaction (Sect. C., Table 2). The rank order, with the approximate factors by which the extravasation of dye into the site had been reduced shown in brackets, was triprolidine (120), chlorpheniramine (21), mepyramine (16), tripelennamine (15), promethazine (7), diphenhydramine (4), chlorcyclizine (3), thenaldine (1.6), antazoline (1.3) (WILHELM and MASON, 1960). The effects of the last two compounds is only slight, if significant. These results are compatible with other findings indicating a release of small amounts of histamine in mild thermal injury (cited in WILHELM and MASON, 1958, 1960).

When in similar experiments the skin was exposed to 54° C for 20 min, the immediate response was represented by only a thin ring of blue at the periphery of the heated site. This too could be abolished by antihistamines. Later, starting at about 30 min, a delayed response followed, being seen as blueing of the whole of the exposed area (Fig. 6). The delayed response was not affected despite elevation of the triprolidine dosage to 10 μg locally or to 1 mg/kg i.v. It was presumed to be due to other mediators.

These results, therefore, support the conclusion that only the early phase of the inflammatory response to heat in the guinea pig is attributable to histamine. It should be noted further that the early phase may only be susceptible to antihistamine action if tissue damage is minimised; protection was not afforded in experiments using higher temperatures (SEVITT, 1958).

Early and late permeability reactions similar to those resulting from direct application of heat are produced by ultraviolet irradiation and likewise the early, but not the late, response was readily suppressed by triprolidine (LOGAN and WILHELM,

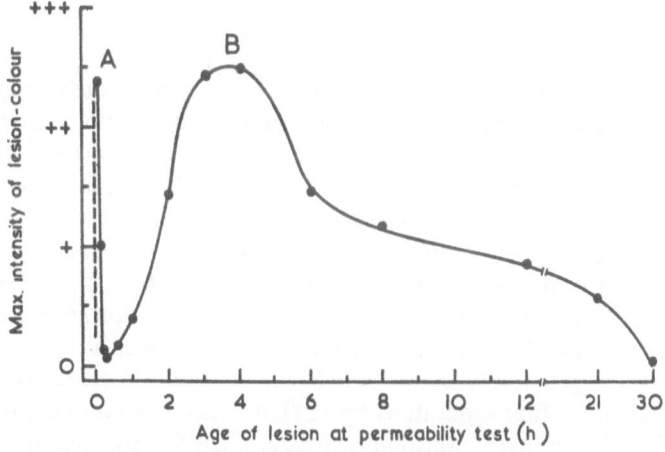

Fig. 6. The diphasic nature of the permeability effect of a moderate heat stimulus in the skin of the guinea-pig. (From WILHELM and MASON, 1958)

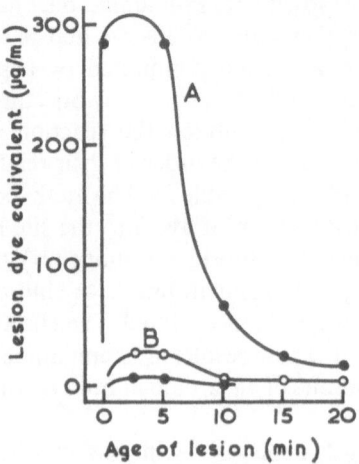

Fig. 7. The suppression by intravenous triprolidine of the early permeability response to ultraviolet injury in the guinea pig. A = control; B = triprolidine, 0.01 mg/kg; bottom response line = triprolidine, 0.1 mg/kg. (From: LOGAN and WILHELM, 1966)

1966). No more than 0.01 mg/kg triprolidine i.v. was required to suppress the early response (Fig. 7). The late response began to develop after about 2 h and developed progressively for at least 12 h. It was insusceptible to repeated administration of triprolidine systemically or to repeated local i.d. injection of triprolidine or mepyramine. The results do not prove that histamine played no part at any time in the delayed permeability response, but they show emphatically that (a) suppression of the immediate response with antihistamine does not materially affect the subsequent development of the delayed response, and (b) that inhibition of histamine by H_1 antagonists does not diminish the increased permeability when inflammation has developed (at 20 h).

2. Local Anaphylaxis

Understanding of local anaphylaxis in the guinea pig is complicated by the ability of this species to produce several different classes of homocytotropic antibody depending upon the sensitizing schedule employed. In early experiments in which unfractionated antiserum was used to sensitize the skin passively, and was followed 4–24 h later by i.v. injection of antigen and blue dye, the extravasation of dye was not inhibited, or only marginally reduced, by antihistamines including triprolidine and mepyramine (OVARY and BIER, 1953; ALBERTY and TAKKUNEN, 1957; OVARY, 1958; HALPERN et al., 1959; CRAIG and WILHELM, 1963). Such reactions may be associated with the release of lysosomal enzymes from polymorphonuclear leucocytes and in particular those using heterologous sera (MOVAT et al., 1967). Recently, PERINI and MOTA (1972) identified four separate types of skin-sensitising antibody in the guinea pig, three of them being "early" antibody fractions identified by their varying persistence in the skin and lability to heat and mercaptoethanol. Each of these early antibodies provoked skin reactions which were inhibited by triprolidine (1 mg/kg i.v.) or mepyramine (5 mg/kg i.v.). Consistent with these findings was the observation that each homocytotropic antibody fraction sensitized mesenteric mast cells in vitro ready for degranulation on antigen challenge. Thus, the skin reactions associated with these antibodies may be mediated entirely by histamine released from mast cells. In contrast, reactions provoked by hyperimmune IgG-type antibodies were only slightly reduced by antihistamines, suggesting that other mediators may be involved. STECHSCHULTE et al. (1967) have reported that guinea pig tissues sensitized with IgG-type antibody release slow-reacting substance of anaphylaxis (SRS-A) as well as histamine on antigen challenge. The part played by histamine in IgG-type reactions may, however, vary depending upon the experimental conditions since, while MOVAT et al. (1967) also found that triprolidine (1 mg/kg i.p./i.v.) partially reduced such a reaction, PHAIR et al. (1970) found that neither this potent antihistamine nor a specific histidine decarboxylase inhibitor (brocresine) had a significant effect. It may, perhaps, be relevant that, whereas MOVAT et al. (1967) measured dye concentration at the site of cutaneous reactions, PHAIR et al. (1970) measured areas of blueing.

In actively sensitized guinea pigs the i.d. injection of *Mycobacterium tuberculosis* produced an immediate phase of increased capillary permeability, that was reduced but not abolished by triprolidine at 0.1 or 1 mg/kg i.v. and a delayed reaction that was insusceptible to the antihistamine (BAUMGARTEN and WILHELM, 1969).

Local cutaneous anaphylactic reactions, both active and passive, were unaffected by LSD in test situations in which these reactions were suppressed by the antihistamines promethazine and mepyramine (HALPERN et al., 1959).

The SCHULTZ-DALE reaction of sensitized isolated guinea pig ileum to antigen challenge is highly sensitive to antihistamines in that low concentrations of these substances delay the onset of anaphylactic contracture. However, much higher concentrations are required to reduce the final extent of anaphylactic contractions and in a study of the highly specific antihistamine, triprolidine, abolition of the response was achieved only by the use of concentrations of the same order as those which nonspecifically suppressed responses to acetylcholine and barium (GREEN, 1953). It was these and similar observations using mepyramine (BROCKLEHURST, 1953) that led to reconsideration of the observation of KELLAWAY and TRETHEWIE (1940) that anaphylactic lungs of guinea pigs released not only histamine but also a slow-reacting substance. This substance, later designated SRS-A (BROCKLEHURST, 1960), is responsible for that part of the anaphylactic contraction of guinea pig ileum that is resistant to antihistamines.

3. Systemic Anaphylaxis

Acute anaphylactic shock such as follows i.v. challenge with antigen of previously sensitized guinea pigs is first seen as asthmatic symptoms associated with bronchospasm; persistence of severe bronchospasm leads to death of the animal. At low dosage, selective antihistamine compounds such as triprolidine and mepyramine protect against the bronchospasm and prevent immediate deaths (GREEN, 1953; BERNAUER et al., 1969). Delayed deaths occur, however, and these are associated not with emphysema but mostly with severe vascular congestion of the intestine (Fig. 8). There are many possible interpretations of these delayed deaths, for similar toxic

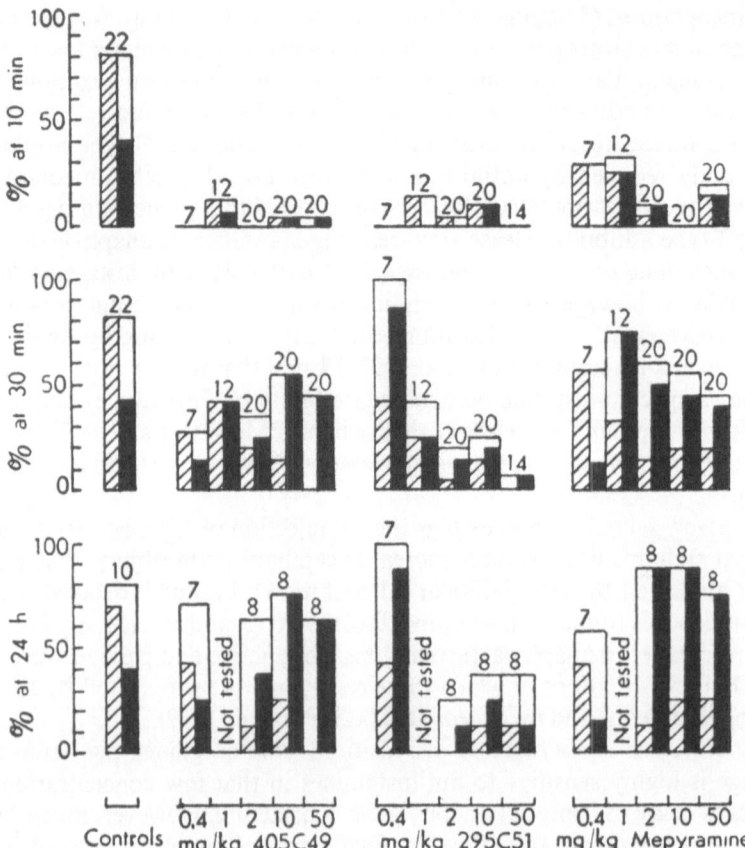

Fig. 8. The percentage mortality in groups of sensitized guinea pigs (number used shown above each column) at intervals after testing with antigen (i.v.), preceded by various doses of antihistamines (i.p. 30 min previously). The heights of the shaded and black portions show respectively the percentages dying with severe emphysema and with severe congestion of the intestine. 295C 51 = triprolidine hydrochloride. (From: GREEN, 1953)

signs in the intestine follow the injection of large doses of histamine, 5-HT, SRS-A or 48/80 in rats (this Sect. II.3.). In view, however, of the known synergistic effect of H_1 and H_2-receptor antagonists in blocking vascular effects of histamine in some species (Sect. E.), it would be pertinent to examine the extent to which a combination of these antagonists is able to protect guinea pigs against anaphylaxis. BERNAUER et al. (1969) have attributed delayed anaphylactic death to heart failure, most likely caused by spasm of the pulmonary and coronary vessels which is not caused by histamine and not inhibited by mepyramine.

In contrast to BERNAUER et al. (1969), who obtained full protection with antihistamines, COLLIER and JAMES (1967) found when recording changes in bronchial tone in urethanised guinea pigs that mepyramine failed to inhibit completely anaphylactic bronchospasm and that the residual bronchoconstriction was largely abolished by meclofenamate. The interpretation of this finding is discussed in Section I.I.

A "microshock" method for studying anaphylactic responses was introduced by ARMITAGE et al. (1952). The antigen challenge is presented at low concentration as an aerosol to sensitized guinea pigs and the same animals can be used on several occasions. Many antihistamines have been shown to antagonise anaphylactic microshock (e.g. ARMITAGE et al., 1952; HERXHEIMER and STRESEMANN, 1963) whereas the 5-HT antagonist, LSD, was ineffective (HERXHEIMER, 1955). Methysergide also failed consistently to protect guinea pigs against anaphylactic bronchospasm, despite its administration in an amount (0.1 mg/kg i.v.) sufficient to diminish greatly sensitivity to 5-HT (COLLIER and JAMES, 1967). That 5-HT is unlikely to be involved in respiratory anaphylaxis is indicated also by the finding of very low concentrations of 5-HT in guinea pig lung and failure to detect its release in the effluent from anaphylactic lung in vitro (SANYAL and WEST, 1958b; AVIADO and SADAVONGVIVAD, 1970; STECHSCHULTE and AUSTEN, 1974).

These results, therefore, support the conclusion that histamine but not 5-HT plays a significant role in the mediation of anaphylactic responses in guinea pigs at least during the early stages.

4. Compound 48/80 and Polymyxin B

Guinea pig mast cells are relatively resistant to disruption by compound 48/80 (BECKER et al., 1968) and higher concentrations of this substance are required to increase cutaneous permeability in guinea pigs than in rats (Table 1; SPARROW and WILHELM, 1957; HALPERN et al., 1959). Antihistamines are much less effective in antagonising cutaneous responses to 48/80 than to histamine (Table 2; HALPERN et al., 1959; ALBERTY and TAKKUNEN, 1957; CARR, 1972) as if some mediator in addition to histamine was contributory to the response. It is uncertain as to whether or not the other mediating substance is 5-HT as might be expected from studies in rats (this Sect. II.4.), as cutaneous reactions to 48/80 in the guinea pig were resistant to pretreatment with LSD (HALPERN et al., 1959). A study of the effects of combined antagonism of 5-HT and histamine would clarify the situation. Cutaneous reactions in guinea pigs to polymyxin B, which are expected by analogy with results in rats to be due exclusively to histamine release (this Sect. II.4.) were virtually abolished by prior treatment with triprolidine at 0.1 mg/kg i.v. (CARR, 1972).

5. Bradykinin

Mepyramine and triprolidine did not reduce increases in capillary permeability caused by bradykinin as they did in some other species according to the report of BECKER et al. (1968) (this Sect. II.8.) but distinct diminution of the responses to high but not low concentrations of bradykinin was found by CARR (1972) in guinea pigs given triprolidine (0.1 mg/kg i.v.).

II. Rat

1. Thermal and Ultraviolet Injury

Permeability studies similar to those described above for guinea pig are reported by WILHELM and MASON (1960). An immediate response to exposing the skin to a temperature of 50–56° C for 5–20 s was seen only occasionally and was slight, by comparison with that in guinea pigs and rabbits; it was unsuitable for studying drug effects. Erythema appeared in 20–30 s and was unaffected by triprolidine (0.5–2 mg/kg i.v.) but swelling which began 1–2 min after heating was reduced by triprolidine. A delayed increase in permeability ensued during the next 6 h and this was unaffected by triprolidine (2 × 1 mg/kg i.v.) or by the 5-HT antagonist brom-LSD (2 × 1 mg/kg i.v.). Similar results were reported by SPECTOR and WILLOUGHBY (1959a) using exposure periods of 27 s at 55° C; mepyramine (1 mg/kg i.v.), slightly delayed the onset of the inflammation but not the final extent of the subsequent inflammation at 6 h. The 5-HT antagonist brom-LSD was ineffective alone and did not increase the inhibitory action of mepyramine. When the thermal injury was more severe (60° C for 45 s), mepyramine failed completely to delay either leakage of circulating dye into the skin or the development of oedema.

Immersion of rats' feet for 30 min in water at 45° C (the rats should be anaesthetised) caused oedema that was insusceptible to either mepyramine or diphenhydramine and barely affected by promethazine (ROCHA E SILVA, 1964). Cyproheptadine, imipramine, and phenoxybenzamine were effective but the 5-HT antagonists LSD, brom-LSD and methysergide were not; the effect was said to correlate better with antagonism of bradykinin than with antagonism of either histamine or 5-HT. In similar studies to these, STARR and WEST (1967) detected no inhibition of thermic oedema with mepyramine (50 mg/kg i.p.) or brom-LSD (10 mg/kg i.p.).

Experiments using UV irradiation of the skin led to different conclusions (LOGAN and WILHELM, 1966). The irradiation produced distinct early and late phases of increased capillary permeability. The early phase was marked following 30 s expo-

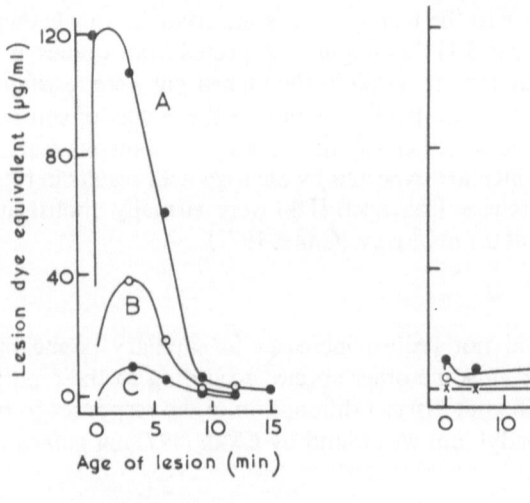

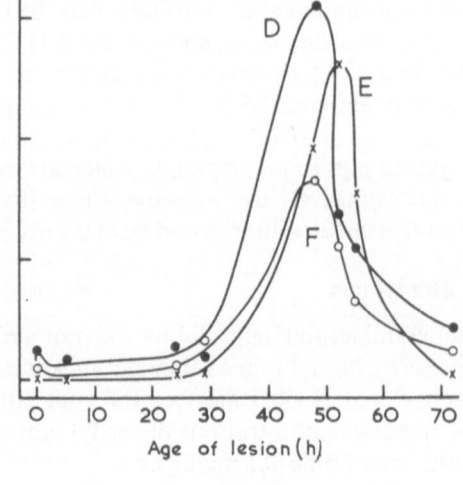

Fig. 9   Fig. 10

Fig. 9. The suppression of the early permeability response to ultraviolet injury in the rat by the 5-HT antagonist, brom-LSD, given intravenously. A = control; B = brom-LSD, 0.1 mg/kg; C = brom-LSD, 1.0 mg/kg. (From: LOGAN and WILHELM, 1966)

Fig. 10. The effects of intravenous brom-LSD and triprolidine on the late permeability response to ultraviolet injury in the rat. D = control; E = brom-LSD, 2 mg/kg; F = triprolidine, 2 mg/kg. (From: LOGAN and WILHELM, 1966)

sure and was highly susceptible to the 5-HT antagonist brom-LSD (Fig. 9) but not to triprolidine (1 mg/kg i.v.). The late phase (studied after exposure to 10 s irradiation) showed a considerably delayed onset after either brom-LSD (2 mg/kg) or triprolidine (2 mg/kg), the latter also markedly reducing the maximal intensity of the reaction (Fig. 10). The antagonists were given immediately before irradiation and again at 5, 24, and 51 h later—not sufficiently often to ensure continued protection against the amines.

The onset of increased capillary permeability following X-irradiation of the intestine was markedly delayed by mepyramine and though there was a tendency towards delay by brom-LSD this was non-significant (WILLOUGHBY, 1959, 1960).

Comment. Factors other than histamine and 5-HT are known to play a major part in the induction of inflammatory responses to thermal injury or irradiation, bradykinin apparently playing a significant role (ROCHA E SILVA, 1964; STARR and WEST, 1967). However, susceptibility to antagonists suggests that either or both of these amines contribute significantly at least during the early phases of inflammation. Minimisation of tissue injury appears to facilitate recognition of this contribution and the greater use of combined antagonists might have revealed effects that were overlooked using specific antagonists separately.

2. Local Anaphylaxis

Reversed passive Arthus type III reactions of skin produced by heterologous precipitating antibody show no damage of mast cells (MOTA, 1963; GOOSE and BLAIR, 1969) and are scarcely affected by high doses of antihistamine (e.g. 50 mg/kg mepyramine i.p.) or by antagonists of 5-HT (e.g. 4 mg/kg LSD s.c.) (BROCKLEHURST et al., 1955, 1960; HALPERN et al., 1959; ORR et al., 1970). Passive cutaneous anaphylaxis (PCA) reactions using homologous precipitating (IgGa-like) antibody also appeared to be resistant to antihistamine and anti-5-HT action when the increase in permeability was measured 20–30 min after antigen challenge (BROCKLEHURST et al., 1960; CRAPS and INDERBITZIN, 1961; ORR et al., 1970) though some diminution in the intensity of the response was observed by BROCKLEHURST et al. (1960) in rats given brom-LSD (2 mg/kg i.v.) and by ORR et al. (1970) in rats given cyproheptadine (10 mg/kg i.p.). On the other hand, when such PCA reactions were examined 5 min after antigen challenge, at which time mast cell degranulation could be seen, cyproheptadine (10 mg/kg i.p. 30 min prior to challenge) abolished the permeability response (ORR et al., 1970). Similarly, PCA reactions mediated by reagin-like antibodies showed mast cell damage and produced vascular changes that were reduced by antihistamines. Thus, MOTA (1964) and GOOSE and BLAIR (1969) found that such responses were reduced by mepyramine (50 mg/kg i.p.) and abolished by combinations of mepyramine (50 mg/kg i.p.) and brom-LSD (2 or 4 mg/kg i.v.); GOOSE and BLAIR (1969) and ORR et al. (1970) found full suppression with cyproheptadine (5–10 mg/kg i.p.). Unfortunately, all the antihistamine doses used in the above experiments exceed those required for antagonism of histamine; their effects might have been non-specific. Using a PCA reaction of the kind described in Chapter 34 (Sect. B.I.) i.v. administration of triprolidine, at the same time as i.v. antigen challenge, reduced the areas of blueing observed at 30 min as follows: 0.1 mg/kg, 47%; 1 mg/kg, 52%; 3 mg/kg, 61% (unpublished observations).

Table 3. PCA reactions provoked by rat IgE and IgG-type antibodies in unfractionated antiserum observed 10 min after intravenous antigen challenge in rats injected with triprolidine (1 mg/kg i.v.) and/or the 5-HT antagonist BW 501C67 (1 mg/kg i.v.) together with antigen. Mean diameters in mm $\pm$ s.e.m.; $n = 4$

	IgE-type	IgG-type
Control	16 $\pm$ 1.0	13 $\pm$ 0.24
Triprolidine	9.1 $\pm$ 1.1	12 $\pm$ 0.65
BW 501C67	12 $\pm$ 1.1	13 $\pm$ 0.54
Triprolidine ⎫ BW 501C67 ⎭	1.9 $\pm$ 1.9	12 $\pm$ 0.60

IgE-type reactions were provoked as described in Chapter 34, Section B.I. IgG-type reactions were provoked by intravenous antigen challenge 1 h after the intradermal injection of heat stable homologous antiserum produced according to the method of ORANGE et al. (1968). (Unpublished results: GARLAND and GREEN, 1975).

The results of a further test, differing in that the observations were made 10 min after antigen challenge and in that the IgE-type PCA reactions were compared with IgGa-type PCA reactions, are shown in Table 3. The test shows a moderate reduction by triprolidine (1 mg/kg i.v.) of the area of the IgE-type provoked reaction (dye intensity was also reduced), no effect with BW 501C67 (1 mg/kg i.v.) alone and almost complete abolition of the response by a combination of these drugs. In contrast these treatments, like cromoglycate in these particular experiments, did not affect the IgG-like reaction. Thus, a parallel can be drawn between results with amine antagonists and those with inhibitors of the release of anaphylactic mediators such as cromoglycate and doxantrazole. These substances affect the IgE-type response, and in experiments by ORR et al. (1970, 1971) the early phase of the IgGa-like response, both of which are associated with mast cell degranulation and amine release. The later phase of IgGa-like response is apparently not mediated by either histamine or 5-HT and may be attributable to release of other inflammatory mediators, perhaps SRS-A from polymorphonucleocytes (Chap. 34, Sections B.III. and C.III.).

Cutaneous anaphylaxis in actively sensitized rats was abolished by mepyramine (50 mg/kg i.p.) in experiments reported by CRAPS and INDERBITZIN (1961) but not appreciably changed in those of BROCKLEHURST et al. (1960). Brom-LSD (4 mg/kg i.p.) had no effect (CRAPS and INDERBITZIN, 1961).

The relative contributions of histamine and 5-HT to anaphylactic reaction in the rat vary in different tissues. For example, both amines were released when antigen was added to peritoneal cell suspensions or the perfusion fluid of the small intestine of sensitized rats, whereas in parallel experiments with minced uterus only 5-HT was released (GARCIA-AROCHA, 1961). Mepyramine and the 5-HT antagonist brom-LSD produced inhibitory effects in keeping with these release studies.

3. Systemic Anaphylaxis

Since severe systemic anaphylaxis in rats is associated with degranulation of mast cells and the release of histamine (MOTA, 1963; ORANGE et al., 1970), it might be expected that antihistamines would influence the response. Nevertheless, no protection against overt anaphylactic symptoms or fatalities was detected by SANYAL and WEST (1958a, 1958b) in rats sensitized with either egg white or a mixture of horse serum and *B. pertussis* vaccine when either mepyramine (10 mg/kg i.p.) and/or brom-LSD (4 mg/kg i.p.) had been administered prior to antigen challenge. Neither was protection found in this situation in animals previously given inhibitors of histamine decarboxylase (RADWAN and WEST, 1967) or polymyxin B to deplete their tissue histamine (SANYAL and WEST, 1958b).

Studies of passive lung anaphylaxis reported by FARMER et al. (1975) in rats sensitized by the i.v. injection of high-titre reaginic antiserum prepared in rats, demonstrate that the bronchoconstrictor response in this species is not antagonised by mepyramine (Fig. 11). They indicate that the anaphylactic bronchoconstriction in the rat is due partly to 5-HT and partly to SRS-A (FPL 55712 is an antagonist of SRS-A, Sect. I.III.). In experiments reported by CHURCH et al. (1972) methysergide (0.1 mg/kg) was sufficient to reduce anaphylactic bronchoconstriction. Rat lungs do contain histamine but, whereas this is released during anaphylactic shock, such release would not be expected to cause bronchoconstriction in the experiments of FARMER et al. (1975); in their studies i.v. injection of histamine at doses up to 100 µg/kg did not cause bronchospasm. Bronchoconstriction was not found with histamine (40 µg/kg–40 mg/kg) in experiments reported by CHURCH (1975), but some increase in pulmonary resistance following histamine administration in rats was reported by AVIADO and SADAVONGVIVAD (1970).

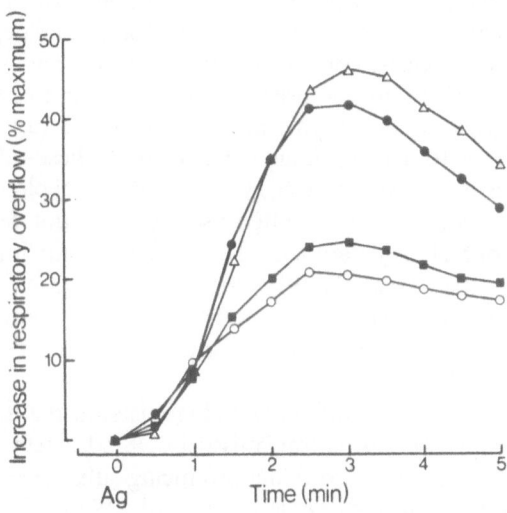

Fig. 11. Time course of anaphylactic bronchoconstriction in passively sentisized rats. (●) Control response; (△) response in animals pretreated with mepyramine (10 mg/kg i.p. 30 min before antigen); (■) methysergide (4 mg/kg i.v. 15 min before antigen) or (○) FPL 55712 (10 mg/kg i.v., immediately before antigen). ($n = 9$.) (From: FARMER et al., 1975)

Antihistamines do, however, appear to influence one major component of the anaphylactic reaction in the rat. Anaphylaxis is characterised by progressive circulatory collapse and the principal organ visibly damaged is the small intestine, which shows oedema and haemorrhagic infiltration (SANYAL and WEST, 1958a; GARCIA-AROCHA, 1961; MOTA, 1963). In studies in which rats were killed 4 h after i.v. antigen challenge, haemorrhagic infiltration of the small intestine was reported to be less severe than in control rats in some animals given mepyramine (8 mg/kg i.v.) or brom-LSD (4 mg/kg i.v.) 20 min prior to antigen challenge, and a combination of the two drugs was more effective, protection being "substantially complete" in 25% of the animals (GARCIA-AROCHA, 1961). MOTA (1963) reported a delayed onset of anaphylactic symptoms and death in animals given antihistamines or antagonists of 5-HT (unspecified). He also reported similar intestinal congestion in rats dying in consequence of shock induced by histamine or 5-HT and by compound 48/80 which releases both these amines. This does not demonstrate that the haemorrhagic infiltration in the intestine that occurs during anaphylaxis is due to the release of these amines; BROCKLEHURST (1967) reported a similar effect in rats dying after large doses of SRS-A.

Inhibition of histamine and 5-HT by promethazine and BW 501 C 67 respectively suppressed the rapid phase of the immune expulsion of parasitic infections with *Nippostrongylus brasiliensis* in rats (MURRAY et al., 1971).

4. Compound 48/80, Polymyxin, Dextran, and Egg White

Among the most powerful of known histamine releasers are compound 48/80 (PATON, 1951, 1958) and polymyxin B and E (BUSHBY and GREEN, 1955). They cause degranulation of mast cells in rats and in other species. An important distinction between their effects in rats is that, whereas 48/80 releases (and depletes) 5-HT as well as histamine, polymyxin releases only histamine (PARRATT and WEST, 1957a; WEST, 1957). Polymyxin can, therefore, be used as a tool to cause release of endogenous histamine or to deplete stores of this amine, and 48/80 can be used to release histamine and 5-HT or to deplete tissue stores of both these amines. A number of examples of their use are presented in this Chapter. When depletion of 5-HT but not of histamine is required, reserpine is often used. It does not disrupt mast cells or cause active release of 5-HT; depletion is slow in onset and attributed to inhibition of granular binding (PLETSCHER et al., 1955, 1956; BHATTACHARYA and LEWIS, 1956). The effect of reserpine is not specific as the noradrenaline content of tissues is also depleted and adrenergic neurone function is suppressed (see Reviews by BEIN, 1956; SCHNEIDER, 1957; GREEN, 1962).

The effects of antihistamines and 5-HT antagonists on the increases in capillary permeability and/or oedema formation caused by 48/80, dextran and egg albumin have been much investigated. The oedema producing substances have been injected i.d. into the abdominal skin (BROCKLEHURST et al., 1955; HALPERN et al., 1959; CRAPS and INDERBITZIN, 1961), s.c. into the dorsum of the foot (ROWLEY and BENDITT, 1956; WEST, 1957; PARRATT and WEST, 1957b; 1958; STONE et al., 1961; GELFAND and WEST, 1961; VOGEL and MAREK, 1961; MALING et al., 1974) or by the i.v. or i.p. routes (PARRATT and WEST, 1957b; BEACH and STEINETZ, 1961; ANKIER and

WEST, 1968). A variety of antagonists at various dosages have been tested and interpretation is in some instances complicated by insufficient information being available on their anti-amine effectiveness or the selectivity of effect of some treatment schedules. However, the overall pattern of results shows clearly that whatever the oedema-producing substance, suppression of 5-HT sensitivity reduces the responses to a greater extent than does suppression of histamine sensitivity and that a combination of the two kinds of antagonist or a single compound which possesses the two effects in combination is best able to abolish the response. In contrast, CRAPS and INDERBITZIN (1961) found that sensitivity to the capillary permeability increasing effect of i.d. polymyxin was unaffected by a 5-HT antagonist (brom-LSD, 4 mg/kg i.p.) but almost abolished after mepyramine (50 mg/kg i.p.).

It has also been demonstrated that depletion of both histamine and 5-HT from tissues by prior administration of 48/80 or depletion of 5-HT by reserpine, but not depletion of histamine alone with polymyxin, reduces greatly the local inflammatory responses to 48/80, dextran and egg white (WEST, 1957; PARRATT and WEST, 1957b; CRAPS and INDERBITZIN, 1961). As expected, depletion of histamine by polymyxin reduced subsequent i.d. responses only to polymyxin (CRAPS and INDERBITZIN, 1961). These results add support to the conclusion that 5-HT release makes a greater contribution to the inflammatory effects produced by 48/80, dextran or egg white than does histamine release.

5. Turpentine Pleurisy

SPECTOR and WILLOUGHBY (1957, 1958, 1959b) studied inflammation produced by injecting turpentine (0.1 ml) into the pleural cavity of the rat. Pleural exudates produced shortly after such injections contained both histamine and 5-HT. The latter appeared not to be a mediator of the fluid formation since the volume was unchanged by the prior administration of brom-LSD (3 mg/kg i.v.) or reserpine (4×5 mg/kg i.p.). Histamine apparently contributed to early but not late oedema formation. Rats pretreated with mepyramine (1 mg/kg) or promethazine (1 mg/kg) i.v. or previously depleted of their tissue amine stores by compound 48/80 (multiple doses of 0.6–1.2 mg/kg i.p.) or polymyxin B (multiple doses of 3–6 mg/kg i.p.), showed virtual suppression of the exudate normally obtainable in 30 min. These effects were due to inhibition of the turpentine-induced increase in capillary permeability. Exudate volumes at 4 h in animals given repeated doses of 48/80 and mepyramine did not differ significantly from control volumes.

Pretreatment with sodium salicylate (660 mg/kg i.p.) alone had no effect on the development of pleural exudate apart from slightly delaying its onset. However salicylate, in conjunction with either mepyramine or prior histamine and 5-HT depletion, suppressed the increased permeability and almost abolished exudate formation for the whole of the 4-h experimental period. This indicated that the delayed oedema formation was due to a component other than histamine. This could be bradykinin. Today's knowledge allows the interpretation of the effect of the salicylate in terms of inhibition of prostaglandin synthetase; prostaglandins are released by bradykinin and potentiate the increased vascular permeability induced by bradykinin in various situations (VANE and FERREIRA, 1975, 1976).

6. Carrageenin Oedema

The injection of carrageenin into the hind feet of rats causes local oedema and this response forms the basis of a commonly used test for non-steroid anti-inflammatory agents. Long after the *first* use of this test, in conjunction with the granuloma assay in the discovery of the anti-inflammatory action of indomethacin (WINTER et al., 1962, 1963), it was appreciated that this oedema-producing substance has an unsuspected advantage in providing a model for the screening of drugs. The inflammation, unlike that of dextran and formalin, is associated with a leucocytic response (DI ROSA and WILLOUGHBY, 1971). The activity of anti-inflammatory agents in this test correlates with inhibition of prostaglandin synthetase (FLOWER et al., 1972) and carrageenin releases PGE_2 when injected s.c. in rats either into the subplantar surface (WILLIS, 1969a) or in the abdominal region (WILLIS, 1969b).

There is divergency in the results relating to the role of histamine and 5-HT in the response. VAN ARMAN (1965), in a detailed study of the time course of the oedema response to carrageenin (0.1 ml of 1% suspension), found that the oedema was not reduced at any time by cyproheptadine (0.5 mg/kg s.c.) whereas this treatment markedly diminished comparable responses to 5-HT. They also failed to show release of histamine by carrageenin from peritoneal cell suspensions. Similarly, VINEGAR et al. (1969), who used 0.05 ml of a 1% carrageenin suspension and uncovered two phases in the foot oedema response, found no inhibition of either phase with chlorpheniramine (10 mg/kg i.p.) and very little inhibition with cyproheptadine (10 mg/kg i.p.). In contrast, DI ROSA et al. (1971) reported that oedema responses to carrageenin (0.1 ml of 1% suspension) were unaffected by either mepyramine (0.25 mg/kg i.v.) or cyproheptadine (0.5 mg/kg s.c.) given alone, but showed delayed onset when a combination of these drugs had been administered. The offered explanation of this finding was that inhibition of both 5-HT and histamine is required. [It has since been found that cyproheptadine is a more powerful antagonist of 5-HT than of histamine using the foot oedema response in the rat (MALING et al., 1974)]. Both rapid and delayed release of histamine from abdominal skin following injection of 2% carrageenin suspension has also been reported (WILLIS, 1969b).

The cause of these variations in results is unknown. The strain of rat is one possibility but it should be noted that carrageenin is not a distinct chemical entity and that variation between different batches of carrageenin, especially from different suppliers, is to be expected. Furthermore, DOHERTY and ROBINSON (1975) have aptly drawn attention to the physical trauma associated with the injection of 0.1 ml volumes of suspensions into the hind feet of rats.

Intrapleural injection of carrageenin provides another useful model for studying non-steroid anti-inflammatory drugs. In this system, pleural effusion was not affected either by triprolidine (1 mg/kg p.o.) or cyproheptadine (5 mg/kg p.o.) (VINEGAR et al., 1973), or by mepyramine (0.25 mg/kg i.v.; DI ROSA et al., 1971). Early pleural effusion caused by carrageenin or turpentine was, however, greatly reduced if rats received prior injections of 48/80 to deplete their tissue contents of histamine and 5-HT, as also were the early foot oedema responses to these same substances (DI ROSA et al., 1971). A contribution of histamine and/or 5-HT to the early stages of carrageenin responses is thereby indicated but not proved.

7. Croton Oil

The volume of inflammatory exudate in granuloma pouches induced by croton oil in rats was decreased in animals pretreated with methysergide (1.5 mg/day for 7 days) (ZILELI et al., 1962).

8. Bradykinin

Mepyramine (0.5 and 5 mg/kg i.v.), triprolidine (0.5 mg/kg i.v.) and chlorpheniramine (6 mg/kg i.v.) reduced significantly the local increase in vascular permeability at the site of i.d. injections of bradykinin (0.04–1 µg) in rats (BECKER et al., 1968). Analogous inhibitory effects were observed in mice and rabbits, but not in guinea pigs. The reductions of the bradykinin responses were substantially less than those of histamine, but BECKER et al. (1968) suggested that part of the action of bradykinin might be due to histamine release and refer to some supporting indications. Alternatively, the inhibitory effect of antihistamines on bradykinin responses might possibly be due to the antihistamine combatting an effect of endogenous histamine that maintains sensitivity to bradykinin.

III. Rabbit

1. Thermal Injury

The skin of rabbits exposed to 54° C showed a biphasic permeability response resembling that illustrated for guinea pigs (Fig. 6) and similarly the immediate response to an exposure period of 5 s was suppressed by triprolidine (0.1 mg/kg i.v.) (WILHELM and MASON, 1960). Greater permeability responses were produced by exposure to 56° C for 20 s and the early but not the delayed phase was suppressed by local injection of 1–10 µg triprolidine but not of 0.1–1 mg/kg i.v. The early release of histamine was also directly identified but the cause of the delayed phase was not discovered. When higher temperatures were applied to the skin (90° C for 10 s), tripelennamine (4 mg/kg i.v.) reduced the early erythema response but not the increased capillary permeability (WEEKS and GUNNAR, 1949). Hence it is concluded that histamine contributes significantly to the early but not the late phase of the permeability response and only when the tissue injury is mild.

In a study of cutaneous responses to UV irradiation of skin, LOGAN and WILHELM (1966) found that the time course of both the early and late permeability responses in rabbits resembled that in the guinea pig. In contrast, however, 0.1 mg/kg of triprolidine i.v. failed to influence either phase of the response despite this amount being sufficient to cause a 35-fold diminution in sensitivity to i.d. histamine. On this account, and because of the low cutaneous sensitivity to 5-HT, it was concluded that neither histamine nor 5-HT was the main mediator of the early permeability response to UV injury in this species.

2. Anaphylactic Reactions

Passive cutaneous anaphylactic reactions caused by an IgE-type heat labile immunoglobulin are associated with mast cell degranulation and histamine release

(Zvaifler et al., 1971) and their areas were reduced by triprolidine, chlorpheniramine, and mepyramine (all at 10 mg/kg i.v.). In contrast, the reaction was not significantly affected by methysergide (2 or 4 mg/kg i.v. or 10 mg/kg i.p.) nor did this 5-HT antagonist enhance the inhibitory effect of mepyramine. A heat stable homocytotropic immunoglobulin prepared by immunising rabbits with tetanus toxoid was investigated by Lindquist (1968); in individual animals, the PCA reactions were suppressed by mepyramine and tripelennamine (large doses) but not by methysergide. Similarly, complement-dependent PCA reactions (Henson and Cochrane, 1969) were suppressed by chlorpheniramine (20 mg/kg i.m.) but not by methysergide (0.5 mg/kg) given 2–4 h before antigen challenge. This inhibitory effect of the antihistamine increased as the interval between sensitization and antigen challenge was prolonged from 20 min to 72 h. Since depletion of platelets was also inhibitory, platelets were the most likely source of the histamine.

Antihistamines (e.g. 40 mg/kg of Antergan) failed, however, to ameloriate the systemic anaphylactic reaction and in particular the rise in pulmonary pressure in the rabbit (Reuse, 1956), suggesting either that the pulmonary effect is not mediated by H_1 receptors or that the reaction involves not only histamine but also other factors such as SRS-A.

3. Inflammation Associated With Bacterial Infections

A deleterious effect of promethazine on infections of *Salmonella typhimurium* in rabbits has been reported by Halpern et al. (1949) and the localisation of infections with *Staphylococcus aureus* was also found to be adversely affected in a study reported by Petri et al. (1952). In this latter study, mepyramine (10 mg/kg s.c.) and promethazine (30 mg/kg s.c.) were administered repeatedly at 6-hourly intervals. Following s.c. inoculation with staphylococci, the antihistamine-treated animals showed a lesser degree of leucocytosis and differential counts showed much smaller increases in juvenile cells (left shift) than did the controls. The accumulation at the site of infection of Indian ink previously administered i.v. was less during the first 12 h in animals given the antihistamine. This was interpreted as inhibition by the antihistamine of a "protective" stimulatory effect of histamine, released by the bacterial activity, on phagocytosis in the infected area. Histological examination revealed that the infected sites were not as well circumscribed in antihistamine treated animals as they were in controls. The "protective" role of released histamine in combatting infection appeared to be greater during the early stages of infection.

IV. Mouse

1. General Anaphylaxis

The behaviour of the mouse mast cell during anaphylaxis in vitro has been reviewed by Vaz and Prouvost-Danon (1969). Degranulation of mast cells and the release in parallel of histamine and 5-HT have been demonstrated. There are also indications of the release in vivo of SRS-A and bradykinin.

The Schultz-Dale reaction of the mouse uterus was not affected by diphenhydramine at 0.4 µg/ml (Fink and Rothlauf, 1955), but it would have been more convincing if higher concentrations or a more active antihistamine had been used. Neither antihistamines nor 5-HT antagonists (GELFAND and WEST, 1961) are very effective in blocking in vivo anaphylactic reactions in mice but antagonism of both histamine and 5-HT is more effective (TOKUDA and WEISER, 1961; HALPERN et al., 1963; VAZ and PROUVOST-DANON, 1969; CASEY and TOKUDA, 1973). Increased capillary permeability of the peritoneum is prominent and only partially reduced by antihistamines alone (TAKAGI and TUKAO, 1971).

Almost complete protection against systemic anaphylactic shock was shown by mepyramine (approx. 75 mg/kg) in studies reported by CAMERON (1956) but not in those reported later by TOKUDA and WEISER (1961). The latter authors used a somewhat smaller dose (40–60 mg/kg), but suggested that the explanation of the difference might lie in the different strain of mouse. It is of interest that in the strain used by TOKUDA and WEISER (1961) significant protection was shown by the 5-HT antagonists, LSD, and brom-LSD, except when the mice had been sensitized to anaphylaxis and to histamine by prior administration of *B. pertussis* organisms. (At the higher dosage of mepyramine used by CAMERON (1956), antagonism of 5-HT would be expected to become more pronounced, and this may have contributed to its protective effect against anaphylaxis; protection against the toxic action of histamine is achieved with lower dosages of mepyramine.)

The finding of HIGGINBOTHAM (1962), that adrenalectomy greatly reduces the resistance of mice to the lethal effects of both 5-HT and anaphylactic shock, without appreciably changing their resistance to either histamine or polymyxin B (a small reduction in resistance to 48/80 was observed), lends support to the conclusion that 5-HT plays a major role in mediating anaphylactic death in mice.

2. Cutaneous Anaphylaxis

Synergism between antagonists of histamine and 5-HT has been clearly demonstrated in studies of PCA. HALPERN et al. (1963) studied the PCA reaction to antigen injected i.v. 3 h after injecting various amounts of mouse anti-egg albumin antibody into the abdominal skin (the antibody was prepared by repeatedly injecting antigen and Freund's adjuvant i.p. and was collected as the ascitic exudate one month or more later). They showed that the PCA reaction was only weakly inhibited by mepyramine (up to 25 mg/kg s.c.) or LSD (up to 25 mg/kg s.c.), but that the simultaneous administration of 6.24 mg/kg of each compound increased the threshold dose of antibody for producing a PCA reaction by about 1800-fold. Similarly, chlorpromazine and promethazine, at dosages that antagonised reaction to both histamine and 5-HT, powerfully inhibited the PCA reaction.

CASEY and TOKUDA (1973) studied PCA reactions provoked by either mouse IgG or rabbit IgG-type antibodies or by rabbit F (ab')$_2$ antibody fragments using varying latent periods. The antagonists examined were brom-LSD (2.5–5 mg/kg i.v.) and mepyramine (25–50 mg/kg i.p.). The mouse IgG-provoked reaction was partially inhibited by each antagonist and suppressed by the combination of antagonists; the release of histamine and 5-HT was not, however, from a system susceptible to inhibition by cromoglycate or diethylcarbamazine. When animals were sensitized by rabbit IgG using a 1-h latent period, the reaction was reduced by mepyramine but not by brom-LSD. The reaction provoked either by rabbit IgG using a 3-h latent period or by rabbit F (ab′)$_2$ antibody fragments was unaffected by either antagonist, indicating that these reactions, unlike those with homologous antibody, were not mediated by the release of 5-HT and histamine.

Local anaphylactic responses provoked in the pinna by horse serum antigen in actively sensitized mice were partially inhibited by both mepyramine and methysergide, at doses that exerted specific antagonism of histamine and 5-HT respectively in the mouse pinna test (CHURCH and MILLER, 1975).

3. Other Local Inflammatory Reactions

Oedema formation provoked by injection of dextran into the hind feet of mice was studied by UDA (1960). Some inhibitory effect was observed with mepyramine but 5-HT appeared to play a more important part than histamine in mediating the oedema response, since marked inhibition was caused by dibenamine and by prior deletion of tissue 5-HT with reserpine.

Mice injected i.v. with dextran (400 mg/kg i.v.) and Pontamine Sky blue show pinnal extravasation of dye, the incidence varying in different strains (ANKIER and NEAT, 1972). This blueing response was reduced when the following substances were administered i.v. 30 min previously: cyproheptadine (1 mg/kg), mepyramine (1 mg/kg), methysergide (0.5 mg/kg), promethazine (2 mg/kg), brom-LSD (1 mg/kg) and chlorpheniramine (5 mg/kg). The treatments are ranked here in order of decreasing mean effectiveness but all produced inhibitions between 36 and 68% and differences between treatments are of unknown statistical significance. Whereas cyproheptadine gave the highest protection, there was no indication that combined antagonism of 5-HT and histamine was advantageous, as inhibition by mepyramine was not enhanced by methysergide or brom-LSD.

Inflammation of the hind feet caused by local injection of formaldehyde was not influenced by antihistamine (mepyramine at 4 mg/kg s.c., NORTHOVER and SUBRAMANIAN, 1962; chloropyramine at 20 mg/kg i.p., WEIS, 1963) by prior depletion of tissue histamine with polymyxin (NORTHOVER and SUBRAMANIAN, 1962) nor by LSD (0.1 mg/kg i.p. WEIS, 1963). Prior administration of cyproheptadine, at doses that fully suppressed responses to both 5-HT and histamine (0.2–0.8 mg/kg), did, however, reduce the reaction to formaldehyde (NORTHOVER and SUBRAMANIAN, 1962). Oedema caused by silver nitrate in mouse foot was unaffected by the antihistamine chloropyramine (20 mg/kg i.p.) or LSD (0.1 mg/kg i.p.) but chloropyramine (which also has a weak anti-5-HT activity) and also LSD weakly reduced reactions to yeast (WEIS, 1963).

4. Systemic Reactions Involving Inflammation

Burns. Partial protection against the lethal effects of burns was found with chlorpheniramine, mepyramine, and cyproheptadine and also with LSD. Cyproheptadine was easily the most effective, presumably in consequence of its antagonism of both histamine and 5-HT (GANLEY, 1962).

Streptolysin "O". Tripelennamine and another antihistamine did not protect mice against the lethal toxic action of streptolysin "O" whereas several 5-HT antagonists of diverse chemical structures did (HALBERT et al., 1963). The significance of this observation is in doubt as activity in protecting against streptolysin "O" in mice was not correlated with anti-5-HT potency estimated in rats. Lack of correlation of anti-5-HT potencies in mice and rats has been reported by GELFAND and WEST (1961).

V. Man

1. Burns

Antihistamines may reduce oedema formation in mild burns in man but they would not be expected to influence the course of severe burns. Antazoline, at a dose that reduced sensitivity to histamine, failed to influence the course of burns following exposure of human skin to 60° C for 15 s (SEVITT et al., 1952), this being a more severe exposure than that influenced by antihistamines in animal studies.

2. Compound 48/80 and Polymyxin

The increased permeability at the site of i.d. injection of histamine, 5-HT, polymyxin and 48/80 has been studied in volunteers injected i.v. with Coomassie blue by KALZ and FEKETE (1961). Histamine, 48/80 and polymyxin all produced spreading weals surrounded by flares; the weals showing marked blueing while the flares were unstained. Sensitivity to 5-HT was less and, despite the use of high concentrations and the production of large flares, only small flat weals were observed. These results, together with the knowledge that human skin contains much more histamine than 5-HT, suggest that the effects of 48/80 and polymyxin were mediated by released histamine rather than by released 5-HT. The weal formation and the blueing reactions representing extravasation of dye at the site of each of the four above substances were suppressed by oral cyproheptadine. Cyproheptadine and promethazine were also effective when applied locally by iontophoresis.

3. Hypersensitivity States

Antihistamines have a useful palliative effect in many allergic states, including urticarias, rhinitis, and angioedema, indicating that histamine plays a significant role as a mediator of these conditions. Histamine is released from human lung during anaphylaxis but antihistamines are poorly effective in controlling asthma, perhaps because other mediators play a more significant role than does histamine. In reviewing this subject, STECHSCHULTE and AUSTEN (1974) concluded that it was probable but unproven that SRS-A makes a contribution to the constriction and presented evidence contra-indicating the participation of 5-HT. Similarly, STACEY (1965) concluded that 5-HT probably plays only a minor role in anaphylaxis in man.

4. Rheumatoid Arthritis and 5-HT Antagonists

Reviews of the effects of 5-HT and its antagonists in man (STACEY, 1965; GYERMEK, 1966; WARNER, 1967) show little connection between 5-HT and inflammation, but there is one set of observations worthy of mention. This concerns a possible relation of 5-HT to rheumatoid arthritis and collagen diseases.

In 1958, SCHERBEL and HARRISON described an abnormal response to intradermal 5-HT in patients with active rheumatoid arthritis or systemic lupus erythematosus, characterised by a rapid onset of erythema, swelling and cyanosis, which was blocked by brom-LSD. These observations were followed by clinical trials and claims of improvements following peri-articular, intra-articular or systemic administration of methysergide and other 5-HT antagonists in patients with rheumatoid arthritis (SCHERBEL and SCHMID, 1962; GRAMAJO and CERVIO, 1965). It was also reported that the excretion of 5-methoxytryptamine, a metabolite of 5-HT, is increased during rheumatic fever (HADDOX and SASLAW, 1963).

If the clinical improvement caused by inhibition of 5-HT is real, might a possible explanation be derived from the effect of 5-HT and some of its metabolites on collagen? At present, such a relationship is tenuous indeed. It has been reported that the shrinkage temperature of collagen in rheumatic nodules is lower than normal (BROWN et al., 1958; STRINGER and HIGHTON, 1960) but whereas HIGHTON and GARRETT (1963) have shown that 5-HT and 5-methoxytryptamine lower the shrinkage temperature of human tendon collagen, high concentrations and prolonged incubation were required.

VI. Bovine Anaphylaxis

Studies of systemic anaphylaxis in calves have been reported by AITKEN and SANFORD (1972a, 1972b) and by EYRE et al. (1973). Comparison with the effects produced by injected histamine and 5-HT and the partial inhibition of anaphylaxis by mepyramine and methysergide indicated that both these amines were involved in anaphylaxis. Meclofenamate and diethylcarbamazine (but not cromoglycate) also reduced the anaphylactic hypotensive response, suggesting a contribution by a prostaglandin and possibly also by bradykinin and SRS-A (EYRE et al., 1973). (The interpretation of results obtained with meclofenamate is discussed in Section I.I.). These same mediators appear also to be involved in the SCHULTZ-DALE reaction of bovine pulmonary artery studied by EYRE (1971a, 1971b). The response was reduced by mepyramine, methysergide, and by meclofenamate. It was also reduced by the two inhibitors of mediator release, cromoglycate and diethylcarbamazine and abolished by a combination of these substances.

On the other hand, there is no evidence for the participation in the bovine PCA reaction of mediators other than histamine and perhaps SRS-A (WELLS and EYRE, 1972). These reactions were reduced by mepyramine and by diethylcarbamazine and the inhibitory effect of the latter was augmented by cromoglycate; methysergide and meclofenamate were ineffective.

I. Antagonists of SRS-A

The structure, distribution and actions of SRS-A, are discussed by LICHTENSTEIN and PLAUT in Chapter 11 and the role of SRS-A in the vascular phenomena of inflammation is reviewed by YOULTEN in Chapter 16. This Section is therefore confined to a brief description of known antagonists of SRS-A.

I. Non-Steroid Anti-Inflammatory Drugs

Non-steroid anti-inflammatory agents are not specific antagonists of SRS-A nor do they antagonise SRS-A by direct receptor competition. They do, however, potently reduce the bronchoconstrictor effects of SRS-A preparations from anaphylactic guinea pig lung (BERRY and COLLIER, 1964) and similarly they inhibit the broncho-constrictor actions of bradykinin and related kinins (COLLIER et al., 1960; COLLIER and SHORLEY, 1960, 1963; COLLIER et al., 1968). The antagonism of SRS-A in guinea pigs resembles the antagonism of kinins in being surmounted by elevation of dosage of agonist and in the relative potencies of different anti-inflammatory agents. However, the receptors of the bronchial muscle for SRS-A appear to be distinct from those for bradykinin as the muscle could be made unresponsive to either spasmogen while remaining sensitive to the other (BERRY and COLLIER, 1964). Anaphylactic bronchospasm in guinea pigs is partially reduced by non-steroid anti-inflammatory agents, partially reduced by mepyramine and further reduced or abolished by administration of a combination of the anti-inflammatory agents with mepyramine (COLLIER and JAMES, 1967; COLLIER et al., 1968). Experiments in which tachyphylaxis had been induced separately to bradykinin and to SRS-A indicated that both kinins and SRS-A contribute to anaphylactic bronchoconstriction in guinea pigs (COLLIER and JAMES, 1967).

Meclofenamate did not, however, reduce the bronchoconstrictor effect of brady-kinin in the rat (CHURCH, 1975) as it did in the guinea pig (COLLIER et al., 1968). Furthermore, whereas it is not known whether meclofenamate affects responses to SRS-A as it does in guinea pigs, anaphylactic bronchospasm in rats is not inhibited by meclofenamate (CHURCH et al., 1972) or by aspirin (FARMER et al., 1975). The bronchoconstrictor action of SRS-A prepared from guinea pig lungs was weak in rats (CHURCH, 1975) but anaphylactic release of SRS-A from rat isolated perfused lungs has been demonstrated (FARMER et al., 1975).

Anaphylactic contractions of bovine pulmonary vein (EYRE, 1971b) and the respiratory and circulatory effects of anaphylaxis in calves (AITKEN and SANFORD, 1972a; EYRE et al., 1973) were powerfully inhibited by meclofenamate, whereas PCA reactions in this species were unaffected by this drug (WELLS and EYRE, 1972). By analogy with the observations in guinea pigs, these effects and the known reduction of responses to bradykinin in the presence of meclofenamate in the bovine (AITKEN and SANFORD, 1972b), suggest that SRS-A and/or bradykinin may be involved in systemic anaphylaxis in the bovine.

Interpretation. The inhibitory effects of non-steroid anti-inflammatory agents on responses to bradykinin can be interpreted on the basis of the known effects of these agents in inhibiting the synthesis of prostaglandins (VANE, 1971; FERREIRA et al., 1971; SMITH and WILLIS, 1971; PIPER and VANE, Chapter 24). The infusion of brady-kinin into isolated guinea pig lungs causes the release of RCS (PIPER and VANE, 1969) and of prostaglandins E_2 and $F_{2\alpha}$ (PALMER et al., 1973), the RCS consisting of prostaglandin endoperoxides and their derivative thromboxane A_2 (FLOWER et al., 1976). It is known that $PGF_{2\alpha}$ is a powerful bronchoconstrictor and lack of its synthesis, because of inhibition of prostaglandin synthetase by an anti-inflammatory agent, would be expected to lead to reduced bronchoconstrictor responses to brady-kinin. This question is discussed further by VANE and FERREIRA (1975, 1976) and by

PIPER and VANE in Chapter 24, who refer to several situations in which bradykinin releases prostaglandins and/or potentiates the intrinsic effects of prostaglandins. The parallelism between the behaviour of SRS-A and bradykinin with respect to antagonism by anti-inflammatory agents, referred to earlier in this section, strongly suggests that the same or a similar mechanism operates for this mediator, i.e. that the effect of SRS-A is dependent upon unimpaired synthesis of prostaglandins or their precursors, and perhaps $PGF_{2\alpha}$ in particular.

COLLIER and SWEATMAN (1968) demonstrated that meclofenamate, flufenamate and phenylbutazone potently, and aspirin less potently, blocked the contraction of human isolated bronchial muscle induced by $PGF_{2\alpha}$. Moreover, the fenamates were many hundred times more active against $PGF_{2\alpha}$ than against SRS-A. These observations do not, however, provide an alternative explanation of the antagonism by non-steroid anti-inflammatory agents of SRS-A, bradykinin or anaphylactic responses in guinea pigs since aspirin and meclofenamate did not antagonise the bronchoconstrictor effects of $PGF_{2\alpha}$ in this species. The significance of the effects of non-steroid anti inflammatory agents on the bronchial responses to prostaglandins was discussed recently by COLLIER (1976) and is referred to also in Chapter 24.

Similar results to those in the guinea pig have been obtained using bovine but not rat tissues. Rats differ from guinea pigs not only in showing undiminished bronchoconstrictor responses in the presence of meclofenamate and aspirin but also in being relatively resistant to the bronchoconstrictor effects of both bradykinin and SRS-A (CHURCH, 1975). CHURCH et al. (1972) draw attention to the analogies between human asthma and rat anaphylaxis, both being relatively insensitive to antagonism by non-steroid anti-inflammatory drugs but sensitive to steroids and inhibited by anti-allergic agents (Chap. 34, Sect. B.I.).

II. Polyphloretin Phosphate (PPP)

Polyphloretin phosphate (mol wt 15000) blocks the responses of human bronchioles to SRS-A as also it blocks the response of this tissue to $PGF_{2\alpha}$ but high concentrations (20 µg/ml) are required (MATHÉ and STRANDBERG, 1971). Infusion of PPP in cats and guinea pigs also antagonises the bronchoconstriction and blood pressure changes caused by both $PGF_{2\alpha}$ and SRS-A but again the amount required is high (40–80 mg/kg) (MATHÉ et al., 1972). A variety of other influences of PPP on prostaglandin action and metabolism have been described (EAKINS et al., 1970; EAKINS and SANNER, 1972; VILLANEUVA et al., 1972; McQUEEN, 1973). These observations provide a further indication of the similarities in structures of $PGF_{2\alpha}$ and SRS-A (STRANDBERG and UVNAS, 1971), although the work of ORANGE et al. (1973, 1974) distinguishes SRS-A from the known prostaglandins.

III. FPL 55712

FPL 55712 inhibits responses to rat, guinea-pig and human SRS-A (AUGSTEIN et al., 1973). It is highly active against spasm of guinea pig ileum caused by SRS-A (IC_{50}, about 5 ng/ml), irrespective of source of SRS-A but has relatively little antagonistic activity towards the spasmogenic actions of histamine ($IC_{50} \approx 21$ µg/ml), 5-HT

(IC$_{50}$≃28 µg/ml), ACh (IC$_{50}$≃20 µg/ml), bradykinin (IC$_{50}$≃9.8 µg/ml), PGE$_1$ (IC$_{50}$≃4.7 µg/ml), PGF$_{2\alpha}$ (IC$_{50}$≃4.9 µg/ml). Studies of the effect of this substance in anaphylactic bronchospasm in passively sensitized rats have been reported by FARMER et al. (1975). As illustrated in Figure 11, FPL 55712 (10 mg/kg i.v.) markedly diminished this bronchospasm. Furthermore, together with methysergide (4 mg/kg i.v.) it almost abolished anaphylactic bronchospasm in the rat. This suggests that the anaphylactic response is due almost completely to the combined release of SRS-A and 5-HT. This should, however, be regarded only as a tentative conclusion as it is known that FPL 55712 has some effect in the rat PCA test, suggesting that it may act to some degree by inhibiting mediator release. Alternatively the anti-PCA effect of FPL 55712 might be attributable to inhibition of a contribution of SRS-A to the PCA response—the release of SRS-A into the peritoneal cavity of rats by antigen-antibody interaction is discussed in Chapter 34.

3 FPL 55712

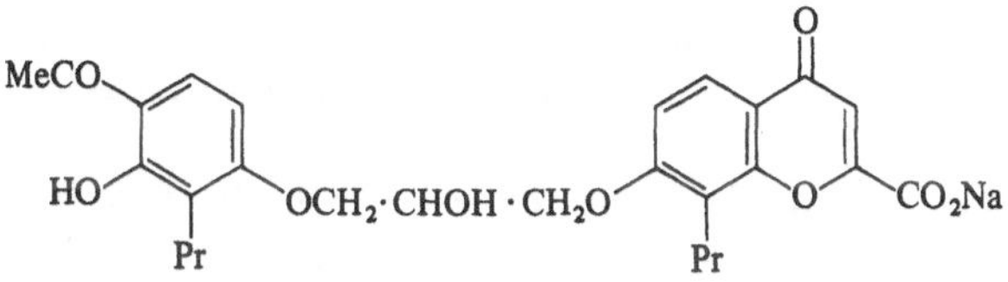

Another interesting effect of FPL 55712 has been described by JONES and KAY (1974). In earlier work they had found an eosinophil chemotactic factor of anaphylaxis (ECF-A) and they proceeded to demonstrate that FPL 55712 was antagonistic towards it. Inhibition of the chemotactic response of guinea pig eosinophils increased linearly with the log concentration of FPL 55712 over the range of 10^{-8}–10^{-6} g/ml, the IC$_{50}$ being about 0.2 µg/ml (3.8×10^{-7} M). Neither cromoglycate nor hydrocortisone inhibited the activity of ECF-A.

IV. Hydratropic Acids

A group of hydratropic acids (I) have recently been reported (GREIG and GRIFFIN, 1975) to be potent antagonists of the spasmogenic action of SRS-A on guinea pig trachea.

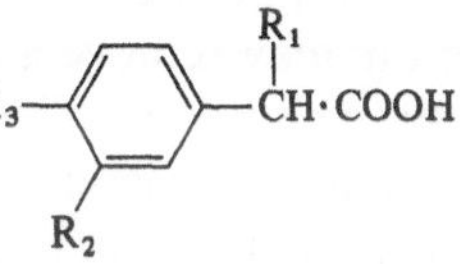

(I)

Activity was high in compounds when R$_1$ was CH$_3$, R$_2$ was F, Cl, or H, and R$_3$ was C$_6$H$_5$, C$_6$H$_{11}$ or 2F-C$_6$H$_4$. The more active compounds inhibited SRS-A concentrations of the order of 1–10 ng/ml. The compound examined in greatest detail was I, R$_1$=CH$_3$; R$_2$=F; R$_3$=C$_6$H$_5$ named flurbiprofen. It blocked tracheal responses to SRS-A at 2–3 ng/ml and at similar concentrations inhibited the response to PGF$_{2\alpha}$ suggesting a similarity in structure of these agonists. Higher concentrations (ca. 20 ng/ml) antagonised bradykinin responses but histamine responses were only slightly antagonised by concentrations 100 times greater than those that blocked SRS-A. Responses to arachidonic acid and linoleic acid were relatively resistant. Anaphylactic bronchospasm, provoked by exposing sensitized guinea pigs to an aerosol of egg albumin antigen, was prevented by prior administration of flurbiprofen (1 mg/kg i.p.) when the challenge was presented at 3–4 weeks but not at 5–8 weeks after sensitization. The results of further studies of these compounds are awaited with interest. They are not to be likened to FPL 55712, for in contrast to it, flurbiprofen, while having a powerful inhibitory action in tracheal preparations, had little or no effect on the stimulating action of SRS-A on guinea pig ileum. This suggests that there may be more than one kind of receptor for SRS-A.

J. Prospects for New Drugs

There is already an abundance of highly potent and specific H_1 antihistamines which in simple or more complex formulations provide good protective effects of appropriate persistence against histamine when they are administered orally in man. The dosage of all these substances is, however, limited by the somnolence and impairment of concentration that they produce (Sect. C.V.). This now being the case for so many compounds of a variety of chemical classes, the expectation of finding an antihistamine whose dosage is not limited by such properties seems small; these properties may be unavoidable with substances that block H_1 receptors. The means of finding an antihistamine that lacks these properties are also limited, since animal tests have so far failed to reveal the CNS depressant effects that are apparently common to all H_1 antagonists in man; they reveal the gross depressant effects that are shown by only some antihistamines such as promethazine. However, an antihistamine that could be given to man, in amounts that suppressed responses to greater concentrations of histamine than do currently available antihistamines, could be advantageous, as high local concentrations of histamine are to be expected at sites of anaphylactic release, for example in the bronchial system of asthmatic subjects.

The value, if any, of histamine H_2 antagonists in inflammatory responses in man has yet to be worked out. Synergism with H_1 histamine antagonism in blocking vasodilator responses to histamine has been demonstrated (Sect. E) and this may point the way to potentially useful properties. On the other hand, the possibility exists that blockade of H_2 receptors may remove a moderating inhibitory effect of released histamine on further histamine release (Chap. 34, Sect. C.II.). Such effects could enhance inflammatory and allergic reactions. Inhibition of gastric secretion would also be an undesirable property in the present context.

It is doubtful whether any antagonist of 5-HT will be found to be of value in the treatment of inflammatory conditions in man, but the coming availability of potent and specific blocking agents that act only on peripheral mechanisms and which can, therefore, be given in less restricted amounts provides added opportunities for investigation.

SRS-A antagonists have only recently been found and their value for man has yet to be demonstrated.

Of the compounds referred to in this chapter, the only class of agents for which there is significant information to base a meaningful opinion as to whether or not the ideal drug of its class is likely to have been found is that of the H_1 histamine antagonists. Such an opinion is only soundly based when a substantial number of compounds of a class of pharmacological agents has been used extensively in man over a long period of time. Furthermore, the lesson indicated from the use of antihistamines is that the ideal compound varies from one subject to another and that there is merit in having available several good drugs of the same class.

References

Adamson,D.W., Barrett,P.A., Billinghurst,J.W., Green,A.F., Jones,T.S.G.: Geometrical isomers in a series of antihistamines. Nature (Lond.) **168**, 204—205 (1951)

Aitken,M.M., Sanford,J.: Modification of acute systemic anaphylaxis in cattle by drugs and by vagotomy. J. comp. Path. **82**, 247—256 (1972a)

Aitken,M.M., Sanford,J.: Effects of histamine, 5-hydroxytryptamine and bradykinin on cattle and their modification by antagonists and by vagotomy. J. comp. Path. **82**, 257—266 (1972b)

Alberty,J., Takkunen,R.: Der Anteil von Histamin an der anaphylaktischen und der durch einen chemischen Histaminfreisetzer hervorgerufenen vasculären Hautreaktion. Int. Arch. Allergy **10**, 285—304 (1957)

Ankier,S.I., Neat,M.L.: Some studies on acute inflammation induced by dextran in the mouse. Int. Arch. Allergy **42**, 264—277 (1972)

Ankier,S.I., West,G.B.: Inhibition of the anaphylactoid reaction in rats. Brit. J. Pharmacol. **33**, 304—311 (1968)

Armitage,P., Herxheimer,H., Rosa,L.: Protective action of antihistamines in the anaphylactic microshock of the guinea pig. Brit. J. Pharmacol. **7**, 625—632 (1952)

Ash,A.S.F., Schild,H.O.: Receptors mediating some actions of histamine. Brit. J. Pharmacol. **27**, 427—439 (1966)

Ashford,C.A., Heller,H., Smart,G.A.: The action of histamine on hydrochloric acid and pepsin secretion in man. Brit. J. Pharmacol. **4**, 153—161 (1949)

Augstein,J., Farmer,J.B., Lee,T.B., Sheard,P., Tattersall,M.L.: Selective inhibitor of slow-reacting substance of anaphylaxis. Nature (New Biol.) **245**, 215—217 (1973)

Austen,K.F., Humphrey,J.H.: In vitro studies of the mechanism of anaphylaxis. In: Dixon,F.J., Humphrey,J.H. (Eds.): Advances in Immunology, Vol. 3, pp. 1—96. New York-London: Academic Press 1963

Aviado,D.M., Sadavongvivad,C.: Pharmacological significance of biogenic amines in the lungs: histamine. Brit. J. Pharmacol. **38**, 366—373 (1970)

Bain,W.A.: Discussion on antihistamine drugs. Proc. roy. Soc. Med. **42**, 615—625 (1949)

Bain,W.A.: The evaluation of drugs in man, with special reference to antihistamines. Analyst. **76**, 573—579 (1951)

Baumgarten,A., Wilhelm,D.L.: Vascular permeability responses in hypersensitivity: I. The tuberculin reaction. Pathology **1**, 301—315 (1969)

Beach,V.L., Steinetz,B.G.: Quantative measurement of Evans blue space in tissue of the rat; influence of 5-hydroxytryptamine antagonists and phenelzine on experimental inflammation. J. Pharmacol. exp. Ther. **131**, 400—406 (1961)

Becker,E.L., Mota,I., Wong,D.: Inhibition by antihistamines of the vascular permeability increase induced by bradykinin. Brit. J. Pharmacol. **34**, 330—336 (1968)

Bein,H.J.: The pharmacology of rauwolfia. Pharmacol. Rev. **8**, 435—483 (1956)

Beretta,C., Ferrini,R., Glässer,A.H.: 1-Methyl-8-β-carbobenzyloxy-aminomethyl 10 α-ergoline, a potent and long-lasting 5-hydroxytryptamine antagonist. Nature (Lond.) **207**, 421—422 (1965)

Bernauer,W., Hahn,F., Giertz,H.: Comparison of the antilethal, broncholytic and antiemphysematous activities of mepyramine in anaphylactic, histamine, and anaphylatoxin shock of guinea pigs. Arch. int. Pharmacodyn. **178**, 137—151 (1969)

Berry,P.A., Collier,H.O.J.: Bronchoconstrictor action and antagonism of a slow reacting substance from anaphylaxis of guinea pig isolated lung. Brit. J. Pharmacol. **23**, 201—216 (1964)

Bhattacharya, B. K., Lewis, G. P.: The effects of reserpine and compound 48/80 on the release of amines from the mast cells of rats. Brit. J. Pharmacol. 11, 411—416 (1956)

Black, J. W., Duncan, W. A. M., Durant, G. J., Ganellin, C. R., Parsons, E. M.: Definition and antagonism of histamine H_2-receptors. Nature (Lond.) 236, 385—390 (1972)

Black, J. W., Duncan, W. A. M., Emmett, J. C., Ganellin, C. R., Hesselbo, T., Parsons, M. E., Wyllie, J. H.: Metiamide—an orally active histamine H_2 receptor antagonist. Agents Actions 3, 133—137 (1973)

Black, J. W., Owen, D. A. A., Parsons, M. E.: An analysis of the depressor responses to histamine in the cat and dog: involvement of both H_1- and H_2-receptors. Brit. J. Pharmacol. 54, 319—324 (1975)

Brimblecombe, R. W., Duncan, W. A. M., Durant, G. J., Emmett, J. C., Ganellin, C. R., Parsons, M. E.: Cimetidine. Nonthiourea histamine H_2-receptor antagonist. J. int. med. Res. 3, 86—92 (1975)

Brittain, R. T., D'Arcy, P. F., Hunt, J. H.: Resolution of chlorpheniramine and the pharmacological properties of its isomers. Nature (Lond.) 183, 734—735 (1959)

Brocklehurst, W. E.: Occurrence of an unidentified substance during anaphylactic shock in cavy lung. J. Physiol. (Lond.) 120, 16 P (1953)

Brocklehurst, W. E.: The release of histamine and formation of a slow-reacting substance (SRS-A) during anaphylactic shock. J. Physiol. (Lond.) 151, 416—435 (1960)

Brocklehurst, W. E.: Pharmacologically active substances in hypersensitivity reactions. In: Cruickshank, R., Weir, D. M. (Eds.): Modern Trends in Immunology, Vol. 2, pp. 235—249. London: Butterworth 1967

Brocklehurst, W. E., Humphrey, J. H., Perry, W. L. M.: The role of histamine in cutaneous antigen-antibody reactions in the rat. J. Physiol. (Lond.) 129, 205—225 (1955)

Brocklehurst, W. E., Humphrey, J. H., Perry, W. L. M.: Cutaneous antigen-antibody reactions in the rat. J. Physiol. (Lond.) 150, 489—500 (1960)

Brown, P. C., Consden, R., Glynn, L. E.: Observations on the shrink temperature of collagen and its variations with age and disease. Ann. rheum. Dis. 17, 196—208 (1958)

Bushby, S. R. M., Green, A. F.: The release of histamine by polymyxin B and polymyxin E. Brit. J. Pharmacol. 10, 215—219 (1955)

Cameron, J.: Anaphylactic shock in mice. Brit. J. exp. Path. 37, 470—476 (1956)

Carr, J.: The effect of anti-inflammatory drugs on increased vascular permeability induced by chemical mediators. J. Path. 108, 1—14 (1972).

Casey, F. B., Tokuda, S.: A comparative study of the mechanisms of passive cutaneous anaphylaxis induced by mouse IgG, rabbit IgG, and rabbit F (ab')$_2$ antibodies. Int. Arch. Allergy 44, 737—744 (1973)

Casy, A. F., Ison, R. R.: Stereochemical influences upon antihistaminic activity. Further studies of isomeric 4-amino-1,2-diarylbutenes. J. Pharm. (Lond.) 22, 270—278 (1970)

Church, M. K.: Response of rat lung to humoral mediators of anaphylaxis and its modification by drugs and sensitization. Brit. J. Pharmacol. 55, 423—430 (1975)

Church, M. K., Collier, H. O. J., James, G. W. L.: The inhibition by dexamethasone and disodium cromoglycate of anaphylactic bronchoconstriction in the rat. Brit. J. Pharmacol. 46, 56—65 (1972)

Church, M. K., Miller, P.: Simple models of anaphylaxis and of histamine and 5-hydroxytryptamine induced inflammation using the mouse pinna. Brit. J. Pharmacol. 55, 315P (1975)

Collier, H. O. J.: Role of kallikrein-kinin system in lung diseases. In: Proc. No. 27 of the Fogerty International Center. Washington, D.C.: U.S. Government Printing Office 1976. In press

Collier, H. O. J., Holgate, J. A., Schachter, M., Shorley, P. G.: The bronchoconstrictor action of bradykinin in the guinea pig. Brit. J. Pharmacol. 15, 290—297 (1960)

Collier, H. O. J., James, G. W. L.: Humoral factors affecting pulmonary inflation during acute anaphylaxis in the guinea pig in vivo. Brit. J. Pharmacol. 30, 283—301 (1967)

Collier, H. O. J., James, G. W. L., Piper, P. J.: Antagonism of fenamates and like-acting drugs of bronchoconstriction induced by bradykinin or antigen in the guinea pig. Brit. J. Pharmacol. 34, 76—87 (1968)

Collier, H. O. J., Shorley, P. G.: Analgesic antipyretic drugs as antagonists of bradykinin. Brit. J. Pharmacol. 15, 601—610 (1960)

Collier, H. O. J., Shorley, P. G.: Antagonism by mefenamic and flufenamic acids of the broncho-constrictor action of kinins in the guinea pig. Brit. J. Pharmacol. **20**, 345—351 (1963)

Collier, H. O. J., Sweatman, W. J. F.: Antagonism by fenamates of prostaglandin $F_{2\alpha}$ and of slow reacting substance on human bronchiole muscle. Nature (Lond.) **219**, 864—865 (1968)

Copp, F. C., Green, A. F., Hodson, H. F., Randall, A. W., Sim, M. F.: New peripheral antagonists of 5-hydroxytryptamine. Nature (Lond.) **214**, 200—201 (1967)

Craig, J. P., Wilhelm, D. L.: Cutaneous anaphylaxis in the guinea pig and its relative insusceptibility to an antihistamine. J. Immunol. **90**, 43—51 (1963)

Craps, L., Inderbitzin, Th.: Anaphylactoid and anaphylactic cutaneous exoserosis in the rat. Int. Arch. Allergy **18**, 268—285 (1961)

Day, M., Vane, J. R.: An analysis of the direct and indirect actions of drugs on the isolated guinea pig ileum. Brit. J. Pharmacol. **20**, 150—170 (1963)

Di Rosa, M., Giroud, J. P., Willoughby, D. A.: Studies of the mediators of the acute inflammatory response induced in rats in different sites by carrageenan and turpentine. J. Path. **104**, 15—29 (1971)

Di Rosa, M., Willoughby, D. A.: Screens for antiinflammatory drugs. J. Pharm. (Lond.) **23**, 297—298 (1971)

Doepfner, W., Cerletti, A.: Comparison of lysergic acid derivatives and antihistamines as inhibitors of the oedema provoked in the rat's paw by serotonin. Int. Arch. Allergy **12**, 89—97 (1958)

Doherty, N. S., Robinson, B. V.: The inflammatory response to carrageenan. J. Pharm. (Lond.) **27**, 701—703 (1975)

Durant, G. J., Ganellin, C. R., Parsons, M. E.: Chemical differentiation of histamine H_1- and H_2-receptor agonists. J. med. Chem. **18**, 905—909 (1975)

Dutta, N. K.: Some pharmacological properties common to antihistamine compounds. Brit. J. Pharmacol. **4**, 281—289 (1949)

Eakins, K. E. S., Karim, S. M. M., Miller, J. D.: Antagonism of some smooth muscle actions of prostaglandins by polyphloretin phosphate. Brit. J. Pharmacol. **39**, 556—563 (1970)

Eakins, K. E., Sanner, J. H.: Prostaglandin antagonists. In: Karim, S. M. M. (Ed.): The Prostaglandins. Progress in Research, pp. 263—292. Oxford: Medical & Technical Publishing Co. Ltd. 1972

El-Ackad, T. M., Meyer, M. J., Sturkie, P. D.: Inotropic and chronotropic actions of histamine on the avian heart. Fed. Proc. **33**, Abst. 2110 (1974)

Ensor, C. R., Russell, D., Chen, G.: A comparative study on some aspects of the pharmacology of diphenhydramine (Benadryl) and chemically related compounds. J. Pharmacol. exp. Ther. **112**, 318—325 (1954)

Erspamer, V. (Ed.): 5-Hydroxytryptamine and Related Indolealkylamines. Handbook of Experimental Pharmacology, Vol. XIX. Berlin-Heidelberg-New York: Springer 1966

Eyre, P.: Histamine release from calf lung in vitro by specific antigen and by compound 48/80. Arch. int. Pharmacodyn. **192**, 347—352 (1971 a)

Eyre, P.: Pharmacology of bovine pulmonary vein anaphylaxis in vitro. Brit. J. Pharmacol. **43**, 302—311 (1971 b)

Eyre, P., Lewis, A. J., Wells, P. W.: Acute systemic anaphylaxis in the calf. Brit. J. Pharmacol. **47**, 504—516 (1973)

Eyre, P., Wells, P. W.: Histamine H_2-receptors modulate systemic anaphylaxis: a dual cardiovascular action of histamine in calves. Brit. J. Pharmacol. **49**, 364—367 (1973)

Fanchamps, A., Doepfner, W., Weidmann, H., Cerletti, A.: Pharmakologische Charakterisierung von Deseril, einem Serotonin-Antagonisten. Schweiz. med. Wschr. **90**, 1040—1046 (1960)

Farmer, J. B., Richards, I. M., Sheard, P., Woods, A. M.: Mediators of passive lung anaphylaxis in the rat. Brit. J. Pharmacol. **55**, 57—64 (1975)

Fastier, F. N.: Structure activity relationships of amidine derivatives. Pharmacol. Rev. **14**, 37—90 (1962)

Feinberg, S. M., Malkiel, S., Feinberg, A. R.: The Antihistamines. Their Clinical Application. Chicago-Illinois: Yearbook Publications Inc. 1950

Feldberg, W., Miles, A. A.: Regional variations of increased permeability of skin capillaries induced by histamine liberator and their relation to the histamine content of the skin. J. Physiol. (Lond.) **120**, 205—213 (1953)

Feldberg, W., Smith, A. N.: Release of histamine by tryptamine and 5-hydroxytryptamine. Brit. J. Pharmacol. **8**, 406—411 (1953)

Ferreira, S. H., Moncada, S., Vane, J. R.: Indomethacin and aspirin abolish prostaglandin release from the spleen. Nature (New Biol.) **231**, 237—239 (1971)

Fink, M. A., Rothlauf, M. V.: In vitro anaphylaxis in the sensitised mouse uterus. Proc. Soc. exp. Biol. (N.Y.) **90**, 477—480 (1955)

Flower, R., Grygleski, R., Herbaczynska-Cedro, K., Vane, J. R.: Effects of anti-inflammatory drugs on prostaglandin biosynthesis. Nature (New Biol.) **238**, 104—106 (1972)

Flower, R. J., Harvey, E. A., Moncada, S., Nijkamp, F., Vane, J. R.: Some properties of rabbit aorta contracting substance-releasing factor (RCS-RF). Brit. J. Pharmacol. 461P—462P (1976)

Flynn, S. B., Owen, D. A. A.: Histamine receptors in peripheral vascular beds in the cat. Brit. J. Pharmacol. **55**, 181—188 (1975)

Fourneau, E., Bovet, D.: The "sympathicolytic" action of a new derivative of dioxane. Arch. int. Pharmacodyn. **46**, 178—191 (1933)

Fowle, A. S. E., Hughes, D. T. D., Knight, G. J.: The evaluation of histamine antagonists in man. Europ. J. clin. Pharmacol. **3**, 215—220 (1971)

Gaddum, J. M., Picarelli, Z. P.: Two kinds of tryptamine receptor. Brit. J. Pharmacol. **12**, 323—328 (1957)

Ganellin, C. R., Port, G. N. J., Richards, W. G.: Conformation of histamine derivatives. II. Molecular orbital calculations of preferred conformations in relation to dual receptor activity. J. med. Chem. **16**, 616—620 (1973)

Ganley, O. H.: Protective effect of cyproheptadine, a new antihistamine antiserotonin compound on lethal burns in the mouse. Arch. int. Pharmacodyn. **138**, 125—132 (1962)

Garattini, S., Valzelli, L.: Serotonin. Amsterdam: Elsevier 1965

Garcia-Arocha, H.: Liberation of 5-hydroxytryptamine and histamine in the anaphylactic reaction of the rat. Canad. J. Biochem. **39**, 403—416 (1961)

Gelfand, M. D., West, G. B.: Experimental studies with the butanolamide and propanolamide of 1-methyl-lysergic acid. Int. Arch. Allergy. **18**, 286—291 (1961)

Goose, J., Blair, A. M. J. N.: Passive cutaneous anaphylaxis in the rat, induced with two homologous reagin-like antibodies and its specific inhibition with disodium cromoglycate. Immunology **16**, 749—760 (1969)

Gramajo, R., Cervio, N.: The use in rheumatology of a synthetic antiserotonin: methysergide. Pren. méd. argent. **52**, 2900—2902 (1965)

Green, A. F.: The antagonism of histamine and the anaphylactic response by phenylpyridylallylamines. Brit. J. Pharmacol. **8**, 171—176 (1953)

Green, A. F.: Antihypertensive drugs. In: Garattini, S., Shaw, P. A. (Eds.): Advances in Pharmacology, Vol. 1, pp. 161—225. New York: Academic Press Inc. 1962

Greig, M. E., Griffin, R. L.: Antagonism of slow reacting substance in anaphylaxis (SRS-A) and other spasmogens on the guinea pig tracheal chain by hydratropic acids and their effects on anaphylaxis. J. med. Chem. **18**, 112—116 (1975)

Gyermek, L.: Drugs which antagonize 5-hydroxytryptamine and related indolealkylamines. In: Erspamer, V. (Ed.): Handbook of Experimental Pharmacology, Vol. 19, pp. 471—528. Berlin-Heidelberg-New York: Springer 1966

Gyermek, L., Nádor, K.: The pharmacology of tropane compounds in relation to their steric structure. J. Pharm. (Lond.) **9**, 209—229 (1957)

Haddox, C. H., Saslaw, M. S.: Urinary 5-methoxytryptamine in patients with rheumatic fever. J. clin. Invest. **42**, 435—441 (1963)

Halbert, S. P., Bircher, R., Dahle, E.: Studies on the mechanism of the lethal toxic action of streptolysin "O" and the protection by certain antiserotonin drugs. J. Lab. clin. Med. **61**, 437—452 (1963)

Halpern, B. N.: Synthetic antihistamine substances. Arch. int. Pharmacodyn. **68**, 339—408 (1942)

Halpern, B. N., Dumas, J., Reber, H.: Rôle favorisant d'un antihistaminique de synthese dans la généralisation de l'infection locale. C.R. Soc. Biol. (Paris) **143**, 1563—1565 (1949)

Halpern, B. N., Liacopoulos, P., Liacopoulos-Briot, M.: Recherches sur les substances exogènes et endogènes agissant sur la permeabilité capillaire et leur antagonists. Arch. int. Pharmacodyn. **119**, 56—101 (1959)

Halpern, B. N., Neveu, T., Spector, S.: On the nature of the chemical mediators involved in anaphylactic reactions in mice. Brit. J. Pharmacol. **20**, 389—398 (1963)

Ham, N. S.: Solution conformation of antihistamines. J. pharm. Sci. **60**, 1764—1765 (1971)

Hanna, P. E., Ahmed, A. E.: Conformationally restricted analogues of histamine H_1 receptor antagonists. *trans* and *cis*-1,5-Diphenyl-3-dimethylaminopyrrolidine. J. med. Chem. **16**, 963—
968 (1973)

Harms, A. F., Nauta, W. T.: The effects of alkyl substitution in drugs. 1. Substituted dimethyl-
aminoethyl benzhydryl ethers. J. med. Chem. **2**, 57—77 (1960)

Henson, P. M., Cochrane, C. G.: Immunological induction of increased vascular permeability. I. A
rabbit passive cutaneous anaphylactic reaction requiring complement, platelets, and neutrophils. J. exp. Med. **129**, 153—165 (1969)

Herxheimer, H.: The 5-hydroxytryptamine shock in the guinea-pig. J. Physiol. (Lond.) **128**, 435—
445 (1955)

Herxheimer, H., Stresemann, E.: The effect of some new antihistamines on the anaphylactic microshock of the guinea pig. Brit. J. Pharmacol. **21**, 414—418 (1963)

Higginbotham, R. D.: Influence of adrenalectomy and cortisol on resistance of mice to histamine,
serotonin, anaphylactic, and endotoxin shocks. J. Allergy **33**, 35—44 (1962)

Highton, T. C., Garrett, M. H.: Some effects of serotonin and related compounds on human collagen. Lancet **1963, I**, 1234—1237

Ison, R. R., Casy, A. F.: Structural influences upon antihistamine activity; 3-amino-L-aryl-L-(2-
pyridyl)propenes and related compounds. J. Pharm. (Lond.) **23**, 848—856 (1971)

Ison, R. R., Franks, F. M., Soh, K. S.: The binding of conformationally restricted antihistamines to
histamine receptors. J. Pharm. (Lond.) **25**, 887—894 (1973)

James, M. N. G., Williams, G. J. B.: Structural studies of histamine H_1 effector molecules: the
crystal structure of the antihistaminic drug (+)-chlorpheniramine maleate; [(+)-S—(p-chlo-
rophenyl)-L-(2-pyridyl)-3-N,N-dimethylamine maleate]. Canad. J. Chem. **52**, 1872—1879
(1974)

Jones, D. G., Kay, A. B.: Inhibition of eosinophil chemotaxis by the antagonist of slow reacting
substance of anaphylaxis—compound FPL 55712. J. Pharm. (Lond.) **26**, 917—918 (1974)

Julou, L., Ducrot, R., Bardone, M. C., Detaille, J. Y., Feo, C., Guyonnet, J. C., Loiseau, G., Pasquet, J.: Etude des propriétés pharmacologiques de la diméthylsulfamido-3 (diméthylamino-
2 propyl)-10 phénothiazine (8,599 R.P.). Arch. int. Pharmacodyn. **159**, 70—86 (1966)

Kalz, F., Fekete, Z.: Studies on capillary permeability using Coomassie blue as indicator. J.
invest. Derm. **36**, 37—46 (1961)

Kellaway, C. H., Trethewie, E. R.: The liberation of a slow-reacting smooth muscle-stimulating
substance in anaphylaxis. Quart. J. exp. Physiol. **30**, 121—145 (1940)

Kier, L. B.: Molecular orbital calculations of the preferred conformations of histamine and a
theory on its dual activity. J. med. Chem. **11**, 441—445 (1968a)

Kier, L. B.: Preferred conformation of serotonin and a postulate on the nature of its receptor from
molecular orbital calculations. J. pharm. Sci. **57**, 1188—1191 (1968b)

Kraft, E., Zimmerman, B. G.: Influence of histamine H_1- and H_2-receptor blockers on sympathetic vasodilator and vasoconstrictor responses in canine paw. Brit. J. Pharmacol. **53**, 51—
58 (1975)

Kutter, E., Hansch, C.: Steric parameters in drug design. Monoamine oxidase inhibitors and
antihistamines. J. med. Chem. **12**, 647—652 (1969)

Levi, R., Lee, C.-H.: Characterization of cardiac histamine receptors by means of selective H_1-
and H_2-agonists and antagonists. Fed. Proc. **33**, Abst. 2109 (1974)

Lindquist, K. J.: A unique class of rabbit immuno-globulins eliciting passive cutaneous anaphylaxis in homologous skin. Immunochemistry **5**, 525—542 (1968)

Loew, E. R.: Pharmacology of antihistamine compounds. Physiol. Rev. **27**, 542—573 (1947)

Logan, G., Wilhelm, D. L.: Vascular permeability changes in inflammation. I. The role of endogenous permeability factors in ultraviolet injury. Brit. J. exp. Path. **47**, 300—314 (1966)

Maling, H. M., Webster, M. E., Williams, M. A., Wilford, S., Anderson, W.: Inflammation induced
by histamine, serotonin, bradykinin and compound 48/80 in the rat: antagonists and the
mechanism of action. J. Pharmacol. exp. Ther. **191**, 300—310 (1974)

Margolin, S., Tislow, R.: Experimental and clinical efficacy of trimeton and chlor-trimeton maleate. Ann. Allergy **8**, 515—518 (1950)

Mathé, A. A., Strandberg, K.: Antagonism of slow reacting substance by polyphloretin phosphate on isolated human bronchi. Acta physiol. scand. **82**, 460—465 (1971)

Mathé, A. A., Strandberg, K., Fredholm, B.: Antagonism of prostaglandin $F_{2\alpha}$ induced broncho-constriction and blood pressure changes by polyphloretin phosphate in the guinea-pig and cat. J. Pharm. (Lond.) **24**, 378—382 (1972)

Mawson, C., Whittington, H.: Evaluation of the peripheral and central antagonistic activities against 5-hydroxytryptamine of some new agents. Brit. J. Pharmacol. **39**, 223 P (1970)

McQueen, D. S.: The effects of prostaglandin E_2, prostaglandin $F_{2\alpha}$ and polyphloretin phosphate on respiration and blood pressure in anaesthetized guinea pigs. Life Sci. **12**, 163—172 (1973)

Miles, A. A., Wilhelm, D. L.: The activation of endogenous substances inducing pathological increases of capillary permeability. Part I. A survey of endogenous permeability factors. In: The Biochemical Response to Injury, pp. 51—83. Oxford: Blackwell 1960

Mota, I.: Mast cells and anaphylaxis. Ann. N.Y. Acad. Sci. **103**, 264—277 (1963)

Mota, I.: The mechanism of anaphylaxis. I. Production and biological properties of mast cell sensitizing antibody. Immunology **7**, 681—699 (1964)

Movat, H. Z., Di Lorenzo, N. L., Taichman, N. S., Berger, S., Stein, H.: Suppression by antihistamine of passive cutaneous anaphylaxis produced with anaphylactic antibody in the guinea pig. J. Immunol. **98**, 230—235 (1967)

Murray, M., Smith, W. D., Waddell, A. H., Jarrett, W. F. H.: *Nippostrongylus brasiliensis*: histamine and 5-hydroxytryptamine inhibition and worm expulsion. Exp. Parasit. **30**, 58—63 (1971)

Nauta, W. T., Bultsma, T., Rekker, R. F., Timmerman, H.: Structure-activity relations in a series of compounds related to diphenhydramine. Med. Chem. Spec. Contrib. Int. Symp. 3 rd., 1972, p. 125 (Pub. 1973). Ed. Pratesi, P. London: Butterworth 1973

Northover, B. J., Subramanian, G.: A study of possible mediators of inflammatory reactions in the mouse foot. Brit. J. Pharmacol. **18**, 346—355 (1962)

Orange, R. P., Murphy, R. C., Austen, K. F.: Inactivation of slow reacting substance of anaphylaxis (SRS-A) by arylsulfatases. J. Immunol. **113**, 316—322 (1974)

Orange, R. P., Murphy, R. C., Karnovsky, M. L., Austen, K. F.: The physicochemical characteristics and purification of slow-reacting substance of anaphylaxis. J. Immunol. **110**, 760—770 (1973)

Orange, R. P., Stechschulte, D. J., Austen, K. F.: Immunochemical and biologic properties of rat IgE. II. Capacity to mediate the immunologic release of histamine and slow reacting substance of anaphylaxis (SRS-A). J. Immunol. **105**, 1087—1095 (1970)

Orange, R. P., Valentine, M. D., Austen, K. F.: Antigen-induced release of slow reacting substance of anaphylaxis (SRS-A^{rat}) in rats prepared with homologous antibody. J. exp. Med. **127**, 767—782 (1968)

Orr, T. S. C., Gwilliam, J., Cox, J. S. G.: Studies on passive cutaneous anaphylaxis in the rat with disodium cromoglycate. Immunology **19**, 469—479 (1970)

Orr, T. S. C., Gwilliam, J., Cox, J. S. G.: Studies on passive cutaneous anaphylaxis in the rat with disodium cromoglycate. II. A comparison of the rat anti-DNP 7 S_{y2} and rat reagin induced cutaneous reactions. Immunology **21**, 405—417 (1971)

Ovary, Z.: Immediate reactions in the skin of experimental animals provoked by antibody-antigen interaction. In: Kallos, P. (Ed.): Progr. Allergy, Vol. 5, pp. 459—508. Basel-New York: S. Karger 1958

Ovary, Z., Bier, O. G.: Quantitative studies on passive cutaneous anaphylaxis in the guinea pig and its relationship to the Arthus phenomenon. J. Immunol. **71**, 6—11 (1953)

Palmer, M. A., Piper, P. J., Vane, J. R.: Release of rabbit aorta contracting substance (RCS) and prostaglandins induced by chemical or mechanical stimulation of guinea-pig lungs. Brit. J. Pharmacol. **49**, 226—242 (1973)

Parratt, J. R., West, G. B.: Release of 5-hydroxytryptamine and histamine from tissues of the rat. J. Physiol. (Lond.) **137**, 179—192 (1957 a)

Parratt, J. R., West, G. B.: 5-Hydroxytryptamine and the anaphylactoid reaction in the rat. J. Physiol. (Lond.) **139**, 27—41 (1957 b)

Parratt, J. R., West, G. B.: Inhibition by various substances of oedema formation in the hind-paw of the rat induced by 5-hydroxytryptamine, histamine, dextran, egg white and compound 48/80. Brit. J. Pharmacol. **13**, 65—70 (1958)

Paton, W. D. M.: Compound 48/80: a potent histamine liberator. Brit. J. Pharmacol. **6**, 499—508 (1951)

Paton, W. D. M.: The release of histamine. In: Kallos, P. (Ed.): Progr. Allergy, Vol. 5, pp. 79—148. Basel-New York: S. Karger 1958

Peck, A. W., Fowle, A. S. E., Bye, C.: A comparison of triprolidine and clemastine on histamine antagonism and performance tests in man: implications for the mechanism of drug induced drowsiness. Europ. J. clin. Pharmacol. **8**, 455—463 (1975)

Perini, A., Mota, I.: Heterogeneity of guinea-pig homocytotropic antibodies. Immunology **22**, 915—923 (1972)

Petri, G., Cspiak, J., Kovacs, A., Bentzik, M.: Data on the pathology of pyogenic inflammation. I. The role of histamine in pyogenic inflammation and the effect of antihistaminics on its course. Acta med. Acad. Sci. hung **3**, 347—368 (1952)

Phair, J. P., Eisenfeld, A. J., Levine, R. J., Kantor, F. S.: Effects of pharmacological inhibition of histamine synthesis upon immunological reactions in guinea-pigs. Immunology **18**, 611—619 (1970)

Piper, P. J., Vane, J. R.: Release of additional factors in anaphylaxis and its antagonism by antiinflammatory drugs. Nature (Lond.) **223**, 29—35 (1969)

Pletscher, A., Shore, P. A., Brodie, B. B.: Serotonin release as a possible mechanism of reserpine action. Science **122**, 374—375 (1955)

Pletscher, A., Shore, P. A., Brodie, B. B.: Serotonin as a mediator of reserpine action in brain. J. Pharmacol. exp. Ther. **116**, 84—89 (1956)

Radwan, A. C., West, G. B.: Alterations in histidine decarboxylase activity during anaphylactic shock in the rat. Brit. J. Pharmacol. **30**, 392—399 (1967)

Rekker, R. F., Nauta, W. T., Bultsma, T., Waringa, C. G.: Integrated QSAR of H_1-receptor antagonists. Europ. J. med. Chem. **10**, 557—562 (1975)

Reuse, J. J.: Antihistamine drugs and histamine release, especially in anaphylaxis. In: Wolstenholme, G. E. W., O'Connor, C. M. (Eds.): Histamine. Ciba Foundation Symposium 1955, pp. 150—154. London: Churchill 1956

Rieveschl, G. R.: Dialkylaminoalkyl benzhydryl ethers. U.S. Patent 2, 421, 714 (1947)

Rocha e Silva, M.: Chemical mediators of the acute inflammatory reaction. Ann. N.Y. Acad. Sci. **116**, 899—911 (1964)

Rocha e Silva, M. Ed.: Handbook of Experimental Pharmacology. Histamine and Antihistaminics. Part 1. Histamine. Its chemistry, metabolism, and physiological and pharmacological actions, Vol. XVIII. Berlin-Heidelberg-New York: Springer 1966

Rocha e Silva, M. (Eds.): Handbook of Experimental Pharmacology, Part 2. Histamine II and Antihistaminics, Vol. XVIII. Berlin-Heidelberg-New York: Springer 1977

Rowley, D. A., Benditt, E. P.: 5-Hydroxytryptamine and histamine as mediators of the vascular injury produced by agents which damage mast cells in rats. J. exp. Med. **103**, 399—411 (1956)

Sanyal, R. K., West, G. B.: Anaphylactic shock in the albino rat. J. Physiol. (Lond.) **142**, 571—584 (1958 a)

Sanyal, R. K., West, G. B.: The relationship of histamine and 5-hydroxytryptamine to anaphylactic shock in different species. J. Physiol. (Lond.) **144**, 525—531 (1958 b)

Schachter, M.: Histamine and Antihistamines, Vol. I. International Encyclopedia of Pharmacology and Therapeutics, Section 74. Oxford-New York-Toronto-Sydney-Braunschweig: Pergamon Press 1973

Scherbel, A. L., Harrison, J. W.: Exaggerated reactivity to serotonin in patients with rheumatoid arthritis and related diseases. Circulation **18**, 777 (1958)

Scherbel, A. L., McKittrick, R. L., Hawk, W. A.: Lesions in rats caused by serotonin and histamine before and after amine oxidase inactivation and serotonin inhibition. J. clin. Invest. **39**, 1025—1026 (1960)

Scherbel, A. L., Schmid, E. A.: Effect of serotonin inhibitors on connective tissue disease. Cleveland Clin. Quart. **29**, 1—15 (1962)

Schneider, J. A.: Pharmacology of Rauwolfia. In: Rauwolfia. Pharmacology of Rauwolfia, pp. 109—143. Boston, Mass.: Little, Brown 1957

Sevitt, S.: Early and delayed oedema and increase in capillary permeability after burns of the skin. J. Path. Bact. **75**, 27—37 (1958)

Sevitt, S., Bull, J. P., Cruickshank, C. N. D., Jackson, D. M., Lowbury, E. J. L.: Failure of an antihistamine drug to influence the course of experimental human burns. Brit. med. J. 1952 II, 57—62

Sicuteri, F., Michelacci, S., Franchi, G.: Antagonism between an antiserotonin—the butanolamide of 1-methyl-lysergic-acid—and the effects of a histamine-liberating substance 48/80 B.W. in man. Int. Arch. Allergy 15, 291—299 (1959)

Shafi'ee, A., Hite, G.: The absolute configurations of the pheniramines, methyl phenidates, and pipradols. J. med. Chem. 12, 266—270 (1969)

Smith, J. B., Willis, A. L.: Aspirin selectively inhibits prostaglandin production in human platelets. Nature (New Biol.) 231, 235—237 (1971)

Sparrow, E. M., Wilhelm, D. L.: Species differences in susceptibility to capillary permeability factors: histamine, 5-hydroxytryptamine, and compound 48/80. J. Physiol. (Lond.) 137, 51—65 (1957)

Spector, W. G., Willoughby, D. A.: Histamine and 5-hydroxytryptamine in acute experimental pleurisy. J. Path. Bact. 74, 57—65 (1957)

Spector, W. G., Willoughby, D. A.: Experimental suppression of the early inflammatory phenomena of turpentine pleurisy in rats. Nature (Lond.) 181, 708—709 (1958)

Spector, W. G., Willoughby, D. A.: Experimental suppression of the acute inflammatory changes of thermal injury. J. Path. Bact. 78, 121—132 (1959 a)

Spector, W. G., Willoughby, D. A.: The demonstration of the role of mediators in turpentine pleurisy in rats by experimental suppression of the inflammatory changes. J. Path. Bact. 77, 1—17 (1959 b)

Spector, W. G., Willoughby, D. A.: The inflammatory response. Bact. Rev. 27, 117—154 (1963)

Stacey, R. S.: Clinical aspects of cerebral and extracerebral 5-hydroxytryptamine. In: Handbook of Experimental Pharmacology. 5-Hydroxytryptamine and related indolealkylamines. Berlin-Heidelberg-New York: Springer-Verlag 1965, Vol. XIX

Starr, M. S., West, G. B.: Bradykinin and oedema formation in heated paws of rats. Brit. J. Pharmacol. 31, 178—187 (1967)

Stechschulte, D. J., Austen, K. F.: Anaphylaxis. In: Zweifach, B. W., Grant, L., McCluskey, R. T. (Eds.): The Inflammatory Process, 2nd Ed., Vol. III, Ch. 5. New York-London: Academic Press 1974

Stechschulte, D. J., Austen, K. F., Bloch, K. J.: Antibodies involved in antigen-induced release of slow reacting substance of anaphylaxis (SRS-A) in the guinea pig and rat. J. exp. Med. 125, 127—147 (1967)

Stewart, P. B., Bliss, J. Q.: The permeability-increasing factor in diluted human plasma. Brit. J. exp. Path. 38, 462—466 (1957)

Stone, C. A., Wenger, H. C., Ludden, C. T., Stavorski, J. M., Ross, C. A.: Antiserotonin-antihistaminic properties of cyproheptadine. J. Pharmacol. exp. Ther. 131, 73—84 (1961)

Strandberg, K., Uvnas, B.: Purification and properties of the slow reacting substance formed in the cat paw perfused with compound 48/80. Acta physiol. scand. 82, 358—374 (1971)

Stringer, H. C. W., Highton, T. C.: The shrinkage temperature of skin collagen. Aust. J. Derm. 5, 230—234 (1960)

Takagi, K., Tukao, T.: Effects of some drugs on capillary permeability in the anaphylaxis of the mouse. Jap. J. Pharmacol. 21, 455—465 (1971)

Tokuda, S., Weiser, R. S.: Studies on the role of serotonin and mast cells in anaphylaxis of the mouse produced with soluble antigen-antibody complexes. J. Immunol. 86, 292—301 (1961)

Toldy, L., Vargha, L., Toth, I., Borsy, J.: Promethazine 1. Acta chim. Acad. Sci. hung. 19, 273—275 (1959)

Trendelenberg, U.: The action of histamine and 5-hydroxytryptamine on isolated mammalian atria. J. Pharmacol. exp. Ther. 130, 450—460 (1960)

Uda, T.: The mode of inhibitory actions of guaiazulene and some other antiinflammatory agents on the anaphylactoid edemas. Nippon Yakurigaku Zasshi 56, 1151—1163 (1960)

Van Arman, C. G., Begany, A. J., Miller, L. M., Pless, H. H.: Some details of the inflammations caused by yeast and carrageenin. J. Pharmacol. exp. Ther. 150, 328—334 (1965)

Vane, J. R.: Inhibition of prostaglandin synthesis as a mechanism for aspirinlike drugs. Nature (New Biol.) 231, 232—235 (1971)

Vane, J. R., Ferreira, S. H.: Interactions between bradykinin and prostaglandins. Life Sci. **16**, 804—805 (1975)

Vane, J. R., Ferreira, S. H.: Interactions between bradykinin and prostaglandins. In: Proc. No. 27 of the Fogerty International Center. Washington, D.C.: U.S. Government Printing Office 1976. In press

Vaz, N. M., Prouvost-Danon, A.: Behaviour of mouse mast cells during anaphylaxis in vitro. In: Kallos, P., Waksman, B. H. (Eds.): Progr. Allergy, Vol. XIII, pp. 111—173. Basel-New York: S. Karger 1969

Villaneuva, R., Hinds, L., Katz, R. L., Eakins, K E.: The effect of polyphloretin phosphate on some smooth muscle actions of prostaglandins in the cat. J. Pharmacol. exp. Ther. **180**, 78—85 (1972)

Vinegar, R., Schreiber, W., Hugo, R.: Biphasic development of carrageenin edema in rats. J. Pharmacol. exp. Ther. **166**, 96—103 (1969)

Vinegar, R., Truax, J. F., Selph, J. L.: Some quantitative temporal characteristics of carrageenin-induced pleurisy in the rat. Proc. Soc. exp. Biol. (N.Y.) **143**, 711—714 (1973)

Vogel, G., Marek, M. L.: Über die Hemmung verschiedener Rattenpfoten-Ödeme durch Serotonin-Antagonisten. Arzneimittel-Forsch. **11**, 1051—1054 (1961)

Warner, R. R. P.: Current status and implications of serotonin in clinical medicine. In: Dock, W., Snapper, I. (Eds.): Advances in Internal Medicine, Vol. XIII, pp. 241—282. Chicago: New Book Medical Publ. Inc. 1967

Weeks, R. E., Gunnar, R. M.: Effect of tripelennamine hydrochloride on acute inflammation. Arch. Path. (Chicago) **48**, 178—182 (1949)

Weis, J.: Investigations on some experimental inflammations in mouse paws. Med. exp. (Basel) **8**, 1—11 (1963)

Wells, P. W., Eyre, P.: The pharmacology of passive cutaneous anaphylaxis in the calf. Canad. J. Physiol. Pharmacol. **50**, 255—262 (1972)

West, G. B.: 5-Hydroxytryptamine, tissue mast cells and skin oedema. Int. Arch. Allergy **10**, 257—275 (1957)

Wilhelm, D. L.: The mediation of increased vascular permeability in inflammation. Pharmacol. Rev. **14**, 251—280 (1962)

Wilhelm, D. L.: Chemical mediators. In: Zweifach, B. W., Grant, L., McCluskey, R. T. (Eds.): The Inflammatory Process, 2nd Ed., Vol. II, pp. 251—301. New York-London: Academic Press 1973

Wilhelm, D. L., Mason, B.: Rationale of antihistaminic therapy in thermal injury. An experimental evaluation in the guinea pig. Brit. med. J. **1958 II**, 1141—1143

Wilhelm, D. L., Mason, B.: Vascular permeability changes in inflammation: the role of endogenous permeability factors in mild thermal injury. Brit. J. exp. Path. **41**, 487—506 (1960)

Willis, A. L.: Parallel assay of prostaglandin-like activity in rat inflammatory exudate by means of cascade superfusion. J. Pharm. (Lond.) **21**, 126—128 (1969 a)

Willis, A. L.: Release of histamine, kinin, and prostaglandins during carrageenin-induced inflammation in the rat. In: Mantegazza, P., Horton, E. W. (Eds.): Prostaglandins, Peptides, and Amines, pp. 31—38. London-New York: Academic Press 1969 b

Willoughby, D. A.: Pharmacological suppression of increased capillary permeability following irradiation of the intestine of rats. Nature (Lond.) **184**, 1156 (1959)

Willoughby, D. A.: Pharmacological aspects of the vascular permeability changes in the rat's intestine following abdominal radiation. Brit. J. Radiol. **33**, 515—519 (1960)

Willoughby, D. A.: Mediation of increased vascular permeability of inflammation. In: Zweifach, B. W., Grant, L., McCluskey, R. T. (Eds.): The Inflammatory Process, 2nd Ed., Vol. II, pp. 303—331. New York-London: Academic Press 1973

Winter, C. A., Risley, E. A., Nuss, G. W.: Carrageenin-induced edema in hind paw of the rat as an assay for antiinflammatory drugs. Proc. Soc. exp. Biol. (N.Y.) **111**, 544—547 (1962)

Winter, C. A., Risley, E. A., Nuss, G. W.: Antiinflammatory and antipyretic activities of indomethacin, 1-(p-chlorobenzyl)-5-methoxy-2-methylindole-3-acetic acid. J. Pharmacol. exp. Ther. **141**, 369—376 (1963)

Witiak, D. T.: Antiallergenic agents. In: Burger, A. (Ed.): Medicinal Chemistry, Vol. 2, 3rd Ed., Ch. 65, pp. 1643—1668. New York: Wiley 1970

Wood, D. R.: The effect on gastric secretion of different rates of histamine infusion and of "Neoantergan". Brit. J. Pharmacol. **3**, 231—236 (1948)

Woolley, D. W., Shaw, E.: Differentiation between receptors for serotonin and tryptamine by means of the exquisite specificity of antimetabolites. J. Pharmacol. exp. Ther. **121**, 13—17 (1957)

Wyllie, J. H., Hesselbo, T., Black, J. W.: Effects in man of histamine H_2-receptor blockade by burimamide. Lancet **1972 II**, (7787), 1117—1120

Zileli, T., Chapman, L., Wolff, H. G.: Antiinflammatory action of UML-491 (1-methyl-D-lysergic acid butanolamide dimaleate) demonstrated by the granuloma pouch technique in rats. Arch. int. Pharmacodyn. **136**, 463—464 (1962)

Zvaifler, N. J., Bauer, H., Robinson, J. O.: IgE immunoglobulin in the rabbit. In: Austen, K. F., Becker, E. L. (Eds.): Biochemistry of the Acute Allergic Reactions, Vol. 2, pp. 33—44. Oxford: Blackwell 1971

CHAPTER 34

Inhibitors of the Release
of Anaphylactic Mediators

L. G. GARLAND, A. F. GREEN, and H. F. HODSON

A. Characteristics of Anti-Allergic Agents Discussed

Cromoglycate inhibits a number of allergic reactions and in particular the allergen-induced bronchospasm in patients with extrinsic asthma; clinical findings which are outside the scope of this chapter have been reviewed by PEPYS (1973) and BROGDEN et al. (1974). Laboratory studies revealed that this compound was neither a bronchodilator nor an antagonist of histamine, 5-hydroxytryptamine (5-HT) nor slow reacting substance of anaphylaxis (SRS-A), the suspected mediators of allergic bronchospasm, but rather prevented the anaphylactic release of these mediators (Cox, 1967; Cox et al., 1970). Lymphocyte functions correlated with the cell-mediated immune response were not inhibited by the drug (WALKER and DOLBY, 1975). In animals and man, cromoglycate inhibits immediate hypersensitivity reactions provoked by several different antigens, suggesting that it does not act by blocking the antibody receptor for antigen. This has been confirmed by ORR et al. (1970a) in studies using double sensitization with two antigenically distinct rat reagins. Furthermore, since the compound is effective in passively sensitized tissues, and in clinical usage does not reduce serum IgE levels (BERG and JOHANSSON, 1971), it does not act by inhibiting antibody production. These observations, together with results described in detail in later sections, suggest that an important part of the clinical efficacy of cromoglycate may be attributed to prevention of exocytosis in mast cells. Cromoglycate together with other more recently developed compounds which inhibit exocytosis and the release of mediators from mast cells have been classified as anti-allergic agents.

This review is concerned only with specific agents of this type and not with β-adrenoceptor stimulants and E-type prostaglandins (PGs) or phosphodiesterase inhibitors such as theophylline. Their anti-allergic properties, attributable to elevation of cAMP levels, have been thoroughly reviewed by KALINER and AUSTEN (1974a), KALINER and AUSTEN (1974b) and LICHTENSTEIN (1974).

B. Cromoglycate and Similar Compounds

I. Identification and Screening

The activity of cromoglycate was identified primarily from observations of asthmatic reactions provoked in man by the deliberate inhalation of specific antigen (ALTOUNYAN, 1967). This unique approach is not repeatable and the laboratory evaluation of potential anti-allergic agents requires the use of animal experimental models of the immediate-type hypersensitivity reaction. Laboratory models of lung anaphylaxis in the intact animal have an obvious and important place in the screening of anti-allergic agents but the rat passive cutaneous anaphylaxis (PCA) reaction is preferred for primary screening because a large number of compounds can be tested more rapidly and efficiently and oral administration is practicable. The selectivity of the rat PCA test is poor, however, (see below) and other tests, including in vitro models of immediate hypersensitivity reactions, are required to confirm that compounds which inhibit the PCA response act by preventing the release of anaphylactic mediators. The final validity of these tests can only be examined by the correlation between the results obtained and the clinical effects subsequently found.

1. The Passive Cutaneous Anaphylaxis Reaction (PCA) in Rats

Following the demonstration by GOOSE and BLAIR (1969) that cromoglycate inhibited the reagin-mediated PCA reaction in rats, this procedure has been used extensively as a primary screen for anti-allergic compounds. In this test, pharmacological mediators released by an immediate hypersensitivity reaction in the skin produce a local increase in capillary permeability, measurement of which provides an estimate of the intensity of the anaphylactic reaction.

a) Preparation of Antibody

Unlike some species of laboratory animal, rats may be stimulated quite readily to produce reagin-like antibodies with properties in common with those of human IgE (MOTA, 1964; JONES and OGILVIE, 1967; BLOCH and WILSON, 1968; BINAGHI et al., 1964) and designated as rat IgE by STECHSCHULTE et al. (1970).

Before being classified as reaginic, antiserum should be checked for the latency and persistence (to 72 h and beyond) of skin sensitizing activity and for the destruction of this activity by heating at 56° C for 1 h.

Three methods have been described for the production of reaginic antibodies in rats.

1. A single injection of antigen together with *Bordetella pertussis* as adjuvant (MOTA, 1964) stimulates the production of reagin-like antibody in low titre[1] (usually < 50) during the period 6–30 days after the injection, peak levels being achieved between 12 and 18 days. The choice of antigen influences the antibody response, ovalbumin being a more effective antigen than human serum albumin, bovine serum albumin, rabbit γ-globulin or bovine γ-globulin. The route of the injection is also important. The highest antibody titres are achieved either by injecting the antigen intramuscularly (i.m.) and *B. pertussis* intraperitoneally (i.p.) or by injecting both the antigen and the adjuvant intradermally (i.d.).

2. Infection with a suitable helminth parasite such as *Nippostrongylus brasiliensis* provokes a high titre (> 100) reagin response of long duration. Antibody to the parasite can be detected in the serum at about 25 days after infection and persists in the circulation for at least 7 months after a single infection. The levels of reagin are enhanced by subsequent infection. *N. brasiliensis* antigen is prepared by extracting adult nematodes into phosphate-buffered saline (OGILVIE, 1964).

---

[1] Titre being defined as the highest dilution of antiserum giving PCA response of at least 5 mm diameter.

3. Infection of rats with *N. brasiliensis* 10 days after the injection of ovalbumin and *B. pertussis*—as (a)—potentiates the primary sensitization yielding reagin-like antisera against ovalbumin with titres often greater than 1000 (ORR and BLAIR, 1969; ORR et al., 1971 c). This method has practical advantages since reagin-like antibody is produced in high titre against a well-defined antigen.

Serum is collected from anaesthetised rats either by cardiac puncture or by bleeding from the neck. Because of the instability of unpurified rat reagin at room temperature (BINAGHI et al., 1964) the blood should be allowed to clot at 4° C and centrifuged in the cold at about 1000 *g* to separate the serum which may then be stored at −20° C for at least 2 years without loss of activity (OGILVIE, 1964).

b) Test Procedure

Descriptions of the rat PCA method vary in detail (OGILVIE, 1964; MOTA, 1964; GOOSE and BLAIR, 1969). Groups of preferably 4 or 5 rats weighing at least 100 g are shaved with electric hair clippers prior to the i.d. injection of a small volume (0.05 or 0.1 ml) of antiserum diluted to produce suitable responses (15–20 mm diameter). After a latent period of 24–72 h each rat is injected intravenously (i.v.) with a mixture of antigen and Evans blue dye (25 mg/kg). They are killed 30 min later and the dorsal skin is reflected to expose the under surface. The size of the blue area at the site of i.d. injection of serum is determined by measuring the diameter. If the shape is irregular, its size may be estimated from either the product of opposing diameters or the mean of the biggest and smallest diameters. Other methods of measuring the PCA reaction have been based on the spectrophotometric determination of the Evans blue dye extracted from skin (TAICHMAN and MOVAT, 1966) and on the use of radioactive tracer substances (UDAKA et al., 1970). However, BLUM and OVARY (1974) have concluded that the added precision offers no real advantage because of the inherent variability of the response itself. Drugs are usually injected either i.v. together with the antigen and blue dye or orally at an appropriate interval beforehand. The percentage inhibition of the PCA reaction is calculated for each animal or group of animals by comparison with saline treated controls.

c) Antibody Concentration

GOOSE and BLAIR (1969) reported that when potent antisera were used undiluted, the effect of cromoglycate in the dosage range 2–10 mg/kg administered i.v. with antigen plateaued at 50% inhibition, but that submaximal reactions could be inhibited completely. Figure 1 shows that the dose-response curves for two anti-allergic compounds, cromoglycate and doxantrazole, were similar at each of five dilutions of sera producing graded responses in the range 11–44 mm diameter.

While a single reaction per rat is sufficient, multiple dilutions of antisera may be used for drug screening so that the PCA reaction may be evaluated either as a quantal response (HALL et al., 1974) or by the shift of the response line relating antibody concentration to the diameter of the blueing reaction (MIELENS et al., 1974).

d) Interpretation of Results

The reagin-mediated rat PCA response is associated with degranulation of subcutaneous mast cells which contain histamine and 5-HT and is prevented either by the

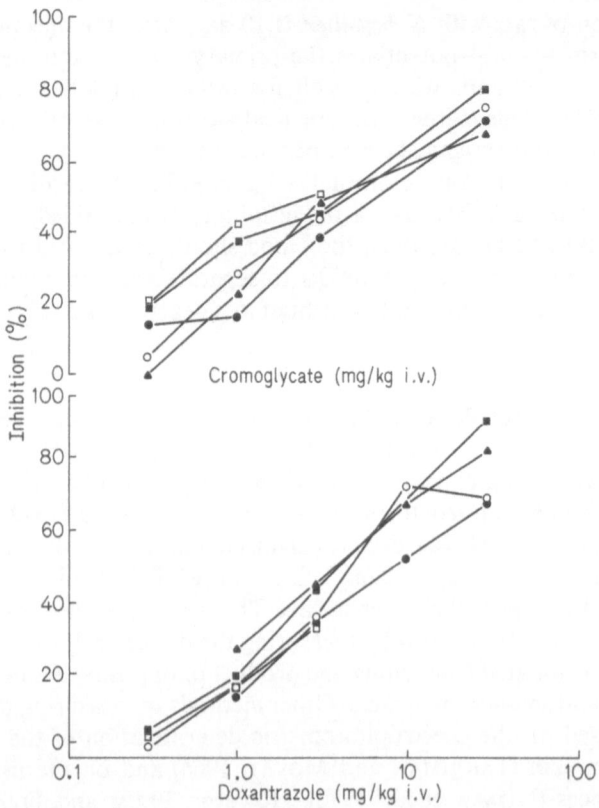

Fig. 1. Inhibition (%) by either cromoglycate or doxantrazole injected i.v. with antigen of reactions caused by dilutions of antiserum provoking various sized reactions as follows control diameters in brackets). ● 1/1 (42 mm); ▲ 1/3 (30 mm); ○ 1/10 (20 mm); ■ 1/30 (16 mm) and □ 1/100 (11 mm). Points plotted are the means from 4–17 rats. (FOLLENFANT, M. J., unpublished observations)

prior administration of a combination of histamine and 5-HT antagonists or by the prior degranulation of mast cells with compound 48/80 or polymyxin B (Chap. 33), indicating that histamine and 5-HT released from skin mast cells are primarily responsible for the local increase in capillary permeability. The role of SRS-A in the rat PCA reaction is not clear. When injected i.d. rat SRS-A weakly increased capillary permeability (ORANGE and AUSTEN, 1969), and FARMER et al. (1975) have reported that the SRS-A antagonist FPL 55712 caused some inhibition of rat PCA reactions. The PCA response is also inhibited by drugs that lower the capillary perfusion pressure. Such "false positive" effects may be readily distinguished by determining the effect of the same compounds on blueing responses to histamine and 5-HT. The anti-allergic activity in the rat PCA test of cromoglycate (COX, 1967) and more recently doxantrazole (BATCHELOR et al., 1975) ICI 74917 (EVANS and THOMSON, 1975) M&B, 22948 (BROUGHTON et al., 1974) and W 8011 (HERZIG et al., 1976) have been verified in this way. However, many compounds have been claimed to have anti-allergic activity in the rat PCA test without evidence of this kind.

The following compounds representing diverse pharmacological classes were reported by ANKIER (1971) to reduce the PCA reaction; polymyxin B sulphate (mast cell degranulation), phentolamine, tripelennamine, tyramine, guanethidine, amitriptyline, imipramine, hydrochlorthiazide, flufenamic acid, and β-adrenoceptor stimulants, though the effect of flufenamic acid was not confirmed (40 mg/kg i.v., TAYLOR et al., 1974a). The effect of β-adrenoceptor stimulants such as isoprenaline is of special interest because low concentrations were required and because such compounds are known to inhibit the anaphylactic release of mediators in other experimental systems (ASSEM and SCHILD, 1969; LICHTENSTEIN and MARGOLIS, 1968). Inhibition by isoprenaline of cutaneous responses to histamine, 5-HT and bradykinin was found by ROESCH and ROESCH (1973) but not by ANKIER (1971).

2. Lung Anaphylaxis in vivo

Respiratory anaphylaxis in subhuman primates has obvious relevance for the identification of anti-allergic agents suitable for the prevention of human asthma. Not only is the correct shock organ under investigation but also monkey lung may be sensitized by human IgE. Respiratory reactions have been described following the inhalation of antigen by rhesus monkeys either actively sensitized (PATTERSON and TALBOT, 1969) or passively sensitized by the prior injection of specific reaginic serum (MIYAMOTO et al., 1968). Furthermore, PATTERSON et al. (1971) found that the respiratory response following inhalation of ascaris antigen by actively sensitized monkey was inhibited, although incompletely, by cromoglycate administered prior to antigen either i.v. or by inhalation as an aerosol. However, due to the risk of handling monkeys, (a proportion of rhesus monkeys are known to carry simian B virus, rabies virus or mycobacteria), and the expense, anaphylactic bronchoconstriction in monkeys has not been widely used to investigate anti-allergic agents. A safer and less expensive alternative is to use the common marmoset *(Callithrix jaccus)*. COX et al. (1970) reported that these animals when passively sensitized by i.v. injection of human serum rich in IgE, responded on subsequent antigen challenge with an increase in airway resistance which was reduced by prior injection of cromoglycate. However, the control response was too small for studying dose-dependence.

In contrast to primates, rats, and guinea pigs have been used extensively to study respiratory anaphylaxis. COX (1967) reported that cromoglycate did not protect actively sensitized guinea pig against antigen-induced bronchoconstriction which suggests that this model of immediate hypersensitivity has little value for screening compounds of this type; the results with anti-allergic agents identified primarily by other methods, are described in Section B.III. In contrast, the rat has proved to be of value for identifying compounds which inhibit anaphylactic bronchoconstriction. FARMER et al. (1973; 1975) have described a lung anaphylaxis reaction in passively sensitized rats (the rat PLA test). Rats are passively sensitized by i.v. injection of 0.5–1 ml antiserum with a high titre raised against a specific antigen by the method of ORR and BLAIR (1969) described in Section B.I.1.a.γ. Twenty-four hours later they are anaesthetised and challenged by i.v. injection of antigen and changes in airways resistance are recorded by the technique of KONZETT and ROSSLER (1940), as modified by BURDEN et al. (1971). Of the anaphylactic mediators released from sensitized rat lung on antigen challenge, 5-HT seems to be most responsible for the resultant

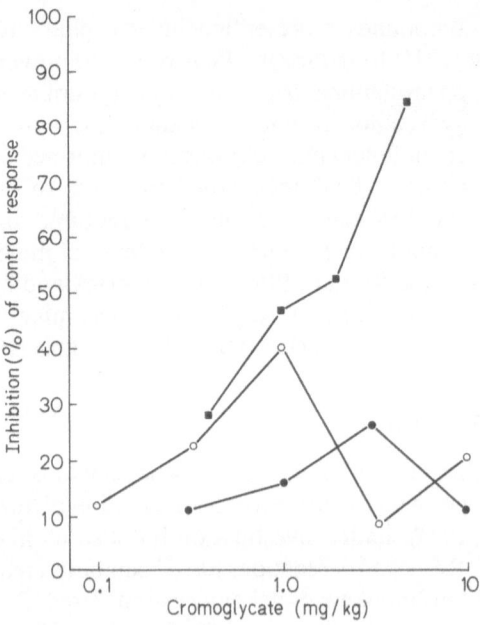

Fig. 2. Inhibition by cromoglycate (i.v. 1–5 minutes prior to antigen) of anaphylactic broncho-spasm in passively sensitized rats *(closed squares)* compared with actively sensitized rats *(open and closed circles)*; the data is taken from (○) CHURCH et al. (1972), (●) STOTLAND and SHARE (1974), (■) FARMER et al. (1975)

bronchoconstriction (CHURCH et al., 1972; STOTLAND and SHARE, 1974; FARMER et al., 1975), although experiments with the SRS-A antagonist FPL 55712 suggest that this mediator may also be involved (FARMER et al., 1975). Anti-allergic agents such as cromoglycate (FARMER et al., 1975) or doxantrazole (BATCHELOR et al., 1975) admin-istered i.v. 1 min before challenge produced a dose-dependent inhibition of the PLA response.

The powerful dose-related inhibition by cromoglycate of lung anaphylaxis in passively sensitized rats contrasts with the low order of activity and bell-shaped dose-response curves (Fig. 2) in actively sensitized rats (CHURCH et al., 1972; STOT-LAND and SHARE, 1974). The reason for this difference is not clear but may be attributed to the presence in actively sensitized rats of antibodies other than IgE which contribute to, or initiate events leading to, bronchoconstriction.

3. Passive Peritoneal Anaphylaxis

The peritoneal cavity of the rat provides a suitable site for the study of immediate hypersensitivity reactions. In the rat, two physicochemically distinct homologous immunoglobulins designated IgGa and IgE can mediate the release of anaphylactic mediators from the peritoneal tissue (BLOCH et al., 1968; STECHSCHULTE et al., 1970). Rat IgGa is a heat stable, 7S, electrophoretically "slow", complement fixing immu-noglobulin whereas rat IgE is a heat labile, 8S, electrophoretically "fast" trace immu-noglobulin. The IgGa antibodies present in whole hyperimmune rat antiserum pre-

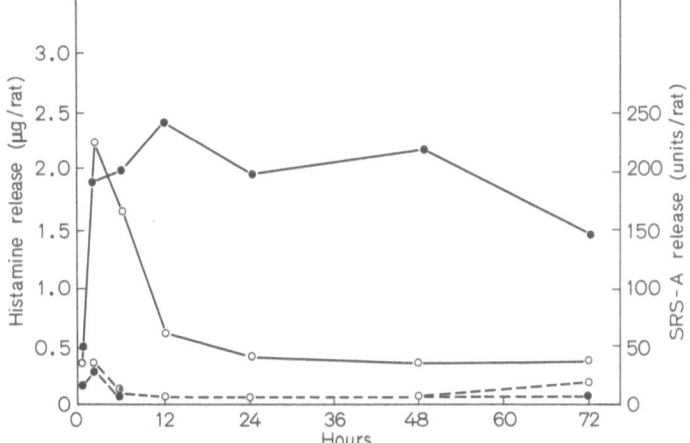

Fig. 3. The effect of varying the latent period between i. p. injection of 0.25 ml of homocytotropic-(anti-DNP-KLH)antiserum (PCA titre at 48 h = 50) on the subsequent antigen-induced release of histamine (●—●) and SRS-A (o—o). The effect of heating the homocytotropic antiserum at 56° C for 4 h is also indicated (-----). (Reproduced from ORANGE et al., 1970)

pare the peritoneum for the release of SRS-A but only negligible amounts of histamine. Polymorphonuclear leucocytes and an intact complement system, but not the peritoneal mast cells or circulating lymphocytes, are required for this reaction (ORANGE et al., 1968). However, hyperimmune rat antiserum can be fractionated by DEAE-cellulose chromatography to yield an IgGa fraction capable of sensitizing the peritoneum to release both histamine and SRS-A; this reaction requires the peritoneal mast cells for optimal release of both mediators and is believed to reflect the interaction of IgGa with peritoneal mast cells in the absence of competing non-specific immunoglobulins present in whole hyperimmune antisera (ORANGE and AUSTEN, 1971). Rat IgE antibody prepares the peritoneum for the release of histamine when a 24-h sensitization period is used as in the PCA reaction but ORANGE et al. (1970) have shown that SRS-A also is released when the latent period between i.p. injection of antiserum and antigen is reduced to 2 h (Fig. 3). Under these conditions, the release of not only histamine but also SRS-A requires the mast cell but not the circulating polymorphonuclear leucocyte or an intact complement system. Thus it differs from the IgGa mediated release of SRS-A.

A suitable method for investigating inhibitors of the IgE-mediated release of both histamine and SRS-A from peritoneal tissues is described by Ross et al. (1976); it also measures the extravasation of blue dye into the peritoneal cavity. Each rat is injected i.p. with 2 ml of an appropriate dilution of rat serum containing antigen-specific IgE, (e.g. 1 in 5 dilution of heat labile serum with a 24 h PCA titre of 1:64) followed 2 h later by 0.3 ml of blue dye (5% Pontamine Sky blue) injected i.v. and antigen (e.g. ovalbumin 0.4 mg/ml in 5 ml Tyrode's solution containing heparin 50 µg/ml) injected i.p. After a suitable interval, usually 5 min, the rats are killed and the peritoneal fluid is poured into ice cold tubes. The peritoneal cells are separated by centrifugation and the supernatants assayed for histamine, SRS-A and blue dye content (samples containing blood should be discarded). Anti-allergic agents such as cromoglycate and

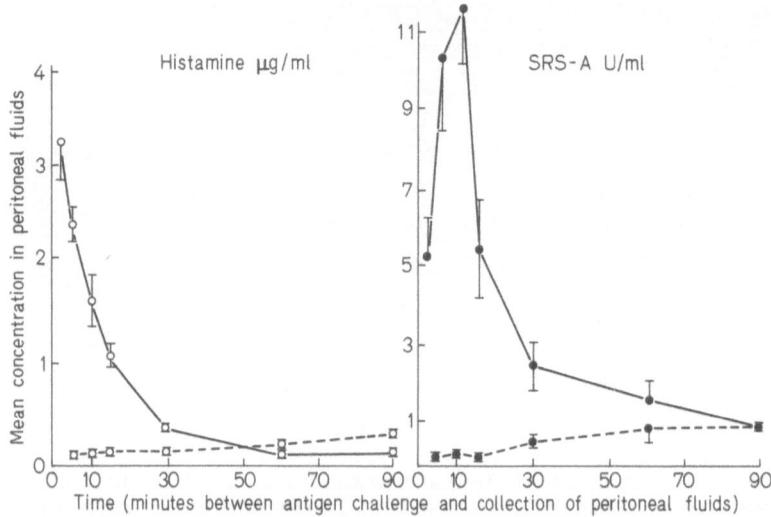

Fig. 4. Rat passive peritoneal anaphylaxis. Changes in the concentrations of histamine and SRS-A in peritoneal fluid following antigen challenge. Rats were passively sensitized by i.p. injection of antiserum containing rat IgE followed 2 h later by either antigen in Tyrode's solution (———) or Tyrode's solution (–––––) i.p. Results are the mean ± s.e. mean and numbers in brackets refer to the numbers of rats used. (Reproduced from Ross et al., 1976 with permission of S. Karger AG, Basel)

the nitro-indandione BRL 10833 cause a graded inhibition of the release of histamine and SRS-A when injected i.p. with antigen.

Changes in the concentrations of histamine and SRS-A in the rat peritoneal fluid in vivo are influenced not only by the rate of release of the mediators but also by the rate of their removal from the peritoneal cavity by absorption and metabolism so that the interval between challenge and sample collection is critical (Fig. 4). This also complicates interpretation but the method has some good points. Firstly, drugs may be identified which inhibit the anaphylactic release of SRS-A as well as histamine from the mast cell or the polymorphonuclear leucocyte, depending upon the class of immunoglobulin used and the sensitizing schedule (see above). Secondly, Ross et al. (1976) have suggested that the extravasation of fluid into the peritoneum, estimated by the concentration of blue dye, may be a model of the serous transudation of fluid into the small airways, prevention of which may account for the apparent therapeutic effectiveness of cromoglycate in short term trials when studies of upper airway resistance have shown no improvement.

4. Human Tissues in vitro

Methods by which human lung tissue, removed at surgery for carcinoma of the bronchus, may be passively sensitized and prepared for the release of anaphylactic mediators have been described by PARISH (1967), SHEARD et al. (1967), ASSEM and SCHILD (1968) and ORANGE et al. (1971).

The lung tissue should be put into cold Tyrode's solution as soon as possible after removal from the patient and chopped into small pieces after removing the large blood vessels and bronchii. The pieces of lung parenchyma are then washed thoroughly in ice cold Tyrode's solution before being cut into smaller fragments. After further washing they are then sensitized by incubation (for about 18 h at room temperature or 0.5 h at 37° C) in human serum rich in IgE antibody of known antigen specificity. After washing to remove excess antiserum, aliquots of tissue are incubated at 37° C in a small volume (e.g. 2 ml) of Tyrode's solution. After 5 min antigen is added and incubation is continued for 15 min during which time anaphylactic mediators are released. The release reaction is stopped by adding ice-cold Tyrode's solution and placing the reaction tubes in ice. The supernatant is separated from the lung fragments using a filter pipette and residual mediators are released from the tissue either by boiling the lung fragments to release histamine or by six cycles of freezing and thawing to release intracellular SRS-A (LEWIS et al., 1974). As a control, antigen is added to tissue incubated previously in Tyrode's solution. Histamine may be assayed either biologically (BOURA et al., 1954) or fluorimetrically (SHORE et al., 1959; EVANS et al., 1973; KUSNER and HERZIG, 1971). Samples may be assayed separately for SRS-A, preferably after separation (ORANGE et al., 1973), using guinea pig terminal ileum bathed in Tyrode's solution containing atropine (0.2 μmol/l) and an antihistamine such as triprolidine (0.2 μmol/l) or mepyramine (1 μmol/l).

Cromoglycate inhibits the anaphylactic release of histamine and SRS-A from human lung (SHEARD and BLAIR, 1970). In early experiments, the dose-response relationship was inconsistent (ASSEM and MONGAR, 1970; ASSEM and RICHTER, 1971) but a graded effect has since been obtained (PIPER and WALKER, 1973; BROUGHTON et al., 1974) using a fairly narrow range of inhibitor concentrations (Fig. 5). However,

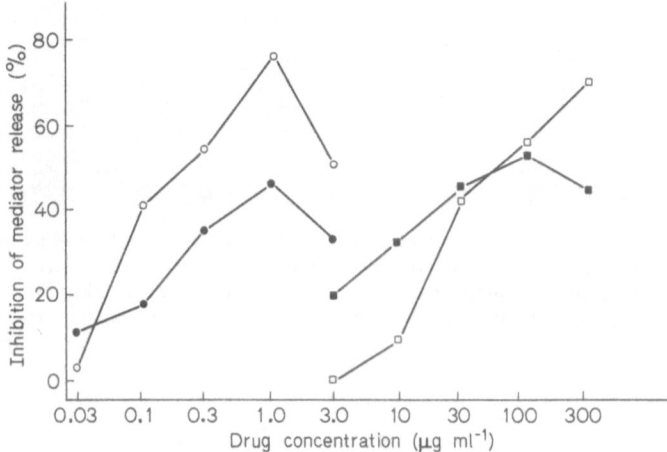

Fig. 5. Inhibition of allergen-induced release of histamine and SRS-A from passively sensitized human lung tissue by M & B 22948 and disodium cromoglycate in two separate experiments. Using M & B 22948: ● histamine: ○ SRS-A. Using disodium cromoglycate: ■ histamine; □ SRS-A. Chopped human lung was incubated for 18 h with serum from asthmatic subjects. Aliquots were challenged with extracts of *Dermatophagoides farinae* (500 μg ml⁻¹) immediately after the addition of graded concentrations of the test compounds. Histamine was assayed fluorimetrically. SRS-A was assayed on the guinea pig ileum in the presence of mepyramine. Points refer to single determinations from three pooled samples at each drug concentration. (Reproduced from BROUGHTON et al., 1974)

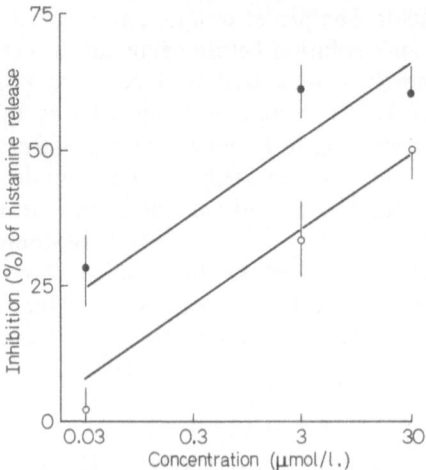

Fig. 6. Inhibition (%) of anaphylactic histamine release from passively sensitized human chopped lung by either cromoglycate (o—o) or fluorene-2,7-dicarboxylic acid (DCF) (●—●) added concomitantly with grass pollen antigen. Each point is the mean from four replicate experiments, vertical bars represent s.e. mean. Deviations from linearity and parallelism were not significant and the potency DCF: cromoglycate was calculated as 18.7 with 95% limits 4–151. (Reproduced from GARLAND, 1975)

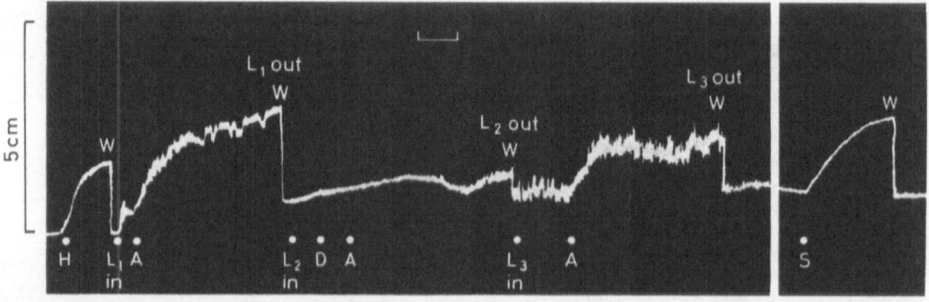

Fig. 7. Contractions of human bronchial strip produced by histamine 4 µg/ml (*H*), SRS-A 3 units/ml (*S*), and antigen-induced release of spasmogens (*A*) from successive portions of passively sensitized human lung (L_1 to L_3). In the presence of disodium cromoglycate 10 µg/ml (*D*), there was inhibition of the contraction of the bronchial strip caused by antigen challenge of the second lung portion (L_2). *W*: wash; time scale: 5 min. (Reproduced from SHEARD and BLAIR, 1970, with permission of S. Karger AG, Basel)

the method is not sufficiently precise to allow reliable quantitative comparison of different compounds (Fig. 6). An adaption of the method (SHEARD and BLAIR, 1970), in which strips of passively sensitized human lung are challenged with antigen while suspended in an organ bath with a strip of human bronchial smooth muscle, is also suitable for semi-quantitative or qualitative tests (Fig. 7).

Alternative human tissues suitable for studying in vitro the release of anaphylactic mediators include circulating basophil leucocytes (LICHTENSTEIN and OSLER, 1964) and skin (GREAVES et al., 1972). However, since cromoglycate is inactive in these tissues (Assem and Mongar, 1970; Lichtenstein and Adkinson, 1969; Pearce et al., 1974) their use has been largely reserved for the further investigation of anti-allergic compounds identified as active in other systems (see Sect. B.III.).

5. Rat Tissues in vitro

From the work of Cox and his colleagues (Cox, 1967; Cox et al., 1970), it is concluded that of the usual laboratory species, the rat provides the most suitable tissues for the identification of cromoglycate-like compounds. The release of anaphylactic mediators (histamine, 5-HT, SRS-A, and occasionally PGs) in vitro from actively or passively sensitized rat lungs is inhibited by cromoglycate at 10 or 100 µg/ml (Sheard and Blair, 1970; Farmer et al., 1975). However, a dose-related effect has not been demonstrated and the technique has not been developed for the quantitative study of anti-allergic agents. By contrast, the anaphylactic release of histamine from rat peritoneal cells has been widely used for this purpose (Garland, 1973; Kusner et al., 1973; Thomson and Evans, 1973; Fullarton et al., 1973a). Cells may be either taken from actively sensitised rats or passively sensitized in vitro. For either method, peritoneal washings are obtained from rats recently killed by decapitation under anaesthesia by injecting into the peritoneal cavity a suitable volume (e.g. 10 ml) of cold physiological medium (Hank's or Tyrode's solution). After massaging the abdomen, the fluid is withdrawn through a midline abdominal incision. Pooled peritoneal washings from several rats are centrifuged at 250 g for 6 min, the supernatant is discarded and the cell pellet resuspended in ice cold medium. At this stage, actively sensitized cells are diluted and divided into experimental aliquots (usually 0.5 ml) containing approximately 10^6 mast cells or 1 µg total histamine. Cells may be passively sensitized by incubating them with an appropriate dilution of antiserum containing rat IgE at 37° C for 60 min. They are washed to remove excess antibody and resuspended in medium (Evans and Thomson, 1972). Aliquots of sensitized cells are then brought to 37° C before adding either antigen or inhibitor/antigen mixtures (Sect. B.III.3.). After between 1 and 5 min, the release reaction is stopped by adding ice-cold medium and cells separated from supernatant after centrifuging at 250 g for 6 min. The cell pellets are resuspended in medium and boiled for 10 min to release residual histamine. Released and residual histamine are assayed biologically or fluorimetrically, that released being expressed as a fraction of the total. In this system, the concentration-effect curve for cromoglycate regularly has an adequate slope and maximum inhibition occurs within the range 1–30 µmol/l (Fig. 8). Very similar results have been obtained by the different laboratories using this method. Several investigators have found that the IC_{50} of cromoglycate is 5–10 µmol/l and that a maximum of 60–80% inhibition can be achieved.

Garland and Mongar (1974) have demonstrated that the release of histamine from rat peritoneal cells in vitro induced by mixtures of dextran and phosphatidyl serine is inhibited by cromoglycate and that the concentration-effect curve is almost coincident with that for inhibition of the anaphylactic release of histamine. This anaphylactoid reaction has been used successfully for the quantitative comparison of inhibitors. It has the advantages that rat peritoneal washings may be used without prior sensitization and that the release of histamine from one experiment to the next is quite consistent.

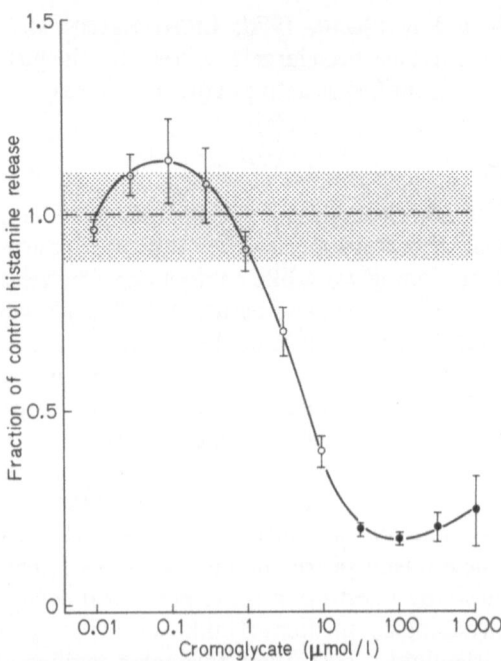

Fig. 8. Inhibition by cromoglycate of anaphylactic histamine release from rat peritoneal cells. Open circles are the mean values (±s.e. mean) from six duplicate experiments, closed circles are the means from two duplicate experiments. Shaded area delineates the 95% fiducial range of control histamine release calculated from the variance within thirty-four experiments. (Reproduced from GARLAND, 1973)

In the above methods, the release of histamine is used as an index of the exocytosis of mast cell granules. Alternatively, estimates can be made of the degree of mast cell degranulation by examining under the light microscope preparations of various tissues, including subcutaneous connective tissue (GOOSE and BLAIR, 1969; COX et al., 1970), rat peritoneal cell suspensions (TAYLOR et al., 1974a, 1974b) and the periosteal membranes of rat calvaria (HERZIG et al., 1976). However, electron microscopic studies show that during exocytosis, granules apparently retained in the cell may be in contact with extracellular fluid and able to release histamine by cation exchange (ANDERSON et al., 1973). Thus, exocytosis should be more sensitively estimated by measuring released histamine rather than degranulation. However, concentration-related inhibition by anti-allergic agents of rat mast cell degranulation has been reported (ORR, 1974; TAYLOR et al., 1974a, 1974b).

II. Structure-Activity Relationships

Inhibition of the PCA reaction in rats may not necessarily be the most relevant to human asthma, but this is the test which for reasons of practicability has been most widely used and for which results are given in almost all discussions of anti-allergic activity. The following consideration of structure activity relationships is, therefore, necessarily based on activity in this test.

The work of the Fisons' group (Cox et al., 1970) leading to cromoglycate (1; the structure here given is that of the free dicarboxylic acid) started from a consideration of the structure of the natural product khellin (2) a bronchodilator and vasodilator which had earlier achieved some status in the treatment of asthma but which was no longer used because of unpleasant side-effects.

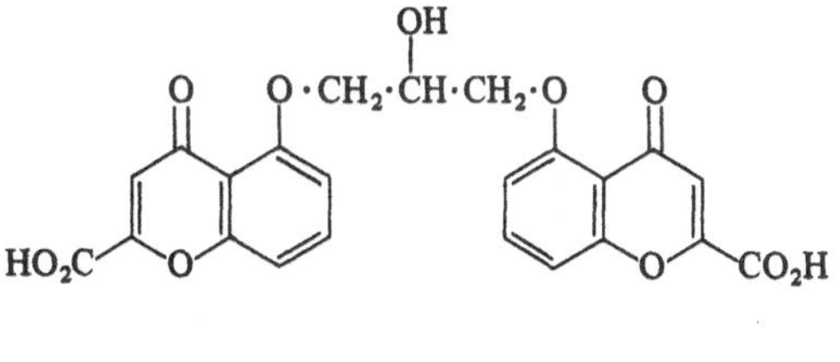

(1) Cromoglycic acid 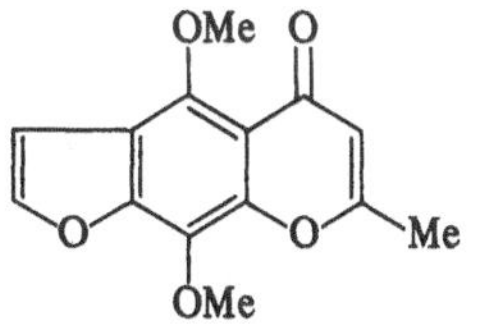   (2) Khellin

Anti-allergic activity due to inhibition of mediator release was first detected in a number of substituted chromone-2-carboxylic acids. The structural relationship between chromone-2-carboxylic acid (3) itself, and khellin is obvious, but it is interesting to note that khellin itself was subsequently shown not to be a potent inhibitor of mediator release. From a perusal of Fisons' patents it appears that activity was compatible with a large variation in the position and nature of substituents in the benzene ring (ring A of 3); this relative insensitivity towards substitution is a characteristic of other anti-allergic series as will be seen later. In many cases, the substitution took a cyclic form giving tricyclic carboxylic acids such as (4).

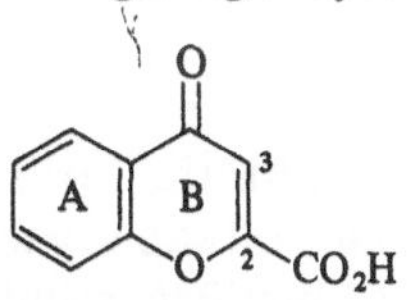

(3) 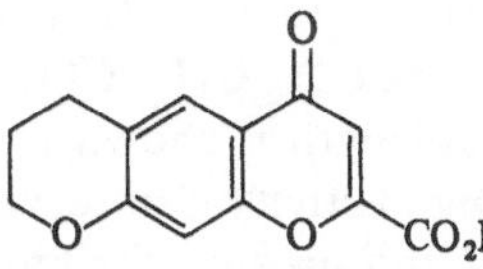   (4)

All the chromone-2-carboxylic acids tested in the early studies were short-acting but a major step forward for the Fisons' group came with the demonstration that compounds in which two chromone-2-carboxylic acid moieties were linked together had a much greater persistence of action (Cox et al., 1970). Cromoglycate is, of course, a specific example of such a compound and was the culmination of an extensive investigation into bis-chromone-2-carboxylic acids (5) with a variety of linking groups, X (CAIRNS et al., 1972).

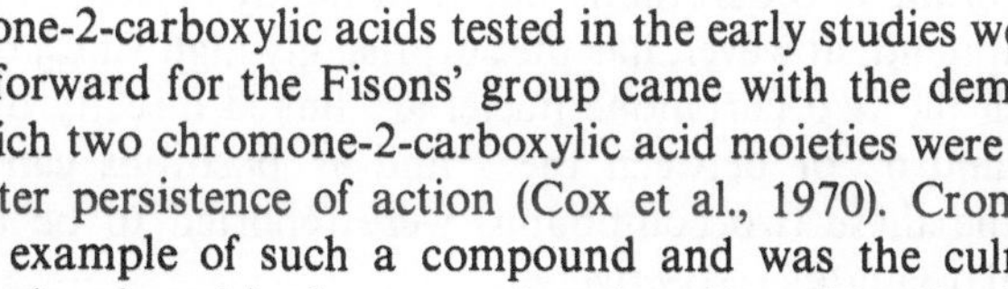

(5)

A notable feature in this series is the general lack of specific influence on activity produced by changes in the positions of linkage and in the nature of the connecting chain X. With one exception the position of the linkage has little effect on activity, as

Table 1. Inhibition of rat PCA reaction; i.v. administration; bischromone carboxylic acids (5)

Compound no.	X	Link	PCA ED_{50} mg/kg
5a (cromoglycate)	$O-CH_2-CHOH-CH_2O$	$5,5^1$	0.7
5b	$O-CH_2-CHOH-CH_2O$	$6,6^1$	0.3
5c	$O-CH_2-CHOH-CH_2O$	$7,7^1$	0.5
5d	$O-CH_2-CHOH-CH_2O$	$5,7^1$	0.2
5e	$O-[CH_2]_5-O$	$5,5^1$	2.9
5f	$O-[CH_2]_5-O$	$6,6^1$	2.4
5g	$O-[CH_2]_5-O$	$7,7^1$	2.0
5h	$O-[CH_2]_5-O$	$5,7^1$	4.5
5i	$O-[CH_2]_5-O$	$8,8^1$	> 10.0

can be seen from Table 1; the four compounds (5a–d) have similar potencies and compounds (5e–h), although less active, are close to each other. The exception is provided by linkage through the $8,8^1$ position, as exemplified by the compound (5i) in Table 1. Although there is no ready explanation for this lack of activity, it must be due to steric factors and it was noted that it is consistent with the low activity observed for 8-substituted monochromone-2-carboxylic acids.

The nature of the connecting link and of the atoms bonded to the chromone-2-carboxylic acid moieties is not critical. Potency comparable with that of cromoglycate is observed with compounds possessing the following links (X in formula 5):

$O·CH_2·CHOH·CH_2O$; $O·[CH_2]$ $·O$; $[CH_2]_3$; $[CH_2]_5$;
$CH_2·CH_2·CHOH·CH_2·CH_2$; CO; NH; O.

The effect of chain length is shown in compounds with the $6,6^1$-O. $[CH_2]$ $·O$ link; where $n=2$ to 6 high activity is observed but this falls off rapidly for the longer chain compounds, $n=7$ and greater. Strikingly, the $6,6^1$-methylene linked compound (5; $x=6,6^1$-CH_2-) is virtually inactive and this result was interpreted as a requirement for coplanarity of the two chromone nuclei in highly active compounds; the $6,6^1$-NH-linked compound, however, has the surprisingly high ED_{50} of 0.5 mg/kg. Compounds in which the two chromone nuclei are linked directly by a covalent bond between the 6 and 6^1 or between the 7 and 7^1 positions can achieve a planar conformation and these two compounds were reported to be highly active with ED_{50}s of 0.2 and 0.3 mg/kg respectively.

Thus, the ability of the bischromones to adopt a coplanar conformation appears to be an important but not the sole factor for high activity in this series. Prompted by this hypothesis the Fisons' workers synthesized the tetracyclic dicarboxylic acid (6) in which the chromone nuclei are necessarily coplanar; its ED_{50} was 0.5 mg/kg (CAIRNS et al., 1972)

(6)

All the chromone-2-carboxylic acids of this study were strongly acidic with pK_a values between 1.3 and 2.0. There was no obvious correlation between pK_a and PCA inhibitory activity.

A later, independent, study on bis-chromones described the preparation of the compound $(5; X = 6,6^1\text{-CO}\cdot\text{NH}\cdot\text{CH}_2\cdot\text{NH}\cdot\text{CO-})$ which had activity "comparable with that of cromoglycate" (BARKER et al., 1973). This example, in which the chromone nuclei are substituted by amide carbonyl groups, reinforces the earlier observations that the nature of substituents on chromone-2-carboxylic acids has little effect on activity.

The therapeutic success and the uniqueness of the activity of cromoglycate ensured that variation of the key structural features of the molecule was quickly and extensively taken up by workers in the pharmaceutical industry and elsewhere. Much of the resulting work has to date appeared only in the patent literature where biological test results are seldom given in detail and where negative results are not discussed. Despite the vast number of patent publications in this area there is a paucity of information which can be used for meaningful discussion of structure-activity relationships.

One of the obvious points for variation of the chromone-2-carboxylic acid structure is the oxygen atom in the chromone ring. Sulphur analogues, e.g. (7) and related bis-thiochromone-2-carboxylic acids, have been described in patents and presumably have good activity. Nitrogen analogues have, however, been investigated more extensively by several groups, with interesting results.

(7)   (8)   (9)

The simple nitrogen analogue of chromone-2-carboxylic acid is the quinoline derivative $(8; R=H)$ with the trivial name of kynurenic acid. Kynurenic acid and its derivatives exist in the tautomeric forms (8) and (9), the relative concentration of which will vary according to the physical environment. Because the 4-oxo form is likely to be predominant under physiological conditions, and because the formal

Table 2. Inhibition of rat PCA reaction, i.v. administration; kynurenic acids (8)

Compound	R	PCA, ED_{50} mg/kg
8a	H	~ 50
8b	6Br	10
8c	6OH	10
8d	6NO_2	10
8e	6NH_2	5
8f	$6p\text{CO--NH--C}_6\text{H}_4\text{--CO}_2\text{H}$	1
8g	$6p\text{O--C}_6\text{H}_4\text{--CO}_2\text{H}$	10
8h	$7\text{NH}_2, 8\text{Me}$	0.1
8i	$5\text{NH}_2, 8\text{Me}$	1

relationship to chromones is obvious, only this form (8) will be referred to here. HALL et al. (1974) described a series of aryl-substituted kynurenic acids (8) some members of which were considerably more active than cromoglycate; it will be apparent from Table 2, which lists a few of these acids, that there is no clear structure-activity relationship. A few bis-kynurenic acids (10) were also described but again there was no obvious correlation between activity and structural features. Some quinolone-3-carboxylic acids (11) were inactive or had only low activity; this correlates well with the lack of activity shown by chromone-3-carboxylic acids.

(11)   (10)

EVANS et al. (1974) also found that some substituted kynurenic acids (cf. 8) were potent inhibitors in the PCA test and extension of this work led to closely related tricyclic compounds of type 12 with exceptionally high activity. For example, ICI 74917 (12, R = butyl) was reported to be 300 times as active as cromoglycate and also to have a wider spectrum of anti-allergic activity (EVANS and THOMSON, 1975).

(12)   (13)

The chromone-2-carboxylic acid system (3) consists of a 4-pyrone-2-carboxylic acid moiety (13) fused to a benzene ring. Polycyclic structures, in which a 4-pyrone-2-carboxylic acid moiety is fused to either aromatic or heterocyclic ring systems have been extensively investigated. Of these compounds, the tricyclic acids (14) and (15) (WRIGHT and JOHNSON, 1973) have activity comparable with cromoglycate while the tetracyclic acid PR-D-92-EA (16) is considerably more active (ED_{50} 0.42 mg/kg) and has been the subject of extensive pharmacological study as a potential anti-asthmatic agent. As well as causing inhibition of mediator release PR-D-92-EA also blocks the responses of isolated guinea pig ileum to bradykinin, 5-HT, SRS-A, PGE_2, and $PGF_{2\alpha}$ but not histamine (POSSANZA et al., 1974).

(14) X = O
(15) X = S   (16)

(17)

Table 3. Inhibition of rat PCA reaction, i.v. administration; values
relative to cromoglycate = 1

Compound	R	PCA assay (cromoglycate = 1)
17a	1 MeO	<1
17b	3 MeO	0.3
17c	4 MeO	~0.1
17d	5 MeO	3
17e	6 MeO	0.3
17f	7 MeO	3
17g	8 MeO	0.4
17h	7 Me	0.5
17i	7 Et	3
17j	7 Me$_2$CH	7
17k	7 Me$_2$CHO	8
17l	7 OH	~1
17m	7 CO$_2$H	2

Anti-allergic activity in a series of xanthone-2-carboxylic acids (17) was discovered independently by several groups. The structural similarity to the chromone-2-
carboxylic acids is not as close as the compounds so far discussed, but is clearly
recognisable. The study of PFISTER et al. (1972) showed that only those xanthones
with the carboxyl group in the 2-position (cf. 17) have significant activity; the xan-
thone-1,3 and 4-carboxylic acids are inactive or have only low activity. The effect of
substitution in the xanthone nucleus is evident from the results in Table 3 which lists
a selection of the compounds described in this study. Substitution in positions 1, 3, 4,
6 or 8 gave compounds which were only as active as or less active than the parent
carboxylic acid. Activity greater than that of xanthone-2-carboxylic acid was observed in compounds with a substituent in the 5- or 7-position (and in 5,7-disubsti-
tuted compounds). Examples (17f, i, j, k, l, and m) show that an exceptionally wide
range of lipophilic-hydrophilic and electronic character is tolerated in the substituent group; this was noted in the chromone-2-carboxylic acids discussed above and
is a striking feature of other anti-allergic drug series; in most other series of biologically active compounds there is a significant correlation between activity and the
physico-chemical characteristics of substituent groups. Patent applications from
Syntex, Allen, and Hanbury, and Wellcome also claim anti-allergic activity for xan-
thone-2-carboxylic acids and the range of compounds covered supports the above
observations on the relationship between structure and activity.

Hitherto in this discussion all quoted inhibitory activities in the rat PCA test
have referred to i.v. administration; none of the compounds showed significant
activity after oral dosing. This is true of cromoglycate which has virtually no oral
activity in the rat PCA test, an observation which parallels the ineffectiveness of
cromoglycate against human asthma when given orally. In the xanthone-2-carbox-
ylic acid series, significant oral anti-allergic activity was noted for the first time.
Several compounds have been studied extensively in anticipation that they might
prove to be effective oral anti-asthmatic drugs; examples are xanoic acid (18) (Rosz-

KOWSKI et al., 1974; SPRENKLE et al., 1975) SMX (19) (FERRARESI et al., 1974) and AH 7725 (20) (ASSEM, 1973; ASSEM et al., 1974).

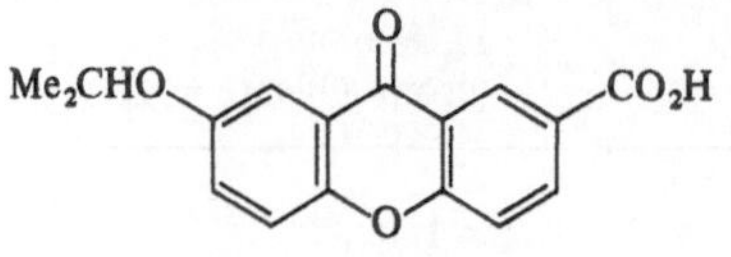

(18) Xanoic acid

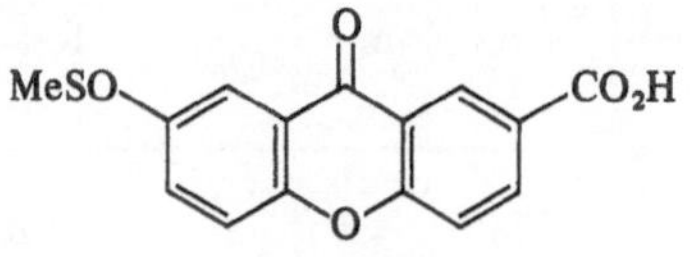

(19) SMX

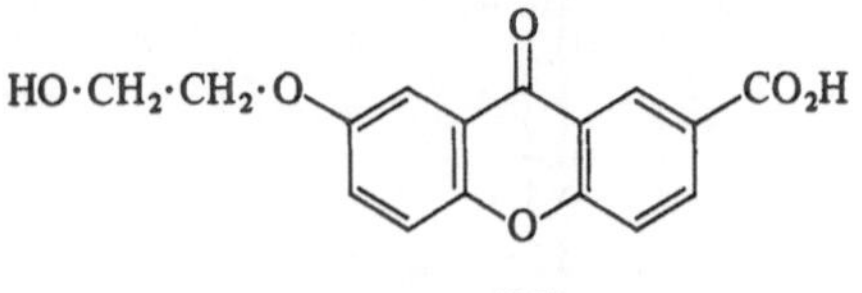

(20)

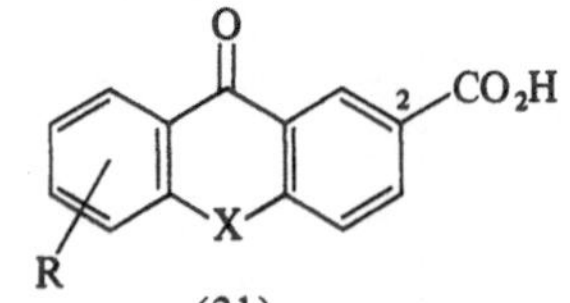

(21)

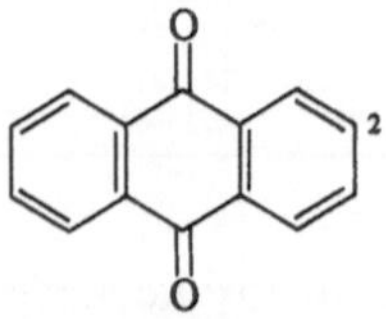

(22)

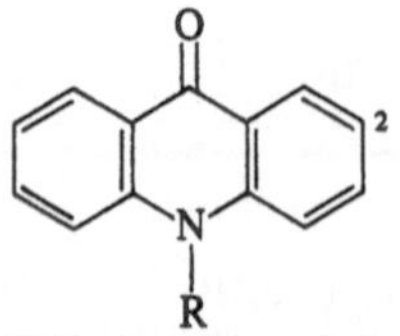

(23)   R = H or alkyl

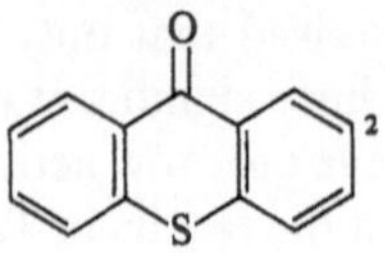

(24)

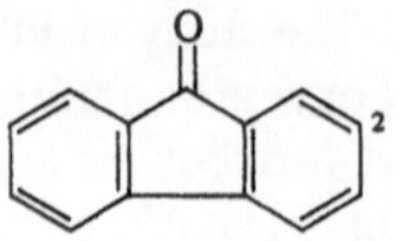

(25)

It is evident from patent applications that anti-allergic activity at least as good as that of the xanthone-2-carboxylic acids is possessed by a range of formally related tricyclic carboxylic acids (21). These include 2-substituted acids of the anthraquinone (22), acridone (23), thioxanthone (24), and fluorenone (25) systems; it appears that in all cases the carboxylic acid function must be located in the 2-position and that the tolerance towards substituent position and character parallels that seen in the xanthone series. The presence of the carbonyl function in these acids seems to be essential for activity. It is worth noting that the nature of the group X (cf. 21) has a marked effect on the chemical character of this carbonyl function and the high activity of derivatives of all the systems (22–25) is a further expression of the tolerance towards substituent type in the tricyclic carboxylic acids.

The carboxyl group is a feature common to all the compounds so far considered in this section. It has been known for many years that the 5-tetrazole group is acidic and that for any given carboxylic acid (26) and tetrazole (27) pair the difference in pK_a is generally less than 0.2 (MIHINA and HERBST, 1950; MCMANUS and HERBST, 1959). Since the overall bulk of the two functions—and even more importantly that of the anions (28) and (29) derived from them—is not dissimilar, it was suggested that in a biologically active molecule with a carboxyl group, that group could be replaced by a 5-tetrazole moiety with retention of biological activity (HERBST, 1956); the resulting compound could have therapeutic advantages. A number of studies have since shown that this hypothesis is valid in a general sense although there are exceptions (e.g. JUBY et al., 1968; DRAIN et al., 1971).

(26) R·C

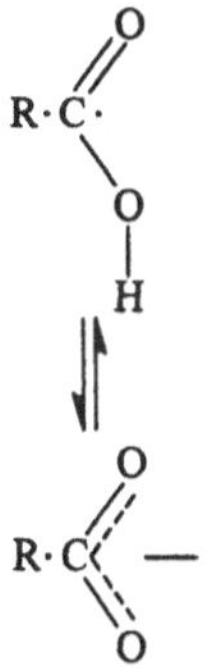

(27) R·C

(28) R·C —

(29) R·C

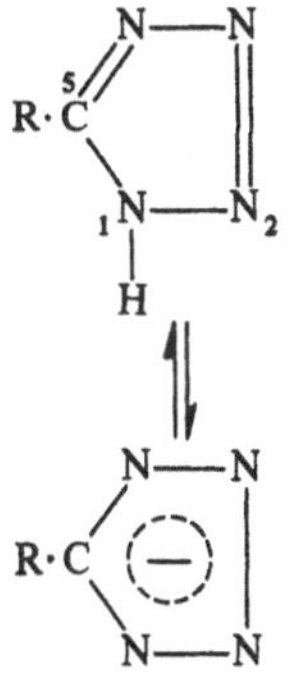

ELLIS and SHAW (1972) described the preparation of a number of 2-(5-tetrazolyl) chromones as analogues of anti-allergic chromone-2-carboxylic acids. The parent compound (30) and several with methyl, chloro, or nitro groups in the 6 or 7 positions were reported to be "comparable with, or better than, cromoglycate" in the rat PCA test. Tetrazole analogues of most of the other anti-allergic carboxylic acid series have been described in the patent literature and the xanthone-tetrazole AH 7079 (31) (ASSEM, 1973), was at one time considered to be worthy of trial in man and was subjected to extensive pharmacological study.

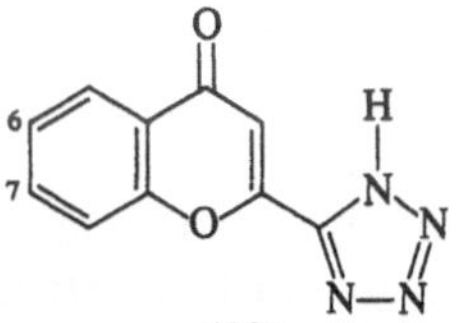

(30)

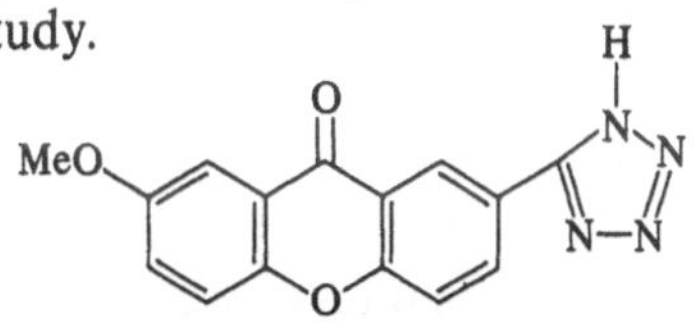

(31) AH 7079

All the anti-allergic compounds discussed above fall into two broad groups represented by the partial formulae (32) and (33) respectively where R is a carboxyl or a 5-tetrazolyl function. The chromone-2-carboxylic acids and related compounds are represented by the partial formula (32) where ring A may be monocyclic, polycyclic or heterocyclic but is usually fully aromatic and, therefore, planar. The second group comprises what are here conveniently referred to as the tricyclic acids, all of which contain the partial structure (33), again embedded in what is an essentially planar polycyclic aromatic ring system. Within each group there is thus a different, but specific requirement for a particular spatial relationship between the carbonyl and acidic functions.

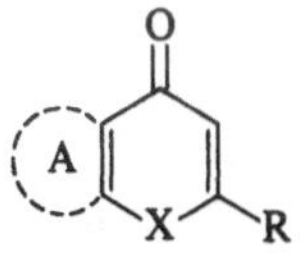

(32)

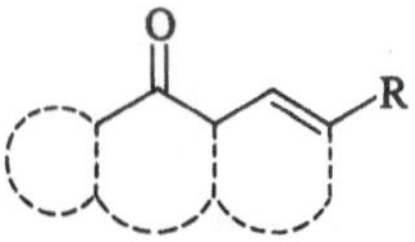

(33)

A study of some chromone acrylic acids by NOHARA et al. (1975) is of particular interest in the light of this classification. These workers discovered high activity in a series of trans-chromone-3-acrylic acids of general formula (34); the best compound (34 R = 6-isopropyl) for example has an ED_{50} in the rat PCA test of less than 1 mg/kg after intravenous i.v. dosing. These trans-acids contain the partial structure (33) in

common with the active tricyclic acid series. Only one *cis*-acid, the *n*-propyl analogue (35) was obtained; its activity (ED_{50} 20 mg/kg) was considerably less than that
of the corresponding 6-*n*-propyl *trans* acid (ED_{50} 1–3 mg/kg). Chromone-2-acrylic
acid (36) (ED_{50} 10–20 mg/kg), which has strong chemical affinities with chromone-2-
carboxylic acid is less active than the unsubstituted chromone-3-acrylic acid (ED_{50}
4–10 mg/kg) (NOHORA et al., 1975). The spatial relationships implied in partial formula (33) seem, therefore, to be more important than any purely chemical relationships.

(34)   (35)

(36)

The tetrazole doxantrazole (37) (BATCHELOR et al., 1975) is a potent anti-allergic
agent which has been selected for trial in man; it has an ED_{50} of 1 mg/kg in the rat
PCA test after i.v. dosing. Doxantrazole does not contain the partial formula (33)
common to the tricyclic acids so far reviewed, and it is interesting to note that the
isomeric tetrazole (38) which does, is less active with an ED_{50} of 3 mg/kg; furthermore, the phenoxathiin derivative (39) which has no carbonyl function is highly
active (ED_{50}, 1.5 mg/kg) (GARLAND, unpublished). Similar relative activities are
shown by the corresponding carboxylic acids. This suggests that doxantrazole (37)
and (39) are members of a new series of compounds in which the structural requirement for high activity is represented by the partial formula (40), which implies a
necessary spatial relationship between the acidic group and a *sulphone* function.
Doxantrazole was selected for possible clinical evaluation because of its relatively
high oral activity ($ED_{50} \simeq$ 10 mg/kg) in the rat PCA test. On the basis of information
currently available, almost nothing meaningful can be said about the structural
prerequisites for oral activity. However, the tetrazole (39) has appreciable oral activity and it does appear that in this series of compounds the partial formula (40)
favours a high oral:i.v. potency ratio.

(37) Doxantrazole   (38)

(39)   (40)

BUCKLE et al. (1973) from Beecham, England, found that the long-known, strongly acidic, 2-nitroindan-1,3-dione (41) has activity very close to that of cromoglycate in the rat PCA test, and they investigated a series of nuclear substituted analogues. No definite correlations emerged although it was noted that the completely substituted 4,5,6,7-tetrachloro compound was devoid of activity and that two 5,6-disubstituted compounds were highly active. These were the tricyclic compound (42) and 5,6-dimethyl-2-nitro-indan-1,3-dione (cf. 41), BRL 10833, with ED_{50} values of 1.1 and 0.17 mg/kg respectively, after i.v. dosing. BRL 10833 was studied further (SPICER et al., 1975) and shown to be as active in the rat PCA test after oral administration as cromoglycate is when given subcutaneously.

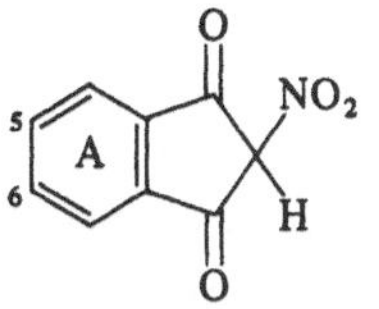

(41) 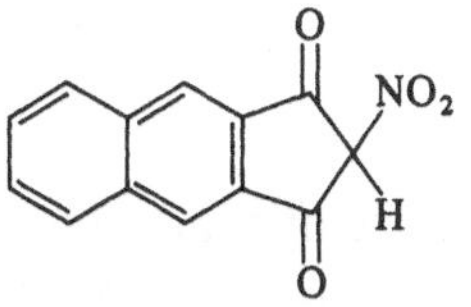   (42)

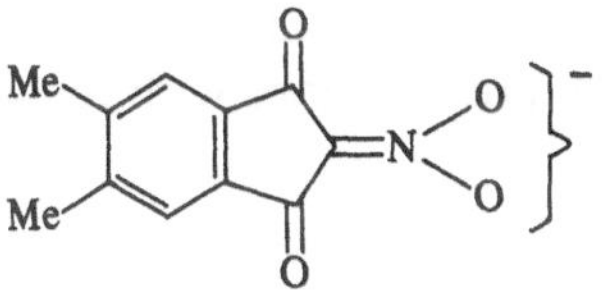

(43)

BRL 10833, like the other 2-nitroindan-1,3-diones, is an acid with pK_a 1, i.e. somewhat stronger than the anti-allergic carboxylic acids and tetrazoles. The derived anion is best represented as (43), in which form the nitroindandiones are seen to be structurally closer to the compounds already discussed than one might expect at first sight. The similarity is heightened when one considers the planarity of (41) and (42) and notes that hydroaromatic (reduced ring A) derivatives of (41), which are no longer planar, are not active (BUCKLE et al., 1975a). Not surprisingly, a free hydrogen atom at position 2 is essential for activity (BUCKLE et al., 1973).

A number of ω-nitroacetophenones (44), prepared by the alcoholic cleavage of 2-nitroindan-1,3-diones, showed good activity. For selected compounds, both in vitro and in vivo conversion back to the nitroindandiones was demonstrated, e.g. the 4,5-dimethyl derivative of (44, R = Me) gave BRL 10833. Convincing evidence was presented to indicate that this in vivo conversion is an essential prerequisite for activity in this series (BUCKLE et al., 1975b).

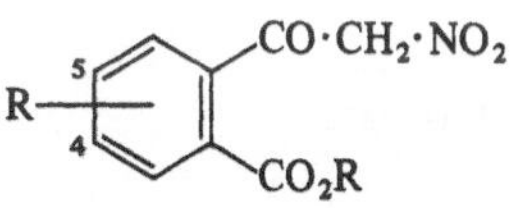

(44) 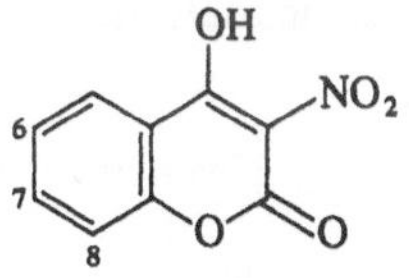   (45) 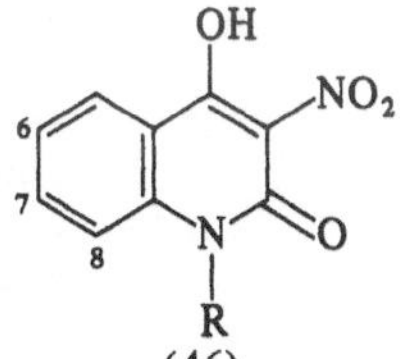   (46)

Other cyclic systems related to (41) were investigated by the Beecham group and compounds with activity similar to that of cromoglycate were found in two series; the 4-hydroxy-3-nitrocoumarins (BUCKLE et al., 1975c) exemplified by the parent compound (45), and the 4-hydroxy-3-nitro-2-quinolones (BUCKLE et al., 1975d) exemplified by (46, R = H or Me). As in the nitroindanedione series, alkyl substitution at position 6, 7, or 6 and 7 in both series gave compounds more active than the parent; substitution at position 8 with either alkyl or halogeno groups gave compounds which are slightly more active. Other substitutions, in general, gave compounds with slightly diminished activity.

(47) W 8011

All highly active compounds discussed hitherto in this section have been either carboxylic acids or compounds with comparable acidity. A notable exception is provided by the chromone W 8011 (47) (HERZIG et al., 1975) which is reported to have an oral ED_{50} of 2 mg/kg as an inhibitor of the rat PCA reaction. W 8011 does, however, have obvious structural affinities with the acidic anti-allergic compounds.

III. Anti-Allergic Properties

1. Tissue and Species Selectivity

a) Cromoglycate

Cromoglycate has shown selectivity between the anaphylactic reactions of different cell types in the rat peritoneal cavity, having inhibited the release of histamine and SRS-A from rat peritoneal mast cells sensitized by homocytotropic antibodies of either the IgE or IgGa class but not the release of SRS-A from polymorphonuclear leucocytes sensitized by IgGa (ORANGE and AUSTEN, 1968; MORSE et al., 1969; ORANGE et al., 1970); see Tables 4 and 5.

Table 4. Inhibition by cromoglycate of the release of histamine and SRS-A from rat peritoneal cells sensitized 2 h previously by injecting i.p. 0.25 ml of an IgE-like fraction (fraction 4 separated by Sephadex G-200 gel filtration) of homocytotropic rat antiserum. Various doses of cromoglycate were injected i.p. 30 s before antigen by the same route. (Reproduced from ORANGE et al., 1970)

Disodium cromoglycate mg/kg	Histamine release µg/rat	SRS-A release units/rat
0	2.9	176
0.0001	3.4	207
0.001	2.6	121
0.01	0.9	69
1.00	0.3	23

Table 5. Effect of cromoglycate on the antigen-induced release of histamine and SRS-A from rat peritoneal cells sensitized 2 h previously by injecting i.p. 1 ml of the IgGa fraction of rat antiserum. Various doses of cromoglycate were injected i.p. 30 s before antigen by the same route. (Reproduced from MORSE et al., 1969)

Disodium cromoglycate	IgGa Fraction	
mg/rat	Mean histamine release μg/rat	Mean SRS-A release units/rat
0	2.4	1395
0.3		
3.0	0.3	1778
12	0.4	1765
50		

In rat skin, the 24-h PCA reaction (mediated by IgE antibody) and concomitant degranulation of subcutaneous mast cells was inhibited by cromoglycate (GOOSE and BLAIR, 1969). Furthermore, GREAVES et al. (1971), using in vitro slices of skin taken from actively sensitized rats, found that cromoglycate added simultaneously with antigen reduced significantly the anaphylactic release of histamine. However, the 4-h PCA reaction (mediated by IgGa antibody, also termed $7S_{\gamma 2}$ antibody by ORR et al., 1970b, 1971a) was only partially inhibited by cromoglycate at dose levels sufficient to inhibit completely the IgE mediated PCA reaction. In fact, the IgGa mediated reaction showed two temporal phases following antigen challenge (Fig. 9), an initial reaction maximal at 5 min which was inhibited by cromoglycate and a more slowly developing reaction maximal at 20 min which was not inhibited (ORR et al., 1970b, 1971a). However, a graded inhibition of the rat PCA reaction mediated by either IgE (24-h latency) or IgGa (4-h latency) was found providing that the reactions were measured 5 min after the injection of antigen and blue dye. The cromoglycate-insensitive reaction was dependent not only upon the concentration of IgGa antibody used to sensitize the skin (Fig. 10), but also upon the dose of antigen (FERRARESI et al., 1974). ORR et al. (1970b) noted that this second phase of the IgGa reaction and the heterologous PCA reaction produced in rats by the i.d. injection of rabbit hyperimmune serum were similar both in their rate of development (Fig. 9) and their resistance to inhibition either by cromoglycate or by antagonists of histamine and 5-HT (GOOSE and BLAIR, 1969; BROCKLEHURST et al., 1955, 1960). These observations are in agreement with the proposal made by COX and ALTOUNYAN (1970) that cromoglycate acts specifically on mast cells, as the PCA reaction provoked in rats by rabbit hyperimmune serum was not accompanied by degranulation of cutaneous mast cells (GOOSE and BLAIR, 1969) but may involve the phagocytosis of antigen-antibody complexes by polymorphonuclear leucocytes which release their lysosomal contents, resulting in increased vascular permeability (ORR et al., 1970b). However, since the cromoglycate-insensitive PCA reaction mediated by homologous IgGa antibody was reduced or abolished by (i) pretreating the rats with compound 48/80, (ii) the concomitant passive sensitization of the skin site with IgE, or (iii) the prior

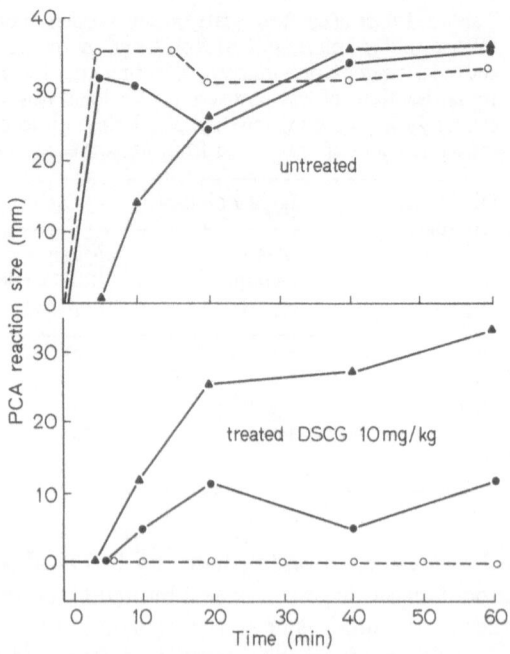

Fig. 9. Sizes of PCA reaction induced in rats by rat reagin (○), rabbit antiovalbumin hyperimmune antibody (▲), and anti-DNP 7S$_{\gamma 2}$ antibody (●) examined at various time intervals following antigen challenge, with and without treatment with cromoglycate (DSCG; 10 mg/kg). Each point is the mean of five results. (Reproduced from ORR et al., 1971a)

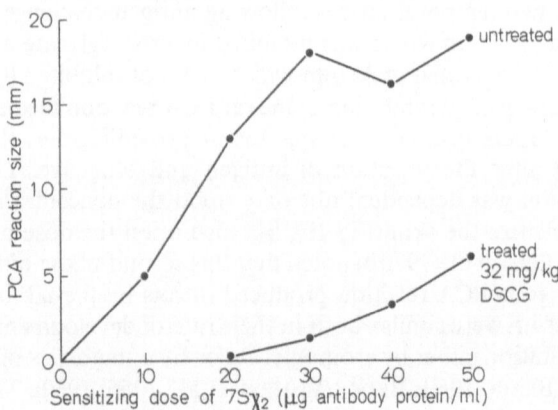

Fig. 10. Concentration of anti-DNP 7S$_{\gamma 2}$ antibody required to elicit a cromoglycate insensitive late PCA reaction as shown by using increasing sensitizing doses of antibody and cromoglycate treatment (DSCG: 32 mg/kg). Each point is the mean of fifteen results. (Reproduction from ORR et al., 1971a)

active sensitization of the rats to produce high tissue levels of IgE, ORR et al. (1971a) suggested that this response may depend at least in part upon biologically reactive mast cells. The interaction between cromoglycate and diethylcarbamazine as inhibitors of the IgGa PCA reaction is described in Section C.III.4.

Table 6. Effect of cromoglycate (DSCG) on 24-h PCA in the rat induced with mouse reagin antibodies and in the mouse induced with rat reagin antibodies. (Reproduced from Cox et al., 1970)

Recipient animal	Serum donor animal	Mean PCA reaction diameters (mm)				
		Control	DSCG (mg/kg) i.v. with antigen			
			0.5	1.0	5.0	10.0
Rat	Mouse	12.0	11.0	4.8		0
Mouse	Rat	23.0		25.0	22.0	21.0

Experiments summarised by Cox et al. (1970) suggest that cutaneous mast cells in the mouse, in contrast to those in the rat, are not susceptible to the effect of cromoglycate. Administered i.v. with antigen, cromoglycate (2–250 mg/kg) did not inhibit the PCA reaction elicited 4, 24 or 72 h after the i.d. injection of homologous antiserum; the 4-h reaction is mediated by a heat stable IgG_1 type antibody, the 24- and 72-h reactions by a heat labile IgE-like (reaginic) antibody. However, the 24-h PCA reaction in rats sensitized with mouse reagin was inhibited by cromoglycate at concentrations which inhibited the rat reagin PCA reaction. Conversely, in mice sensitized with rat reagin, the 24-h PCA reaction was not inhibited by cromoglycate (Table 6). EVANS and THOMSON (1975) have confirmed that in mice cromoglycate, at doses of 40 mg/kg administered i.v. with antigen, did not inhibit the 48-h PCA reaction mediated by an homologous IgE-like antibody produced according to the method of MOTA (1967). Furthermore, mice actively sensitized to egg albumin with B. pertussis as adjuvant were not protected from fatal systemic anaphylaxis by cromoglycate (1, 5, 20, or 100 mg/kg) administered either i.p. at 30 min or i.v. 5 min before the i.v. injection of antigen. However, in preliminary experiments, cromoglycate (5–50 mg/kg) given 30–60 min prior to antigen challenge produced partial inhibition of the 72-h but not the 4-h PCA reaction induced by homologous antiserum (Cox et al., 1970). Other species which exhibit reagin-mediated reactions apparently resistant to the anti-allergic effect of cromoglycate are the rabbit (ASSEM and MONGAR, 1970; ZVAIFLER et al., 1971) and the bovine (WELLS and EYRE, 1972; BURKA and EYRE, 1975).

In guinea pigs, neither the PCA reaction provoked by purified IgG_1 antibody (Cox et al., 1970; LOPEZ and BLOCH, 1969) nor anaphylactic bronchoconstriction in microshock experiments (Cox et al., 1970) was inhibited by cromoglycate, although in the latter test high doses of the compound (40–160 mg/kg), administered i.p. 15 min before exposure to antigen aerosol, enhanced the protection afforded by mepyramine (1 mg/kg i.m.) given 1 h previously. Generally, it has been found either that the anaphylactic release of mediators from guinea pig lung tissue in vitro is not inhibited by cromoglycate or that millimolar concentrations are required (Cox et al., 1970; ASSEM and MONGAR, 1970; ASSEM and RICHTER, 1971; SCHMUTZLER et al., 1973; DAWSON and TOMLINSON, 1974), although ASSEM (1973) reported inhibition at lower concentrations. Furthermore, the release of histamine from unsensitized perfused guinea pig lung by soluble immune complexes containing rabbit antibody, a response with many properties in common with the anaphylactic release reaction, was not inhibited by cromoglycate (0.1 and 1 mmol/l) included in the perfusion fluid (BRODER and TAICHMAN, 1971). While concentrations of this order did not prevent the antigen-induced release of histamine from the skin of actively sensitized guinea pigs (TAY et al., 1972), the reaction in guinea pig bone marrow basophils was inhibited (GREAVES, 1969).

In each of the above experiments, guinea pig tissues were either passively sensitized with IgG$_1$ antibodies or taken from animals actively sensitized by methods likely to produce a predominance of this class of antibody. Thus, it was not clear whether the relative inactivity of cromoglycate was due to the nature of guinea pig mast cells or the sensitizing antibody. When MARTIN (1971) reported that in guinea pigs cromoglycate (40 mg/kg i.v.), administered just prior to antigen and blue dye, did not inhibit the PCA reaction provoked by antiserum containing IgE-like antibody, it seemed likely that skin mast cells in this species, as in mice, were not susceptible to the effect of cromoglycate. However, several authors have since published results to the contrary. A thorough investigation by TAYLOR and ROITT (1973) demonstrated a graded inhibition by cromoglycate (Fig. 11) of the guinea pig PCA reaction, mediated by antisera containing homocytotropic antibody which was IgE-like, being heat and mercaptoethanol sensitive, persistent in the skin for more than 4 days and capable of inducing a 24-h PCA reaction in response to relatively low doses of antigen. Furthermore, they suggested that the variable effect of cromoglycate in actively sensitized guinea pigs, for example as an inhibitor of ocular sensitivity (Fig. 12) or of the anaphylactic release of histamine in vitro, might be attributed to the specificity of the drug for reactions mediated by IgE-like antibodies which tend to predominate during the early stages of an immune response. The subsequent loss of activity of cromoglycate might have been due to a change in the class of antibody in the tissues from IgE to IgG$_1$. BROUGHTON et al. (1974), WATANABE et al. (1975) and HERZIG et al. (1976) have each described the inhibition by cromoglycate of anaphylactic reactions in guinea pigs mediated by homologous antisera containing reagin-like antibody (identified primarily by persistent skin fixation and heat lability). Dose-response relationships for the inhibitor have not always been described but generally large doses of cromoglycate were used to inhibit these reactions. For example, BROUGHTON et al. (1974), found that cromoglycate (100 mg/kg) administered i.v. 1 min prior to exposure to an allergen aerosol, increased by 50% the mean preconvulsion time of groups of guinea pigs passively, systemically sensitized with *Trichinella spiralis* antiserum and premedicated with propranolol. Similarly, WATANABE et al. (1975) found that cromoglycate at 50 mg/kg i.v. 10 min prior to the i.v. injection of antigen inhibited respiratory anaphylaxis in anaesthetised guinea pigs passively sensitized 48 h previously with homocytotropic antiserum (LEVINE et al., 1971). The same dose administered 5 min prior to antigen inhibited PCA reactions induced by this antiserum, the 7 day (IgE-like) reactions being reduced more than the 4-h (IgG$_1$) reactions.

The weight of this evidence supports the hypothesis that in the guinea pig, as in the rat, cromoglycate inhibits anaphylactic reactions caused by IgE-like antibodies. This is supported by observations that the anti-allergic compounds W 8011 (HERZIG et al., 1976) and N-(3',4'-dimethoxycinnamoyl)anthranilic acid (WATANABE et al., 1975) have each been found to inhibit anaphylactic bronchoconstriction in such models, usually more effectively than cromoglycate. It remains to be determined

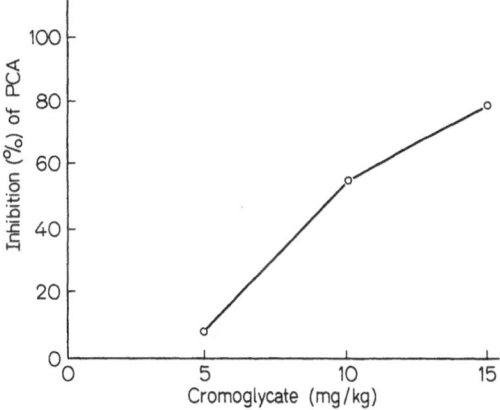

Fig. 11. Inhibition (%) by cromoglycate of 48-h PCA reactions in guinea pigs. Each point represents a comparison of the mean weal diameter of five drug-treated animals with that of five controls. (Reproduced from TAYLOR and ROITT, 1973, with permission of S. Karger AG, Basel)

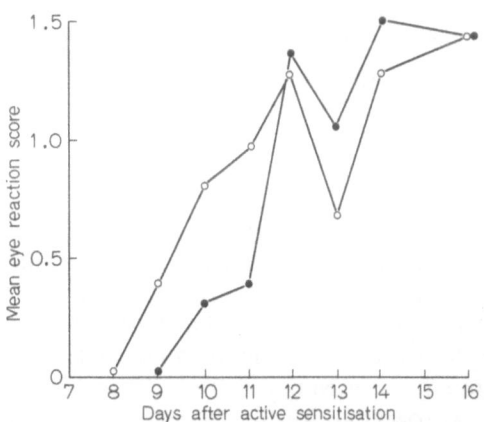

Fig. 12. The effect of cromoglycate on the development of ocular sensitivity to egg albumin in guinea pigs. Each point represents the mean score* for a group of 10 animals. A different group of animals was tested on each day. Each animal served as its own control with two drops of 4 mg/ml egg albumin solution in one eye (o) and two drops of the same solution containing 10 mg/ml cromoglycate in the other eye (•). (Reproduced from TAYLOR and ROITT, 1973, with permission of S. Karger AG, Basel, which should be consulted for details of scoring eye reaction*)

whether guinea pig PCA reactions mediated by IgG_1 antibodies have an early cromoglycate sensitive phase developing within 5 min after antigen challenge similar to that described for IgGa reactions in the rat by ORR et al. (1970b, 1971a).

Two populations of mast cells in human tissues may be distinguished by their susceptibility to cromoglycate. This compound has consistently been found to inhibit in vitro the anaphylactic release of mediators from passively sensitized human lung (SHEARD and BLAIR, 1970; ASSEM and MONGAR, 1970; PIPER and WALKER, 1973; BROUGHTON et al., 1974; see also Figs. 5–7). However, neither the Prausnitz-Küstner reaction in human skin (ASSEM and MONGAR, 1970) nor the anaphylactic release of histamine from human skin in vitro (PEARCE et al., 1974) was consistently inhibited by cromoglycate even though concentrations of up to 500 µmol/l were used in the latter experiments. This difference cannot be attributed to sensitization by a different antibody class since both skin and lung tissue were passively sensitized with human IgE. Similarly, the weal and flare induced in atopic individuals by direct skin tests were not inhibited but enhanced by introducing cromoglycate with the antigen (HADDAD and GILLMAN, 1973). A distinction has also been made between different monkey tissues passively sensitized in vitro with human IgE (STEWART et al., 1973); cromoglycate consistently inhibited the antigen-induced release of histamine from chopped lung tissue but did not reduce release from chopped skin. The same conclusion may be reached from results of in vivo experiments (PATTERSON et al., 1971). Cromoglycate administered either i.v. or into the bronchioles by aerosol with antigen partially inhibited the respiratory response of ascaris-sensitive rhesus monkeys but, given i.v., did not inhibit the skin reactions produced by i.d. injection of either specific antigen or rabbit antihuman IgE. The results of these more recent experiments confirm previous findings that cromoglycate inhibits the antigen-induced release of mediators in vitro from primate lung tissue (COX et al., 1970; ASSEM and MONGAR, 1970) but serve to emphasise that the inconsistent inhibition of reversed PCA reactions in monkeys described by Cox et al. (1970) was probably due to the high local concentrations of inhibitor achieved by injecting either 0.5 or 1 mg cromoglycate i.d. with antigen. In contrast to the skin, human conjunctiva and nasal mucosa may be classed together with the lung since clinically the topical application of cromoglycate ameliorates immediate hypersensitivity reactions in these tissues (TAYLOR and SHIVALKAR, 1971; EASTY et al., 1972).

ASSEM and MONGAR (1970) reported that the antigen-induced release of histamine in vitro from leucocytes of allergic patients was not significantly inhibited by the addition of high concentrations of cromoglycate (30, 90, and 600 µmol/l) and, whereas KIMURA et al. (1975) have reported that cromoglycate inhibits degranulation of basophil leucocytes induced by antihuman IgE, only a single high concentration of the drug (70 mmol/l) was used in this study. Since others (LICHTENSTEIN and ADKINSON, 1969; FULLARTON et al., 1973b; ASSEM, 1973) have confirmed that cromoglycate at concentrations effective in lung tissue does not impair histamine release from human leucocytes, it seems that these cells differ from lung mast cells in susceptibility to cromoglycate.

The results of experiments described in this section indicate that cromoglycate exhibits tissue specificity in the rat and in primates including man, while skin from the mouse, rabbit, and bovine does not respond to the drug. Furthermore, in guinea pigs and rats anaphylactic reactions mediated by IgE-like antibodies appear to be inhibited more readily than those mediated by IgG homocytotropic antibodies. This is in keeping with clinical observation made by BRYANT et al. (1973; 1975) that within a group of 21 asthmatic patients, those who were unresponsive to cromoglycate correlated significantly with those having in their serum heat stable, short latency (IgG) skin sensitizing antibodies; the possible role in asthma of a short term sensitizing IgG antibody is discussed by PARISH (1973; 1975) and by ISHIZAKA and ISHIZAKA (1973). Since the inhibitor exhibits selectivity between the mast cells of different tissues in primates, it should be established that IgE and IgG homocytotropic antibodies interact with the same population of mast cells, before concluding that the two classes of antibody trigger separate reactions in the same cell that differ in sensitivity to cromoglycate.

b) Other Compounds

With a few exceptions, most of the recently developed cromoglycate-like anti-allergic compounds have so far been investigated using only reactions in which cromoglycate has been found to be effective. In particular, the PCA reaction induced in rats by IgE-like antibody has been used for screening purposes and investigating structure-activity relationships (Sections B.I., B.II.). Other experimental systems which have been used to confirm anti-allergic activity are described below.

Doxantrazole. The antigen-induced release of histamine in vitro from peritoneal cells of rats actively sensitized to ovalbumin (MOTA, 1964) was suppressed by up to 80% by doxantrazole (0.1–3 μmol/l). Comparable effects were also observed using passively sensitized human chopped lung challenged with an extract of grass pollen. In addition, the antigen-induced release of histamine from actively sensitized guinea pig lung in vitro was inhibited by doxantrazole but at concentrations ($IC_{50} = 420$ μmol/l) far greater than those found effective in either rat peritoneal cells or human lung. Cromoglycate in the same experiments was not inhibitory.

Apart from cromoglycate, only doxantrazole has been reported to inhibit rat anaphylactic bronchoconstriction; 1–30 mg/kg i.v. given 1 min prior to antigen was effective (BATCHELOR et al., 1975).

AH 6556, AH 7079, and AH 7725. AH 7725 ($IC_{50} = 20$ ng/ml) was more active than cromoglycate (5 μg/ml) in suppressing the release of histamine from passively sensitized rat mast cells in vitro, and the passive peritoneal anaphylaxis reaction in vivo was inhibited by a smaller dose of AH 7725 ($ED_{50} = 20$ μg/kg i.v.) than of cromoglycate ($ED_{50} = 120$ μg/kg) (FULLARTON et al., 1973a). The effect of AH 7079 on histamine release in vitro showed a biphasic relationship to concentration, an optimum of about 60% inhibition being found with 100 μmol/l; cromoglycate had a comparable effect in the same experiment. Anaphylactic release of histamine from passively sensitized chopped human lung was inhibited by AH 7079 and AH 6556, the effective concentrations (1–100 μmol/l) being similar to those for cromoglycate. However, inhibition was often inconsistently concentration-related and relative potencies could not be estimated (ASSEM, 1973). In passively sensitized guinea pig lung these xanthones showed similar activity to cromoglycate in suppressing anaphylactic histamine release but cromoglycate was unusually active in these experiments (ASSEM, 1973) by comparison with those reported elsewhere. The three xanthone derivatives have also been compared with cromoglycate as inhibitors of the anaphylactic release of histamine from human leucocytes but with inconsistent results. ASSEM (1973) has reported the results of two experiments testing cromoglycate, AH 7079 and AH 6556. In both experiments, cromoglycate (1–100 μmol/l) was inactive whereas these xanthones (1–100 μmol/l) were inhibitory in one experiment but not in the other. FULLARTON et al. (1973b) have reported that the closely related analogue AH 7725 was, like cromoglycate, relatively ineffective in this tissue.

ICI 74917. The substituted kynurenic acid ICI 74917 (bufrolin) has a broad spectrum of anti-allergic activity (EVANS and THOMSON, 1975). When present at antigen challenge, this compound produced a graded inhibition of the anaphylactic

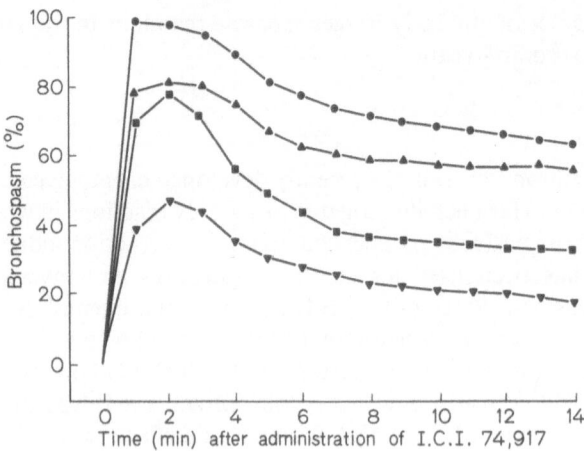

Fig. 13. Allergic bronchospasm in anaesthetised guinea pigs. Results are the mean from a group of 20 control animals (●) and animals (10 per group) treated with I.C.I. 74917 at 2.5 µg/kg i.v. (▲), 5 µg/kg i.v. (■) and 10 µg/kg i.v. (▼). (Reproduced from EVANS and THOMSON, 1975)

release of histamine from passively sensitized rat peritoneal cells but maximum inhibition (50% at between 1 to 10 µg/ml) was less than with cromoglycate. Whilst having no bronchodilator activity in the guinea pig, ICI 74917 conferred some protection against systemic anaphylaxis and produced a graded inhibition of allergic bronchospasm in guinea pigs passively sensitized with a heat stable antibody preparation (Fig. 13). The compound also partially inhibited anaphylactic histamine release from passively sensitized chopped guinea pig lung but at high concentrations (5–20 µg/ml) compared with those effective in vivo. Guinea pig PCA reactions provoked by heat stable antibody were inhibited by ICI 74917 (0.25–1 mg/kg i.v.) but not by cromoglycate at doses of up to 50 mg/kg i.v. However, since the doses required to inhibit the PCA reaction were much higher than those which inhibited anaphylactic bronchospasm, it was suggested that ICI 74917 exhibits specificity towards lung tissue in the guinea pig. In experiments which confirmed clearly that cromoglycate did not inhibit PCA reactions induced by IgE-like antibody in the mouse, ICI 74917 produced a graded inhibition but with doses 100 times higher than were required for similar effects in the rat. Like cromoglycate, ICI 74917 did not produce a marked dose-dependent inhibition of PCA reactions induced by homologous heat stable (IgGa) antibody or by heterologous (guinea pig) antibodies in the rat. Inhibition of the early phase of the homologous IgGa reaction was not investigated.

    BRL 10833. In rat passive peritoneal anaphylaxis experiments, both cromoglycate (20 µmol/l) and BRL 10833 (2 µmol/l) inhibited the antigen-induced release of histamine more than the production of SRS-A (SPICER et al., 1975). This difference may have been due to the production of SRS-A provoked by IgGa from polymorphonuclear leucocytes since the cells were sensitized with *unfractionated* serum containing homocytotropic antibody 2 h prior to antigen challenge.

    PR-D-92-EA. The benzopyranobenzopyran PR-D-92-EA (Sect.B.II. compound number 16) has been reported by POSSANZA et al. (1975) to inhibit degranulation of rat mast cells in vivo ($ED_{50} = 0.6$ mg/kg i.v.). This compound also shows tissue selectivity in primates similar to that described for cromoglycate. By i.v. injection in sensitive rhesus monkeys *(Maccaca mulatta)*, it inhibited the increase in airway resistance caused by inhalation of an aerosol of *Ascaris suum* antigen but not the skin reaction provoked by i.d. injection of antigen. Similarly, PR-D-92-EA prevented the release of histamine induced by antigen challenge from chopped monkey lung but not from chopped monkey skin (STEWART et al., 1974). This compound also inhibits the anaphylactic release of SRS-A from bovine lung in vitro (BURKA and EYRE, 1975).

2. Inhibition of Mast Cell Reactions Provoked by Stimuli Other Than Antigen-Antibody Interactions

Results presented in Sect. B.III.1.a. show that cromoglycate inhibits degranulation and release of mediators from mast cells of the rat sensitized by IgE and IgGa antibodies. Other agents known to stimulate degranulation and mediator release from rat mast cells have been investigated for two main reasons (i) the development of convenient screening techniques, (ii) to investigate the mode of action of anti-allergic agents.

a) Compound 48/80

It was reported by COX (1967) and subsequently confirmed by others (TAYLOR, 1973; EVANS and THOMSON, 1975) that in rats the submaximal extravasation of blue dye following i.d. injection of Compound 48/80 (0.1–1 µg per site) was not inhibited by the concomitant i.v. injection of cromoglycate, even at doses ten times those required to inhibit the IgE-PCA response. The recently developed anti-allergic compounds W 8011 and ICI 74917 were also ineffective against dermal blueing reactions provoked by compound 48/80 in the rat (HERZIG et al., 1976; EVANS and THOMSON, 1975). Furthermore, cromoglycate (10 mg/kg i.v.) did not inhibit blueing reactions provoked by Compound 48/80 (0.75 µg per site) in the guinea pig (TAYLOR, 1973). However, in the rat, dermal blueing reactions were inhibited in a dose-related manner when high local concentrations of either cromoglycate or ICI 74917 were achieved by injecting the inhibitor i.d. at the same site as Compound 48/80 (EVANS and THOMSON, 1975).

The above findings conflict with the results of ORR et al. (1971b) that cromoglycate at i.v. doses of 10 and 100 mg/kg inhibited the degranulation of subcutaneous mast cells induced by i.d. injections of Compound 48/80 (0.125, 0.25, and 0.5 µg per site). This discrepancy could be due to the different end points employed, as GOOSE and BLAIR (1969) have described an apparent inhibition of mast cell degranulation, assessed under the light microscope at the site of a PCA reaction in rat skin, when the extravasation of blue dye was not reduced (see Sect. B.I.5.). This is unlikely to be the entire explanation, however, since the release of histamine by Compound 48/80 from rat peritoneal cells was inhibited by cromoglycate (ORR et al., 1971b; MARSHALL, 1972), although this effect was poorly dose-related and the concentrations required for inhibition (10–500 µmol/l) were higher than for inhibition of release by antigen from sensitized cells (GARLAND, 1973; KUSNER et al., 1973). A further explanation may be derived from the observations of ORR et al. (1971b) and ORR (1974) that the inhibitory effect of cromoglycate is reduced with increasing concentrations of Com-

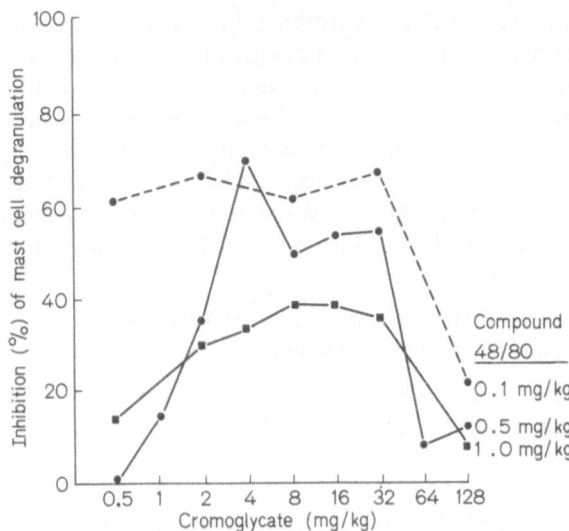

Fig. 14. Inhibition by cromoglycate of rat mast cell degranulation induced by Compound 48/80 at 3 concentrations. (Reproduced from ORR, 1974)

pound 48/80 (Fig. 14). While low concentrations of Compound 48/80 release histamine by a mechanism comparable in many ways to the anaphylactic release reaction (JOHNSON and MORAN, 1969), differences between the reactions have been found (GOTH et al., 1971), particularly when the concentration of Compound 48/80 is increased (ROTHSCHILD, 1970).

b) Phospholipase A₂

Phospholipase A_2 (phosphatide acyl-hydrolase) is an enzyme which occurs in the venoms of some snakes, bees, and wasps and also in mammalian tissues. It cleaves one fatty acid from the β position of phosphatides producing a lysophosphatide (TATTRIE, 1959). It has been reported to disrupt rat mesenteric mast cells (HÖBERG and UVNÄS, 1957) and to release histamine and 5-HT from isolated rat mast cells (MORAN et al., 1962). In a study of this release process, UVNÄS and ANTONSSON (1963) found it to be temperature and calcium dependent and prevented by either previously warming the cells to 45° C or by inhibition of energy metabolism. In these respects, the release process resembles antigen-induced release of histamine.

The effect of cromoglycate on the response of mast cells to phospholipase A_2 has been investigated but results show some inconsistencies. ORR and COX (1969) found that the disruption in vitro of rat subcutaneous mast cells and the concomitant release of histamine induced by phospholipase A_2 were inhibited by cromoglycate (10 µg/ml) to about the same degree as the reaction induced by antigen challenge of passively sensitized tissue. In agreement with this finding, TAYLOR et al. (1974a, b) reported that the degranulation of rat peritoneal mast cells by phospholipase A_2 (25 µg/ml) was inhibited by several agents including cromoglycate (0.1–10 µg/ml). ORR and COX (1969) suggested that the anti-allergic action of cromoglycate might be through inhibition of this enzyme but in later investigations by the same group

(HINES et al., 1972), cromoglycate (0.1–1000 µmol/l) did not inhibit hydrolysis of lecithin in egg yolk emulsion by purified snake venom phospholipase A_2. Furthermore, purified snake venom enzyme did not significantly release histamine from isolated rat peritoneal mast cells, confirming the observations of others (ROTHSCHILD, 1965; FREDHOLM, 1966; MARSHALL, 1972). Phospholipase A_2 enhances release by chymotrypsin of histamine from isolated rat mast cells (AMUNDSEN et al., 1969), but HINES et al. (1972) found that cromoglycate (1–1000 µmol/l) did not inhibit release induced by either chymotrypsin alone or in combination with phospholipase A_2.

Degranulation by phospholipase A_2 of tissue fixed mast cells observed by ORR and COX (1969) may have been indirectly through one of the products resulting from enzymic hydrolysis of phospholipids such as lysolecithin or PGs (KUNZE and VOGT, 1971). While cromoglycate (1–1000 µmol/l) did not inhibit the disruption of isolated rat peritoneal mast cells by lysolecithin (HINES et al., 1972), TAYLOR (1973) confirmed the observation of CRUNKHORN and WILLIS (1971) that PGE_1 (15 ng per site) provoked the extravasation of blue dye in rat skin and described the inhibition of this response by cromoglycate (10 mg/kg i.v.) Thus, the original observations of ORR and COX (1969) may have been due to inhibition by cromoglycate of mast cell degranulation triggered by PGE rather than by the phospholipase A_2 enzyme (COX, 1971).

c) Polypeptides

Whereas the phospholipase A_2 enzyme purified from bee venom failed to release histamine from rat peritoneal mast cells (TATESON, unpublished), a peptide comprising 22 amino acid residues isolated from the same source (BREITHAUPT and HABERMANN, 1968), known as peptide 401 or mast cell degranulating peptide (MCDP), stimulated directly the release of histamine from rat peritoneal mast cells but not human leucocytes (ASSEM and ATKINSON, 1973). Cromoglycate and the xanthone derivatives AH 7079 and AH 7725 at concentrations of 1 and 10 µmol/l inhibited the mast cell reaction by between 30 and 70% (ASSEM and ATKINSON, 1973; ASSEM, 1973). JASANI and STANWORTH (1973) have confirmed the inhibition by cromoglycate of the mast cell triggering action of several basic peptides and polypeptides including MCDP.

d) Dextran

The anaphylactoid reaction provoked in some rat strains by dextran (VOORHEES et al., 1951) represents an unusual vascular response, similar in many ways to an immediate hypersensitivity reaction but occurring after the first injection of this foreign substance. There is evidence that the reaction is provoked following the interaction of the polysaccharide, probably through the terminal glucose units, with receptors on tissue mast cells to release anaphylactic mediators, in particular histamine and 5-HT (PARRATT and WEST, 1957a, b, c; BONACCORSI and WEST, 1963; POYSER and WEST, 1968). In view of this, the release of histamine by dextran from, for example, rat peritoneal mast cells has been investigated as a model of the anaphylactic reaction (BAXTER, 1972, 1973; BAXTER and ADAMICK, 1974, 1975; GARLAND and MONGAR, 1974; FOREMAN and GARLAND, 1974; FOREMAN et al., 1976; GARLAND and MONGAR, 1976).

ASSEM and RICHTER (1971) found that the extravasation of albumin-bound dye in rats following i.d. injection of dextran was inhibited by cromoglycate, but only with i.v. doses of the order of 100 mg/kg. Acute inflammation of the pinna produced in mice by i.v. injection of dextran, was also inhibited by cromoglycate (ANKIER and NEAT, 1972) but again the effect required large doses ($ED_{50} \geqq 50$ mg/kg i.v.) and could be non-specific. HANAHOE et al. (1972) investigated inhibition by cromoglycate of the dextran response in three types of experiment in rats. (1) In the anaphylactoid reaction of the whole rat, poor and irregular inhibition (maximum 20%) was obtained when the drug (5 mg/kg) was given i.p. along with the dextran. (2) Increased vascular permeability following i.d. injection of dextran was reduced by cromoglycate administered either i.v. immediately prior to the dextran ($ED_{50} \simeq 10$ mg/kg) or i.d. mixed with the dextran. (3) The release of histamine by i.p. injection of dextran was inhibited by the concomitant i.p. injection of cromoglycate ($ED_{50} = 25$ μg/kg).

The release of histamine from rat peritoneal cells in vitro induced by mixtures of dextran and phosphatidyl serine was inhibited by cromoglycate and by doxantrazole, the concentration-effect curves being almost coincident with those for inhibition of the anaphylactic release of histamine (GARLAND and MONGAR, 1974; BATCHELOR et al., 1975). This dextran-induced release of histamine from rat peritoneal cells in vitro has also been employed to investigate the mode of action of antiallergic agents (Sect. B.IV.).

3. Time Course Studies

In the rat PCA test, i.v. cromoglycate is more effective when administered at the same time as antigen challenge than at earlier times (Cox et al., 1970; FULLARTON et al., 1973a; THOMSON and EVANS, 1973; SPICER et al., 1975; GARLAND, 1975). The decline of effect with time at least for moderate dosage is not, however, monophasic as had been supposed from the studies of high doses by THOMSON and EVANS (1973). Close examination of the time course of effect of cromoglycate revealed a biphasic sequence as illustrated in Figure 15 (GARLAND, 1975). A similar result was obtained with doxantrazole (1 mg/kg i.v.). These results indicate that there are two ongoing processes. The overall loss of effect when drug is given at moderate dosage 30 min before antigen challenge is not explained by tachyphylaxis to cromoglycate, since the effect of a second dose given at the same time as antigen challenge is undiminished (EVANS et al., 1975; GARLAND, unpublished). The loss of effect in 30 min can, however, be explained by cromoglycate's short (2-min) plasma half-life (Moss et al., 1970). Superimposed upon the relatively gradual decline of effect is a highly significant and transient loss of effect within the first 5 min. This is seen not only after i.v. injection but also when an anti-allergic agent is injected directly into the PCA site (Fig. 16).

Analogous effects have been found in vitro using rat peritoneal cells. Experiments using a mixture of dextran and phosphatidyl serine as the releasing stimulus are illustrated in Figure 17 (GARLAND, 1975). The release of histamine was inhibited maximally only when cromoglycate was added to the cells simultaneously with the dextran phosphatidyl serine mixture (phase I inhibition); preincubation with the drug resulted in the loss of inhibitory effect which partially recovered when preincubation was extended beyond 20 min (phase II inhibition). Two phases of inhibition

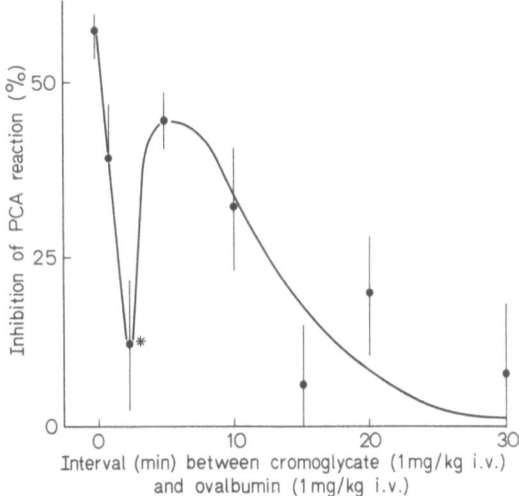

Fig. 15. Time course of the anti-allergic effect of cromoglycate: inhibition of the PCA reaction by cromoglycate (1 mg/kg) administered i.v. at intervals of up to 30 min prior to i.v. antigen challenge. Each point is the mean (±s.e. mean) of three separate experiments. In each experiment, a treated and control group (4 rats in each) were compared at each time interval. Average control PCA reaction from 96 rats, measured as multiples of opposing diameters, was 215 mm, s.e. mean = 7. (*$p < 0.001$) (Reproduced from GARLAND, 1975)

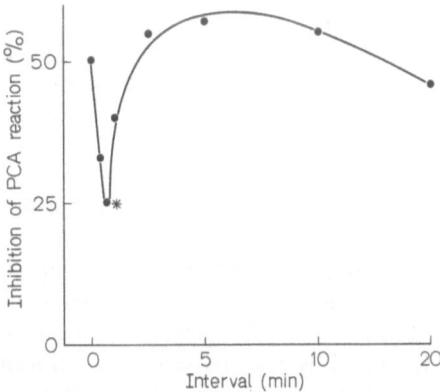

Fig. 16. Inhibition (%) of the rat PCA reaction by doxantrazole (0.05 ml of 1 mg/ml solution) injected i.d. into the region of the PCA site at intervals of between 20 s and 20 min prior to i.v. antigen challenge (ovalbumin 1 mg/kg i.v.). Each point is the mean from a group of four rats. (*$p \leq 0.01$). (Reproduced from GARLAND, 1975)

were also observed using doxantrazole and, as with cromoglycate, both phases were related to drug concentration (Fig. 18). Using antigen, Compound 48/80 or phospholipase A_2 to release histamine, others have observed the decline of inhibitory effect following preincubation with cromoglycate (ORR et al., 1971b; KUSNER et al., 1973; THOMSON and EVANS, 1973; JOHNSON and VAN HOUT, 1974). The second phase of

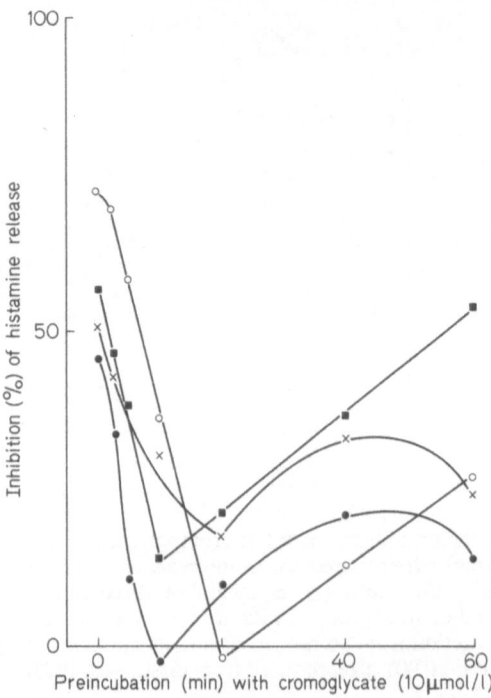

Fig. 17. Inhibition (%) of histamine release from rat peritoneal cells by cromoglycate (10 μmol/l) added to cells either together with or at various intervals prior to adding a mixture of dextran (6 mg/ml) and phosphatidyl serine (10 μg/ml). Results from four separate experiments are shown, each point being the mean of duplicates. (Reproduced from GARLAND, 1975)

inhibition has not previously been reported, but TAYLOR et al. (1974b) found that substantial inhibition remained after 30 or 60 min preincubation (intervals between 10 and 30 min were not investigated). Failure to detect two phases might be accountable to the use of either too few time intervals or excessive concentrations of cromoglycate. The release of histamine from rat peritoneal mast cells induced by the ionophore A 23187 is not inhibited by cromoglycate-like anti-allergic agents (Sect.-B.IV.) but when cells were incubated with cromoglycate prior to adding the ionophore, there was a significant and transient enhancement of histamine release. The time course of this enhancement was strikingly similar to the transient loss of inhibition when dextran was used to release histamine (Fig. 19). These various observations, therefore, suggest that when rat peritoneal cells are preincubated with a modest concentration of cromoglycate for up to 40 min prior to adding a releaser such as antigen or dextran, the effect observed represents a balance between release-inhibiting and release-enhancing activities of the drug.

Mast cells in human lung parenchyma do not appear to behave like those in the rat peritoneal cavity; when passively sensitised human lung fragments were incubated in vitro at 37° C for up to 15 min with cromoglycate, inhibition of the anaphylactic reaction was maintained (ASSEM and MONGAR, 1970; GARLAND, 1975).

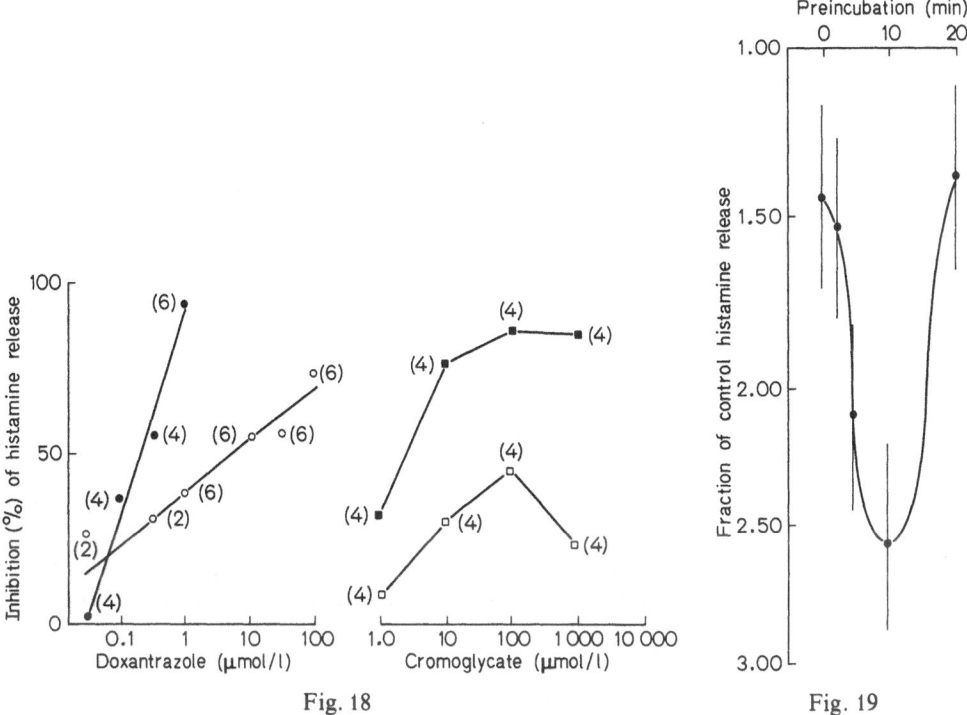

Fig. 18. Inhibition (%) of histamine release from rat peritoneal cells by either doxantrazole or cromoglycate. Various concentrations of each inhibitor were added to the cell suspension either together with (*closed symbols*) or 40 min prior to (*open symbols*) adding a mixture of dextran (6 mg/ml) and phosphatidyl serine (10 µg/ml). Number of experiments contributing to each point is shown in brackets. (Reproduced from GARLAND, 1975)

Fig. 19. The release of histamine, expressed as a fraction of the control release (20.6±4.5% of total histamine), from rat peritoneal cells incubated at 37° C with cromoglycate (60 µmol/l) for various times prior to the addition of the calcium ionophore A23187 (1 µmol/l). Each point is the mean of four experiments, vertical bars represent s.e. mean calculated from pooled error mean square. Time scale (*abscissa*) compares with Figure 17. (Reproduced from GARLAND, 1975)

Like cromoglycate and doxantrazole, AH 7725, ICI 74917 and BRL 10833 are maximally effective in the rat PCA test by the i.v. route when injected at the same time as antigen (FULLARTON et al., 1973a; EVANS and THOMSON, 1975; SPICER et al., 1975). By the s.c. route, peak inhibition was attained when BRL 10833 (0.5 mg/kg) was injected 10 min prior to antigen i.v. and declined substantially when the interval was increased to 30 min; similar results were obtained with cromoglycate, 20 mg/kg s.c., and isoprenaline, 0.02 mg/kg s.c. (SPICER et al., 1975). The comparison between AH 7725 and cromoglycate was extended to in vitro experiments in which a time-related loss of inhibition of anaphylactic histamine release occurred when passively sensitized rat peritoneal cells were preincubated at 37° C with each inhibitor. This effect was contrasted with sustained inhibition of the anaphylactic reaction when cells were preincubated with either salbutamol or the phosphodiesterase inhibitor ICI 30966 (FULLARTON et al., 1973a).

4. Tachyphylaxis

Tachyphylaxis has been observed with cromoglycate in the sense that pretreatment with the drug reduced the effect of a second dose given together with antigen challenge. This effect has been observed using two experimental systems in the rat, the PCA reaction and the anaphylactic release of histamine from peritoneal mast cells in vitro.

Figure 20 illustrates the development of tachyphylaxis to cromoglycate in the PCA reaction. Groups of sensitized rats received a large dose of cromoglycate (40 mg/kg i.v.) followed after various intervals of time by a second dose (40 mg/kg i.v.) injected with antigen. Control animals received only the second dose of cromoglycate mixed with antigen (THOMSON and EVANS, 1973). Using an interval of 30 min between doses EVANS et al. (1975) found that the degree of tachyphylaxis varied with the size of the first dose of cromoglycate, being absent with 1 mg/kg, threshold with 10 mg/kg and marked with either 20 or 40 mg/kg. Tachyphylaxis to cromoglycate has been confirmed by others and extended to include AH 7725, ICI 74917, and BRL 10833 which also show cross-tachyphylaxis with cromoglycate, suggesting a common site of action. Furthermore, time courses for tachyphylaxis with ICI 74917 and cromoglycate were comparable (FULLARTON et al., 1973a; EVANS et al., 1975; SPICER et al., 1975). In contrast, inhibition of the PCA reaction by isoprenaline injected i.v. with antigen challenge was not diminished by i.v. injection 30 min previously of cromoglycate 40 mg/kg (SPICER et al., 1975).

The pretreatment of sensitised rat peritoneal mast cells in vitro with cromoglycate reduces the inhibitory activity of the drug administrated for a second time together with antigen challenge (THOMSON and EVANS, 1973; KUSNER et al., 1973). Similar findings have been reported with AH 7725 (FULLARTON et al., 1973a) and this in vitro system has been employed to investigate the tachyphylaxis which devel-

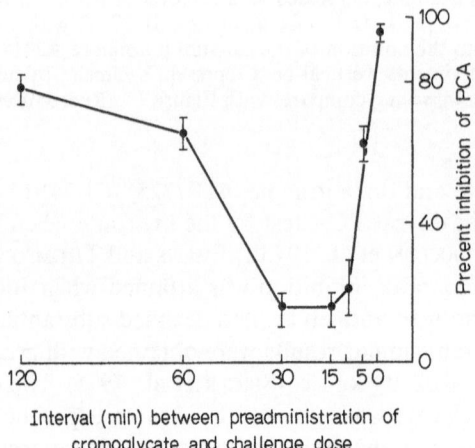

Interval (min) between preadministration of
cromoglycate and challenge dose

Fig. 20. Tachyphylaxis to the inhibitory activity of cromoglycate in rat PCA following prior administration of the drug. Results are the mean ±s.e. mean from groups of fifteen animals. (Reproduced from THOMSON and EVANS, 1973, with permission of the Editor of Clinical and Experimental Immunology)

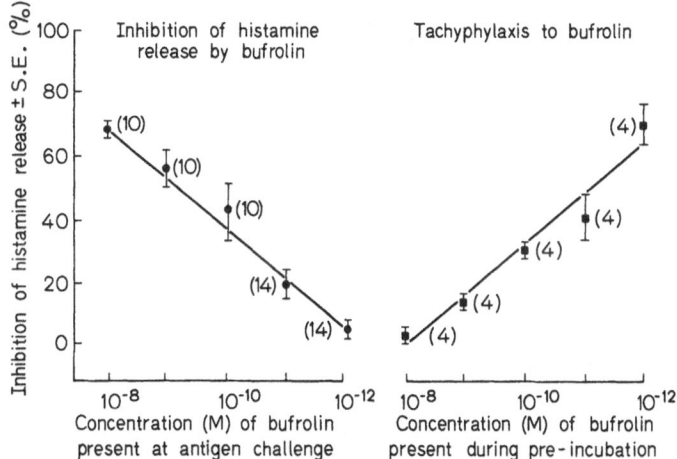

Fig. 21. Inhibition by bufrolin (I.C.I. 74, 917) of anaphylactic release of histamine from rat peritoneal cells and tachyphylaxis to the inhibitory action of 10^{-6} M bufrolin when the cells had been preincubated for 10 min with various concentrations of bufrolin. Control release of histamine by antigen alone was $48 \pm 3.1\%$ ($n=20$) and has not been corrected for non-specific release ($8.3 \pm 0.7\%$, $n=18$). Drug concentrations (*abscissa*) refer either to the concentration present at antigenic challenge (●) and no preincubation with drug, or to the preincubation concentration (■) with a constant challenge concentration (10^{-6} M). Each point represents the mean $\pm$ s.e. mean, with the number of observations in brackets. Solid lines are regression lines calculated on these data by the method of least squares. (Reproduced from MARSHALL et al., 1976, with permission of S. Karger AG, Basel)

ops to ICI 74917 as well as to cromoglycate (EVANS et al., 1975; MARSHALL et al., 1976). The results of these investigations may be summarised as follows:

1. Tachyphylaxis caused by incubating cells with either cromoglycate (1 mmol/l) or ICI 74917 (1 nmol/l) for 10 min at 37° C was reversed by washing the cells, whereas tachyphylaxis to ICI 74917 at the higher concentration of 10 µmol/l persisted.

2. The degree of tachyphylaxis was related to the preincubation concentration of ICI 74917. Both tachyphylaxis and inhibition of the anaphylactic release of histamine occurred over the same concentration range (Fig. 21). KUSNER et al. (1973) have reported similar findings with cromoglycate.

3. The ease of reversibility of tachyphylaxis by washing was associated with both the length of preincubation with and the concentration of ICI 74917.

4. When cells were incubated with a maximal effective concentration (10 nmol/l) of ICI 74917, tachyphylaxis was well developed within 5 min and complete by 30 min.

It is generally agreed from studies of the time course of action and tachyphylaxis that cromoglycate-like anti-allergic agents have an effect on the mast cells which is temporally independent of the mediator-releasing stimulus, inhibition of release being maximal only when this stimulus occurs simultaneously with the initial effect of the inhibitor. Two explanations of tachyphylaxis have been offered. One is that cromoglycate promotes the production of labile intracellular inhibitor product from a limited supply of substrate, the lability of the factor accounting for the reduced inhibition after preincubation (KUSNER et al., 1973; THOMSON and EVANS, 1973). The alternative explanation is that the initial effective drug-receptor interaction is followed by ineffective receptor occupation. This is supported by the observations that tachyphylaxis is reversed either in vitro by washing the cells free of inhibitor or in vivo at a time when tissue levels would be expected to have fallen as the consequence of urinary excretion (THOMSON and EVANS, 1973; MARSHALL et al., 1976).

When mast cells are preincubated with high concentrations of inhibitor, the time-dependent loss of effect may be due entirely to tachyphylaxis. However, with low concentrations a release enhancing phenomenon unrelated to tachyphylaxis may account for this effect.

In contrast to tachyphylaxis, JOHNSON and VAN HOUT (1973; 1974) reported that in rats, inhibition of the PCA reaction by a dose of cromoglycate given with antigen challenge was enhanced by predosing. However, others have been unable to repeat their observations (EVANS et al., 1975; RILEY et al., 1975; GARLAND, unpublished).

IV. Studies of the Mechanism of Anti-Allergic Action

Cromoglycate-like compounds inhibit exocytosis in mast cells triggered by several different stimuli. This should not be regarded as a non-specific stabilisation of the mast cell membrane but rather as an anti-secretory action, since neither the spontaneous release of histamine from rat mast cells nor the cytotoxic reaction induced by rabbit anti-rat mast cell serum are inhibited (KUSNER et al., 1973; ORANGE and AUSTEN, 1968). The biochemical processes linking the antigen-antibody reaction on the cell membrane with the release of mediators is not fully understood but it has been known for some years that for release to occur calcium is required in the extracellular medium and that metabolic processes within the mast cell must be intact (MONGAR and SCHILD, 1962; FOREMAN and MONGAR, 1972). Furthermore, by the use of a calcium ionophore (a substance which transports calcium across biological membranes and other organic phases) known as A 23187 it has been shown that the movement of calcium ions from the extracellular to the intracellular compartment of mast cells stimulates metabolically intact cells to secrete histamine (FOREMAN et al., 1973). There is also increased association of isotopic calcium with rat mast cells following antigen stimulation. Therefore, it has been suggested that an early event following the union of antigen with mast cell-fixed antibody is an increase in the mast cell membrane permeability to calcium (i.e. "opening of calcium gates" in the membrane), promoting entry of calcium into the cell (FOREMAN et al., 1973, 1975). Dextran also promotes the apparent influx of calcium ions into rat mast cells (HALLETT, unpublished observations) and thus may trigger exocytosis by a similar mechanism (FOREMAN et al., 1976).

The calcium ionophore, A 23187, has been valuable in studies of the action of anti-allergic agents. By providing an alternative route for calcium to enter into the mast cell, the ionophore bypasses the calcium-gating mechanism operated by the antigen-antibody reaction (Fig. 22). A drug which acts by inhibiting calcium transport through gates in the mast cell membrane opened by the antigen-antibody reaction should not inhibit the calcium transport function of the ionophore. Thus, drugs inhibiting histamine secretion by blocking antigen-induced calcium transport will not inhibit ionophore-mediated calcium transport and histamine secretion,

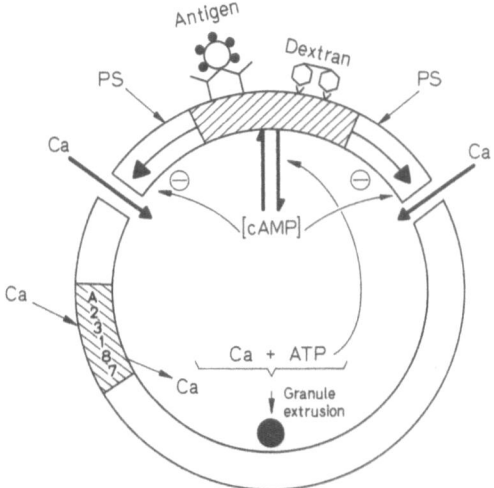

Fig. 22. A model for the mechanism of histamine release from mast cells. The stimuli are shown acting on a common membrane site (*hatched area*) which, when activated is considered to mediate the opening of membrane calcium-channels and a transient fall in the intracellular cAMP level. cAMP reduces calcium influx and thus the degree of release is controlled by the return of the cAMP levels towards the resting value after the transient fall induced by the stimulus. Phosphatidyl serine (*PS*) is shown acting on the opening of the calcium channels. The calcium ionophore bypasses the stimulus-operated, physiological calcium-channels. Influx of calcium into the cell triggers the extrusion of histamine containing granules, a process which also utilises a source of ATP within the cell. (Reproduced from FOREMAN et al., 1976)

whereas drugs such as metabolic inhibitors which act after the entry of calcium into the cell will inhibit equally the release of histamine induced either by antigen or by ionophore. A preliminary study by JOHNSON and BACH (1975) suggested that ionophore-induced release of histamine from rat mast cells could be inhibited by cromoglycate. However, extensive experiments in which ionophore- and dextran-induced histamine release from rat peritoneal cells were used in parallel to differentiate the actions of several inhibitors (GARLAND and MONGAR, 1975, 1976) showed that the anti-allergic agents cromoglycate and doxantrazole and also ICI 74917 (GARLAND, unpublished observation) inhibited the anaphylactic-type reaction but not that induced by the ionophore. The uncoupler of oxidative phosphorylation, 2,4-dinitrophenol, was included as a positive control and in each experiment inhibited almost equally both release reactions (Fig. 23).

Thus, each of these anti-allergic drugs probably acts by blocking the transport of calcium across the mast cell membrane triggered by stimuli such as the interaction of dextran with its receptor on rat mast cells or the combination of antigen with cell-fixed antibodies. This site of action may be considered to correspond to the antigen-dependent, calcium-independent first stage of the anaphylactic reaction which in human leucocytes may be separated from the calcium-dependent, antigen-independent second stage (LICHTENSTEIN, 1971). Membrane activation, which may be thought of as calcium-gate opening, occurs in the first stage while in the second stage the secretory mechanism is triggered by movement of calcium ions into the cell.

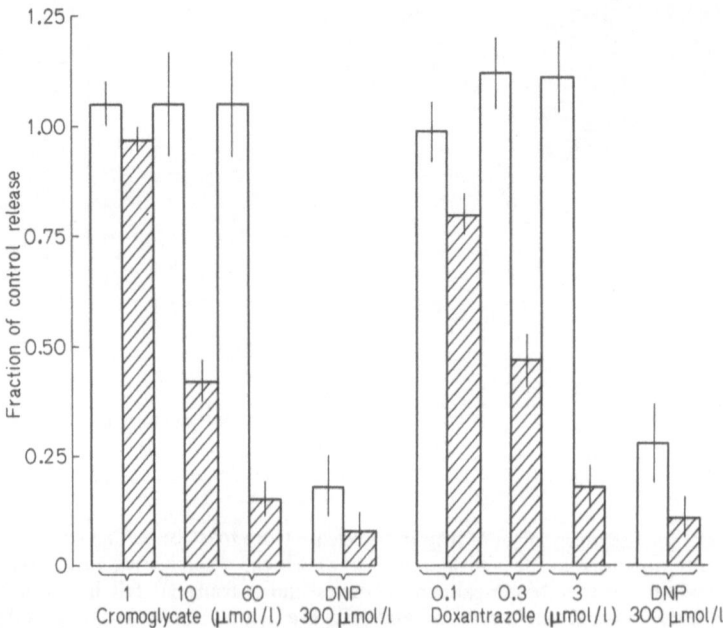

Fig. 23. The effect of cromoglycate (eight experiments) and doxantrazole (six experiments) on histamine release from rat peritoneal cells induced either by dextran (*shaded colums*) or ionophore (*open colums*). 2,4-dinitrophenol (DNP, 300 μmol/l) which inhibits release induced by dextran and by ionophore, has been included as a positive control in each experiment. Vertical bars represent s.e. mean. In these experiments the control release of histamine by dextran and phosphatidyl serine was $44.6 \pm 2.3\%$ (range 31–58.5%) and by ionophore was $25.3 \pm 3.1\%$ (range 9–42%). (Reproduced from GARLAND and MONGAR, 1976, with permission of S. Karger AG Basel)

Since cromoglycate is inactive in human leucocytes, subdivision of the release reaction in rat mast cells was examined but it was impracticable. The activated state following antigen challenge in calcium-free medium decayed rapidly, possibly due to the closure of calcium gates in the cell membrane (FOREMAN and GARLAND, 1974). By contrast, phospholipase A_2 from *Vipera russeli* in the absence of calcium appears to induce in rat mast cells an activated state which is stable for longer than 30 min. The addition of calcium then triggers degranulation even though the cells had been washed free of enzyme (TAYLOR et al., 1974b). In this system, cromoglycate (100 μg/ml) was a more effective inhibitor of the activation stage than the secretory stage, an observation consistent with results from the above comparisons of dextran- and ionophore-induced histamine release. Phosphatidyl serine, which enhances the release of histamine from rat peritoneal mast cells by either antigen or dextran (GOTH et al., 1971; MONGAR and SVEC, 1972; GARLAND and MONGAR, 1974) and increases the level of isotopic calcium associated with mast cells following antigen challenge (FOREMAN et al., 1973), not only acts as if to slow the rate of calcium gate closure following antigen challenge (FOREMAN and GARLAND, 1974) but also overcomes the inhibition by cromoglycate of dextran-induced release of histamine (GARLAND and MONGAR, 1974). These findings are consistent with the hypothesis that cromoglycate, directly or indirectly, inhibits the opening of calcium gates in the mast cell membrane. This hypothesis is not supported by the observation that degranulation of rat mast cells in calcium-free medium induced by Compound 48/80 was inhibited by cromoglycate (TAYLOR et al., 1974b). However, the mechanism of action of Compound 48/80 is not thoroughly understood.

A primary event which may occur prior to calcium entry into the mast cell is the activation of a serine-esterase, that is inhibited irreversibly by diisopropyl-phosphofluoridate (DFP) (KALINER and AUSTEN, 1973) and reversibly by amino acid esters (AUSTEN and BROCKLEHURST, 1960, 1961). There is little firm information but two observations suggest that cromoglycate may not act at this stage. Firstly, the compound did not inhibit histamine release from rat peritoneal mast cells induced by chymotrypsin (HINES et al., 1972). Secondly, whereas cromoglycate inhibited release induced by Compound 48/80 from mast cells in calcium-free medium, DFP did not (TAYLOR and SHELDON, 1974).

In view of the recent advances of knowledge about modulation of the anaphylactic release of mediators by agents which influence intracellular levels of cyclic nucleotides (see reviews by KALINER and AUSTEN, 1974a, b; LICHTENSTEIN, 1974), it is not surprising that a role has been sought for cyclic 3',5' adenosine monophosphate (cAMP) in the mechanism of action of cromoglycate-like agents. Cromoglycate does not act by stimulating adenylate cyclase through β-adrenoceptors (MARTIN, 1971) but has been reported to inhibit cAMP phosphodiesterase isolated from several tissues (ROY and WARREN, 1974; NEWMAN et al., 1975; RACHELEFSKY et al., 1975; TATESON and TRIST, 1976). However, there is not complete agreement about its inhibitory activity. In particular, TATESON and TRIST (1976) found that cromoglycate only weakly inhibited cAMP phosphodiesterase from human lung, whereas ROY and WARREN (1974) found it to be particularly active against an enzyme isolated from this tissue. Another point of difference was that where ROY and WARREN (1974) reported that cromoglycate was a competitive inhibitor, recent work has suggested that the inhibition kinetics are more complex (TATESON and TRIST, 1976). Furthermore, the tissue selectivity shown by cromoglycate as an anti-allergic agent (Sect. B.III.1.) has not been paralleled by its activity as a cAMP phosphodiesterase inhibitor. However, the enzyme preparations used have so far been isolated from heterogeneous tissues and no data has been reported for inhibition of cAMP phosphodiesterase enzymes isolated from purified mast cells.

Table 7. Inhibition of the anaphylactic release of histamine from passively sensitized human chopped lung by salbutamol (0.1, 1 or 10 nmol/l), doxantrazole (1 µmol/l) or by combinations of the two compounds. Each value represents the mean from three separate experiments each carried out in duplicate. (Reproduced from GARLAND, 1975). (Percent inhibition of anaphylactic histamine release)

	Salbutamol, nmol/l			
	0	0.1	1	10
Alone	—	5	27	47
+Doxantrazole 1 µmol/l	−14	30	75	76

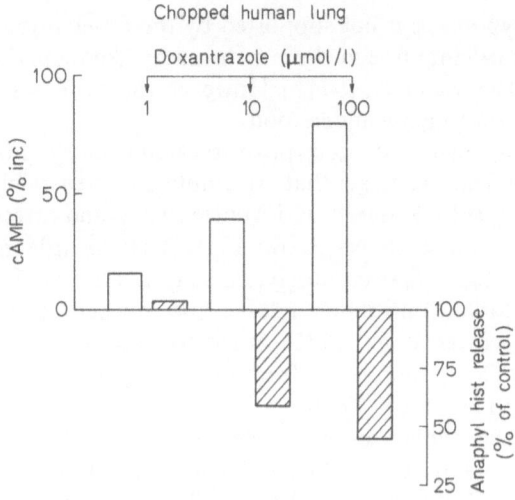

Fig. 24. The effect of doxantrazole on levels of cAMP in human lung tissue expressed as percent increase above control level (*open colums*), and on the anaphylactic release of histamine from passively sensitized human chopped lung (*hatched colums*). (GARLAND and TATESON, unpublished)

In comparisons of histamine release by dextran and ionophore, the profiles of activity of cromoglycate and doxantrazole have similarities with those of dibutyryl cAMP and theophylline, but contrast with those of inhibitors of energy metabolism such as uncouplers of oxidative phosphorylation and oligomycin (GARLAND and MONGAR, 1976). Furthermore, the anti-allergic actions of both cromoglycate and doxantrazole (Table 7) were augmented by β-adrenoceptor stimulants (TAYLOR et al., 1974a; FOLLENFANT et al., 1975b) and the level of cAMP in human lung tissue was elevated by doxantrazole at concentrations which inhibit the anaphylactic release of histamine (Fig. 24). SCHMUTZLER et al. (1973) have also reported that in sensitized guinea pig lungs cromoglycate (1 mmol/l) inhibited histamine release and elevated cAMP. Similarly, RACHELEFSKY et al. (1975) found that cromoglycate (10 μg/ml) elevated levels of cAMP in normal human lymphocytes. Taken together, this evidence confirms that cromoglycate and doxantrazole inhibit cAMP phosphodiesterase activity and tends to support the suggestion first made by TAYLOR et al. (1974a) that the anti-allergic activity of cromoglycate may be attributed to this property. TAYLOR (1975) has since speculated about how phosphodiesterase inhibition might account for some of the anti-allergic properties of cromoglycate described in Section B.III. Nevertheless, this hypothesis must be viewed cautiously because of the lack of synergism between cromoglycate and isoprenaline as inhibitors of the release of SRS-A from mast cells in the rat peritoneum (KOOPMAN et al., 1970a) and because of the inactivity of cromoglycate in human leucocytes (ASSEM and MONGAR, 1970) from which theophylline effectively inhibits anaphylactic release of histamine (LICHTENSTEIN and MARGOLIS, 1968). The second of these anomalies might possibly be attributed to the variation in the sensitivities to blockade of cAMP phosphodiesterase at different sites (SHEPPARD and WIGGAN, 1971; CHASIN et al., 1972). In conclusion, evidence for the role of cAMP in the mechanism of anti-allergic activity of cromoglycate-like compounds remains indirect and incomplete. Future studies designed to investigate the relative activities of several compounds with respect to both inhibition of histamine release and elevation of cAMP levels using a purified suspension of mast cells would be informative.

In several experimental systems, a biphasic dose-response curve has been found with cromoglycate (Fig. 14), inhibition of exocytosis reaching an optimum and then declining with increasing dosage. A similar finding has also been reported for inhibition of the rat PCA reaction by M&B 22948 (BROUGHTON et al., 1974). It is interesting to note that inhibition of cAMP phosphodiesterase declined below an optimum with increasing concentrations of cromoglycate (TATESON and TRIST, 1976). The reason for this remains unclear but two explanations deserve consideration: (1) To be effective, each drug molecule has to occupy at least two sites on each receptor. Beyond an optimum drug concentration, the tendency will be for each of these sites to be competed for by multiple drug molecules resulting in reduced ability of molecules to occupy both sites, i.e. ineffective drug-receptor interaction. A similar explanation has been proposed for inhibition of acetylcholinesterase at high substrate concentrations (ZELLER and BISSEGGER, 1943; BARLOW, 1964). (2) Cromoglycate may have not only an inhibitory effect on mediator release but also an augmenting effect, either by enhancing the anaphylactic reaction (HADDAD and GILLMAN, 1973; GARLAND, 1973; PEARCE et al., 1974) or by a direct releasing effect in the absence of an allergic stimulus (GREAVES, 1969).

V. Other Pharmacological Effects

Such information as is available concerning the general pharmacology of the above anti-allergic compounds indicates relative freedom from effects on a variety of physiological systems; moreover, the additional effects described for individual compounds do not reveal a consistent pattern among them. Smooth muscle relaxant or fairly non-specific anti-spasmodic properties are shown in vitro but not importantly in vivo by doxantrazole (BATCHELOR et al., 1975; FOLLENFANT et al., 1975a), M&B 22948 (BROUGHTON et al., 1974) and PR-D-92-EA (POSSANZA et al., 1975) but not by cromoglycate (COX et al., 1970). In contrast, ICI 74917 showed a bronchoconstrictor action in guinea pigs that was insusceptible to mepyramine, atropine, and methysergide. Cromoglycate and doxantrazole produced brief hypotension and bradycardia when injected i.v. in dogs but not in other species and these effects were abolished by vagotomy or chilling the cervical vagi and were reduced by atropine (COX et al., 1970; BATCHELOR et al., 1975). It is not known whether or not the other anti-allergic drugs produce analogous effects. Cromoglycate is the only compound known to have been examined in marmosets. This species was unique in showing brief but marked hypertension and tachycardia with i.v. doses of cromoglycate at 1 to 20 µg/kg. These responses were attributed to catecholamine release as they were enhanced by ganglion blockade and suppressed by cocaine and guanethidine or a combination of phenoxybenzamine and propranolol (COX et al., 1970).

VI. Pharmacokinetics

This discussion will be limited to studies of the distribution and metabolism of cromoglycate in laboratory animals although studies have been carried out in man, particularly with respect to absorption following inhalation of the drug in various particle sizes (Moss et al., 1971; WALKER et al., 1972; BENSON et al., 1973; CURRY et al., 1974). Pharmacokinetic data for other anti-allergic agents described in previous sections have yet to be published.

The plasma concentrations and excretion of cromoglycate have been studied in the mouse, rat, rabbit, dog, and five species of primate (Moss et al., 1970; ASHTON et al., 1973). In each species, the decline of plasma concentration was rapid, e.g. with a half-life of approximately 2 min in the rat. The compound was excreted in the bile and urine in all species studied but the major route of excretion varied among them, biliary excretion being more dominant in squirrel monkeys and urinary excretion being more pronounced in rabbits. Levels of residual drug in the tissues were low and no metabolites were detected in any species. In rats, metabolism was not induced by either phenobarbitone or methylcholanthrene but phenobarbitone reduced biliary excretion and increased urinary excretion, possibly by competing with cromoglycate for uptake into hepatic cells (NEALE and Moss, 1972). These studies also showed that pretreatment with cromoglycate did not alter the metabolism and excretion patterns of a subsequently administered dose.

Poor absorption of cromoglycate after oral administration has been found in each of the species studied (ASHTON et al., 1973). By contrast, the drug was rapidly absorbed when instilled into the trachea, either as a fine powder in rabbits and monkeys or as a solution in rats (Moss and RITCHIE, 1970). GARDINER and SCHANKER (1974) found that cromoglycate was absorbed from rat lungs partly by a saturable carrier-transport mechanism and partly by diffusion. Once absorbed from the lung, it was excreted unchanged as after i.v. administration (Moss and RITCHIE, 1970; ASHTON et al., 1973).

C. Other Inhibitors of Mediator Release

I. Isosteres of Theophylline

1. Structure-Activity Relationships

Theophylline (48) and closely related methylxanthines exhibit some inhibitory activity in the rat PCA test, but this is of a low order (0.02–0.05 x cromoglycate). However, replacement of the imidazo-CH by N gave a series of compounds, the so-called 8-azaxanthines, (49) with greatly increased PCA inhibitory activity: 8-azatheophylline (49, $R^1 = R^2 = Me$) for example is ten times as active as theophylline. The best compounds in this series, (49, $R^1 = Me$, $R^2 = benzyl$) and (49, $R^1 = Me$, $R^2 = p$-nitrobenzyl) have activity approaching that of cromoglycate; highest activity is associated with those compounds in which R^2 is a bulky group (COULSON et al., 1974).

(48)   (49)

Continued investigation of compounds related to (49) led to a series of triazolo-pyrimidine derivatives, the 8-azapurinones, one of which M & B 22948 (50) is of particular interest (BROUGHTON et al., 1974). M & B 22948 is 35–50 times as active as cromoglycate after intravenous dosing; complete inhibition of the rat PCA reaction is achieved at a dose of 0.1 mg/kg. More significantly, M & B 22948 has appreciable oral activity; complete inhibition of the PCA reaction is rarely obtained, but a maximal inhibition is seen with oral doses of 2–5 mg/kg.

(50) M & B 22,948   (51)

M & B 22948 is the most active compound of the series of monosubstituted 2-phenyl-8-azapurin-6-ones (51) the optimal substitution of this compound having been predicted by an interesting application of extrathermodynamic correlation techniques to the initial series (BROUGHTON et al., 1975). No significant correlations were evident employing the usual partition, electronic and steric parameters but it appeared that intramolecular hydrogen bonding between an ortho (2^1) substituent and the hydrogen atom in position 1 might be implicated. This was strikingly confirmed by the introduction of a parameter ΔI relating to this hydrogen bonding; the infrared ^{1}N-H stretching frequency gives a measure of the hydrogen bonding and $\Delta\lambda$ is defined as the difference between the position of the NH stretching frequency in a substituted compound (51) and that in the unsubstituted compound (51, R=H). Regression analysis incorporating this parameter gave a statistically highly significant ($p<0.0001$) equation which correlated high PCA inhibitory activity with an ortho (2^1) substituent of low bulk and with a high tendency to form hydrogen bonds.

Powerful support for the importance of hydrogen bonding comes from a further study in which 2-heteroaryl analogues of (51) were examined (HOLLAND et al., 1975). The pyridyl analogue (52) which cannot form an intramolecular hydrogen bond is of low potency, but its N-oxide derivative (53) in which hydrogen bonding is possible has 100 times the activity and is comparable with cromoglycate.

The intramolecular hydrogen bond ensures that the phenyl ring in (51) is co-planar with the heterocyclic system and thus, although the azapurinones are structurally so remote they do have some features in common with the compounds discussed in the preceding section; they are essentially planar polycyclic systems with an acidic centre.

(52)   (53)

Independent studies on isosteres of purine bases led to two series of compounds, triazolo-pyrazines and triazolo-pyrimidines, with inhibitory activity against histamine-induced bronchospasm in guinea pigs. Representative compounds from each series are ICI 58301 (54) and ICI 63197 (55) (DAVIES, 1973). Although both compounds are potent inhibitors of 3',5'-cAMP phosphodiesterase, only (55) inhibits the PCA reaction in rats (DAVIES and EVANS, 1973).

(54) ICI 58301　　　　　　　　　　(55) ICI 63197

2. Anti-Allergic Properties

The azapurinone M & B 22948 inhibited the anaphylactic release of histamine and SRS-A from passively sensitized chopped human lung and in comparable experiments was more active than cromoglycate, although neither compound was completely inhibitory (Fig. 5). By contrast, the IgE-mediated PCA reaction in rats was completely inhibited by either M & B 22948 (0.1 mg/kg) or cromoglycate (2–5 mg/ kg) administered i.v. with antigen (BROUGHTON et al., 1974). In this test, the azapurinone was active orally, the dose-response curve by this route being biphasic with an optimum of approximately 90% inhibition with 1 mg/kg administered 15 min prior to antigen. This degree of oral activity contrasted with the negligible effect of cromoglycate and poor activity of theophylline by this route. Inhibition of the rat PCA reaction by M & B 22948 was shown to be an action against the release of mediators, since large i.v. doses were required to reduce the effects on capillary permeability of i.d. histamine or 5-HT. Reagin-mediated anaphylactic bronchospasm in guinea pigs which was sensitive to cromoglycate ($ED_{50} = 100$ mg/kg i.v.) was also inhibited by M & B 22948 but at one-tenth of the cromoglycate dose i.v. and also after oral administration (Table 8). This effect also may be attributed to inhibition of the release of mediators since in vivo the compound was neither a bronchodilator nor an inhibitor of bronchoconstriction induced by histamine or 5-HT. However, in vitro it antagonised the contractions of either human bronchial muscle or guinea pig ileum in response to several spasmogens. In addition to the above anti-allergic properties, M & B 22948 (0.3–30 μmol/l) inhibited the anaphylactic release of SRS-A from bovine lung, a reaction in which cromoglycate (2–200 μmol/l) was inactive (BURKA and EYRE, 1975).

ICI 63197 by oral administration shortened the duration of anaphylactic shock in guinea pigs and reduced the anaphylactic release of histamine from isolated perfused guinea pig lungs. However, it is not clear what part of the in vivo activity is attributable to inhibition of mediator release, since the compound also inhibited lethal bronchoconstriction induced by histamine aerosol, reduced bronchospasm caused by various agents in isolated perfused lungs and enhanced the bronchodilator activity of catecholamines (DAVIES, 1973; DAVIES and EVANS, 1973). Other properties

Table 8. Inhibition of reagin-mediated anaphylactic bronchospasm in the guinea pig by M & B 22, 948 administered i.v., orally or by the inhalation of an aqueous aerosol. The % protection was $100\,[1-(C/T)]$ where C and T were the preconvulsion times of control and treated groups

Route of drug administration	Dose $(mg\ kg^{-1})$	Time (min) between dose and bronchial allergen challenge	Mean % protection
Intravenous	5	1	19 (4)[a]
	10	1	50 (4)
	20	1	69 (4)
		15	62 (4)
		40	54 (2)
Oral	200	60	48 (6)
		120	43 (3)
		240	42 (3)
Inhalation	50[b] $(mg\ ml^{-1})$	1	34 (11)

[a] Figures in parentheses refer to the number of experiments.
[b] Concentration of aerosol generating solution. Animals exposed to aerosol for 2 min. (Reproduced from BROUGHTON et al., 1974).

of ICI 63 197 include the partial inhibition of PCA reactions in guinea pigs and protection of mice from systemic anaphylaxis. The compound also inhibited PCA reactions in rats provoked by either IgE-like or heterologous antibodies but had no effect on late (30-min) IgGa PCA responses. Propranolol blocked the effect against IgE-mediated PCA responses but not that against the heterologous reactions. Again, it is not clear what part inhibition of mediator release played in these activities; the compound may alternatively have interfered with the effects of mediators on the target organ. Furthermore, causal relationship between the reported cAMP phosphodiesterase inhibitory activity and any of the anti-anaphylactic properties of ICI 63 197 remains to be proven (DAVIES and EVANS, 1973).

II. Antihistamines and Histamine

MOTA and DIAS DA SILVA (1960) demonstrated that antihistamines (H_1) acted in three different ways in guinea pig and rat tissues: (a) by the known competition with histamine at the level of the effector cell, (b) by destroying mast cells and releasing histamine, and (c) by preventing anaphylactic histamine release. The effects were not correlated with one another and the concentrations for producing the effects (b) and (c) were vastly greater (of the order of 1000 times) than those for producing the known competitive effects on end organ responses. Release of histamine by high concentrations of certain antihistamines (4 mmol/l) has been reported by MALING et al. (1974). The same compounds and others also antagonised the release of histamine and 5-HT by Compound 48/80. These are likely to be non-specific effects. The studies were extended to human leucocytes by LICHTENSTEIN and GILLESPIE (1975) who found the release of histamine by high concentrations of diphenhydramine, promethazine, and cyclizine (about 1 mmol/l) but not by mepyramine or chlorpheniramine (up to 6 mmol/l). These compounds also suppressed the anaphylactic release

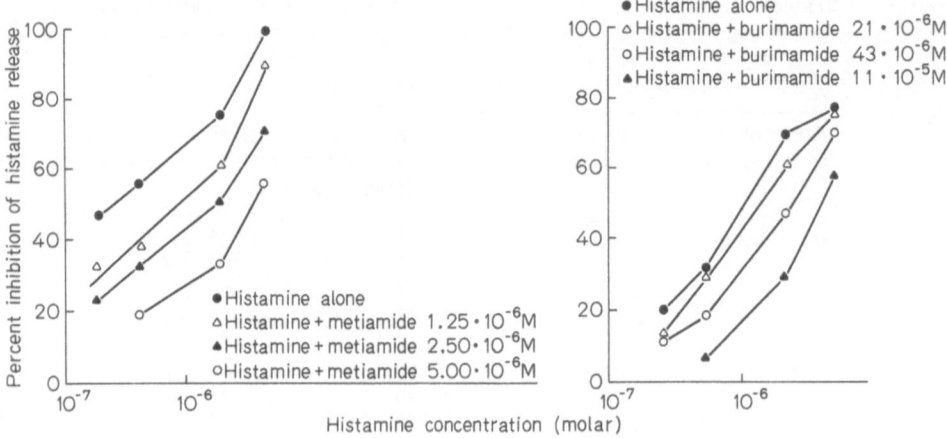

Fig. 25. Inhibition of antigen-induced release of histamine from human leucocytes by histamine either alone or in the presence of the designated concentrations of burimamide (*right-hand graph*) and in the presence of the designated concentrations of metiamide (*left-hand graph*). (Reproduced from LICHTENSTEIN and GILLESPIE, 1975)

of histamine to various degrees, at concentrations in the range of 0.1 to 1 mmol/l and promethazine at 10–100 μmol/l abolished histamine release. The action of promethazine is shared by other phenothiazines such as chlorpromazine and imipramine. Such effects are unrelated to antihistamine activity but may be attributable to a general stabilizing effect on cell membranes as the lysis of dog erythrocytes was inhibited by chlorpromazine and imipramine at 20 μmol/l (DESPOPOULOS, 1970).

KOOPMAN et al. (1970b) have reported inhibition by antihistamines of the release of SRS-A into the rat peritoneal cavity prepared with rat IgE and challenged by i.p. injection of antigen. The significance of these observations in terms of antihistamine action is doubtful. A concentration of mepyramine in excess of 10 μmol/l was required to produce 50% inhibition of SRS-A release and only one other antihistamine was tested (brompheniramine, 12 μmol/l). Specificity of action cannot be assumed with such concentrations.

Histamine, like other substances that stimulate adenylate cyclase, suppresses the anaphylactic release of histamine from human leucocytes (LICHTENSTEIN and BOURNE, 1971; BOURNE et al., 1972). The effect is predominantly on the first stage of the reaction (Sect. B.IV.) and requires concentrations in the range of 0.1–1 μmol/l. These amounts are within physiological limits and released histamine may therefore play some part in modulating subsequent histamine release. This inhibitory action of histamine on histamine release was not consistently reduced by mepyramine, pyribenzamine or antazoline, even at concentrations 100 times that at which histamine was inhibitory. Neither did these antihistamines block the stimulatory effect of histamine on cAMP formation. Some inhibitory action was produced by diphenhydramine but the concentrations used were high (0.1–1 mmol/l) and interpretation was further complicated by diphenhydramine itself releasing histamine. The histamine releasing effect of this antihistamine was prominent in the studies of MOTA and DIAS DA SILVA (1960).

LICHTENSTEIN and GILLESPIE (1973, 1975) found that in contrast to antagonists of histamine at H_1 receptors, antagonists at H_2 receptors blocked the inhibitory action of histamine on histamine release. This is illustrated for metiamide and burimamide in Figure 25. These H_2 antagonists also abolished the increase in cAMP caused by incubating human leucocytes (basophils) with histamine. It seems, therefore, that released histamine can moderate further histamine release by activating H_2 receptors.

In keeping with these observations, CHAKRIN et al. (1974) reported that metiamide (40–400 µmol/l) enhanced anaphylactic histamine release in passively sensitized chopped monkey lung and skin. The release of SRS-A from anaphylactic monkey lung was less affected by metiamide and in contrast with the results in monkey tissues, metiamide failed to enhance antigen-induced release of histamine from passively sensitized rat lung.

III. Diethylcarbamazine

Diethylcarbamazine, an antifilarial agent which has also therapeutic value in tropical eosinophilia (DANARAJ, 1958) was reported to relieve intractable asthma (MALLEN, 1965) but this has not been a consistent finding (BENNER and LOWELL, 1970). The compound has, however, been extensively studied as an inhibitor of the release of anaphylactic mediators.

1. Rat Peritoneal Cells in vivo

Diethylcarbamazine (30 mg/kg i.p.) administered 30 s prior to antigen inhibited the complement-dependent release of SRS-A from rat peritoneal polymorphonuclear leucocytes prepared with homologous hyperimmune antiserum. Since tissues became desensitized to subsequent antigen challenge when exposed to antigen in the presence of diethylcarbamazine the drug did not interfere with the antigen-antibody interaction (ORANGE and AUSTEN, 1968). In subsequent studies, diethylcarbamazine was found also to inhibit the release of SRS-A from polymorphonuclear leucocytes prepared with rat IgGa, or from mast cells prepared with rat IgE, without suppressing the concomitant release of histamine (ORANGE et al., 1970; ORANGE and AUSTEN, 1969). By contrast, cromoglycate inhibited the release of both histamine and SRS-A from rat mast cells sensitized by rat IgE (Table 4) and was more potent than diethylcarbamazine as an inhibitor of SRS-A release (ORANGE et al., 1970). Inhibition by diethylcarbamazine of the release of SRS-A from rat peritoneal cells prepared with rat IgE was not augmented by aminophylline at non-inhibitory concentrations or blocked by propranolol. However, diethylcarbamazine augmented the inhibitory effect of isoprenaline and adrenaline and prevented the enhancement of release by noradrenaline (Table 9). These findings led KOOPMAN et al. (1970a) to contrast diethylcarbamazine with β-adrenoceptor stimulants and compare it with aminophylline. Similar observations have been made using primate lung tissue (see below).

Apart from diethylcarbamazine, ORANGE and AUSTEN (1968) tested 13 compounds of which only pipecolamide and isonicotinic acid hydrazide had activity comparable with diethylcarbamazine. The range of compounds considered was too narrow for a meaningful structure-activity relationship to be established.

Table 9. Inhibition of the antigen-induced release of SRS-A from rat peritoneal cells in vivo prepared with IgE-like antibody by diethylcarbamazine either alone or in combination with isoprenaline, adrenaline or noradrenaline. (Reproduced from KOOPMAN et al., 1970a)

Expt.	Diethylcarbamazine	Isoprenaline	Mean SRS-A release	% Inhibition
	mmol/l	nmol/l	units/rat	
A	—[a]	—	410	—
	0.42	—	438	7
	—	3.8	400	3
	0.42	3.8	178	57
		Adrenaline nmol/l		
B	—	—	362	—
	0.42	—	335	7
	—	16.0	314	13
	0.42	16.0	72	80
		Noradrenaline nmol/l		
C	—	—	410	—
	0.42	—	438	+ 7
	—	58.4	799	+94
	0.42	58.4	332	− 19

[a] —: none.

2. Lung Tissue

The anaphylactic release of histamine and SRS-A from monkey lung in vitro passively sensitized with human IgE was inhibited by high concentrations of diethylcarbamazine added with antigen challenge, the IC_{50} for inhibition of release being comparable for the two mediators (Fig. 26). The inhibition was augmented by isoprenaline (Fig. 26) but not by theophylline and was unaffected by propranolol (ISHI-

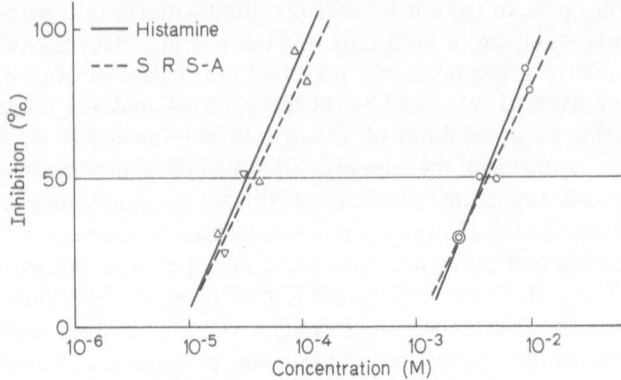

Fig. 26. Inhibition of the anaphylactic release of histamine (——) and SRS-A (−−−−) from passively sensitized monkey lung by diethylcarbamazine (*concentrations on abscissa*) either alone (*circles*) or in the presence of isoprenaline 0.4 µmol/l (*triangles*). (Reproduced from ISHIZAKA et al., 1971b)

ZAKA et al., 1971 b). Similar results were obtained by ORANGE et al. (1971) who used passively sensitized human lung. A graded inhibition of the release of SRS-A was also found when calf lung was incubated in vitro with diethylcarbamazine (0.3–3 mmol/l) but was significant only with the highest concentration (BURKA and EYRE, 1975). Acute anaphylaxis in actively sensitized calves was partially inhibited by diethylcarbamazine (20 mg/kg i.v. 2–3 min prior to antigen), this effect being additive with that of cromoglycate (10 mg/kg i.v.) given simultaneously (EYRE et al., 1973). However, the action of diethylcarbamazine in vivo may not be due entirely to inhibition of the release of SRS-A as the compound also antagonised the effects of injected mediators (histamine, 5-HT, PGE_1, and PGE_2) and the role of SRS-A as a mediator of anaphylaxis in the calf is unknown (BURKA and EYRE, 1974, 1975).

3. Human Leucocytes

Diethylcarbamazine inhibited the release of histamine from human leucocytes stimulated either by anti-IgE (ISHIZAKA et al., 1971 a) or by specific antigen (LICHTENSTEIN and DE BERNARDO, 1971). The high concentrations required ($IC_{50} \simeq 3$ mmol/l) were not cytotoxic as estimated by potassium efflux studies. In studies of the two stages of the anaphylactic release reaction diethylcarbamazine was found approximately equi-effective in the calcium-independent, membrane activation (first) stage and the calcium-dependent, secretory (second) stage (LICHTENSTEIN and DE BERNARDO, 1971). Recently, it has been shown that the release of histamine triggered by concanavallin A was inhibited by diethylcarbamazine at concentrations comparable with those required to inhibit the anaphylactic reaction (SIRAGANIAN and SIRAGANIAN, 1974).

4. Passive Cutaneous Anaphylaxis Reactions

In rats, neither the 48-h (IgE) PCA reaction nor the 4-h (IgGa) PCA reaction was inhibited by diethylcarbamazine (20 mg/kg i.v.) injected 30 s prior to antigen, but this dose augmented the partial inhibition by cromoglycate (50 mg/kg i.v.) of the IgGa reaction (ORANGE and AUSTEN, 1968, 1969). ORR et al. (1970 b) confirmed that diethylcarbamazine (20 mg/kg i.v.) was ineffective but when cyproheptadine (10 mg/kg i.v.) was used instead of cromoglycate to inhibit the early phase of the rat IgGa PCA reaction, they found no enhancement of the effect by diethylcarbamazine (20 mg/kg i.v.). Insufficient information is available for meaningful interpretation. A higher dose of diethylcarbamazine (100 mg/kg i.v.) suppressed non-specifically both the IgGa and IgE PCA reactions.

The 72-h PCA reaction in calves was reduced by diethylcarbamazine (20 mg/kg), unaffected by cromoglycate (10 mg/kg) and more strongly inhibited by a combination of these drugs (WELLS and EYRE, 1972). Since the response was inhibited by mepyramine but not by methysergide, the indications are that histamine and perhaps also SRS-A are the most significant mediators of this reaction.

IV. Chlorphenesin

BERGER et al. (1967) reported that chlorphenesin (100 mg/kg i.p.) inhibited guinea pig PCA reactions provoked by antisera to penicillin but not those provoked by antisera to bovine serum albumin. This specific anti-allergic effect seemed to be due to receptor blockade of penicillin antibodies; the compound had no antihistamine, anti-5-HT or other anti-inflammatory properties. In addition, chlorphenesin was later found to inhibit the release of histamine in vitro from human leucocytes induced by specific antigen, anti-IgE or concanavalin A and had comparable activity ($IC_{50} \simeq 600$ μmol/l) whichever stimulus was employed (LICHTENSTEIN and ADKINSON, 1969; SIRAGANIAN and SIRAGANIAN, 1974). LICHTENSTEIN and ADKINSON (1969) showed that inhibition of histamine release was unchanged by preincubating leucocytes with chlorphenesin and was reversed by washing. In two-stage release experiments the compound was effective in the second (secretory) stage.

Chlorphenesin has been studied as an inhibitor of the release of histamine and SRS-A from rat peritoneal cells in vivo mediated by rat antibody of either the IgGa or IgE class. A dose of approximately 1 mg per rat i.p. just prior to antigen (also i.p.) inhibited by 50% the release of SRS-A but not the release of histamine mediated by either class of immunoglobulin (ORANGE and AUSTEN, 1971). By contrast, the release of both histamine and SRS-A from passively sensitised monkey lung was inhibited by chlorphenesin (50–400 μg/ml), an effect which may have been associated with the observed elevation of tissue cAMP levels (MALLEY and BAECHER, 1971). This again emphasises the variation of effects of mediator release inhibitors in different test situations and underlines the present impracticability of generalisation in this rapidly developing field of knowledge and ignorance.

D. Prospects for New Drugs

The techniques described in Section B.I. are at present being used extensively in an attempt to develop potent cromoglycate-like compounds effective by the oral route. While some progress appears to have been made towards this objective, very little clinical information on orally active compounds is available and the techniques described have therefore yet to be validated by correlating experimental and clinical results.

Cromoglycate-like drugs are not, however, expected to be the ideal anti-allergic agents. It would be useful to have a wider spectrum of activity, probably extending, for example, to reactions in man mediated by anaphylactic IgG antibody. Non-steroid prophylactic inhibitors of skin allergy would also be of value. Whether or not a wide spectrum of anti-allergic effects is likely to be found in a single chemical entity is a matter of conjecture.

References

Altounyan, R. E. C.: Inhibition of experimental asthma by a new compound—disodium cromoglycate "Intal". Acta allerg. (Kbh.) **22**, 487 (1967)

Amundsen, E., Ofstad, E., Hagen, P.-O.: Histamine release induced by synergistic action of kallikrein and phospholipase A. Arch. int. Pharmacodyn. **178**, 104—114 (1969)

Anderson, P., Slorach, S. A., Uvnäs, B.: Sequential exocytosis of storage granules during antigen-induced histamine release from sensitized rat mast cells in vitro. An electron microscopic study. Acta physiol. scand. **88**, 359—372 (1973)

Ankier, S. I.: Disodium cromoglycate and inhibition of passive cutaneous anaphylaxis. Int. Arch. Allergy **41**, 163—165 (1971)

Ankier, S. I., Neat, M. L.: Some studies on acute inflammation induced by dextran in the mouse. Int. Arch. Allergy **42**, 264—277 (1972)

Ashton, M. J., Clark, B., Jones, K. M., Moss, G. F., Neale, M. G., Ritchie, J. T.: The absorption, metabolism, and excretion of disodium cromoglycate in nine animal species. Toxicol. appl. Pharmacol. **26**, 319—328 (1973)

Assem, E. S. K.: Inhibition of allergic reactions by cromoglycate and by a new series of compounds (AH 6556, AH 7079, and AH 7725). Int. Arch. Allergy **45**, 708—718 (1973)

Assem, E. S. K., Atkinson, G.: Histamine release by MCDP (401), a peptide from the venom of the honey bee. Brit. J. Pharmacol. **48**, 337 P—338 P (1973)

Assem, E. S. K., Evans, J. A., McAllen, M.: Inhibition of experimental asthma in man by a new drug (AH 7725) active when given by mouth. Brit. med. J. **2**, 93—94 (1974)

Assem, E. S. K., Mongar, J. L.: Inhibition of allergic reactions in man and other species by cromoglycate. Int. Arch. Allergy. **38**, 68—77 (1970)

Assem, E. S. K., Richter, A. W.: Comparison of in vivo and in vitro inhibition of the anaphylactic mechanism by β-adrenergic stimulants and disodium cromoglycate. Immunology **21**, 729—739 (1971)

Assem, E. S. K., Schild, H. O.: Detection of allergy to penicillin and other antigens by in vitro passive sensitization and histamine release from human and monkey lung. Brit. med. J. **1968 III**, 272—276

Assem, E. S. K., Schild, H. O.: Inhibition by sympathomimetic amines of histamine release by antigen in passively sensitised human lung. Nature (Lond.) **224**, 1028—1029 (1969)

Austen, K. F., Brocklehurst, W. E.: Inhibition of the anaphylactic release of histamine from chopped guinea-pig lung by chymotrypsin substrates and inhibitors. Nature (Lond.) **186**, 866—868 (1960)

Austen, K. F., Brocklehurst, W. E.: Anaphylaxis in chopped guinea-pig lung. I. Effect of peptidase substrates and inhibitors. J. exp. Med. **113**, 521—539 (1961)

Barker, G., Ellis, G. P., Shaw, D.: Benzopyrones. 9. Synthesis and pharmacology of some novel bischromones. J. med. Chem. **16**, 87—89 (1973)

Barlow, R. B.: Introduction to Chemical Pharmacology, 2nd Ed., p. 270. London: Methuen 1964

Batchelor, J. F., Follenfant, M. J., Garland, L. G., Gorvin, J. H., Green, A. F., Hodson, H. F., Hughes, D. T. D., Tateson, J. E.: Doxantrazole, an antiallergic agent orally effective in man. Lancet **1975 I**, 1169—1170

Baxter, J. H.: Histamine release from rat mast cells by dextran: Effects of adrenergic agents, theophylline and other drugs. Proc. Soc. exp. Biol. (N.Y.) **141**, 576—581 (1972)

Baxter, J. H.: Role of Ca^{++} in mast cell activation, desensitization, and histamine release by dextran. J. Immunol. **111**, 1470—1473 (1973)

Baxter, J. H., Adamik, R.: Temperature dependence of histamine release from rat mast cells by dextran. Proc. Soc. exp. Biol. (N.Y.) **146**, 71—74 (1974)

Baxter, J. H., Adamik, R.: Control of histamine release: effects of various conditions on rate of release and rate of cell desensitization. J. Immunol. **114**, 1034—1041 (1975)

Benner, M., Lowell, F. C.: Failure of diethylcarbamazine citrate (Hetrazan) in the treatment of asthma. J. Allergy **46**, 29—31 (1970)

Benson, M. K., Curry, S. H., D'A Mills, G. G., Hughes, D. T. D.: Uptake of disodium cromoglycate in obstructive airways disease. Clin. Allergy **3**, 389—394 (1973)

Berg, T., Johansson, S. G. O.: In vitro diagnosis of atopic allergy. Int. Arch. Allergy **41**, 452—462 (1971)

Berger, F. M., Fukui, G., Ludwig, B. J., Margolin, S.: Selective suppression of penicillin hypersensitivity by certain phenoxy propanediols. Proc. Soc. exp. Biol. (N.Y.) **124**, 303—310 (1967)

Binaghi, R. A., Benacerraf, B., Bloch, K. J., Kourilsky, F. M.: Properties of rat anaphylactic antibody. J. Immunol. **92**, 927—933 (1964)

Bloch, K. J., Morse, H. C., Austen, K. F.: Biologic properties of rat antibodies. I. Antigen-binding by four classes of anti-DNP antibodies. J. Immunol. **101**, 650—657 (1968)

Bloch, K. J., Wilson, R. J. M.: Homocytotropic antibody response in the rat infected with the nematode, *Nippostrongylus brasiliensis*. III. Characteristics of the antibody. J. Immunol. **100**, 629—636 (1968)

Blum, J., Ovary, Z.: Evaluation of methods of measurements of permeability increases. Int. Arch. Allergy **46**, 121—127 (1974)

Bonaccorsi, A., West, G. B.: Absence of capillary permeability response in rats to dextran and egg-white. J. Pharm. (Lond.) **15**, 372—378 (1963)

Boura, A. L. A., Mongar, J. L., Schild, H. O.: Improved automatic apparatus for pharmacological assays on isolated preparations. Brit. J. Pharmacol. **9**, 24—30 (1954)

Bourne, H. R., Lichtenstein, L. M., Melmon, K. L.: Pharmacologic control of allergic histamine release in vitro: evidence for an inhibitory role of 3′,5′-adenosine monophosphate in human leukocytes. J. Immunol. **108**, 695—705 (1972)

Breithaupt, H., Habermann, E.: Mastzelldegranulierendes Peptid (MCD-Peptid) aus Bienengift: Isolierung, biochemische und pharmakologische Eigenschaften. Naunyn-Schmiedeberg's Arch. exp. Path. Pharmak. **261**, 252—270 (1968)

Brocklehurst, W. E., Humphrey, J. H., Perry, W. L. M.: The role of histamine in cutaneous antigen-antibody reactions in the rat. J. Physiol. (Lond.) **129**, 205—224 (1955)

Brocklehurst, W. E., Humphrey, J. H., Perry, W. L. M.: Cutaneous antigen-antibody reactions in the rat. J. Physiol. (Lond.) **150**, 489—500 (1960)

Broder, I., Taichman, N. S.: Mechanism of histamine release from perfused guinea-pig lung by soluble immune complexes. Immunology **21**, 193—205 (1971)

Brogden, R. M., Speight, T. M., Avery, G. S.: Sodium cromoglycate (Cromolyn Sodium): a review of its mode of action, pharmacology, therapeutic efficacy and use. Drugs **7**, 164—282 (1974)

Broughton, B. J., Chaplen, P., Knowles, P., Lunt, E., Pain, D. L., Wooldridge, K. R. H., Ford, R., Marshall, S., Walker, J. L., Maxwell, D. R.: New inhibitor of reagin-mediated anaphylaxis. Nature (Lond.) **251**, 650—652 (1974)

Broughton, B. J., Chaplen, P., Knowles, P., Lunt, E., Marshall, S. M., Pain, D. L., Wooldridge, K. R. H.: Antiallergic activity of 2-phenyl-8-azapurin-6-ones. J. med. Chem. **18**, 1117—1122 (1975)

Bryant, D. H., Burns, M. W., Lazarus, L.: New type of allergic asthma due to IgG "reaginic" antibody. Brit. med. J. **1973 IV**, 589—592

Bryant, D. H., Burns, M. W., Lazarus, L.: Identification of IgG antibody as a carrier of reaginic activity in asthmatic patients. J. Allergy clin. Immunol. **56**, 417—428 (1975)

Buckle, D. R., Cantello, B. C. C., Morgan, N. J., Smith, H., Spicer, B. A.: Antiallergic activity of ω-nitroacetophenones. J. med. Chem. **18**, 733—736 (1975 b)

Buckle, D. R., Cantello, B. C. C., Smith, H., Spicer, B. A.: Antiallergic activity of 4-hydroxy-3-nitro-coumarins. J. med. Chem. **18**, 391—394 (1975 c)

Buckle, D. R., Cantello, B. C. C., Smith, H., Spicer, B. A.: 4-Hydroxy-3-nitro-2-quinolones and related compounds as inhibitors of allergic reactions. J. med. Chem. **18**, 726—732 (1975 d)

Buckle, D. R., Morgan, N. J., Ross, J. W., Smith, H., Spicer, B. A.: Antiallergic activity of 2-nitroindan-1,3-diones. J. med. Chem. **16**, 1334—1339 (1973)

Buckle, D. R., Morgan, N. J., Smith, H.: Hydroaromatic analogues of 2-nitro-1,3-indandiones. J. med. Chem. **18**, 203—206 (1975 a)

Burden, D. T., Parkes, M. W., Gardiner, D. G.: Effect of β-adrenoceptive blocking agents on the response to bronchoconstrictor drugs in the guinea-pig air over-flow preparation. Appendix describing a new modification of the air overflow method. Brit. J. Pharmacol. **41**, 122—131 (1971)

Burka, J. F., Eyre, P.: A study of prostaglandins and prostaglandin antagonists in relation to anaphylaxis in calves. Canad. J. Physiol. Pharmacol. **52**, 942—951 (1974)

Burka, J. F., Eyre, P.: Modulation of the formation and release of bovine SRS-A in vitro by several anti-anaphylactic drugs. Int. Arch. Allergy **49**, 774—781 (1975)

Cairns, H., Fitzmaurice, C., Hunter, D., Johnson, P. B., King, J., Lee, T. B., Lord, G. H., Minshull, R., Cox, J. S. G.: Synthesis and structure-activity relationships of disodium cromoglycate and some related compounds. J. med. Chem. **15**, 583—589 (1972)

Chakrin, L. W., Mengel, J., Young, D., Zaher, C., Krell, R. D., Wardell, J. R.: Enhancement of immediate-type hypersensitivity reactions by N-methyl-N′ {2[(4-methyl-5-imidazolyl)methylthio]ethyl} thio urea (SK & F 92058), a histamine H_2-receptor antagonist. Fed. Proc. **33**, 585 (1974)

Chasin, M., Harris, D. N., Phillips, M. B., Hess, S. M.: 1-Ethyl-4-(isopropylidenehydrazino)-1 H-pyrazolo(3,4-b)-pyridine-5-carboxylic acid, ethyl ester, hydrochloride (SQ 20009): a potent new inhibitor of cyclic 3′,5′-nucleotide phosphodiesterases. Biochem. Pharmacol. **21**, 2443—2450 (1972)

Church, M. K., Collier, H. O. J., James, G. W. L.: The inhibition by dexamethasone and disodium cromoglycate of anaphylactic bronchoconstriction in the rat. Brit. J. Pharmacol. **46**, 56—65 (1972)

Coulson, C. J., Ford, R. E., Lunt, E., Marshall, S., Pain, D. L., Rogers, I. H., Wooldridge, K. R. H.: Antiallergic activity of a series of 8-azaxanthines. Europ. J. med. Chem. Chim. Ther. **9**, 313—317 (1974)

Cox, J. S. G.: Disodium cromoglycate (FPL 670) ("Intal"): a specific inhibitor of reaginic antibody—antigen mechanisms. Nature (Lond.) **216**, 1328—1329 (1967)

Cox, J. S. G.: Disodium cromoglycate. Mode of action and its possible relevance to the clinical use of the drug. Brit. J. Dis. Chest **65**, 189—204 (1971)

Cox, J. S. G., Altounyan, R. E. C.: Nature and modes of action of disodium cromoglycate (Lomudal). Respiration **27** (Suppl.), 292—309 (1970)

Cox, J. S. G., Beach, J. E., Blair, A. M. J. N., Clarke, A. J., King, J., Lee, T. B., Loveday, D. E. E., Moss, G. F., Orr, T. S. C., Ritchie, J. T., Sheard, P.: Disodium cromoglycate (Intal). In: Advances in Drug Research, Vol. V, pp. 115—196. London-New York: Academic Press 1970

Crunkhorn, P., Willis, A. L.: Cutaneous reactions to intradermal prostaglandins. Brit. J. Pharmacol. **41**, 49—56 (1971)

Curry, S. H., Taylor, A. J., Evans, S., Godfrey, S., Zeidifard, E.: Disposition of disodium cromoglycate administered in three particle sizes. J. Pharm. (Lond.) **26** Suppl., 79 P (1974)

Danaraj, T. J.: The treatment of eosinophilic lung (tropical eosinophilia) with diethylcarbamazine. Quart. J. Med. **27**, 243—263 (1958)

Davies, G. E.: Antibronchoconstrictor activity of two new phosphodiesterase inhibitors, a triazolopyrazine (ICI 58 301) and a triazolopyrimidine (ICI 63 197). J. Pharm. (Lond.) **25**, 681—689 (1973)

Davies, G. E., Evans, D. P.: Studies with two new phosphodiesterase inhibitors (ICI 58 301 and ICI 63 197) on anaphylaxis in guinea-pigs, mice, and rats. Int. Arch. Allergy **45**, 467—478 (1973)

Dawson, W., Tomlinson, R.: Effect of cromoglycate and eicosatetraynoic acid on the release of prostaglandins and SRS-A from immunologically challenged guinea-pig lungs. Brit. J. Pharmacol. **52**, 107 P—108 P (1974)

Despopoulos, A.: Antihemolytic actions of tricyclic tranquilizers. Structural correlations. Biochem. Pharmacol. **19**, 2907—2914 (1970)

Drain, D. J., Davy, B., Horlington, M., Howes, J. G. B., Scruton, J. M., Selway, R. A.: The effects of substituting tetrazole for carboxyl in two series of anti-inflammatory phenoxyacetic acids. J. Pharm. (Lond.) **23**, 857—864 (1971)

Easty, D. L., Rice, N. S. C., Jones, B. R.: Clinical trial of topical disodium cromoglycate in vernal kerato-conjunctivitis. Clin. Allergy **2**, 99—107 (1972)

Ellis, G. P., Shaw, D.: Benzopyrones. 7. Synthesis and antiallergic activity of some 2-(5-Tetrazolyl) chromones. J. med. Chem. **15**, 865—867 (1972)

Evans, D. P., Gilman, D. J., Thomson, D. S., Waring, W. S.: Inhibition of allergic reactions by a novel phenanthroline ICI 74917. Nature (Lond.) **250**, 592—593 (1974)

Evans, D. P., Lewis, J. A., Thomson, D. S.: An automated fluorimetric assay for the rapid determination of histamine in biological fluids. Life Sci. **12**, 327—336 (1973)

Evans, D. P., Marshall, P. W., Thomson, D. S.: Inhibition of immediate hypersensitivity reactions in the rat by ICI 74917 and disodium cromoglycate. Int. Arch. Allergy **49**, 417—427 (1975)

Evans, D. P., Thomson, D. S.: Histamine release from rat mast cells passively sensitised with homocytotropic (IgE) antibody. Int. Arch. Allergy **43**, 217—231 (1972)

Evans, D. P., Thomson, D. S.: Inhibition of immediate hypersensitivity reactions in laboratory animals by a phenanthroline salt (ICI 74917). Brit. J. Pharmacol. **53**, 409—418 (1975)

Eyre, P., Lewis, A. J., Wells, P. W.: Acute systemic anaphylaxis in the calf. Brit. J. Pharmacol. **47**, 504—516 (1973)

Farmer, J. B., Richards, I. M., Sheard, P., Woods, A. M.: Passive lung anaphylaxis in the rat. Inhibition by disodium cromoglycate (Die Hemmung der passiven Lungen-Anaphylaxis in der Ratte durch di-Natrium Cromoglycate). Naunyn-Schmiedebergs Arch. Pharmacol. **279** Suppl., R 35 (1973)

Farmer, J. B., Richards, I. M., Sheard, P., Woods, A. M.: Mediators of passive lung anaphylaxis in the rat. Brit. J. Pharmacol. **55**, 57—64 (1975)

Ferraresi, R. W., Roszkowski, A. P., Kepel, E.: Sodium 7-methylsulfinylxanthone-2-carboxylate (SMX), a potent inhibitor of rat reaginic-mediated inflammation. Fed. Proc. **33**, 762 (1974)

Follenfant, M. J., Garland, L. G., Green, A. F., Tateson, J. E.: 3-(5-tetrazolyl) thioxanthone 10,10-dioxide (TTD) a new orally effective antiallergic. In: Proceedings Sixth International Congress of Pharmacology, Helsinki: p. 360. Sanomaprint (1975a)

Follenfant, M. J., Garland, L. G., Green, A. F., Tateson, J. E.: Some properties of the antiallergic agent 3-(5-tetrazolyl) thioxanthone 10,10-dioxide (TTD) related to its possible mechanism of action. In: Proceedings Sixth International Congress of Pharmacology, Helsinki: p. 360. Sanomaprint (1975b)

Foreman, J. C., Garland, L. G.: Desensitization in the process of histamine secretion induced by antigen and dextran. J. Physiol. (Lond.) **239**, 381—391 (1974)

Foreman, J. C., Garland, L. G., Mongar, J. L.: The role of calcium in secretory processes: model studies in mast cells. In: Duncan, C. J. (Ed.): Calcium in Biological Systems, Society of Experimental Biology Symposium, pp. 193—218. Cambridge: Cambridge University Press 1976

Foreman, J. C., Hallett, M. B., Mongar, J. L.: 45-Calcium uptake in rat peritoneal mast cells. Brit. J. Pharmacol. **55**, 283 P—284 P (1975)

Foreman, J. C., Mongar, J. L.: The role of the alkaline earth ions in anaphylactic histamine secretion. J. Physiol. (Lond.) **224**, 753—769 (1972)

Foreman, J. C., Mongar, J. L., Gomperts, B. D.: Calcium ionophores and movement of calcium ions following the physiological stimulus to a secretory process. Nature (Lond.) **245**, 249—251 (1973)

Fredholm, B.: Studies on a mast cell degranulating factor in bee venom. Biochem. Pharmacol. **15**, 2037—2043 (1966)

Fullarton, J., Martin, L. E., Vardey, C.: Studies on the inhibition of cellular anaphylaxis. Int. Arch. Allergy **45**, 84—86 (1973a)

Fullarton, J., Vardey, C. J., Atkinson, J.: Comparison of the release of histamine from rat mast cells and human basophil leucocytes. Paper read to the British Society for Immunology, Autumn Meeting (1973b)

Gardiner, T. H., Schanker, L. S.: Absorption of disodium cromoglycate (DSCG) from the rat lung: evidence of carrier transport. Fed. Proc. **33**, 513 (1974)

Garland, L. G.: Effect of cromoglycate on anaphylactic histamine release from rat peritoneal mast cells. Brit. J. Pharmacol. **49**, 128—130 (1973)

Garland, L. G.: The action of drugs that suppress histamine release from mast cells. University of London: Ph.D. Thesis 1975

Garland, L. G., Mongar, J. L.: Inhibition by cromoglycate of histamine release from rat peritoneal mast cells induced by mixtures of dextran, phosphatidyl serine and calcium ions. Brit. J. Pharmacol. **50**, 137—143 (1974)

Garland, L. G., Mongar, J. L.: Differentiation by inhibitors between histamine release induced by dextran and by the ionophore A 23187. Proceedings Sixth International Congress of Pharmacology, p. 361. Helsinki: Samonaprint 1975

Garland, L. G., Mongar, J. L.: Differential histamine release by dextran and the ionophore A 23187: the actions of inhibitors. Int. Arch. Allergy **50**, 27—42 (1976)

Goose, J., Blair, A. M. J. N.: Passive cutaneous anaphylaxis in the rat, induced with two homologous reagin-like antibodies and its specific inhibition with disodium cromoglycate. Immunology **16**, 749—760 (1969)

Goth, A., Adams, H. R., Knoohuizen, M.: Phosphatidylserine: selective enhancer of histamine release. Science **173**, 1034—1035 (1971)

Greaves, M. W.: The effect of disodium cromoglycate and other inhibitors on in vitro anaphylactic histamine release from guinea-pig basophil leucocytes. Int. Arch. Allergy **36**, 497—505 (1969)

Greaves, M. W., Fairley, V. M., Yamamoto, S.: Release of histamine from skin during in vitro anaphylaxis. Int. Arch. Allergy **41**, 932—939 (1971)

Greaves, M. W., Yamamoto, S., Fairley, V. M.: IgE-mediated hypersensitivity in human skin studied using a new in vitro method. Immunology **23**, 239—248 (1972)

Haddad, Z. H., Gillman, S. A.: Disodium cromoglycate and human reagin (IgE) mediated reactions. Int. Arch. Allergy **45**, 439—446 (1973)

Hall, C. M., Johnson, H. G., Wright, J. B.: Quinoline derivatives as antiallergy agents. J. med. Chem. **17**, 685—690 (1974)

Hanahoe, T. H. P., Holliman, A., Gordon, D., Wieczorek, W.: Disodium cromoglycate and the dextran response in rats. J. Pharm. (Lond.) **24**, 666—667 (1972)

Herbst, R. M.: Tetrazoles as carboxylic acid analogs. In: Graff, S. (Ed.): Essays in Biochemistry, pp. 141—155. New York: John Wiley and Sons Inc. 1956

Herzig, D. J., Giles, R. E., Schumann, P. R., Kusner, E. J., Dubnick, B.: 3-(Hydroxymethyl)-8-methoxychromone: a new, orally active specific prophylactic inhibitor of reaginic anaphylaxis. Fed. Proc. **34**, 760 (1975)

Herzig, D. J., Schumann, P. R., Kusner, E. J., Robichaud, L., Giles, R. E., Dubnick, B., von Strandtmann, M., Klutchko, S., Cohen, M. P., Shavel, J. Jr.: The search for specific inhibitors of immediate hypersensitivity reactions. The activity of some chromones in various laboratory models. In: Immunopharmacology, pp. 103—124. New York: Spectrum Press 1975. In press

Hines, M. C., Moss, G. F., Cox, J. S. G.: Effect of disodium cromoglycate on phospholipase A activity. Studies with egg yolk and isolated mast cell systems. Biochem. Pharmacol. **21**, 171—179 (1972)

Högberg, B., Uvnäs, B.: The mechanism of the disruption of mast cells produced by Compound 48/80. Acta physiol. scand. **41**, 345—369 (1957)

Holland, A., Jackson, D., Chaplen, P., Lunt, E., Marshall, S. M., Pain, D. L., Wooldridge, K.: Antiallergic activity of 8-azapurin-6-ones with heterocyclic 2-substituents. Europ. J. Med. Chem-Chim. Ther. **10**, 447—449 (1975)

Ishizaka, K., Ishizaka, T.: Role of IgE and IgG antibodies in reaginic hypersensitivity in the respiratory tract. In: Austen, K. F., Lichtenstein, L. M. (Eds.): Asthma: Physiology, Immunopharmacology, and Treatment, pp. 55—68. New York: Academic Press 1973

Ishizaka, T., Ishizaka, K., Lichtenstein, L. M.: Antibody-induced histamine release and degranulation of human basophil leukocytes. Fed. Proc. **30**, 654 (1971 a)

Ishizaka, T., Ishizaka, K., Orange, R. P., Austen, K. F.: Pharmacologic inhibition of the antigen-induced release of histamine and slow reacting substance of anaphylaxis (SRS-A) from monkey lung tissues mediated by human IgE. J. Immunol. **106**, 1267—1273 (1971 b)

Jasani, B., Stanworth, D. R.: Studies on the mast cell triggering action of certain artificial histamine liberators. Int. Arch. Allergy **45**, 74—81 (1973)

Johnson, A. R., Moran, N. C.: Release of histamine from rat mast cells: a comparison of the effects of 48/80 and two antigen-antibody systems. Fed. Proc. **28**, 1716—1720 (1969)

Johnson, H. G., Bach, M. K.: Prevention of calcium ionophore-induced release of histamine in rat mast cells by disodium cromoglycate. J. Immunol. **114**, 514—516 (1975)

Johnson, H. G., Vanhout, C. A.: The enhanced efficacy of disodium cromoglycate (DSCG) in DSCG predosed rats. Proc. Soc. exp. Biol. (N.Y.) **143**, 427—432 (1973)

Johnson, H. G., Vanhout, C. A.: Studies on the mode of action of disodium cromoglycate (DSCG). Enhanced efficacy in predosed rats. Allergol. Immunopath. (Madr.) **2**, 33—40 (1974)

Jones, V. E., Ogilvie, B. M.: Reaginic antibodies and immunity to *Nippostrongylus brasiliensis* in the rat. II. Some properties of the antibodies and antigens. Immunology **12**, 583—597 (1967)

Juby, P. F., Hudyma, T. W., Brown, M.: Preparation and antiinflammatory properties of some 5-(2-anilinophenyl) tetrazoles. J. med. Chem. **11**, 111—117 (1968)

Kaliner, M., Austen, K. F.: A sequence of biochemical events in the antigen-induced release of chemical mediators from sensitised human lung tissue. J. exp. Med. **138**, 1077—1094 (1973)

Kaliner, M., Austen, K. F.: Cyclic nucleotides and modulations of effector systems of inflammation. Biochem. Pharmacol. **23**, 763—771 (1974 a)

Kaliner, M., Austen, K. F.: Hormonal control of the immunologic release of histamine and slow-reacting substance of anaphylaxis from human lung. In: Braun, W., Lichtenstein, L. M., Parker, C. W. (Eds.): Cyclic AMP, Cell Growth and the Immune Response, pp. 163—175. Berlin-Heidelberg-New York: Springer 1974 b

Kimura, I., Tanizaki, Y., Sato, S., Takahashi, K., Saito, K., Ueda, N.: Morphological changes of basophils in immunological reactions—effect of sodium cromoglycate. Clin. Allergy **5**, 181—187 (1975)

Konzett, H., Rossler, R.: Versuchsanordnung zu Untersuchungen an der Bronchialmuskulatur. Naunyn-Schmiedeberg's Arch. exp. Path. Pharmak. **195**, 71—74 (1940)

Koopman, W. J., Orange, R. P., Austen, K. F.: Immunochemical and biologic properties of rat IgE. III. Modulation of the IgE-mediated release of slow-reacting substance of anaphylaxis by agents influencing the level of cyclic 3',5'-adenosine monophosphate. J. Immunol. **105**, 1096—1102 (1970a)

Koopman, W. J., Orange, R. P., Austen, K. F.: Inhibition by antihistamines of the immunologic release of slow reacting substance of anaphylaxis (SRS-A) in the rat. Trans. Ass. Amer. Phycns **83**, 225—234 (1970b)

Kunze, H., Vogt, W.: Significance of phospholipase A for prostaglandin formation. Ann. N.Y. Acad. Sci. **180**, 123—125 (1971)

Kusner, E. J., Dubnick, B., Herzig, D. J.: The inhibition by disodium cromoglycate in vitro of anaphylactically induced histamine release from rat peritoneal mast cells. J. Pharmacol. exp. Ther. **184**, 41—46 (1973)

Kusner, E. J., Herzig, D. J.: An automated fluorimetric method for the determination of histamine from mast cell suspension. In: Advances in Automated Analysis, Vol. II, pp. 429—433. Miami; Thurman Associates 1971

Levine, B. B., Chang, H., Vaz, N. M.: The production of hapten-specific reaginic antibodies in the guinea-pig. J. Immunol. **106**, 29—33 (1971)

Lewis, R. A., Wasserman, S. I., Goetzl, E. J., Austen, K. F.: Formation of slowreacting substance of anaphylaxis in human lung tissue and cells before release. J. exp. Med. **140**, 1133—1146 (1974)

Lichtenstein, L. M.: The immediate allergic response: in vitro separation of antigen activation, decay and histamine release. J. Immunol. **107**, 1122—1130 (1971)

Lichtenstein, L. M.: The role of the cyclic AMP system in inflammation: An introduction. In: Braun, W., Lichtenstein, L. M., Parker, C. W. (Eds.): Cyclic AMP, Cell Growth and the Immune Response, pp. 147—162. Berlin-Heidelberg-New York: Springer 1974

Lichtenstein, L. M., Adkinson, N. F.: Chlorphenesin: a new inhibitor of IgE-mediated histamine release. J. Immunol. **103**, 866—868 (1969)

Lichtenstein, L. M., Bourne, H. R.: Inhibition of allergic histamine release by histamine and other agents which stimulate adenyl cyclase. In: Austen, K. F., Becker, E. L. (Eds.): Biochemistry of the Acute Allergic Reactions, pp. 161—173. Oxford: Blackwell 1971

Lichtenstein, L. M., Debernardo, R.: The immediate allergic response: in vitro action of cyclic AMP-active and other drugs on the two stages of histamine release. J. Immunol. **107**, 1131—1136 (1971)

Lichtenstein, L. M., Gillespie, E.: Inhibition of histamine release by histamine controlled by H_2 receptor. Nature (Lond.) **244**, 287—288 (1973)

Lichtenstein, L. M., Gillespie, E.: The effects of the H_1 and H_2 antihistamines on "allergic" histamine release and its inhibition by histamine. J. Pharmacol. exp. Ther. **192**, 441—450 (1975)

Lichtenstein, L. M., Margolis, S.: Histamine release in vitro: Inhibition by catecholamines and methylxanthines. Science **161**, 902—903 (1968)

Lichtenstein, L. M., Osler, A. G.: Studies on the mechanisms of hypersensitivity phenomena. IX. Histamine release from human leukocytes by ragweed pollen antigen. J. exp. Med. **120**, 507—530 (1964)

Lopez, M., Bloch, K. J.: Effect of disodium cromoglycate on certain passive cutaneous anaphylactic reactions. J. Immunol. **103**, 1428—1430 (1969)

McManus, J. M., Herbst, R. M.: Tetrazole analogues of amino acids. J. org. Chem. **24**, 1643—1649 (1959)

Maling, H. M., Webster, M. E., Williams, M. A., Saul, W., Anderson, W.: Inflammation induced by histamine, serotonin, bradykinin, and compound 48/80 in the rat: antagonists and the mechanism of action. J. Pharmacol. exp. Ther. **191**, 300—310 (1974)

Mallen, M. S.: Treatment of intractable asthma with diethylcarbamazine citrate. Ann. Allergy **23**, 534—537 (1965)

Malley, A., Baecher, L.: Inhibition of histamine and SRS-A from monkey lung tissue by chlorphenesin. J. Immunol. **107**, 586—588 (1971)

Marshall, P. W., Thomson, D. S., Evans, D. P.: The mechanism of tachyphylaxis to ICI 74917 and disodium cromoglycate. Int. Arch. Allergy **51**, 274—283 (1976)

Marshall, R.: Protective effect of disodium cromoglycate on rat peritoneal mast cells. Thorax **27**, 38—43 (1972)

Martin, L. E.: Inhibition of cellular anaphylaxis by beta-stimulants. Postgrad. med. J. **47**, suppl., 26—30 (1971)

Mielens, Z. E., Ferguson, E. W., Rosenberg, F. J.: Effects of anti-anaphylactic drugs upon passive cutaneous anaphylaxis mediated by graded doses of reaginic or non-reaginic antibodies in rats. Int. Arch. Allergy **47**, 633—649 (1974)

Mihina, J. S., Herbst, R. M.: The reaction of nitriles with hydrazoic acid: synthesis of monosubstituted tetrazoles. J. org. Chem. **15**, 1082—1092 (1950)

Miyamoto, T., Reynolds, L. B., Patterson, R., Cugell, P. W., Kettel, L. J.: Respiratory changes in passively sensitised dogs and monkeys as models of allergic asthma. Amer. Rev. resp. Dis. **97**, 76—88 (1968)

Mongar, J. L., Schild, H. O.: Cellular mechanisms in anaphylaxis. Physiol. Rev. **42**, 226—270 (1962)

Mongar, J. L., Svec, P.: The effect of phospholipids on anaphylactic histamine release. Brit. J. Pharmacol. **46**, 741—752 (1972)

Moran, N. C., Uvnäs, B., Westerholm, B.: Release of 5-hydroxytryptamine and histamine from rat mast cells. Acta physiol. scand. **56**, 26—41 (1962)

Morse, H. C., Austen, K. F., Bloch, K. J.: Biological properties of rat antibodies. III. Histamine release mediated by two classes of antibodies. J. Immunol. **102**, 327—337 (1969)

Moss, G. F., Jones, K. M., Ritchie, J. T., Cox, J. S. G.: Distribution and metabolism of disodium cromoglycate in rats. Toxicol. appl. Pharmacol. **17**, 691—698 (1970)

Moss, G. F., Jones, K. M., Ritchie, J. T., Cox, J. S. G.: Plasma levels and urinary excretion of disodium cromoglycate after inhalation by human volunteers. Toxicol. appl. Pharmacol. **20**, 147—156 (1971)

Moss, G. F., Ritchie, J. T.: The absorption and clearance of disodium cromoglycate from the lung in rat, rabbit, and monkey. Toxicol. appl. Pharmacol. **17**, 699—707 (1970)

Mota, I.: The mechanism of anaphylaxis. I. Production and biological properties of "mast cell sensitizing" antibody. Immunology **7**, 681—699 (1964)

Mota, I.: Biological characterisation of mouse "early" antibodies. Immunology **12**, 343—348 (1967)

Mota, I., Dias da Silva, W.: The anti-anaphylactic and histamine-releasing properties of the antihistamines. Their effect on the mast cells. Brit. J. Pharmacol. **15**, 396—404 (1960)

Neale, M. G., Moss, G. F.: Effect of inducers on the metabolism and excretion of disodium cromoglycate in rats. Biochem. J. **130**, 85 P—86 P (1972)

Newman, D. J., Spainhour, Jr., C. B., Brann, E. G.: Partial purification and properties of cAMP-phosphodiesterase isolated from guinea pig tracheal muscle. Fed. Proc. **34**, 261 Abstr. (1975)

Nohara, A., Kuriki, H., Saijo, T., Ukawa, K., Murata, T., Kanno, M., Sanno, Y.: Studies on anti-anaphylactic agents. 4. Synthesis and structure-activity relationships of 3-(4-oxo-4H-1-benzopyran-3) acrylic acids, a new series of antiallergic substances, and some related compounds. J. med. Chem. **18**, 34—37 (1975)

Ogilvie, B. M.: Reagin-like antibodies in animals immune to helminth parasites. Nature (Lond.) **204**, 91—92 (1964)

Orange, R. P., Austen, K. F.: Pharmacologic dissociation of immunologic release of histamine and slow reacting substance of anaphylaxis in rats. Proc. Soc. exp. Biol. (N.Y.) **129**, 836—841 (1968)

Orange, R. P., Austen, K. F.: Slow reacting substance of anaphylaxis in the rat. In: Cellular and Humoral Mechanisms in Anaphylaxis and Allergy, pp. 196—206. Basel-New York: Karger 1969

Orange, R. P., Austen, K. F.: Drug-induced modulation of the immunologic release of histamine and slow reacting substance of anaphylaxis. Int. Arch. Allergy **41**, 79—85 (1971)

Orange, R. P., Austen, W. G., Austen, K. F.: Immunological release of histamine and slow reacting substance of anaphylaxis from human lung. J. exp. Med. **134**, 136—148 (1971)

Orange, R. P., Murphy, R. C., Karnovsky, M. L., Austen, K. F.: The physicochemical characteristics and purification of slow reacting substance of anaphylaxis. J. Immunol. **110**, 760—770 (1973)

Orange, R. P., Stechschulte, D. J., Austen, K. F.: Immunochemical and biological properties of rat IgE. II. Capacity to mediate the immunologic release of histamine and slow reacting substance of anaphylaxis (SRS-A). J. Immunol. **105**, 1087—1095 (1970)

Orange, R. P., Valentine, M. D., Austen, K. F.: Antigen-induced release of slow reacting substance of anaphylaxis (SRS-A rat) in rats prepared with homologous antibody. J. exp. Med. **127**, 767—782 (1968)

Orr, T. S. C.: The mast cell and disodium cromoglycate in immediate type reactions. Acta tuberc. pneumol. belg. **65**, 300—307 (1974)

Orr, T. S. C., Blair, A. M. J. N.: Potentiated reagin response to egg albumin and conalbumin in *Nippostrongylus brasiliensis* infected rats. Life Sci. **8**, 1073—1077 (1969)

Orr, T. S. C., Cox, J. S. G.: Disodium cromoglycate, an inhibitor of mast cell degranulation and histamine release induced by phospholipase A. Nature (Lond.) **223**, 197—198 (1969)

Orr, T. S. C., Gwilliam, J., Cox, J. S. G.: Studies on passive cutaneous anaphylaxis in the rat with disodium cromoglycate. I. Cutaneous reactions induced by an anti-DNP $7S_{y2}$ antibody. Immunology **19**, 469—479 (1970 b)

Orr, T. S. C., Gwilliam, J., Cox, J. S. G.: Studies on passive cutaneous anaphylaxis in the rat with disodium cromoglycate. II. A comparison of the rat anti-DNP $7S_{y2}$ and rat reagin induced cutaneous reactions. Immunology **21**, 405—417 (1971 a)

Orr, T. S. C., Hall, D. E., Gwilliam, J. M., Cox, J. S. G.: The effect of disodium cromoglycate on the release of histamine and degranulation of rat mast cells induced by compound 48/80. Life Sci. **10**, 805—812 (1971 b)

Orr, T. S. C., Pollard, M. C., Gwilliam, J., Cox, J. S. G.: Mode of action of disodium cromoglycate studies on immediate type hypersensitivity reactions using "double sensitization" with two antigenically distinct rat reagins. Clin. exp. Immunol. **7**, 745—757 (1970 a)

Orr, T. S. C., Riley, P., Doe, J. E.: Potentiated reagin response to egg albumin in *Nippostrongylus brasiliensis* infected rats. II. Time course of the reagin response. Immunology **20**, 185—189 (1971 c)

Parish, W. E.: Release of histamine and slow reacting substance with mast cell changes after challenge of human lung sensitized passively with reagin in vitro. Nature (Lond.) **215**, 738—739 (1967)

Parish, W. E.: A human heat-stable anaphylactic or anaphylactoid antibody which may participate in pulmonary disorders. In: Austen, K. F., Lichtenstein, L. M. (Eds.): Asthma: Physiology, Immunopharmacology, and Treatment, pp. 71—89. New York: Academic Press 1973

Parish, W. E.: Some biological activities of IgG subclass antibodies after inoculation and in disease. In: Ganderton, M. A., Frankland, A. W. (Eds.): Allergy '74, Proceedings of the Ninth European Congress of Allergology and Clinical Immunology, pp. 153—175. New York: Pitman Medical Publ. 1975

Parratt, J. R., West, G. B.: 5-Hydroxytryptamine and tissue mast cells. J. Physiol. (Lond.) **137**, 169—178 (1957 a)

Parratt, J. R., West, G. B.: Release of 5-hydroxytryptamine and histamine from tissues of the rat. J. Physiol. (Lond.) **137**, 179—192 (1957 b)

Parratt, J. R., West, G. B.: 5-Hydroxytryptamine and the anaphylactoid reaction in the rat. J. Physiol. (Lond.) **139**, 27—41 (1957 c)

Patterson, R., Talbot, C. H.: Respiratory responses in sub-human primates with immediate-type hypersensitivity. J. Lab. clin. Med. **73**, 924—933 (1969)

Patterson, R., Talbot, C. H., Brandfonbrener, M.: The use of IgE mediated responses as a pharmacologic test system. The effect of disodium cromoglycate in respiratory and cutaneous reactions and on the electrocardiograms of rhesus monkeys. Int. Arch. Allergy **41**, 592—603 (1971)

Pearce, C. A., Greaves, M. W., Plummer, V. M., Yamamoto, S.: Effect of disodium cromoglycate on antigen-evoked histamine release from human skin. Clin. exp. Immunol. **17**, 437—440 (1974)

Pepys, J.: Disodium cromoglycate in clinical and experimental asthma. In: Austen, K. F., Lichtenstein, L. M. (Eds.): Asthma: Physiology, Immunopharmacology, and Treatment, pp. 279—292. New York: Academic Press 1973

Piper, P. J., Walker, J. L.: The release of spasmogenic substances from human chopped lung tissue and its inhibition. Brit. J. Pharmacol. **47**, 291—304 (1973)

Pfister, J. R., Ferraresi, R. W., Harrison, I. T., Rooks, W. H., Roszkowski, A. P., Van Horn, A.: Xanthone-2-carboxylic acids, a new series of antiallergic substances. J. med. Chem. **15**, 1032—1035 (1972)

Possanza, G. J., Bauen, A., Stewart, P. B.: Effect of a benzopyrano benzopyran (PR-D-92-EA) on the mediators of allergy in vitro. Pharmacologist 16, 198 (1974)

Possanza, G. J., Bauen, A., Stewart, P. B.: In vitro antagonism of the mediators of allergy by a benzopyrano-benzopyran carboxylic acid PR-D-92-EA. Int. Arch. Allergy 49, 789—795 (1975)

Poyser, R. H., West, G. B.: Structural requirements of sugars as antagonists of the vascular response to dextran in rat skin. Brit. J. Pharmacol. 32, 219—226 (1968)

Rachelefsky, G. S., Lavin, N., Kaplan, S. A.: An action of cromolyn sodium (CS): Inhibition of cyclic 3',5'-adenosine monophosphate (cAMP) phosphodiesterase (PDE). J. Allergy 55, 117—118 (1975)

Riley, P. A., Sheard, P., Clarke, A. J., Orr, T. S. C.: The effect of predosage with disodium cromoglycate (DSCG) on the dose-related inhibition of rat passive cutaneous anaphylaxis by DSCG. Life Sci. 17, 793—802 (1975)

Roesch, E., Roesch, A.: The local dextran reaction in skin of rats as influenced by beta-adrenergic mechanisms and the cyclic AMP-system. Naunyn Schmiedeberg's Arch. Pharmacol. 279, R 15 (1973)

Ross, J. W., Smith, H., Spicer, B. A.: Increased vascular permeability during passive peritoneal anaphylaxis (PPA) in the rat. The effects of disodium cromoglycate and a nitroindandione. Int. Arch. Allergy 51, 226—237 (1976)

Roszkowski, A. P., Ferraresi, R. W., Schuler, M. E., Sullivan, B. J.: Pharmacological properties of sodium 7-isopropoxy-xanthone 2-carboxylate (IXC). Fed. Proc. 33, 569 (1974)

Rothschild, A. M.: Histamine release by bee venom phospholipase A and mellitin in the rat. Brit. J. Pharmacol. 25, 59—66 (1965)

Rothschild, A. M.: Mechanisms of histamine release by compound 48/80. Brit. J. Pharmacol. 38, 253—262 (1970)

Roy, A. C., Warren, B. T.: Inhibition of cAMP phosphodiesterase by disodium cromoglycate. Biochem. Pharmacol. 23, 917—920 (1974)

Schmutzler, W., Derwall, R., Poblete Freundt, G.: The effects of catecholamines and of disodium cromoglycate (DSCG) on the cyclic AMP and the anaphylactic release of histamine in the guinea pig lung. Naunyn Schmiedeberg's Arch. Pharmacol. 277, R 67 (1973)

Sheard, P., Blair, A. M. J. N.: Disodium cromoglycate. Activity in three in vitro models of the immediate hypersensitivity reaction in lung. Int. Arch. Allergy 38, 217—224 (1970)

Sheard, P., Killingback, P. G., Blair, A. M. J. N.: Antigen induced release of histamine and SRS-A from human lung passively sensitized with reaginic serum. Nature (Lond.) 216, 283—284 (1967)

Sheppard, H., Wiggan, G.: Different sensitivities of the phosphodiesterases (adenosine-3',5'-cyclic phosphate 3'-phosphohydrolase) of dog cerebral cortex and erythrocytes to inhibition by synthetic agents and cold. Biochem. Pharmacol. 20, 2128—2130 (1971)

Shore, P. A., Burkhalter, A., Cohn, V. H.: A method for the fluorometric assay of histamine in tissues. J. Pharmacol. exp. Ther. 127, 182—186 (1959)

Siraganian, P. A., Siraganian, R. P.: Basophil activation by concanavalin A: characteristics of the reaction. J. Immunol. 112, 2117—2125 (1974)

Spicer, B. A., Ross, J. W., Smith, H.: Inhibition of immediate hypersensitivity reactions in the rat by disodium cromoglycate and a nitroindanedione. Clin. exp. Immunol. 21, 419—429 (1975)

Sprenkle, A. C., Van Arsdel, P. P., Bierman, C. W.: New class of antiallergic compounds effective in man. J. Allergy 55, 118 (1975)

Stechschulte, D. J., Orange, R. P., Austen, K. F.: Immunochemical and biologic properties of rat IgE. I. Immunochemical identification of rat IgE. J. Immunol. 105, 1082—1086 (1970)

Stewart, P. B., Bell, R., Goodfriend, L.: Pharmacological differentiation of monkey lung and skin mast cell—reagin reactions in vitro. In: Goodfriend, L., Sehon, A. H., Orange, R. P. (Eds.): Mechanisms in Allergy. Reagin-Mediated Hypersensitivity, pp. 457—466. New York: Marcel Dekker Inc. 1973

Stewart, P. B., Devlin, J. P., Freter, K. R.: Anti-allergic activity of a benzopyrano benzopyran PR-D-92-EA. Fed. Proc. 33, 762 (1974)

Stotland, L. M., Share, N. N.: Pharmacological studies on active bronchial anaphylaxis in the rat. Canad. J. Physiol. Pharmacol. 52, 1119—1125 (1974)

Taichman, N. S., Movat, H. Z.: Do polymorphonuclear leukocytes play a role in passive cutaneous anaphylaxis of the guinea-pig? Int. Arch. Allergy **30**, 97—102 (1966)

Tateson, J. E., Trist, D. G.: Inhibition of adenosine-3′,5′-cyclic monophosphate phosphodiesterase by potential antiallergic compounds. Life Sci. **18**, 153—162 (1976)

Tattrie, N. H.: Positional distribution of saturated and unsaturated fatty acids on egg lecithin. J. Lipid Res. **1**, 60—65 (1959)

Tay, C. H., Yeoh, T. S., Greaves, M. W.: Spontaneous and evoked histamine release from guinea pig skin in vitro in presence of disodium cromoglycate. Int. Arch. Allergy **43**, 390—394 (1972)

Taylor, G., Shivalkar, P. R.: Disodium cromoglycate: laboratory studies and clinical trial in allergic rhinitis. Clin. Allergy **1**, 189—198 (1971)

Taylor, W. A.: The effect of disodium cromoglycate and $PGF_{2\alpha}$ on acute cutaneous reactions of the guinea pig and rat. Int. Arch. Allergy **45**, 82—83 (1973)

Taylor, W. A.: Control of mast cell degranulation. In: Ganderton, M. A., Frankland, A. W. (Eds.): Allergy '74. Proceedings of the Ninth European Congress of Allergology and Clinical Immunology, pp. 256—266. New York: Pitman Medical Publishers 1975

Taylor, W. A., Francis, D. H., Sheldon, D., Roitt, I. M.: The anti-anaphylactic actions of disodium cromoglycate, theophylline, isoprenaline, and prostaglandins. Int. Arch. Allergy **46**, 104—120 (1974 a)

Taylor, W. A., Francis, D. H., Sheldon, D., Roitt, I. M.: Anti-allergic actions of disodium cromoglycate and other drugs known to inhibit cyclic 3′,5′-nucleotide phosphodiesterase. Int. Arch. Allergy **47**, 175—193 (1974 b)

Taylor, W. A., Roitt, I. M.: Effect of disodium cromoglycate on various types of anaphylactic reaction in the guinea pig. Int. Arch. Allergy **45**, 795—807 (1973)

Taylor, W. A., Sheldon, D.: Mast cell degranulation. A comparison of the inhibitory actions of disodium cromoglycate, drugs known to influence the level of intracellular cyclic nucleotide and diisopropylfluorophosphate (DFP). Int. Arch. Allergy **47**, 696—707 (1974)

Thomson, D. S., Evans, D. P.: Inhibition of immediate hypersensitivity reactions by disodium cromoglycate. Requirements for activity in two laboratory models. Clin. exp. Immunol. **13**, 537—544 (1973)

Udaka, K., Takeuchi, Y., Movat, H. Z.: Simple method for quantitation of enhanced vascular permeability. Proc. Soc. exp. Biol. (N.Y.) **133**, 1384—1387 (1970)

Uvnäs, B., Antonsson, J.: Triggering action of phosphatidase A and chymotrypsins on degranulation of rat mesentery mast cells. Biochem. Pharmacol. **12**, 867—873 (1963)

Voorhees, A. B., Baker, H. J., Pulaski, E. J.: Reactions of albino rats to injections of dextran. Proc. Soc. exp. Biol. (N.Y.) **76**, 254—256 (1951)

Walker, D. M., Dolby, A. E.: Effect of disodium cromoglycate on lymphocyte response to antigen and mitogen. Int. Arch. Allergy **49**, 303—309 (1975)

Walker, S. R., Evans, M. E., Richards, A. J., Paterson, J. W.: The fate of [^{14}C] disodium cromoglycate in man. J. Pharm. (Lond.) **24**, 525—531 (1972)

Watanabe, S., Nakamura, K., Koda, A.: Experimental asthma caused by homocytotropic antibody in guinea pigs. Proceedings Sixth International Congress of Pharmacology, p. 494. Helsinki: Sanomaprint 1975

Wells, P. W., Eyre, P.: The pharmacology of passive cutaneous anaphylaxis in the calf. Canad. J. Physiol. Pharmacol. **50**, 255—262 (1972)

Wright, J. B., Johnson, H. G.: Antiasthma agents. I. 4-Oxo-4 H-[1]benzothieno[3,2-b]pyran-2-carboxylic acid and 4-oxo-4 H-[1]benzofuro[3,2-b]pyran-2-carboxylic acid. J. med. Chem. **16**, 861—862 (1973)

Zeller, E. A., Bissegger, A.: Über die Cholin-esterase des Gehirns und der Erythrocyten. Helv. chim. Acta **26**, 1619—1630 (1943)

Zvaifler, N. J., Bauer, H., Robinson, J. O.: IgE immunoglobulin in the rabbit. In: Austen, K. F., Becker, E. L. (Eds.): Biochemistry of the Acute Allergic Reactions, pp. 34—42. Oxford: Blackwell 1971

CHAPTER 35

Cytostats With Effects in Chronic Inflammation

K. BRUNE and M. W. WHITEHOUSE

A. Introduction

A number of toxic agents happen to exhibit therapeutic side-effects including the suppression of inflammatory disease. Obviously, those used in the clinic have a tolerable therapeutic index. The acceptability of some of these toxic drugs may be due to any one or more of the following reasons: (1) they have a reversible effect on cell populations that turn over slowly; (2) they mainly delete cells from populations with a high rate of generation; (3) their toxicity is not incompatible with maintenance of cell vitality.

Drugs exhibiting this latter property (cell deactivating agents) are designated *cytostats*, to distinguish them from grossly toxic, cytolytic agents. A cytostat will desensitize "irritable"/reactive cells and/or retard cellular proliferation, without necessarily being cytotoxic.

The right hand column of Table 1 lists a number of drugs and antibiotics which suppress inflammatory disease. This listing covers a wide range of chemical species. This same table also shows that cellular stasis can be induced by drugs acting fairly selectively on a number of different cellular structures or receptors. If these receptors or structures are not present in all cells, then a certain restriction of drug activity can be anticipated. So for example, at low doses, cholinomimetic quaternary nitrogen compounds bind preferentially to the neuromuscular junction (acetylcholine receptors) and oral contraceptives at the progestagen-binding receptor(s) in the hypophysis. Ideally, an anti-inflammatory cytostatic drug would distribute to just those cells located in, or specifically attached to, an inflammatory focus. This selective distribution might be achieved by at least three means: (1) local bioactivation of an inert precursor drug; (2) "trapping" in a restricted compartment, e.g. whenever the pH is appreciably different from that of the plasma or lymph; (3) uptake by receptors that are not uniformly distributed on most cells of the body but are certainly enriched on others, e.g. the characteristic surface components by which T-lymphocytes are distinguished from B-lymphocytes.

We can only discuss here some drugs which approximate to these conditions. As Table 1 indicates, a number of drugs fairly selectively inhibit cell surface phenomena or cellular proliferation (acting either on the nucleus or the microtubular apparatus) in dividing cells that are intimately associated with *chronic* inflammation. Chronicity often derives from persistence of an immunogen or an otherwise prolonged immune response. Other chronic inflammatory conditions, e.g. pneumonoconiosis, arise from persistent fibrogenesis due to prolonged irritant action of an indigestible particle. Where the drug action is primarily directed against a component of the immune

Table 1. Cellular stasis induced by (anti-inflammatory–immunosuppressive) drugs

Locus of action	Process affected	Type of agent	Examples
a) Cell surface[a]	Secretion/ingestion	Unspecific blocking, specific blocking, exoalkylating, anti-metabolites, enzymes	NSAID, local anaesthetics, ALS, lectins, cromoglycate, counterstimuli[b], chalones, CxPA, Pt (II), HN-2, cyclo-leucine, RNA-ase, asparaginase
b) Cytoskeleton/ endocontractile elements	Exocytosis/endo-cytosis	Myofibril binding	Cytochalasin-B
	Conveying of infor-mation, organelles	Tubulin binding	Vinblastin, PEH, Col.
c) Endocellular membranes:			
—reticulum	Biopolymer synthesis, compartmentalisa-tion (e. g. hydrolases within lysosome)	Inhibitors of protein synthesis	Cycloheximide, rifampicins
—mitochondria	Energy transduc-tion/ATP-secretion	Cell poisons, uncoupling agents	Chloramphenicol, NSAID
d) Nucleus	mRNA excretion, DNA-replication	Anti-metabolites, antibiotics: alkylating, nucleolytic	Ara-C actinomycin, daunorubicin phosphoramide mustard (from CP), HN-2, PCZ, HC.
e) Cytosol/lyso-some-interior	Premitochondrial catabolisation of foodstuffs	Anti-metabolic, SH-blocking	MTX, thioinosonate (from 6-MP) Gold (I) drugs

[a] Target cells would be leucocytes (lc), phagocytic cells, platelets, fixed cells of the reticulo-endothelial system, vascular endothelium, connective tissue cells.
[b] Counterstimuli would be e. g.: prostaglandins modulating certain lymphocyte populations.

Abbreviations used: ALS = anti-lymphocyte sera; ara-c = cytosine arabinoside; Col = colchicine; CP = cyclophosphamide; CxPA = carboxyphosphamide; HC = hydrocortisone (cortisol); HN-2 = mechlorethamine (Nitrogen mustard); MTX = methotrexate; 6-MP = 6-mercaptopurine; NSAID = non-steroid anti-inflammatory drugs (e.g. salicylate, indomethacin); PEH = podo-phyllotoxinethylhydrazide PCZ = procarbazine.

system in an immunologically induced inflammation it is appropriate to describe it as "immunosuppressive." However, the same drug may still be "anti-inflammatory" when acting by the *same* molecular mechanism(s) on non-lymphoid cells. One exam-ple would be the proliferating synovial lining in the early stages of pannus formation that accompanies joint inflammation in rheumatoid arthritis; another example would be the proliferation of dermal tissue in psoriasis. For this reason we prefer to use the designation "cytostat" to embrace both immunosuppressants and tubular inhibitors, and yet other classes of fairly toxic drugs, which have in common the property of regulating the signs of inflammatory disease.

In this chapter, we will consider only drugs acting primarily at one of the follow-ing loci: (1) nucleus; (2) cell surface; (3) tubular apparatus.

Processes:

Antigen (Ag) sensitizes T- and B-lymphocytes (*Tc, Bc*); Tc- and B-interaction controls degree of sensitization. Tc proliferate, transform to killer (K) cells and influence macrophages (*Mac*) by lymphokines (*Lk*). Both may then destroy antigen-carrying connective tissue cells (*Ctc*). Bc proliferate, transform to plasma cells (*Pl*) which release e. g. complement fixing antibodies (*AbC*). Ab also sensitize mast cells (*Mc*), and interact with Ag and complement (C). Interaction leads to release of: lysosomal enzymes, prostaglandins, histamine, 5-HT, complement fragments, etc.

Chronic (immunologic) inflammation

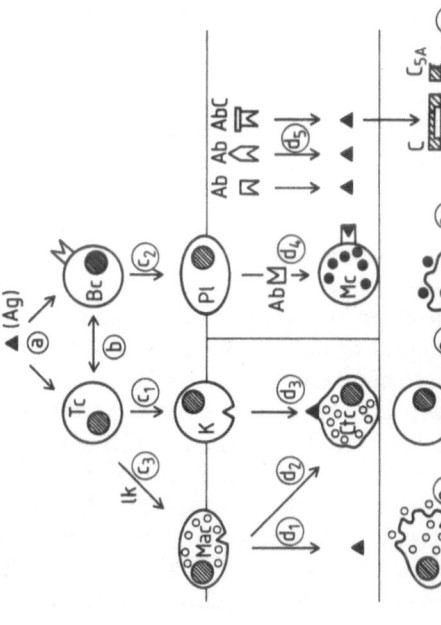

Phases:

1. Induction of immunologic Reactivity

2. Interaction with antigen or antigen-carying cells

3. Release of mediators of inflammation

Resulting inflammatory symptoms:

Tissue destruction   Vascular dilation
and inadequate repair (f_1)   and increased exudation (f_2).

Impaired function, pain, erythema, oedema, warmth

Fig. 1. Processes which might be inhibited by immunosuppressants in inflammation. From the theoretical point of view, the optimal pharmacological armament would be by selectively inhibiting all the processes indicated (a—f_2). In fact, we have at present only non-specific means which interfere not only with many of the processes shown above but also with other body functions as well. The most important effect of current immunosuppressant drugs is the inhibition of the two proliferative steps namely c_1, c_2, and f_1

Whilst the importance of the nucleus and cell surface are well known, the essential functions of the endocellular microtubules are eventually overlooked. They are: (1) to preserve the arrangement of membrane receptors; (2) to divert the flux of vesicle-enclosed material (e.g. phagosomes) from the cell surface to lysosomal or reticular organelles within the cell; (3) to direct a counterflux of cell products (e.g. synthesized in the endoplasmic reticulum) to the cell exterior; and (4) to transform into "spindles" which attach to both the poles and the chromosomes and organize the binary fission of a cell at mitosis. We must emphasize the fact that paralysing the tubular apparatus often has quite far-reaching effects on the behaviour of a cell, beyond just restricting proliferation.

The multiplicity of events which might be blocked or modulated in inflammation by drug-induced cellular stasis is illustrated in Figure 1. In this figure we chose to exemplify possible targets of the action of cytostats in a chronic immunological inflammation, in which persistence of antigenic material is likely to perpetuate the inflammatory process (for details see Chapter 8 of this volume). Even in this type of inflammation, cells that are not immunologically committed will still participate in the inflammatory process. Also, it is obvious from the schema that cytostats may either (1) act by selectively blocking *one* crucial process, e.g. the recruitment of committed "killer cells" which will otherwise destroy both antigen-carrying cells and "innocent bystander" cells, or (2) they could interfere with a *variety* of processes and thus modulate the final outcome of all events, namely one or several of the classical signs of inflammation.

For good reasons it has always been the aim of pharmacologists to develop selective drugs. To achieve this goal in chronic inflammation a variety of in vitro (Table 2) and in vivo (Table 3) assay systems have been developed. They allow one to measure the effects of cytostats on isolated immunological reactions (top of the tables) and also in complex immunological or non-immunological cellular interactions (bottom) which might be relevant to human inflammatory diseases. Using these and other models, a broad variety of cytostats have been tested and were effective in most of the assays listed here (for details see Rosenthale, 1974). These findings enable us to draw two conclusions: (1) the availability of virtually specific assay systems does not immediately lead to the discovery of selective drugs, and (2) all the drugs which will be discussed here exert a wide variety of activities in the human body, of which only some are of therapeutic value. Most of them show side-effects that are only tolerable in serious cases of recurrent or chronic inflammation that resist treatment with less potent or toxic agents.

B. General Pharmacology of Cytostats Effective in Chronic Inflammation

Two previous volumes (XXXVIII/1 and 2) of this handbook deal with antineoplastic/immunosuppressive drugs *in extenso*. It is, therefore, not necessary to detail here the general pharmacodynamics, pharmacokinetics, and toxicology of many of the cytostats, since these aspects are adequately discussed in these earlier volumes. In this section, we shall concentrate on some properties of these drugs, used systemical-

Table 2. Some in vitro assay systems for measuring effects of cytostats

Test system	Cells involved	Literature	Compounds tested	Literature
Lymphocyte stimulation	T-lymphocytes	JANOSSY and GRAVES (1972)	Ara-C, 6-MP, MTX	FARROW and VAN-DYKE (1971) CARON (1969)
Lymphokine production	T-lymphocytes	DUMONDE et al. (1969)	HC	WAHL (1975)
Rosette formation with erythrocytes	T-lymphocytes	JONDAL et al. (1972)	Several immunosuppressants	BACH et al. (1969), BACH and DARDENNE (1971)
Rosette formation with erythrocytes coated with complement	B-lymphocytes	JONDAL et al. (1972)	Several immunosuppressants	MUNRO et al. (1971)
Migration (chemotaxis) of (PMN)	PMN	BOYDEN (1962) KELLER et al. (1972)	Col, vinca alcaloids, 6-MP, AThP	WARD (1971)
Phagocytosis and intracellular killing by PMN	PMN	LEHRER and CLINE (1969) SCHMID and BRUNE (1974)	Col HC	KVARSTEIN and STORMORKEN (1971)
Macrophage (monocyte) migration inhibition	Macrophages	STASTNY et al. (1976)	Ara-C 6-MP 5-FUdR	KAPLAN and CALABRESI (1965)
Counting of ϑ-antigen-bearing lymphocytes	Mainly T-lymphocytes	RAFF (1969)	AThP CP PCZ	QUAGLIATA et al. (1972), YU et al. (1974), HURD and ZIFF (1974)
Counting of antibody-bearing lymphocytes	Mainly B-lymphocytes	PERNIS et al. (1970)	AThP CP	YU et al. (1974), HURD and ZIFF (1974)
Antibody response to diphteria and tetanus toxoids	Mainly B-lymphocytes	CAMPBELL et al. (1964)	6-MP	ROSENBERG and CALABRESI (1963)
Antibody-forming cell-plaque test	Mainly B-lymphocytes	JERNE et al. (1963) KALISS (1971)	AThP CP 6-MP MTX	BERENBAUM (1969) BERENBAUM (1971)
Lymphocyte cytotoxicity	T-, (B-) lymphocytes and complement-producing cells	BACH (1975)	AThP FUdR Cycloheximide ALS	WILSON (1965) MAUEL et al. (1970)
Antigen-induced mediator release from sensitized leucocytes	B-lymphocytes, PMN, mast cells	SHEARD et al. (1967) LEVY (1969)	Col, disodium cromoglycate	LEVY (1969)

Abbreviations: AThP=azathioprine, FUdR=S-fluoro-2'-deoxyuridine, PMN=polymorphonuclear leucocytes (otherwise as in Table 1).

Table 3. Some in vivo assay systems for measuring effects of cytostats in inflammatory reactions

Test systems	Cells of mecha-nisms of main importance	Literature	Compounds tested	Literature
Delayed hypersensitivity:				
1. Graft-vs.-host	T-cell activity	ELKINS (1971)	All important immuno-suppressants	BRUNE (1970) BECK et al. (1973)
2. Homograft	T-cell activity	BILLINGHAM et al. (1971)	All important immuno-suppressants	BERENBAUM (1965)
3. Tuberculin	T-cell activity +monocytes	FLOERSHEIM (1965)	PCZ and other cytostats	FLOERSHEIM (1965)
4. Contact dermatitis	T-cell activity +monocytes	OORT and TURK (1965)	CP MTX	TURK (1964), MAIBACH and MAGUIRE (1969)
5. Experimental allergic en-cephalomyelitis	T-cell activity + other leucocytes	ROSE (1974)	AThP, CP, 6-MP, PCZ, cycloleucine, gold compounds	KOMAREK and DIETRICH (1971), BECK and WHITE-HOUSE (1976)
6. Experimental allergic thyroiditis	T-cell activity + other leucocytes	ROSE (1974)	CP, MTX	SPIEGELBERG and MIESCHER (1963), PATERSON et al. (1971)
7. Adjuvant arthritis, immune arthritis	Lymphocytes + other leucocytes	SWINGLE (1974)	Most anti-inflam-matory drugs	ROSENTHALE (1974) see Chapter 23
"Lupus-like" syndrome in New Zealand black mice	T-cell deficiency (?)	LAMBERT and DIXON (1968)	AThP, CP, 6-MP	LEMMEL et al. (1971), HAHN et al. (1975)
Immediate hypersensitivity:				
1. Arthus-type a) Generalized b) Localized c) Passive d) Reverse passive	Antigen-antibody interaction with leucocytes, the reti-culoentoendothe-lial system and complement	COCHRANE and JANOFF (1974)	All important immuno-suppressants	BOREL and SCHWARZT (1964), AISENBERG and WILKES (1964), ASSEM and MONGAR (1970), GOLDLUST and SCHREIBER (1975)
2. Schwarzmann type a) Generalized b) Localized	Endotoxin inter-action with leuco-cytes, platelets, complement and the reticuloendo-thelial system	LEE and STETSON (1965)	HN-2	HORN and COLLINS (1968)
Irritant inflammations: 1. Heat, UV-light 2. Microcrystals 3. Chemical agents	Non-immunolo-gical reactions, platelets, PMN, monocytes, com-plement, etc.)	SWINGLE (1974)	All important immuno-suppressants	STEVENS and WIL-LOUGHBY (1969), FLOERSHEIM et al. (1973), CURREY (1971b), DUKES et al. (1973), TSU-KADA et al. (1974)

Abbreviatious as in Table 1 and 2

ly, which may be more relevant to their clinical efficacy in treating the inflammatory states, rather than curbing tumours, or the pretreatment of patients for tissue transplantation.

I. "Immunosuppressants"

Several classes of anti-inflammatory drugs are currently believed to exert their anti-inflammatory action, at least in part, by inhibiting immunological processes. Some of these drugs are discussed extensively in other chapters of this volume (see Chap. 32 and 36). By contrast, there are many compounds which both decrease immunological reactivity and impair certain aspects of the inflammatory process in selected experimental systems. However, their clinical effectiveness in chronic inflammatory states in man still remains to be demonstrated. Therefore, the action of these compounds will not be discussed here. What remains is a small group of so-called immunosuppressive drugs which have proved useful in controlled clinical trials to counteract symptoms of chronic inflammation as, for example, in rheumatoid arthritis. These drugs do not appear, however, to act merely by inhibiting some immunological mechanisms alone, since there are several indications that they might interfere with inflammatory processes by other means.

The chemical structures of immunosuppressants, of therapeutic value in the treatment of chronic or relapsing inflammatory states in man, are given in Table 4. It is significant that all of these drugs interfere with cell proliferation. For some, one very distinct site of action has been identified; others may have several sites of action (Table 4). Because these agents cause a generalized depression of cell proliferation, it is inevitable that they will impair a variety of cellular reactions and cell-dependent humoral events in inflammation. Hence these drugs are all potentially toxic, because of their damaging effects on cells and tissues which are not involved in the inflammatory reaction; this would appear to be the basis of their serious side-effects. Although it has been pointed out that several immunosuppressants can at the same time inhibit immunological and non-immunological inflammation in the same person (JOHNSON et al., 1971) there are indications that, for example, some of the alkylating agents (such as cyclophosphamide—CP) predominantly interfere with the immune system and thus exert a major part of their therapeutic effects by inhibiting the recruitment and function of committed lymphocytes in chronic (immunological) inflammation (BACH, 1975).

Since the first report of a successful treatment of patients suffering from rheumatoid arthritis with immunosuppressants more than 20 years ago (DIAZ et al., 1951), numerous clinical reports have appeared (some without appropriate control data) which have generally claimed success with these agents in the management of arthritis (see reviews by CURREY, 1971a; SKINNER and SCHWARTZ, 1974; LEVY and WHITE-HOUSE, 1975). For convenience in discussing them further, these immunosuppressant anti-arthritic drugs will be considered as (1) alkylating agents or (2) anti-metabolites. Immunosuppression with anti-lymphocytic sera (ALS) BACH, 1975) has, as yet, been little explored in arthritis clinics though it is very effective in one anti-arthritic assay in rats (CURREY and ZIFF, 1966, 1968). The corresponding non-pharmacological means of depleting circulating T-lymphocytes (that is achieved with ALS), by removing these cells from the lymph after thoracic duct drainage, has led to dramatic but

Table 4. Structure and action of insert in steads: cytotoxic drugs used to treat inflammation in man

Structure[a]	Mode of action[b]	Side-effects[b]
Alkylating agents Chlorambucil (CBC) Cyclophosphamide (CP)	Transfer of alkyl groups to important cell constituents (such as amino, carboxyl phosphate or sulphhydryl groups thus impairing cell functions. Alkylation of N^7 of guanine in DNA is a crucial reaction leading to: (a) alteration of guanine, forming abnormal base pairs with thymine (miscoding); (b) cleavage of the imidazole ring of guanine (destroying); (c) linking of guanine pairs, (cross-linked DNA strands which cannot replicate); (d) depurination of DNA	Bone marrow depression, gastrointestinal distress, herpes zoster, infections, sterility, alopecia.
 Procarbazine (PCZ)	Uncertain. Inhibitory effects on synthesis of proteins, RNA and DNA in cells. Oxydative breakdown products degrade DNA. They may liberate formaldehyde, azomethine, N-hydroxymethyl derivatives and hydrogen peroxide, responsible for the inhibitory effects? N-methylated PCZ could inhibit methylation of transfer RNA and thus contribute to carcinostatic activity	Alopecia, gastro-intestinal distress, cystitis, sterility, alopecia, predisposition to infections, carcinomas of the bladder (?) Gastrointestinal distress, leuco- and thrombopenic allergic reactions, CNS-depression, interaction with psychotropic substances

Anti-metabolites		
Azathioprine (AThP)	Direct inhibition of T-lymphocytes appears possible. Both agents metabolized intracellularly to their ribonucleotide (6-thioinosinic acid) causing: (a) suppression of purine biosynthesis via 'pseudo-feedback inhibition'; (b) inhibition of formation of adenylic and guanylic acid from iosinic acid; (c) inhibition of interconversion of purine derivatives	Gastro-intestinal distress, allergy, infections, hepatic damage (sarcomas?). Interactions with inhibitors of xanthine oxidase. Leucopenia, hepatitis, gastro-intestinal distress, infections.
6–Mercaptopurine (6–MP)		
Methotrexate (MTX)	Inhibits dihydrofolate reductase, decreases the availability of tetrahydrofolic acid (THF). THF is important for transfer of one-carbon units in biochemical reactions including biosynthesis of thymidylic acid from deoxyuridine 5'-monophosphate and the biosynthesis of inosinic acid, the precursor of adenine and guanine nucleotides	Gastro-intestinal distress, oral and gastro-intestinal ulcerations, diarrhoe, hepatic necrosis. Increased toxicity in patients with impaired renal function. Leucovorin 'rescue' possible

[a] CBC: Chlorambucil, CP: Cyclophosphamide, PCZ: Procarbazine, AThP: Azathioprine, 6-MP: 6-Mercaptopurine, MTX: Methotrexate.
[b] From: GEREBTZOFF et al. (1972), CARTER and SLAVIC (1974), Volume XXXVIII this Handbook series (ELION and HITCHINGS (1975) and REED (1975)).

short-lived reductions in the signs of rheumatoid arthritis (Paulus et al., 1973; Pearson et al., 1975).

1. Alkylating Agents

a) Clinical Effects of Alkylating Agents

Among the alkylating agents chlorambucil (CBC), procarbazine (PCZ), and CP have been employed against chronic inflammatory states (mainly rheumatoid arthritis) in humans. All of these compounds appear to have been highly effective in controlled (see Table 5) and/or uncontrolled trials (see footnote). These drugs improved to some extent the observed clinical parameters of the inflammatory state (such as duration of morning stiffness, number of painful and/or swollen joints, grip strength, time required for a short walk and additional analgesic and/or steroid requirements). Also, in many cases, a reduction of the erythrocyte sedimentation rate and rheumatoid factor titre was observed (Table 5). Two controlled trials with CBC were also performed and both showed uniformly positive results. With CP, six controlled studies (Table 5) have been reported of which five showed clearly positive results whilst one was negative. However, in this study (Lidsky et al., 1972), comparatively low doses were administered; doses which in another study (Cooperating Clinics Committee of the A.R.A., 1972) were only marginally effective. In the same study (Lidsky et al., 1972), no side-effects were reported (as noted by others) indicating that the doses might have been too low for causing clinical measurable improvement. This also stresses the real difficulty in treating chronic inflammatory states with immunosuppressants, namely, that serious side-effects inevitably occur with effective doses. In this context, it is worth mentioning that the two alkylating agents, CP and CBC[1], are almost equally effective in rheumatoid arthritis although they differ considerably in their main side-effects: Whilst hair loss (Decker, 1973) and cystitis (Worth, 1971; Aptekar et al., 1973) are characteristic for treatment with CP, CBC does not cause these effects (Snaith et al., 1973). However, CBC facilitates the development of infections (especially herpes zoster) more frequently than CP (Kahn et al., 1971). When present, these and other side-effects (Tables 4 and 5) necessitated the cessation of therapy in up to 50% of the patients in the trials. This would appear to limit immunosuppressive therapy with these compounds almost exclusively to desperate cases (Gifford, 1973). The side-effect most feared, namely the increased incidence of malignancy which might be expected both from animal studies (Allison, 1970) and from observations of organ transplant patients undergoing immunosuppressive treatment (Penn and Starzle, 1972), has not been observed to the extend feared to date (Kahn and de Seze, 1974).

b) Mode of Action of Alkylating Agents

Aside from the well-known chemical actions of the alkylating agents (see Table 4), attention is directed to drug-sensitive reactions that are (1) probably involved in

---

[1] See for results with the following compounds: CBC; Kahn et al. (1971), Thumb (1972); CP and derivatives: Maldyk and Chwalinska-Sadowska (1970), Alepa et al. (1970), Rau (1971), Weigl et al. (1971), Fricke (1972), Miehlke and Kafarnik (1972), Wawszynska-Pagowska et al. (1973), Hurd and Ziff (1974); PCZ: Thumb (1972); for earlier studies see Currey (1971a).

Table 5. Controlled trials using cyclophosphamide (CP) or chlorambucil (CBC) in rheumatic patients

Drug	Type of study	No. of patients (controls: drugged)	Doses	Administration	Clinical success	Side-effects	Changes in lab. data	Literature
CP	Double-blind. High dose (HD) vs. low doses (LD)	(28:20)	150 mg 15 mg	Daily for 32 weeks	About 40% improvement in LD group about 80% in high dose, radiological examination reveals arrested progression in HD group	LD: 40% experienced minor problems HD: 90% had side-effects: gastrointestinal distress, hair loss, dysuria, haemeturia, hemmorhagic cystitis, herpes zoster	Leucopenia but no correlation with clinical success; greater reduction of immunoglobulins and rheumatoid-factor titres in HD	Cooperating Clinics Committee of the American Rheumatism Association (1970)
CP	Double-blind, high dose (HD) vs. low doses (LD) and medium dose (MD)	54 (No. per group not given)	HD 150 mg MD 75 mg LD 10 mg	Daily for 32 weeks	Dose-related improvement of all clinical parameters	As above plus: convulsions and pneumonia (HD)	Leucopenia in HD correlating with clinical success	Cooperating Clinics Committee of the American Rheumatism Association (1972)
CP	Double-blind cross-over	(11:11)	average: 118 mg (according to WBC)	Daily for 9 months	100% improvement in CP-treated patients	Hair loss in all CP-treated patients, 30% experienced haematuria and 15% cystitis	Antibody responses normal, skin reaction to dinitro-chlorobenzene reduced	Townes et al. (1972)
CP	Double-blind vs. placebo	(11:10)	50 or 75 mg according to weight	Daily for 1 year	No significant improvement	No side-effects	No changes in immunological reactivity but at the beginning B-cell reduction, later T-cell reduction	Curtis et al. (1973) Lidsky et al. (1973)

Table 5 (continued)

Drug	Type of study	No. of patients (controls: drugged)	Doses	Administration	Clinical success	Side-effects	Changes in lab. data	Literature
CP	Double-blind vs. AThP or gold	CP (39): AThP (44): gold (38)	1.5 mg/kg	Daily for more than 48 weeks in 55% of patients	65% improvement as compared to status at the beginning of the trial, CP was more effective than AThP or gold	51% withdrawal due to side-effects as above plus: allergic reactions, amenorrhoea and azoospermia	ESR-improvement, less steroids required	Currey et al. (1974) Woodland (1974)
CP	Double-blind vs. gold	67 (No. per group not specified)	up to 150 mg until leucopenia	Daily (duration not specified)	Significant improvement (not significant for gold)	Few side-effects, did not lead to drug withdrawal	ESR improvement as compared to status at beginning of trial	Gumpel et al. (1974)
CBC	Controlled high dose (HD) vs. low dose (LD); *not double-blind*	(20:20)	0.2 mg/kg (HD) then 0.1 mg/kg (LD)	Daily for 6–12 months Daily for 1 month Daily for 2–3 months	Evaluation (single blind) after 1 year: 90% improvement (HD) 60% improvement (LD)	Infections (herpes zoster)	Significant improvement of ESR and reduced immunoglobulins in HD	Kahn et al. (1971)
CBC	Double-blind vs. placebo	(24:25)	0.2 mg/kg	Daily for 3–4 months	60% improvement (30% improvement in controls)	Not specified	Improved ESR, reduced immunoglobulins, delayed skin reactions unchanged	Hatchuel et al. (1972) quoted from De Seze and Kahn (1974)

Abbreviations: ESR = erythrocyte sedimentation rate, WBC = white blood cell count.

immunologically sustained inflammations (see Fig. 1), and (2) other pathways of the inflammatory response which might be selectively or predominantly suppressed by different alkylating agents. However, claims for a clearly selective effect of these compounds on one specific receptor, mediator or cell system have not been clearly established. CP and CBC (and many other compounds which have not been extensively used in the clinic) interfered with a wide variety of cellular processes (HILL, 1975) and exerted inhibitory actions as assessed by a variety of in vivo and in vitro systems used to detect immunosuppressive and/or anti-inflammatory effects (see Tables 2 and 3). They were also found, in effective doses, to suppress not only the (clearly immunological) inflammatory response to antigens but also to simple irritants (JOHNSON et al., 1971). However, several authors have noted the absence of any impairment of immunological reactivity (both cellular and humoural) in patients showing clear signs of the remission of inflammation (DENMAN et al., 1970; LIDSKY et al., 1972; CURTIS et al., 1973). In general, effective treatment with alkylating agents causes a certain degree of leucopenia. Nevertheless selective and lasting reduction in the number of either T or B cells has not been observed even though at some stages of treatment a comparatively high degree of T (or B) cell reduction or dysfunction was noted by several authors (WINKELSTEIN et al., 1972; STRONG et al., 1973; HURD and GUILIANO, 1975).

Although the mode of action of alkylating agents is essentially non-specific, the therapeutic ratios of CBC and CP compare favourably with other alkylating agents, e.g. nitrogen mustard. This could be mainly due to a specific metabolic pattern and/or pharmacokinetic behaviour by these compounds. A later section (B.II) discusses the formation of pharmaco-active metabolites of CP and distribution of relatively high concentrations of the active metabolite to inflamed tissues.

Regretably little information is available concerning the metabolism or distribution of CBC or PCZ (see also Vol. XXXVIII in this series) which might explain the therapeutic effectiveness of these drugs (THUMB, 1972).

In summary, the alkylating agents probably have multifactorial actions in inflammation, with only some selectivity towards immunologically-committed cell populations. Their anti-proliferative effect on other types of leucocytes and connective tissue cells probably also contributes towards the beneficial effects of these drugs observed in chronic inflammation.

c) Loci of Action of Alkylating Agents

At least two sites of action of these drugs can be distinguished—(1) within the cell nucleus, and (2) at the cell periphery—depending on how the physicochemical properties of a given drug or reactive metabolite restrict its penetration into the cell interior. Those acting on the cell nucleus may show some, perhaps not very marked, cellular selectivity. Since cell-penetrant metabolites alkylate nuclear proteins and DNA with little specificity, the degree of cellular activity attained is primarily due to the differing capacities of different cells to "buffer" or neutralise the alkylating mustards and their aldehyde metabolites whilst in transit between the cellular envelope and the chromosomal/nucleolar nucleoproteins. Thus, cells with ample reserves of thiols, e.g. glutathione, will inactivate both nitrogen mustards and cytotoxic aldehydes, especially acrolein. Cells lacking such a thiol reserve or alternative inactivating systems (e.g. oxidative enzymes), will be the first to be affected by these cytotoxic products. Obviously repeated drug dosing may annihilate this differential intercellar sensitivity as the thiol resources of even the most thiol-abundant cells become exhausted.

Nuclear intoxications may not be expressed until the cell is stimulated to divide, so there may be a "memory" of the drug action, i.e. no immediate response to the drug/metabolite while an appreciable amount of the active drug or its precursor is maintained in the circulation. It is important to understand this "hit and run" property of these alkylating drugs, largely based on their irreversible interaction with the receptor's functional groups, forming covalent linkages with the receptor. By contrast, most of the other types of anti-inflammatory drugs now used in the clinic, including the steroids, associate reversibly with their receptors (forming mainly hydrophobic or ionic bonds therewith) and their efficacy and duration of action is chiefly governed by the pool of unmetabolised drug in the circulation or other labile stores.

Alkylation of the cell exterior (exoalkylation) is another possible site of drug action, which differs from nuclear alkylation (endoalkylation) in at least two respects: (1) the drug action may be apparent very soon after the active metabolite is distributed to the blood and lymph; (2) the drug action may be highly restricted, particularly if the receptor happens to have a limited distribution on the surface of different cell types. Where it is uniquely associated with the disease, e.g. virus adsorbed to the surface of certain cells, but not to others, then EHRLICH's ideal drug (which he likened to a magic bullet) may be realised.

There is some evidence that portions of DNA may be present at the exterior of certain cell types, especially lymphoid cells, in leukemia and rheumatoid arthritis—presenting a suitable "target" for therapy with platinum drugs and CP metabolites (WHITEHOUSE, 1975). Both CBC itself and carboxyphosphamide, a polar metabolite of CP (see Sect. C.II.1.), have some affinity for cell surface receptors but do not readily penetrate into the cell interior (LINFORD et al., 1963; WHITEHOUSE et al., 1974b; DRÄGER and HOHORST, 1976) and would appear to fall into this category of exoalkylating drugs.

One consequence of exoalkylation is that the cell exterior is primarily compromised by the drug and, provided the essential selective barriers of the cell membrane are not affected, then cell vitality may be unimpaired while the exoalkylated receptor is functional/non-functional vis à vis its former non-functional/functional status (see e.g. GUTTMANN, 1974). Thus, a cryptic viral infection or tumour that was formerly tolerated may now be recognised by the immune defences because the affected cell surface acquires a higher immunogenic profile through alkylation. Conversely, a pathogenic DNA or protein sequence at the cell surface may be sufficiently "scrambled" by alkylation that it can no longer participate in, or sustain, a cell-cell or cell-messenger molecule interaction that was formerly a pacemaker event in the overall pathology. Alternatively, a rather specific membrane function of one cell class may be affected. Thus, CBC inhibits the uptake and transport of exogenous pyrimidine and purines into leucemic lymphocytes by blocking base/nucleoside permeation; a property shared with certain non-alkylating cytostats, e.g. procarbazine and cortisol (KUMMER and OCHS, 1970).

2. Anti-Metabolites

a) Clinical Effects of Anti-Metabolites

A number of anti-metabolites have been employed for the treatment of chronic inflammatory states. Methotrexate (MTX), formerly a drug used extensively to treat psoriasis, has been employed in the treatment of psoriatic arthritis, but with little success (FELDGES and BARNES, 1974). Azathioprine (AThP) and its metabolite 6-mercaptopurine (6-MP) have proved very useful in rheumatoid arthritis (CURREY, 1971a). In the past few years, AThP has been used in a series of uncontrolled (MIEHLKE and KOHLHARDT, 1970; CURREY, 1971a; KÖLLE et al., 1972; FRICKE, 1972; THUMB, 1972; APOSTOLOFF et al., 1974) and controlled trials (Table 6). With one exception, a measurable clinical improvement was noted in the controlled trials—not to the same degree as that seen with CP but quite comparable to the positive effects seen with gold therapy in a control group (CURREY et al., 1974). With the doses employed, the side-effects were less frequent and/or less serious than those in CPA-treated patients or in patients receiving gold therapy. However, this cannot be taken as proof against the effectiveness of AThP in rheumatoid arthritis (NICHOLS et al., 1973): only 14 patients with advanced stages of rheumatoid arthritis with vasculitis were investigated in this study. Hence, any generalizations from these observations obtained from such a small, selected group of patients are probably not justified.

Controlled trials using 6-MP or MTX have not been reported. This is probably a consequence of claims that the therapeutic ratio is more favourable for AThP in comparison with its (active) metabolite 6-MP (BACH, 1975), although this claim is not universally accepted (BERTINO, 1973). On the other hand, the characteristic serious side effects of MTX in humans, namely development of oral and gastrointestinal ulcerations and hepatic damage (DECKER, 1973), limits the use of this compound in inflammation to otherwise unresponsive cases of psoriasis.

It may, therefore, be concluded that AThP among the anti-metabolites comprises a relatively safe and effective compound for the treatment of chronic inflammatory states in humans. It should be borne in mind that AThP facilitates the development of reticulum sarcomas, at least in immunosuppressed recipients for renal transplants (WALKER et al., 1971).

b) Mode of Action of Anti-Metabolites

In searching for an explanation for the beneficial effects of anti-metabolites, especially AThP, one is tempted to attribute this effect to the non-specific anti-proliferative potency of these compounds. This effect, in contrast to the immunosuppressive activity, is even more evident with anti-metabolites than with alkylating agents (see above). Although AThP in clinically effective doses caused some reduction of the number of T- and B-lymphocytes along with a generalized leucopenia, the functions of these immunological competent cells (as assessed in vitro and in vivo) are essentially unchanged (YU et al., 1974; LEVY et al., 1972). This latter observation has been confirmed in studies from experimental animals. ARINOVICHE and LOEWI (1970) tested the potency of AThP in the suppression of a variety of immunological and non-immunological inflammations. They found that AThP, in contrast to CPA and anti-lymphocytic globulins, suppressed only the non-immunological inflammations

Table 6. Controlled trials using azathioprine in rheumatic patients

Type of study	No. of patients (controls:drugged)	Doses	Administration	Clinical successs	Side-Effects	Changes in lab. data	Literature
Double-blind crossover	(24:24)	3 mg/kg	Daily for 6 months either placebo or AThP	83% improvement	Leucopenia, Gastro-intestinal diseases	Reduced immuno-globulin levels, delayed hypersensitivity to different agents unchanged, reduced number of B and T cells	LEVY et al. (1972) Compiled by YU et al. (1974)
Double-blind vs. placebo	(8:7)	2.5 mg/kg	Daily, for an average of 27 weeks	No improvement (of vasculitis)	3 deaths in AThP-group, 2 deaths in control group unrelated to treatment, 1 withdrawal due to vomiting	No change in PHA-stimulation lymphocytes, no change in number of platelets	NICHOLS et al. (1973)
Double-blind crossover	(17:17)	2–2.5 mg/kg	Daily for 16 weeks either placebo or AThP then up to 40 weeks	60% improvement	Gastro-intestinal distress, thrombocytopenia, herpes zoster, chromosomal breaks	ESR and rheumatoid factor titer unchanged	UROWITZ (1973) HUNTER (1975)
Double-blind vs. CP or gold	AThP (44): CP (39): gold (38)	2.5 mg/kg	Daily for more than 48 weeks in 50% of patients	55% improvement	Leucopenia, allergies, gastro-intestinal distress	ESR improvement, smaler amounts of steroid required	CURREY et al. (1974) WOODLAND et al. (1974)

Abbreviations: PHA = phytohaemagglutinin. Otherwise as in Table 5.

but left the immunologic reactions unimpaired. Also PERINGS et al. (1971) observed an even more pronounced inhibition of exudate formation after croton-oil injection with high doses of AThP than with corticocosteroids. Correspondingly, CPA was clearly more effective in prolonging the survival or preventing the development of glomerulonephritis of NZB/NZW-mice suffering from immuno-deficiency diseases than AThP (STEINBERG et al., 1975). It appears that AThP (and other anti-metabolites) owe their effectiveness in inflammation mostly to their anti-proliferative activity and only in a minor degree to their immunosuppressive potency.

c) Pharmacokinetics of Anti-Metabolites

It is generally assumed that 6-thioinosinic acid is the most active anti-metabolite derived from AThP and 6-MP (Table 6). However, it is not entirely clear to what extent AThP and 6-MP serve only as precursors of 6-thioinosinic acid or have anti-proliferative/immunosuppressive potency of their own. It is well established in selected immunological systems that AThP is superior in potency compared with 6-MP (BACH, 1975). On the other hand, in man, AThP is no more potent as a cytostatic drug (RUNDLES et al., 1961) but it appears to have fewer side-effects than 6-MP (ELION and HITCHINGS, 1975). This could be a consequence of the slow and prolonged release of 6-MP from AThP mediated by sulphhydryl-groups in plasma and cells. Claims that AThP might be preferentially transformed in lymphocytes, thus causing selective immunosuppressive effects, have not been substantiated by either clinical observations or experimental findings (ELION, 1972).

As long as it is not entirely clear which compound (AThP, 6-MP or one of its metabolites) is the active principle in suppressing chronic inflammations, one cannot gain much further insight into the mode of action of these anti-metabolites in chronic inflammation. It is known that the rate-limiting step in the bio-inactivation of both AThP and 6-MP is the transformation of the latter to thiouric acid by the enzyme xanthine oxidase. Simultaneous administration of inhibitors of this enzyme, to decrease uric acid formation in gouty persons, requires reduction of the dose of AThP or 6-MP to about one-quarter (BERTINO, 1973).

In contrast to AThP and 6-MP the mode of action, pharmacokinetics and toxicology of MTX is fairly clear (see BERTINO, 1975). Of interest is the fact that accumulation of MTX, due to the presence of specific transport mechanisms, was observed in the liver, kidney and intestinal mucosa. This may explain the high incidence of liver necrosis and intestinal ulcerations observed in patients treated with MTX (DECKER, 1973; BERTINO, 1975). Also, the almost exclusive elimination of MTX via the kidney may lead to inappropriate dosage and severe toxicity in patients with impaired renal function. If MTX is used in patients with kidney dysfunction, leucovorin "rescue" should be utilized if drug excretion is delayed significantly (BERTINO, 1975).

II. Microtubular Inhibitors

Of the microtubular inhibitors, only one compound and its analogues is of great interest, namely colchicine (Col). Vinblastin and its analogues have not been used extensively in chronic inflammatory states (see Vol. XXXVIII of this Handbook series). A derivative of podophyllotoxin could be effective in relieving the symptoms of rheumatoid arthritis (WAWRZYNSKA-PAGOWSKA et al., 1973), but it is still not clear whether this agent appears superior to the alkylating agents because of the absence of appropriate controls in this trial.

1. Colchicine

a) Clinical Effects

The beneficial effect of Col and its analogues in the treatment of acute attacks of gouty arthritis is well known. However, less well known are the therapeutic effects of Col and other microtubular inhibitors in (1) *preventing* regularly relapsing inflammatory events like gout and Familial Mediterranean Fever, and (2) inflammatory episodes connected with chronic degenerative disease, such as osteoarthritis or delayed-type inflammatory reactions as in erythema nodosum or chronic (immunological) inflammatory diseases such as sarcoid arthritis. Since we believe the effectiveness of microtubular inhibitors under these conditions offers some clue not only to the understanding of these diseases but also to the mode of action of microtubular inhibitors in inflammation, some aspects of their pharmacology should be considered (see Table 7; WALLACE, 1974; FITZGERALD, 1974; SPILBERG, 1975; SOIFER, 1975). Recent studies indicate that Col appears still to be a valuable drug in preventing gouty attacks, especially at the beginning of treatment of tophaceous gout, even when used together with allopurinol and/or probenecid (or other inhibitors of generation or reabsorption of uric acid in the human body) (see Table 8). It also appears to have the unique property of preventing the regularly occuring relapses of Familial Mediterranean Fever but it does not cure these episodes (WALLACE, 1974) (see Table 8). The effectiveness of Col in these situations cannot be explained by the popular concept that it acts in preventing these inflammatory conditions by interfering with granulocyte function (SPILBERG, 1975; CHANG and MALAWISTA, 1975), although the impairment of granulocyte functions may explain why Col alleviates the symptoms of gout. There is no indication that these cells precipitate an attack of either gout or Familial Mediterranean Fever. Also, Col has been shown to be effective in reducing swelling and pain in degenerative and immunologic inflammation such as in osteoarthritis or sarcoid arthritis (Table 8), inflammatory events which are generally believed to take place without the major involvement of granulocytes. Furthermore, a recent report describes an attack of gout and its cure by Col in a patient suffering from almost complete granulocytopenia (ORTEL and NEWCOMBE, 1974). Finally, another microtubular inhibitor, podophyllic acid ethylhydrazide (Proresid) has been reported to have outstanding effects in severe cases of rheumatoid arthritis (WAWRZYNSKA-PAGOWSKA et al., 1973) and, in these cases, to be superior to other cytostats or immunosuppressants, causing less serious side effects than CP. The above evidence indicates that microtubules, in a wide variety of cellular systems, might be involved and correspondingly inhibited by microtubular inhibitors in inflammation (BRUNE et al., 1975).

b) Mode of Action

Microtubular inhibitors such as Col show a variety of effects in experimental systems which could help to explain their therapeutic actions in different inflammatory

Table 7. Structure and action of microtubular inhibitors used to treat inflammation in man

Structure	Mode of action[a]	Side-effects[a]
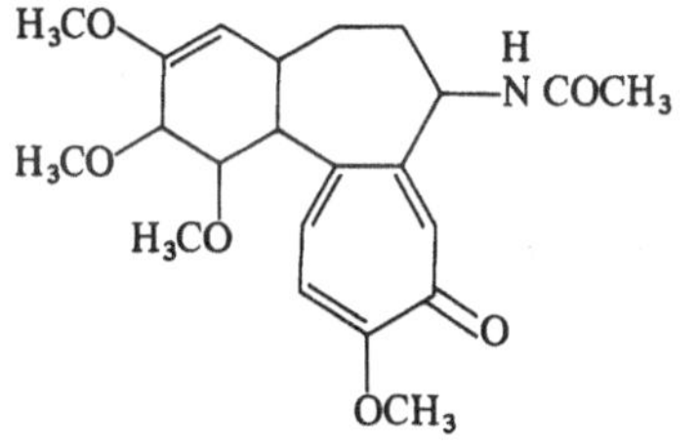 Anti-tubulins	Interferes with microtubule assembly, causes: 1. Impaired locomotion of cells 2. Inhibited membrane functions 3. Reduced (or increased) mediator release 4. Reduced transcellular transport 5. Mitotic arrest	p.o. administration: diarrhoea, nausea, vomiting, malabsorption; i.v.: venous irritation; long term administration: bone marrow depression, sterility (?), alopecia, increased incidence of Down's syndrome (?)

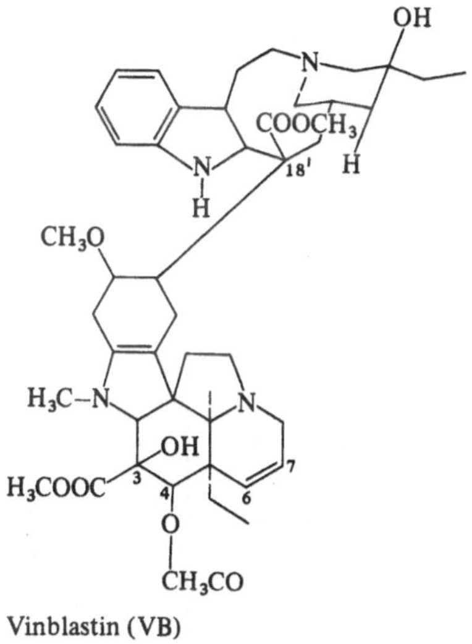

H$_3$CO, H$_3$CO, H$_3$CO, —N COCH$_3$, H, O, OCH$_3$

Colchicine (Col)

OH, N, COOCH$_3$, 18', H, N, H, CH$_3$O, H$_3$C—N, N, OH, H$_3$COOC, 3, 4, 6, 7, O, CH$_3$CO

Vinblastin (VB)

| | Destroys assembled microtubules and causes: the same effects as Col, but impairment of some functions, e.g. inhibition of mitosis and DNA-RNA assembly is more prominent | As with Col, plus-neurotoxicity |

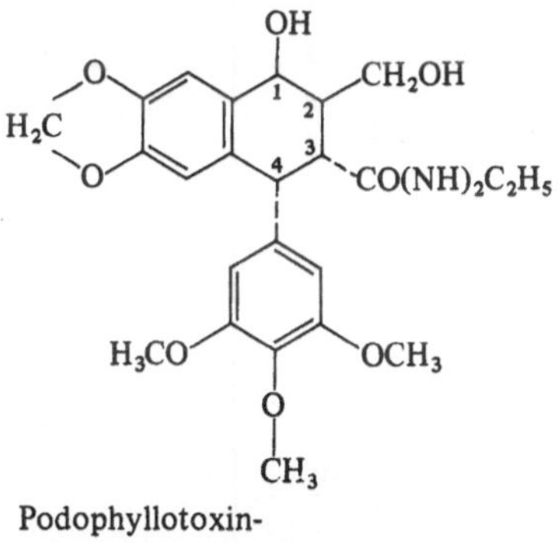

OH, CH$_2$OH, H$_2$C, O, O, 1, 2, 3, 4, CO(NH)$_2$C$_2$H$_5$, H$_3$CO, OCH$_3$, O, CH$_3$

Podophyllotoxin-ethylhydrazide(PEH)

| | Interferes with microtubule assembly (and destroys) assembled microtubules. Effects similar to Col, and vinblastin | As with Col, plus: increased incidence of infections |

[a] From: GEREBTZOFF et al. (1972), CARTER and SLAVIC (1974), Volume *XXXVIII* this Handbook series and literature quoted in the text.

Table 8. Effects of colchicine in different clinical inflammatory states

Disease	Dose/administration	Clinical effects	Assumed mode of action	References
Gouty arthritis	Curative: p.o.: 0.5 mg/h until relieved or 8 mg total i.v.: 3 mg/day Prophylactic: p.o.: 1 mg/day	Dramatic relief within 48 h, gastrointestinal side-effects. Dramatic relief within 24 h, almost no side-effects; reduces incidence of attacks	Interference with leucocyte function + interference with synovial lining cells + interference with endo- thelia; unexplained	Spilberg (1975) Wallace (1974) Brune et al. (1975)
Familial Mediterranean Fever (periodic polyserositis)	Curative: as in gout Prophylactic: as in gout	No effect Dramatic reduction in incidence of attacks	Unexplained Unexplained	Ehrlich (1973) Goldfinger (1972) Goldfinger (1973)
Sarcoid arthritis	Curative: as in gout Prophylactic: as in gout	Dramatic relief (not in all cases) Reduction in incidence of attacks	Unexplained Unexplained	Kaplan (1960) Kaplan (1963) Wallace et al. (1967)
Pseudogout	Curative: as in gout	Dramatic or moderate response	Unexplained (possibly as in gout)	McCarty and Gatter (1966) Thompson et al. (1968)
Erythema nodosum	Curative: as in gout	Good response	Unexplained	Wallace et al. (1967)
Rheumatoid arthritis Osteoarthritis	Curative: as in gout	Some good responses	Unexplained	Wallace (1974) (review of several trials)

states. Firstly, they change the organization and function of receptors and/or transport mechanisms located on the cell surface (BERLIN, 1975a). These effects on the outer cell membrane might be responsible for some cytostatic effects by affecting the uptake of essential nutritents, e.g. uridine, adenosine, lysine (MIZEL and WILSON, 1972). Any inhibition of essential transport mechanisms could lead to reduced cellular performance and division in inflammatory states. Secondly, microtubules channel the transport of extracellular material wrapped in vesicles towards lysosomes and other intracellular compartments (WRIGHT and MALAWISTA, 1972). Drug-induced tubulostasis may lead to reduced digestion of phagocytized material. On the other hand, it could prevent metabolic transformation of this material or the metabolism-associated energy transduction (MALAWISTA and BODEL, 1967). These events are assumed to play a role in the generation of inflammatory mediators. They could also perpetuate the persistence of inflammatory stimuli by, for example, the de novo precipitation of urate crystals in gout (compare Chap. 35a of this volume). Thirdly, microtubules control the excretion of secretory vacuole-bound material (e.g. histamine) and also probably interfere with the transcellular transport of high molecular weight molecules. The movement of plasma proteins across endothelial membrane in experimental inflammations (GLATT et al., 1974), during attacks of gouty arthritis or Familial Mediterrenean Fever, may thus be inhibited by these drugs and the resulting oedema then reduced.

Finally, microtubular inhibitors interfere with the generation of the spindle apparatus required for mitosis and thus have a direct anti-proliferative effect. This property might be of considerable importance for the reduction of pannus, after local administration of podophyllic acid ethylhydrazide into rheumatic joints (chemical synovectomy) (CHLUD et al., 1972).

In conclusion, microtubular inhibitors may exert anti-inflammatory actions acting along a variety of pathways. It seems that this old and enigmatic drug, Col, may serve as a very useful tool for elucidating cellular events in inflammation while it still retains its position in modern medicine as a selective therapeutic agent. A better understanding of the cytostatic events following administration of Col would certainly help the development of other microtubular inhibitors specifically designed to modulate pathophysiological processes originating in certain other compartments in human disease. Our present knowledge of the pharmacodynamics and pharmacokinetics of Col is rather incomplete and much more experimental work on these topics is still needed.

c) Pharmacokinetics and Side-Effects

Extensive information on the pharmacokinetics and side-effects of Col may be obtained from the recent review by WALLACE (1974). The toxic reactions following the clinical use of microtubular inhibitors are listed in Tables 7 and 8. Gastro-intestinal side-effects are only observed after oral administration. This points to some peculiarities of the pharmacokinetics of Col (and possibly other microtubular inhibitors) of which the main features are:

1. Col is taken up avidly by almost all cells of the body. As a consequence, the plasma concentration falls rapidly and does not reflect any enhanced excretion of the compounds.

2. Col is distributed unequally throughout the body. It appears as if cells which have been in early contact with Col take up large quantities of the drug. Thus, after oral administration, high concentrations are found in the cells of the small intestine and the drug persists in this tissue for long periods of time. After i.v. administration, the liver, spleen, and leucocytes (i.e. organs or cells which are "blood-bathed") take up large amounts of Col. Although detailed information is lacking, it can be assumed that vascular endothelia also take up relatively large quantities of Col, which might explain the inhibition of increased vascular permeability normally seen in inflamed tissue (GLATT et al., 1974). These observations offer a plausible explanation for the action of Col in so many different types of inflammation.

C. Some Properties of Selected Compounds

I. Microtubular Inhibitors

Recent reviews and monographs have intensively reviewed the biology (SOIFER, 1975), biochemistry (FITZGERALD, 1974), pharmacology (FITZGERALD, 1974; CHANG and MALAWISTA, 1975) and clinical importance (WALLACE, 1974) of these compounds. We shall, therefore, concentrate on a few aspects of their pharmacology and mode of action which appear somewhat neglected.

Vinblastin is not an acceptable anti-inflammatory drug, (for details of the pharmacological properties of this compound see CREASEY, 1975; Vol. XXXVIII of this Handbook). Podophyllotoxin and its derivatives appear to have a variety of properties of which the cytotoxic effects are more pronounced than with Col; this may be responsible for some very encouraging results in the treatment of rheumatoid arthritis (WAWRZYNSKA-PAGOWSKA et al., 1973). However, very little pharmacological data on this compound has yet been published. It is, therefore, too early to speculate why podophyllic acid ethylhydrazide is more effective than other microtubular inhibitors. What remains is the fact that one of the oldest and most enigmatic agents, namely Col (or its analogues and derivatives) is so effective in a variety of chronic or recurrent inflammatory states.

1. Cytostatic Effects of Colchicine

a) Locomotion of Cells

It is well documented that Col inhibits the locomotion of granulocytes. On the other hand, there are claims that it does not interfere with the appearance of monocytes in an inflamed tissue (PERPER et al., 1974). However, nothing is known about any comparable effect on other inflammatory cells, e.g. lymphocytes and mast cells. Since all cells contain microtubules it would appear that inhibition of motility by Col (1) is more apparent in only one specific cell type, or (2) under different circumstances precludes all motile cells from entering into inflamed areas.

b) Membrane Effects of Colchicine

Col inhibits a variety of uptake mechanisms which supply the cell with essential nutritients (UKENA and BERLIN, 1972; MIZEL and WILSON, 1972). This effect, however, may not entirely be due to inhibition of microtubules because lumicolchicine, being devoid of antitubular action, is also effective (MIZEL and WILSON, 1972), although only in somewhat higher concentrations. In low (μM) concentrations Col also changes the arrangement of cell surface receptors which are essential for information transmission from the surface to the cell interior and thus suppresses the usual cell reaction towards different message molecules (YAHARA and EDELMAN, 1975). At the same low concentrations, the amount of membrane lipids containing unsaturated essential fatty acids translocated from the cell surface to the cell interior with phagocytic vacuoles during phagocytosis is increased. This results in decreased fluidity of the outer cell membrane (BERLIN, 1975b) and may explain two effects observed with Col in inflammation: Col decreases oedema formation and increases prostaglandin release in inflamed tissue (BRUNE et al., 1975). Whilst the changes of the cell membrane might contribute to the alteration of transport of materials across cells (see Sect. C.I.1.c below) and thus contribute to the anti-inflammatory action, the increased incorporation of unsaturated fatty acids may cause the increased release of prostaglandins. The latter effect is possibly not causally related to the anti-inflammatory action of Col.

c) Channelling of Ingested Material

Col interferes with the uptake of ingested material within the cells and so inhibits the fusion of phagocytic vacuoles with lysosomes (MALAWISTA and BODEL, 1967; HOFF-STEIN et al., 1974). Together with the increased transformation of vacuolar components by cytoplasmic enzymes and so forth, this effect points to a poorly understood field of cellular biology. We do not know which role this intracellular transport and metabolism plays in inflammation. It may well be that it regulates the generation of inflammatory mediators which after release result in inflammatory symptoms.

d) Release of Mediators

Col inhibits the release of mediators as, for example, cortisol, thyroxin, catecholamines etc. (WALLACE, 1974). It also increases the liberation of prostaglandins from as yet uncertain sources (GLATT et al., 1976). Both these Col-sensitive events, and probably a variety of other release processes, may play key roles in inflammation.

e) Transcellular Transport

Col, partly together with other pharmacological agents, blocks not only the transcellular movement of macromolecules—as for example in intestinal absorption—but also the movement of water and salts across cells (TAYLOR et al., 1975). These effects, at present little understood, could explain the malabsorption syndrome seen in patients treated with oral Col (WALLACE and ERTEL, 1969) and also the almost complete inhibition of oedema formation in experimental inflammations (GLATT et al., 1974).

II. Cyclophosphamide

1. Metabolism

a) Bioactivation

The general pharmacology of this very potent pro-drug has been extensively reviewed by HILL (1975). It is not actually a drug per se but must first be bioactivated to generate a range of metabolic products with varying degrees of cytotoxic, cyto-static and anti-inflammatory activity. This complicates the description of the compound's pharmacological profile, for of necessity we must actually consider the overall sum of the individual activities of each pharmaco-active metabolite. Some of these only exert their action in specific compartments, whilst others are more ubiquitous in their distribution and drug action. The effective half-lives of the different active metabolites, as well as their differing bio-distribution, must also be taken into account in any attempt to describe how CP can, when administered over different time schedules, promote or break tolerance, suppress or enhance an immune response, facilitate tissue grafting, depress the bone marrow or stimulate haemopoietic recovery, suppress tumour growth or promote the establishment of tumours and also suppress the very same inflammatory processes which may permit the establishment of a tumour. This list of ambivalent effects of CP can be extended to include tissue irritancy, as well as anti-inflammatory activity, engendered by its metabolites (Whitehouse and Beck, 1975).

This pro-drug is also remarkably versatile for quite another reason; its action is not particularly dependent upon the stage in the cell cycle that the target cell may have reached. For this reason, it is potentially toxic to a large number of tissues, regardless of how rapidly the individual cells of that tissue may be turning over. In the whole animal, therefore, it is extremely difficult to assign the activity to a specific effect upon a given cell population, to the exclusion of many other cell populations. What is conveniently designated the toxic effects of the drug may be no more than a fairly accurate reflection of the actual therapeutic effects of the drug, albeit perhaps on another tissue or cell population that is more intimately associated with the inflammatory disease. Perhaps the most remarkable feature of this pro-drug is the fact that it can be used with confidence in man outside the context of a terminal disease. Its therapeutic index, relative to other alkylating agents, is fairly high—probably because the unchanged pro-drug and its principal metabolites are readily cleared from the body, principally through the kidneys.

b) Pathways

This has been the subject of several recent reviews (Montgomery and Struck, 1973; Connors, 1974; Torkelson et al., 1974; Hill, 1975) and will only be outlined here. The hepatic endoplasmic reticulum is the prime site of drug activation. The principal products of this process are the 4-oxyderivatives: 4-hydroxycyclophosphamide II (which is actually the cyclic aldehyde-ammonia compound in tautomeric equilibrium with the acyclic aldehyde, aldophosphamide III), and possibly also the 4-hydroperoxy compound I (which may be an intermediate in the formation of II) (see Table 9).

In the context of inflammation, it would be valuable to know if there were any local drug bioactivation within an inflammatory cell population. Lymphocytes stimulated by aryl hydrocarbons or lectins are known to contain cytochrome P_{450} and to hydroxylate xenobiotics, e.g. benzo(a)pyrene (Kellerman et al., 1973) including CP (Singer and Brody, 1972), while the unstimulated cells lack this activity. The raised level of superoxide ion and other oxygenating species in certain leucocyte populations (De Chatelet et al., 1974; Fridovich, 1974) might provide another initiator of local drug activation within an inflammatory focus.

Table 9. Some biotransformations of cyclophosphamide in mammals

The hydroxymetabolite (aldophosphamide) formed in the liver then enters into at least three different metabolic pathways: (1) the acyclic form III is detoxified in situ by aldehyde oxidases, yielding the corresponding carboxylate, carboxyphosphamide IV, a principal metabolite of CP in the urine and bile; (2) the cyclic form, with which it is in equilibrium (4-hydroxycyclophosphamide, III) may be oxidised by a dehydrogenase in the hepatic cytosol to the corresponding 4-oxocyclophosphamide (V), a minor urinary and biliary metabolite of CP that is devoid of cytostatic activity. Thus, this is another pathway of aldophosphamide detoxication; (3) it spontaneously decomposes by β elimination of acrolein (VI) generating the phosphoramide mustard VII (N,N-bis(2-chloroethyl)phosphorodiamidic acid) (COLVIN et al., 1973; CONNORS et al., 1974), which has been detected in human blood and urine (FENSELAU et al., 1975); (4) it is exported from the liver and carried in the blood as a latent or masked type, from which it can be obtained by trapping with semicarbazide to form the relatively stable semicarbazone (SLADEK, 1973a). This transport form of (IV) is probably an aldimine or thiohemiacetal, formed by reversible combination of the -CHO group with plasma (albumin)-NH_2 or SH groups. Decomposition of this masked product in the peripheral tissues then liberates the reactive lipophilic aldehyde (IV), which can enter into the cells of the peripheral tissues, decompose irreversibly therein by pathway (3), thereby generating both acrolein (VI) and the reactive phosphoramide mustard (VII) within the cell. The charged phosphate group on (VII) minimises its egress and effectively traps this mustard intracellularly. 3-Hydroxypropylmercapturic acid, a known metabolite of acrolein (KAYE, 1973) is present in the urine of rats or humans receiving CP (KAYE and YOUNG, 1974).

Studies of the metabolism and in vivo pharmaco-activity of some simple CP derivatives have substantiated the essential accuracy of this concept of CP activation via 4-hydroxylation. Thus, 4-monomethyl-CP is readily oxidised in vivo (or in vitro) and is an effective drug precursor, generating (VII) and 3-buten-2-one (in place of acrolein) (THOMSON and COLVIN, 1974). Since pathways (1) and (2), above, cannot be followed by the 4-hydroxymetabolite of 4-methyl CP, it was predicted and verified that 4-methyl CP would have to be more toxic than CP, i.e. exhibit a lower therapeutic index (Cox et al., 1975). Both 4,4-dimethyl CP and 5,5-dimethyl CP are however devoid of CP-like activity in vivo; the former because it cannot be hydroxylated at position C_4 (essential for rupturing the cyclic oxazaphorane ring); the latter because the corresponding dimethyl analogue of (III) cannot undergo β elimination to liberate (VII) as it lacks a hydrogen atom at C_5 (Cox et al., 1976). Likewise, CP derivatives in which both the 4 and 5, or 5 and 6, positions have been blocked by fusion with a benzene ring, fail to show CP-like activity (LUDEMAN and ZOM, 1975).

There is another pathway of CP decomposition that does yield some bioreactive metabolites, by oxidative alkylation of the side-chain, yielding chloracetaldehyde (VIII) and deschlorethyl-CP (IX). The experimental evidence for this alternative pathway is at present far less abundant and its existence has been chiefly inferred from the known biological transformations of related nitrogen mustards (CONNORS et al., 1973; NORPOTH et al., 1975; NORPOTH, 1976; Cox et al., 1976), the cytotoxic/immunosuppressant activity of chloracetaldehyde (VIII) (WHITEHOUSE et al., 1974a), chemical oxidation of CP (JARMAN, 1973) and the detection of (IX) as a minor metabolite of CP in sheep and mouse plasma (BAKKE et al., 1972; STRUCK et al., 1975; STRUCK, 1976), and in incubations of CP with rat liver microsomes (CONNORS et al., 1974). Even if it is only a minor pathway of CP metabolism in the liver, its occurrence in peripheral tissue would still be very important for understanding the pharmacology of CP.

The most obvious potential pathway of CP decomposition, involving hydrolysis of the P-N bond and liberation of bis(chloroethyl)amine (X) = "nor-nitrogen mustard", was formerly considered to be of little significance in determining the overall pharmacological activity of CP in vivo. However, the recent isolation of not only (X) but also two of its further transformation products, the piperazine mustard (XI) and 3-(2-chloroethyl)-1,3-oxazolidone (XII) from the urine of patients treated with CP (Cox and LEVIN, 1975) or mice treated with phosphoramide mustard (STRUCK et al., 1975), clearly establishes that bis(chloroethyl)amine is a true metabolite of CP— though probably derived from the breakdown of other CP metabolites, rather than from CP itself. This piperazine mustard displays quite powerful anti-tumour activity (Cox and LEVIN, 1975) and immunosuppressant activity in vitro (WHITEHOUSE, 1976), and must certainly be considered as yet another potential pharmaco-active metabolite. The oxazole derivative (XII) may be regarded as a detoxification product of (X).

These simple mustard metabolites (X, XI) may differ quite sharply in cytostatic/immunosuppressant potency from the nitrogen mustard, HN-2 (= N-methyl X) that is still occasionally used in chemotherapy where the local action of the drug is required, without requiring hepatic bioactivation. HN-2 can enter some cells by a carrier that recognises choline and some other tertiary bases, whereas the secondary amine (X) and other N mustards are not transported into the cell by this route (GOLDENBERG, 1975).

Other biotransformations of CP metabolites, involving dechlorination and the formation of hydroxyethyl amines, may not concern us here since these products are certainly not cytotoxic. However, further oxidation of these alcohols yielding N-substituted glycines or the formation of other carboxylates, e.g. hydracrylic acid after ring opening, might yield products that can act on the inflammatory process, even though they lack conventional cytostatic/anti-tumour properties.

Destruction of the reactive metabolites varies considerably within the peripheral tissues and undoubtedly accounts for why certain tissues are more affected than others by a given dose of CP. Thus, ability to deactivate aldophosphamide by NAD^+-dependent aldehyde dehydrogenases is greatest in the liver cytosol and least in spleen extracts (SLADEK, 1973a; Cox et al., 1975), and explains why CP causes rapid splenic involution but has little effect at low doses on the liver tissue which activates it. Presumably, of the cells participating in a chronic inflammatory response, those which most lack the means to detoxify the toxic metabolites will be the most prominently affected by the pro-drug. This offers further scope to sharpen the focus of CP metabolites. Parallel treatment with inhibitors of in vivo aldehyde oxidation/detoxication, that do not distribute uniformly to all tissues, might selectively potentiate the action of the aldehyde-derived metabolites of CP, including acrolein and chloracetaldehyde, within certain tissues only.

In experimental animals with severe inflammatory disease (e.g. adjuvant-induced arthritis in rats) or a tumour burden, the oxidative activation of CP by the liver may be severely compromised (BECK and WHITEHOUSE, 1973; BARTOSEK et al., 1975) and the anti-inflammatory activity of the drug cannot be assayed readily. Repeated dosing of animals with CP may inhibit liver microsomal hydroxylases and consequently CP metabolism/bioactivation can be profoundly modified by prior dosing. Experimental induction of the cytochrome P_{450}-drug metabolising system increases blood levels of alkylating metabolites (SLADEK, 1972a; OHIRA et al., 1974) but may have little effect on the therapeutic index (SLADEK, 1972a, b). Hepatotoxic agents, e.g. CCl_4 or ethanol, may not only depress CP bioactivation but also depress the metabolic detoxification of the active metabolites (BRAUN and SCHOENEICH, 1975). Also, large inter-individual variations have been noted in the rates of CP metabolism in human subjects (MOURIDSEN et al., 1974).

The considerable advances in our understanding of CP metabolism owe much to recent developments in analytical methods. Gas-liquid chromatography is useful for determining unmetabolised drug in biological specimens (PANTAROTTO et al., 1974). Very careful thin layer chromatographic methods have been developed for separating the metabolites (SLADEK, 1973a; VÖLKER et al., 1974; NORPOTH et al., 1975) in sufficient quantity for direct bioassay (PHILLIPS, 1974) but their actual identification may still be complicated by the existence of stereoisomers. Field desorption mass spectrometry has proved particularly useful for characterising the most labile metabolites such as 4-hydroxy-CP and aldophosphamide, since this technique avoids the evaporation (and degradation) of samples to be studied by their induced ionisation.

Electron impact mass spectrometry has also been of considerable value for identifying structurally diagnostic ion fragments of the various CP metabolites (see Struck et al., 1975; Cox et al., 1976).

2. Properties of Some Metabolites

As discussed earlier (Sect. B.II.3.), two sites of alkylation must be considered—within the nucleus (and throughout the cell) or a restricted action at the exterior of the cell. The endo-alkylating CP metabolites are readily recognised by their powerful cytotoxic activity in vitro, especially to lymphoid cells; they include the first metabolic transformation product, aldophosphamide (Sladek, 1973b; Van der Steen et al., 1973; Whitehouse et al., 1974b; Takamizawa et al., 1975). The next decomposition product, phosphoramide mustard (Connors et al., 1974; Phillips, 1974) is also cytotoxic, as are some further and alternative breakdown products, namely chloracetaldehyde (Lawrence et al., 1972; Whitehouse et al., 1974a), bis(chloroethyl)amine = nor HN-2 (Sladek, 1973b; Whitehouse et al., 1974b; Cox and Levin, 1975) and piperazine mustard (Cox and Levin, 1975). Acrolein per se may not be truly cytotoxic (Thomson and Colvin, 1974; Van der Steen et al., 1973—but see Connors et al., 1974; Phillips, 1974; Whitehouse and Beck, 1975) though its ability to deplete cell thiols, through the nucleophilic addition of thiols to the highly reactive (-C = C-CO-), undoubtedly depresses cellular resistance to concurrently applied or liberated mustards.

By this experimental criterion of direct cytoxicity when applied in vitro, exogenously applied phosphoramide mustard is not a particularly reactive endoalkylating agent; being ionised and hydrophilic it is not readily taken up by most of the cells/tumour lines that are susceptible to the metabolites indicated above (or to reference alkylating agents, e.g. HN-2) and its ED_{50} (cytotoxicity) in vitro is therefore relatively high (Whitehouse et al., 1974b—but see Colvin et al., 1973). Cells provoked to engage in vigorous pinocytosis might, however, demonstrate a greater susceptibility to phosphoramide mustard if they took up this drug with the ambient medium in the pinocytic vacuoles. This may account for the greater susceptibility of certain tumour cells.

By contrast, endogenously-generated phosphoramide mustard is a very powerful cytostatic drug and the same properties of low lipophilicity and complete ionisation at pH 7 (Whitehouse et al., 1974b), which minimise its entry into cells when applied exogenously, also ensure its entrapment in cellulo when formed therein by the decomposition of 4-hydroxy CP. This latter metabolite is highly lipophilic, readily penetrates the cell walls of lymphoid and tumour cells and can, therefore, be likened to the Trojan horse in the Homeric legend.

Hydrophilic mustards have almost uniformly proved to have little anti-tumour or cytotoxic activity (though there are certain notable exceptions to this generalisation, e.g. HN-2). Nonetheless, they may exhibit exoalkylating activity especially in their interactions with lymphoid cells. Thus mannomustine, carboxyphosphamide (IV) and phosphoramide mustard (VII) all deactivate lymphoid cells that will cause inflammatory disease in rats after passive transfer to tolerant recipients (Whitehouse et al., 1974b). Carboxyphosphamide has negligible anti-tumour activity (Struck et al., 1971; Takamizawa et al., 1972; Sladek, 1973b).

CP itself is almost inert in all these in vitro assays with the exception of its effects on isolated liver cells (GRAYZEL and BECK, 1975; WALTON and BUCKLEY, 1975) and lectin-stimulated lymphocytes (SINGER and BRODY, 1972) in which it is activated in situ. The lactam metabolite (V) is also almost devoid of alkylating, cytotoxic, and potential immunosuppressant activity (STRUCK et al., 1971; TAKAMIZAWA et al., 1972; SLADEK, 1973b; WHITEHOUSE et al., 1974b). The monodeschlorethyl derivative of CP (IX) is not cytotoxic in vitro (CONNORS et al., 1974; PHILLIPS, 1974).

This brief summary of the pharmacological activity of some of the CP biotransformation products clearly shows how nearly all the research interest (and support) has centered on the cytotoxic anti-tumour potential of this pro-drug. What is still needed is a systematic study of the anti-inflammatory and non-cytotoxic immunosuppressant profile of all these various CP-derived products. Their chemical instability is one impediment to such a study. Artefacts are readily introduced, e.g. use of phosphate buffers which are alkylating substrates (see e.g. LINFORD et al., 1963), competing with the natural receptors. Fortunately, recent improvements in synthetic methods for activating CP non-enzymically, for example with H_2O_2 plus Fe^{++}, i.e. Fenton's reagent (VAN DER STEEN, 1973; STRUCK, 1974; STRUCK et al., 1974; THOMSON and COLVIN, 1974; TAKAMIZAWA et al., 1975), or permanganate ions (JARMAN, 1973), make it possible to study the properties of aldophosphamide or its homologues without having to use liver extracts. Stabilisation of the labile 4-hydroxy CP/ aldophosphamide is possible by forming a semicarbazide (STRUCK, 1974) or the isomeric semiacetals, 4-ethoxy CP="alcophosphamide" (CONNORS et al., 1974). These isomers differ in their stability to hydrolysis but are both highly cytotoxic (PHILLIPS, 1974).

3. Site of Action

Considerable discussion has centered on this question, especially in the context of immunosuppression and induction of tolerance to transplanted organs (AISENBERG, 1973; MÜLLER-RUCHHOLTZ, 1974). As the previous section has shown, a whole family of potent metabolites may "execute" the therapeutic effects of CP with different half-lives and efficacy in different tissues of the body, differing in their alkylating potential and ability to penetrate dividing cells; these target cells in turn differing in their capacity to repair or resist the drug damage.

In experimental immunopathies, e.g. adjuvant arthritis, allergic encephalomyelitis, CP treatment can be withheld to much later stages in the development of these diseases (ARRIGONI-MARTELLI and BRAMM, 1975; BECK and WHITEHOUSE, 1976) than is the case with most cytostatic/immunosuppressant drugs. The latter are chiefly effective by interfering with an antigen-priming process, including perhaps deletion of a virgin population of lymphocytes with short half-lives (B cells) that may be required for immunogen recognition. Many reports have indicated the suppression or deletion of B cell populations by CP in mice, guinea pigs, and human subjects, but T cells are reduced in numbers as well (CLEMENTS et al., 1974; DUMONT, 1974; HOWARD and COURTENAY, 1974; HORWITZ, 1974; REVELL, 1974; ZIFF et al., 1974; HURD and GIULIANO, 1975). Effects of CP on acute inflammation (STEVENS and WILLOUGHBY, 1969; LEVY, 1974; VAN ARMAN, 1974) have been ascribed to a decrease in the white blood cells, other than the polymorphs. Lymphocyte circulation streams are not adversely affected by CP or its metabolites (Yu and Whitehouse, 1974) but the cytotoxic activity of sensitised lymphocytes may be compromised by serum metabolites of CP (Petranyi et al., 1973). Other immunological functions of the lymphocyte membrane may be altered by CP pre-treatment in vivo (Guttmann, 1974).

4. Some Side-Effects

An important corollary of these studies of the pharmacology of the various individual CP metabolites is an assessment of their individual capacity for producing some of the well-known side-effects of CP administration, e.g. alopecia, cystitis, sterility, etc.

Investigations of wool loss in sheep, induced by CP (Reis and Chapman, 1974) and some of its congeners (Feil and Lamoureux, 1974), suggest that aldophosphamide is the probable defleecing agent formed by CP metabolism, since phosphoramide mustard applied i.v. was inactive. It seems reasonable to suppose that this same metabolite is primarily responsible for hair loss in man, until comparable studies on the drug sensitivity of the isolated wool follicle and human hair follicles prove otherwise. Such comparative studies are still badly needed, even though the metabolic pathway of CP activation in sheep is identical with that in man (Bakke et al., 1972), because the drug-resistance mechanisms may differ appreciably even in the same target cells taken from different animal species. This same caveat also applies to extrapolating from toxicity and efficacy studies conducted with cells from laboratory animals to understanding the overall drug action in human disease.

The bladder injury induced by the presence of CP metabolites in the urine (Schultz and Weldon, 1974) is efficiently prevented by a high fluid intake to ensure copious urination and dilution of the urinary metabolites or by oral dosing with N-acetylcysteine (NAC) (Botta et al., 1973; Harris et al., 1975; Tolley and Castro, 1975). This latter treatment is effective even after CP dosage and may not block the therapeutic effects of CP (Devlin et al., 1974). NAC neutralises the irritant potential of both the CP-derived aldehydes and reactive mustards (Whitehouse and Beck, 1975), so it is a fairly widespread antidote. The prime irritant of the bladder following CP administration has not yet been identified but piperazine mustard has recently been suggested as a candidate (Cox and Levin, 1975).

The potential risk of chemical sterilisation in both sexes has been investigated by studying the effects of CP on fertility and general reproductive performance in rats (Botta et al., 1974).

Before CP can be confidently used generally in the wider context of anti-inflammatory therapy, it will be important to know how the various individual tissue toxicities can be modulated or amplified by exogenous agents, as well as by the disease. Competitive blockade of aldehyde dehydrogenases, e.g. with glyceraldehyde, chloral, and disulfiram, enhances the cytotoxicity of aldophosphamide by suppressing one pathway of metabolic inactivation. Ethanol ingestion must obviously be considered one potential complication of CP therapy, though with judicious prescription it might perhaps be a means to lower the total CP dosage required for effective therapy.

III. Chlorambucil

CBC (4-bischlorethylaminophenylbutanoic acid) has been considered to be a direct-acting drug not requiring prior bioactivation—in contrast to CP.

1. Metabolism

In rats, the butyric acid side-chain of CBC undergoes β-oxidation with eventual elimination of the original carboxyl group and α-carbon as CO_2. At least three urinary metabolites have been detected containing the carbon atoms derived from the mustard moiety (GODENECHE et al., 1975). In common with other mustards, CBC also suffers dechlorethylation and chlorine atoms are removed in vivo engendering a variety of hydrolysis products. Preparation of tritium-labelled aromatic mustards by iodination of the unlabelled compound in oleum, followed by catalytic deiodination with tritium gas ($^3H_2$), now offers the opportunity to explore CBC metabolism with radioactive materials of high specific activity (JARMAN et al., 1974).

Comparison of the doses of CBC required to kill tumour cells in vitro and in vivo indicate that, in contrast to CP, CBC does not have to be extensively modified by liver metabolism to be directly cytotoxic (CONNORS and PHILLIPS, 1975), though relatively high doses (approximately 50 times those of HN-2) are required to kill the Walker tumour in vitro. Evidence has been presented that tumour cells may metabolise CBC and the cytotoxicity of CBC can be enhanced by pretreating these tumour cells in vitro (or in vivo) with other drugs which induce microsomal drug metabolism (HILL et al., 1973). These findings would indicate that (local) metabolic activation may also be involved in determining cytotoxicity.

2. Anti-Inflammatory Effects

In rats, repeated dosing with CBC prevents the development of adjuvant-induced arthritis (CURREY, 1973), a local graft-vs.-host reaction (BECK et al., 1973; SWINGLE et al., 1973) and the acute paw oedema elicited by carrageenin (DUKES et al., 1973). CBC mimics the non-steroid anti-inflammatory drugs in depleting the number of mononuclear leucocytes in the carrageenin-inflamed paw.

3. Mode of Action

CBC very rapidly inhibits the high affinity form of cyclic 3',5'-nucleotide phosphodiesterase, a membrane-associated enzyme, in susceptible tumours, rat bone marrow and intestinal mucosa (TISDALE and PHILLIPS, 1975). As a consequence, the cell levels of cAMP are increased; a phenomenon that has been correlated with both growth inhibition and suppression of the immune response.

The CBC anion (carboxylate) readily aggregates in vitro without loss of alkylating activity. This aggregate ($MW \geq 2 \times 10^5$) is not very toxic to mouse tumour cells but is evidently taken up by mouse macrophages since it is toxic to these latter cells (BLAKESLEE et al., 1975). Thus, cells engaging in active endocytosis might be selectively intoxicated by micellar forms of detergent-like mustards. Other models of focussing the drug action have been explored, including chemically conjugating CBC to IgG molecules (ROSS, 1975), concurrently applying CBC with antibodies that are specific for a given target cell (Fleschner, 1973; Rubens and Dulbecco, 1974) or with a lectin (Lozzio and Cawein, 1972). Differences between cells in their binding of CBC, especially by nuclear proteins, may be one determinant of drug sensitivity (Riches and Harrap, 1975). Alkylation and inactivation of certain proteases, particularly at an alkaline pH, by CBC in vitro (Brecher and Stephens, 1972; Griffiths and Brecher, 1973) points to a possible extracellular effect of the drug in inflammation.

In mice, CBC induces lymphocytolysis and increases (lysosomal) membrane permeability of spleen and lymphoid tissues, resembling that caused by irradiation or corticosteroids (Aikman and Will, 1974). Phytohaemaglutinin stimulation of both mouse and human lymphocytes (Lozzio and Cawein, 1972; Stevenson and Patel, 1973) enhances their susceptibility to CBC.

IV. Methotrexate

In current medical practice, folate antagonists do not play a very important role in the treatment of inflammatory states. Their use is almost exclusively confined to the treatment of otherwise resistant cases of psoriasis (Weinstein, 1971). The effectiveness of MTX in curing the inflammatory/proliferative destruction of skin is, interestingly enough, not paralleled by a comparable activity in psoriatic arthritis (Feldges and Barnes, 1974) or in other inflammatory states in man. This is a good reason to discuss some aspects of MTX pharmacology, in that it may help in understanding the requirements for anti-inflammatory activity.

MTX apparently displays a certain degree of specificity in its action. MTX inhibits nucleic acid formation and hence protein synthesis in all cells and tissues in vitro, via inhibition of dihydrofolate reductase (Table 4). It is apparent, however, that MTX exerts its activity in vivo predominantly upon epithelial cell systems, implying either a selective bio-distribution to epithelial cells, or rapid acquisition of MTX resistance by other cell types. These inhibitory effects in epithelial cells result in the following characteristic side-effects: (1) erythema and ulcerations of the mucosa of the oralintestinal tract;(2) maculopapular skin rashes and herpetiform skin eruptions; (3) hepatic damage, ranging from transient enzyme release to liver necrosis and/or cirrhosis; (4) impairment of the function of tubular cells in the kidney.

This selective action on epithelial cells also accounts for the effectiveness of MTX-treatment against certain carcinomas and non-malignant skin diseases, such as: choriocarcinomas, epidermoid carcinomas of the head and neck, mycosis fungoides and generalized psoriasis.

An explanation for the role of distribution in selective actions of MTX comes from the observations that after oral administration of labelled MTX, high concentrations are observed in intestinal mucosa, liver, kidney, and skin (Grignani et al., 1967; Anderson et al., 1970; Bischoff et al., 1970) whilst other cell or organ systems such as CNS, muscle and fat, take up and retain very little of this compound. This specific pharmacokinetic behaviour can be explained by the fact that MTX is essentially of polar character (i.e. hydrophilic) and under normal physiological conditions it is wholly ionized estimated pK_a 3:5, 3.0 (COOH), 5.0 (N-CH$_3$), 5.3 (Pterid), and so does not easily cross biological membranes, e.g. the so-called blood-brain barrier. On the other hand, there is evidence that a variety of epithelial cells contain active transport systems for MTX which could cause high intracellular concentrations of the drug which persist for long periods of time. Such transport mechanisms, together with high levels of dihydrofolate reductase which bind MTX strongly, probably exist in the liver, kidney and skin cells.

In conclusion, MTX apparently is another example of a cytostat with a non-specific (biochemical) mode of action, which achieves a degree of therapeutic selectivity through its unequal bio-distribution. This effectively transforms an otherwise quite toxic compound into a valuable drug for treating, e.g. psoriasis or epidermoid carcinomas of the head and neck (CAPIZZI et al., 1970).

V. Azathioprine

This substance is essentially a drug precursor, being transformed to 6-MP and methylnitroimidazole (MNI). The contribution of MNI to the overall clinical activity of AThP has not been clearly defined.

In animal studies, especially those using rats, it has been difficult to discern anti-inflammatory/immunosuppressant activity with 6-MP or AThP (BECK et al., 1973; DUKES et al., 1973; SWINGLE et al., 1973; BECK and WHITEHOUSE, 1974; LEVY, 1974; TSUKADA et al., 1974; SOFIA et al., 1975). An anti-arthritic activity can be demonstrated by inhibition of the adjuvant disease in rats (CURREY, 1973) but it is far from dramatic. Either we must assume that rodents are a poor guide to the pharmacology of thiopurines in man, or that these purine analogues are indeed a unique class of drug that act quite differently from alkylating drugs, steroids, and non-steroid anti-inflammatory agents in regulating (immuno-)inflammatory disease. Human tissues certainly have a higher capacity than those of dogs, mice, etc., to cleave rapidly AThP to generate 6-MP (BACH, 1975). Exogenous 6-MP may be rapidly destroyed by S-methylation, oxidation to thiouric acid (high in mouse, low in man) etc., so that a direct comparison of the pharmacological activity of 6-MP and AThP in laboratory animals may not adequately answer the question as to how important the cleavage of the S-nitroimidazole linkage may be in conferring overall drug activity in man. Local metabolism of AThP in an inflammatory focus, duly colonised with invading leucocytes, pannus, etc., could certainly be a significant factor in determining overall anti-inflammatory activity.

At least three lines of evidence suggest that 6-MP and AThP are rather unique drugs:

1. The synthesis of antibodies (especially rheumatoid factor, RF) is slowed down in patients receiving AThP; the actual levels of serum antibodies may not fall significantly but their overall turnover is certainly reduced by the drug (see LEVY and WHITEHOUSE, 1975) so that the net production of RF etc. is inhibited. This drug effect is not accompanied by gross leucopenia (contrast CP). In vitro, AThP is a more potent inhibitor of protein synthesis in lymphoid cells than 6-MP (SMITH and FORBES, 1970).

2. A characteristic liver lesion develops in rodents with severe inflammation, that is a central response to peripheral injury. This lesion (depression in hepatic drug metabolism) is largely prevented by 6-thiopurines or steroids (BECK and WHITE-HOUSE, 1974). The former drugs have little effect on the magnitude of the acute (extrahepatic) inflammation but they evidently "protect" the liver from responding to

a stimulus provided by the tissue injury within the inflammatory focus. The production of acute-phase reactants (fibrinogen and serum glycoproteins), which is a characteristic of trauma, infection or inflammation in animals and man, is much reduced by AThP in rats with acute inflammation (Whitehouse, 1976). True anti-arthritic agents reduce these acute-phase reactants in rheumatoid patients (McConkey, 1976). The acute-phase reactants are primarily synthesized in the liver but it is not clear whether the drugs which affect their production (including penicillamine, gold compounds and steroids in man), are normalising the liver response to peripheral injury by primarily acting upon the liver itself, or upon the affected peripheral tissues (including leucocytes).

3. In mice, AThP has a direct effect upon certain populations of T-lymphocytes (Fournier et al., 1973; Bach, 1975), affecting their function but not their numbers. The drug has no effect on the lymphocyte count in rats but does decrease the number of circulating polymorphs (Baardsen et al., 1975). (Effects on monocyte production are discussed by Van Furth, Chap. 3.)

Liver disease may prevent AThP transformation to serum metabolites which depress rosette formation with erythrocytes, or the mixed lymphocyte reaction, by mouse lymphocytes (Bach, 1975). AThP sensitivity is conferred by thymosin, an immunopotentiating hormone prepared from the thymus (Bach et al., 1971).

D. Current Problems

The overriding problem which arises out of the studies to date is the unsatisfactory state of knowledge concerning the use and desirability of cytostats in inflammation, their present toxicity and how much has still to be learned before such powerful drugs can be confidently introduced into general use, if ever, for anti-inflammatory therapy. Because of the low therapeutic index of all compounds discussed so far, their use in humans at present must be restricted to desperate cases and very cautious guidelines have been formulated to try to prevent the uncontrolled and inappropriate use of these agents; see e.g. Decker and Healey (1973).

However, any real breakthrough towards "curative" agents, for rheumatoid arthritis, psoriasis etc., can only be expected after adequate animal models have been developed which are both relevant to (1) the human inflammatory diseases (reflecting the pathophysiological conditions of these diseases), and (2) the disposition of drugs in humans with these diseases. Besides unexpected luck, only the unravelling of these underlying pathogenetic mechanism(s) on the one hand, and factors determining drug distribution and efficacy in situ on the other, will help to develop such models. The pharmacologist may perhaps have to wait for the first of these events to be elucidated by others but she or he can surely assist in the development of models that reflect drug distribution and behaviour in diseased (vs. normal) people.

In the meantime, much could be achieved by using the approaches of contemporary pharmacology to sharpen the action and focus the distribution of drugs we have on hand. Specificity, and thus acceptable therapeutic indices, cannot only be obtained by finding the optimal drug for a certain (as yet undefined) "receptor": it can also be achieved by directing or confining known but fairly unspecific agents to act within the appropriate compartment. If these compartments are known and if they show morphological, biochemical, and/or biophysical characteristics which distinguish them from others throughout the body, it should be possible to distribute cytostats preferentially thereto or release these agents therein. From all we know at present, it can be reasonably assumed that the inflamed tissue itself comprises a specialist compartment differing from the normal tissue in at least three aspects. Firstly, inflamed tissues are often characterized by extensive cell destruction, which causes high concentrations of catabolic enzymes to be released from lysosomal and other membrane-bounded organelles into the extracellular milieu. These enzymes could possibly be exploited as activators of otherwise inactive precursor forms of cytostats (i.e. pre-drugs), within the inflammatory compartment. In such a manner the inactive sodium salt of diethylstilboestrol-diphosphate is hydrolysed to the active drug, diethylstilboestrol, in situ by the abundant phosphatases in the prostate gland to control the local cell growth in prostatic cancer (DUCKREY and RAABES, 1952). Secondly, inflamed tissue usually has a relatively low extracellular pH which is not accompanied by lowered intracellular pH, while cell viability is maintained. This can provide a pH gradient across the local cell membranes that is suitable for trapping the anions of weakly acidic drugs in the intracellular space, after the uptake of the (non-ionised) drug has been facilitated by the low local pH. In normal tissue on the other hand, the pH (and drug concentration) gradient across the cell membrane may be much less, as the pH of the ambient medium will be much nearer to the intracellular pH. There are now good indications that this phenomenon is important not only in determining, for example, the anti-inflammatory action, but also the gastric and renal side effects of non-steroid anti-inflammatory drugs (BRUNE et al., 1976). Thirdly, the mediators of immunological reactivity, the small (T-) lymphocytes, appear to exhibit surface characteristics (DNA-patches(?)) not shared by other cells. These surface markers can apparently be recognized and bind certain chemicals, e.g. bivalent platinum complexes, which interfere with the function of these lymphocytes and may render them incapable of mounting an inflammation (WHITEHOUSE, 1975).

We believe that all three approaches to sharpen and focus the action of cytostats have—perhaps unwittingly—already been used in practical therapeutics even in the context of inflammatory disorders. The endogenous biotransformation of CP, which has first to be metabolized to release breakdown products having fairly selective effects, e.g. hair loss or lymphocyte inactivation, appears to be responsible for the clinical advantages this agent has over, for example, HN-2. CBC can be assumed to behave like a weak acid (est. pK_a's 2.8 (tert.N), 4.8 (COOH), and thus may selectively accumulate in the (acidic) inflamed tissue. This would perhaps explain the relatively high efficacy and the low incidence of side effects of these two particular agents in treating rheumatoid arthritis. However, these speculations require confirmation by further studies. It is hoped that further experimentation will be based on these concepts and will concentrate on the development of less toxic cytostats which are mainly therapeutic agents with only a few, acceptable, side-effects.

Appendix

Synovectomy and Destruction of Pannus

The proliferation of the synovial tissue in joint inflammation and overgrowth and destruction of articular cartilage by pannus (a degenerate, invasive, extension of the synovium) in advanced rheumatoid disease, are barely affected by many non-steroid anti-inflammatory drugs. These tissue-destroying events are legitimate targets for drug therapy as an alternative to surgical synovectomy. Currently, the intra-articular injection of radioisotopes, e.g. ^{90}Ym ^{198}Au, is the preferred alternative to surgery as a means of medical synovectomy (ANON, 1974). Cytostats such as corticosteroids, osmic acid, nitrogen mustards, thiotepa, etc., have been applied intra-articularly to achieve "chemical synovectomy". Inevitably some destruction of the cartilage tissue accompanies the use of either local radiation or toxic agents in attempts to regulate synovium/pannus proliferation. These approaches to "medical synovectomy" must be considered fairly blunt. They can, however, be sharpened by at least two strategies:

1. Selective uptake of toxic, particulate, radiochemicals or cytotoxic drugs by the phagocytic cells in the synovium. However, these are not always the cells that are proliferating and thereby pathogenic to the normal cartilage.

2. Using natural regulators of lymphoid/fibroblast proliferation, namely chalones, that are specific for their respective tissues but are not species-specific (and can therefore be supplied from animal sources).

Considerable progress has been made in recent years towards characterising fibroblast and lymphocyte chalones (FLORENTIN et al., 1973; HOUCK, 1973; HOUCK and IRAUSQUIN, 1973; HOUCK et al., 1973a, b, c; KIGER et al., 1973; BULLOUGH, 1975; LOZZIO et al., 1975). It will be very interesting to learn what value they may have when injected intra-articularly either in lieu of, or together with, other agents now employed to procure a medical synovectomy.

References

Aikman,A.A., Will,E.D.: Lysosomes after irradiation. II. Lysosomal membrane permeability and acid phosphatase activity of lymphoid and other tissues of the whole-body irradiation. Radiat. Res. 57, 416—430 (1974)

Aisenberg,A.C.: Immunosuppression by alkylating agents. Tolerance induction. Transplant. Proc. 5, 1221—1226 (1973)

Aisenberg,A.C., Wilkes,B.: Studies on the suppression of immune responses by the periwinkle alkaloids vincristine and vinbalstine. J. clin. Invest. 43, 2394—2403 (1964)

Alepa,F.P., Zvaifler,N.J., Sliwinski,A.J.: Immunologic effects of cyclophosphamide treatment in rheumatoid arthritis. Arthr. Rheum. 13, 754—760 (1970)

Allison,A.C.: Tumour development following immunosuppression. Proc. roy. Soc. Med. 63, 1077—1080 (1970)

Anderson,L.L., Collins,G.J., Ojima,Y., Sullivan,R.D.: A study of the distribution of methotrexate in human tissues and tumors. Cancer Res. 30, 1344—1348 (1970)

Anon: Medical synovectomy (Editorial). Brit. med. J. 1974 II, 682

Apostoloff,E., Reitzig,P., Jendrusch,C., Apostloff,G.: Experiences with long-term immunosuppressive therapy of connective tissue diseases. Z. inn. Med. 29, 26—30 (1974)

Aptekar,R.G., Atkinson,J.P., Decker,J.L., Wolff,S.M., Chu,E.W.: Bladder toxicity with chronic oral cyclophosphamide therapy in nonmalignant disease. Arthr. Rheum. 16, 461—467 (1973)

Arinoviche,R., Loewi,G.: Comparison of the effects of two cytotoxic drugs and of antilymphocytic serum. On immune and non-immune inflammation in experimental animals. Ann. rheum. Dis. 29, 32—39 (1970)

Arrigoni-Martelli,E., Bramm,E.: Investigations in the influence of cyclophosphamide, gold sodium thiomalate and D-penicillamine on nystatin oedema and adjuvant arthritis. Agents Actions 5, 264—267 (1975)

Assem, E. S. K., Mongar, J. L.: Inhibition of allergic reactions in man and other species by cromoglycate. Int. Arch. Allergy **38**, 68—77 (1970)

Baardsen, A., Midtvedt, T., Trippestad, A.: Influence of methylprednisolone and azathioprine on polymorphonuclear neutrophils (PMN) and lymphocytes in germ free, monocontaminated and conventional rats. Acta path. microbiol. scand. Sect. C. **83 C**, 210—214 (1975)

Bach, J. F.: The mode of action of immunosuppressive agents. Amsterdam: North-Holland 1975

Bach, J. F., Dardenne, M.: Activities of immunosuppressive agents in vitro. I. Rosette inhibition by azathioprine. Rev. europ. Et. clin. biol. **16**, 770—777 (1971)

Bach, J. F., Dardenne, M., Fournier, C.: In vitro evaluation of immunosuppressive drugs. Nature (Lond.) **222**, 998—999 (1969)

Bach, J. F., Dardenne, M., Goldstein, A. L., Guha, A., White, A.: Appearance of T-cell markers in bone marrow rosette-forming cells after incubation with thymosin, a thymic hormone. Proc. nat. Acad. Sci. (Wash.) **68**, 2734—2738 (1971)

Bakke, J. E., Feil, V. J., Fjelstul, C. J., Thacker, E. J.: Metabolism of cyclophosphamide by sheep. Agric. Food Chem. **20**, 384—388 (1972)

Bartosek, I., Donelli, M. G., Guaitani, A., Colombo, T., Russo, R., Garattini, S.: Differences of cyclophosphamide and 6-mercaptopurine metabolic rates in perfused livers of normal and tumourbearing animals. Biochem. Pharmacol. **24**, 289—291 (1975)

Beck, F. J., Levy, L., Whitehouse, M. W.: Local graft-versus-host reaction in rat as a tool for drug mechanism studies. Brit. J. Pharmacol. **49**, 293—302 (1973)

Beck, F. J., Whitehouse, M. W.: Effect of adjuvant disease in rats on cyclophosphamide and isophosphamide metabolism. Biochem. Pharmacol. **22**, 2453—2468 (1973)

Beck, F. W. J., Whitehouse, M. W.: Impaired drug metabolism in rats associated with acute inflammation: a possible assay for anti-injury agents. Proc. Soc. exp. Biol. (N.Y.) **145**, 135—140 (1974)

Beck, F. W. J., Whitehouse, M. W.: Modification in the establishment of allergic encephalomyelitis (EAE) in rats: An improved assay for immunosuppressant drugs. Agents Actions **6**, 460—467 (1976)

Berenbaum, M. C.: Immunosuppressive agents. Brit. med. Bull. **21**, 140—146 (1965)

Berenbaum, M. C.: Dose-response curves for agents that impair cell reproductive integrity; fundamental difference between dose-response curves of antimetabolites and those for radiation and alkylating agents. Brit. J. Cancer **23**, 426—433 (1969)

Berenbaum, M. C.: Is azathioprine a better immunosuppressive than 6-mercaptopurine? Clin. exp. Immunol. **8**, 1—8 (1971)

Berlin, R. D.: Microtubules and the fluidity of the cell surface. Ann. N.Y. Acad. Sci. **253**, 445—454 (1975a)

Berlin, R. D.: Microtubule membrane interactions fluorescence techniques. In: Borgers, M., De Brabander, M. (Eds.): Microtubules and Microtubule Inhibitors, pp. 327—339. Amsterdam: North-Holland Publ. 1975b

Bertino, J. R.: Chemical action and pharmacology of methotrexate, azathioprine, and cyclophosphamide in man. Arthr. Rheum. **16**, 79—83 (1973)

Bertino, J. R.: Folate antagonists. In: Sartorelli, A. C., Johns, D. G. (Eds.): Antineoplastic and Immunosuppressive Agents, Part II, Handbook of experimental Pharmacology, pp. 468—483. Berlin-Heidelberg-New York: Springer 1975

Billingham, R. E., Streiblein, J. W., Zakarian, S.: Specificity of the homograft reaction. In: Forscher, B. K., Houck, J. C. (Eds.): Immunopathology of Inflammation, pp. 161—175. Amsterdam: Excerpta Medica Found. 1971

Bischoff, K. B., Dedrick, R. L., Zaharko, D. S.: Preliminary model for methotrexate pharmacokinetics. J. pharm. Sci. **59**, 149—153 (1970)

Blakeslee, D., Chen, M., Kennedy, J. C.: Aggregation of chlorambucil in vitro may cause misinterpretation of protein-binding data. Brit. J. Cancer **31**, 689—902 (1975)

Borel, Y., Schwartz, R. J.: Inhibition of immediate and delayed hypersensitivity in the rabbit by 6-mercaptopurine. J. Immunol. **92**, 754—761 (1964)

Botta, J. A., Hawkins, H. C., Weikel, J. H.: Effects of cyclophosphamide on fertility and general reproductive performance of rats. Toxicol. appl. Pharmacol. **27**, 602—611 (1974)

Botta, J. A., Nelson, L. W., Weikel, J. H.: Acetylcysteine in the prevention of cyclophosphamide-induced cystitis in rats. J. nat. Cancer Inst. **51**, 1051—1057 (1973)

Boyden, S.: The chemotactic effect of mixtures of antibody and antigen on polymorphonuclear leukocytes. J. exp. Med. **115**, 453—466 (1962)

Braun, R., Schoeneich, J.: Influence of ethanol and carbon tetrachloride on the mutagenic effectivity of cyclophosphamide in the host-mediated assay with *Salmonella typhimurium*. Mutat. Res. **31**, 191—194 (1975)

Brecher, A. S., Stephens, L. E.: Kinetics of inactivation of chymotrypsins by chlormabucil. Enzymologia **42**, 115—121 (1972)

Brune, K.: Graft-versus-Host-Reaktionen: Modelle, Beeinflußbarkeit und klinische Analogien. Schweiz. med. Wschr. **100**, 49—58 (1970)

Brune, K., Glatt, M., Graf, P.: Mechanism of action anti-inflammatory drugs. Gen. Pharmacol. **7**, 27—33 (1976)

Brune, K., Graf, P., Glatt, M.: Anti-inflammatory action of colchicine. In: Borgers, M., DeBrabander, M. (Eds.): Microtubules and Microtubule Inhibitors, pp. 471—481. Amsterdam: North-Holland 1975

Bullough, W. S.: Chalone control mechanisms. Life Sci. **16**, 323—330 (1975)

Campbell, D. H., Garvey, J. S., Cremer, N. E., Sussdorf, D. H.: Methods in Immunology, pp. 69—70. New York: Benjamin 1964

Capizzi, R. L., De Conti, R. C., Marsh, J. C., Bertino, J. R.: Methotrexate therapy of head and neck cancer: improvement in therapeutic index by the use of leucovorin "rescue". Cancer Res. **30**, 1782—1788 (1970)

Caron, G. A.: Effect of antimetabolites and corticosteroids on lymphocyte transformation in vitro. In: Rieke, W. O. (Ed.): Proceedings of the Third Annual Leucocyte Cultur Conference, pp. 287—305. New York: Appleton 1969

Carter, S. K., Slavik, M.: Chemotherapy of cancer. Ann. Rev. Pharmacol. **14**, 157—183 (1974)

Chang, Y.-H., Malawista, St. E.: Mechanism of action of colchicine. IV. The failure of nonleukopenic doses of colchicine to supress urate crystal-induced canine joint inflammation. Inflammation **1**, 143—153 (1975)

Chlud, K., Kotz, R., Zeitlhofer, J.: Die intraartikuläre Zytostatikaanwendung bei chronischer Polyarthritis. Therapiewoche **22**, 2740—2750 (1972)

Clements, P. J., Yu, D. T., Levy, J., Paulus, H. E., Barnett, E. V.: Effects of cyclophosphamide on B- and T-lymphocytes in rheumatoid arthritis. Arthr. Rheum. **17**, 347—353 (1974)

Cochrane, C. G., Janoff, A.: The Arthus Reaction: A model of neutrophil and complement—mediated injury. In: Zweifach, B. W., Grant, L., McCluskey, R. T. (Eds.): The Inflammatory Process, Vol. III, pp. 86—162. New York: Academic Press 1974

Colvin, M., Padgett, C. A., Fenselau, C.: A biologically active metabolite of cyclophosphamide. Cancer Res. **33**, 915—918 (1973)

Connors, T. A.: Alkylating agents in "Topics in Current Chemistry" **52**, 141—171. Berlin-Heidelberg-New York: Springer 1974

Connors, T. A., Cox, P. J., Farmer, P. B., Foster, A. B., Jarman, M.: Some studies of the active intermediates formed in the microsomal metabolism of cyclophosphamide and isophosphamide. Biochem. Pharmacol. **23**, 115—129 (1974)

Connors, T. A., Farmer, P. B., Foster, A. B., Gilsenan, A. M., Jarman, M., Tisdale, M. J.: Metabolism of aniline mustard. Biochem. Pharmacol. **22**, 1971—1980 (1973)

Connors, T. A., Phillips, B. J.: Screening for anti-cancer agents: the relative merits of in vitro and in vivo techniques. Biochem. Pharmacol. **24**, 2217—2224 (1975)

Cooperating Clinics Committee of the American Rheumatism Association: A controlled trial of cyclophosphamide in rheumatoid arthritis. New Engl. J. Med. **283**, 883—889 (1970)

Cooperating Clinics Committee of the American Rheumatism Association: A controlled trial of high and low doses of cyclophosphamide in 82 patients with rheumatoid arthritis. Arthr. Rheum. **15**, 434 (1972)

Cox, P. J., Farmer, P. B., Jarman, M.: The microsomal metabolism of some analogues of cyclophosphamide: 4-methylcyclophosphamide and 6-methylcyclophosphamide. Biochem. Pharmacol. **24**, 599—606 (1975)

Cox, P. J., Farmer, P. B., Jarman, M.: The use of cyclophosphamide analogues in mechanistic studies of the metabolism of cyclophosphamide. In: Frigerio, A., Castagnoli, N. (Eds.): Advances in Mass Spectrometry in Biochemistry and Medicine. New York: Spectrum Publications 1976

Cox, P. J., Levin, L.: Novel metabolic products of cyclophosphamide in human urine. Biochem. Pharmacol. **24**, 1233—1235 (1975)

Cox, P. J., Phillips, B. J., Thomas, P.: The enzymatic basis of the selective action of cyclophosphamide. Cancer Res. **35**, 3755—3761 (1975)

Creasey, W. A.: Vinca alkaloids and colchicine. In: Sartorelli, A. C., Johns, D. G. (Eds.): Antineoplastic and Immunosuppressive Agents, Handbook of experimental Pharmacology, Part II, pp. 670—694. Berlin-Heidelberg-New York: Springer 1975

Currey, H. L.: Immunosuppressive drugs in rheumatoid arthritis. Mod. Trends Rheum. **2**, 174—198 (1971 a)

Currey, H. L.: A comparison of immunosuppressive and anti-inflammatory agents in the rat. Clin. exp. Immunol. **9**, 879—887 (1971 b)

Currey, H. L.: Comparison of immunosuppressive and anti-inflammatory agents in the rat. Rheumatologie (Paris) **3**, 293—300 (1973)

Currey, H. L., Harris, J., Mason, R. M., Woodland, J., Beveridge, T., Roberts, C. J., Vere, D. W., Dixon, A. S., Davies, J., Owen-Smith, B.: Comparison of azathioprine, cyclophosphamide, and gold in treatment of rheumatoid arthritis. Brit. med. J. **1974 III**, 763—766

Currey, H. L. F., Ziff, M.: Suppression of experimentally induced polyarthritis in the rat by heterologous anti-lymphocyte serum. Lancet **1966 II**, 889—891

Currey, H. L. F., Ziff, M.: Suppression of adjuvant disease in the rat by heterologous anti-lymphocyte globulin. J. exp. Med. **127**, 185—203 (1968)

Curtis, J. E., Sharp, J. T., Lidsky, M. D., Hersh, E. M.: Immune response of patients with rheumatoid arthritis during cyclophosphamide treatment. Arthr. Rheum. **16**, 34—42 (1973)

De Chatelet, L. R., McCall, C. E., McPhail, L. C., Johnston, R. B.: Superoxide dismutase activity in leukocytes. J. clin. Invest. **53**, 1197—1201 (1974)

Decker, J. L.: Toxicity of immunosuppressive drugs in man. Arthr. Rheum. **16**, 89—91 (1973)

Decker, J. L., Healey, L. A.: When to use cytotoxic drugs in rheumatoid arthritis. Geriatrics **28**, 103—106 (1973)

Denman, E. J., Denman, A. M., Greenwood, B. M., Gall, D., Heath, R. B.: Failure of cytotoxic drugs to suppress immune responses of patients with rheumatoid arthritis. Ann. rheum. Dis. **29**, 220—231 (1970)

Devlin, R. G., Schwartz, N. L., Mackey, H. K., Baronowsky, P. E.: Effects of cyclophosphamide and cyclophosphamide plus acetylcysteine on the in vivo—in vitro mixed lymphocyte reaction. Transplantation **17**, 70—74 (1974)

Diaz, C. J., Garzia, E. L., Merchante, A., Perianes, J.: Treatment of rheumatoid arthritis with nitrogen mustard: Preliminary report. J. Amer. med. Ass. **147**, 1418—1419 (1951)

Dräger, U., Hohorst, H.-J.: Permeation of cyclophosphamide metabolites into tumour cells. Cancer Treat. Rep. **60**, 423—427 (1976)

Druckrey, H., Raabes, S.: Organspezifische Chemotherapie des Krebses. (Prostata-Karzinom) Klin. Wschr. **30**, 882—884 (1952)

Dukes, M., Chan, W. C., Willoughby, D. A.: Effect of various immunosuppressive agents on the vascular and cellular response to carrageenan in the rat. J. Path. **109**, 151—161 (1973)

Dumonde, D. C., Wolstencroft, R. A., Panayi, G. S., Matthew, M., Morley, J., Hoson, W. T.: Lymphokines: non-antibody mediators of cellular immunity generated by lamphocyte activation. Nature (Lond.) **224**, 38—42 (1969)

Dumont, F.: Destruction and regeneration of lymphocyte populations in the mouse spleen after cyclophosphamide treatment. Int. Arch. Allergy **47**, 110—123 (1974)

Ehrlich, G.: Colchicine for familial Mediterranean fever. New Engl. J. Med. **288**, 798 (1973)

Elion, G. B.: The significance of azathioprine metabolites. Proc. roy. Soc. Med. **65**, 257—260 (1972)

Elion, G. B., Hitchings, G. H.: Azathioprine. In: Sartorelli, A. C., Johns, D. G. (Eds.): Antineoplastic and Immunosuppressive Agents, Part II, Handbook of experimental Pharmacology, Vol. XXXVIII/2, pp. 404—425. Berlin-Heidelberg-New York: Springer 1975

Elkins, W. L.: Cellular immunology and the pathogenesis of the graft-versus-host reactions. Progr. Allergy **15**, 78—187 (1971)

Farrow, M. G., Van Dyke, K.: Micro-system for screening antileukemic drugs utilizing human whole blood. Chemotherapy (Basel) **16**, 76—84 (1971)

Feil, V. J., Lamoureux, C. J. H.: Alopecia activity of cyclophosphamide metabolites and related compounds in sheep. Cancer Res. **34**, 2596—2598 (1974)

Feldges, D. H., Barnes, C. G.: Treatment of arthropathy with either azathioprine or methotrexate. Rheum. Rehabil. **13**, 120—124 (1974)

Fenselau, C., Kan, M.-N., Billets, S., Colvin, M.: Identification of phosphorodiamidic acid mustard as a human metabolite of cyclophosphamide. Cancer Res. **35**, 1453—1457 (1975)

Fitzgerald, T. J.: Colchicine and allopurinol. In: Scherrer, R. A., Whitehouse, M. W. (Eds.): Antiinflammatory Agents, Vol. I, pp. 295—361. New York: Academic Press 1974

Fleschner, I.: Cure and concomitant immunisation of mice bearing Ehrlich ascites tumors by treatment with an antibody-alkylating complex. Europ. J. Cancer **9**, 741—745 (1973)

Floersheim, G. L.: Pharmakologische Beeinflußbarkeit cellulärer Immunität. Z. naturwiss.-med. Grundlagenforschung **2**, 307—360 (1965)

Floersheim, G. L., Brune, K., Seiler, K.: Cytotoxic drugs in an avian urate microcrystal arthritis. Agents Actions **3**, 24—27 (1973)

Florentin, I., Kiger, N., Mathé, G.: T lymphocyte specificity of a lymphocyte-inhibiting factor (chalone) extracted from the thymus. Europ. J. Immunol. **3**, 624—627 (1973)

Fournier, C., Bach, M. A., Dardenne, M., Bach, J. F.: Selective action of azathioprine on T cells. Transplant. Proc. **5**, 523—526 (1973)

Fricke, R.: Cytostatic long-term therapy of rheumatoid arthritis. Verh. dtsch. Ges. Rheum. **2**, 382—386 (1972)

Fridovich, I.: Superoxide radical and the bactericidal action of phagocytes. New Engl. J. Med. **290**, 624—625 (1974)

Gerebtzoff, A., Lambert, P. H., Miescher, P. A.: Immunosuppressive agents. Ann. Rev. Pharmacol. **12**, 287—316 (1972)

Gifford, R. H.: Chemotherapy for rheumatoid arthritis. Ration. Drug Ther. **7**, 1—7 (1973)

Glatt, M., Peskar, B., Brune, K.: Leukocytes and prostaglandins in acute inflammation. Experientia (Basel) **30**, 1257—1259 (1974)

Glatt, M., Wagner, K., Brune, K.: The effects of antiinflammatory doses of colchicine on prostaglandin content inflamed tissue. In: Samuelson, B., Paoletti, R. (Eds.): Advances in Prostaglandin and Thromboxane Research, Vol. 1, pp. 111—115. New York: Raven Press 1976

Godeneche, D., Madelmont, J. C., Sauvezne, B., Billaud, A.: Etude de la cinetique d'absorption, de distribution et d'élimination de l'acide N,N-dichloro-2, ethyl, p-aminophenyl-4-butyrique (chloraminophene) marque au ^{14}C chez le rat. Biochem. Pharmacol. **24**, 1303—1308 (1975)

Goldenberg, G. J.: The role of drug transport in resistance to nitrogen mustard and other alkylating agents in L 5178 Y lymphoblasts. Cancer Res. **35**, 1687—1692 (1975)

Goldfinger, S. E.: Colchicine for Familial Mediterranean Fever. New Engl. J. Med. **287**, 1302 (1972)

Goldfinger, S. E.: Colchicine for Familial Mediterranean Fever. New Engl. J. Med. **288**, 1301 (1973)

Goldlust, M. B., Schreiber, W. F.: Use of the reversed passive Arthus Reaction as a test for antiinflammatory agents. Agents Actions **5**, 39—47 (1975)

Grayzel, A. I., Beck, C.: Activation of cyclophosphamide by liver cell cultures. Biochem. Pharmacol. **24**, 645—646 (1975)

Griffiths, A. E., Brecher, A. J.: Protection afforded to trypsin and trypsinogen by calcium ion from inactivation by chlorambucil. Proc. Soc. exp. Biol. (N.Y.) **142**, 1045—1047 (1973)

Grignani, F., Martinelli, M. F., Tonato, M., Finzi, A. F.: Folate dependent enzymes in human epidermis. Arch. Derm. **96**, 577—585 (1967)

Gumpel, J. M., Hall, A., Ansell, B.: A double-blind comparative trial of cyclophosphamide and gold in rheumatoid arthritis. Ann. rheum. Dis. **33**, 574 (1974)

Guttmann, R.: Membrane properties and functional activity of lymphocytes from cyclophosphamide-pretreated rats. J. Immunol. **112**, 1594—1601 (1974)

Hahn, B. H., Knotts, L., Mary, N. G., Hamilton, T. R.: Influence of cyclophosphamide and other immunosuppressive drugs on immune disorders and neoplasia in NZB/NZW mice. Arthr. Rheum. **18**, 145—152 (1975)

Harris, E. R., Levy, L., Levy, J.: Inhibition of cyclophosphamide-induced bladder toxicity by N-acetylcysteine in rats. Proc. W. pharmacol. Soc. **18**, 354—357 (1975)

Hill, B. T., Douglas, I. D. C., Grover, P. L.: Increased antitumour activity of chlorambucil following pretreatment with inducers of drug-metabolizing enzymes. Biochem. Pharmacol. **22**, 1083—1089 (1973)

Hill, D. L.: A Review of Cyclophosphamide. Springfield, Illinois: C. C. Thomas 1975

Hoffstein, S., Zurier, R. B., Weissmann, G.: Mechanisms of lysosomal enzyme release from human leukocytes. III. Quantitative morphologic evidence for an effect of cyclic nucleotides and colchicine on degranulation. Clin. Immunol. Immunopath. **3**, 201—217 (1974)

Horn, R. G., Collins, R. D.: Studies on the pathogenesis of the generalized Schwartzmann reaction. The role of granulocytes. Lab. Invest. **18**, 101—107 (1968)

Horwitz, D. A.: Selective depletion of Ig-bearing lymphocytes by cyclophosphamide in rheumatoid arthritis and systemic lupus erythematosus. Guidelines for dosage. Arthr. Rheum. **17**, 363—374 (1974)

Houck, J. C.: General introduction to the chalone concept. Nat. Cancer Inst. Monogr. **38**, 1—4 (1973)

Houck, J. C., Attallah, A. M., Lilly, J. R.: Immunosuppressive properties of the lymphocyte chalone. Nature (Lond.) **245**, 148—150 (1973 a)

Houck, J. C., Cheng, R. F., Sharma, V. K.: Control of fibroblast proliferation. Nat. Cancer Inst. Monogr. **38**, 161—170 (1973 b)

Houck, J. C., Irausquine, H.: Some properties of the lymphocyte chalone. Nat. Cancer Inst. Monogr. **38**, 117—122 (1973)

Houck, J. C., Sharma, V. K., Cheng, R. F.: Fibroblast chalone and serum nitrogen (anti-chalone). Nature (New Biol.) **246**, 111—113 (1973 c)

Howard, J. G., Courtenay, E. M.: Induction of B cell tolerance to polysaccharides by exhaustive immunization and during immunosuppression with cyclophosphamide. Europ. J. Immunol. **4**, 603—608 (1974)

Hunter, T., Urowitz, M. B., Gordon, D. A., Smythe, H. A., Ogryzlo, M. A.: Azathioprine in rheumatoid arthritis: A long-term follow-up study. Arthr. Rheum. **18**, 15—20 (1975)

Hurd, E. R., Giuliano, V. J.: The effect of cyclophosphamide on B and T lymphocytes in patients with connective tissue diseases. Arthr. Rheum. **18**, 67—75 (1975)

Hurd, E. R., Ziff, M.: Parameters of improvement in patients with rheumatoid arthritis treated with cyclophosphamide. Arthr. Rheum. **17**, 72—78 (1974)

Janossy, G., Graeves, M. F.: Lymphocyte activation. II. Discriminating stimulation of lymphocytes subpopulations by phytomitogens and heterologous antilymphocyte sera. Clin. exp. Immunol. **10**, 525 (1972)

Jarman, M.: Formation of 4-oxocyclophosphamide by the oxidation of cyclophosphamide with potassium permanganate. Experientia (Basel) **29**, 812—814 (1973)

Jarman, M., Griggs, L. J., Tisdale, M. J.: Synthesis of tritium-labelled chlorambucil and aniline mustards of high specific activity. J. med. Chem. **17**, 194—197 (1974)

Jerne, N. K., Nordin, A. A., Henry, C.: The agar plaque technique tor recognizing antibody-producing cells. In: Amos, B., Koprowski, H. (Eds.): Cell-Bound Antibodies, pp. 109—122. Philadelphia: Wistar Institute Press 1963

Johnson, M. W., Maibach, H. I., Salmon, S. E.: Skin reactivity in patients with cancer. Impaired delayed hypersensitivity or faulty inflammatory response? New Engl. J. Med. **284**, 1255—1257 (1971)

Jondal, M., Holm, G., Wigzell, H.: Surface markers on human T and B lymphocytes. A large population of lymphocytes forming non-immune rosettes with sheep red blood cells. J. exp. Med. **136**, 207—215 (1972)

Kahn, M. F., Bedoiseau, M., Six, B., Le Goff, P., De Seze, S.: Le chlorambucil dans la polyarthrite rhumatoide. Rev. Rhum. **38**, 741—748 (1971)

Kahn, M. F., De Seze, S.: The immunosuppressive agents in rheumatology. Indications, results and problems of long-term surveillance. Ann. Med. interne (Paris) **125**, 497—506 (1974)

Kaliss, N.: Jerne plague assay for antibody—forming spleen cells: some technical modifications. Transplantation **12**, 146—147 (1971)

Kaplan, H.: Sarcoid arthritis with a response to colchicine. New Engl. J. Med. **263**, 778—781 (1960)

Kaplan, H.: Further experiences with colchicine in the treatment of sarcoid arthritis. New Engl. J. Med. **268**, 761—764 (1963)

Kaplan, S. R., Calabresi, P.: Suppression of delayed hypersensitivity in vivo and in vitro by cytosin arabinoside. Clin. Res. **13**, 543—548 (1965)

Kaye, C. M.: Biosynthesis of mercapturic acids from allyl alcohol. Allyl Esters and acrolein. Biochem. J. **134**, 1093—1101 (1973)

Kaye, C. M., Young, L.: Acrolein as a possible metabolite of cyclophosphamide in man. Biochem. Soc. Trans. **2**, 308—310 (1974)

Keller, H. U., Borel, J. F., Wilkinson, P. C., Hess, M. W., Cottier, H.: Reassessment of Boyden's technique for measuring chemotaxis. J. immunol. Methods **1**, 165—168 (1972)

Kellermann, G., Cantrell, E., Shaw, C. R.: Variations in extent of aryl hydrocarbon hydroxylase induction in cultured human lymphocytes. Cancer Res. **33**, 1654—1656 (1973)

Kiger, N., Florentin, I., Mathé, G.: Inhibition of graft-versus-host reaction by preincubation of the graft with a thymic extract (lymphocyte chalone). Transplantation **16**, 393—397 (1973)

Kölle, G., Stöber, E., Schöntag, W.: Immunosuppressive agents in the basic therapy of visceral forms of rheumatoid arthritis in children. Med. Klin. **67**, 603—607 (1972)

Komarek, A., Dietrich, M. F.: Chemical prevention of experimental allergic encephalomyelitis in rats: A quantitative evaluation of steroids and various non-steroid drugs. Arch. int. Pharmacodyn. **193**, 249—257 (1971)

Kummer, D., Ochs, H. D.: Differenzierung der Wirkungsmechanismen alkylierender Cytostatika an Ehrlich-Ascitescarcinom- und lymphatischen Leukamiezellen. Z. Krebsforsch. **73**, 315—328 (1970)

Kvarstein, B., Stormorken, H.: Influence of acetylsalicylic acid, butazolidine, colchicine, hydrocortisone, chlorpromazine, and imipramine on the phagocytosis of polystyrene latex particles by human leucocytes. Biochem. Pharmacol. **20**, 119—124 (1971)

Lambert, P. H., Dixon, F. J.: Pathogenesis of the glomerulonephritis of NZB/W mice. J. exp. Med. **127**, 507—521 (1968)

Lawrence, W. H., Dillingham, E. O., Turner, J. E., Autian, J.: Toxicity profile of chloracetaldehyde. J. pharm. Sci. **61**, 19—25 (1972)

Lee, L., Stetson, C. A.: The local and generalized Schwartzman phenomena. In: Zweifach, B. W., Grant, Z., McClushey, R. T. (Eds.): The Inflammatory Process, pp. 791—818. New York: Academic Press 1965

Lehrer, R. I., Cline, M. J.: Interaction of Candida albicans with Human Leukocytes and Serum. J. Bact. **98**, 996—1004 (1969)

Lemmel, E., Hurd, E. R., Ziff, M.: Differential effect of 6-mercaptopurine and cyclophosphamide on autoimmune phenomena in NZB mice. Clin. exp. Immunol. **8**, 355—362 (1971)

Levy, D. A.: Studies of histamine release from human leukocytes. (Review) Ann. Allergy **27**, 511—518 (1969)

Levy, J., Paulus, H. E., Barnett, E. V., Sokoloff, M., Bangert, R., Pearson, C. M.: A double-blind controlled evaluation of azathioprine treatment in rheumatoid arthritis and psoriatic arthritis. Arthr. Rheum. **15**, 116—117 (1972)

Levy, J., Whitehouse, M. W.: Experimental evaluation of immunosuppressive durgs in the context of connective tissue diseases. In: Buchanan, W. W., Dick, W. C. (Eds.): Recent Advances in Rheumatology. Edinburgh: Churchill Livingston 1975

Levy, L.: Effect on pre-dosing animals with immunosuppressive drugs on immune and non-immune induced inflammatory responses. Arch. int. Pharmacodyn. **211**, 8—17 (1974)

Lidsky, M. D., Sharp, J. T., Billings, S.: Double-blind study of cyclophosphamide in rheumatoid arthritis. Arthr. Rheum. **16**, 148—153 (1973)

Lidsky, M. D., Sharp, J. T., Billings, S., Curtis, J. E.: Double-blind study of cyclophosphamide in rheumatoid arthritis. Arthr. Rheum. **15**, 117 (1972)

Linford, J. H., Froese, A., Israels, L. G.: Interaction of chlorambucil with cell surface. Nature (Lond.) **197**, 1068—1070 (1963)

Lozzio, B. B., Cawein, M. J.: Effects of phytohaemagglutinin on the depression of hematopoiesis by cytotoxic drugs. Advances Antimicrobial and Antineoplastic Chemotherapy, Proceeding 7th International Congress Chemotherapy 1971 **2**, 13—15 (1972)

Lozzio, B. B., Lozzio, C. B., Bamberger, E. G., Lair, S. V.: Regulators of cell division: Endogenous mitotic inhibitors of mammalian cells. Int. Rev. Cytol. **42**, 1—47 (1975)

McCarty, D. J., Gatter, R. A.: Recurrent acute inflammation associated with focal apatite crystal deposition. Arthr. Rheum. **9**, 804—809 (1966)

McConkey, B.: New drugs for inflammation—a clinical viewpoint for their assessment. Agents Actions **6**, 593—595 (1976)

Maibach, H. I., Maguire, H. C.: Interchangeability of methotrexate and cyclophosphamide as inhibitors of allergic contact dermatitis in the guinea pig. Int. Arch. Allergy **35**, 535—543 (1969)

Malawista, S. E., Bodel, P. T.: The dissociation by colchicine of phagocytosis from increased oxygen consumption in human leukocytes. J. clin. Invest. **46**, 786—796 (1967)

Maldyk, H., Chwalinska-Sadowska, H.: Results of endoxan therapy of psoriatic arthropathy and rheumatoid arthritis. Med. Welt **6**, 236—240 (1970)

Mauel, J., Rudolph, H., Chapuis, B., Brunner, K. T.: Allograft immunity in mice. II. Mechanism of target cell inactivation in vitro by sensitized lymphocytes. Immunology **18**, 517—535 (1970)

Miehlke, K., Kafarnik, U.: Clinical experiences in the therapy of rheumatoid arthritis using isophosphamide. Verh. dtsch. Ges. Rheum. **2**, 415—418 (1972)

Miehlke, K., Kohlhardt, I.: Basic therapy in chronic polyarthritis. Med. Klin. **65**, 1065—1072 (1970)

Mizel, S. B., Wilson, L.: Nucleosidetransport in mammalian cells. Inhibition by colchicine. Biochemistry **11**, 2573—2578 (1972)

Montgomery, J. A., Struck, R. F.: The relationship of the metabolism of anticancer agents to their activity. Progr. Drug Res. **17**, 320—409 (1973)

Mouridsen, H. T., Faber, O., Skovsted, L.: Biotransformation of cyclophosphamide in man. Analysis of the variation in normal subjects. Acta pharmacol. (Kbh.) **35**, 98—106 (1974)

Müller-Ruchholtz, W.: Beeinflussung transplantations-immunologischer Reaktionen durch Cyclophosphamid und andere homologe Oxazaphosphorin-2-oxide. Arzneimittel-Forsch. **24**, 1160—1167 (1974)

Munro, A., Bewick, M., Manuel, L., Cameron, J. S., Ellis, F. G., Boulten-Jones, M., Ogg, G. S.: Clinical evaluation of a rosette inhibition test in renal allotransplantation. Brit. med. J. **1971 III**, 271—276

Nicholls, A., Snaith, M. L., Maini, R. N., Scott, J. T.: Proceedings: controlled trial of azathioprine in rheumatoid vasculitis. Ann. rheum. Dis. **32**, 589—591 (1973)

Norpoth, K.: Studies on the metabolism of Ifosfamide in man. Cancer Treat. Rep. **60**, 437—443 (1976)

Norpoth, K., Addicks, H. W., Witting, U., Müller, G., Raidt, H.: Quantitative Bestimmung von Cyclophosphamid, Ifosfamid und Trofosfamid sowie ihrer stabilen Metabolite auf der DC-Platte mit 4-Pyridinaldehyd-2-benzothiazoylhydrazon PBH. Arzneimittel-Forsch. **25**, 1331—1336 (1975)

Ohira, S., Maezawa, S., Irinoda, Y., Watanabe, K., Kitada, K., Saito, T.: Increased antitumour activity of cyclophosphamide (Endoxan) following pretreatment with an inducer of drug-metabolizing enzymes. Tuhoku J. exp. Med. **114**, 55—60 (1974)

Oort, J., Turk, J. L.: A histological and autoradiographic study of lymphnodes during the development of contact sensitivity in the guinea-pig. J. exp. Path. **46**, 147—154 (1965)

Ortel, R. W., Newcombe, D. S.: Acute gouty arthritis and response to colchicine in the virtual absence of synovial-fluid leukocytes. New Engl. J. Med. **290**, 1363—1364 (1974)

Pantarotto, C., Bossi, A., Belvedere, G., Martini, A., Donelli, M. G., Frigerio, A.: Quantitative GLC determination of cyclophosphamide and isophosphamide in biological specimens. J. pharm. Sci. **63**, 1554—1558 (1974)

Paterson, P. Y., Drobish, D. G., Biddick, A. S.: Cyclophosphamide inhibition of experimental allergic thyroditis and thyroid antibody production in rats. J. Immunol. **106**, 570—572 (1971)

Paterson, A. R. P., Tidd, D. M.: 6-Thiopurines. In: Sartorelli, A. C., Johns, D. G. (Eds.): Antineoplastic and Immunosuppressive Agents, Part II, Handbook of Experimental Pharmacology, pp. 384—403. Berlin-Heidelberg-New York: Springer-Verlag 1975

Paulus, H. E., Machleder, H., Bangert, R., Stratton, J. A., Goldberg, L., Whitehouse, M. W., Yu, D., Pearson, C. M.: A case report: thoracic duct lymphocyte drainage in rheumatoid arthritis. Clin. Immunol. Immunopath. **1**, 173—181 (1973)

Pearson, C. M., Paulus, H. E., Machleder, H. T.: The role of the lymphocyte and its products in the propagation of joint disease: Ann. N.Y. Acad. Sci. **256**, 150—168 (1975)

Penn, I., Starzle, T. E.: A summary of the status of de novo cancer in transplant patients. Transplant. Proc. **4**, 719—732 (1972)

Perings, E., Reisert, P. E., Kraft, H. G.: Studies on the anti-inflammatory effect of azathioprine. Int. Z. klin. Pharmakol. Ther. Toxikol. **5**, 200—202 (1971)

Pernis, B., Farris, L., Awante, L.: Immunoglobulin spots on the surface of rabbit lymphocytes. J. exp. Med **132**, 1001—1018 (1970)

Perper, R. J., Sanda, M., Chinea, G., Oronsky, A. L.: Leukocyte chemotaxis in vivo. II. Analysis of the selective inhibition of neutrophil a mononuclear cell accumulation. J. Lab. clin. Med. **84**, 394—406 (1974)

Petranyi, G. G., Benczur, M., Onody, K., Alfoldy, P., Institoris, L.: Dose- and time-dependent suppressive and enhancing effect of cytostatics in vitro on the target cell killing activity of lymphocytes. Folia biol. (Krakow) **19**, 420—423 (1973)

Phillips, B. J.: A simple, small scale cytotoxicity test, and its uses in drug metabolism studies. Biochem. Pharmacol. **23**, 131—138 (1974)

Quagliata, F., Phillips-Quagliata, J. M., Floersheim, G. L.: Immunosuppression by procarbazine. I. Sites of action of the drug and effect on adjuvant arthritis and circulating antibody response. Cell. Immunol. **3**, 198—212 (1972)

Raff, M. G.: Theta antigen, a marker for thymusderived lymphocytes. Nature (Lond.) **244**, 378—380 (1969)

Rau, R.: Cyclophosphamide therapy of progredient chronic polyarthritis with special reference to acid alpha 1-proteins and immunoglobulins. Dtsch. med. Wschr. **96**, 992 (1971)

Reed, D. J.: Procarbazine. In: Sartorelli, A. C., Johns, D. G. (Eds.): Antineoplastic and immunosuppressive agents, Part II, Handbook of Experimental Pharmacology, pp. 747—765. Berlin-Heidelberg-New York: Springer 1975

Reis, P. J., Chapman, R. E.: Changes in wool growth and skin of Merino sheep following administration of cyclophosphamide. Aust. J. agric. Res. **25**, 931—943 (1974)

Revell, P. A.: Studies on the effect of cyclophosphamide on T and B lymphocytes in the blood, lymph nodes, and thymus or normal guinea-pig. Int. Arch. Allergy **47**, 864—874 (1974)

Riches, P. G., Harrap, K. R.: The binding of (^{3}H) chlorambucil to nuclear proteins of the Yoshida ascites sarcoma. Chem. biol. Interact. **11**, 291—299 (1975)

Rose, N. R.: Autoimmune diseases. In: Zweifach, B. W., Grant, L., McCluskey, R. T. (Eds.): The Inflammatory Process, Volume III, pp. 347—400. New York: Academic Press 1974

Rosenberg, S., Calabresi, P.: Enhanced suppression of secondary immune response by combination of 6-mercaptopurine "duazomycin A". Nature (Lond.) **199**, 1101—1102 (1963)

Rosenthale, M. E.: Evaluation for immunosuppressive and antiallergic activity. In: Scherrer, R. A., Whitehouse, M. W. (Eds.): Antiinflammatory Agents, Chemistry and Pharmacology, Vol. II, pp. 123—182. New York: Academic Press 1974

Ross, W. C. J.: Conjugation of chlorambucil with human γ-globulin. Confirmation that the drug is bound in an active form. Chem. biol. Interactions **10**, 169—172; **11**, 139—143 (1975)

Rubens, R. D., Dulbecco, R.: Augmentation of cytotoxic drug action of antibodies directed at cell surface. Nature (Lond.) **248**, 81—82 (1974)

Rundles, R. W., Laszlo, J., Itoga, T., Hobson, J. B., Garrison, F. E.: Clinical and hematologic study of 6(/1-methyl-4-nitro-5-imidazolyl/thio)-purine and related compounds. Cancer Chemother. Rep. **14**, 99—115 (1961)

Schmid, L., Brune, K.: Assessement of phagocytic and antimicrobial activity of human granulocytes. Infect. Immun. **10**, 1120—1126 (1974)

Schultz, M. E., Weldon, M. W.: Initial effects of cyclophosphamide on urinary bladder epithelium in the rat. Pathology **6**, 343—350 (1974)

Sheard, P., Killingback, P. G., Blair, A. M.: Antigen induced release of histamine and SRS-A from human lung passively sensitized with reaginic serum. Nature (Lond.) **216**, 283—284 (1967)

Singer, B. L., Brody, J. L.: In vitro activation of cyclophosphamide by phytohaemagglutinin-stimulated lymphocytes. Amer. J. med. Sci. **264**, 307—312 (1972)

Skinner, M. D., Schwartz, R. S.: Immunosuppressive therapy of immuno inflammatory diseases. Rheumatology **5**, 1—48 (1974)

Sladek, N. E.: Therapeutic efficacy of cyclophosphamide as a function of its metabolism. Cancer Res. **32**, 535—542 (1972a)

Sladek, N. E.: Therapeutic efficacy of cyclophosphamide as a function of inhibition of its metabolism. Cancer Res. **32**, 1848—1854 (1972b)

Sladek, N. E.: Evidence for an aldehyde possessing alkylating activity as the primary metabolite of cyclophosphamide. Cancer Res. **33**, 651—658 (1973a)

Sladek, N. E.: Bioassay and relative cytotoxic potency of cyclophosphamide metabolites generated in vitro and in vivo. Cancer Res. **33**, 1150—1158 (1973b)

Smith, J. L., Forbes, I. J.: Inhibition of protein synthesis in human lymphocytes by thiopurines. Aust. J. exp. Biol. med. Sci. **48**, 267—276 (1970)

Snaith, M. L., Holt, J. M., Oliver, D. O., Dunnill, M. S., Halley, W., Stephonson, A. C.: Treatment of patients with systemic lupus erythematosus including nephritis with chlorambucil. Brit. med. J. **1973 II**, 197—201

Sofia, R. D., Knobloch, L. C., Vassar, H. B.: Inhibition of the primary lesion of adjuvant-induced polyarthritis in rats (18-hr-arthritis test) for specific detection of clinically effective antiarthritic drugs. J. Pharmacol. exp. Ther. **193**, 918—931 (1975)

Soifer, D. (Ed.): The biology of cytoplasmic microtubules. Ann. N.Y. Acad. Sci. **253** (1975)

Spiegelberg, H. L., Miescher, P. A.: The effect of 6-mercaptopurine and aminopterin on experimental immune thyroiditis in guinea pigs. J. exp. Med. **118**, 869—890 (1963)

Spilberg, I.: Current concepts of the mechanisme of acute inflammation in gouty arthritis. Arthr. Rheum. **18**, 129—134 (1975)

Stastny, P., Rosenthal, M., Andreis, M., Cooke, D., Ziff, M.: Lymphokines in rheumatoid synovitis. Ann. N.Y. Acad. Sci. **256**, 117—131 (1975)

Steinberg, A. D., Gelfand, M. C., Hardin, J. A., Lowenthal, D. T.: Therapeutic studies in NZB/W mice. III. Relationship between renal status and efficacy of immunosuppressive drug therapie. Arthr. Rheum. **18**, 9—14 (1975)

Stevens, J. E., Willoughby, D. A.: The anti-inflammatory effect of some immunosuppressive agents. J. Path. **97**, 367—373 (1969)

Stevenson, A. C., Patel, C.: Effects of chlorambucil on human chromosomes. Mutation Res. **18**, 333—351 (1973)

Strong, J. S., Bartholomew, P. A., Smyth, C. J.: Immunoresponsiveness of patients with rheumatoid arthritis receiving cyclophosphamide or gold salts. Ann. rheum. Dis. **32**, 233—237 (1973)

Struck, R. F.: Isolation and identification of a stabilised derivative of aldophosphamide, a major metabolite of cyclophosphamide. Cancer Res. **34**, 2933—2935 (1974)

Struck, R. F.: Aldophosphamide: Synthesis, characterization, and comparison with "Hohorst's aldophosphamide". Cancer Treat. Rep. **60**, 317—319 (1976)

Struck, R. F., Kirk, M. C., Mellett, L. B., El Dareer, S., Hill, D. L.: Urinary metabolites of the antitumour agent cyclophosphamide. Molec. Pharmacol. **7**, 519—529 (1971)

Struck, R. F., Kirk, M. C., Witt, M. H., Laster, W. R.: Isolation and mass spectral identification of blood metabolites of cyclophosphamide: evidence for phosphoramide mustard as the biologically active metabolite. Biomed. Mass Spectr. **2**, 46—52 (1975)

Struck, R. F., Thorpe, M. C., Coburn, W. C., Laster, W. R.: Cyclophosphamide. Complete inhibition of murine leukemia L 1210 in vivo by a Fenton oxidation product. J. Amer. chem. Soc. **96**, 313—315 (1974)

Swingle, K. F., Grant, T. J., Valle, P. M.: Effect of immunosuppressive drugs on a localised graft-versus-host reaction in the rat. Proc. Soc. exp. Biol. (N.Y.) **142**, 1329—1331 (1973)

Swingle, K. F.: Evaluation for anti-inflammatory activity. In: Scherrer, R. A., Whitehouse, M. W. (Eds.): Anti-Inflammatory Agents, Chemistry and Pharmacology, Vol. II, pp. 34—110. New York: Academic Press 1974

Takamizawa, A., Matsumoto, S., Iwata, T., Tochino, Y., Katagiri, K., Yamaguchi, K., Shiratori, O.: Preparation of an active species of cyclophosphamide and related compounds. J. med. Chem. **18**, 376—383 (1975)

Takamizawa, A., Tochino, Y., Hamashima, Y., Iwata, T.: Studies on cyclophosphamide metabolites and their related compounds I. Chem. pharm. Bull. **20**, 1612—1616 (1972)

Taylor, A., Maffly, R., Wilson, L., Raven, E.: Evidence for involvement of microtubules in the action of vasopressin. The biology of cytoplasmic microtubules. Ann. N.Y. Acad. Sci. **253**, 723—737 (1975)

Thompson, G. R., Ting, J. M., Riggs, G. A.: Calcific tendinitis and soft-tissue calcification resembling gout. J. Amer. med. Soc. **203**, 464 (1968)

Thomson, M., Colvin, M.: Chemical oxidation of cyclophosphamide and 4-methylcyclophosphamide. Cancer Res. **34**, 981—985 (1974)

Thumb, N.: Immunosuppressive therapy of chronic polyarthritis. Wien Z. inn. Med. Suppl., 1—52 (1972)

Tisdale, M. J., Phillips, B. J.: Comparative effects of alkylating agents and other anti-tumour agents on the intracellular level of adenosine-3',5'-monophosphate in Walker carcinoma. Biochem. Pharmacol. **24**, 1271—1276 (1975)

Tolley, D. A., Castro, J. E.: Cyclophosphamide-induced cystitis of the urinary bladder of rats and its pretreatment. Proc. roy. soc. Med. **68**, 169—170 (1975)

Torkelson, A. R., La Budde, J. A., Weikel, J. H.: The metabolic fate of cyclophosphamide. Drug Metab. Rev. **3**, 131—165 (1974)

Townes, A. S., Sowa, J. M., Shulman, L. E.: Controlled trial of cyclophosphamide in rheumatoid arthritis (RA): An 18-month double-blind cross-over study. Arthr. Rheum. **15**, 129—130 (1972)

Tsukada, W., Akimoto, T., Mizushima, Y.: Some aspects of anti-inflammatory action of immunosuppressive drugs. Jap. J. Pharmacol. **24**, 583—588 (1974)

Turk, J. L.: Studies on the mechanism of action of methotrexate and cyclophosphamide on contact sensitivity in the guinea pig. Int. Arch. Allergy **24**, 191—200 (1964)

Ukena, T. E., Berlin, R. D.: Effect of colchicine and vinblastine on the topographical separation of membrane functions. J. exp. Med. **136**, 1—7 (1972)

Urowitz, M. B., Gordon, D. A., Smythe, H. A., Pruzanski, W., Ogryzio, M. A.: Azathioprine in rheumatoid arthritis. A double-blind, cross over study. Arthr. Rheum. **16**, 411—418 (1973)

Van Arman, C. G.: Anti-inflammatory drugs. Clin. Pharmacol. Ther. **16**, 900—904 (1974)

Van der Steen, J., Timmer, E. C., Westra, J. G., Benckhuysen, C.: 4-Hydroperoxidation in the Fenton oxidation of the anti-tumour agent cyclophosphamide. J. Amer. chem. Soc. **95**, 7535—7536 (1973)

Völker, G., Dräger, U., Peter, G., Hohorst, H. J.: Studien zum Spontanzerfall von 4-Hydroxycyclophosphamid and 4-Hydroperoxycyclophosphamid mit Hilfe der Dünnschichtchromatographie. Arzneimittel-Forsch. **24**, 1172—1176 (1974)

Wahl, S. M.: Corticosteroid inhibition of chemotactic lymphokine production by T and B lymphocytes. Mechanism of Tissue Injury with Reference to Rheumatoid Arthritis. Ann. N.Y. Acad. Sci. **256**, 375—385 (1975)

Walker, D., Gill, J. J., Carson, J. M.: Leiomyosarcoma in a renal allograft recipient treated with immunosuppressive drugs. J. Amer. med. Ass. **215**, 2084—2086 (1971)

Wallace, S. L.: Colchicine. Semin. Arthr. J. Amer. med. Ass. Rheum. **3**, 369—381 (1974)

Wallace, S. L., Bernstein, D., Diamond, H.: Diagnostic value of the colchicine therapeutic trial. J. Amer. med. Ass. **199**, 525 (1967)

Wallace, S. L., Ertel, N. H.: Colchicine: Current Problems. Bull. rheum. Dis. **20**(4), 582—587, Dec. 1969

Walton, J. R., Buckley, I. K.: Cell models in the study of mechanisms of toxicity. Agents Actions **5**, 69—88 (1975)

Ward, P. A.: Leukotactic factors in health and disease. Amer. J. Path. **64**, 521—530 (1971)

Wawrzynska-Pagowska, J., Graff-Wroblewska, T., Juszczozyk, T., Michalski, J., Pakula, A., Piotrowska, D., Scislowska, M.: Results of clinical management of patients with very active rheumatoid arthritis. Comparative demonstration of therapy with non-steroid antiphlogistics, gold salts and the immunosuppressive agents proresid and endoxan. Z. Rheumaforsch. **32**, 32—39 (1973)

Weigl, E., Lehmann, G., Krieg, D.: Immunosuppressive therapy in rheumatoid arthritis. Z. ges. inn. Med. **26**, 561—563 (1971)

Weinstein, G. D.: Biochemical and pathophysiological rationale for amethopterin in psoriasis. Ann. N.Y. Acad. Sci. **186**, 452—466 (1971)

Whitehouse, M. W.: Timely appraisal: Ectopic (excellular) nucleic acid as a drug target, especially in rheumatoid arthritis and certain cancers(?). Agents Actions **5**, 508—511 (1975)

Whitehouse, M. W.: Unpublished observations (1976)

Whitehouse, M. W., Beck, F. W. J.: Irritancy of cyclophosphamide-derived aldehydes (acrolein, chloracetaldehyde) and their effects on lymphocyte distribution in vivo: protective effect of thiols and bisulphite ions. Agents Actions **5**, 541—548 (1975)

Whitehouse, M. W., Beck, F. W. J., Dröge, M. M., Struck, R. F.: Lymphocyte deactivation by (potential immunosuppressant) alkylating metabolites of cyclophosphamide. Agents Actions **4**, 117—124 (1974 b)

Whitehouse, M. W., Beck, F. J., Kacena, A.: Some (pharmacological) properties of chloracetaldehyde, an oxidation product and potential metabolite of cyclophosphamide. Agents Actions **4**, 34—43 (1974 a)

Wilson, D. B.: Quantitative studies on the behavior of sensitized lymphocytes in vitro. II. Inhibitory influence of the immunosuppressor, Imuran, on the destructive reaction of sensitized lymphoid cells against homologous target cells. J. exp. Med. **122**, 167—172 (1965)

Winkelstein, A., Mikulla, J. M., Nankin, H. R., Pollock, B. H., Stolzer, B. L.: Mechanisms of immunosuppression: effects of cyclophosphamide on lymphocytes. J. Lab. clin. Med. **80**, 506—513 (1972)

Woodland, J., Mason, R. M., Harris, J., Dixon, A. S., Currey, H. L., Brownjohn, A. M., Davies, J., Owen-Smith, B. D.: Trial of azathioprine, cyclophosphamide, and gold in rheumatoid arthritis. Ann. rheum. Dis. **33**, 399—401 (1974)

Worth, P. N. L.: Cyclophosphamide and the bladder. Brit. med. J. **1971 III**, 182

Wright, D. G., Malawista, S. E.: The mobilization and extracellular release of granular enzymes from phagocytizing human leukocytes. J. Cell Biol. **53**, 788—797 (1972)

Yahara, I., Edelman, G. M.: Modulation of lymphocyte receptor mobility by concanavalin A and colchicine. Ann. N. Y. Acad. Sci. **253**, 454—469 (1975)

Yu, D. T., Clements, P. J., Peter, J. B., Levy, J., Paulus, H. E., Barnett, E. V.: Lymphocyte characteristics in rheumatic patients and the effect of azathioprine therapy. Arthr. Rheum. **17**, 37—45 (1974)

Yu, D. T. Y., Whitehouse, M. W.: Effect of some nitrogen mustards and thoracic duct drainage on lymphocyte distribution in rats. Int. Arch. Allergy **46**, 172—182 (1974)

Ziff, M., Hurd, E. R., Stastny, P.: B- and T-lymphocytes in rheumatoid synovitis and the effect of cyclophosphamide. Proc. roy. soc. Med. **67**, 536—540 (1974)

Addendum

The following papers which have appeared after completion of this manuscript are of relevance to the topics discussed:

Side-Effects of Cytostats:

Kahn, M. F., Vitale, C., Grimaldi, A.: Infections et immunod'epresseurs en rhumatologie. Sem. Hop. Paris **52**, 1374—1376 (1976)

Pinals, R. S.: Azathioprine in the treatment of chronic polyarthritis: Longterm results and adverse effects in 25 patients. J. Rheumatol. **3**, 140—144 (1976)

Thorpe, P.: Rheumatoid arthritis treated with chlorambucil: A five-year follow-up. Med. J. Aust. **2**, 197—199 (1976)

Seidenfeld, A. M., Smythe, H. A., Ogryzlo, M. A., Urowitz, M. B., Dotten, D. A.: Acute leukemia in rheumatoid arthritis treated with cytotoxic agents. J. Rheumatol. **3**, 295—304 (1976)

Controled Studies:

Berry, H., Liyanage, S. P., Durance, R. A., Barnes, C. G., Berger, L. A., Evans, S.: Azathioprine and penicillamine in treatment of rheumatoid arthritis: A controlled trial. Brit. Med. J. **1**, 1052—1054 (1976)

Dwosh, I. L., Stein, H. B., Urowitz, M. B., Smythe, H. A., Hunter, T., Ogryzlo, M. A.: Azathioprine in early rheumatoid arthritis: Comparison with gold and chloroquine. Arthritis Rheum. **20**, 685—692 (1977)

Cade, R., Stein, G., Pickering, M., Schlein, E., Spooner, G.: Low dose, long-term treatment of rheumatoid arthritis with azathioprine. South. Med. J. **69**, 388—392 (1976)

Goebel, K. M., Janzen, R., Joseph, K., Börngen, U.: Disparity between clinical and immune responses in a controlled trial of azathioprine in rheumatoid arthritis. Eur. J. Clin. Pharmacol. **9**, 405—410 (1976)

Townes, A. S., Sowa, J. M., Shulman, L. E.: Controlled trial of cyclophosphamide in rheumatoid arthritis. Arthritis Rheum. **19**, 563—573 (1976)

Immunologic Status of Patients during Therapy:

Ziegler, J. B., Hansen, P., Cooper, D. A., Penny, R.: Monitoring immune function during immunosuppressive therapy. Aust. NZ. J. Med. **6**, 136—141 (1976)

CHAPTER 36

Control of Hyperuricemia

J. KOVARSKY and E. W. HOLMES*

A. Introduction

Gout is a disorder of diverse aetiologies characterized by recurrent episodes of acute and chronic inflammation of the joints. Several groups of investigators have shown that the acute attack of gouty arthritis is due to the deposition of monosodium urate crystals in the synovial fluid (PHELPS et al., 1968; SEEGMILLER et al., 1963; ZWAIFLER and PEKIN, 1963). Other clinical manifestations of this disorder may include relatively painless tophaceous deposits, renal calculi and renal insufficiency.

Hyperuricemia, the biochemical hallmark of gout, was first demonstrated in 1848 by Sir Alfred GARROD. Defined by stastical analysis of normal populations, hyperuricemia exists when the serum urate concentration exceeds 7 mg/100 ml in males or 6 mg/100 ml in females, as measured by the enzymic spectrophotometric method (BROCHNER-MORTENSEN et al., 1963). Serum is supersaturated with urate when the concentration is greater than 6.4 mg/100 ml (PETERS and VAN SLYKE, 1946). The conditions leading to urate crystallization are not fully understood at the present time. Crystallization may be influenced by factors other than urate concentration, such as salt concentration (KIPPEN et al., 1974a), protein binding of urate (BLUE-STONE et al., 1974), glycosoaminoglycan binding of urate (KATZ and SCHUBERT, 1970), calcium concentration (WILCOX and KHALAF, 1975) and other factors (reviewed in WYNGAARDEN and KELLEY, 1976).

Reduction of serum urate below the saturation level for extracellular fluid is effective in the long term control of the "gouty diathesis", i.e. acute arthritis, tophi and renal complications. The primary objective of hypouricemic therapy is the reduction of the total body urate pool. In the absence of tophi, the serum urate is generally a reliable index of the miscible urate pool (SORENSEN, 1959, 1962). Drugs used clinically for reduction of the urate pool fall into two major categories: agents inhibiting uric acid synthesis and uricosuric agents. Pharmacological uricolysis has been used although it is not in general clinical use. Before discussing specific pharmacological agents in more detail, a brief review of uric acid metabolism in order.

B. Uric Acid Metabolism

In all mammals, except man and some of the higher apes, the endproduct of purine metabolism is allantoin. Uricase, the enzyme responsible for oxidizing uric acid to allantoin, is functionally absent in man. As a consequence the endproduct of purine metabolism is uric acid, a compound $^1/_{10}$–$^1/_{100}$ as soluble as allantoin, predisposing man to the development of hyperuricemia and gout. Hyperuricemia may result from an increase in the rate of synthesis of uric acid, a decrease in the renal excretion of uric acid or a combination of both of these processes.

Figure 1 illustrates the metabolic sequences leading to the synthesis of uric acid. Because of the high activity of xanthine oxidase in the liver, and the limited tissue distribution of xanthine oxidase, uric acid synthesis appears to be largely a hepatic process in man (reviewed in WYNGAARDEN and KELLEY, 1976). Since plasma contains only small amounts of the uric acid precursors hypoxanthine and xanthine (HOFFMAN et al., 1951; JORGENSEN and POULSEN, 1955; SEGAL and WYNGAARDEN, 1955), the major source of these oxypurines (hypoxanthine and xanthine) derives from the intracellular catabolism of purine ribonucleotides. There are three pathways leading to the synthesis of purine ribonucleotides: catabolism of nucleic acids, re-utilization of purine bases and purine biosynthesis de novo. Abnormalities in each of these pathways have been reported to produce hyperuricemia and gout (reviewed in WYNGAARDEN and KELLEY, 1976). The common feature of each of these abnormalities is an increase in the rate of purine biosynthesis de novo (Fig. 1). Recent studies have begun to elucidate the factors controlling the activity of this pathway (reviewed in HOLMES et al., 1976). An increase in the intracellular concentration of PP-ribose-P or a decrease in purine ribonucleotides may accelerate the rate of purine biosynthesis de novo by increasing the activity of the first enzyme unique to this pathway, amidophosphoribosyltransferase (Fig. 1).

The major route of uric acid elimination in man is the kidney. Approximately 75% of an intravenous dose of radiolabelled uric acid can be recovered in the urine (BUZARD et al., 1952; GEREN et al., 1950; SORENSEN, 1959, 1960; WYNGAARDEN, 1955). The remaining 25% is excreted into the gastro-intestinal tract where it may be degraded by bacteria in the gut (SORENSEN, 1959). Trivial amounts of uricolysis may also occur in human tissues, via two enzyme systems shown to degrade uric acid in vitro at physiological pH: verdoperoxidase (CANELLAKIS et al., 1955) and cytochrome-cytochrome oxidase (GRIFFITHS, 1952).

The renal excretion of uric acid in man is regulated by a three-component system, originally described by GUTMAN and YU (1961). These include glomerular filtration, tubular secretion and tubular reabsorption. Most reviews of renal urate handling state that urate is freely filtrable at the glomerulus. Investigations of urate binding to plasma proteins, which may influence urate availability for glomerular filtration, have yielded conflicting but generally negative results (ALVSAKER, 1965; CAMPION et al., 1973; FARRELL et al., 1971; KOVARSKY et al., 1976; SHEIKH and MOLLER, 1968). While it is clear that urate is both reabsorbed and secreted, it is not clear what relative role each of these processes play in the final excretion of uric acid. Recent evaluations of the "pyrazinamide suppression test" have cast some doubt on the validity of this technique for differentiation of secretion and reabsorption of uric acid (HOLMES et al., 1972). Likewise, it is not possible to state with certainty the site(s) at which urate is reabsorbed and secreted in the human nephron. Studies have been interpreted to indicate that urate is secreted in the proximal nephron, and there may be multiple sites for urate reabsorption in the proximal and distal nephron (reviewed in RIESELBACH and STEELE, 1975).

Although it is not possible to quantitate urate reabsorption and secretion with current techniques, there are reliable measures of uric acid excretion in man. Under

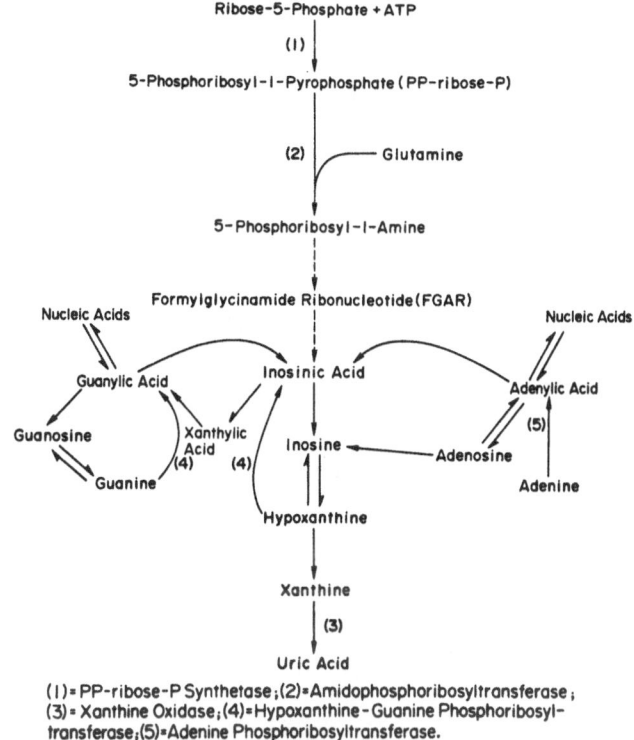

Fig. 1. Formation of uric acid in man. *(1)* = PP-ribose-P synthetase; *(2)* = Amidophosphoribosyl-transferase; *(3)* = Xanthine oxidase; *(4)* = Hypoxanthine-guanine phosphoribosyltransferase; *(5)* = Adenine phosphoribosyltransferase

normal circumstances, a 24-h urine sample contains up to 600 mg of uric acid in a person ingesting a purine-free diet (GUTMAN and YU, 1957a; SEEGMILLER et al., 1961). When ingesting a regular diet, daily excretion of uric acid may reach 800 to 1000 mg of uric acid. The clearance ratio of urate of inulin is 7 to 10% in normal humans (reviewed in WYNGAARDEN and KELLEY, 1976).

C. Biochemical Pharmacology of Hypouricemic Drugs

I. Drugs Reducing Uric Acid Synthesis

1. Allopurinol and Oxipurinol

Allopurinol [4-hydroxy-pyrazolo(3,4-d)-pyrimidine] was initially developed as a chemotherapeutic agent, but proved largely ineffective on experimental tumors (SHAW et al., 1960; WHITE, 1959). Other studies demonstrated that it was a potent xanthine oxidase inhibitor in vitro (FEIGELSON et al., 1957), leading to its initial clinical use as a therapeutic adjunct in leukaemic patients receiving 6-thiopurine (RUNDLES et al., 1963). During the course of these studies it was observed that serum

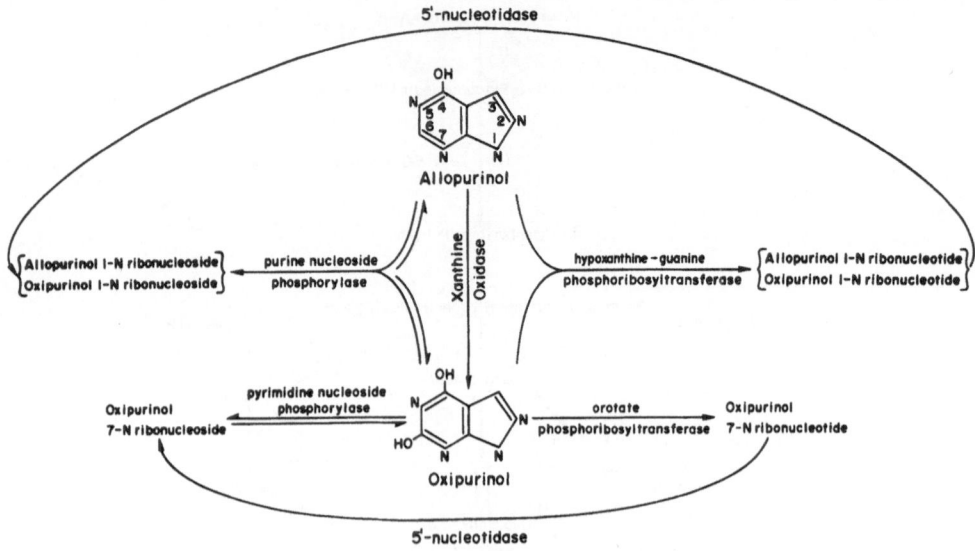

Fig. 2. Metabolism of allopurinol and oxipurinol

and urinary urate values were lowered, leading to a therapeutic trial of allopurinol in gouty patients (RUNDLES et al., 1963; WYNGAARDEN et al., 1963). Within a few years, allopurinol was demonstrated to be an effective form of therapy for interval gout (DELBARRE et al., 1966; KLINENBERG et al., 1965; RUNDLES et al., 1964, 1966; WYN-GAARDEN et al., 1965; YU and GUTMAN, 1964).

Figure 2 shows the metabolic fate of allopurinol. Only 3–10% of the allopurinol administered is excreted unchanged in the urine. Most of the absorbed allopurinol is rapidly oxidized to oxipurinol [4,6-dihydroxypyrazolo (3,4-d)-pyrimidine] (ELION, 1966). This reaction is predominantly catalyzed by xanthine oxidase in vitro, but another aldehyde oxidase may also play a role in this oxidation (KRENITSKY et al., 1972). A small portion of the allopurinol is metabolized to allopurinol ribonucleoside (KRENITSKY et al., 1967) and ribonucleotide (FOX et al., 1970a). Allopurinol metabolite incorporation into nucleic acids has not been demonstrated (NELSON and ELION, 1975). Most of the oxipurinol is excreted unchanged in the urine, with small amounts being converted to oxipurinol ribonucleosides (BEARDMORE and KELLEY, 1971) and ribonucleotides (ELION et al., 1968). The biological half-life of allopurinol is only 2–3 h, whereas that of oxipurinol is approximately 28 h (ELION et al., 1966).

Both allopurinol and oxipurinol produce pseudo-irreversible inactivation of xanthine oxidase in vitro, although experimental data suggest their inhibitory mechanisms may differ. The in vitro affinity of xanthine oxidase for allopurinol is 15–200 times greater than for oxipurinol (ELION, 1966). While allopurinol inhibits xanthine oxidase in the absence of substrate, oxipurinol reportedly has no effect on xanthine oxidase activity in the absence of xanthine (ELION, 1966; RUNDLES et al., 1969). The inhibition produced by allopurinol can be reversed by prolonged dialysis (ELION, 1966), and that produced by oxipurinol by prolonged exposure to oxygen (MASSEY et al., 1970).

In addition to the inhibition of xanthine oxidase, allopurinol administration decreases total purine production (RUNDLES et al., 1963). This effect of allopurinol in decreasing purine biosynthesis de novo requires the presence of hypoxanthine-guanine phosphoribosyltransferase (HGPRT) activity (Fig. 1), since Lesch-Nyhan patients do not demonstrate this phenomenon (KELLEY et al., 1968). Following allopurinol administration there is an increase in the availability of substrates (hypoxanthine and allopurinol) for the HGPRT reaction. An increase in the utilization of these substrates by HGPRT could account for the observed PP-ribose-P depletion in patients receiving allopurinol (Fox et al., 1970a). This same reaction sequence could lead to an increase in the synthesis of purine and allopurinol ribonucleotides. Since the rate of purine biosynthesis de novo may be regulated by the relative intracellular concentrations of PP-ribose-P and purine ribonucleotides (reviewed in HOLMES et al., 1976), the above observations provide a potential explanation for the observed decrease in purine biosynthesis de novo in patients receiving allopurinol.

Allopurinol has a number of additional metabolic effects. The clinical significance of each remains to be determined. The orotate phosphoribosyltransferase and orotidylic decarboxylase reactions of pyrimidine metabolism are inhibited (BEARD-MORE et al., 1972; Fox et al., 1970b; GROBNER and KELLEY, 1975; KELLEY and BEARDMORE, 1970; KROOTH et al., 1974). Several hepatic microsomal enzymes important in drug metabolism are inhibited by allopurinol (VESELL et al., 1970), and drugs metabolized by this system should be used with caution in patients receiving allopurinol. Several other enzyme systems are inhibited by allopurinol in vitro, but in vivo activity remains to be demonstrated. These include tryptophan pyrrolase (CHYTIL, 1968; GHOSH and FORREST, 1967; JULIAN and CHYTIL, 1970), purine nucleoside phosphorylase (KRENITSKY et al, 1967, 1968), pyrimidine deoxyribosyltransferase (GALLO et al., 1968) and urate oxidase (TRUSCOE and WILLIAMS, 1968).

2. Thiopurinol

The actions of thiopurinol [mercapto-4-pyrazolo-(3,4d)-pyrimidine] will be discussed here, although the mechanism of its hypouricemic action remains to be elucidated. Thiopurinol is the 4-thio analogue of allopurinol. Over 70% of this compound is oxidized to oxithiopurinol and excreted in the urine (AUSCHER et al., 1974a). While oxithiopurinol is a potent inhibitor of mouse xanthine oxidase in vitro (cited in SIMMONDS et al., 1974), it does not inhibit xanthine oxidase in vivo, since the urinary excretion of hypoxanthine and xanthine is unchanged in patients receiving thiopurinol (DELBARRE et al., 1968; GRAHAME et al., 1974; SERRE et al., 1970). To account for these observations it has been suggested that thiopurinol, unlike allopurinol, is not oxidized by xanthine oxidase in vivo, but by another aldehyde oxidase (KRENITSKY et al., 1972). Because of the lack of increase in xanthine excretion during thiopurinol administration, it was thought to be of potential value as a hypouricemic agent in patients markedly overproducing uric acid and prone to develop xanthine stones on allopurinol (cited in SIMMONDS et al., 1974). However, thiopurinol is not an effective hypouricemic agent in patients with HGPRT deficiency (AUSCHER et al., 1974b).

No single theory currently advanced adequately explains the mode of action of thiopurinol. Since its hypouricemic effect requires the presence of HGPRT activity, it has been postulated to inhibit purine biosynthesis de novo through conversion to its ribonucleotide and/or depletion of PP-ribose-P (Auscher et al., 1974b; Cartier and Hamet, 1973; Delbarre et al., 1968; Serre et al., 1970). However, thiopurinol and oxithiopurinol ribonucleotides have not been demonstrated in vivo (Grahame et al., 1974). No effects on orotate phosphoribosyltransferase or orotidylic decarboxylase activities have been noted in patients receiving thiopurinol (Fox et al., 1971; Nelson et al., 1973), as opposed to patients receiving allopurinol. Furthermore, the mode of action of thiopurinol may not be the same in all groups of hyperuricemic patients. Only serum urate levels are lowered in normoexcretors of uric acid, while both serum and urinary urate levels are lowered in hyperexcretors (Delbarre et al., 1968; Grahame et al., 1974; Serre et al., 1970). Based on in vitro data demonstrating that thiopurinol displaces urate bound to serum proteins, it has been postulated that this agent might be uricosuric (Dean et al., 1974). However, the above clinical studies have failed to document that thiopurinol is uricosuric. Further studies are needed to determine the mechanism of the observed hypouricemic effect.

3. Other Inhibitors of Uric Acid Synthesis

A large number of compounds may produce hypouricemia by inhibiting purine biosynthesis de novo (cited in Henderson, 1972). Among these are the glutamine antagonists azaserine and diazonorleucine, and a wide variety of purine analogues. The latter include diaminopurine, 6-methylpurine, 6-mercaptopurine, 6-methylthiopurine and 6-thioguanine. These agents are not currently in clinical use for the control of hyperuricemia and will not be discussed further here.

II. Uricosuric Agents

These are the oldest of the clinically useful hypouricemic agents. The uricosuric properties of high dose salicylate were known before 1900, and salicylate continued to be used for this purpose until the mid 1950s when more effective uricosuric agents became available (cited in Kippen et al., 1974b). In the late 1940s, Beyer et al. (1947) introduced the drug caronamide to retard the renal excretion of penicillin. Caronamide was subsequently found to increase uric acid excretion (Wolfson et al., 1948), and was soon replaced by its structural analogue, probenecid, which was an effective uricosuric at much lower doses (Gutman and Yu, 1951; Gutman and Yu, 1957b). Sulphinpyrazone, another commonly used uricosuric agent, was identified in the late 1950s (Burns et al., 1957; Yu et al., 1958). Sulphinpyrazone is 2–6 times more potent on a weight basis than probenecid (Beyer et al., 1951; Burns et al., 1957).

Table 1 lists the agents shown to be uricosuric in man. Besides probenecid and sulphinpyrazone, benzbromarone (Zollner et al., 1968; Zollner et al., 1970) and zoxazolamine (Burns et al., 1958) are employed in Europe for the treatment of interval gout. All of the agents in this table are organic acids except the outdated tetracyclines, chlorprothixene, glycopyrrolate and sodium bicarbonate. The mechanism by which these agents increase the renal excretion of uric acid is not well understood, since the factors controlling the renal handling of uric acid in man have not been well characterized (see above). Uric acid excretion could be increased by these drugs through one of three mechanisms acting alone or in combination: (1)

Table 1. Drugs shown to be uricosuric in man

Acetazolamide	Iopanoic acid
Acetoheximide	Meclofenanine acid
ACTH	Meglumine iodipamide
Azauridine	Mersalyl
Benzbromarone	Metiazinine acid
Benziodarone	p-Nitrophenylbutazone
Calcium ipodate	Oestrogens
Caronamide	Orotic acid
Chlorprothixene	Outdated tetracyclines
Cincophen	Phenolsulphonphthalein
Citrate	Phenoxyisobutyric acid
Dicumarol	Phenylbutazone
Diflumidone	Phenylindandione
Diuretics (in absence of volume contraction)	Potassium indoxyl sulphate
Ethyl biscoumacetate	Probenecid
Ethyl p-chlorophenoxyisobutyric acid	Salicylates (high dose)
Glyceryl guaiacolate	Sodium bicarbonate
Glycine	Sodium diatrizoate
Glycopyrrolate	Sulphaethylthiadiazole
Halofenate	Sulphinpyrazone
Hippuric acid	W 2354 (5-chlorosalicylic acid)
Iodopyracet	Zoxazolamine

decrease in urate binding to serum proteins (2) increase in urate secretion and (3) decrease in urate reabsorption. Some in vitro studies suggest that a number of these agents decrease urate binding to serum proteins (WHITEHOUSE et al., 1973), although the physiological significance of in vitro binding of urate is questionable (see above). There are no data to suggest that these agents increase urate secretion, and in the case of probenecid there are studies that suggest this uricosuric drug inhibits urate secretion (MOLLER, 1965). The majority of the studies would seem to indicate that the organic acid uricosurics increase uric acid excretion through an inhibition of urate reabsorption (KELLEY, 1975b).

Probenecid is readily absorbed from the gastrointestinal tract. Its half-life, which is dose dependent, ranges from 6 to 12 h (DAYTON et al., 1963). Approximately 90% of probenecid is bound to plasma proteins and hence confined to the extracellular fluid. Less than 5% of an administered dose is recovered unchanged in the urine within 24 h. Probenecid acylmonoglucuronide, the major urinary metabolite, accounts for about 40% of the administered dose. Other probenecid metabolites, which retain their uricosuric activity in animals (ISRAILI et al., 1972), result from oxidative attack on the n-propyl side chain and account for 20–35% of the administered dose (BEYER et al., 1951; DAYTON et al., 1973).

Table 2 lists several metabolic effects of probenecid in addition to its uricosuric properties. Of particular note is its tendency to interfere with a number of transport systems.

Sulphinpyrazone was specifically developed as a uricosuric agent. It is rapidly and completely absorbed from the gastrointestinal tract, with a serum half-life of 1–3 h (BURNS et al., 1957; DAYTON et al., 1961). At therapeutic concentrations, it is almost completely bound to plasma proteins and is largely confined to the extracel-

Table 2. Metabolic effects of probenecid

Clinical effect	Reference(s)
1. Inhibits renal organic acid transport (para-aminohippurate, phenolsulphon-phthalein, salicylate, phlorizin, acetazol-amide, dapsone, sulphinpyrazone, indomethacin)	DeSeze et al., 1964; Boger et al., 1951; Mudge, 1971; Newcombe and Cohen, 1963; Peck and Beyer, 1954; Gutman et al., 1955; Schacter and Manis, 1958; Weiner et al., 1959; Yu and Gutman, 1959; Braun et al., 1957; Goodwin and Sparell, 1969; Perel et al., 1969; Skeith et al., 1968
2. Inhibits renal excretion and reduces volume of distribution of several antibiotics (ampicillin, nafcillin, cephaloridine, penicillin)	Gibaldi and Schwartz, 1968; Kampmann et al., 1973
3. Impairs hepatic uptake of certain agents (bromosulphthalein and rifampin)	Blondheim, 1955; Goetzee et al., 1960; Kenwright and Levi, 1973
4. Delays heparin metabolism	Sanchez, 1975
5. Blocks transport of 5-hydroxytryptamine and dopamine out of the CSF (5-hydroxy-indole acetic acid and homovanillic acid in spinal fluid)	Bowers, 1970; Tamarkin et al., 1970; Van Praag et al., 1970
6. Inhibits renal excretion of pantothenic acid, androsterone, corticotropin and diiodotyrosine	Boger et al., 1953; Markkanen et al., 1963; Gardner et al., 1951; Bonar and Perkins, 1962; Huang, 1961
7. Reduces serum phosphorus in patients with hyperparathyroidism (no effect in normals)	Kolb and Rukes, 1954; Dubin et al., 1956; Persellin and Schmid, 1961
8. Inhibits conjugation of benzoic derivatives with glycine	Beyer et al., 1950

lular fluid (Dayton et al., 1961; Gutman et al., 1960). Approximately 20–45% of an administered dose is excreted unchanged in the urine within 24 h (Burns et al., 1957; Gutman et al., 1960). Sulphinpyrazone is mostly excreted as the parahydroxyl metabolite, which is also uricosuric in man.

Sulphinpyrazone may inhibit the metabolism and excretion of many of the same compounds as probenecid, but these effects have been less well characterized for sulphinpyrazone. Sulphinpyrazone may enhance uricosuria in patients on full doses of probenecid, and the combination of these two agents may be useful in refractory patients. A reduction in platelet function has been observed during sulphinpyrazone administration. This property has been used to decrease thrombosis of a–v shunts (Kaegi et al., 1974) and to prolong platelet survival in patients with prosthetic heart valves, rheumatic heart disease and recurrent venous thrombosis (Steele et al., 1973; Weily and Genton, 1970).

Benziodarone was introduced in 1965 as a hypouricemic agent (Delbarre et al., 1965a, and 1965b; Nivet et al., 1965). Because of problems with hypothyroidism (Harrison and Cameron, 1965) and hyperthyroidism (Camus et al., 1973), both apparently related to the iodine content, the bromine analogue of benziodarone was evaluated for use as a hypouricemic agent (Delbarre et al., 1967). Benzbromarone was demonstrated to be an effective hypouricemic agent, and on a weight basis is a more effective uricosuric than either probenecid or sulphinpyrazone (BROEKHUYSEN et al., 1972; LEVINSON, 1975). The extent to which it reduces the serum urate cannot be explained entirely by its uricosuric effect (cited in BROEKHUYSEN et al., 1972). Benzbromarone has been reported to inhibit xanthine oxidase in vitro (DELTOUR et al., 1967). It was postulated that this latter effect might contribute to its hypouricemic action; however benzbromarone does not increase the urinary excretion of hypoxanthine or xanthine in man (DE GERY et al., 1974; DELBARRE et al., 1967). It has also been speculated that benzbromarone might activate HGPRT and decrease uric acid production through this mechanism, but in vitro studies have demonstrated that HGPRT is inhibited by benzbromarone (cited in GREILING and KANEKO, 1974). Further studies are necessary to clarify the mechanism(s) by which this agent produces hypouricemia.

Approximately 50% of a single oral dose of benzbromarone is excreted unchanged in the faeces within 3 days, probably not having been absorbed (BROEKHUYSEN et al., 1972). The principal route of elimination of benzbromarone is the gastrointestinal tract, with only 8% being excreted unchanged in the urine. The serum half-life of a single oral dose is approximately 1.2 days, with peak blood levels occurring within 6 h. After 6 h there is a small decline, followed by a sustained plateau for 12–48 h. At the 6 h peak, approximately 50% of the administered benzbromarone has been metabolized to dehalogenated derivates and other unidentified substances. By 48 h, approximately 75% of the benzbromarone has been dehalogenated to benzarone. Dehalogenation occurs largely in the liver, and the benzarone thus formed is conjugated with glucuronic acid. Benzarone itself exhibits some hypouricemic activity (DELBARRE et al., 1965a, 1967).

III. Uricolytic Agents

The intravenous infusion of purified uricase has been shown to cause a transient reduction of the serum urate in man (ALTMAN et al., 1949; KISSEL et al., 1968; LONDON and HUDSON, 1957; ROYER et al., 1968). In addition to uricolysis, an increase in uric acid clearance seems at least partly responsible for the decrease in serum urate (ROYER et al., 1968). The effectiveness of this form of hypouricemic therapy decreases rapidly with the development of antibodies to uricase (FITZGERALD et al., 1975). The use of glass bead immobilized uricase, in an extracorporeal shunt system, has been suggested as a potential means of circumventing problems with antibody formation (VENTER et al., 1975).

D. Clinical Use of Hypouricemic Drugs

I. Criteria for Selecting a Hypouricemic Drug

The major purpose of hypouricemic therapy is reduction of the total body pool of urate. As discussed above, the serum urate is usually a good reflection of this pool size and the end point of therapy is to achieve a serum urate of less than 6.4 mg per 100 ml, the concentration above which supersaturation occurs. Ideally, the choice of hypouricemic agent should be individualized on the basis of the pathogenic mecha-

Table 3. Indications for allopurinol

1. Tophaceous gout
2. Gout complicated by renal insufficiency (GFR < 30 ml/min)
3. Uric acid excretion greater than 800 to 1000 mg/day (on regular diet)
4. History of uric acid calculi
5. HGPRT deficiency and PP-ribose-P synthetase overactivity
6. Secondary hyperuricemia with overproduction of uric acid
7. Prior to the use of cytotoxic agents or extensive radiation therapy
8. Allergy to uricosurics
9. Uricosurics ineffective or poorly tolerated

nism responsible for gouty arthritis, i.e. increase in uric acid synthesis, decrease in the renal clearance of uric acid or a combination of these two. Patients exhibiting an increase in uric acid production are candidates for treatment with allopurinol; those with decreased uric acid clearances and normal glomerular filtration rates are candidates for a uricosuric. In the absence of radioisotopic incorporation studies, it may be difficult to distinguish between these two groups of gouty patients. One test that may be helpful in this regard is a 24-h urine uric acid. Any patient who excretes more than 800 to 1000 mg of uric acid per day on a regular diet is almost certainly an overproducer, and should be treated with allopurinol. Other indications for allopurinol therapy are listed in Table 3. Patients who excrete less than 800–1000 mg in 24 h may have a component of uric acid overproduction as well as decreased clearance, but these parameters cannot be adequately evaluated without radioisotopic incorporation techniques. Since this is not feasible under routine clinical situations, we feel that either a uricosuric or allopurinol may be used in these patients, unless there are specific indications for choosing allopurinol (Table 3).

II. Use of Individual Hypouricemic Drugs

Allopurinol, in a dose of 200–400 mg per day, is an effective hypouricemic agent in most patients. Occasionally, higher doses may be necessary, particularly in patients with marked overproduction of urate. In all patients the dose of allopurinol should be adjusted to achieve the desired serum urate, which is less than 6.4 mg per 100 ml in most patients (see above). Once control is obtained, adequate therapy may be maintained with a single daily dose of allopurinol (Brewis et al., 1975; Rodnan and Robin, 1975). The occurrence of acute gouty arthritis may be increased during the initiation of allopurinol therapy (Yu and Gutman, 1964). This may be controlled by the concomitant administration of colchicine during the first several months of allopurinol therapy. The progression of gouty nephropathy seems to halt in most patients receiving allopurinol (Emmerson, 1967; Levin and Abrahams, 1966; Ogryzlo et al., 1966; Rundles, 1966a; Rundles et al., 1966; Stoberg, 1966; Wilson et al., 1967), and extensive resolution of tophi occurs within 12 months in most patients (Rundles et al., 1966; Wyngaarden et al., 1965).

Therapy with uricosuric agents should be initiated slowly to avoid the sudden mobilization of large amounts of urate. This can lead to the formation of uric acid calculi, as well as a flare of acute gouty arthritis. The incidence of the former complication may be reduced by initiation of uricosuric therapy at a low dose, maintenance of a urine output of one litre per day and temporary maintenance of urine pH above 6.5 with sodium bicarbonate or sodium citrate. In patients where sodium overload may be a problem, combined low dose sodium biscarbonate and acetazolamide may be of benefit (FREED, 1975). Once the hyperuricemia has been controlled, these precautions are no longer necessary in most patients.

Probenecid therapy can be initiated at a dosage of 250 mg, two or three times a day. This dosage is slowly increased to the required maintenance dose, which may range from 500 mg to 3 gm per day (GUTMAN and YU, 1957b). Sulphinpyrazone therapy is usually initiated at 100 mg per day, and then increased to 200–400 mg per day for maintenance therapy. Occasionally it is necessary to use 800 mg per day of sulphinpyrazone for maximal effect (cited in KELLEY, 1975a). Rarely, allopurinol is used in combination with a uricosuric drug when patients are refractory to allopurinol alone. It should be recognized that the uricosuric response is accompanied by an increased clearance of oxipurinol (ELION et al., 1968), and may necessitate a higher dose of allopurinol. Also, the half-life of probenecid is prolonged by about 50% in patients receiving allopurinol, probably due to the inhibitory effect of allopurinol on hepatic microsomal drug metabolizing systems (TJANDRAMAGA et al., 1972). Benzbromarone, although not in general use in the United States, has been shown to be an effective uricosuric in doses of 40–100 mg (BROEKHUYSEN et al., 1972; LEVINSON, 1975).

A word of caution should be injected concerning the initiation of hypouricemic therapy with allopurinol or a uricosuric agent. Just as an acute attack of gouty arthritis may be precipitated with these drugs, an acute attack may be aggravated by the initiation of hypouricemic therapy during the attack. Therefore, we recommend that hypouricemic therapy should not be begun during an acute attack, but during the intercritical period when the patient is on maintenance colchicine therapy.

III. Toxicity of Hypouricemic Agents

Serious side-effects of allopurinol are unusual, although the overall incidence of reactions may be about 20% (KUZELL et al., 1966). It is not clear whether these reactions are related to direct toxic effects of the drug or hypersensitivity reactions. Side-effects include gastrointestinal intolerance (YU and GUTMAN, 1964), hepatitis (SIMMONS et al., 1972), skin rash and fever (KLINENBERG et al., 1965), leucopenia, thrombocytopenia, vasculitis (JARZOBSKI et al., 1970) and agranulocytosis (GREENBERG and ZAMBRANO, 1972). Renal insufficiency with linear glomerular deposition of IgG has been reported in association with systemic vasculitis in a small group of patients receiving allopurinol (YOUNG et al., 1974). These reactions may be more prominent in patients receiving thiazide diuretics. A three-fold higher incidence of ampicillin-related skin rashes has been reported in patients receiving allopurinol, although it is unclear whether this is related to allopurinol or the presence of hyperuricemia (*Boston Collaborative Drug Surveillance Program*, 1972). Increased cyclophosphamide toxicity appears to occur in patients simultaneously receiving allopurinol, but the mechanism of action is not known (*Boston Collaborative Drug Surveillance Program*, 1974). Toxic epidermal necrolysis has been associated with allopurinol therapy (ELLMAN et al., 1975), as has granular deposition of IgM at the dermo-epidermal junction (Utsinger and Yount, 1976). Xanthine stones are only found in patients with markedly excessive uric acid excretion, such as the Lesch-Nyhan syndrome (Greene et al., 1969) and lymphosarcoma (Band et al., 1970). Even under these circumstances, this is a rare complication. Renal stone and urinary sludge formation due to oxipurinol have been reported in an 8-year-old boy receiving allopurinol and oxipurinol (Landgrebe et al., 1975). Crystals of xanthine, hypoxanthine and oxipurinol have been found in skeletal muscle from gouty patients treated with allopurinol (Watts et al., 1971 a), although the degree of hypoxanthine and xanthine crystal deposition was substantially less than that seen in patients with xanthinuria (Watts et al., 1971 b).

Allopurinol has been reported to potentiate the action of purine analogues, such as 6-mercaptopurine (6-MP) and azathioprine, which are also metabolized by xanthine oxidase (Rundles, 1966 b). Although toxicity data are not conclusive, it may be warranted to reduce the dose of purine analogue in patients simultaneously receiving allopurinol. As discussed above, allopurinol should be used with caution in patients receiving drugs such as antipyrine, coumadin derivatives or hydantoins, which are metabolized by hepatic microsomal enzymes.

Serious side-effects of probenecid are unusual. Hepatic necrosis (Reynolds et al., 1957), nephrotic syndrome (Ferris et al., 1961) and seizures (cited in Kelley, 1975 a) have all been reported in a single patient. There is a 10–15% incidence of gastrointestinal complaints, 5% incidence of hypersensitivity and rash, and a 10–20% incidence of acute gouty arthritis. Despite careful management, a significant number of patients may not be brought under ideal control on probenecid. In one large series, 27% of patients receiving probenecid did not reduce their serum urate below 7 mg/100 ml (Gutman and Yu, 1957 b). The incidence of gastro-intestinal symptoms with sulphinpyrazone is about the same as with probenecid (Deseze and Ryckewaert, 1960; Emmerson, 1963; Kuzell et al., 1964; Yu et al., 1958). A higher incidence of bone marrow changes occurs with sulphinpyrazone, as compared with probenecid (Glick, 1961; Persellin and Schmid, 1961; Yu et al., 1958). Uric acid stone formation has been reported in approximately 10% of patients receiving probenecid and sulphinpyrazone (Gutman and Yu, 1957 b). This latter complication is largely preventable, as discussed above.

References

Altman, K. I., Smull, K., Guzman-Barron, E. S.: A new method for the preparation of uricase and the effect of uricase on the blood uric acid levels of the chicken. Arch. Biochem. **21**, 158—165 (1949)

Alvsaker, J. O.: Uric acid in human plasma. III. Investigations on the interaction between urate ion and human albumin. Scand. J. clin. Lab. Invest. **17**, 467—475 (1965)

Auscher, C., Mercier, N., Masquier, C., Delbarre, F.: Allopurinol and thiopurinol: effect on oxypurine excretion and on rate of in vitro synthesis of ribonucleotides. Advanc. exp. Med. Biol. **41 B**, 657—662 (1974 b)

Auscher, C., Pasquier, C., Mercier, N., Delbarre, F.: Oxidation of pyrazolo (3,4-d) pyrimidine in a xanthinuric man. Advanc. exp. Med. Biol. **41 B**, 663—667 (1974 a)

Band, P. R., Silverberg, D. S., Henderson, J. F., Ulan, R. A., Wensel, R. N., Benerjee, T. K., Little, A. S.: Xanthine nephropathy in a patient with lymphosarcoma treated with allopurinol. New Engl. J. Med. **283**, 354—357 (1970)

Beardmore,T.D., Cashman,J.S., Kelley,W.N.: Mechanism of allopurinol-mediated increase in enzyme activity in man. J. clin. Invest. **51**, 1823—1832 (1972)

Beardmore,T.D., Kelley,W.N.: Mechanism of allopurinol-mediated inhibition of pyrimidine biosyntheses. J. Lab. clin. Med. **78**, 696—704 (1971)

Beyer,K.H., Miller,A.K., Russo,H.F., Patch,E.A., Verwey,W.F.: The inhibitory effect of caronamide on the renal elimination of penicillin. Amer. J. Physiol. **149**, 355—368 (1947)

Beyer,K.H., Russo,H.F., Tillson,E.K., Miller,A.K., Verwey,W.F., Gass,S.R.: 'Benemid', p-(di-n-propylsulfamyl)-benzoic acid: its renal affinity and its elimination. Amer. J. Physiol. **166**, 625—640 (1951)

Beyer,K.H., Wiebelhaus,V.D., Tillson,E.K., Russon,H.F., Wilhoyte,K.M.: 'Benemid', p-(di-n-propylsulfamyl)-benzoic acid; inhibition of glycine conjugative reactions. Proc. Soc. exp. Biol. (N.Y.) **74**, 772—775 (1950)

Blondheim,S.H.: Effect of probenecid on excretion of bromosulphthalein. J. appl. Physiol. **7**, 529—532 (1955)

Bluestone,R., Kippen,I., Campion,D., Klinenberg,J., Whitehouse,M.: Urate binding: a clue to the pathogenesis of gout. J. Rheum. **1**, 230—235 (1974)

Boger,W.P., Bayne,G.M., Gylfe,J., Wright,L.D.: Renal clearance of pantothenic acid in man: inhibition by probenecid ('benemid'). Proc. Soc. exp. Biol. (N.Y.) **82**, 604—608 (1953)

Boger,W.P., Matteucci,W.V., Schimmel,N.H.: Renal clearances of penicillin, phenolsulfonphthalein (PSP) and paraaminohippurate (PAH) modified by 'benemid' (abstract). Amer. J. Med. **11**, 517 (1951)

Bonar,J.A., Perkins,W.H.: Inhibition of urinary excretion of iodine[131]-labeled corticotropin by probenecid. J. clin. Endocr. **22**, 38—42 (1962)

Boston Collaborative Drug Surveillance Program: Excess of ampicillin skin rashes associated with allopurinol or hyperuricemia. New Engl. J. Med. **286**, 505—507 (1972)

Boston Collaborative Drug Surveillance Program: Allopurinol and cytotoxic drugs. Interaction in relation to bone marrow depression. J. Amer. med. Ass. **227**, 1036—1040 (1974)

Bowers,M.B., Jr.: CSF homovanillic acid: effects of probenecid and alpha-methyl tyrosine. Life Sci. **9**, 691—694 (1970)

Braun,W., Whittaker,V.P., Lotspeich,W.D.: Renal excretion of phlorizin and phlorizin glucuronide. Amer. J. Physiol. **190**, 563—569 (1957)

Brewis,I., Ellis,R.M., Scott,J.T.: Single daily dose of allopurinol. Ann. rheum. Dis. **34**, 256—259 (1975)

Brochner-Mortensen,K., Cobb,S., Rose,B.S.: Review of diagnostic criteria and known etiological factors in gout. In: Kellgren,J. (Ed.): The Epidemiology of Chronic Rheumatism, Vol. 1, p. 295. Philadelphia: F.A. Davies 1963

Broekhuysen,J., Paco,M., Sion,R., Demeulenaere,L., Van Hee,W.: Metabolism of benzbromarone in man. Europ. J. clin. Pharmacol. **4**, 125—130 (1972)

Burns,J.J., Yu,T.-F., Berger,L., Gutman,A.B.: Zoxazolamine: physiological disposition, uricosuric properties. Amer. J. Med. **25**, 401—408 (1958)

Burns,J.J., Yu,T.-F., Perel,J.M., Gutman,A.B., Brodie,B.B.: A potent new uricosuric agent, the sulfoxide metabolite of the phenylbutazone analogue, G-25761. J. Pharmacol. exp. Ther. **119**, 418—426 (1957)

Buzard,J., Bishop,C., Talbott,J.H.: Recovery in humans of intravenously injected isotopic uric acid. J. biol. Chem. **196**, 179—184 (1952)

Campion,D.S., Bluestone,R., Klinenberg,J.R.: Uric acid: characterization of its interaction with human serum albumin. J. clin. Invest. **52**, 2383—2387 (1973)

Camus,J.P., Prier,A., Kartun,P., Maugeis de Bourguesdon,J.: Thyretoxicose et benziodarone. Rev. Rhum. **40**(2), 148—150 (1973)

Canellakis,E.S., Tuttle,A.L., Cohen,P.P.: A comparative study of the end-products of uric acid oxidation by peroxidases. J. biol. Chem. **213**, 397—404 (1955)

Cartier,P.H., Hamet,M.: Mechanism of action of 4-oxy- and 4-thiopyrazole pyrimidines. Biochem. Pharmacol. **22**, 3061—3075 (1973)

Chytil,F.: Activation of liver tryptophan oxygenase by adenosine 3',5'-phosphate and other purine derivatives. J. biol. Chem. **243**, 893—899 (1968)

Dayton,P.G., Perel,J.M., Cunningham,R.F., Israili,Z.H., Weiner,I.M.: Studies on the fate of metabolites and analogues of probenecid. The significance of metabolic sites, especially lack of ring hydroxylation. Drug Metab. Dispos. **1**, 742—751 (1973)

Dayton, P. G., Sicam, L. E., Landrau, M., Burns, J. J.: Metabolism of sulfinpyrazone (Anturane) and other thio analogues of phenylbutazone in man. J. Pharmacol. exp. Ther. **132**, 287—290 (1961)

Dayton, P. G., Yu, T.-F., Chen, W., Berger, L., West, L. A., Gutman, A. B.: The physiological disposition of probenecid, including renal clearance, in man, studied by an improved method for its estimation in biological materials. J. Pharmacol. exp. Ther. **140**, 278—286 (1963)

Dean, B. M., Perrett, D., Simmonds, H. A., Grahame, R.: Thiopurinol: comparative enzyme inhibition and protein binding studies with allopurinol, oxipurinol and 6-mercaptopurine. Brit. J. clin. Pharmacol. **1**, 119—127 (1974)

De Gery, A., Auscher, C., Saporta, L., Delbarre, F.: Treatment of gout and hyperuricemia by benzbromarone, ethyl 2 (dibromo-3,5 hydroxy-4 benzoyl)-3 benzofuran. Advanc. exp. Med. Biol. **41 B**, 683—689 (1974)

Delbarre, F., Amor, B., Auscher, C., De Gery, A.: Treatment of gout with allopurinol. A study of 106 cases. Ann. rheum. Dis. **25**, 627—633 (1966)

Delbarre, F., Auscher, C., Amor, B.: Action uricosurique et antigoutteuse de certain derives du benzofuranne. Presse méd. **73**, 2725—2726 (1965 a)

Delbarre, F., Auscher, C., Amor, B.: Action uricosurique de certains derives du benzofuranne. Bull. Soc. Med. Hôp. Paris **116**, 1193—1196 (1965 b)

Delbarre, F., Auscher, C., De Gery, A., Brouilhet, H., Olivier, J. L.: Le traitement de la dyspurinurie goutteuse par la mercapto-pyrazolo-pyrimidine (M.P.P.: thiopurinol). Presse méd. **76**, 2329—2332 (1968)

Delbarre, F., Auscher, C., Olivier, J. L., Rose, A.: Traitement des hyperuricemies et de la goutte par les derives du benzofuranne. Sem. Hôp. Paris **43**, 1127—1133 (1967)

Deltour, G., Broekhuysen, J., Ghislain, M., Bourgeois, F., Binon, F.: Recherches dans la serie des benzofurannes. XXI. Effet inhibiteur de derives benzofuranniques phenoliques et des quelques analogues sur la xanthine oxydase hepatique du rat in vitro. Arch. int. Pharmacodyn. **165**, 25—30 (1967)

Deseze, S., Ryckewaert, A.: Gout (in French). Paris: Expansion Sci. Franc. (1960)

Deseze, S., Ryckewaert, A., Cariot, M., Kahn, M. F., D'Anglejan, G.: Le traitement uricosurique de la goutte. In: Congres International de la Goutte et de la Lithiase Urique, p. 297. Evian: 1964

Dubin, A., Kushner, D. S., Bronsky, D., Pascale, L. R.: Hyperuricemia in hypoparathyroidism. Metabolism **5**, 703—709 (1956)

Elion, G. B.: Enzymatic and metabolic studies with allopurinol. Ann. rheum. Dis. **25**, 608—614 (1966)

Elion, G. B., Kovensky, A., Hitchings, G. H., Metz, E., Rundles, E. W.: Metabolic studies of allopurinol, an inhibitor of xanthine oxidase. Biochem. Pharmacol. **15**, 863—880 (1966)

Elion, G. B., Yu, T.-F., Gutman, A. B., Hitchings, G. H.: Renal clearance of oxipurinol, the chief metabolite of allopurinol. Amer. J. Med. **45**, 69—77 (1968)

Ellman, M. H., Fretzin, D. F., Olson, W.: Toxic epidermal necrolysis associated with allopurinol administration. Arch. Derm. **111**, 986—990 (1975)

Emmerson, B. T.: A comparison of uricosuric agents in gout, with special reference to sulfinpyrazone. Med. J. Aust. **50**, 839—844 (1963)

Emmerson, B. T.: The use of the xanthine oxidase inhibitor, allopurinol, in the control of hyperuricemia, gout and uric acid calculi. Aust. Ann. Med. **16**, 205—214 (1967)

Farrell, P. C., Popovich, R. P., Babb, A. L.: Binding levels of urate ions in human serum albumin and plasma. Biochim. biophys. Acta **243**, 49—52 (1971)

Feigelson, P., Davidson, J. D., Robins, P. K.: Pyrazolopyrimidines as inhibitors and substrates of xanthine oxidase. J. biol. Chem. **226**, 993—1000 (1957)

Ferris, T. F., Morgan, W. S., Levitin, H.: Nephrotic syndrome caused by probenecid. New Engl. J. Med. **265**, 381—383 (1961)

Fitzgerald, O., Fitzpatrick, D. A., McGeeny, K. F.: Urate-oxidase treatment for hyperuricemia. Lancet **1975 I**, 525

Fox, I. H., Wyngaarden, J. B., Kelley, W. N.: Depletion of erythrocyte phosphoribosylpyrophosphate in man, a newly observed effect of allopurinol. New Engl. J. Med. **283**, 1177—1182 (1970 a)

Fox, R. M., Royse-Smith, D., O'Sullivan, W. J.: Orotidinuria induced by allopurinol. Science **168**, 861—862 (1970 b)

Fox, R. M., Wood, M. H., O'Sullivan, W. H.: Studies on the coordinate activity and lability of orotidylate phosphoribosyltransferase and decarboxylase in human erythrocytes, and the effects of allopurinol administration. J. clin. Invest. **50**, 1050—1060 (1971)

Freed, S. Z.: The alternating use of an alkalinizing salt and acetazolamide in the management of cystine and uric acid stones. J. Urol. (Baltimore) **113**, 96—99 (1975)

Gallo, R. C., Perry, S., Breitman, T. R.: Inhibition of human leukocyte pyrimidine deoxynucleoside synthesis by allopurinol and 6-mercaptopurine. Biochem. Pharmacol. **17**, 2185—2191 (1968)

Gardner, L. I., Crigler, J. R., Jr., Migeon, C. J.: Inhibition of 17-keto-steroid excretion produced by 'benemid'. Proc. Soc. exp. Biol. (N.Y.) **78**, 460—463 (1951)

Garrod, A. B.: Observations on certain pathological conditions of the blood and urine in gout, rheumatism and Bright's disease. Med.-chir. Soc. Trans. **31**, 83—98 (1848)

Geren, W., Bendich, A., Bodansky, O., Brown, G. B.: Fate of uric acid in man. J. biol. Chem. **183**, 21—31 (1950)

Ghosh, D., Forrest, H. S.: Inhibition of tryptophan pyrrolase by some naturally occurring pteridines. Arch. Biochem. **120**, 578—582 (1967)

Gibaldi, M., Schwartz, M. A.: Apparent effect of probenecid on the distribution of penicillins in man. Clin. Pharmacol. Ther. **9**, 345—349 (1968)

Glick, E. N.: Sulfinpyrazone in the treatment of arthritis associated with hyperuricaemia. Proc. roy. Soc. Med. **54**, 423—426 (1961)

Goetzee, A. E., Richards, T. G., Tindall, V. R.: Experimental changes in liver function induced by probenecid. Clin. Sci. **19**, 63—78 (1960)

Goodwin, C. S., Sparell, G.: Inhibition of dapsone excretion by probenecid. Lancet **1969 II**, 884—885

Grahame, R., Simmonds, H. A., Cadenhead, A., Dean, B. M.: Metabolic studies of thiopurinol in man and pig. Advanc. exp. Med. Biol. **41 B**, 597—605 (1974)

Greenberg, M. S., Zambrano, S. S.: Aplastic agranulocytosis after allopurinol therapy. Arthr. Rheum. **15**, 413—416 (1972)

Greene, M. L., Fujimoto, W. Y., Seegmiller, J. E.: Urinary xanthine stones—a rare complication of allopurinol therapy. New Engl. J. Med. **280**, 426—427 (1969)

Greiling, H., Kaneko, M.: Influence of a uricosuric drug on connective tissue metabolism. Advanc. exp. Med. Biol. **41 B**, 693—698 (1974)

Griffiths, M.: Oxidation of uric acid catalyzed by copper and by the cytochrome-cytochrome oxidase system. J. biol. Chem. **197**, 399—407 (1952)

Grobner, W., Kelley, W. N.: Effect of allopurinol and its metabolic derivatives on the configuration of human orotate phosphoribosyltransferase and orotidine-5'-phosphate decarboxylase. Biochem. Pharmacol. **24**, 379—384 (1975)

Gutman, A. B., Dayton, P. G., Yu, T.-F., Berger, L., Chen, W., Sicam, L. E., Burns, J. J.: A study of the inverse relationship between pKa and rate of renal excretion of phenylbutazone analogs in man and dog. Amer. J. Med. **29**, 1017—1033 (1960)

Gutman, A. B., Yu, T.-F.: Benemid [(p-di-n-propylsulfamyl)-benzoic acid] as a uricosuric agent in chronic gouty arthritis. Trans. Ass. Amer. Phycns **64**, 279—288 (1951)

Gutman, A. B., Yu, T.-F.: Renal function in gout, with a commentary on the renal regulation of urate excretion and the role of the kidney in the pathogenesis of gout. Amer. J. Med. **23**, 600—622 (1957a)

Gutman, A. B., Yu, T.-F.: Protracted uricosuric therapy in tophaceous gout. Lancet **1957 II**, 1258—1260 (1957b)

Gutman, A. B., Yu, T.-F.: A three component system for regulation of renal excretion of uric acid in man. Trans. Ass. Amer. Phycns **74**, 353—365 (1961)

Gutman, A. B., Yu, T.-F., Sirota, J. H.: A study, by simultaneous clearance techniques, of salicylate excretion in man. Effect of alkalinization of the urine by bicarbonate administration; effect of probenecid. J. clin. Invest. **34**, 711—721 (1955)

Harrison, M. T., Cameron, A. J. V.: Iodine induced hypothyroidism due to benziodarone (cardivix). Brit. med. J. **1**, 840 (1965)

Henderson, J. F.: Regulation of purine biosynthesis. Washington: American Chemical Society Monograph 170, 1972

Hoffmann, G. T., Rottino, A., Albaum, H. G.: Levels of nucleotide in the blood during shock. Science **114**, 188—189 (1951)

Holmes, E. W., Kelley, W. N., Wyngaarden, J. B.: The kidney and uric acid excretion in man. Kidney Int. **2**, 115—118 (1972)

Holmes, E. W., Kelley, W. N., Wyngaarden, J. B.: Control of purine biosynthesis in normal and pathological states. Bull. rheum. Dis. **26**, 848—853 (1976)

Huang, K. C.: Renal excretion of L-tyrosine and its derivatives. J. Pharmacol. exp. Ther. **134**, 257—265 (1961)

Israili, Z. H., Percel, J. M., Cunningham, R. F., Dayton, P. G., Yu, T.-F., Gutman, A. B., Long, K. R., Long, R. C., Goldstein, J. H.: Metabolites of probenecid. Chemical, physical and pharmacological studies. J. med. Chem. **15**, 709—713 (1972)

Jarzobski, A. B., Jr., Ferry, J., Wombolt, D., Fitch, D. M., Egan, J. D.: Vasculitis with allopurinol therapy. Amer. Heart J. **79**, 116—121 (1970)

Jorgensen, S., Poulsen, H. E.: Enzymic determination of hypoxanthine and xanthine in human plasma and urine. Acta pharmacol. (Kbh.) **11**, 223—243 (1955)

Julian, J., Chytil, F.: Participation of xanthine oxidase in the activation of liver tryptophan pyrrolase. J. biol. Chem. **245**, 1161—1168 (1970)

Kaegi, A., Pineo, G. F., Shimizu, A., Trivedi, H., Hirsh, J., Gent, M.: Arteriovenous shunt thrombosis. Prevention by sulfinpyrazone. New Engl. J. Med. **290**, 304—306 (1974)

Kampmann, J., Lindahl, F., Hansen, J. M., Siersback-Nielsen, K.: Effect of probenecid on the excretion of ampicillin in human bile. Brit. J. Pharmacol. **47**, 782—786 (1973)

Katz, W. A., Schubert, M.: The interaction of monosodium urate with connective tissue components. J. clin. Invest. **49**, 1783—1789 (1970)

Kelley, W. N.: Effects of drugs on uric acid in man. Ann. Rev. Pharmacol. **15**, 327—350 (1975a)

Kelley, W. N.: Pharmacologic approach to the maintenance of urate homeostasis. Nephron **14**, 99—115 (1975b)

Kelley, W. N., Beardmore, T.: Allopurinol: alteration in pyrimidine metabolism in man. Science **169**, 388—390 (1970)

Kelley, W. N., Rosenbloom, F. M., Miller, J., Seegmiller, J. E.: An enzymatic basis for variation in response to allopurinol. New Engl. J. Med. **278**, 287—293 (1968)

Kenwright, S., Levi, A. J.: Impairment of hepatic uptake of rifamycin antibiotics by probenecid, and its therapeutic implications. Lancet **1973 II**, 1401—1405

Kippen, I., Klinenberg, J. R., Weinberger, A., Wilcox, W. R.: Factors affecting urate solubility in vitro. Ann. rheum. Dis. **33**, 313—317 (1974a)

Kippen, I., Whitehouse, M. W., Klinenberg, J. R.: Pharmacology of uricosuric drugs. Ann. rheum. Dis. **33**, 391—396 (1974b)

Kissel, P., Lamarche, M., Royer, R.: Modification of uricemia and the excretion of uric acid nitrogen by an enzyme of fungal origin. Nature (Lond.) **217**, 72—74 (1968)

Klinenberg, J. R., Goldfinger, S. E., Seegmiller, J. E.: The effectiveness of the xanthine oxidase inhibitor allopurinol in the treatment of gout. Ann. intern. Med. **62**, 639—647 (1965)

Kolb, F. O., Rukes, J. M.: Effects of benemid (probenecid) in the treatment of hypoparathyroidism and pseudohypoparathyroidism (abstract). J. clin. Endocr. **14**, 785 (1954)

Kovarsky, J., Holmes, E. W., Kelley, W. N.: Absence of significant urate binding to human serum proteins (abstract). Clin. Res. **24**, 21A (1976)

Krenitsky, T. A., Elion, G. B., Henderson, A. M., Hitchings, G. H.: Inhibition of human purine nucleoside phosphorylase. Studies with intact erythrocytes and the purified enzyme. J. biol. Chem. **243**, 2876—2881 (1968)

Krenitsky, T. A., Elion, G. B., Strelitz, R. A., Hitchings, G. H.: Ribonucleotides of allopurinol and oxoallopurinol. Isolation from human urine, enzymatic synthesis and characterization. J. biol. Chem. **242**, 2675—2682 (1967)

Krenitsky, T. A., Neil, S. M., Elion, G. B., Hitchings, G. H.: A comparison of the specifities of xanthine oxidase and aldehyde oxidase. Arch. Biochem. **150**, 585—589 (1972)

Krooth, R. S., Lam, G. F. M., Kiang, S. Y. C.: Oxipurinol and orotic aciduria: effect on orotidine-5'-monophosphate decarboxylase activity of cultured human fibroblasts. Cell **3**, 55—57 (1974)

Kuzell, W., Glover, R., Gibbs, J., Blau, R.: Effect of anturane on serum uric acid and cholesterol in gout. A long-term study. Acta rheum. scand. Suppl. **8**, 31—40 (1964)

Kuzell, W., Seebach, L. M., Glover, R. P., Jackman, A. E.: Treatment of gout with allopurinol and sulfinpyrazone in combination and with allopurinol alone. Ann. rheum. Dis. **25**, 634—642 (1966)

Landgrebe, A. R., Nyhan, W. L., Coleman, M.: Urinary tract stones resulting from excretion of oxypurinol. New Engl. J. Med. **292**, 626—627 (1975)

Levin, N. W., Abrahams, O. L.: Allopurinol in patients with impaired renal function. Ann. rheum. Dis. **25**, 681—687 (1966)

Levinson, D. L.: Clinical experience with benzbromarone in gout. A potent uricosuric agent (abstract). Arthr. Rheum. **18**, 412 (1975)

London, M., Hudson, P. B.: Uricolytic activity of purified uricase in two human beings. Science **125**, 937—938 (1957)

Markkanen, T., Toivanen, P., Toivanen, A., Sotaneimi, E.: The effect of probenecid (p-[di-n-propylsulfamyl]-benzoic acid) on the spontaneous renal excretion of biologically active metabolites of thiamine, riboflavin and pantothenic acid. Scand. J. clin. Lab. Invest. **15**, 511—516 (1963)

Massey, V., Komai, H., Palmer, G., Elion, G. B.: On the mechanism of inactivation of xanthine oxidase by allopurinol and other pyrazolo (3,4-d) pyrimidines. J. biol. Chem. **245**, 2837—2844 (1970)

Moller, J. U.: The rubular site of urate transport in the rabbit kidney and the effect of probenecid on urate secretion. Acta pharmacol. (Kbh.) **23**, 329—336 (1965)

Mudge, G. H.: Uricosuric action of cholecystographic agents. A possible factor in nephrotoxicity. New Engl. J. Med. **284**, 929—933 (1971)

Nelson, D. J., Bugge, C. J. L., Krasny, H. C., Elion, G. B.: Formation of nucleotides of (6-^{14}C) allopurinol and (6-^{14}C) oxipurinol in rat tissues and effects on uridine nucleotide pools. Biochem. Pharmacol. **22**, 2003—2022 (1973)

Nelson, D. J., Elion, G. B.: Metabolism of (6-^{14}C) allopurinol-lack of incorporation of allopurinol into nucleic acids. Biochem. Pharmacol. **24**, 1235—1237 (1975)

Newcombe, D. S., Cohen, A. S.: Uricosuric agents and phenolsulfonphthalein excretion. Arch. intern. Med. **112**, 738—741 (1963)

Nivet, M., Marcovici, J., Laurelle, P., Farah, M.: Note preliminaire sur l'action d'un benzofuranne sur l'uricemie. Bull. Soc. Med. Hôp. Paris **73**, 1187—1192 (1965)

Ogryzlo, M. A., Urowitz, M., Weber, H. M., Haupt, J. B.: Effects of allopurinol on gouty and nongouty uric acid nephropathy. Ann. rheum. Dis. **25**, 673—680 (1966)

Peck, H. M., Beyer, K. H.: Renal function: excretion of phenolsulfonphthalein by the amphibian *(Rana pipiens)* kidney (abstract). Fed. Proc. 393—394 (1954)

Perel, J. M., Dayton, P. G., Snell, M. M., Yu, T.-F., Gutman, A. B.: Studies of interactions among drugs in man at the renal level: probenecid and sulfinpyrazone. Clin. Pharmacol. Ther. **10**, 834—840 (1969)

Persellin, R. H., Schmid, F. R.: The use of sulfinpyrazone in the treatment of gout. J. Amer. med. Ass. **75**, 971—975 (1961)

Peters, J. P., van Slyke, K. K.: Quantitative Clinical Chemistry, 2nd Ed., Vol. 1. Baltimore: Williams and Wilkins 1946

Phelps, P., Steele, A. D., McCarty, D. J., Jr.: Compensated polarized light microscopy. Identification of crystals in synovial fluids from gout and pseudogout. J. Amer. med. Ass. **203**, 508—512 (1968)

Reynolds, E. S., Schlant, R. C., Gonick, H. C., Dammin, G. J.: Fatal massive necrosis of the liver as a manifestation of hypersensitivity to probenecid. New Engl. J. Med. **256**, 592—596 (1957)

Rieselbach, R. E., Steele, T. H. (eds.): Symposium on influence of the kidney upon urate homeostasis in man. Nephron **14**, 5—115 (1975)

Rodnan, G. P., Robin, J. A.: Allopurinol and gouty hyperuricemia: efficacy of a single daily dose. J. Amer. med. Ass. **231**, 1143—1147 (1975)

Royer, R., Vindel, J., Lamarche, M., Kissel, P.: Modalités d'elimination des purines au cours du traitement enzymatique de la goutte et des ètats hyperuricemiques par une urate-oxydase. Presse. med. **76**, 2325—2328 (1968)

Rundles, R. W.: Allopurinol in gouty nephropathy and renal dialysis. Ann. rheum. Dis. **25**, 694—696 (1966 a)

Rundles, R. W.: Effect of allopurinol on 6-mercaptopurine therapy in neoplastic diseases. Ann. rheum. Dis. **25**, 655—656 (1966 b)

Rundles, R. W., Metz, E. N., Silberman, H. R.: Allopurinol in the treatment of gout. Ann. intern. Med. **64**, 229—258 (1966)

Rundles, R. W., Silberman, H. R., Hitchings, G. H., Elion, G. B.: Effects of xanthine oxidase inhibitor on clinical manifestations and purine metabolism in gout (abstract). Ann. intern. Med. **60**, 717—718 (1964)

Rundles, R. W., Wyngaarden, J. B., Hitchings, G. H., Elion, G. B.: Drugs and uric acid. Ann. Rev. Pharmacol. **9**, 345—362 (1969)

Rundles, R. W., Wyngaarden, J. B., Hitchings, G. H., Elion, G. B., Silberman, H. R.: Effects of a xanthine oxidase inhibitor on thiopurine metabolism, hyperuricemia and gout. Trans. Ass. Amer. Phycns **76**, 126—140 (1963)

Sanchez, G.: Enhancement of heparin effect by probenecid. New Engl. J. Med. **292**, 48 (1975)

Schacter, D., Manis, J. D.: Salicylate and salicyl conjugates: fluorometric estimation, biosynthesis and renal excretion in man. J. clin. Invest. **37**, 800—807 (1958)

Seegmiller, J. E., Grayzel, A. I., Laster, L., Liddle, L.: Uric acid production in gout. J. clin. Invest. **40**, 1304—1314 (1961)

Seegmiller, J. E., Laster, L., Howell, R. R.: Biochemistry of uric acid and its relation to gout (part I). New Engl. J. Med. **268**, 712—716 (1963)

Segal, S., Wyngaarden, J. B.: Plasma glutamine and oxypurine content in patients with gout. Proc. Soc. exp. Biol. (N.Y.) **88**, 342—345 (1955)

Serre, H., Simon, L., Claustre, J.: Les urico-frenateurs dans le traitement de la goutte. A propos de 126 cas. Sem. Hôp. Paris **46**, 3295—3301 (1970)

Shaw, R. K., Shullman, R. N., Davidson, J. D., Rall, D. P., Frei, E. III: Studies with the experimental antitumor agent 4-aminopyrazolo (3,4-d) pyrimidine. Cancer (Philad.) **13**, 482—489 (1960)

Sheikh, M. I., Moller, J. V.: Binding of urate to proteins of human and rabbit plasma. Biochim. biophys. Acta **158**, 456—458 (1968)

Simmonds, H. A., Cadenhead, A., Cameron, J. S., Rising, T. J., Grahame, R., Dean, B. M.: Thiopurinol and purine metabolism: metabolic and radioisotope studies. Ann. rheum. Dis. **33**, 548—553 (1974)

Simmons, F., Feldman, B., Gerenty, D.: Granulomatous hepatitis in patients receiving allopurinol. Gastroenterology **62**, 101—104 (1972)

Skeith, M. D., Simkin, P. A., Healey, L. A.: The renal excretion of indomethacin and its inhibition by probenecid. Clin. Pharmacol. Ther. **9**, 89—93 (1968)

Sorensen, L. B.: Degradation of uric acid in man. Metabolism **8**, 687—703 (1959)

Sorensen, L. B.: The elimination of uric acid in man studied by menas of C^{14}-labeled uric acid. Uricolysis. Scand. J. clin. Lab. Invest. **12 (suppl. 54)**, 1—214 (1960)

Sorensen, L. B.: The pathogenesis of gout. Arch. intern. Med. **109**, 379—390 (1962)

Steele, P. P., Weily, H. S., Genton, E.: Platelet survival and adhesiveness in recurrent venous thrombosis. New Engl. J. Med. **288**, 1148—1152 (1973)

Stoberg, K.-H.: Allopurinol therapy of gout with renal complications. Ann. rheum. Dis. **25**, 688—690 (1966)

Tamarkin, N. R., Goodwin, F. K., Axelrod, J.: Rapid elevation of biogenic amine metabolites in human CSF following probenecid. Life Sci. **9**, 1397—1408 (1970)

Tjandramaga, T. B., Cucinell, S. A., Israili, Z. H., Perel, J. M., Dayton, P. G., Yu, T.-F., Gutman, A. B.: Observation on the disposition of probenecid in patients receiving allopurinol. Pharmacology (Basel) **8**, 259—272 (1972)

Truscoe, R., Williams, V.: The effect of allopurinol on urate oxidase activity. Biochem. Pharmacol. **17**, 165—167 (1968)

Utsinger, P. D., Yount, W. J.: Granular deposition of IgM at the dermo-epidermal junction in allopurinol hypersensitivity (abstract). Clin. Res. **24**, 23A (1976)

Van Praag, H. M., Korf, J., Puite, J.: 5-Hydroxyindolacetic acid levels in the cerebrospinal fluid of depressive patients treated with probenecid. Nature (Lond.) **225**, 1259—1260 (1970)

Venter, J. C., Venter, B. R., Dixon, J. E., Kaplan, N. O.: A possible role for glass bead immobilized enzymes as therapeutic agents (immobilized uricase as enzyme therapy for hyperuricemia). Biochem. Med. **12**, 79—91 (1975)

Vesell, E. W., Passananti, G. T., Greene, F. E.: Impairment of drug metabolism in man by allopurinol and nortriptyline. New Engl. J. Med. **283**, 1484—1488 (1970)

Watts, R. W. E., Scott, J. T., Chalmers, R. A., Bitensky, L., Chayen, J.: Microscopic studies on skeletal muscle in gout patients treated with allopurinol. Quart. J. Med. **40**, 1—14 (1971 a)

Watts, R. W. E., Snedden, W., Parker, R. A.: A quantitative study of skeletal muscle purines and pyrazolo (3,4-d) pyrimidines in gout patients treated with allopurinol. Clin. Sci. **41**, 153—158 (1971 b)

Weily, H. S., Genton, E.: Altered platelet function in patients with prosthetic mitral valves. Effects of sulfinpyrazone therapy. Circulation **42**, 967—972 (1970)

Weiner, I. M., Washington, J. A. II., Mudge, G. H.: Studies on the renal excretion of salicylate in the dog. Bull. Johns Hopk. Hosp. **105**, 284—297 (1959)

White, F. R.: 4-Aminopyrazolo (3,4-d) pyrimidine and three derivatives. Cancer Chemother. Rep. **3**, 26—36 (1959)

Whitehouse, M. W., Kippen, I., Klinenberg, J. R., Schlosstein, L., Campion, D. S., Bluestone, R.: Increasing excretion of urate with displacing agents in man. Ann. N. Y. Acad. Sci. **226**, 309—318 (1973)

Wilcox, W. R., Khalaf, A. R.: Nucleation of monosodium urate crystals. Ann. rheum. Dis. **34**, 332—339 (1975)

Wilson, J. D., Simmonds, H. A., North, J. D. K.: Allopurinol in the treatment of uraemic patients with gout. Ann. rheum. Dis. **26**, 136—141 (1967)

Wolfson, W. Q., Cohn, C., Levine, R., Huddlestun, B.: Transport and excretion of uric acid in man. III. Physiologic significance of the uricosuric effect of caronamide (abstract). Amer. J. Med. **4**, 774 (1948)

Wyngaarden, J. B.: The effect of phenylbutazone on uric acid metabolism in two normal subjects. J. clin. Invest. **34**, 256—262 (1955)

Wyngaarden, J. B., Kelley, W. N.: Gout and hyperuricemia. New York: Grune and Stratton 1976. In press

Wyngaarden, J. B., Rundles, R. W., Metz, E. N.: Allopurinol in the treatment of gout. Ann. intern. Med. **62**, 842—847 (1965)

Wyngaarden, J. B., Rundles, R. W., Silberman, H. R., Hunter, S.: Control of hyperuricemia with hydroxypyrazolopyrimidine, a purine analogue which inhibits uric acid synthesis (abstract). Arthr. Rheum. **6**, 306—307 (1963)

Young, J. L., Jr., Boswell, R. B., Nies, A. S.: Severe allopurinol hypersensitivity. Association with thiazides and prior renal compromise. Arch. intern. Med. **134**, 553—558 (1974)

Yu, T.-F., Burns, J. J., Gutman, A. B.: Results of a clinical trial of G-28315, a sulfoxide analogue of phenylbutazone, as a uricosuric agent in gouty subjects. Arthr. Rheum. **1**, 532—543 (1958)

Yu, T.-F., Gutman, A. B.: Study of the paradoxical effects of salicylate in low, intermediate and high dosage on the renal mechanisms for excretion of urate in man. J. clin. Invest. **38**, 1298—1315 (1959)

Yu, T.-F., Gutman, A. B.: Effects of allopurinol [4-hydroxypyrazolo (3,4-d) pyrimidine] on serum and urinary uric acid in primary and secondary gout. Amer. J. Med. **37**, 885—898 (1964)

Zollner, N., Dofel, W., Grobner, W.: Die Wirkung Benzbromaronum auf die renale Harnsäureausscheidung Gesunder. Klin. Wschr. **48**, 426—432 (1970)

Zollner, N., Stern, G., Grobner, W., Dofel, W.: Über die Senkung des Harnsäurespiegels im Plasma durch Benzbromaronum. Klin. Wschr. **46**, 1318—1319 (1968)

Zwaifler, N. J., Pekin, T. J.: Significance of urate crystals in synovial fluids. Arch. intern. Med. **111**, 99—102 (1963)

CHAPTER 37

Anti-Inflammatory Steroids: Mode of Action in Rheumatoid Arthritis and Homograft Reaction

M. K. JASANI

A. General Considerations

Chemically, the anti-inflammatory steroids are closely related to the predominant human adrenocortical hormone cortisol or hydrocortisone (17-hydroxycorticosterone). They have the basic structural formula shown in Figure 1. The central skeleton of three interconnected rings each of six carbon atoms, and the other ring of five carbon atoms, feature also in oestrogens, progesterone, testosterone and aldosterone, all of which, though devoid of anti-inflammatory action, exhibit other highly specific biological activities (KAPPAS and PALMER, 1963).

The various steroids are structurally similar, all being synthesised from the same chemical precursor, cholesterol. Biosynthesis of the steroid hormones involves alteration of the side groups of cholesterol with the aid of specific enzymes present in cells of the appropriate endocrine glands; the adrenal glands in case of the naturally-occurring anti-inflammatory steroids and aldosterone (see RINGOLD and BOWERS, 1963). The differences between the biological activity of various steroids are determined by the pattern of chemical bonds within the rings and by the nature and orientation of the side groups attached to the rings (O'MALLEY and SCHRADER, 1976). Although the differences may appear to be superficial, they alter the molecule's shape (see also BUSH, 1962) and can thereby completely change their biological activity.

Because of their chemical similarity to cortisol, the anti-inflammatory steroids exert important metabolic and endocrine effects in addition to the anti-inflammatory action. Like cortisol, their metabolic effects tend to be wide-spread, affecting many organs and tissues including, for example, the liver, kidneys, heart and brain, lymphoid organs, skeletal muscle, bones, skin and adipose tissue. The cellular elements of all these different responsive tissues have one especially important macromolecular constituent in common, namely the presence of a cytoplasmic protein (molecular weight 50000–150000) that has a high affinity for cortisol and other anti-inflammatory steroids (BALLARD et al., 1974): This will be referred to as the cytoplasmic cortisol receptor.

Contrary to the general rule for various hormonal agents, the diseases that respond favourably to cortisol and other anti-inflammatory steroids are not characterised by a deficiency of cortisol or other evidence of impaired adrenocortical function (HENCH, 1925; JASANI, 1975); the only important exception being Addison's disease in which the adrenal glands themselves are the seat of inflammation. Instead, the diseases which improve with the use of anti-inflammatory steroids are characterised by a prominent pathogenetic role for antibodies or the type of sensitised lym-

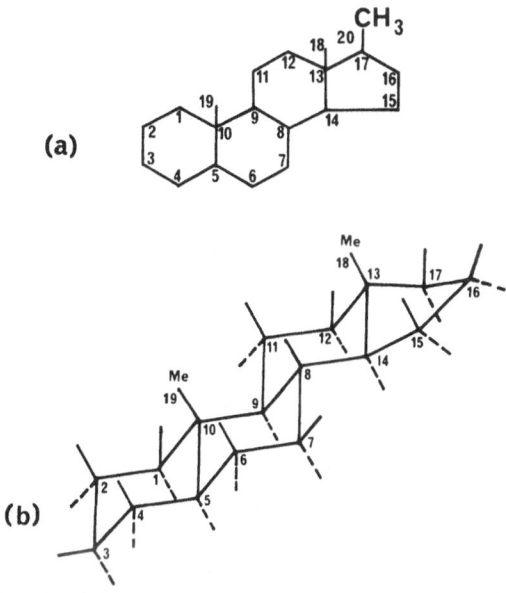

(a)

(b)

Fig. 1. (a) Core structure of steroid hormones consists of four interconnected rings of carbon atoms, three of which are cyclohexane rings. Each ring in the steroid molecule is in the "chair" form. (b) The multiplicity of bonding within the rings as well as the side groups attached to them differ from one hormone to another. The structural differences subtly alter the shapes of hormone molecules (see BUSH, 1962; O'MALLEY and SHRADER, 1976). It is principally on the basis of shape that hormones are recognised by their receptors. Axial bonds are shown without hydrogen; α-bonds dashed; β-bonds solid; angular methyl groups, Me

phocytes that mediate cellular hypersensitivity (BLOOM et al., 1974; CHESS et al., 1974; HALL, 1974; WILSON, 1974). Such conditions are collectively referred to as allergic diseases because the affected individuals show altered reactivity, or allergy (VON PIRQUET, 1968) to some environmental or endogenous constituents recognised as allergen(s) or antigen(s). This includes even rheumatoid arthritis, the condition for which cortisone (see Fig. 1) was first administered as a therapeutic agent (HENCH et al., 1949) and in which there is not only a definite pathogenetic role for auto-antibodies (ZVAIFLER, 1970) but also for elements of cellular hypersensitivity (GLEN and JASANI, 1968; PEARSON et al., 1975; STASTNY et al., 1975; VON BOXAL and PA-GET, 1975).

Ideally, an anti-inflammatory agent should be capable of reversing all the clinical manifestations of inflammation; namely pain, redness, heat, and swelling. In addition, its prolonged use should prevent loss of function. Of the presently available chemotherapeutic agents, only the anti-inflammatory steroids fulfil all these criteria. However, their therapeutic usefulness is severely limited by three sets of pharmacological complications.

Firstly, the amount of anti-inflammatory steroid required for maximal depression of subjective phenomenon *(stiffness, soreness and tenderness)* as well as objective signs *(joint swelling, flexion contractures, if not long established, and histopathological features)*, for example in rheumatoid arthritis (HENCH et al., 1950; HENCH,

1952), is so high as to result in many side-effects and even some life-threatening complications. Side-effects are common also with the use of non-steroid anti-inflammatory agents, even when they are used in doses inadequate to depress the objective signs of rheumatoid arthritis. However, side-effects are particularly troublesome in the case of anti-inflammatory steroids because, owing to their chemical resemblance to cortisol, they induce more profound metabolic and endocrine aberrations than those encountered with the use of non-steroid agents.

Secondly, although fully effective against all types of inflammation, anti-inflammatory steroids are not therapeutically beneficial in most instances of non-allergic inflammation. If anything, they prove to be positively harmful in conditions associated with the persistence of viable pathogenic micro-organisms such as tubercle bacilli and pyogenic bacteria, or the continued influence of chemical irritants such as acid gastric juice. For instance, both tuberculosis and peptic ulcer are exacerabated and may even be reactivated once healed (STEPHANOPOULOS and KAMAROULAS, 1961; MEADOR, 1962; JANOWITZ et al., 1958; SKORYNA et al., 1958).

Thirdly, they lower the host's resistance to microbial infection (see DAVID et al., 1970). Such an effect may account for the increased incidence of unusual fungal, viral and protozoal infections in patients receiving immunosuppressive doses of anti-inflammatory steroids as, for example, following renal homotransplantation (RIF-KIND et al., 1967; PARKHURST and VLAHIDES, 1967; GOLDSTEIN and RAMBO, 1962).

To avoid such complications, new agents must be developed which differ from cortisol-like anti-inflammatory steroids in being relatively devoid of: (a) metabolic activity in non-diseased tissues, (b) activity against cellular and vascular changes characteristic of non-specific inflammation such as that found during wound healing, and (c) activity against vascular or cellular mechanisms which defend the individual against microbial infection. However, that cannot be achieved until we have: (1) better understanding of the probable influence which currently available anti-inflammatory steroids exert against the pathophysiological mechanism underlying allergic inflammation in general and rheumatoid synovial inflammation in particular; (2) test models which differ from the currently employed methods such as the cotton pellet granuloma test of MEIER et al. (1950), the cutaneous vasoconstriction test of McKENZIE and STOUGHTON (1962), or the in vitro tests based on stabilisation of lysosomes (WEISSMANN and THOMAS, 1964; IGNARRO and COLOMBO, 1972) in that they involve a role for antibodies or sensitised lymphocytes, or both. The fullest exploitation of the potential which exists for variation of the biological activity of steroid compounds through subtle alterations in their structure, cannot in fact be achieved until we have test models which allow simultaneous recognition of the therapeutically useful as well as harmful effects of newly synthesised steroids.

B. Scope of the Review

Detailed analysis of the effect of structural alteration on the anti-inflammatory properties of cortisol-like molecules is beyond the scope of the present review because, but for a few exceptions, enhancement of the anti-inflammatory activity measured by the cotton pellet granuloma test or the cutaneous vasoconstriction test has resulted in a proportional augmentation of the undesirable metabolic and endocrine effects of the naturally occurring anti-inflammatory steroids. The few exceptions, including especially the attenuation of sodium-retaining activity, have received considerable attention because they underline the paramount need for utilisation of test systems that can recognise specifically the pharmacological effect under study. The interested reader may, however, find valuable background information on this aspect in the authoritative reviews by LIDDLE (1961), BUSH (1962), SARRETT et al. (1963), RINGLER (1964) and POPPER and WATNIK (1974).

It is customary to view the biological activity of anti-inflammatory steroids as being physiological if it can be elicited using cortisol concentrations in the region of 10^{-10}–10^{-7} M (MUNCK, 1968). Therefore, their anti-inflammatory, anti-rheumatic and anti-allergic effects requiring concentrations equal to or higher than 10^{-6} M are relegated to the pharmacological category, and regarded by implication as being unrelated to the metabolic and other physiological effects of the natural hormones. This view has gained additional strength from the good correlation which exists between the anti-rheumatic potency of cortisol-like steroids and their inhibitory action on in vitro lysis of isolated lysosomes and erythrocytes (WEISSMANN and THOMAS, 1964; WEISSMANN, 1972; IGNARRO, 1974; AGARWAL and GARBY, 1964). The in vitro observations have tended also to foster the idea that the anti-inflammatory, anti-rheumatic and anti-allergic effects of cortisol-like hormones may arise from molecular mechanisms not requiring a role for the cytoplasmic cortisol receptor.

However, the above view may require to be modified considerably in the light of evidence which indicates that physiological amounts of at least one naturally occurring cortisol-like hormone, corticosterone, can be fully anti-inflammatory if administered with adrenaline (see SENDELBECK and YATES, 1970). Even more to the point, such anti-inflammatory action of the steroid may derive in part from hormonally induced provision of glucose to the injured tissue. As described later, adrenaline is essential for both the glycogenolytic as well as lipolytic effects of the naturally occurring cortisol-like steroids.

Therefore, in the present review, the mode of action of cortisol-like steroids in allergic diseases in general and rheumatoid arthritis in particular, is not discussed as a separate section but is outlined in terms of biological activities observed with physiological amounts of cortisol-like steroids.

Throughout the present account, inflammation is viewed, irrespective of its cause, as a vascular response consisting of vasodilatation, increased vascular permeability and emigration of inflammatory cells. Further, irrespective of the dose employed, the effectiveness of anti-inflammatory steroids against allergic inflammation is analysed in terms of activity that may either interfere with the response of the vessels, or the intermediary role of non-lymphocytic factors, or inhibit directly the formation and release of lymphocytic factors themselves. Such an analysis is imperative because of the increasing realisation that although antibodies as well as specifically sensitised lymphocytes may initiate allergic inflammation, the non-lymphocytic cellular elements such as monocytic and polymorphonuclear (PMN) phagocytes, as well as non-antibody macromolecular plasma constituents such as complement components, are essential for the maximal development of its vascular manifestations.

The exercise reveals that, although currently available anti-inflammatory steroids can inhibit the antigen-induced metabolic activation of previously non-sensitized lymphocytes, they are almost completely ineffective against similar activation of specifically sensitized lymphocytes. As antigen-induced metabolic activation results in synthesis of antibodies or lymphokines (see Chap. 10), this implies that currently available anti-inflammatory steroids are ineffective against formation and release of lymphocytic mediators in fully sensitized, i.e. allergic, individuals. Instead, the experimental data support the previously made suggestion (see GERMUTH, 1956; JASANI, 1972) that the beneficial effects of even the fully anti-allergic doses of anti-inflammatory steroids (300 mg cortisone, intramuscularly (i.m.) daily) such as those employed by HENCH et al., 1950, in their initial clinical trials (see JASANI, 1975) may derive chiefly from the ability of the drugs to depress the local tissue reactivity, i.e. the response of the vessels to inflammatory mediators released during antibody-mediated as well as lymphocyte-initiated allergic reactions.

Results of a systematic study of the effect of a topical anti-inflammatory steroid against lymphocyte-initiated inflammatory component in rabbit skin homografts, reported in Section F, suggest that the beneficial effects of high doses of anti-inflammatory steroids currently advocated for the management of rejection crises in patients who have received kidney homotransplants, may derive mainly from the ability of the drug to alter the microcirculatory response to factors released from specifically sensitized lymphocytes. Anti-inflammatory steroids exert a more pronounced depressive effect against the role of non-lymphocytic inflammatory cells such as the monocytic and PMN phagocytes than do most non-steroid anti-rheumatic drugs. However, the results of homograft experiments show that in the fully sensitized, i.e. allergic, individual this action of anti-inflammatory steroids may not prove to be as important a basis for their therapeutically beneficial effects as their ability to make vessels less responsive to mediators released from lymphocytes.

If anything, the data reviewed in this chapter tends instead to favour strongly the possibility that the steroid-induced depression of circulating monocytes, as well as inhibition of the biological response of macrophages to lymphokines (CLAMAN, 1974; BALOW and ROSENTHAL, 1973), may contribute to the following harmful effects of the drugs: (a) delay or failure of wound healing, (b) inability to withstand microbial infection, (c) increased susceptibility to and lowering of resistance against infection by low-grade pathogens such as commensal bacteria, fungi and viruses, and (d) immunosuppression.

C. Naturally Occurring Anti-Inflammatory Steroids

The three naturally occurring mammalian anti-inflammatory steroids are corticosterone (11β-21-dihydroxy-4-pregnone-3,20-dione, Fig. 2a), cortisol (17-hydroxy-corticosterone; hydrocortisone, Fig. 2b) and cortisone (17-hydroxy-11-dehydrocorticosterone, Fig. 2c). All three are synthesised from cholesterol and secreted by the adrenal glands in response to stimulation by adrenocorticotrophic hormone (ACTH).

Cortisol constitutes almost 90% of the adrenocortical steroid output of man. Cortisone, which was the first adrenocortical hormone to be isolated (KENDALL et al., 1934) and used in the treatment of rheumatoid arthritis (HENCH et al., 1950), is not, however, secreted to any significant extent in many species including man. As shown by Table 1, there is a considerable variation in the relative proportion of the three anti-inflammatory steroids in the adrenal venous effluent of commonly employed laboratory animals (guinea pig, dog and golden hamster) resembling man.

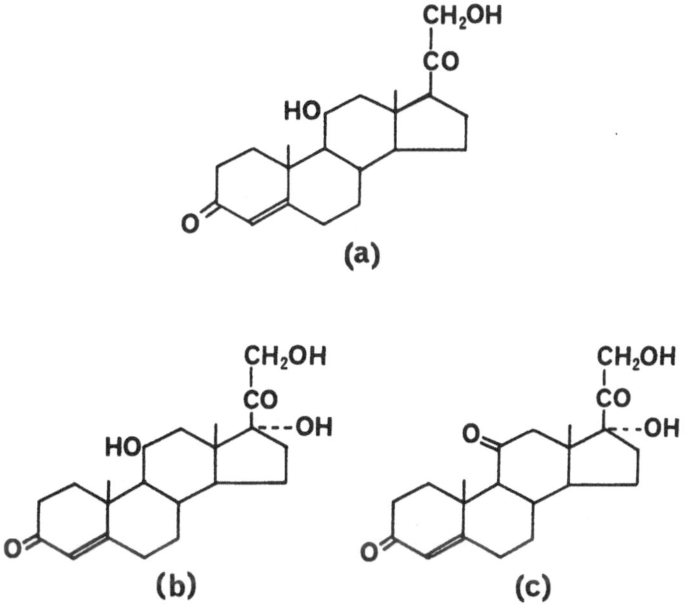

Fig. 2a—c. Structural formulae: (a) common to anti-inflammatory steroids; (b) cortisol (17-hydroxy-corticosterone); (c) cortisone (17-hydroxy, 11-dehydro-corticosterone)

Table 1. Principal adrenocortical steroids in the venous effluent of some mammalian adrenal glands. Data based on the report of BRAVERMAN and DAVIS (1973). Values shown are mean secretion rate ($\pm$S.E.) expressed in appropriate units per minute except where stated otherwise

	Anti-inflammatory steroids		Mineralocorticoids
	Cortisol µg/min	Corticosterone µg/min	Aldosterone µg/min
Man basal (range)	6.60–20.30	1.00– 2.70	104 – 229
Dog basal	0.20±0.10	0.29±0.20	0.20± 0.10
Rabbit stressed	0.12±0.03	5.00±0.40	2.20± 0.50
Rat stressed (range)	—	0.80±1.50	1.7 – 3.3
Sheep basal (±S.D.)	2.68±2.02	0.17±0.18	10.5 ± 0.5

Corticosterone which is the predominant circulating anti-inflammatory steroid in the rat (SENDELBECK and YATES, 1970) as well as in the rabbit (BUSH, 1953; BRAVERMAN and DAVIS, 1973) has no detectable anti-allergic or anti-rheumatic effect in man (WARD and HENCH, 1955). Aldosterone, which has a potent sodium-retaining effect in all the species, does not exert anti-inflammatory, or anti-allergic effects (WARD and HENCH, 1955). The possible significance of the remaining 37 steroid compounds found in the adrenal cortex (see RINGOLD and BOWERS, 1963), including minute amounts of androgens, oestrogens and progesterone, is largely unresolved (see BAKER and ADAMS, 1955; VOGT and SCHROEDER, 1955).

D. Synthetic Anti-Inflammatory Steroids

An idea of the enormous scope that exists for chemical substitutions in the cortisol molecule, as well as the vast amount of effort that has already been lavished world-wide to obtain more potent but less hazardous analogues of the naturally occurring anti-inflammatory steroids, can be obtained from the excellent reviews by BUSH (1962), SARRETT et al. (1963) and POPPER and WATNIK (1974).

Chemical congeners of naturally occurring anti-inflammatory steroids can be classified into three broad categories depending upon the site of chemical substitution, namely: (1) those in which the hydrogen is replaced at one or more carbon positions on the cyclopentane or cyclohexane rings; (2) those which are derivatives of one of the hydroxyl functions of cortisol; and (3) those which are mixed examples of types one and two. Representative examples of these three types of compound that are either in common use today or referred to in the text, are listed in Tables 2 and 3.

Table 2. Effect of single and multiple substitutions on anti-inflammatory and anti-rheumatic activity of hydrocortisone (all information except that on cortisone based on ARTH et al., reprinted with permission from J. Amer. chem. Soc. **80**, 3161–3163, 1958, copyright by the American Chemical Society; details for cortisone are from Table 4 of SARRETT et al., Progr. Drug. Res. **5**, 11–153, 1963)

	Δ	C6	C9	C11	C16	Anti-in-flammatory activity in rat	Anti-rheumatic activity in man (oral route)
Cortisone	4,5	H	H	O	H	0.7–0.8	Inactive
Hydrocortisone	4,5	H	H	β-OH	H	1.0	1.0
Prednisolone	1,2; 4,5	H	H	β-OH	H	3–4	3–4
Methylprednisolone	1,2; 4,5	CH$_3$	H	β-OH	H	5	3–5
Triamcinolone	1,2; 4,5	H	F	β-OH	α-OH	5	3–5
Dexamethasone	1,2; 4,5	H	F	β-OH	α-CH$_3$	190	28–40

E. Biological Activities Observed With Physiological Amounts of Cortisol-Like Steroids

Physiological amounts of cortisol have important metabolic, endocrine and cardio-vascular effects essential for survival, growth and general well-being.

Table 3. Effect of single and multiple substitutions on the vasoconstrictor activity of hydrocortisone (data of SUTTON et al., J. invest. Derm. **57**, 371–376, 1971, copyright 1971 The Williams & Wilkins Co., Baltimore; McKENZIE, 1962). Data also show the effect of derivatization of one or more of the hydroxyl functions of cortisol

	Δ	C6	C9	C16	R'	R"	R'''	Relative vasoconstrictor activity in man	
								Intradermal injection	External application
Hydrocortisone	4,5	H	H	H	H	H	H	1.0	1.0
Prednisolone	1,2; 4,5	H	H	H	H	H	H	1.7	1.0
Triamcinolone	1,2; 4,5	H	F	OH	H	H	H	6.5	0.1
Dexamethasone	1,2; 4,5	H	F	CH_3	H	H	H	10.2	10.0
Dexamethasone acetate	1,2; 4,5	H	F	CH_3	H	H	OCH_3	8.7	—
Triamcinolone acetonide	1,2; 4,5	H	F	O	O—C(CH_3)(CH_3)—O	H	H	18.9	1000
Fluocinolone acetonide	1,2; 4,5	F	F	O	O—C(CH_3)(CH_3)—O	H	H	58.2	1000

I. Metabolic Effects

For descriptive purposes, the metabolic effects of cortisol-like steroids may be considered under several sub-headings—gluconeogenesis, protein metabolism, glycogenolysis and lipolysis—provided that it is remembered that in the intact animal they are closely inter-related. Their inclusion in a discussion of the anti-inflammatory action of cortisol-like steroids is justifiable not only on the grounds that they might account for the clinically undesirable effects of supraphysiological amounts of the steroids (LIDDLE, 1961), but on the even more important grounds that now, as compared with earlier (see JASANI, 1972), it appears probable rather than possible that they could constitute a basis for the anti-inflammatory, anti-allergic and anti-rheumatic effects of the drugs.

1. Gluconeogenesis

Cortisol influences gluconeogenesis which is essential for life of mammals and many vertebrates in that it maintains the supply of glucose to the brain at times when the intake of food is restricted and the liver glycogen stores are depleted. Gluconeogenesis comprises the synthesis of glucose and glycogen from lactate, pyruvate, certain amino acids such as alanine, serine, threonine and glycine, and to a less significant extent from glycerol and free fatty acids (EXTON, 1972). The liver is the major site of gluconeogenesis, with the kidney becoming an important site during starvation and acidosis. Cortisone, being intrinsically devoid of metabolic activity is less potent than cortisol with regard to glycogen deposition in the liver—by a factor of almost 0.7 (NELSON, 1962), which roughly corresponds to the extent to which it is converted in vivo to cortisol (see PETERSON et al., 1957; Fig. 2b).

Gluconeogenesis appears to be intimately associated with, if not actually dependent upon, changes in protein synthesis that can be induced even in vitro with the aid of physiological concentrations of cortisol-like steroids. Apart from a twofold rise in general protein synthesis measured as increased incorporation of radio-labelled amino acids, cortisol-like steroids induce synthesis de novo of immunoprecipitable enzymes (ROSEN and NICHOL, 1963; FEIGELSON et al., 1971). A number of such enzymes have a key role in intermediary carbohydrate metabolism. For example, increased synthesis of glucose from lactate is related mainly to induction of the enzyme p-enolpyruvate cocarboxinase (EXTON and HARPER, 1972), whereas cortisol-induced synthesis of glycogen appears to result from induction of phosphorylase phosphatase (STALMANS et al., 1971).

The effects of cortisol-like steroids on carbohydrate metabolism are not confined to the liver alone but prevail in all tissues containing cells that possess the specific cytoplasmic receptor proteins. However, the net result varies considerably depending upon the type of tissue. For instance, the uptake of glucose is inhibited in most non-hepatic tissues except the brain and skeletal muscle (see LEUNG and MUNCK, 1975). The possible relevance of these observations to anti-inflammatory action of cortisol-like steroids is discussed in Section E.I.9.

2. Protein Metabolism

Injection of cortisol-like steroids potentiates the excretion of nitrogen in the urine of animals either fasting or feeding normally. In rats administered cortisone acetate

(3 mg subcutaneously (s.c.) daily for 5 days), this effect was found to be mainly due to inhibition of protein synthesis rather than increased breakdown of tissue proteins (CLARK, 1953).

Direct evidence for cortisol-induced decrease in the rate of incorporation of ^{14}C-labelled amino acids into cellular proteins is now available for most of the cortisol-responsive non-hepatic tissues and cells including, for example, skeletal muscle (MUNCK, 1968), diaphragm and heart (MANCHESTER et al., 1959; WOOL and WEIN-SHELBAUM, 1960; WEINSHELBAUM and WOOL, 1961), skin (OVERELL et al., 1960), lymphoid organs (RAUCH et al., 1961; MORITA and MUNCK, 1964; MAKMAN et al., 1967), bone (REYNOLDS, 1966; PECK et al., 1967), fibroblasts (RUHMANN and BERLI-NER, 1965; ISHII et al., 1972), PMN leucocytes (RAUCH et al., 1961; SIMONSEN, 1972) and pituitary cells (BIRGE et al., 1967; FLEISCHER and VALE, 1968). The experiments referred to above involved either (a) treatment of the animals with steroid for a specified length of time, administration of the labelled amino acid shortly before sacrifice and comparison of the protein-bound radioactivity in tissues of the steroid-treated and control animals; or (b) the removal of tissues from steroid-treated animal and incubation in vitro with amino acid.

The depressive effect on protein synthesis tends to be specific, since it is often associated with increased synthesis of some enzymes or protein. For example, in cultured neurogenic cells, cortisol was found to induce glycerophosphate dehydroge-nase (ROCKSTEIN, 1973), glutamine synthetase (SHIMIDA et al., 1967; PIDDINGTON, 1971), RNA polymerase and $Na^+K^+ATPase$, but not $Mg^{++}ATPase$ (STASTNY, 1971). In bone rudiments taken from 7-day-old chick embryos, cultured for 6 days, cortisol (30 nM–3 µM) added on day 0 decreased polysaccharide synthesis, inhibited growth but increased collagen content (REYNOLDS, 1966). In cultured fibroblasts, cortisol at physiological concentrations inhibited RNA synthesis per surviving cell without decreasing protein synthesis (PRATT and ARONOW, 1966). In addition, the depressive effect of cortisol-like steroids upon protein synthesis depends, paradoxi-cally enough, on the prior synthesis of trace (although functionally significant) amounts of some other protein (see THOMSON and LIPPMAN, 1974). The requirement is equally essential for initiation of the increased rate of protein synthesis, such as that found in the hepatocytes. In fact, it constitutes the basis for: (a) the characteris-tic susceptibility of cortisol-induced biological effects to the inhibitory action of actinomycin D, the antibiotic which inhibits DNA-dependent RNA synthesis (REICH and GOLDBERG, 1964), and (b) a time lag which usually varies from 1 to 2 h, but may extend even up to 24 h (for example, see THOMPSON and LIPPMAN, 1974).

3. DNA Synthesis

When measured as incorporation of $[^3H]$-thymidine, DNA synthesis is depressed by cortisol-like steroids in virtually all cell types including even the regenerating liver and infant brain (KIMBERG and LOEB, 1971; HOWARD, 1965).

Insight into the molecular basis for the action of cortisol emerging with use of techniques pioneered by SAMUELS and TOMKINS (1970) and ROUSSEAU et al. (1972), may eventually explain how the various physiological effects of cortisol occur more or less independently of one another in different animal systems.

4. Molecular Basis for Metabolic Effects

Contrary to the previously held belief (see WILLMER, 1961; WILLIAMS-ASHMAN, 1965; JANOSKY et al., 1968; GRANT, 1969), the physiological effects of cortisol require penetration of the steroid into the cell (LEVINSON et al., 1972) and its binding to specific intracellular protein receptors found in the cytosol of cortisol-responsive tissues (HACKNEY et al., 1970; MUNCK, 1971; BAXTER and TOMKINS, 1970). The cell is freely permeable to cortisol and related steroids (SCHAEFFER et al., 1969a; BAXTER and FORSHAM, 1972). Specific protein receptors for cortisol and related anti-inflammatory steroids have now been identified in the liver (ROUSSEAU et al., 1973) and in a variety of extra-hepatic tissues including the brain (McEWEN et al., 1970; GERLACH and McEWEN, 1972; McEWEN and PALPINGER, 1970), fibroblasts (HACKNEY et al.,

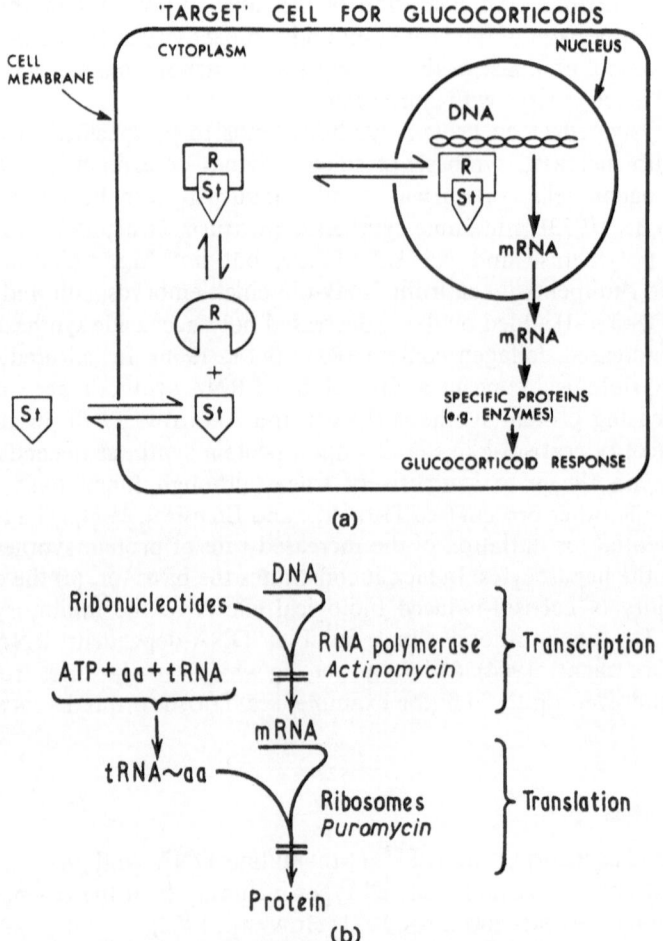

Fig. 3a and b. *Molecular basis for biological effects of cortisol and other anti-inflammatory steroids:* R in Figure 3a represents cytoplasmic specific receptor protein and St represents steroid (scheme according to BAXTER and FORSHAM, 1972). aa in Figure 3b represents amino acids. Outline of pathways in the control of protein synthesis according to MUNCK (1968)

1970), lung (GIANOPOULOS et al., 1972; BALLARD and BALLARD, 1972), retina (CHADER et al., 1972), kidney (BALLARD et al., 1974), lymphoid tissue (MUNCK and BRINK-JOHNSEN, 1968; BAXTER et al., 1971; KIRKPATRICK et al., 1971) and heart, intestine skeletal muscle, smooth muscle, stomach and testes (BALLARD et al., 1974; MUNCK, 1971).

A widely accepted view, outlined schematically in Figure 3, envisages that cortisol binds to the cytoplasmic receptors and is translocated to a nuclear acceptor site, the chromatin (BAXTER and FORSHAM, 1972), resulting in activation of the genome, increase in RNA synthesis and induction of new protein synthesis (Fig.3). The induced protein, usually an enzyme, mediates the biological effect of the hormone. Current indications are that the presence of cytosol receptors, and not the nuclear acceptor sites, determines the responsiveness of a particular cell type to cortisol. The nuclear acceptor sites would appear to be ubiquitous (BAXTER and FORSHAM, 1972). The binding of cortisol to the cytoplasmic receptor proteins (molecular weight 50000–150000) is stereospecific, of high affinity but non-covalent, and of low capacity, i.e. saturable (O'MALLEY, 1971; FELDMAN et al., 1972).

A temperature-dependent configurational change in the cytosol receptor-cortisol complex observed by ISHII et al. (1972), MUNCK et al. (1972), and ROUSSEAU et al. (1973) appears essential for translocation of the complex into the nucleus. It is quite rapid, the half-time in thymic cells being of the order of 30 s at 37° C (WIRA and MUNCK, 1974). After activation of the genome, the cortisol-receptor complex dissociates from the chromatin and reappears in the cytoplasm (Fig.3a). The half-time for receptor regeneration in the case of mouse fibroblasts is about 30 min (ISHII et al., 1972). The regeneration process is also temperature- and energy-dependent but does not require protein synthesis (ISHII et al., 1972; MUNCK et al., 1972; ROUSSEAU et al., 1973). The half-time for dissociation of cortisol from the specific receptor in thymic and hepatoma cells is about 15 min (MUNCK and BRINK-JOHNSEN, 1968; BAXTER and TOMKINS, 1970).

5. Onset and Duration of Cortisol Action

Most physiological effects of cortisol can be detected within two hours, some within 10–30 min and a few (see KIDSON, 1965, 1967; STEVENS et al., 1967) within 1 minute. The duration of various effects is probably dependent on the half-life of products involved in steps of cortisol action that follow nuclear binding (see Fig.3b). They include, for instance, the newly synthesised RNA, specific enzyme proteins or other molecules (BAXTER and FORSHAM, 1972). The probable role of these factors in determination of the temporal features as well as the specificity of physiological response in a particular tissue or cells is discussed below under mechanisms.

6. Mechanism of Action of Cortisol

Although similarity between the cytosol receptors, as well as nuclear acceptor sites of cortisol-responsive cells of different types of organ and tissues, can be expected to lead to similar physiological effects, it cannot account for the specificity of biological response so characteristic of, for example, the hepatocytes as compared with that of the leucocytes, thymic or neurogenic cells (retina), or skeletal muscle. A detailed consideration of the factors that may determine the phenotypic differences between cortisol-responsive cells is not as yet possible owing to lack of information (see THOMPSON and LIPMANN, 1974). The information that is available concerning the induction of three *biochemical* effects; namely, increased synthesis of tyrosine amino-transferase, glutamine synthetase and alkaline phosphatase (reviewed by THOMPSON and LIPMANN, 1974), suggests that the mechanism for cortisol-induced *metabolic* effects may prove to be extremely complex at the molecular level. Encouragingly though, experimental techniques are available for unravelling of the molecular complexity (see THOMPSON and LIPMANN, 1974). It is felt that their fullest exploitation may explain why supraphysiological amounts of cortisol-like steroids are required for mediation of metabolic effects underlying the anti-allergic and anti-rheumatic effects of cortisol-like steroids.

The extent to which some of the molecular complexities arise from concomittant action of other hormones, e.g. growth hormone, insulin, glucagon and especially adrenaline, has also to be defined more fully. Evidence for a close inter-relationship which exists between adrenaline and cortisol-like steroids in the mediation of some metabolic effects is reviewed below.

7. Glycogenolysis

Not unlike lipolysis described below, glycogenolysis in muscle and liver represents the so-called permissive effect of cortisol-like steroids. The term signifies that physiological concentrations of cortisol-like steroids are necessary for metabolic effects mediated by other hormones to occur.

In contradistinction to gluconeogenesis discussed earlier, glycogenolysis leads to increased production of glucose in the liver, heart and skeletal muscle through breakdown of glycogen. Although inducible with adrenaline in the normal state, glycogenolysis cannot be thus induced in the adrenalectonised state without the availability of physiological concentrations of cortisol-like steroids.

At the molecular level, impairment of hepatic glycogenolysis in the rat is due mainly to a greatly diminished level of inactive liver glycogen phosphorylase (SCHAEFFER et al., 1969a). Cortisol replacement therapy (1 mg/100 g per 12 h for 3 days) results in replenishment of inactive phosphorylase to physiological levels allowing return of the glycogenolytic (hyperglycaemic) effect of adrenaline and cAMP. Replenishment is due in all likelihood to de novo synthesis of the enzyme protein (SCHAEFFER et al., 1969a).

The effect of adrenalectomy on muscle (gastrocnemius) phosphorylase of rat differs from that on the liver enzyme. Adrenalectomy does not result in any change in the levels of active or inactive muscle glycogen phosphorylase (SCHAEFFER et al., 1969b). Despite that, however, adrenaline-induced glycogenolysis is impaired. Administration of cortisol (1 mg/100 g per 12 h for 3 days) restores glycogenolysis and results also in an increase in the muscle glycogen phosphorylase to twice the level observed in untreated, normal or adrenalectomised rats. The larger increase in the muscle as compared to the liver enzyme may be due to a slower rate of degradation of the muscle enzyme (SCHAEFFER et al., 1969b).

8. Lipolysis

Physiological concentrations of cortisol-like steroids are essential also for lipolysis induced by adrenaline (GOODMAN and KNOBIL, 1961). In vitro observations suggest that the permissive effect may involve the stimulation of synthesis of a protein that can increase the formation of cAMP in rat adipose tissue (FAIN, 1968).

9. Relationship to Anti-Inflammatory, Anti-Allergic and Anti-Rheumatic Action

The metabolic effects of cortisol-like steroids could prove to be therapeutically beneficial either through provision of glucose to the inflamed tissue via stimulation of gluconeogenesis or glycogenolysis or both, or through inhibition of the formation of chemical mediators of inflammation via depression of protein synthesis or lipolysis, or both.

The measurement of glucose uptake in the inflamed tissue has provided somewhat contradictory results. For instance, EICHORN (1963) reported a tendency for cortisol (administered variously) to increase rather than decrease glucose uptake in rat cotton pellet granuloma induced by the method of DESAULLE et al. (1954), whereas GLENN et al. (1963) found cortisol to inhibit the glucose uptake by rat granuloma pouch.

Histochemical observations have revealed consistent accumulation of glycogen in the injured epidermal cells (LOBITZ et al., 1962). According to BILSKI and GOD-LEWSKI (1965), inactivity of phosphorylase a, low content of phosphorylase b, and partial inactivation of uridine diphosphate glucose dehydrogenase (UDPG-dehydrogenase) may be responsible for such accumulation. The effect of cortisol-like steroids on these metabolic complications of cellular injury was not investigated in either study.

Metabolic studies show that synovial tissue of patients with long-standing rheumatoid arthritis uses more oxygen and produces more lactate than that of control knee joints. Physiological concentrations of cortisol were found to decrease lactate production and oxygen consumption by rheumatoid synovium in vitro (DINGLE and PAGE THOMAS, 1956; PAGE THOMAS and DINGLE, 1958), although intra-articularly administered methyl prednisolone (40 mg per joint) or triamcinolone hexacetonide (24 mg per joint) reduced the production of lactate but left unchanged the uptake of oxygen (GOETZL et al., 1971). Both abnormalities were attributed to the presence of leucocytes. In terms of the well-known morphological appearance of rheumatoid synovium, this implies predominant involvement of lymphocytes and macrophages rather than PMN leucocytes.

Depending upon its cause, initiation as well as maintenance of the inflammatory process requires the constant availability, through synthesis de novo, of hydrolytic and lysosomal enzymes (Chaps. 8 and 9), histamine, 5-hydroxytryptamine (5-HT), and SRS-A (Chap. 11), prostaglandins and related compounds (Chap. 12), complement components and anaphylatoxin (Chap. 13), and bradykinin-like peptides (Chap. 14). Allergic inflammation would require additionally the constant formation of lymphokines (Chap. 10) and of antibodies.

Cortisol-like steroids have been reported to depress or retard the formation of *lysosomal enzymes* in monocytic phagocytes (WIENER and MARMARY, 1969), *collagenase* in human skin, rheumatoid synovium and rat uterus (KOOB et al., 1974), *histamine* as well as *5-HT* (GOTH et al., 1951; TELFORD and WEST, 1960; SCHAYER, 1963, 1967; AVIADO and CARILLO, 1970), *prostaglandins* in synovial explants, fibroblasts and monocytes (KANTROWITZ et al., 1975; TASHJIAN et al., 1975; BRAY and GORDON, 1976) and *antibodies* in the previously immunised as well as non-immunised animals, or lymph nodes and spleen cells of such animals (GERMUTH and OTTINGER, 1950; FAGREUS, 1952; MOUNTAIN, 1955; BERGLUND and FAGREUS, 1956; BERGLUND, 1956a, 1956b; STEVENS and MCKENNA, 1958; DUKOR and DIETRICH, 1968; BECKER and GUTMAN, 1972; SEGAL et al., 1972). Contrary to some claims (CLAMAN, 1974), cortisol-like steroids can depress in vitro formation of *lymphokines* from human lymphocytes, at least under well-defined experimental conditions (LUNDGREN, 1970; BUTTERWORTH, 1975; THONG et al., 1975).

An additional mechanism through which cortisol-like steroids can impair the availability of many of the above factors is discussed in greater detail under the cardiovascular effects of the drugs (Sec. E.IV.3.c). It involves the reduction of the population of inflammatory cells (monocytic and PMN leucocytes) in the inflamed tissue through suppression of their intra- and extravascular accumulation. However, three especially important points to note are that: (a) depressive effect of cortisol-like steroids on formation of histamine and prostaglandins may largely account for their hypoalgesic rather than anti-inflammatory effect (see JASANI, 1975), (b) steroids are more inhibitory against formation of antibodies in previously non-immunised as compared with immunised animals (see JASANI, 1972), and (c) prednisolone inhibits the non-specific cytotoxic potential of human lymphocytes, even at concentrations as low as 10^{-8} M, if added at the beginning of the culture but not once lymphocytes have been transformed by the antigen (BUTTERWORTH, 1975)..

The role of lipolytic effect of cortisol-like steroids during inflammation remains to be established. In contrast to their effect in vitro, intra-arterial (i.a.) administration of hydrocortisone (10–30 µg/ml) or dexamethasone (2–5 µg/ml) inhibits noradrenaline-induced changes in phospholipid metabolism resulting in the abolition of prostaglandin release from contracting mesenteric vessels (GRYGLEWSKI et al., 1975). The observations resemble those of NIJKAMP et al. (1976) who found a variety of cortisol-like steroids to inhibit the formation of arachidonate which occurs when a purified though as yet unidentified peptide (rabbit aorta contracting substance releasing factor: RCS-RF; m.w. < 5000) is administered i.a. into isolated unsensitized guinea pig lungs.

As arachidonate is the rate-limiting substrate for the formation of RCS, a mixture consisting of prostaglandin endoperoxides (PGG_2 and PGH_2) and thromboxane A_2 (TXA_2) that contracts rabbit aortic strips (NIJKAMP et al., 1976), it becomes more clearly understandable why cortisol-like steroids inhibit the vasomotor and other smooth muscle responses associated with allergic conditions including guinea pig anaphylaxis, the allergic reaction which VANE and his group utilised to obtain the peptide RCS-RF. In fact, they found the I_{50} dose for this activity of various steroids to correlate well with the relative anti-inflammatory potency. For instance, the dose of hydrocortisone (1207.0 nmol min^{-1}) required in the infusate to inhibit by 50% the amount of arachidonate released in the lung perfusate, was 6.8 times that of prednisolone, 11.4 times that of triamcinolone, 33.1 times that of betamethasone and 35 times that of dexamethasone (see NIJKAMP et al., 1976), giving a relative potency favourably comparable with those for the anti-rheumatic action shown in Table 2.

Interestingly, the steroid-induced inhibition of arachidonate release from the guinea pig lung was maximal only if the compound was administered intra-arterially 10–20 min before the peptide (NIJKAMP et al., 1976). Secondly, the inhibitory effect of the steroids was reversed if exogenous arachidonate was supplied in the infusate, a feature which has now been reported in a variety of other experimental situations as well (GRYGLEWSKI et al., 1975; FLOMAN et al., 1976; HONG and LEVINE, 1976).

The effect of cortisol-like steroids against large scale lipolysis occurring in the adipocytes has been examined by LEWIS and PIPER (1975). They found close-arterial infusion of hydrocortisone (600 nmol min^{-1}) to be ineffective against ACTH-induced lipolysis in the epigastric fat pad of rabbits. However, LEWIS and PIPER (1975) found that hydrocortisone as well as betamethasone inhibits the vasodilatation accompanying ACTH-induced lipolysis. Since neither steroid antagonised vasodilatation caused by exogenous PGE_2, and because both were ineffective against the increase which occurred in the PGE_2 content of ACTH-activated fat pads, LEWIS and PIPER (1975) concluded that the steroids inhibited the vasodilatation accompanying lipolysis through interference with the transport of prostaglandins from inside the fat cells to an extracellular space. If, however, the effect of i.a. infused ACTH were to resemble that of RCS-RF referred to above, or that of bradykinin (VARGAFTIG and DAO HAI, 1972), the question arises as of whether the inhibition of vasodilatation in the fat pad by cortisol-like steroids may not be due to prevention of changes in the phospholipid metabolism of the vasculature rather than in that of the adipocytes.

10. Relationship to Clinically Undesirable Effects

If impairment of gluconeogenesis were regarded as being the principal metabolic disturbance arising from cortisol deficiency, inhibition of synthesis of protein can be viewed as being the cardinal abnormality resulting from supraphysiological amounts of cortisol-like steroids. The abnormality is, of course, confined mainly to extrahepatic cortisol-responsive organs, tissues and cells, although the presence of morphological changes in the liver (WIENER et al., 1968) resembling those described in the skeletal muscles (BULLOCK et al., 1971) suggests that the effect may be more widespread.

The biological consequences vary both qualitatively and quantitatively depending upon the dose and type of steroid employed, but in general they reflect the consequences of disturbance of the predominant function of the tissue or cell concerned. Taking the list of mammalian tissues known to possess the cytoplasmic cortisol-receptors (BAXTER and FORSHAM, 1972; BALLARD et al., 1974; MAYER et al., 1975) we note the following in published reports.

a) Brain

Corticosterone (0.08–0.6 mg per day) prevents the increase in forebrain DNA and retards that in RNA/DNA ratio observed in untreated infant mice. Reduction in brain growth of mice is proportional to that in body growth (HOWARD, 1965). Adult rats show increased excitability of brain. The electroshock seizure threshold (EST) of animals receiving 2 mg of cortisol (s.c.) daily for 20 days, was only 15% of the control value (WOODBURY, 1952). Clinically, such changes become apparent not only as electroencephelographic abnormalities (GLASER et al., 1955; WAYNE, 1954) but also as frank convulsive seizures (see WOODBURY, 1952). For a more detailed account of other functional as well as morphological abnormalities the reader is referred to the review by JANOSKY et al. (1968) and DAVID et al. (1970).

b) Skeletal Muscle

Protein synthesis measured as incorporation of $[^{14}C]$ glycine uptake into the rat adductor muscle protein was depressed profoundly by cortisol 10 mg (but not 0.1 mg) given daily for 3 days (DE LOCKER and REDDY, 1962). Reported biological accompaniments of such treatment include metabolic (BULLOCK et al., 1972) electrophysiological (FALUDE et al., 1964) and histological (TUNCBAY et al., 1965) changes, muscle weakness and wasting (ENGEL, 1966). The reported clinical incidence of muscle wasting has been greater following administration of supraphysiological concentration of halogenated cortisol-like steroids such as triamcinolone or dexamethasone than cortisol, cortisone or corticosterone. Although largely unexplained until recently, the difference may turn out to be mainly related to the presence in some groups of muscles of a subclass of cytoplasmic receptors that exhibit a higher affinity for the halogenated as compared with the naturally occurring cortisol-like steroids (MAYER et al., 1974, 1975).

c) Bone

Multiple biochemical abnormalities, including (a) diminution of incorporation of ^{35}S into mucopolysaccharides (BOSTRÖM and ODEBLAD, 1953; KAPLAN and FISHER, 1964; SZIGETTI et al., 1965), (b) decrease in the amount of hexosamine and collagen content (KOWALEWSKI, 1962), and (c) increased bone resorption (EISENBERG, 1964) induced by cortisol-like steroids, result in osteoporosis and retardation of healing of bone fractures in the adult (BLUNT et al., 1950; EISENBERG, 1964). On the other hand, in children or in certain growing animals e.g. weanling rats, there is arrest of linear growth (WELLS and KENDALL, 1940; SOYKA and CRAWFORD, 1965). Cortisol receptors have now been identified in foetal bone tissue (see FELDMAN, 1975). Finally, focal necrosis of the femoral head or other bone extremities found with considerable regularity in patients receiving high doses of cortisol-like steroids may be due to fat emboli resulting from increased lipolysis (JANOSKY et al., 1968).

d) Stomach

Although clinical observations leave some doubt as to the aetiologic link between the administration of cortisol-like steroids and gastric ulceration (see SPIRO and MILES, 1960; CREAN, 1963), experimental data indicate clearly that steroids can induce ulcers with regularity in properly prepared animals such as rats (ROBERTS and NEZAMIS, 1957; GASS and PFEIFFER, 1963) or dogs (NICOLOFF et al., 1963; CHAIKOF et al., 1961; WELBOURN et al., 1960; FOLEY and GLICK, 1962). Elucidation of the metabolic basis for this complication may depend upon the anatomical localisation of cortisol-receptor, known to be present (see BALLARD et al., 1974) in this organ. If they were found to be localised mainly within the vessels, reduction of blood flow may prove to be a pathogenetic factor as in case of indomethacin-induced lesions (see WHITTLE, 1976; see also under ulcerogenesis, Section E.IV.4.b).

11. Implications for the Future

More research needs to be directed towards a study in depth of the cortisol receptors in various tissues with a view to identifying the cell types responsible for the beneficial, as opposed to the clinically undesirable effect, of cortisol-like steroids. Such information could next be utilised for selection of more appropriate biological test systems.

Secondly, if future studies can establish whether facilitation of glycogenolysis, or potentiation of gluconeogenesis or the impairment of glucose uptake by peripheral tissues is essential for the beneficial effects of cortisol-like steroids, newer pharmacological agents could be developed to subserve a specific function, and hence avoid the deleterious consequences of global suppression of extra-hepatic protein synthesis.

If, on the other hand, depression of protein synthesis were found to the cardinal basis for the beneficial effects of cortisol-like steroids in the allergic diseases, our attention could be focussed towards identification of the metabolic processes singularly important to perpetuation of the antibody- or lymphocyte-initiated inflammation. Once identified, modification of the cortisol molecule could be directed towards fulfilment of the required goal. As described in the next section, such a goal appears to have been achieved in respect of attenuation of the sodium-retaining activity of the naturally occurring cortisol-like steroids through modification of their chemical structure.

II. Sodium Retaining Activity

Also referred to as the mineralocorticoid effect, the term sodium retaining activity arose from: (a) the in vivo effect *(sodium retention, potassium depletion, oedema, hypertension, muscular weakness, and cardiac arrythmias)* of supraphysiological doses of cortisone that were administered to rheumatoid patients during the initial trials (SPRAGUE et al., 1950); and (b) the lowering of urinary Na^+/K^+ ratio observed following administration of the naturally occurring cortisol-like steroids to adrenalectomised rats (SIMPSON and TAIT, 1952) and dogs (LIDDLE, 1959).

The naturally occurring cortisol-like steroids promote renal tubular reabsorption of sodium through two different mechanisms. The first, which is sited in the proximal renal tubule and is ouabain insensitive, but which depends on changes in glomerular filtration rate (GFR), is responsible for reabsorption of Na^+, Cl^- and free water (LANDON and FORTE, 1971). The second, which is confined to the distal tubule, is referred to as the aldosterone effect because it does not occur with physiological concentrations of any of the other principal naturally occurring adrenocortical steroids, including cortisol. The aldosterone effect is ouabain sensitive, occurs independently of changes in GFR, and leads to increased reabsorption of Na^+ (2–3 times resting level) and excretion of K^+ in the adrenalectomised state (LIDDLE, 1959; LANDON and FORTE, 1971). In the intact animal, however, it results in a significant increase in K^+ excretion alone (see BARGER et al., 1958; GANONG and MULROW, 1958; MORRIS et al., 1973).

Both electrolyte effects occur following a latent period which, for the aldosterone effect, differs further in respect of the two cations. Latency for Na^+ reabsorption is of the order of 30 to 45 min, as compared with 90 min for the excretion of K^+ (MORRIS et al., 1973). The aldosterone effect is inducible (FIMOGNARI et al., 1967) and depends on RNA and protein synthesis (WILLIAMSON, 1963; FIMOGNARI et al., 1967). All these

Table 4. Effect of single and multiple substitutions on the electrolyte and antirheumatic activity of hydrocortisone (cortisol) molecule. Note that hydrocortisone causes loss of sodium in adrenalectomised dog

Entry	Δ	C2	C6	C9	C16	Effect in adrenalectomised dog[a]			Effect in man[b]	
						Sodium	Potassium Effect	Potency	Sodium retention	Antirheumatic activity
Cortisol	4,5	H	H	H	H	Loss	Loss	0.04	1	1
2	4,5	CH₃	H	H	H	Variable	Loss	1.00		
3	4,5	H	CH₃	H	H	Loss	Loss	0.08		
4	4,5	H	H	F	α-OH	Variable	Loss	5.50	>1	10
5	4,5	H	H	F	H	Loss	Loss	0.30	<1	3-4
6	1,2; 4,5	H	H	H	H	Loss	Loss	0.03	<1	3-4
7[d]	1,2; 4,5	H	CH₃	H	H	Loss	Loss	0.08	<1	3-5
8	1,2; 4,5	H	H	F	H	Variable	Loss	8.00	>1	20
9[e]	1,2; 4,5	H	H	F	α-CH₃	Loss	Loss	0.50	<1	28-40

[a] Reprinted with permission from Liddle, G.W., Ann. N.Y. Acad. Sci. **82**, 854-867 (1959).
[b] Reprinted with permission from Arth et al., J. Amer. Chem. Soc. **80**, 3161-3163 (1958). Copyright by the American Chemical Society.
[c] Details for Triamcinolone are from Sarrett et al., Progr. Drug Res. **5**, 11-153 (1963).
[d] Medrol.
[e] Dexamethasone.

features imply a role for cytoplasmic receptors and their interaction with the genome, as in the case of hepatic effects of cortisol-like steroids.

As revealed by the data in Table 4, structural modification of the hydrocortisone molecules on purely empirical grounds results in several instances either in the potentiation or the attenuation of sodium retaining activity without a parallel change in the anti-rheumatic potency. The mineralocorticoid activity is potentiated by the introduction of any of the following substituents: 2α-methyl (if 11-β-hydroxyl is present) 9α-halogen and 21-hydroxyl. It is attenuated, on the other hand, by the presence of 16α-hydroxyl, 16α-methyl and 17-hydroxyl substituents (see LIDDLE, 1959; ARTH et al., 1958).

The quantitative differences between the ability of aldosterone and cortisol-like steroids to induce electrolyte effects may be explained using a model proposed by EDELMAN and FIMOGNARI (1968). Based on observations of the response of the toad bladder to aldosterone and methyl prednisolone, it envisaged the possibility that the potency of the steroids to induce the electrolyte effect in the isolated organ was proportional to their binding affinity for the specific receptors present in the tissue. Attenuation of electrolyte effect through structural modification of the steroid molecule was then explicable on the basis of reduction of its affinity for specific receptors.

According to further extension of this concept (see ROUSSEAU et al., 1972), cortisol-like steroids may be envisaged as suboptimal inducers whilst spironolactone should be regarded as an anti-inducer of the aldosterone effect. The view is based on the possibility that steroids interact with either, or both, of two conformational states of the receptors, the uncomplexed receptors being present predominantly in one (inactive) form. Binding by inducers, but not by anti-inducers, increases the concentration of the other (active) conformation, the rate and extent of the increase being greater in presence of the inducer as compared with the suboptimal inducers.

Although the quantitative differences between the effect of various steroid drugs on the mammalian kidney, as opposed to the isolated toad bladder, may depend additionally upon many other factors (see BUSH, 1962; HENDLER et al., 1972; FUNDER et al., 1973a, b); the fact that at least one biological effect of the naturally occurring cortisol-like hormones can be attenuated through chemical substitution is not only theoretically important but strengthens the hope that therapeutic agents of increasingly specific action might yet be developed. A prime requirement for fulfilment of such a goal would appear to be the availability of a biological test which could recognise accurately the desired pharmacological activity, as for instance the measurement of urinary Na^+/K^+ ratio (SIMPSON and TAIT, 1952) helped recognition of the mineralocorticoid effect.

III. Control of Adrenocorticotrophic Hormone (ACTH) Synthesis and Secretion

ACTH exerts, as its name implies, a stimulatory action on the adrenal cortex, one manifestation of which is an increase in the circulating level of naturally occurring cortisol-like hormones. Prolonged stimulation by ACTH results additionally in adrenocortical cell hyperplasia as well as increase in the size and weight of adrenal glands.

1. Neuroendrocrine Control

As outlined in Figure 4, a neuroendocrine mechanism situated in the hypothalamus regulates the release of pituitary ACTH. Fairly well-defined groups of neurones situated mainly in the median eminence (see TRAVIS and SAYERS, 1965) are especially sensitive to positive neurogenic impulses relayed from the cerebral cortex and other areas of the brain (Fig. 4). Their excitation by neurogenic impulses results in the accumulation and release of a small peptide, corticotrophin releasing factor (CRF).

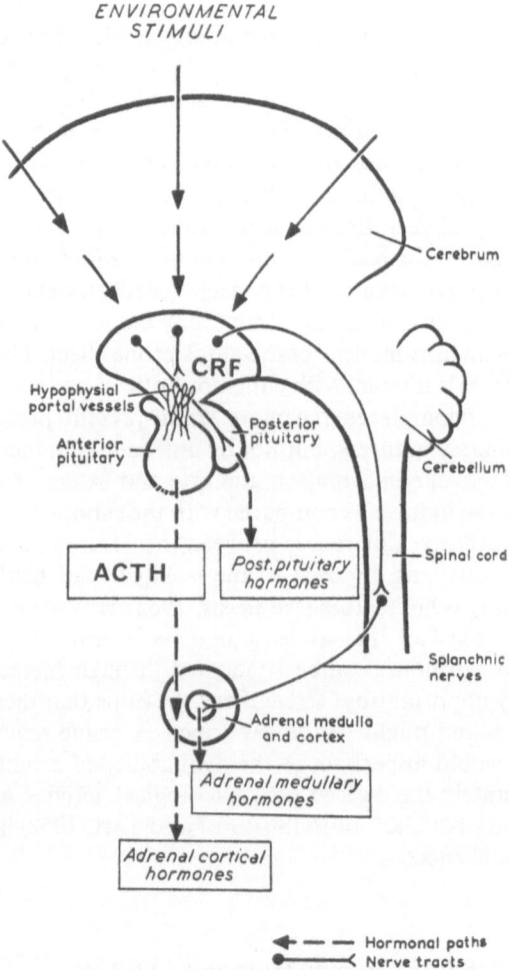

Fig. 4. Neuroendocrine control of synthesis and release of pituitary ACTH. Environmental stimuli acting through reflex pathways in the CNS modulate the synthesis and release of a small peptide, corticotrophin releasing factor (CRF), by an appropriate effect on groups of well defined neurones in the median eminence. CRF regulates synthesis as well as release of pituitary ACTH. It is conveyed to the ACTH cells of the anterior pituitary via the hypothalamico-hypophysial portal vessels. ACTH, passing via the general circulation, stimulates synthesis of naturally occurring cortisol-like steroids by cells of the adrenal cortex (Schematic diagram according to a report in Brit. med. J. (1963)II, 230

CRF constitutes the efferent humoral impulse. It is transported from the capillary network in the region of the medial eminence to the anterior pituitary by the hypothalamico-hypophyseal portal vessels (see YATES et al., 1971). Synthesis and release of CRF can change independently, so that the content of CRF in hypothalamic tissue can increase following noxious stimuli (HIROSHIGE et al., 1969a), or vary with the diurnal variations in the plasma concentration of corticosterone (HIROSHIGE et al., 1969b; DAVID-NELSON and BRODISH, 1969).

2. Negative Feedback Control

The regulatory influence of circulating cortisol-like steroids upon the synthesis and release of ACTH has long been recognised (GEMZELL et al., 1951), although the manner in which the steroids exert the negative feedback control still remains debatable. The traditional view has entertained a dual mechanism, one involving a role for the neuroendrocrine axis described above, and the other emphasising a direct effect of the steroid upon the anterior pituitary as illustrated in Figure 5.

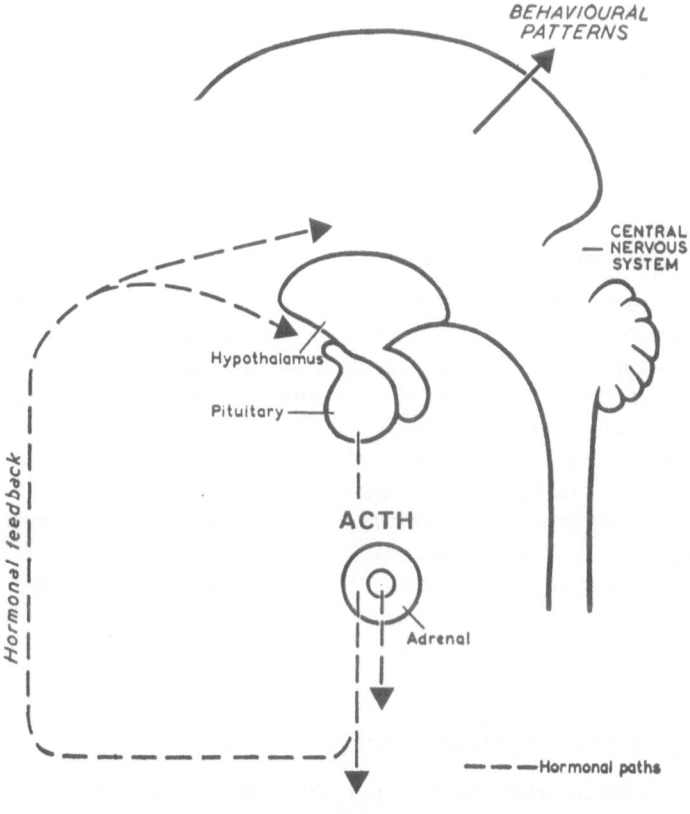

Fig. 5. Negative feedback control of synthesis and release of pituitary ACTH. Cortisol-like steroids, passing via the general circulation, inhibit the release and synthesis of pituitary ACTH by either a direct effect on the ACTH cells of the anterior pituitary, or indirectly via an effect on the synthesis and release of CRF, or by both the mechanisms. (Schematic diagram based on a report in Brit. med. J. **(1963)**II, 231

When cortisol is given (ca. 5 mg/100 g, orally) to adrenalectomised animals (SI-PERSTEIN and MILLER, 1970), its initial effect is to decrease the release, but not the synthesis, of ACTH. Cortisol also prevents the development of the 'adrenalectomy cells' which have the same morphological features and functional attributes as the 'ACTH cell' of the anterior pituitary (NAKAYAMA et al., 1969; BAKER et al., 1970).

3. Basis for Negative Feedback Control

Experiments involving the implantation of cortisol-like steroids directly into the rat or dog pituitary (ARIMURA et al., 1969; GONZALEZ-LUQUE et al., 1970) leave little doubt as to the ability of anti-inflammatory steroids to inhibit directly the CRF-induced synthesis of ACTH. The blockade occurs equally well following addition in vitro of relatively small concentrations (2 μg/ml) of dexamethasone (ARIMURA et al., 1969). Dexamethasone-induced inhibition of ACTH formation requires DNA-dependent RNA synthesis. It occurs only if the steroid is added to the medium 2 h before the addition of hypothalamic extract containing CRF. Both features suggest a role for molecular processes initiated by interaction of the steroid with cytoplasmic cortisol receptors.

CRF-induced release of the hormone does not, on the other hand, appear to be dependent upon a metabolic effect of the anti-inflammatory steroids, for it is inhibited by dexamethasone even if added simultaneously with the hypothalamic extract (ARIMURA et al., 1969).

4. Role of Cytoplasmic Steroid Receptors

In the in vitro study of WATANBE et al. (1973), the inhibitory effect of various steroids including corticosterone and dexamethasone correlated well with their ability to compete for triamcinolone-binding receptors found in cultured mouse pituitary tumour cells. Cortisol and aldosterone showed only a minimal inhibitory effect against such binding as well as synthesis of ACTH.

A higher affinity for corticosterone instead of cortisol has also been reported for binding proteins isolated from rat brain cytosol (MCEWEN and WALLACH, 1973). Cytoplasmic binding proteins, possibly the same as those which bind corticosterone, have been demonstrated in rat brain with triamcinolone (CHYTIL and TOFT, 1972) and with dexamethasone (ROTH, 1974). The preponderance of such receptors in the hippocampus suggests that these receptor sites may prove to be related to steroid effects on behaviour (FELDMAN, 1975).

5. Relationship to Clinically Desirable Effects

Presently available information does not allow us to assess reliably whether the negative feedback effect of supraphysiological concentrations of cortisol-like steroids on the release of pituitary ACTH can account for the beneficial effects of anti-inflammatory steroids in rheumatoid arthritis or other allergic diseases. The possibility should not, however, be overlooked in any scheme to establish the mode of anti-allergic and anti-rheumatic action of these agents.

6. Relationship to Clinically Undesirable Effects

Prolonged suppression of ACTH release by anti-inflammatory steroids is associated with degenerative changes in the hypothalamus (CASTOR et al., 1951) as well as in the anterior pituitary (KILBY et al., 1957), and results in histopathological changes in the adrenal glands (KILBY et al., 1957). Functional assessment of the hypothalamo-pituitary-adrenal (HPA) axis reveals a sequential impairment of the reserve secretory capacity of the hypothalamus initially, subsequently the pituitary and finally the adrenal cortex (JASANI et al., 1967). A detailed account of the factors governing the development of this complication of oral steroid therapy may be found in the reviews by DAVID et al. (1970), NUKI and DOWNIE (1973) and MYLES and DALY (1974).

The clinically undesirable effects of long-standing endocrine suppression do not become apparent either until the patient receiving oral steroid therapy suffers stress of acute infection or surgery, or until 24 to 48 h after abrupt discontinuation of therapy. Taking each of these points separately:

1. Patients who suffer stress of acute infection or surgery show signs of acute cardiovascular collapse characterised by severe hypotension which do not respond to usual resuscitative measures, but which respond promptly to rapid intravenous

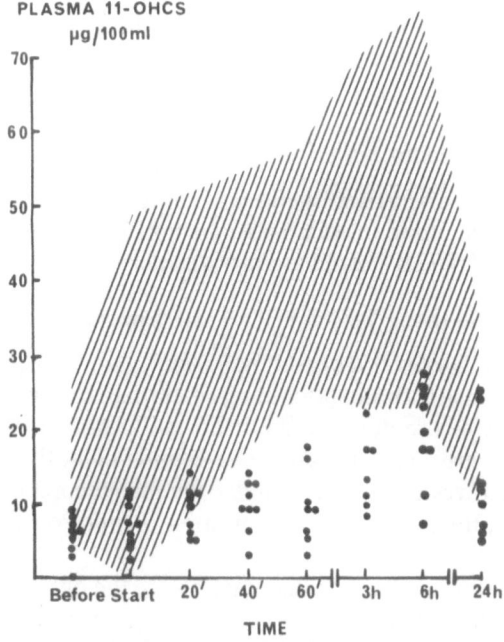

Fig. 6. Plasma cortisol (11-OHCS) response to synovectomy of knee in patients with rheumatoid arthritis (JASANI et al., 1968). The shaded area shows the range of plasma 11-OHCS levels during surgery in 20 patients who had not received corticosteroids previously. Note that the individual plasma 11-OHCS response (●) of 9 corticosteroid-treated patients, who had shown subnormal adrenocortical response to β1-24 ACTH (Synacthen, 250 µg i.m.) several days before operation, was consistently below that of the non-treated patients. One of these patients developed hypotension (B.P. 70/40 mm Hg) at 60 min after the start of operation. His 11-OHCS level was 6 µg/100 ml at the time of collapse; blood sugar 102 mg/100 ml and electrolyte values were normal. His B.P. responded well to hydrocortisone hemisuccinate sodium (100 mg i.v. hourly)

(i.v.) infusion of large doses of cortisol. Although the reported incidence of genuine examples of this complication, i.e. patients who had clear-cut evidence of low plasma cortisol concentration preceding or in association with cardiovascular collapse, is very low (SAMPSON et al., 1961; ROBINSON et al., 1962), the danger is not only ever present, but the complication can prove to be fatal, as is well exemplified by the reports of FRASER et al. (1952) and SALASSA et al. (1953). In a prospective study of the rise in plasma cortisol (11-hydroxycortico-steroids) during synovectomy of the knee (results illustrated in Fig. 6), all nine patients showing biochemical evidence of impaired adrenocortical functional reserve before operations were found to have a grossly subnormal adrenocortical response to the real-life stress of surgery. In addition, one patient was found to develop during the operation a fall in blood pressure sufficiently serious to require rapid infusion of cortisol.

2. Less severe manifestations of the hypoadrenocortical state precipitated by abrupt discontinuation of therapy may go largely unnoticed because of their similarity to clinical features of the disease itself (HENNEMAN et al., 1955; ROTSTEIN and GOOD, 1957; AMATRUDA et al., 1960). Some of the manifestations may be attributable to tissue effects resulting from a rapid change in the concentration of cortisol-like steroids, rather than due to an absolute deficiency of the hormone itself (GOOD et al., 1959).

Anti-rheumatic steroids which do not interfere with the synthesis and secretion of ACTH will be clinically more desirable than the currently available cortisol-like steroids.

IV. Cardiovascular Effects

The physiological role of cortisol-like steroids in the regulation of cardiac output and peripheral vascular tone in man and common laboratory mammals does not become evident until 48–72 h after bilateral adrenalectomy.

1. Heart and Peripheral Blood Vessels in Adrenalectomised State

As recounted well by SAYERS (1950) and by BROWN and REMINGTON (1955), animals in or near to adrenal crisis show: (a) a lowered cardiac output; (b) a lowered mean systemic and pulse pressure; (c) a raised or normal venous pressure; (d) pooling of blood in splanchnic area in cats; and (e) a failure of both the systemic arterial pressure, and of small vessels observed under the microscope in the meso-appendix of rat, to respond in the normal way to injection or infusion of noradrenaline and adrenaline.

Of particular interest to allergic inflammation are the observations that the blood pressure–lowering effect of histamine is 10 times greater in the adrenalectomised than in normal cats (DALE, 1920), and 30 times greater in adrenalectomised dogs than in control animals (BANTING and GAIRNS, 1926). That the increased toxicity is due to loss of the adrenal cortex rather than the medulla was established by KELLAWAY and COWELL (1923).

2. Microcirculation

Cortisol-like steroids have a profound effect on all the components of the microvascular network (see Fig. 7) found in various anatomical sites. The effects are manifest not only in the adrenalectomised but also in the intact animal.

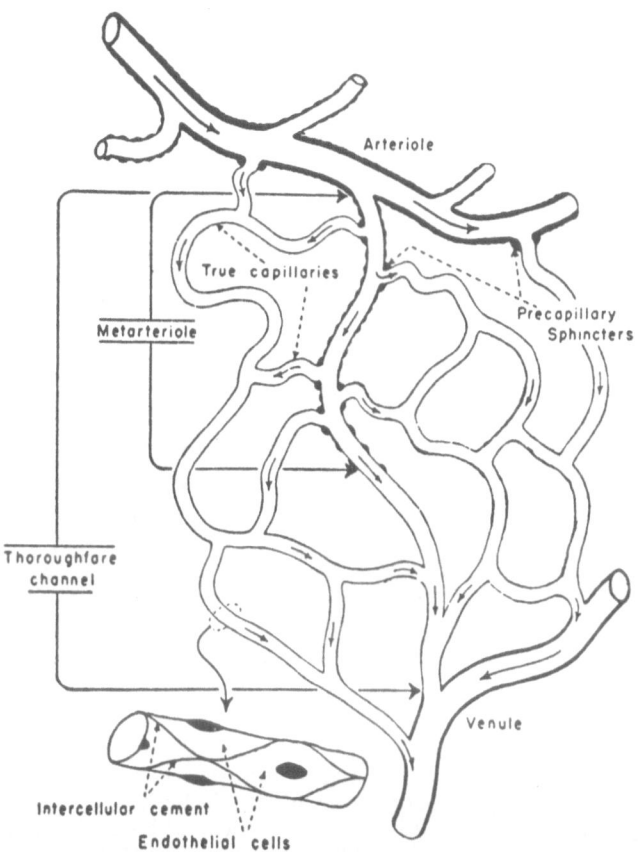

Fig. 7. Schematic representation of microvascular network in rat mesentery (ZWEIFACH et al., Ann. N.Y. Acad. Sci. **56**, 1953)

a) In the Adrenalectomised State

The changes which can be observed under a microscope in the rabbit ear (EBERT and WISSLER, 1951) or in the hamster cheek pouch (WYMAN et al., 1953), have been well documented by ZWEIFACH et al. (1953) who made a detailed study of vessels of rat mesoappendix. They found adrenalectomy to result in loss of spontaneous vasomotion, capillary dilatation and gradual loss of arteriolar tone. The venules likewise became more distended (48–72 h later). The changes were reversed by administration of cortisone (1–2 mg per day) or deoxycorticosterone acetate, DOCA (1 mg per day). Restoration of vascular tone and integrity in the rat mesoappendix did not appear to be due solely to the electrolyte effect of the hormones since treatment of adrenalectomised animals with sodium chloride alone was insufficient to provide protection against even the simple expedient of increasing the temperature of the drip solution that bathed the mesentery from 37.5° C to 39° C (ZWEIFACH et al., 1953). Even such mild stress resulted in the appearance of numerous haemorrhages. A systemic stress such as that associated with exposure to cold or loss of blood through venesection proved to be deleterious in a similar way even in animals receiving the hormonal

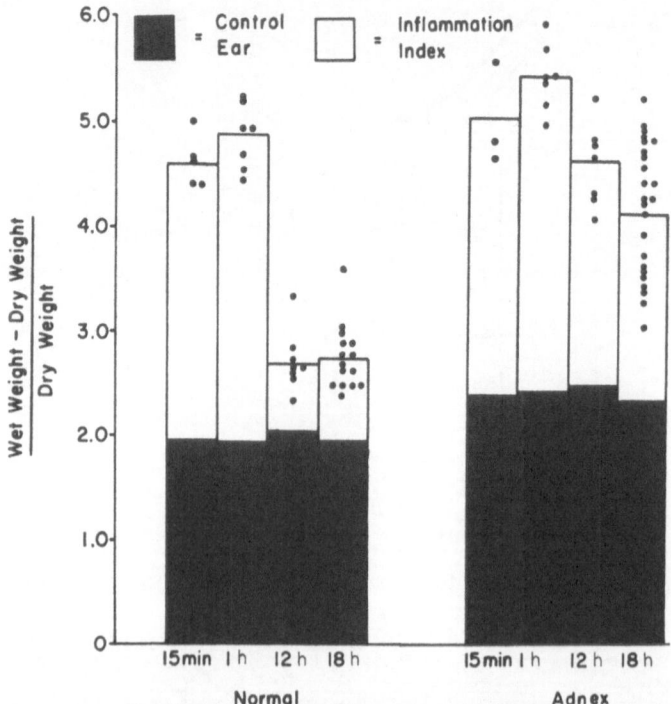

Fig. 8. Recovery from inflammation in normal and adrenalectomised animals deprived of food for 18–24 h before application of xylene (SENDELBECK, and YATES, 1970). Vertical axis shows dimensionless water content per unit dry weight for ears. Values for control ears are represented by black bars and for xylene-inflamed ears by total height of black plus white bars. For each animal difference between control ear and inflamed ear was calculated. Mean differences (inflammation indices) for populations are plotted as white bars

replacement therapy (ZWEIFACH et al., 1953)—observations which imply that the amount of cortisol-like steroids essential for the maintenance of microvascular integrity may be virtually proportional to the severity of systemic or local tissue injury.

The question therefore arises whether the brisk rise in circulating level of cortisol-like steroids found in response to local trauma in man (Fig. 6) and most animals (YATES and URQUHART, 1962) is vital for the subsequent recovery from minor injury, or whether it is merely an accidental, or incidental, physiologically irrelevant coupling of a neuroendrocrine process to other responses, such as the emotional reactions to pain, that are associated with local trauma.

A vital role for physiological amounts of corticosterone in restoration of integrity following local vascular injury, is highlighted most clearly by the elegant experiments of SENDELBECK and YATES (1970). They studied the acute chemical injury of the ear produced in fasted, unanaesthetised female rats by application of xylene to the skin (ear). The progress of swelling and recovery was followed by determining changes in water content of the ear, referred to unit dry weight. They found that although the rate of onset and extent of swelling were the same in fasted normal and adrenalectomised animals (Fig. 8), the recovery was substantially impaired in the fasted adrenalectomised animals, as shown in the right-half of the diagram. Neither corticosterone (0.75 µg/min) nor adrenaline HCl (1 µg/h) alone restored the rate of recovery to normal, although the combination was entirely effective. Their additional observations of: (a) the recovery rate of fed as opposed to fasted adrenalectomised animals, (b) blood glucose levels in the various experimental groups, and (c) the effect of sucrose feeding alone, indicate that the hormonal support of recovery was in probably mediated through effects on carbohydrate metabolism.

The results of SENDELBECK and YATES (1970) leave unanswered the important question whether the restorative effect of the hormones on the vascular integrity of the rat ear was due to changes in the carbohydrate metabolism at the inflamed site, e.g. in the inflamed vessels themselves or in mesenchymal or other cells surrounding them, or whether they were indirectly related to the gluconeogenic and glycogenolytic effect of the hormones on the liver, heart and muscle. Direct measurements of uptake of glucose by *avascular* skin in vitro showed up to 50% inhibition with cortisol concentrations of 10 µg/ml (OVERELL et al., 1960). By contrast, the uptake of glucose by rat cotton pellet granuloma was if anything, increased slightly (EICHORN, 1963). The principal limitation of the in vitro observations lies, however, in the fact that they provide no insight into metabolic changes induced by the hormones in the cellular constituents of the microvascular aparatus itself (see Fig. 7).

Although the observations of SENDELBECK and YATES (1970) leave unanswered the question as to whether supraphysiological concentrations of cortisol-like steroids may prove adequate by themselves (see ZWEIFACH et al 1953), and whether the hormonal requirements for antibody- and lymphocyte-initiated inflammation may be similar or higher than those of the non-specific inflammatory process, they open up a very promising direct experimental approach for elucidation of the metabolic basis for anti-inflammatory, anti-allergic and anti-rheumatic action of parenterally administered steroids.

b) In the Intact Animal

ZWEIFACH et al. (1953) studied also the effect of cortisol-like steroids in normal rats. Administration of ACTH (200–600 µg) was accompanied within 2–3 h by increased vascular reactivity to adrenaline (1:4 M to 1:100 M), augmentation of vasomotion and a definite narrowing of the terminal arterioles and meta-arterioles. The capillary circulation became restricted to preferential channels and was extremely rapid. A similar sequence of changes in the mesoappendix was also found following administration of comparatively large doses of cortisone (3–5 mg) for several days; but injection of DOCA (either acute or chronic), into normal rats had no demonstrable effect on the reactivity of the terminal vascular bed.

Is the vasoconstriction induced by circulating cortisol-like steroids due to their local effect on the microvascular network itself, or can it be, as was once suggested (ZWEIFACH et al., 1953), the indirect result of a systemic action of the hormone, as for example on the kidneys? A direct answer to this question is provided by the observations of several clinical investigators on the effect of cortisol-like steroids on cutaneous microvasculature following local external application (McKENZIE, 1962) or intradermal instillation (SUTTON et al., 1971). The intradermal method revealed even corticosterone to be vasoconstrictor, though less effective than hydrocortisone. Corticosteroid-induced blanching of the skin is associated with a definite reduction in cutaneous blood flow through the blanched area (GREESON et al., 1973). Total skin blood flow was measured by monitoring the clearance rates for epicutaneously applied ^{133}xenon.

3. Relationship to Anti-Inflammatory, Anti-Allergic, and Anti-Rheumatic Action

An intimate relationship between the vascular effects of cortisol-like steroids and their effectiveness against non-specific inflammation, i.e. anti-inflammatory action, is well illustrated by the observations of BANGHAM (1951), HUMPHREY (1951), ASHTON et al. (1951), ASHTON and COOK (1952), SCOTT and KALZ (1956) and KALZ and SCOTT (1956), in addition to those of ZWEIFACH et al. (1953) and SENDELBECK and YATES (1970) that were described earlier. BANGHAM as well as HUMPHREY found that cortisone (7.5 mg/kg) reduced cutaneous vascular permeability induced by intradermal injection of histamine, whereas KALZ and SCOTT found *prior* treatment with topical steroids to reduce the effects of an erythema producing dose of ultraviolet light.

The relationship to the anti-allergic and anti-rheumatic action of cortisol-like steroids is best illustrated by the visual observations made by EBERT and WISSLER (1951), BARCLAY and EBERT (1953) and WILLIAMS et al. (1954) of the effect of cortisone upon antibody-mediated as well as lymphocyte-initiated inflammation in the rabbit.

a) Antibody-Mediated Inflammation

Figure 9 illustrates the experimental protocol employed by BARCLAY and EBERT (1953). They found that cortisone (5 mg i.m. daily) not only prevented the gross dilatation of arterioles that occurred otherwise, e.g. when the animals were challenged on day 39, but also reversed completely the arteriolar changes, even if treatment was reinstituted as late as day 46. Interestingly though, reinstitution of cortisone treatment reversed only partially the dilatation of venules and capillaries; thus implying that the antibody-mediated inflammation might in some way be more permanently injurious to venules and capillaries than to the arterioles.

b) Lymphocyte-Initiated Inflammation

To study the effect of cortisone on this type of inflammation, EBERT and his colleagues selected active tuberculous infection (see Chap. 7). It is characterised by a necrotic avascular area around which the arterioles are dilated, the venules are tortuous and many capillary channels are open. Margination of leucocytes is confined mainly to the venules instead of the arterioles, as in case of the antibody-mediated inflammation. There is also evidence of haemoconcentration, free fluid and leucocytes in the interstitial space.

Cortisone (5 mg i.m. daily) restored the arteriolar tone to normal but was only partially effective against dilatation of the venules, as for antibody-mediated inflammation. It failed to arrest thrombosis and margination of leucocytes in the venules, and its effect on capillaries differed from that observed in antibody-mediated inflammation in that it closed off many of the channels so that the hyperaemic appearance was eliminated.

Discontinuation of cortisone treatment resulted in a flare-up of the inflammation around the area of caseous necrosis, venous thrombosis recurred on a wider scale and there was return of exudation of fluid and extravasation of blood (haemorrhages).

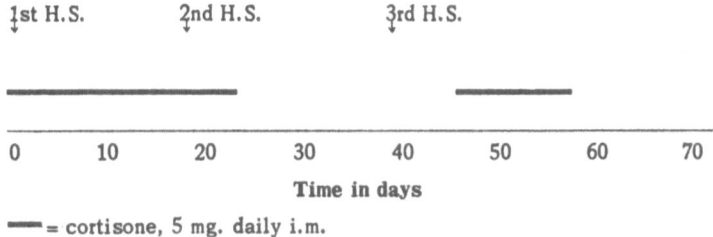

Fig. 9. Experimental protocol of BARCLAY and EBERT (Ann. N.Y. Acad. Sci. **56**, 1953). H.S. denotes horse serum

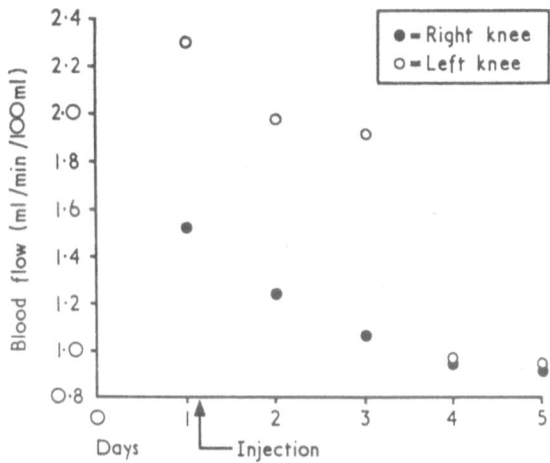

Fig. 10. Blood flow in a patient with rheumatoid arthritis with painful left knee (o) before and after local administration of methylprednisolone (80 mg, i.a.), VADASZ (1971). With the strain-gauge around the joint, venous return from the limb was occluded several times for periods of 10 s. Increase in circumference of joint during venous occlusion was recorded. After calibration, rate of increase in circumference and hence in volume was calculated, and a measure of the blood flow obtained. Note that treatment was followed after an initial difference by a return of blood flow to about the same level on both sides, presumably due to systemic absorption of intraarticular dose

Indirect confirmation of such vasomotor effects of cortisone-like steroids in the active lesions of rheumatoid arthritis in which there is a pathogenetic role for both antibodies and lymphocytes of the type that mediate tuberculous inflammation, is available in several forms. For instance, VADASZ (1971) found that intra-articular injection of methyl-prednisolone (80 mg) abolished differences between the blood flow through painfully active and contralateral quiescent knee joints (Fig. 10). A similar result was observed following injection of hydrocortisone (50 mg) by DICK et al. (1970) who estimated the blood flow before and after treatment of the affected knee by monitoring the rate of clearance of intra-articularly instilled [133]xenon.

c) Effect on the Transvascular Migration of Inflammatory Cells

Whether administered topically, orally or parenterally, cortisol-like steroids have a profound depressive effect upon extravascular accumulation of blood-borne non-lymphocytic inflammatory cells. For example, cortisol-like steroids have been shown

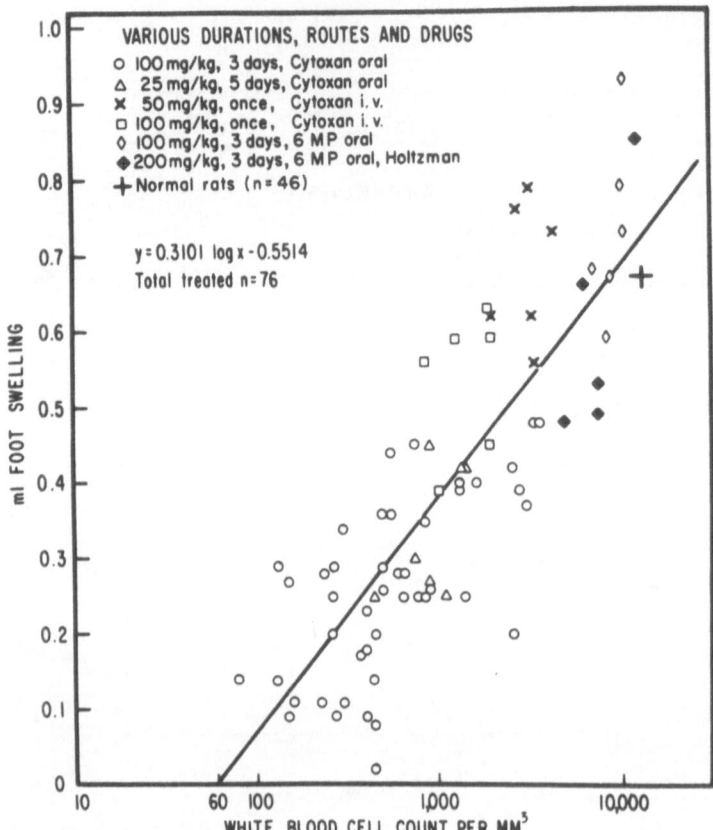

Fig. 11. Dependence of carrageenin-induced swelling of the rat's hind paw on total white blood cell counts (VAN ARMAN et al., 1971)

in vivo to inhibit the infiltration of PMN leucocytes during inflammation of different tissues including the skin (GERMUTH et al., 1951; GELL and HINDE, 1951, 1954) synovium (BERTINO et al., 1963; CHERNEY, 1971) cornea (LEIBOWITZ and KUPFERMAN, 1974; LEIBOWITZ et al., 1974) and lung (GLASER et al., 1951). They also inhibit in vitro migration of PMN leucocytes with various experimental models of chemotaxis (WARD, 1966, 1971). The accumulation of monocytic phagocytes is depressed more severely than that of PMN leucocytes (REBUCK and MELLINGER, 1953; JESSOP et al., 1973).

Inhibition of the extravascular migration of inflammatory cells is associated with significant alterations in their circulating levels. The effect differs, however, in respect of the two types of cells: the level of PMN leucocytes is elevated in most species as a result of steroid therapy (GERMUTH et al., 1951; BOGGS et al., 1964; BISHOP et al., 1968), whereas that of the monocytes is depressed (Chapter 3; YU et al., 1974). Depression of the extravascular accumulation and degranulation of PMN leucocytes can result in: (a) hypoalgesia and analgesia, (b) depression of inflammatory swelling (Fig. 11), (c) lowered incidence of haemorrhages (GERMUTH et al., 1951; GELL and

HINDE, 1954; COCHRANE and AIKEN, 1966), and (d) persistence of fibrin (RIDDLE et al., 1965; JASANI, 1975). Depression of the extravascular accumulation of monocytic phagocytes can result in reduction of the availability of prostaglandins (KANTRO-WITZ et al., 1975; GORDON and BRAY, 1976) and that should afford hypoalgesia or analgesia in patients with rheumatoid arthritis (Chap. 27). Its effect on inflammatory swelling may differ, however, depending upon a number of factors. For instance, in allergic inflammation characterised by a predominant role for thymus derived T-lymphocytes, in vivo depression of the availability of monocytes to the inflamed site could result in partial, if not complete, depression of lymphocyte-initiated inflammatory swelling. This is because monocyte-derived macrophages are essential for the in vitro formation of lymphokines by T- but not by thymus independent B-lymphocytes (WAHL et al., 1975). Secondly, if the dose employed proves to be insufficient for depression of lymphokine synthesis but sufficient for the depression of extravascular migration of monocytes, the swelling may persist, or even enlarge, as for example in rheumatoid arthritis, because of the persistence of fibrin and lymphatic blockage (see JASANI, 1975). Monocyte-derived macrophages are essential for phagocytosis and intracellular degradation of extravascularly deposited fibrin (RIDDLE et al., 1965; LEIBOVICH and ROSS, 1975).

Cortisol-like steroids can also depress the circulating level of lymphocytes in mice, rats and man (COHEN and CLAMAN, 1971; SPRY, 1972; YU et al., 1974); they depress the level of T-lymphocytes to a greater extent than that of B-lymphocytes. The oral dose of prednisolone required to depress lymphocytes to a level (32% of presteroid level) comparable with that of monocytes, was found to be about sixfold in a group of volunteers (see YU et al., 1974). The functional significance of changes in lymphocyte subpopulations in relation to the severity and duration of on-going lymphocyte-initiated inflammation remains to be clarified.

4. Relationship to Clinically Undesirable Effects

The major complications which may result from various pharmacological effects of cortisol-like steroids upom the microcirculation would appear to be (a) retardation of cutaneous wound healing and healing of mucosal ulcers, and (b) lowering of the host's resistance to infection.

a) Effect on Wound Healing

In a well-designed study of wound repair following multiple linear incisions in the dorsal skin of guinea pigs, LEIBOVICH and ROSS (1975) found that macrophages were the principal cell type responsible for wound debridement. Severe depression of circulating levels of monocytes using hydrocortisone (0.6 mg/g body weight, s.c.) when coupled with local injection of anti-macrophage serum around the wounds resulted in impaired clearance of fibrin, neutrophils, erythrocytes and other debris. There was also significant diminution of the collagen content and reduction of the number of fibroblasts. The morphometric abnormalities did not occur if hydrocortisone was administered alone, or if only the anti-macrophage serum was injected locally around the cutaneous wounds. However, when the anti-inflammatory steroid (prednisolone phosphate or acetate; 0.125% and 1% suspension) was instilled sub-conjunctivally, there is a significant effect on corneal inflammation (LEIBOWITZ and

KUPFERMAN, 1974). The remarkable effectiveness of topically applied steroid probably reflects the greater importance of the depression of transvascular migration rather than that of the circulating levels of phagocytes as a basis for depression of the inflammatory response, as well as for impairment of wound debridement and healing by anti-inflammatory steroids. Impairment of extravascular availability of PMN leucocytes was without discernible effect on cutaneous wound healing except in those instances where bacterial infection had intervened (LEIBOWICH and ROSS, 1975).

b) Effect on Healing of Ulcers

Ulceration implies loss of surface continuity. Anti-inflammatory steroids do not retard healing of cutaneous or mucosal, e.g. gastric, ulcers unless the wound involves loss of supporting connective tissue as, for example, in case of biopsy wounds (RAGAN et al., 1949a), or punched out, or excision gastric ulcers (SKORYNA et al., 1958; JANOWITZ et al., 1958). The effect on cutaneous wounds is dose-dependent when the steroid is administered parenterally (RAGAN et al., 1949b), but may be even greater when they are applied topically. Administration of anti-inflammatory steroids orally can therefore, be expected to aggravate gastrointestinal ulcers more than administration by the parenteral route.

Microscopic study of ulcerating wounds reveals that anti-inflammatory steroids retard formation of new vessels, proliferation of fibroblasts and deposition of collagen (RAGAN et al., 1949b; LEIBOWICH and ROSS, 1975). Recent observations of FROMER and KLINTWORTH (1975) indicate that the formation of new vessels in conjunctival ulcers may depend upon the availability of PMN rather than monocytic phagocytes, which raises the question whether the clinically undesirable effects of anti-inflammatory steroids on wound-healing are largely, if not exclusively, attributable to their effects on the transvascular migration and other effects on non-lymphocytic inflammatory cells.

c) Lowering of Host's Resistance to Infection

According to the evidence reviewed below, anti-inflammatory steroids can lower the host's resistance to microbial infection through: (a) reduction of the bactericidal and fungicidal potential of non-lymphocytic inflammatory cells such as the PMN and monocytic phagocytes; (b) interference with the development of systemic immunity, i.e. the aquisition of specifically sensitized lymphocytes that can synthesize and release antibodies or soluble lymphokine-like factors capable of promoting destruction of the micro-organisms; (c) interference with the expression of systemic immunity, e.g. by blockage of the effect of soluble lymphokine-like factors on monocyte-derived macrophages.

The bactericidal potential of PMN phagocytes may be impaired principally through depression of migration of such cells into the sites of microbial invasion (REBUCK and MELLINGER, 1953; GERMUTH, 1956; FRUHMAN, 1962; BOGGS et al., 1964). Circulating PMN leucocytes taken from subjects treated with prednisolone (ALLISON and ADCOCK, 1965) or methylprednisolone (WEBEL et al., 1974) exhibit normal phagocytic and bactericidal activity. Hydrocortisone succinate is, on the other hand, reported to impair the in vitro bactericidal activity of human PMN leucocytes when added directly to the medium. The concentration for the effect, however, has differed greatly, having been approximately 16 µg/ml in the study of RINEHART et al. (1974) and about 1200 µg/ml in that of MANDELL et al. (1970).

The bactericidal capacity of monocytic phagocytes may also be reduced through depression of migration of such cells into the inflammatory exudate. Direct evidence for in vivo inhibition of migration of monocytic phagocytes is provided by the study of JESSOP et al. (1973), whereas the in vitro inhibition of the chemotactic response to Ercherichia coli filtrate has been demonstrated by RINEHART et al. (1974). Impairment of monocytic function was definitely greater than that of PMN phagocytes in the study of JESSOP et al. (1973) as well as RINEHART et al. (1974). Additional observations of RINEHART et al. (1974) indicate that hydrocortisone succinate (16 µg/ml) can impair significantly the in vitro bactericidal (Staphylococeus aureus) as well as phagocytic activity of human monocytes. Impairment of phagocytic activity was demonstrable with the use of Cryptococeus neoformans but not with that of latex particles. The inhibition of in vitro chemotaxis, bactericidal and phagocytic activities was regarded to be due to some intracellular action of the steroid, which did not impair their viability, or modify their membrane characteristics.

In a further study involving removal of circulating leucocytes from healthy volunteers treated with prednisolone (50 mg every 12 h for 3 days), RINEHART et al. (1975) have demonstrated that steroid therapy, using doses as high as those employed for kidney transplant patients, can impair the fungicidal (Candida tropicalis) action of human monocytes. A metabolic basis was postulated for this effect as the same monocytes showed normal or increased chemotactic response, phagocytic rate of cryptococci and ultrastructural characteristics of normal phagocytic process. Evidence of normal chemotaxis, with monocytes isolated from steroid-treated subjects but not with monocytes to which the steroid is added in vitro (RINEHART et al., 1974), was taken to imply a need for the continuous presence of anti-inflammatory steroid for depression of chemotaxis. Interference with the development of systemic immunity implies failure of development of specifically sensitised lymphocytes capable of synthesising antibodies or soluble lymphokine-like factors that can promote destruction of the micro-organisms.

Convincing evidence in respect of a protective role for circulating specifically sensitized lymphocytes against infection due to the facultative intracellular parasite Listeria monocytogenes, has now been established by MCGREGOR and LOGIE (1974). Their experiments involved detection of the presence of protective cells in peritoneal exudates stimulated by intraperitoneal (i.p.) injection of L.monocytogenes into rats previously immunised to the microbe via the subcutaneous route (hind paws). The protective cells were specifically sensitized lymphocytes because: (a) as illustrated in Figure 12, they appeared in the peritoneal exudate soon after they could be detected in the thoracic lymph duct of the immunised animal; (b) their protective capacity paralleled the performance of cells removed from the thoracic duct (Fig. 12); and (c) they could not be detected amongst the residential phagocytic cells harvested from the peritoneal cavity of previously immunised animals without injection (i.p.) of L.monocytogenes.

Cortisone acetate (2.5 mg or more per animal) given to mice within 1 h of initiating infection with a standard dose of L.monocytogenes ($10^3 - 2 \times 10^3$ organisms, i.v.), inhibits completely the development of immunity as judged by unrestricted intracellular growth of the parasite in the liver and spleen and the eventual death of the host.

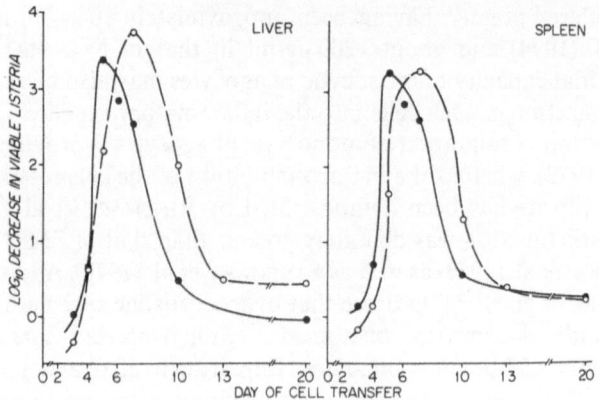

(MacKaness, 1970). Viewed in this light, the observations of North (1971) could imply that cortisone acetate inhibits either the development of specifically sensitized lymphocytes in the spleen of intravenously infected mice, or the activation and assembly of macrophages in the infective foci. Three observations tend to favour the possibility that cortisone acetate inhibits the activation and assembly of macrophages rather than the development of specifically sensitized lymphocytes. Firstly, North (1971) observed that a greater number of PMN leucocytes accumulated at the site of invasion of *L.monocytogenes*. This can be accounted for on the basis not only of drug-induced prolongation of the life-span of emigrated PMN leucocytes, but also of the fact that specifically sensitized lymphocytes release soluble factors chemotactic for PMN leucocytes (see Fig. 13a). Secondly, cortisol (10^{-5} M) can inhibit in vitro the aggregation of macrophages induced by interaction between specifically sensitised lymphocytes and tuberculoprotein, PPD (Weston et al., 1973a). Thirdly, in experiments involving the adoptive transfer of specifically sensitised lymphocytes from fully immunised to non-immune recipients, Weston et al. (1973b) have shown that lymph node lymphocytes taken from cortisol-treated donor guinea pigs (10 mg daily × 4, i.p.) elicit a 'normal' PPD-skin test in non-treated recipients but not in recipients which receive cortisol before (10 mg daily × 2, i.p.) and after (10 mg daily × 2, s.c.) the transfer. On the basis of these observations, Claman (1974) has postulated that cortisol blocks the response of macrophages to soluble factors released from sensitised lymphocytes.

The observations of Weston et al. are important in another respect, namely that they can explain the reactivation of healed tuberculous lesions in patients receiving high doses of cortisol-like steroids. They do not, however, rule out the possibility that cortisol-like steroids can also suppress the development of specifically sensitized lymphocytes. For this to occur, however, the anti-inflammatory steroids have to be administered 24–48 h before the initiation of infection of *L.monocytogenes* (see North, 1971).

Although detailed analysis of the effect of cortisol-like steroids on acquired antibody-dependent immunity against microbial infection are not available, studies of the effect of such steroids on antibody formation in response to injection of bacterial antigens (see Germuth, 1956) suggest that the increased susceptibility to acute infections with streptococci, pneumococci and many viruses may also be mainly due to steroid-induced interference with the defensive role of PMN and monocytic phagocytes, rather than with antibody production.

5. Pharmacological Implications

The data reviewed under Section E.IV support the possibility that the clinically beneficial effects of cortisol-like steroids may be the end result of an action which makes the microvascular network less responsive to chemical mediators released from non-lymphocytic as well as lymphocytic inflammatory cells. Apart from the observations of Sendelbeck and Yates (1970), a major weakness of the available evidence is that it is largely visual in character and so inevitably subject to an interpretative bias.

The harmful effects of therapeutic doses of cortisol-like steroids appear, on the other hand, to be mainly due to interference with the function of monocyte-derived macrophages. This realisation has two broad implications. Firstly, if physiological concentrations of cortisol-like steroids are adequate for a vaso-constrictive effect upon non-injured vessels, and if they are also adequate in the presence of adrenaline to restore vascular integrity following injury, why is it that allergic inflammation pursues a relentless course in patients who do not have adrenocortical insufficiency? Is it because allergic patients have adrenomedullary rather than adrenocortical insufficiency, or is it possible that the clinical inflammatory states are associated with greater degradation of adrenaline-like substances in a manner analogous to that reported for some experimentally induced states (SPECTOR and WILLOUGHBY, 1960)? The usefulness of both adrenaline and isoprenaline in allergic airways obstruction would tend to favour such an inference. Alternatively, is it possible that the involvement of antibodies and lymphocytes of the type which mediate cellular hypersensitivity results in end-organ failure, i.e. partial or complete loss of responsiveness of the terminal vascular bed through, for instance, destruction of receptors for cortisol-like steroids, or catecholamines, or both types of vasoactive hormones? Such destruction could result either from denudation of the endothelial cells (CHERNEY, 1971) or intracellular release of proteolytic lysosomal enzymes (COCHRANE and AIKIN, 1966), or both. The visual observations of BARCLAY and EBERT (1953) described above, lend considerable support to such a possibility. Quantitative support is provided by results described in Section F.

The second important question which arises is whether the ability of cortisol to interfere with the protective and homeostatic role of monocyte-derived macrophages in wound healing can be attenuated through chemical substitution without concomitant loss of the beneficial anti-inflammatory, anti-allergic and anti-rheumatic action of the naturally occurring steroid. In this context, the observations of FAUVE and PIERCE-CHASE (1967) are highly relevant as they show that 6α-methylprednisolone, 21 sodium hemisuccinate (s.c.), despite being a more potent anti-inflammatory steroid than hydrocortisone acetate (s.c.), differed from hydrocortisone acetate in failing to evoke progressive and fatal corynebacterial pseudotuberculosis in mice. Furthermore, like three other steroids which also lacked the ability to evoke fatal bacterial infection, 6α-methylprednisolone, 21 sodium hemisuccinate did not inhibit the in vitro spreading property of macrophages harvested from the peritoneum, even though all four steroids reduced by about 50% the number of cells recoverable in the peritoneal exudate of comparable non-treated controls. By contrast, the five steroids which provoked the fatal infection, inhibited grossly the in vitro spreading power of peritoneal macrophages.

F. Mode of Action in Homograft Reaction

Tissues transplanted from one individual (donor) to another (recipient) of the same species, i.e. homografts, elicit a lymphocyte-initiated inflammatory response which results in the necrosis of the donor cells and the eventual rejection of the homograft. The fate of autografts, i.e. the individual's own tissue transplanted back onto itself, differs from that of the homografts in that they undergo only a transient non-specific inflammatory reaction caused by the trauma of surgery before being incorporated into the surrounding tissue. Lymphocyte-initiated inflammation occurs only in the

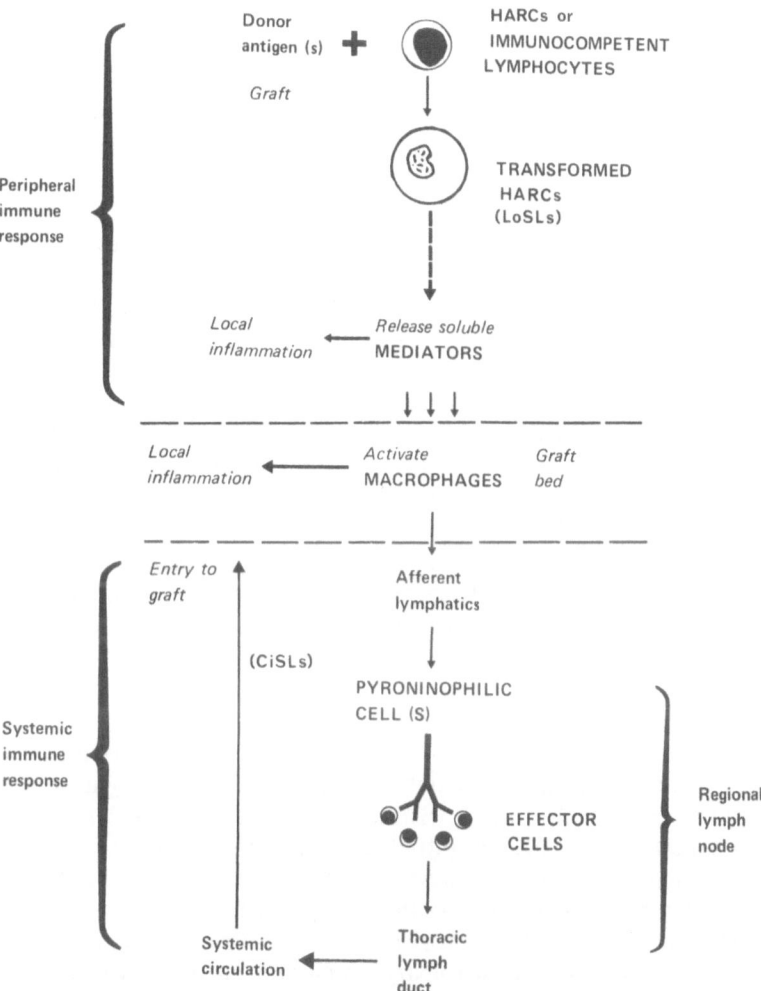

Fig. 13. A scheme to explain the origin of specifically sensitized lymphocytes. Based after MEDA-WAR (1963), GOWANS (1965) and WILSON (1974). HARCs denotes histo-incompatibility antigen recognition cells, LoSLs are locally sensitized lymphocytes, and CiSLs are circulating effector cells, i.e. specifically sensitized lymphocytes

homografts because their cellular constituents differ from those of the recipient. Such constituents are referred to as histo-incompatibility antigens.

Currently available evidence (see HALL, 1974; WILSON, 1974) suggests that lymphocytes may play a dual role during the response of an animal to skin homografts (GOWANS, 1965). As depicted in Figure 13, the circulating immunologically competent lymphocytes (MEDAWAR, 1963) or histo-incompatibility antigen recognition cells (HARCs) (WILSON, 1974) enter the graft via the blood vessels, react with the vascular antigen (WIENER et al., 1969) and undergo metabolic as well as morphological transformation: the transformed HARCs will be referred to as the locally sensitized lymphocytes (LoSLs). LoSLs synthesize and release soluble factors (lympho-kines, Chapter 10), some of which induce local inflammation in the graft itself, whereas others activate the macrophages in the graft bed. Beyond that stage, the antigenic stimulus is conveyed somehow (see HALL, 1974) to the regional lymph node where large pyroninophilic (PNP) cells appear (SCOTHORNE, 1957) and give rise to a new generation of cells which have come to be known as effector cells (WILSON, 1974). On reaching the systemic circulation via the thoracic lymph duct, the effector cells become widely distributed througout the body: these effector cells will be referred to as the circulating sensitized lymphocytes (CiSLs). Those CiSLs that enter the homograft become metabolically activated, and synthesise and release a new set of mediators (see Fig. 14), giving rise to a second wave of inflammation which can be distinguished outwardly from the first wave by the appearance of cyanosis in erst-while hyperaemic grafts. Cyanosis represents an important prelude to necrosis of the grafted donor cells. Figure 14 outlines also the pathophysiological basis for the development of cyanosis as well as the inflammatory swelling accompanying the rejection of homografts. The entire sequence of cellular and vascular events com-mencing from the time of transplantation to epidermal necrosis in the skin homo-graft may be conveniently referred to as the *homograft reaction* (MEDAWAR, 1958). Cortisol-like steroids have long been recognised to exert a profound effect on the homograft reaction in man as well as in a variety of animals (BILLINGHAM et al., 1951; SPARROW, 1954; MEDAWAR and SPARROW, 1956; WOODRUFF and LLAURADO, 1956; FRENKEL and HAVENHILL, 1963; MURRAY et al., 1968), although their mode of action remains largely ill-understood.

Information acquired newly in our laboratory using rabbit skin homografts is reported briefly in this chapter, not only because it sheds some light on this impor-tant area, but also because the experimental observations may prove relevant to future evaluation of more effective anti-allergic and anti-rheumatic drugs. Our exper-imental approach (BITTERLI and JASANI, 1972; JASANI, 1973b; JASANI et al., 1974) has differed from all previous studies on the homograft reaction in one important re-spect. It has involved quantitation of the inflammatory vascular changes in skin homografts in addition to the customary visual and histological assessment of the grafts. Visual assessment of rejection was based on the appearance of cyanosis ac-companying stagnation of blood flow through the homograft (TAYLOR and LEHR-FELD, 1953; EDGERTON et al., 1957; LEWIS et al., 1976). Histological assessment of rejection was based on recognition of epithelial cell necrosis using criteria defined by MEDAWAR (1944).

Skin dissected free of its neurovascular connections during transplantation un-dergoes post-operatively a transudative, exudative and proliferative phase (see RU-DOLPH and KLEIN, 1973) as in the case of *non-lymphocytic* inflammation found in the cotton pellet granuloma (SWINGLE and SHIDEMAN, 1972). Homografts of skin are no exception to this general rule. In fact, a comparison of the degree of inflammation in homografts with that in skin autografts transplanted simultaneously onto identical anatomical sites on the opposite leg of the same recipient reveals, as shown in Figure 15, that in the absence of infiltration of lymphocytes the increase in tissue weight of homografts due to the non-specific inflammatory reaction itself *equals* that of the autografts. In other words the balance, i.e. the gap between changes in the weight of auto- and comparable homografts, represents the swelling due to the

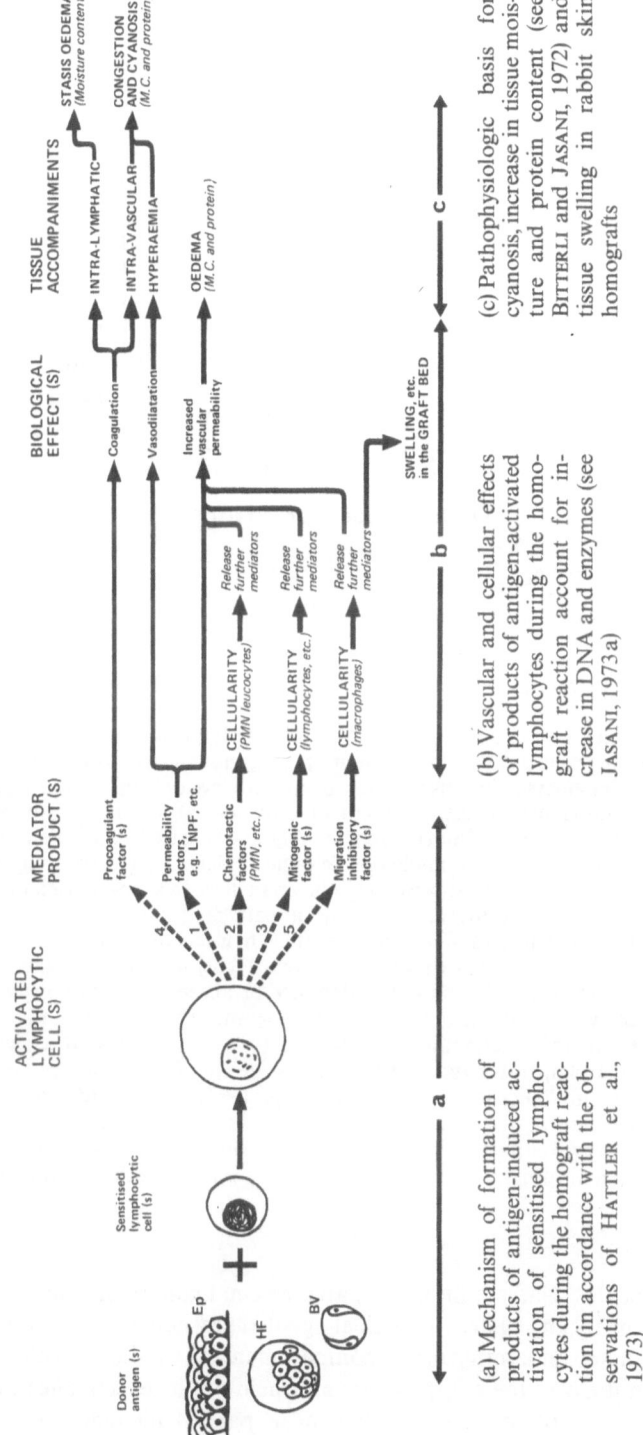

Fig. 14a—c. Vascular basis of cyanosis and tissue swelling due to antigen-induced activation of specifically sensitised lymphocytes (based on a scheme by JASANI, 1975, reproduced by permission from Current Management of R.A. Edited by PEARSON and CARSON DICK, 1975

(a) Mechanism of formation of products of antigen-induced activation of sensitised lymphocytes during the homograft reaction (in accordance with the observations of HATTLER et al., 1973)

(b) Vascular and cellular effects of products of antigen-activated lymphocytes during the homograft reaction account for increase in DNA and enzymes (see JASANI, 1973a)

(c) Pathophysiologic basis for cyanosis, increase in tissue moisture and protein content (see BITTERLI and JASANI, 1972) and tissue swelling in rabbit skin homografts

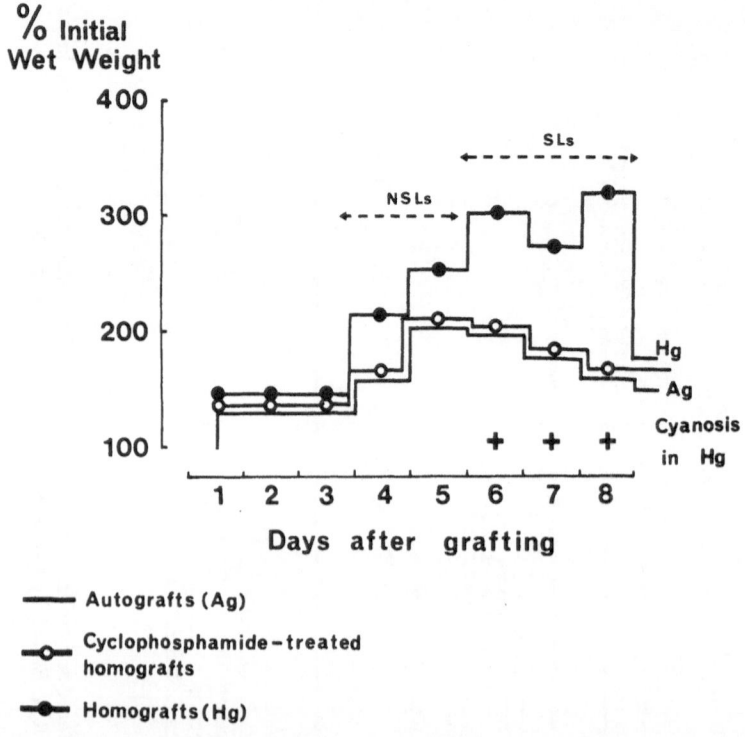

- —— Autografts (Ag)
- —o— Cyclophosphamide–treated homografts
- —●— Homografts (Hg)

Fig. 15. Degree of inflammation in homografts not containing lymphocytes. Results shown are mean per cent increase in tissue wet weight of autografts (*Ag*), homografts (*Hg*) and homografts (—o) not containing lymphocytes because of treatment with cyclophosphamide (750 mg per animal) as described previously (JASANI, 1973a, b). On day 0, with the animals fully anaesthetised using pentobarbitone sodium (i.v.) six homografts were transplanted on to right leg and an equal number of autografts were made on the opposite leg. Grafts were weighed before transplantation (initial wet weight). Postoperatively, the animals were anaesthetised daily, grafts inspected and from the first or third day onwards a pair of grafts belonging to similar anatomical sites in the opposite legs was removed at 24 h intervals until the end of each experiment. After removal each graft was weighed (final wet weight) and a biopsy taken to obtain histological evidence of presence of lymphocytes. Presence or absence of CiSLs in homografts based on appearance of cyanosis and necrosis in the homografts. The data show that although the tissue weight of homografts containing lymphocytes (—●—) increases to a significantly greater extent than that of comparable autografts; the tissue weight of homografts not containing lymphocytes (—o—) does not differ from that of the autografts. In other words, in the absence of lymphocytes, the increase in tissue weight of homografts soley due to the non-specific inflammatory reaction provoked by the trauma of surgery *equals* that of the autografts; and therefore, the gap between the weights of the two types of graft represents the swelling due to the presence of lymphocytes

presence of lymphocytes. Narrowing of the gap between changes in tissue weight of the two types of graft by any pharmacological agent represents effectiveness against the lymphocyte-initiated inflammatory accompaniment of the homograft reaction. The extent to which it closes the gap provides a measure of its effectiveness, the fully effective dose being capable of reducing the mean paired difference between the weight of the grafts to a value not statistically significantly greater than zero.

Depression of increase in tissue weight of autografts reflects the anti-inflammatory action of the drug and, in view of the results of Figure 15 *(vide supra)*, provides an indirect measure of the extent to which the steroid can depress the increase in tissue weight of homografts due to activity against the non-specific inflammatory component preceding the homograft reaction. The quantitative data summarised in Figures 16–19, if analysed as above, show that topical fluocinolone acetonide (FA; 6α, 9α-difluoro-16α-hydroxy-prednisolone 16,17-acetonide, see Table 3) can depress the inflammatory swelling accompanying the homograft reaction even though it does not interfere with (a) the emergence of LoSLs (Fig. 13), (b) the activation of CiSLs (Fig. 14a). The effect varies with the dose and is maximal only if the drug is applied before the emergence of LoSLs or the entry of CiSLs. FA is more effective against inflammation due to LoSLs than against that due to CiSLs. Although it allows the emergence of LoSLs, FA interferes with the development of CiSLs, presumably through an effect upon the intermediary role of macrophages.

I. Interference With the Development of Circulating Sensitized Lymphocytes

Data in Figure 16b show that the tissue swelling of homografts receiving topical FA (0.0025% wt/vol, 1 mg ointment per mg dry weight tissue transplanted) applied once daily from day 0, does not differ significantly from that of the corresponding autografts except on day 7, when the mean difference between the increase in the weights of the two types of graft is significantly greater than zero ($p < 0.05$).

Results of visual and histological observations shown in Figure 16 reveal that although FA does not delay significantly the accumulation of lymphocytes in the homografts, it suppresses not only the hyperaemia which accompanies their presence on day 5 in homografts of the control animals, but much more importantly also prevents the necrosis of grafted cells which occurs from day 6 onwards in the homografts of an increasing proportion of control animals. Failure of development of epithelial necrosis implies prolongation of survival of the grafted tissue (see BILLINGHAM et al., 1951). Since necrosis of the grafted cells depends, as in the case of host resistance against *L. monocytogenes* (McGREGOR and LOGIE, 1974), upon entry of CiSLs (COE et al., 1966; WEISS, 1968; DELORME et al., 1969; DENHAM et al., 1969), its failure in homografts receiving FA may be viewed as indicating that the drug interferes with the development of CiSLs.

1. Basis for the Effect. Topical FA could interfere with the development of CiSLs either at the level of the skin grafts themselves or in the regional lymph node (Fig. 13). SCOTHORNE (1957) has established clearly that cortisone acetate injected (s.c.) between the skin graft and regional lymph node does not prevent the appearance of PNP cells in the regional lymph node. Necrosis of the grafted cells occurred at the expected time in homografts borne by such animals. Therefore, it seems safe to conclude that the prevention of necrosis of the grafted cells by FA in the experiments of Figure 16 is in all likelihood the end result of an effect of the drug upon some cellular or vascular event in or intimately close to the graft itself.

Histological evidence of reduced though definite intravascular accumulation of mononuclear cells from day 5 onwards in the drug-treated homografts (Fig. 16) tends to exclude the possibility that FA prevented physical interaction between the histoin-

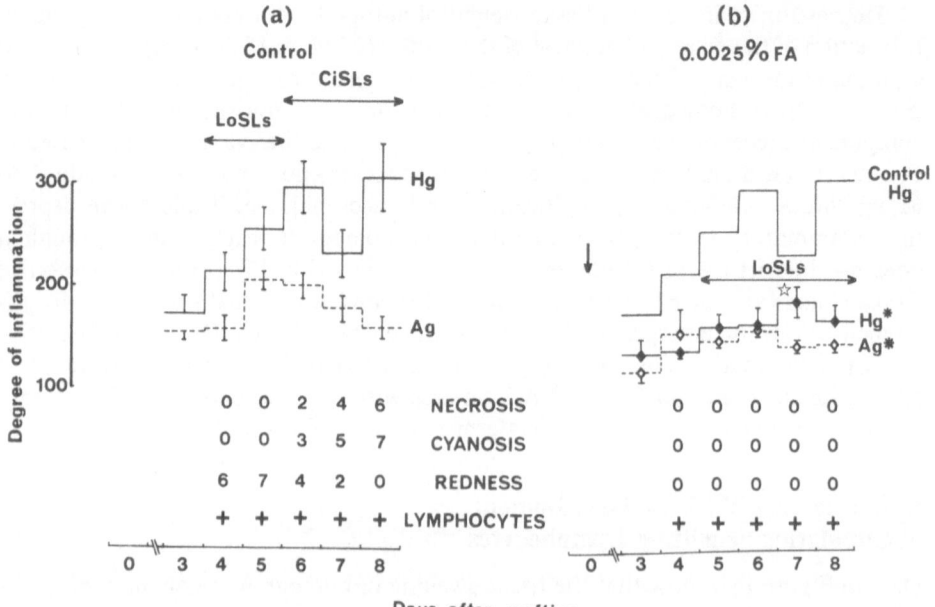

Days after grafting

Fig. 16. (a) Degree of inflammation in comparable auto- and homografts. Results shown are mean per cent increase in tissue wet weight ($\pm$ S.E.): Ag for autografts; Hg, for homografts of control group of 7 rabbits. Operative and other experimental details were as in the experiment of Figure 15; grafts were removed from day 3. The data show that the increase in tissue weight of the two types of graft, similar at first, began to differ from day 4 onwards in association with the presence of lymphocytes; that of the homografts increasing to a significantly greater extent than that of the autografts. LoSLs denote presence of locally sensitized and CiSLs that of circulating sensitized lymphocytes. Presence of CiSLs judged on basis of the appearance of cyanosis and necrosis in homograft

Fig. 16b. Effect of 0.0025% topical fluocinolone acetonide (FA) on inflammation in comparable auto- and homografts. Results shown are mean percent increase in tissue wet weight ($\pm$S.E.): autograft (Ag*) and homografts (Hg*) receiving FA and homografts (Hg) of control group shown in Figure 16a. Operative and other details were as in Figure 16a. Postopratively, grafts on each leg received topical FA on day 0 (1 mg ointment per mg dry weight tissue grafted) and 24 hourly thereafter until the end of each experiment. Results show that although lymphocytes were present in homografts of all drug-treated animals, redness was absent and this was associated with a complete loss of the gap between the two types of graft except on day 7. * $p < 0.05$ for mean paired difference being greater than zero indicates FA was less than fully effective

compatibility antigen recognition cells (HARCs) and the graft antigen. The occurrence of a significantly greater degree of swelling in day 7 homografts as compared with the corresponding drug-treated autografts (Fig. 16) militates against inhibition of antigen-induced synthesis and release of lymphokines by HARCs. That leaves interference with transmission of the antigenic stimulus from the graft to the regional lymph node (Fig. 13), e.g. through inhibition of the metabolic activation of macrophages in the graft bed, as the only other major explanation for the failure of development of CiSLs. The eventuality, although requiring direct proof in case of the homograft reaction, does not appear improbable from a pharmacological angle in view of the observations of (a) NORTH (1971) referred to earlier, and (b) WESTON et al.

(1973a), as well as BALOW and ROSENTHAL (1973) in respect of the effect of cortisol-like steroids (hydrocortisone sodium succin thisate and dexamethasone sodium phosphate; each 10 µg/ml in culline fluid) on macrophages during the interaction of guinea pig lymphocytes with the tuberculoprotein PPD.

II. Effectiveness Against Inflammation Due to Locally Sensitized Lymphocytes

Comparison of the results of control and drug-treated homografts shown in Figure 16b reveals that topical FA (0.0025%) applied once daily from day 0 depresses profoundly the increase in tissue weight of homografts during the non-lymphocytic (days 0–4), as well as the lymphocyte-initiated inflammatory phase (days 5–8) of the homograft reaction. However, as it fails to depress the increase in tissue weight of homografts containing lymphocytes to the same level as that of the comparable autografts, e.g. on day 7, it is judged to be highly active, though less than fully effective against inflammation due to LoSLs.

To distinguish more clearly the effectiveness of FA against inflammation due to LoSLs from that against the non-specific inflammatory component, application of the drug was witheld until the 4th post-operative day. This particular interval was chosen because by that time the blood flow is fully established through both types of skin graft (JASANI and LEWIS, 1971). It was hoped that this would allow intravascular accumulation of HARCs throughout the homograft before application of the first dose of FA, an expectation that was fulfilled as judged by histological examination.

Results of Figure 17a show that topical FA (0.0025%) applied once daily from day 4 is virtually ineffective against inflammation due to LoSLs in spite of the fact that, as judged by its effect on the autografts, it is capable of arresting the increase in tissue weight due to the non-specific inflammatory component. An equivalent amount of FA (0.025%), i.e. a tenfold higher concentration, applied once daily from day 4 is, however, highly active against inflammation due to LoSLs, as can be seen from the results of Figure 17b. Histological observations summarised in Figure 17 are noteworthy in that they show evidence of epithelial necrosis not only in homografts receiving 0.0025% FA but also in those of 2 out of 3 animals receiving the higher concentrations (0.025%) of the drug. Evidence of development of epithelial necrosis despite maximal depression of the increase in tissue weight of homografts receiving 0.025% FA raises the following interesting possibilities: (a) Postponement of topical application of the drug to day 4 permits the development of CiSLs, or (b) a sufficiently large number of LoSLs are capable of securing the necrosis of epithelial cells without the intervention of CiSLs. Commencement of topical treatment of homografts from day 4 instead of day 0 can permit the development of a sufficiently large number of LoSLs if it allowed a more widespread intravascular localisation of HARCs, or HARCs as well as monocytic phagocytes. The concomittant presence of monocytic phagocytes would appear to be essential for expression of the biological effects of LoSLs (CLINE and SVETT, 1968; WAHL et al., 1975). Whichever mechanism may eventually happen to account for the development of necrosis of epithelial cells, the data of Figure 17 leave little doubt as to the ability of FA to depress the inflammatory vascular accompaniments of the homograft reaction despite its failure to inhibit the necrotic effect of LoSLs.

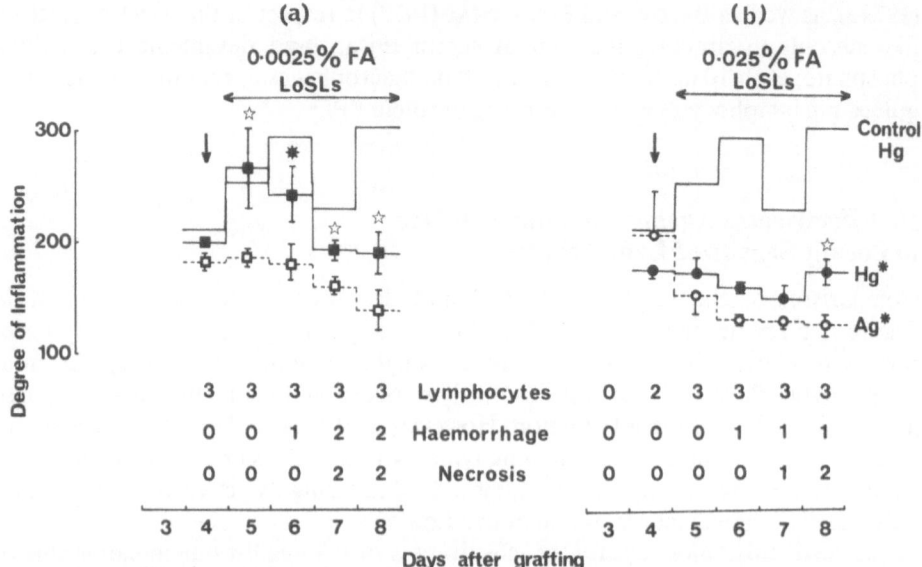

Fig. 17. Effect of FA on inflammation due to presence of locally sensitised lymphocytes (LoSLs) in rabbit skin homografts (Hg*/Ag*) experiments. Apart from application of the first dose of topical FA from day 4 instead of day 0 (see Fig. 16b), experimental and other details were as in Fig. 16b. Depression of the increase in weight of drug-treated homografts (Hg*) to levels as low as that of the corresponding autografts (Ag*) indicates that the steroid is fully effective against lymphocyte-initiated inflammation; whereas a statistically significant difference between the weights of the two types of graft indicates that the drug is less than fully effective, even if it lowers significantly the Hg* value in comparison with that of the placebo-treated control Hg (probability that mean difference between Hg* and Ag* is greater than zero, $\star P < 0.05$; $*P < 0.001$)

1. Basis for the Effect. The development of cyanosis implies that the steroid does not prevent local sensitization of HARCs, whereas the histological presence of epithelial necrosis indicates that the steroid fails to inhibit the synthesis and release of cytotoxic factors such as those reported by WILSON (1965a, b), WEISS (1968), LUNDGREN (1970) and BUTTERWORTH (1975).

An important clue into the physiological basis for the profound depression of inflammatory tissue swelling is provided by the prevention of hyperaemia (redness) by FA (see Fig. 16b). If that were to represent the end-result of the well-known multiple pharmacological effects which cortisol-like steroids exert on the microcirculation (see Sect. E.IV.2), can it be possible that FA depresses inflammation initiated by LoSLs through a metabolic effect which makes the blood vessels less responsive to soluble lymphokine-like factors released from LoSLs?

III. Effectiveness Against Inflammation Due to Circulating Sensitized Lymphocytes

Development of CiSLs in topically-treated animals can be secured through inclusion of a placebo-treated set of homografts on the opposite leg of each recipient rabbit (Hg*/Hg experiments; the asterisk denotes topical application of FA to one set). The

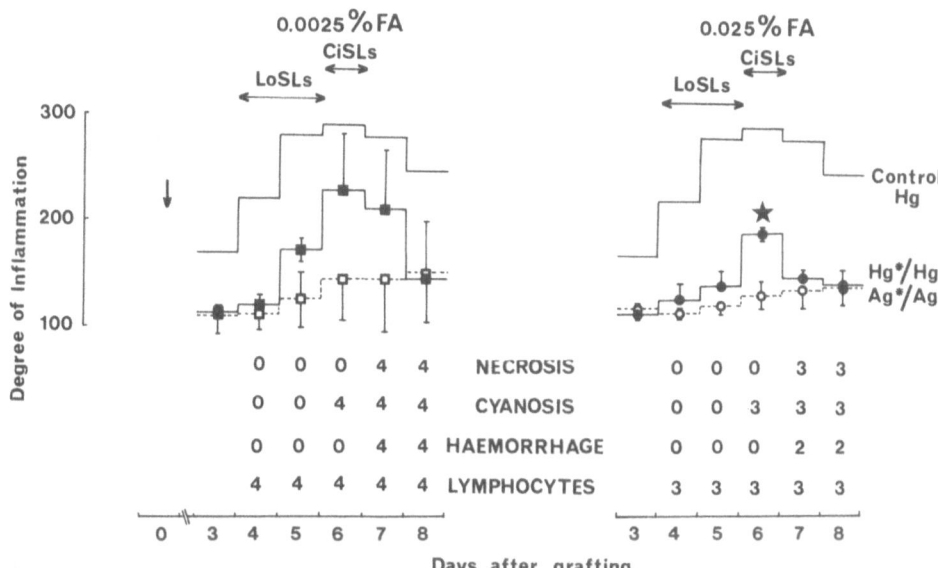

Fig. 18. Effect of FA on inflammation due to presence of circulating sensitized lymphocytes (CiSLs) in rabbit skin homografts (Hg*/Hg experiments). Apart from substitution of six contralateral autografts (Ag*) with six placebo-treated homografts (Hg), experimental and other details were as in Figure 16b. Depression of the increase in weight of drug-treated homografts (Hg*) to levels as low as that of comparable autografts (Ag*) of Ag*/Ag animals indicates that the steroid is fully effective against lymphocyte-initiated inflammation; whereas a statistically significant difference between the weights of the two types of graft indicates that the drug is less than fully effective, even if it lowers significantly the Hg* value in comparison with that of the placebo-treated control Hg. (Probability that the difference between mean percent increase in tissue weight of Hg* and Ag* is greater than zero is: *$P<0.01$

approach, employed originally by BILLINGHAM et al. (1951), is to be preferred to topical application of the steroid to homografts transplanted on to previously immunised animals as it allows re-establishment of blood flow through the skin homografts before onset of rejection due to entry of CiSLs (MEDAWAR, 1958).

The results of Figure 18a contrast sharply with those of Figure 16b; they show that when the animals are concomittantly immunised by inclusion of a placebo-treated set of homografts on the opposite leg, FA (0.0025%) cannot prevent the onset of cyanosis, even if applied from day 0 as in the experiment of Figure 16b, nor can it delay significantly the development of necrosis of the grafted cells as compared with the observations for the non-treated controls reported in Figure 16a. Further, although FA (0.0025%) depresses the inflammatory swelling in homografts, the results of Figure 18a differ from those of Figure 16b in that they show not only a widening of the gap between the weights of drug-treated homo- and autografts on day 7, but the appearance of an even larger gap between them on day 6, the day of onset of cyanosis. The observations suggest that the drug is less effective against the vascular effects of factors released from CiSLs than against those released from LoSLs.

Results of Figure 18b leave no doubt as to the fact that the steroid, if applied in an adequate dose, can depress significantly the inflammatory swelling despite being ineffective against both the onset of cyanosis and necrosis of the grafted cells induced

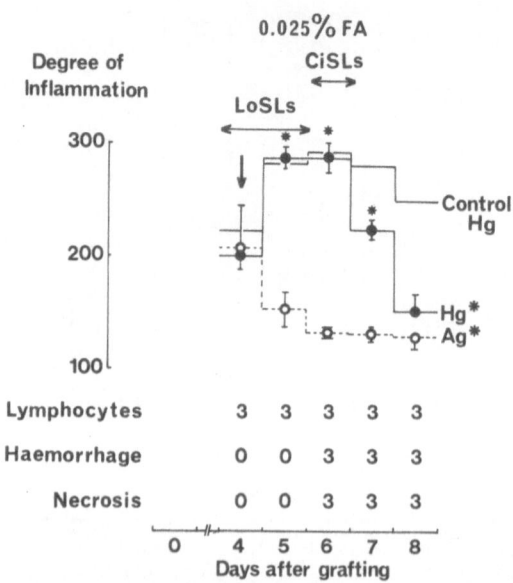

Fig. 19. Effect of FA on inflammation due to presence of circulating sensitized lymphocytes (CiSLs) in rabbit skin homografts (Hg*/Hg) experiments. Apart from application of the first dose of topical FA from day 4 instead of day 0 (see Figure 18), experimental and other details were as in Figure 18. Probability that the difference between the mean percent increase in tissue weight of Hg* and Ag* is greater than zero is: * $P<0.001$

by CiSLs. However, as even the higher dose is only partially effective against swelling due to CiSLs, whilst fully effective against that due to LoSLs, it has to be concluded that the drug is less effective against the vascular effects of factors released from CiSLs than against those released from LoSLs. This impression is further reinforced by results of treatment from day 4 shown in Figure 19.

Results of Figure 19 show that FA (0.025%) is ineffective against swelling of homografts of concomitantly immunised animals on days 5 and 6 but not after day 6 onwards. The data contrast sharply with results of Figure 17b which indicate that a similar concentration of FA applied in a similar manner from day 4 onwards was fully effective against swelling due to LoSLs until day 8.

1. Basis for the Effect. The fact that FA depresses the swelling of homografts of concomitantly immunised animals despite onset of cyanosis and even in spite of failure to protect the epithelial cells against necrosis, suggests that the steroid is effective against inflammation due to CiSLs through an action which makes the blood vessels less responsive to lymphokine-like factors released by such lympho-cytes. In other words, the basis for effectiveness of FA against inflammation due to CiSLs does not differ from that against inflammation due to LoSLs. If so, why is FA less effective against inflammation due to CiSLs than against that due to LoSLs, irrespective of whether the steroid is applied from day 0 or day 4?

A striking feature of the steroid-treated homografts of concomitantly immunised animals was the preponderance of PMN leucocytes in histological sections showing evidence of cellular necrosis. As the rabbit PMNs contain factors which can not only induce necrosis of homologous target cells (CLARK and KLEBANOFF, 1975), but also digest vascular basement proteins (CHOCHRANE and AIKIN, 1966), the question arises whether the lesser effectiveness of FA in the presence of CiSLs may be attributable to end-organ failure. Physical dislodgement and necrosis of endothelial cells in rabbit synovial vessels during immunologically induced arthritis has been attributed to PMN leucocytes by CHERNEY (1971). However, since anti-inflammatory steroids are known to prevent degranulation of rabbit, guinea pig and human PMNs (WRIGHT and MALAWISTA, 1973) in addition to the stabilisation of their lysosomes (IGNARRO, 1974), it does not seem reasonable at first sight to attribute the pathogenesis of end-organ failure in steroid-treated homografts to the prominent involvement of PMN leucocytes.

The situation looks quite different, however, when due account is taken of the fact that the experiments of WRIGHT and MALAWISTA (1973) and IGNARRO (1974) did not involve a role for CiSLs. Accepting the involvement of CiSLs in homografts of concomitantly immunised animals, the question arises whether the lymphokine-like factors released by such lymphocytes are responsible for the poor effectiveness of FA against both the chemotaxis of PMN leucocytes, as well as increase in tissue weight due to hyperaemia and exudation of fluid. As the effects of the steroid hormones can now be visualised via the involvement of the specific receptor proteins, an interesting explanation of the lesser effectiveness of FA against inflammation initiated by CiSLs may involve the stability of the hormone-receptor complex in the PMN leucocytes themselves, or in the endothelial cells, or both types of cell. Lymphokines released by CiSLs may promote the dissociation of such complexes.

Cells containing hormone-receptor complexes that dissociate rapidly must be bathed continuously in a high concentration of hormone if the response is to be maintained (O'MALLEY and SCHRADER, 1976). The protocol employed for the experiments of Figures 18 and 19 leaves considerable room for such a possibility as the steroid was applied only once every 24 h. The explanation fails, however, to account satisfactorily for the greater effectiveness of prophylactically applied dose (Fig. 18) as compared with the dose administered from day 4 onwards (Fig. 19).

As the magnitude of a cell's response to steroids appears to be related to the intracellular concentration of receptor proteins (O'MALLEY and SCHRADER, 1976), decreased effectiveness of FA applied from day 4 as compared with the dose applied from day 0 could imply a depressed level of receptors: either on account of proteolytic degradation, or through some other means. Prophylactically applied steroid may stabilise the hormone receptors of PMN leucocytes, endothelial cells, or both types of cell, against proteolytic degradation.

The fact that after day 6 the tissue weight of steroid-treated homografts returns rapidly towards that of comparable autografts, whereas the tissue weight of control homografts remains elevated, lends strong support to the suggestion that the ineffectiveness of the steroid in homografts of concomitantly immunised animals is limited to lymphokines released from CiSLs. The suggestion is strengthened by the striking similarity between the onset and duration of the biological response elicited by such cells in the experiments of Figure 19 with those of Figure 12.

IV. Clinical Relevance of Experimental Observations

These observations suggest that massive doses of orally or parenterally administered anti-inflammatory steroids to patients receiving organ homotransplants will not prevent the development of LoSLs, nor the necrosis of the grafted parenchymatous cells that such lymphocytes can induce through release of lymphokine-like factors. However, the steroid therapy would maintain the integrity of the microcirulation not only against factors released by LoSLs but even against those released by CiSLs.

Ability of anti-inflammatory steroids to maintain the integrity of the microcirculation against attack by both types of lymphocytes may account for the proven exclusive effectiveness of anti-inflammatory steroids against the clinical manifestations of acute rejection crises in patients with renal homotransplants. This property may also be expected to depress profoundly the transvascular migration of T-lymphocytes and as a consequence their dynamics in the circulation too, a physiological aspect which may facilitate interpretation of many immunological studies including, for example, those of TURSZ et al. (1976). The inability of anti-inflammatory steroids to prevent, on the other hand, the necrosis of parenchymatous elements may explain the disappointing clinical experience in respect of steroid therapy in patients with heart transplants.

Finally, interference by anti-inflammatory steroids with the vital intermediary role of macrophages in the expression of systemic immunity, the aspect which has received most attention in the past, might help to account for the deleterious rather than the beneficial effects of the steroids in patients with organ transplants. It may prevent expression of established immunity against: (a) microbial invasion, allowing opportunistic infections; (b) aberrant cell clones, allowing greater incidence of malignancy.

V. Relevance to Evaluation of More Effective Anti-Rejection and Anti-Rheumatic Drugs

The experimental observations strongly suggest that the priority for the type of pharmacological action desirable in a particular chemical configuration will vary according to the clinical condition for which it is to be used.

For instance, the existing anti-inflammatory steroids selected without exception on the basis of their effectiveness against non-lymphocytic inflammatory granulomata or constrictive potency in respect of non-injured vessels, have a low therapeutic value for patients with heart transplants for they cannot prevent necrosis of the myocardial muscle. Agents which can inhibit the synthesis and release of lymphokine-like factors from both LoSLs and CiSLs can, on the other hand, be expected to prove more worthwile for them.

Steroid drugs useful in heart transplant cases would prove ideal for patients with renal homotransplants for they could ensure the preservation of the secretory function in addition to that of the excretory role of the kidney. However, failing that, anti-inflammatory steroids devoid of interference with the role of macrophages in the expression of systemic immunity, and with or without greater effectiveness against vascular damage induced by lymphokine-activated PMN leucocytes, would prove to be quite acceptable. Steroid drugs of any of these three categories could also prove more effective and desirable than the existing cortisol-like drugs for patients with rheumatoid arthritis because: (a) the vascular changes underlying rheumatoid synovial inflammation bear a striking resemblance to those characteristic of the homograft reaction (TAYLOR and LEHRFELD, 1953; EDGERTON et al., 1957; KULKA, 1964); and (b) CiSLs as well as LoSLs have a role in rheumatoid arthritis (GLEN and JASANI, 1968; PEARSON et al., 1975; ISHIKAWA and ZIFF, 1976).

The mode of action of anti-inflammatory steroids in antibody-mediated inflammation has received less prominence in the present chapter because of lack of further progress since the previous review (JASANI, 1972). It may not prove to be different from that against inflammation due to CiSLs owing to the fact that substances released from PMN leucocytes constitute the final common pathway and the microcirculation is the common target in both types of inflammation.

G. Concluding Remarks

Cortisol-like steroids do not inhibit antigen-induced activation of either the immunologically competent or the specifically sensitized lymphocytes. No species difference exists in respect of this inability; the rabbit, which is normally regarded as being cortisol-sensitive, resembles man, who is generally considered to be cortisol-resistant.

Yet, cortisol-like steroids are specifically beneficial to inflammatory conditions, such as rheumatoid arthritis or allograft rejection, that involve a role for immunologically competent as well as specifically sensitized lymphocytes. The beneficial effect appears to be related to the ability of steroids to make vessels less responsive to the action of pharmacological mediators, lymphokines, that are formed and released after the antigen-induced activation of such lymphocytes. The effect is not species specific. The metabolic basis of this effect may prove to be similar to that underlying the potent vasoconstrictor effect of cortisol-like steroids on non-injured vessels.

The degree to which a constant amount of an anti-inflammatory steroid can depress inflammatory swelling differs considerably depending upon the nature of the cells initiating the inflammation. For example, the inflammatory reactions involving a role for PMN or monocyte-derived phagocytes only are depressed more profoundly than those which incorporate in addition a role for the immunologically competent lymphocytes. Inflammatory reactions due to antigen-induced activation LoSLs alone are depressed to a greater extent than those which involve in addition a role for CiSLs. This may explain the need for supraphysiological concentrations of cortisol for suppression of the clinical manifestations of rheumatoid arthritis and many allergic diseases.

The effectiveness of cortisol-like steroids varies also with the time of commencement of treatment: a fixed amount of the drugs being more effective if applied prophylactically, i.e. before the exposure of vessels to mediators released from the inflammatory cells. This property may reflect either the characteristic latent period essential for initiation of the metabolic effect of cortisol-like steroids or the harmful effect which the mediators of inflammation can exert against the cortisol-free cytoplasmic cortisol receptors.

The inability of currently available cortisol-like steroids to inhibit the antigen-induced formation and release of lymphokines, including especially those that are cytotoxic, may account for the relatively poor therapeutic usefulness of such drugs in patients with cardiac as compared with kidney allografts. The progressive deterioration of renal function may be largely explicable on a similar basis. The identity of the target cell in rheumatoid arthritis remains ill defined. However, if it were to turn out to be the chondrocytes, we might have a satisfactory explanation for the progressive erosion of articular cartilage despite the continued administration of adequate doses of cortisol-like steroids.

Cortisol-like steroids make the monocyte-derived macrophages unresponsive to the biological effects of lymphokines released from specifically sensitized lymphocytes. The metabolic effect depresses profoundly the auxiliary role of such macrophages in the immune response. The effect can prevent both the development and expression of systemic immunity, but it cannot prevent the emergence of LoSLs, at least in case of immunologically competent cells capable of recognising the histo-incompatibility antigens. This may explain why even the massive doses of cortisol-like steroids cannot abrogate the immune response to organ allotransplants.

The profound depression of the bone-marrow dynamics, circulating level and metabolic function of monocyte-derived macrophages by cortisol-like steroids may, however, be chiefly responsible for the harmful rather than the beneficial effects of the drugs. It may account not only for lowering of the host's resistance to microbial infection, but also for: (a) delayed wound healing, (b) ulcerogenesis, (c) re-activation of healed tuberculosis, and (d) failure to resist spread of tumours.

Since the deleterious effect of cortisol upon the auxiliary role of monocyte-derived macrophages in the immune response is not essential for effectiveness of the hormone against lymphocyte-initiated inflammation, it should be possible to attenuate it through skeletal and/or stereochemical changes in the parent molecule. If that could be achieved without loss of the beneficial effect of the hormone, cortisol-like steroids might well regain widespread therapeutic usefulness in the management of patients with allergic diseases.

Acknowledgements. The author is grateful to Miss Julie Benger, Miss Julie Knott, Mrs. Sharon Parker, R.R.Parsons, A.I.I.P., and M.F.Tweed for invaluable assistance in the preparation of bibliography, illustrations and the manuscript. He is also thankful to Dr. R.Wade for advice concerning the stereochemistry of anti-inflammatory steroids.

References

Agarwal, K.N., Garby, L.: Inhibition by corticosteroids of red cell lysis in vitro. Acta endocr. (Kbh.) **93**, Suppl., 3—27 (1964)

Allison, F., Jr., Adcock, M.H.: Failure of pretreatment with glucocorticoids to modify the phagocytic and bactericidal capacity of human leukocytes for encapsulated Type I pneumococcus. J. Bact. **89**, 1256—1261 (1965)

Amatruda, T.T., Jr., Hollingsworth, D.R., D'Esopo, N.D., Upton, G.V., Bondy, P.K.: Study of the mechanism of the steroid withdrawal syndrome. J. clin. Endocr. **20**, 339—354 (1960)

Arimura, A., Bowers, C.T., Schally, A.V., Saito, M., Miller, M.C.: III. Effect of corticotrophin-releasing factor, dexamethasone and actinomycin D on the release of ACTH from rat pituitaries in vivo and in vitro. Endocrinology **85**, 300—311 (1969)

Arth, G.E., Fried, J., Johnston, D.B.R., Hoff, D.R., Sarett, L.H., Silber, R.H., Storek, H.C., Winter, C.A.: 16-methylated steroids. II. 16-α-methyl analogs of cortisone, a new group of anti-inflammatory steroids. 9α-halo derivatives. J. Amer. chem. Soc. **80**, 3161—3163 (1958)

Ashton, N., Cook, C.: In vivo observations of the effects of cortisone upon the blood vessels in rabbit ear chambers. Brit. J. exp. Path. **33**, 445—450 (1952)

Ashton, N., Cook, C., Langham, M.E.: Effect of cortisone on vascularisation and opacification of cornea induced by alloxan. Brit. J. Ophthal. **35**, 718—724 (1951)

Aviado, D.M., Carillo, L.R.: Anti-asthmatic action of corticosteroids: a review of the literature on their mechanism of action. J. clin. Pharmacol. **10**, 3—11 (1970)

Baker, B.L., Adams, G.D.: The physiology of connective tissue. Ann. Rev. Physiol. **17**, 61—78 (1955)

Baker, B.L., Pek, S., Midgley, A.R., Jr., Gersten, B.E.: Identification of the corticotropin cell in rat hypophyses with peroxidase-labelled antibody. Anat. Rec. **166**, 557—567 (1970)

Ballard, P.L., Ballard, R.A.: Glucocorticoid receptors and role of glucocorticoids in foetal lung development. Proc. nat. Acad. Sci. (Wash.) **69**, 2668—2672 (1972)

Ballard,P.L., Baxter,J.D., Higgins,S.J., Rousseau,G.G., Tomkins,G.M.: General presence of glucocorticoid receptors in mammalian tissues. Endocrinology 94, 998—1002 (1974)

Balow,J.E., Rosenthal,A.S.: Glucocorticoid suppression of macrophage migration inhibitory factor. J. exp. Med. 137, 1031—1041 (1973)

Bangham,A.D.: The effect of cortisone on wound healing. Brit. J. exp. Path. 32, 77—84 (1951)

Banting,F.G., Gairns,S.: Suprarenal insufficiency. Amer. J. Physiol. 77, 100—107 (1926)

Barclay,W.R., Ebert,R.H.: The effect of cortisone on the vascular reactions to serum sickness and tuberculosis. Ann. N.Y. Acad. Sci. 56, 634—636 (1953)

Barger,A.C., Berlin,R.D., Tulenko,J.F.: Infusion of aldosterone, 9-α-fluorohydrocortisone and anti-diuretic hormone into the renal artery of normal and adrenalectomised, unanaesthetised dogs: effect on electrolyte and water excretion. Endocrinology 62, 804—815 (1958)

Baxter,J.D., Forsham,P.H.: Tissue effects of glucocorticoids. Amer. J. Med. 53, 573—589 (1972)

Baxter,J.D., Harris,A.W., Tomkins,G.M., Cohn,M.: Glucocorticoid receptors in lymphoma cells in culture: relationship to glucocorticoid killing activity. Science 171, 189—191 (1971)

Baxter,J.D., Tomkins,G.M.: The relationship between glucocorticoid binding and tyrosine aminotransferase induction in hepatoma tissue culture cells. Proc. nat. Acad. Sci. (Wash.) 65, 709—715 (1970)

Becker,M.J., Guttman,H.N.: Differential in vivo effects of dexamethasone on antibody and non-antibody protein synthesis in rabbit lymph nodes. Cell. Immunol. 5, 122—129 (1972)

Bennett,W.A.: Histopathologic alterations of adrenal and anterior pituitary in patients treated with cortisone. J. Bone Jt. Surg. 36 A, 867 (1954)

Berglund,K.: Studies on factors which condition the effect of cortisone on antibody production. I. The significance of time of hormone administration in primary haemolysis response. Acta path. microbiol. scand. 38, 311—328 (1956a)

Berglund,K.: Studies on factors which condition the effect of cortisone on antibody production. III. The significance of time of hormone administration in primary agglutinin response to S. typhi. H. Acta path. microbiol. scand. 38, 403—415 (1956b)

Berglund,K., Fagraeus,A.: A biological factor inhibiting the effect of cortisone on antibody formation. Nature (Lond.) 177, 233—234 (1956)

Bertino,J.R., Hollingsworth,J.W., Cashmore,A.R.: Granulocyte kinetics in rheumatoid effusions studied by a biochemical label. Trans. Ass. Amer. Phycns. 76, 63—67 (1963)

Billingham,R.E., Krohn,P.L., Medawar,P.B.: Effect of locally applied cortisone acetate on survival of skin homografts in rabbits. Brit. med. J. 11, 1049—1053 (1951)

Bilski,R., Godlewski,H.G.: Histochemistry of glycogen, phosphorylases, and UDPG-dehydrogenase in the epidermis of healing scald wound in guinea-pigs. Histochem. Epiderm. 3, 225—232 (1965)

Birge,C.A., Peake,G.T., Mariz,I.K., Daughaday,W.H.: Effects of cortisol and diethylstilbestrol on growth hormone release by rat pituitary in vitro. Proc. Soc. exp. Biol. (N.Y.) 126, 342—345 (1967)

Bishop,C.F., Athiens,J.W., Boggs,D.R., Warner,H.R., Cartwright,G.E., Wintrobe,M.M.: Leukokinetic studies. XIII. A non-steady-state kinetic evaluation of the mechanism of cortisone-induced granulocytosis. J. clin. Invest. 47, 249—260 (1968)

Bitterli,E., Jasani,M.K.: A quantitative assessment of tissue changes accompanying homograft reaction: changes in tissue dry weight, DNA and moisture content in rabbit skin homografts. Brit. J. Pharmacol. 45, 138—139 P (1972)

Bloom,B.R., Stoner,G., Fischetti,V., Nowakowski,M., Mushel,R., Rubenstein,A.: Products of activated lymphocytes (PALs) and the virus plaque assay. In: Brent,L., Holborow,J. (Eds.): Progress in Immunology, Vol. II, Ch. 3, pp. 133—144. Amsterdam: North-Holland 1974

Blunt,J.W., Jr., Plotz,C.M., Lattes,R., Howes,E.L., Meyer,K., Ragan,C.: Effect of cortisone on experimental fractures in the rabbit. Proc. Soc. exp. Biol. (N.Y.) 73, 678—681 (1950)

Boggs,D.R., Athiens,J.W., Cartwright,G.E., Wintrobe,M.M.: The effect of adrenal glucocorticosteroids upon the cellular composition of inflammatory exudates. Amer. J. Path. 44, 763—773 (1964)

Boström,H., Odeblad,E.: The influence of cortisone upon the sulphate exchange of chondroitin sulphuric acid. Ark. Kemi 6, 39—42 (1953)

Braverman,B., Davis,J.O.: Adrenal steroid secretion in the rabbit: sodium depletion, angiotensin II and ACTH. Amer. J. Physiol. 225, 1306—1310 (1973)

Bray,M.A., Gordon,D.: Effects of anti-inflammatory drugs on macrophage prostaglandin biosynthesis. Brit. J. Pharmacol. 57, 466 P. (1976)

Brown, F. K., Remington, J. W.: Arteriolar responsiveness in adrenal crisis in the dog. Amer. J. Physiol. **182**, 279—284 (1955)

Bullock, G. R., Carter, E. E., Elliott, P., Peters, R. F., Simpson, P., White, A. M.: Relative changes in the function of muscle ribosomes and mitochondria during the early phase of steroid-induced catabolism. Biochem. J. **127**, 881—892 (1972)

Bullock, G. R., Christian, R. A., Peters, R. F., White, A. M.: Rapid mitochondrial enlargement in muscle as a response to triamcinolone acetonide and its relationship to the ribosomal defect. Biochem. Pharmacol. **2**, 943—953 (1971)

Bush, I. E.: Species differences in adrenocortical secretion. Endocrinology **9**, 95—100 (1953)

Bush, I. E.: Chemical and biological factors in the activity of adrenocortical steroids. Pharmacol. Rev. **14**, 317—444 (1962)

Butterworth, A. E.: Non-specific cytotoxic effects of antigen-transformed lymphocytes. Cell. Immunol. **16**, 60—73 (1975)

Castor, C. W., Baker, B. L., Ingle, D. J., Li, C. H.: Effect of treatment with ACTH or cortisone on the anatomy of the brain. Proc. Soc. exp. Biol. (N.Y.) **76**, 353—357 (1951)

Chader, G. J., Meltzer, R., Silver, J.: A soluble receptor for corticoids in the neural retina of the chick embryo. Biochem. biophys. Res. Commun. **46**, 2026—2033 (1972)

Chaikof, L., Janke, W. H., Pesaros, P. C., Ponka, J. L., Brush, B. E.: Effects of prednisone and corticotropin on gastric secretion. Experiments in Heidenhain pouch dogs. Arch. Surg. (Chicago) **83**, 32—41 (1961)

Cherney, D. D.: Fine structure of the rabbit synovial membrane during an immunologically-induced arthritis treated with methylprednisolone acetate. J. submicrosc. Cytol. **3**, 217—229 (1971)

Chess, L., MacDermott, R. P., Sondel, P. M., Schlossman, S. F.: Isolation and characterisation of cells involved in human cellular hypersensitivity. In: Brent, L., Holborow, J. (Eds.): Progress in Immunology, Vol. II, pp. 125—132. Amsterdam: North-Holland 1974

Chytil, F., Toft, D.: Corticoid binding component in rat brain. J. Neurochem. **19**, 2877—2880 (1972)

Claman, H. N.: How corticosteroids work. J. Allergy clin. Immunol. **55**, 145—151 (1974)

Clark, I.: The effect of cortisone upon protein synthesis. J. biol. Chem. **200**, 69—76 (1953)

Clark, R. A., Klebanoff, S. J.: Neutrophil-mediated tumour cell cytotoxicity: role of the peroxidase system. J. exp. Med. **141**, 1442—1447 (1975)

Cline, M. J., Svett, V. C.: The interaction of human monocytes and lymphocytes. J. exp. Med. **128**, 1309—1325 (1968)

Cochrane, C. G., Aiken, B. S.: Polymorphonuclear leucocytes in immunological reactions. The destruction of vascular basement membrane in vivo and in vitro. J. exp. Med. **124**, 733—752 (1966)

Coe, J. E., Feldman, J. D., Sun Lee: Immunologic competance of thoracic duct cells. J. exp. Med. **123**, 267—281 (1966)

Cohen, J. J., Claman, H. N.: Hydrocortisone resistance of activated initiator cells in graft versus host reactions. Nature (Lond.) **229**, 274—275 (1971)

Crean, G. P.: The endocrine system and the stomach. Vitam. and Horm. **21**, 213—280 (1963)

Dale, H. H.: Conditions which are conducive to the production of shock by histamine. Brit. J. exp. Path. **1**, 103—107 (1920)

David, D. S., Grieco, M. H., Cushman, P., Jr.: Adrenal glucocorticoids after twenty years: a review of their clinically relevant consequences. J. chron. Dis. **22**, 637—711 (1970)

David-Nelson, M. A., Brodish, A.: Evidence for a diurnal rhythm of corticotrophin-releasing factor (CRF) in the hypothalamus. Endocrinology **85**, 861—866 (1969)

Delorme, E. J., Hodgett, J., Hall, J. G., Alexander, P.: The cellular immune response to primary sarcomata in rats. I. The significance of large basophilic cells in the thoracic duct lymph following antigenic challenge. Proc. roy. Soc. B **174**, 229—236 (1969)

Denham, S., Hall, w J. G., Wolf, A., Alexander, P.: The nature of the cytotoxic cells in lymph following primary antigenic challenge. Transplantation **7**, 194—203 (1969)

Desaulles, P., Schuler, W., Meier, R.: Inhibition of effects of cortisone on experimental granuloma of the rat. Helv. physiol. pharmacol. Acta **19**, C64—66 (1954)

Dick, C., Whaley, K., Stonge, R. A., Downie, W. W., Boyle, J. A., Nuki, G., Gillespie, F. C., Buchanan, W. W.: Clinical studies on inflammation in human knee joints: Xenon (^{133}Xe) clearances correlated with clinical assessment in various arthritides and studies on the effect of intra-articularly administered hydrocortisone in rheumatoid arthritis. Clin. Sci. **38**, 123—133 (1970)

Dingle, J. T. M., Page Thomas, D. P.: In vitro studies on human synovial membrane. A metabolic comparison of normal and rheumatoid tissue. Brit. J. exp. Path. 37, 318—323 (1956)

Dukor, P., Dietrich, F.: Characteristic features by immuno-suppression by steroids and cytotoxic drugs. Int. Arch. Allergy 34, 32—48 (1968)

Ebert, R. H., Wissler, R. W.: In vivo observations of the effects of cortisone on the vascular reaction to large doses of horse serum using the rabbit ear chamber technique. J. Lab. clin. Med. 38, 497—510 (1951)

Edelman, I. S., Fimognari, G. M.: On the biochemical mechanism of action of adolsterone. Recent Progr. Hormone Res. 24, 1—44 (1968)

Edgerton, M. T., Peterson, H. A., Edgerton, P. J.: The homograft rejection mechanism. A.M.A. Arch. Surg. 74, 238—243 (1957)

Eichhorn, J.: Failure of cortisol to reduced glucose uptake in granuloma tissue. Proc. Soc. exp. Biol. (N.Y.) 114, 429—432 (1963)

Eisenberg, E.: Effects of corticoids on bone. In: Pearson, O. H., Joplin, G. F. (Eds.): Dynamic Studies of Metabolic Bone Disease, pp. 119—125. Philadelphia: F. A. Davis Co, 1964

Engel, A. G.: Electron microscopic observations in thyrotoxic and corticosteroid induced myopathies. Proc. Mayo Clin. 41, 785—787 (1966)

Exton, J. H.: Gluconeogenesis. Metabolism 21, 945—990 (1972)

Exton, J. H., Harper, S. C.: Role of cyclic AMP and glucocorticoids in the activation of hepatic gluconeogenesis by diabetes. Fed. Proc. 31, 243—247 (1972)

Fagreus, A.: Role of ACTH and cortisone in resistance and immunity. Acta path. microbiol. scand. 93, Suppl., 20—28 (1952)

Fain, J. N.: Effect of dibutyryl 3',5'-AMP, theophylline and norepinephrine on lipolytic action of growth hormone and glucocorticoids in white fat cells. Endocrinology 82, 825—830 (1968)

Falude, G., Mills, L. C., Chayes, Z. W.: Effects of steroids on muscle. Acta endocr. (Kbh.) 45, 68—78 (1964)

Fauve, R. M., Pierce-Chase, C. H.: Comparative effects of corticosteroids on host resistance to infection in relation to chemical structure. J. exp. Med. 125, 807—821 (1967)

Feigelson, P., Yu, F.-L., Hanoune, J.: Effect of glucocorticoids on hepatic enzyme induction and purine nucleotide and RNA metabolism. In: Christy, N. P. (Ed.): The Human Adrenal Cortex, pp. 257. New York: Harper and Row 1971

Feldman, D.: The role of hormone receptor in the action of adrenal steroids. Ann. Rev. Med. 26, 83—90 (1975)

Feldman, D., Funder, J. W., Edelman, I. S.: Subcellular mechanisms in the action of adrenal steroids. Amer. J. Med. 53, 545—560 (1972)

Fimognari, G. M., Fanestil, D. D., Edelman, I. S.: Induction of RNA and protein synthesis in the action of aldosterone in the rat. Amer. J. Physiol. 213, 954—962 (1967)

Fleischer, N., Vale, W.: Inhibition of vasopressin-induced ACTH release from the pituitary by glucocorticoids in vitro. Endocrinology 83, 1232—1236 (1968)

Floman, Y., Floman, N., Zur, U.: Inhibition of prostaglandin E release by anti-inflammatory steroids. Prostaglandins 11, 591—594 (1976)

Foley, W. A., Glick, D.: Studies in histochemistry. LXVI. Histamine, mast, and parietal cells in stomachs of rats and effects of cortisone treatment. Gastroenterology 43, 425—529 (1962)

Fraser, C. G., Preuss, F. S., Bigford, W. D.: Adrenal atrophy and irreversible shock associated with cortisone therapy. J. Amer. med. Ass. 149, 1542—1543 (1952)

Frenkel, J. K., Havenhill, M. A.: The corticoid sensitivity of golden hamsters, rats and mice. Lab. Invest. 12, 1204—1220 (1963)

Fromer, C. H., Klintworth, G. K.: An evaluation of the role of leukocytes in the pathogenesis of experimentally induced corneal vascularisation. II. Studies on the effect of leukocyte elimination on corneal vascularisation. Amer. J. Path. 81, 531—540 (1975)

Fruhman, G. J.: Adrenal steroids and neutrophil mobilization. Blood 20, 355—363 (1962)

Funder, J. W., Feldman, D., Edelman, I. S.: Glucocorticoid receptors in rat kidney: the binding of tritiated-dexamethasone. Endocrinology 92, 1005—1013 (1973 a)

Funder, J. W., Feldman, D., Edelman, I. S.: The role of plasma binding and receptor specificity in the mineralocorticoid action of aldosterone. Endocrinology 92, 994—1004 (1973 b)

Ganong, W. F., Mulrow, P. J.: Rate of change in sodium and potassium after injection of aldosterone into the aorta and renal artery of the dog. Amer. J. Physiol. 195, 337—342 (1958)

Gass, G. H., Pfeiffer, C. J.: Hydrocortisone-acetylsalicyclic acid synergism in gastric ulcergenesis. Steroids 1, 63—75 (1963)

Gell, P. G. H., Hinde, I. T.: The histology of tuberculin reaction and its modification by cortisone. Brit. J. exp. Path. **32**, 516—529 (1951)

Gell, P. G. H., Hinde, I. T.: Observations on the histology of the Arthus reaction and its relation to other known types of skin hypersensitivity. Int. Arch. Allergy **5**, 23—46 (1954)

Gemzell, C. A., Van Dyke, D. C., Tobias, C. A., Evans, H. M.: Increase in formation and secretion of ACTH following adrenalectomy. Endocrinology **49**, 325—336 (1951)

Gerlach, J. L., McEwen, B. S.: Rat brain binds adrenal steroid hormone: radioautography of hippocampus with corticosterone. Science **175**, 1133—1136 (1972)

Germuth, F. G.: The role of adrenocortical steroids in infection, immunity and hypersensitivity. Pharmacol. Rev. **8**, 1—24 (1956)

Germuth, F. G., Jr., Nedzel, G. A., Ottinger, B., Oyama, J.: Anatomic and histologic changes in rabbits with experimental hypersensitivity treated with compound E and ACTH. Proc. Soc. exp. Biol. (N.Y.) **76**, 177—182 (1951)

Germuth, F. G., Jr., Ottinger, B.: Effect of 17-hydroxy-11-dehydrocorticosterone (Compound E) and of ACTH on Arthus reaction and antibody formation in the rabbit. Proc. Soc. exp. Biol. (N.Y.) **74**, 815—823 (1950)

Giannopoulos, G., Mulay, S., Solomon, S.: Cortisol receptor in rabbit foetal lung. Biochem. biophys. Res. Commun. **47**, 411—418 (1972)

Glaser, G. H., Kornfeld, D. S., Knight, R. P., Jr.: Intravenous hydrocortisone, corticotropin and the electroencephalogram. Arch. Neurol. Psychiat. (Chicago) **73**, 338—344 (1955)

Glaser, R. J., Berry, J. W., Loeb, L. H., Wood, W. B.: The effect of cortisone in streptococcal lymphadenitis and pneumonia. J. Lab. clin. Med. **38**, 363—373 (1951)

Glen, A. C. A., Jasani, M. K.: Lymphocyte DNA and RNA content in rheumatoid arthritis. Ann. rheum. Dis. **27**, 170—174 (1968)

Glenn, E. M., Miller, W. L., Schlagel, C. A.: Metabolic effects of adrenocortical steroids in vivo and in vitro: relationship to anti-inflammatory effects. Recent Progr. Hormone Res. **20**, 107—199 (1963)

Goetzl, E. J., Falchuk, K. H., Zeiger, L. S., Sullivan, A. L., Hebert, C. L., Adams, J. P., Decker, J. L.: A physiological approach to the assessment of disease activity in rheumatoid arthritis. J. clin. Invest. **50**, 1167—1180 (1971)

Goldstein, E., Rambo, O. N.: Cryptococcal infection following steroid therapy. Ann. intern. Med. **56**, 114—120 (1962)

Gonzalez-Luque, A., L'Age, M., Dhariwal, A. P. S., Yates, F. G.: Stimulation of corticotrophin release by corticotrophin-releasing factor (CRF) or by vasopressin following intrapituitary infusions in unaesthetised dogs: inhibition of the responses by dexamethasone. Endocrinology **86**, 1134—1142 (1970)

Good, T. A., Benton, J. W., Kelley, V. C.: Symptomatology resulting from withdrawal of steroid hormone therapy. Arthr. Rheum. **2**, 299—303 (1959)

Goodman, H. M., Knobil, E.: Some endocrine factors in regulation of fatty acid mobilisation during fasting. Amer. J. Physiol. **201**, 1—3 (1961)

Goth, A., Allman, R. M., Merritt, B. C., Holman, J.: Effect of cortisone on histamine liberation induced by Tween in the dog. Proc. Soc. exp. Biol. (N.Y.) **78**, 848—852 (1951)

Gowans, J. L.: The role of lymphocytes in the destruction of homografts. Brit. med. Bull. **21**, 106—110 (1965)

Grant, J. K.: Action of steroid hormones at cellular and molecular levels. Essays Biochem. **5**, 1—58 (1969)

Greeson, J. P., Levan, N. E., Freedman, R. I., Wong, W. H.: Corticosteroid-induced vasoconstriction studied by xenon^{-133} clearance. J. invest. Derm. **61**, 242—244 (1973)

Gryglewski, R. J., Panczenko, B., Korbut, R., Grodzinska, L., Ocetkiewicz, A.: Corticosteroids inhibit prostaglandin release from perfused mesenteric blood vessels of rabbit and from perfused lungs of sensitized guinea pig. Prostaglandins **10**, 343—355 (1975)

Hackney, J. F., Gross, S. R., Aronow, L., Pratt, W. B.: Specific glucocorticoid binding macromolecules from mouse fibroblasts growing in vitro. Molec. Pharmacol. **6**, 500—512 (1970)

Hall, J. G.: Observations on the migration and localisation of lymphoid cells. In: Brent, L., Holborow, J. (Eds.): Progress in Immunology, Vol. II, pp. 15—24. Amsterdam: North-Holland 1974

Hattler, B. G., Rocklin, R. E., Jr., Ward, P. A., Rickles, F. R.: Functional features of lymphocytes recovered from a human renal allograft. Cell. Immunol. **9**, 289—296 (1973)

Hench, P. S.: The protean manifestations of chronic infectious arthritis (with a note on treatment). Med. Clin. N. Amer. **8**, 1295—1304 (1925)

Hench, P. S.: The reversibility of certain rheumatic and non-rheumatic conditions by the use of cortisone or of the pituitary adrenocorticotrophic hormone. Ann. intern. Med. **36**, 1—72 (1952)

Hench, P. S., Kendall, E. C., Slocumb, C. H., Polley, H. F.: The effect of a hormone of the adrenal cortex (17-hydroxy-11-dehydrocortisone: Compound E) and of pituitary adreno-corticotrophic hormone on rheumatoid arthritis. Preliminary report. Proc. Mayo Clin. **24**, 181—197 (1949)

Hench, P. S., Slocumb, C. H., Polley, H. F., Kendall, E. C.: Effect of cortisone and pituitary adreno-corticotrophic hormone (ACTH) on rheumatic diseases. J. Amer. med. Ass. **144**, 1327—1335 (1950)

Hendler, E. O., Torretti, J., Kupor, L., Epstein, F. H.: Effects of adrenalectomy and hormone replacement on Na-K-ATPase in renal tissue. Amer. J. Physiol. **222**, 754—760 (1972)

Henneman, P. H., Wang, D. M. K., Irwin, J. W., Burrage, W. S.: Syndrome following abrupt cessation of prolonged cortisone therapy. J. Amer. med. Ass. **158**, 384—386 (1955)

Hiroshige, T., Sakakura, M., Itoh, S.: Diurnal variation of corticotropin-releasing activity in the rat hypothalamus. Endocr. jap. **16**, 465—469 (1969 b)

Hiroshige, T., Sato, T., Ohta, R., Itoh, S.: Increase of corticotropin-releasing activity in the rat hypothalamus following noxious stimuli. Jap. J. Physiol. **19**, 866—875 (1969 a)

Hong, S. L., Levine, L.: Inhibition of arachidonic acid release from cells as the biochemical action of anti-inflammatory steroids. Proc. nat. Acad. Sci. (Wash.) **73**, 1730—1734 (1976)

Howard, E.: Effects of corticosterone and food restriction on growth and on DNA, RNA and cholesterol contents of the brain and liver in infact mice. J. Neurochem. **12**, 181—191 (1965)

Humphrey, J. H.: The effect of cortisone upon some experimental hypersensitivity reactions. Brit. J. exp. Path. **32**, 274—283 (1951)

Ignarro, L. J.: Regulation of lysosomal enzyme secretion: role in inflammation. Agents Actions **4**, 241—258 (1974)

Ignarro, L. J., Colombo, C.: Enzyme release from guinea pig polymorphonuclear leucocyte lysosomes inhibited in vitro by anti-inflammatory drugs. Nature (Lond.) **239**, 155—157 (1972)

Ishii, D. N., Pratt, W. B., Aronow, L.: Steady-state level of the specific glucocorticoid binding component in mouse fibroblasts. Biochemistry **11**, 3896—3904 (1972)

Ishikawa, H., Ziff, M.: Electron microscopic observations of immunoreactive cells in the rheumatoid synovial membrane. Arthr. Rheum. **19**, 1—14 (1976)

Janoski, A. H., Shaver, J. C., Christy, N. P., Rosner, W.: On the pharmacologic actions of 21-carbon hormonal steroids (glucocorticoids) of the adrenal cortex in mammals. In: Deane, H. W., Rubin, B. L. (Eds.): The Adrenocortical Hormones, Vol. XIV, pp. 256—339. Handbook of Experimental Pharmacology. Berlin-Heidelberg-New York: Springer 1968

Janowitz, H. B., Weinstein, V. A., Shaer, R. G., Cereghini, J. F., Hollander, F.: Effect of cortisone and corticotropin on healing of gastric ulcer: experimental study. Gastroenterology **34**, 11—20 (1958)

Jasani, M. K.: Possible modes of action of ACTH and glucocorticoids in allergic diseases. Clin. Allergy **2**, 1—41 (1972)

Jasani, M. K.: The usefulness of enzyme measurements for evaluation of pharmacological agents which modify the homograft reaction. Biochem. Soc. Trans. **1**, 1043—1048 (1973 a)

Jasani, M. K.: A new approach for studying the influence of cyclophosphamide upon the rejection of rabbit skin homografts. Brit. J. Pharmacol. **48**, 334 P (1973 b)

Jasani, M. K.: The importance of ACTH and glucocorticoids in rheumatoid arthritis. Clin. rheum. Dis. **1**, 335—365 (1975)

Jasani, M. K., Boyle, J. A., Greig, W. R., Dalakos, T. G., Browning, M. C. K., Thomson, A., Buchanan, W. W.: Corticosteroid-induced suppression of the hypothalamo-pituitary-adrenal axis: observations on patients given oral corticosteroids for rheumatoid arthritis. Quart. J. Med. **143**, 261—276 (1967)

Jasani, M. K., Freeman, P. A., Boyle, J. A., Reid, A. M., Diver, M. J., Buchanan, W. W.: Studies of the rise in plasma 11-hydroxycorticosteroids (11-OHCS) in corticosteroid-treated patients with rheumatoid arthritis during surgery: correlations with the functional integrity of the hypothalamo-pituitary-adrenal axis. Quart. J. Med. **147**, 407—421 (1968)

Jasani, M. K., Lewis, G. P.: Lymph flow and changes in intracellular enzymes during rejection of rabbit skin homografts. J. Physiol. (Lond.) 219, 525—554 (1971)

Jasani, M. K., Parsons, R., Roberts, J., Tweed, M. F.: The usefulness of homologous pairs of rabbit skin grafts for studying the pharmacology of anti-rheumatic agents. Brit. J. Pharmacol. 51, 152 P (1974)

Jessop, J. D., Vernon-Roberts, B., Harris, J.: Effects of gold salts and prednisolone on inflammatory cells. I. Phagocytic activity of macrophages and polymorphs in inflammatory exudates studied by a 'skin-window' technique in rheumatoid and control patients. Ann. rheum. Dis. 32, 294—300 (1973)

Kalz, F., Scott, A.: Inhibition of Grenz Ray erythema by one single topical hormone application. J. invest. Derm. 26, 165—168 (1956)

Kantrowitz, F., Robinson, D. R., McGuire, M. B., Levine, L.: Corticosteroids inhibit prostaglandin production by rheumatoid synovia. Nature (Lond.) 258, 737—739 (1975)

Kaplan, D., Fisher, B.: The effect of methylprednisolone on mucopolysaccharides of rabbit vitreous humor and costal cartilage. Biochim. biophys. Acta 83, 102—112 (1964)

Kappas, A., Palmer, R. H.: Selected aspects of steroid pharmacology. Pharmacol. Rev. 15, 123—167 (1963)

Kellaway, C. H., Cowell, S. J.: On the concentration of the blood and the effects of histamine in adrenal insufficiency. J. Physiol. (Lond.) 55, 82—87 (1923)

Kendall, E. C., Masson, J. L., McKenzie, B. F., Myres, C. S.: Isolation in crystalline form of hormone essential to life from suppressed cortex: its chemical nature and physiologic properties. Trans. Ass. Amer. Phycus 49, 147—152 (1934)

Kidson, C.: Kinetics of cortisol action on RNA synthesis. Biochem. biophys. Res. Commun. 21, 283—289 (1965)

Kidson, C.: Cortisol in the regulation of RNA and protein synthesis. Nature (Lond.) 213, 779—782 (1967)

Kilby, R. A., Bennett, W. A., Sprague, R. A.: Anterior pituitary glands in patients treated with cortisone and corticotropin. Amer. J. Path. 33, 155—173 (1957)

Kimberg, D. V., Loeb, J. N.: Differential sensitivity of nuclear and mitochondrial DNA synthesis to suppression by cortisone treatment. Biochim. biophys. Acta 246, 412—420 (1971)

Kirkpatrick, A. F., Milholland, R. J., Rosen, F.: Stereospecific glucocorticoid binding to subcellular fractions of sensitive and resistant lympho-sarcoma P 1798. Nature (New Biol.) 232, 216—218 (1971)

Koob, T. J., Jeffrey, J. J., Eisen, A. Z.: Regulation of human skin collagenase activity by hydrocortisone and dexamethasone in organ culture. Biochem. biophys. Res. Commun. 61, (3) 1083—1088 (1974)

Kowalewski, K.: Effects of steroids on bone formation. In: Gross, F. (Ed.): Protein Metabolism, pp. 238—262. Berlin-Göttingen-Heidelberg: Springer 1962

Kulka, J. P.: Microcirculatory impairmental factor in inflammatory tissue damage. Ann. N.Y. Acad. Sci. (Wash.) 116, 1018—1044 (1964)

Landon, E. J., Forte, L. R.: Cellular mechanisms in renal pharmacology. Ann. Rev. Pharmacol. 11, 171—188 (1971)

Leibowitz, H. M., Kupferman, A.: Anti-inflammatory effectiveness in the cornea of topically administered prednisolone. Invest. Ophthal. 13, 757—763 (1974)

Leibowitz, H. M., Lass, J. H., Kupferman, A.: Quantitation of inflammation in the cornea. Arch. Ophthal. (Chicago) 92, 427—430 (1974)

Leibovich, S. J., Ross, R.: The role of the macrophage in wound repair: A study with hydrocortisone and anti-macrophage serum. Amer. J. Path. 78, 71—100 (1975)

Leung, K., Munck, A.: Peripheral actions of glucocorticoids. Ann. Rev. Physiol. 37, 245—262 (1975)

Levinson, B. B., Baxter, J. D., Rousseau, G. G., Tomkins, G. M.: Cellular site of glucocorticoid-receptor complex formation. Science 175, 189—190 (1972)

Lewis, G. P., Peck, M. J., Williams, T. J., Young, B. A.: Measurement of blood flow in rabbit skin homografts and autografts using a ^{133}Xe clearance technique. J. Physiol. (Lond.) 254, 32—33 (1976)

Lewis, G. P., Piper, P. J.: Inhibition of release of prostaglandins as an explanation of some of the actions of anti-inflammatory corticosteroids. Nature (Lond.) 254, 308—311 (1975)

Liddle, G. W.: Effects of anti-inflammatory steroids on electrolyte metabolism. Ann. N.Y. Acad. Sci. 82, 854—867 (1959)

Liddle, G. W.: Clinical pharmacology of the anti-inflammatory steroids. Clin. Pharmacol. Ther. **2**, 615—635 (1961)

Lobitz, W. C., Brophy, D., Larner, A. E., Ore, P., Daniels, F.: Glycogen response in human epidermal basal cells. Arch. Derm. **86**, 207—211 (1962)

Locker, W. de, Reddy, W. J.: Effect of hydrocortisone on the incorporation of glycine-U-C^{14}. Fed. Proc. **21**, 187 (1962)

Lundgren, G.: In vitro cytotoxicity by human lymphocytes from individuals immunized against histocompatibility antigens. Clin. exp. Immunol. **6**, 661—670 (1970)

McEwen, B. S., Palpinger, L.: Association of ^{3}H corticosterone-1,2 with macromolecules extracted from brain cell nuclei. Nature (Lond.) **226**, 263—265 (1970)

McEwen, B. S., Wallach, G.: Corticosterone binding to hippocampus: nuclear and cytosol binding in vitro. Brain Res. **57**, 373—386 (1973)

McEwen, B. S., Weiss, J. M., Schwartz, L. S.: Retention of corticosterone by cell nuclei from brain regions of adrenalectomised rats. Brain Res. **17**, 471—482 (1970)

McGregor, D. D., Logie, P. S.: The mediator of cellular immunity. VIII. Localisation of sensitised lymphocytes in inflammatory exudates. J. exp. Med. **139**, 1415—1430 (1974)

McGregor, D. D., Logie, P. S.: The mediator of cellular immunity. VIII. Effect of mitomycin C on specifically sensitised lymphocytes. Cell. Immunol. **15**, 69—81 (1975)

MacKaness, G. B.: The influence of immunologically committed lymphoid cells on macrophage activity in vivo. J. exp. Med. **129**, 973—992 (1969)

MacKaness, G. B.: The monocyte in cellular immunity. Semin. Haematol. **7**, 172—184 (1970)

McKenzie, A. W.: Percutaneous absorption of steroids. Arch. Derm. **86**, 611—614 (1962)

McKenzie, A. W., Stoughton, R. B.: Method for comparing percutaneous absorption of steroids. Arch. Derm. **86**, 608—610 (1962)

Makman, M. H., Nakagawa, S., White, A.: Studies on the mode of action of adrenal steroids on lymphocytes. Recent Progr. Hormone Res. **23**, 195—227 (1967)

Manchester, K. L., Randle, P. J., Young, F. G.: The effect of growth hormone and of cortisol on the response of isolated rat diaphragm to the stimulating effect of insulin on glucose uptake and on incorporation of amino acids in protein. J. Endocr. **18**, 395—408 (1959)

Mandell, G. L., Rubin, W., Hook, E. W.: The effect of an NADH oxidase inhibitor (hydrocortisone) on polymorphonuclear leucocyte bactericidal activity. J. clin. Invest. **49**, 1381—1388 (1970)

Mayer, M., Kaiser, N., Milholland, J., Rosen, F.: The binding of dexamethasone and triamcinolone acetonide to glucocorticoid receptors in rat skeletal muscle. J. biol. Chem. **249**, 5236—5240 (1974)

Mayer, M., Kaiser, N., Milholland, R. J., Rosen, F.: Cortisol binding in rat skeletal muscle. J. biol. Chem. **250**, 1207—1211 (1975)

Meador, R. S.: Development of pulmonary tuberculosis during adrenal steroid therapy. Postgrad. Med. **31**, 178—182 (1962)

Medawar, P. B.: The behaviour and fate of skin autografts and skin homografts in rabbits. J. Anat. **78**, 176—199 (1944)

Medawar, P. B.: The homograft reaction. Proc. roy. Soc. B **149**, 145—166 (1958)

Medawar, P. B.: Introduction: definition of the immunologically competent cell. In: Wolstenholme, G. E. W., Knight, J. (Eds.): The Immunologically Competent Cell, pp. 1—4. London: Churchill 1963

Medawar, P. B., Sparrow, E. M.: The effect of adrenocortical hormones, adrenocorticotrophic hormone and pregnancy on skin transplantation immunity in mice. J. Endocr. **14**, 240—256 (1956)

Meier, R., Schuler, W., Desaulles, P.: Zur Frage des Mechanismus der Hemmung des Bindegewebswachstums durch Cortisone. Experientia (Basel) **6**, 469—471 (1950)

Morita, Y., Munck, A.: Effect of glucocorticoids in vivo and in vitro on net glucose uptake and amino acid incorporation by rat thymus cells. Biochim. biophys. Acta **93**, 150—157 (1964)

Morris, D. J., Berek, J. S., Davis, R. P.: The physiological response to aldosterone in adrenalectomised and intact rats and its sex dependence. Endocrinology **92**, 989—993 (1973)

Mountain, I. M.: Antibody production by spleen in vitro. I. Influence of cortisone and other chemicals. J. Immunol. **74**, 270—277 (1955)

Munck, A.: The effects of hormones at the cellular level. In: James, V. H. T. (Ed.): Recent Advances in Endocrinology, pp. 139—180. London: J & A Churchill 1968

Munck, A.: Glucocorticoid inhibition of glucose uptake by peripheral tissues: old and new evidence, molecular mechanism, and physiological significance. Perspect. Biol. Med. **14**, 265—289 (1971)

Munck, A., Brink-Johnsen, T.: Specific and non-specific physiochemical interactions of glucocorticoids and related steroids with rat thymus cells in vitro. J. biol. Chem. **243**, 5556—5565 (1968)

Munck, A., Wira, C., Young, D. A., Mosher, K. M., Hallahan, C., Bell, P. A.: Glucocorticoid-receptor complexes and the earliest steps in the action of glucocorticoids on thymus cells. J. Steroid Biochem. **3**, 567—578 (1972)

Murray, J. E., Wilson, R. E., Tilney, N. O.: Five years' experience in renal transplantation with immunosuppressive drugs, survival, function, complications and the role of lymphocyte depletion by thoracic duct fistula. Ann. Surg. **168**, 416—435 (1968)

Myles, A. B., Daly, J. R.: Effect of corticosteroids and adrenocorticotrophic hormone on the hypothalamo-pituitary-adrenal axis. In: Myles, A. B., Daly, J. R. (Eds.): Corticosteroid and ACTH treatment. Principles and Problems, pp. 66—81. London: Edward Arnold 1974

Nakayama, I., Nickerson, P. A., Skelton, F. R.: An ultrastructural study of the adrenocorticotrophic hormone-secreting cell in the rat adrenohypophysis during adrenal cortical regeneration. Lab. Invest. **21**, 169—178 (1969)

Nelson, D. H.: Relative merits of the adrenocorticosteroids. Ann. Rev. Med. **13**, 241—248 (1962)

Nicoloff, D. M., Sosin, H., Peter, E. T., Leonard, A. S., Wagensteen, O. H.: The effect of cortisone on peptic ulcer formation; an experimental study. J. Amer. med. Ass. **183**, 1019—1021 (1963)

Nijkamp, F. P., Flower, R. J., Moncada, S., Vane, J. R.: Partial purification of rabbit aorta contracting substance-releasing factor and inhibition of its activity by anti-inflammatory steroids. Nature (Lond.) **263**, 479—482 (1976)

North, R. J.: The action of cortisone acetate on cell-mediated immunity to infection. Suppression of host cell proliferation and alteration of cellular composition of infective foci. J. exp. Med. **134**, 1485—1500 (1971)

Nuki, G., Downie, W. W.: Corticosteroid-induced suppression of the cerebro-hypothalamo-pituitary-adrenal axis. Mod. Trends Rheum. **2**, 199—239 (1973)

O'Malley, B. W.: Mechanisms of action of steroid hormones. New Engl. J. Med. **284**, 370—377 (1971)

O'Malley, B. W., Schrader, W. T.: The receptors of steroid hormones. Sci. Amer. **234**, 32—43 (1976)

Overell, B. G., Condon, S. E., Petrow, V.: The effect of hormones and their analogues upon the uptake of glucose by mouse skin in vitro. J. Pharm. (Lond.) **12**, 150—153 (1960)

Page Thomas, D. P., Dingle, J. T. M.: Studies on human synovial membrane in vitro. The metabolism of normal and rheumatoid synovium and the effect of hydrocortisone. Biochem. J. **68**, 231—238 (1958)

Parkhurst, G. F., Vlahides, G. D.: Fatal opportunistic fungus disease. J. Amer. med. Ass. **202**, 279—281 (1967)

Pearson, C. M., Paulus, H. E., Machleder, H. I.: The role of the lymphocyte and its product in the propagation of joint disease. Ann. N.Y. Acad. Sci. **256**, 150—168 (1975)

Pearson, C. M., Carson Dick, W. (Eds.): Clinics in rheumatic diseases. Vol. **1**:2, 335—365. London: W. B. Saunders 1975

Peck, W. A., Brandt, J., Miller, I.: Hydrocortisone-induced inhibition of protein synthesis and uridine incorporation in isolated bone cells in vitro. Proc. nat. Acad. Sci. (Wash.) **57**, 1599—1606 (1967)

Peterson, R. E., Pierce, C. E., Wyngaarden, J. B., Bunim, J. J., Brodie, B. B.: The physiological disposition and metabolic fate of cortisone in man. J. clin. Invest. **36**, 1301—1312 (1957)

Piddington, R.: Distribution and development of glutamine synthetase in the embryonic cerebral hemisphere. J. exp. Zool. **177**, 219—228 (1971)

Popper, T. L., Watnick, A. S.: Anti-inflammatory steroids. In: Scherrer, R. A., Whitehouse, M. W. (Eds.): Anti-inflammatory Agents, pp. 245—294. New York: Academic Press 1974

Pratt, W. B., Aronow, L.: The effect of glucocorticoids on protein and nucleic acid synthesis in mouse fibroblasts growing in vitro. J. biol. Chem. **241**, 5244—5250 (1966)

Ragan, C., Grokoest, A. W., Boots, R. H.: Effect of adrenocorticotrophic hormone (ACTH) on rheumatoid arthritis. Amer. J. Med. **7**, 741—750 (1949a)

Ragan, C., Howes, E. L., Plotz, C. M., Meyer, K., Blunt, J. W.: Effect of cortisone on production of granulation tissue in the rabbit. Proc. Soc. exp. Biol. (N.Y.) **72**, 718—721 (1949b)

Rauch, H. C., Loomis, M. E., Johnson, M. E., Favour, C. B.: In vitro suppression of polymorphonuclear leukocyte and lymphocyte glycolysis by cortisol. Endocrinology **68**, 375—385 (1961)

Rebuck,J.W., Mellinger,R.C.: Interruption by topical cortisone of leukocytic cycles in acute inflammation in man. Ann. N.Y. Acad. Sci. **56**, 715—732 (1953)

Reich,E., Goldberg,I.H.: Actinomycin and nucleic acid function. Progr. nucleic acid Res. molec. Biol. **3**, 183—234 (1964)

Reynolds,J.J.: The effect of hydrocortisone on the growth of chick bone rudiments in chemically defined medium. Exp. Cell Res. **41**, 174—189 (1966)

Riddle,J.M., Bluhm,G.B., Barnhart,M.I.: Inter-relationships between fibrin, neutrophils and rheumatoid synovitis. J. reticuloendoth. Soc. **2**, 420—436 (1965)

Rifkind,D., Goodman,N., Hill,R.B., Jr.: The clinical significance of cytomegalovirus infection in renal transplant recipients. Ann. intern. Med. **66**, 1116—1128 (1967)

Rinehart,J.J., Balcerzak,S.P., Sagone,A.L., Lobuglio,A.F.: Effects of corticosteroids on human monocytic function. J. clin. Invest. **54**, 1337—1343 (1974)

Rinehart,J.J., Sagone,A.L., Balcerzak,S.P., Ackerman,G.A., Lobuglio,A.F.: Effects of corticosteroid therapy on human monocytic function. New Engl. J. Med. **292**, 236—241 (1975)

Ringler,I.: Activities of adrenocorticosteroids in experimental animals and man. Meth. Hormone Res. **3**, 227—350 (1964)

Ringold,H.J., Bowers,A.: Adrenal hormones. In: Florkin,M., Stotz,E.H. (Eds.): Comprehensive Biochemistry, pp. 79—159. Amsterdam-London: Elsevier 1963

Roberts,A., Nezamis,J.E.: The granuloma pouch as a routine assay for anti-phlogistic compounds. Acta endocr. (Kbh.) **25**, 105—112 (1957)

Robinson,B.H.B., Mattingly,D., Cope,C.L.: Adrenal function after prolonged corticosteroid therapy. Brit. med. J. **1**, 1579—1584 (1962)

Rockstein,M.: Development and Aging in the Nervous System, pp.172—198. New York: Academic Press 1973

Rosen,F., Nichol,C.A.: Corticosteroids and enzyme activity. Vitam. and Horm. **21**, 135—214 (1963)

Roth,G.S.: Age-related changes in specific glucocorticoid binding by steroid-responsive tissues of rats. Endocrinology **94**, 82—90 (1974)

Rotstein,J., Good,R.A.: Steroid pseudorheumatism. Arch. intern. Med. **99**, 545—555 (1957)

Rousseau,G.G., Baxter,J.D., Higgins,S.J., Tomkins,G.M.: Steroid induced nuclear binding of glucocorticoids receptors in intact hepatoma cells. J. molec. Biol. **79**, 539—554 (1973)

Rousseau,G.G., Baxter,J.D., Tomkins,G.M.: Glucocorticoid receptors: relations between steroid binding and biological effects. J. molec. Biol. **67**, 99—115 (1972)

Rudolph,R., Klein,L.: Healing processes in skin grafts. Surg. Gynec. Obstet. **136**, 641—654 (1973)

Ruhmann,A.G., Berliner,D.L.: Effect of steroids on growth of mouse fibroblasts in vitro. Endocrinology **76**, 916—927 (1965)

Salassa,R.M., Bennett,W.A., Keating,F.R., Jr., Sprague,R.G.: Postoperative adrenal cortical insufficiency occurring in patients previously treated with cortisone. J. Amer. med. Ass. **152**, 1509—1515 (1953)

Sampson,P.A., Brooke,B.N., Winstone,N.E.: Biochemical confirmation of collapse due to adrenal failure. Lancet **1961I**, 1377

Samuels,H.H., Tomkins,G.M.: Relation of steroid structure to enzyme induction in hepatoma tissue culture cells. J. molec. Biol. **52**, 57—74 (1970)

Sarrett,L.H., Patchett,A.A., Steelman,S.: The effect of structural alteration on the anti-inflammatory properties of hydrocortisone. Progr. Drug Res. **5**, 11—153 (1963)

Sayers,G.: The adrenal cortex and homeostasis. Physiol. Rev. **30**, 241—320 (1950)

Schaeffer,L.D., Chenoweth,M., Dunn,A.: Adrenal corticosteroid involvement in the control of liver glycogen phosphorylase activity. Biochim. biophys. Acta **192**, 292—303 (1969a)

Schaeffer,L.D., Chenoweth,M., Dunn,A.: Adrenal corticosteroid involvement in the control of phosphorylase in muscle. Biochim. biophys. Acta **192**, 304—309 (1969b)

Schayer,R.W.: Induced synthesis of histamine, microcirculating regulation, and the mechanism of action of the adrenal glucocorticoid hormone. Progr. Allergy **7**, 187—212 (1963)

Schayer,R.W.: A unified theory of glucocorticoid action. II. On a circulatory basis for the metabolic effects of glucocorticoids. Perspect. Biol. Med. **10**, 409—417 (1967)

Scothorne,R.J.: Studies of the response of the regional lymph node to skin homografts. Ann. N.Y. Acad. Sci. **64**, 1028—1038 (1957)

Scott,A., Kalz,F.: The effect of the topical application of corticotrophin, hydrocortisone, and fluorocortisone on the process of cutaneous inflammation. J. invest. Derm. **26**, 361—376 (1956)

Segal, S., Cohen, I. R., Feldman, M.: Thymus-derived lymphocytes: Humoral and cellular reactions distinguished by hydrocortisone. Science 175, 1126—1128 (1972)

Sendelbeck, L. R., Yates, F. E.: Adrenal cortical and medullary hormones in recovery of tissues from local injury. Amer. J. Physiol. 219, 845—853 (1970)

Shimida, Y., Piddington, R., Moscona, A. A.: Experimentally induced increases in glutamine synthetase in the optic tectum in the embryo and in culture. Exp. Cell Res. 48, 240—243 (1967)

Simonsson, B.: Depression of ^{3}H-glucose uptake into rabbit polymorphonuclear leukocytes by glucocorticoids in concentrations partly saturating the specific glucocorticoid uptake. Evidence for a glucocorticoid receptor. Acta physiol. scand. 86, 398—409 (1972)

Simpson, S. A., Tait, J. F.: A quantitative method for the bioassay of the effect of adrenal cortical steroids on mineral metabolism. Endocrinology 50, 150—161 (1952)

Siperstein, E. R., Miller, K. J.: Further cytophysiologic evidence for the identity of cells that produce adrenocorticotrophic hormone. Endocrinology 86, 451—486 (1970)

Skoryna, S. G., Webster, D. R., Kahn, D. S.: A new method of production of experimental gastric ulcer: effects of hormone factors on healing. Gastroenterology 34, 1—10 (1958)

Soyka, L. F., Crawford, J. D.: Antagonism by cortisone of the linear growth induced in hypopituitary patients and hypophysectomised rats by human growth hormone. J. clin. Endocr. 25, 469—475 (1965)

Sparrow, E. M.: Effect of cortisone alcohol and ACTH (adrenocorticotrophin hormone) on skin homografts in guinea pigs. J. Endocr. (Kbh.) 11, 57—65 (1954)

Spector, W. G., Willoughby, D. A.: The enzyme inactivation of an adrenaline-like substance in inflammation. J. Path. Bact. 80, 271—280 (1960)

Spiro, H. M., Miles, S. S.: Clinical and physiologic implications of the steroid-induced peptic ulcer. New Engl. J. Med. 263, 286—294 (1960)

Sprague, R. G., Power, M. H., Mason, H. L., Albert, A., Mathieson, D. R., Hench, P. S., Kendall, E. C., Slocumb, Polley, H. F.: Observations on the physiologic effects of cortisone and ACTH in man. Arch. intern. Med. 85, 199—258 (1950)

Spry, C. J. F.: Inhibition of lymphocyte recirculation by stress and corticotropin. Cell. Immunol. 4, 86—92 (1972)

Stalmans, W., Dewulf, H., Hers, H. G.: The control of liver glycogen synthetase phosphatase by phosphorylase. Europ. J. Biochem. 18, 582—587 (1971)

Stastny, F.: Hydrocortisone as a possible inductor of Na$^+$-K$^+$-ATPase in the chick embryo cerebral hemispheres. Brain Res. 25, 397—410 (1971)

Stastny, P., Rosenthal, M., Andreis, M., Cooke, D., Ziff, M.: Lymphokines in rheumatoid synovitis. Ann. N. Y. Acad. Sci. 256, 117—131 (1975)

Stephanopoulos, C., Kamaroulais, D.: The effect of prednisolone on the tuberculin test and on the Middlebrook-Dubos test. Acta tuberc. scand. 41, 19—27 (1961)

Stevens, K. M., McKenna, J. M.: Studies on antibody synthesis initiated in vitro. J. exp. Med. 107, 537—559 (1958)

Stevens, W., Bedke, C., Dougherty, T. F.: Effects of cortisol acetate on various aspects of cellular metabolism in mouse lymphatic tissue. J. reticuloendoth. Soc. 4, 254—283 (1967)

Sutton, P. M., Feldmann, R. J., Maibach, H. I.: Vasoconstrictor potency of corticoids: Intradermal injection. J. invest. Derm. 57, 371—376 (1971)

Swingle, K. F., Shideman, F. E.: Phases of the inflammatory response to subcutaneous implantation of a cotton pellet and their modification by certain anti-inflammatory agents. J. Pharmacol. exp. Ther. 183, 226—234 (1972)

Szigeti, M., Ezer, E., Szporny, L., Kete, F. E.: Acute inhibitory action of glucocorticoids on the uptake of sulphur by bone tissue in vivo. Steroids 5, 729—736 (1965)

Tashjian, A. H. Jr., Voelkel, E. F., McDonough, J.: Hydrocortisone inhibits prostaglandin production by mouse fibrosarcoma cells. Nature (Lond.) 258, 739—741 (1975)

Taylor, A. C., Lehrfeld, J. W.: Determination of survival time of skin homografts in rat by observation of vascular changes in graft. Plast. reconstr. Surg. 12, 423—431 (1953)

Telford, J. M., West, G. B.: The effects of corticosteroids and related compounds on the histamine and 5-hydroxy-tryptamine content of rat tissue. Brit. J. Pharmacol. 15, 532—539 (1960)

Thompson, E. B., Lippman, M. E.: Mechanism of action of glucocorticoids. Metabolism 23, 159—202 (1974)

Thong, Y. H., Hensen, S. A., Vincent, M. M., Rola-Pleszczynski, M., Walser, J. B., Bellanti, J. A.: Effect of hydrocortisone on in vitro cellular immunity to viruses in man. Clin. Immunol. Immunopath. **3**, 363—368 (1975)

Travis, R. H., Sayers, G.: Adrenocorticotrophic hormone: adrenocortical steroids and their synthetic analogues. In: Goodman, L. S., Gilman, A. (Eds.): The Pharmacological Basis of Therapeutics, pp. 1608—1648. New York: MacMillan 1965

Tuncbay, T. O., Ketel, W. B., Boshes, B.: Cortisone effects of myoneural junction. Neurology (Minneap.) **15**, 314—320 (1965)

Tursz, T., Fournier, C., Kreis, H., Crosnier, J., Bach, J. F.: T lymphocytes in kidney allograft recipients. Brit. med. J. **(1976) I**, 799—801

Vadasz, I.: Straingauge plethysmography in the assessment of joint inflammation. Ann. rheum. Dis. **30**, 194—198 (1971)

Van Arman, C. G., Risley, E. A., Kling, P. T.: Correlation between white—cell count and inflammatory swelling induced by carrageenan in the rats foot. Pharmacologist **13**, 284 (1971)

Van Boxal, J. A., Paget, S. A.: Predominantly T-cell infiltrate in rheumatoid synovial membranes. New Engl. J. Med. **293**, 517—520 (1975)

Vargaftig, B. B., Dao Hai, N.: Selective inhibition by nepacrine of the release of "rabbit aorta contracting substance" evoked by the administration of bradykinin. J. Pharm. (Lond.) **24**, 159—161 (1972)

Vogt, K. D., Schroeder, W.: Nitrogen-containing steroids in aqeous cortical extracts. Nature (Lond.) **176**, 599—600 (1955)

Von Pirquet, C.: Allergy. In: Gell, P. G. H., Coombs, R. R. A. (Eds.): Clinical Aspects of Immunology, pp. 1293—1297. Oxford: 1968 Blackwell Sci. Publ.

Wahl, S. M., Wilton, J. M., Rosenstreich, D. L., Oppenheim, J. J.: The role of macrophages in the production of lymphokines by T and B lymphocytes. J. Immunol. **114**, 1296—1301 (1975)

Ward, L. E., Hench, P. S.: Effects of aldosterone (electrocortin) 9-alpha-fluorohydrocortisone acetate and l-dehydrocortisone (metacortandacin) in rheumatoid arthritis. Ann. N.Y. Acad. Sci. **61**, 620—635 (1955)

Ward, P. A.: The chemosuppression of chemotaxis. J. exp. Med. **124**, 209—226 (1966)

Ward, P. A.: Leukotactic factors in health and disease. Amer. J. Path. **64**, 521—530 (1971)

Watanbe, H., Orth, D. N., Toft, D. O.: Glucocorticoid receptors in pituitary cells. I. Cytosol receptors. J. biol. Chem. **248**, 7625—7630 (1973)

Wayne, H. L.: Convulsive seizures complicating cortisone and ACTH therapy: clinical and electro-encephalographic observations. J. clin. Endocr. **14**, 1039—1045 (1954)

Webel, M. L., Ritts, R. E. Jr., Taswell, H. F.: Cellular immunity after intravenous administration of methylprednisolone. J. Lab. clin. Med. **83**, 383—392 (1974)

Weinshelbaum, E. J., Wool, I. G.: Effect of adrenalectomy and croticosteroids on distribution of radioactivity in protein of cell fractions from myocardial slices. Nature (Lond.) **191**, 1401—1402 (1961)

Weiss, L.: Interactions of sensitised lymphoid cells and homologous target cells in tissue culture and in grafts: an electron microscopic and immunofluorescence study. J. Immunol. **101**, 1346—1362 (1968)

Weissman, G.: Lysosomal mechanism of tissue injury in arthritis. New Engl. J. Med. **286**, 141—147 (1972)

Weissmann, G., Thomas, L.: The effects of corticosteroids upon connective tissue and lysosomes. Recent Progr. Hormone Res. **20**, 215—239 (1964)

Welbourn, R. B., Clarke, S. D., Neill, D. W.: The effects of ACTH and corticosteroids on gastric secretion in the dog. Gut **1**, 82—83 (1960)

Wells, B. B., Kendall, E. C.: Influence of corticosterone and 17-hydroxydehydrocorticosterone (compound E) on somatic growth. Proc. Mayo Clin. **15**, 324—328 (1940).

Weston, W. L., Claman, H. N., Krueger, G. G.: Site of action of cortisol in cellular immunity. J. Immunol. **110**, 880—883 (1973 a)

Weston, W. L., Mandel, M. J., Yeckley, J. A., Krueger, G. G., Claman, H. N.: Mechanism of cortisol inhibition of adoptive transfer to tuberculin sensitivity. J. Lab. clin. Med. **82**, 366—371 (1973 b)

Whittle, B. J. R.: Prostaglandins and changes in the gastric mucosal barrier and blood flow during indomethacin and bile salt-induced mucosal damage. Brit. J. Pharmacol. **56**, 340 P (1976)

Wiener, J., Lattes, R. G., Pearl, J. S.: Vascular permeability and leukocyte emigration in allograft rejection. Amer. J. Path. 55, 295—327 (1969)

Wiener, J., Loud, A. V., Kimberg, D. V., Saro, D.: A quantitative description of cortisone-induced alterations in the ultrastructure of rat liver parenchymal cells. J. Cell Biol. 37, 47—61 (1968)

Wiener, E., Marmary, Y.: The in vitro effect of hydrocortisone on cultures of peritoneal monocytes. Lab. Invest. 21, 505—511 (1969)

Williams, C. D. Jr., Heiple, K. G., Ebert, R. H.: The effect of cortisone on vascular reactivity: in vivo observations using the rabbit ear chamber technique. J. Lab. clin. Med. 44, 210—218 (1954)

Williams-Ashman, H. G.: New facets of the biochemistry of steroid hormone action. Cancer Res. 25, 1096—1124 (1965)

Williamson, H. E.: Mechanism of the anti-natriuretic action of aldosterone. Biochem. Pharmacol. 12, 1449—1450 (1963)

Willmer, E. N.: Steroids and cell surfaces. Biol. Rev. 36, 368—398 (1961)

Wilson, D. B.: Quantitative studies on the behaviour of sensitised lymphocytes in vitro. I. Relationship of the degree of destruction of homologous target cells to the number of lymphocytes and to the time of contact in culture and consideration of the effects of isoimmune serum. J. exp. Med. 122, 143—166 (1965 a)

Wilson, D. B.: Quantitative studies on the behaviour of sensitised lymphocytes in vitro. II. Inhibitory influence of the immune suppressor, Imuran, on the destructive reaction of sensitised lymphoid cells against homologous target cells. J. exp. Med. 122, 167—172 (1965 b)

Wilson, D. B.: Immunologic reactivity to major histo-compatibility alloantigens: HARC, effector cells and the problems of memory. In: Brent, L., Holborow, J. (Eds.): Progress in Immunology, Vol. II, Ch. 2, pp. 145—156. Amsterdam: North Holland Publ. Co. 1974

Wira, C. R., Munck, A.: Glucocorticoid-receptor complexes in rat thymus cells. Cytoplasmic-nuclear transformations. J. biol. Chem. 249, 5328—5336 (1974)

Woodbury, D. M.: Effect of adrenocortical steroids and adrenocorticotrophic hormone on electroshock seizure threshold. J. Pharmacol. exp. Ther. 105, 27—36 (1952)

Woodruff, M. F. A., Llaurado, J. G.: The effect of systemic administration of fluoro- and chloro-cortisol and prednisone, and local application of fluoro-cortisol, on skin homografts in rabbits. Plast. reconstr. Surg. 18, 251—259 (1956)

Wool, I. G., Weinshelbaum, E. I.: Corticosteroids and incorporation of ^{14}C-phenylalanine into protein of isolated rat diaphragm. Amer. J. Physiol. 198, 1111—1114 (1960)

Wright, D. G., Malawista, S. E.: Mobilization and extra-cellular release of granular enzymes from human leukocytes during phagocytosis: Inhibition by colchicine and cortisol but not by salicylate. Arthr. Rheum. 16, 749—758 (1973)

Wyman, L. C., Fulton, G. P., Shulman, M. H.: Direct observations on the circulation in the hamster cheek pouch in adrenal insufficiency and experimental hypercorticalism. Ann. N.Y. Acad. Sci. 56, 643—656 (1953)

Yates, F. E., Russell, S. M., Maran, J. W.: Brain-adenohypophysical communication in mammals. Ann. Rev. Physiol. 33, 393—444 (1971)

Yates, F. E., Urquhart, J.: Control of plasma concentrations of adrenocortical hormones. Physiol. Rev. 42, 359—443 (1962)

Yu, D. T. Y., Clements, P. J., Paulus, H. E., Peter, J. B., Levy, J., Barnett, E. V.: Human lymphocyte subpopulations. J. clin. Invest. 53, 565—571 (1974)

Zvaifler, N.: Further speculation of the pathogenesis of joint inflammation in rheumatoid arthritis. Arthr. Rheum. 13, 894—901 (1970)

Zweifach, B. W., Shorr, E., Black, M. M.: The influence of the adrenal cortex on behaviour of terminal vascular bed. Ann. N.Y. Acad. Sci. 56, 626—633 (1953)

CHAPTER 38

Anti-Inflammatory Agents of Animal Origin

M. J. H. SMITH and A. W. FORD-HUTCHINSON

A. Introduction

The purpose of the present chapter is to review anti-inflammatory substances of animal origin. Some degree of selection has been inevitable and preference has been given to those preparations which have been sufficiently characterised in terms of either provenance, structure, range of anti-inflammatory activity or mechanism of action, for a provisional assessment of their potential to be made.

There are two good reasons why naturally occurring anti-inflammatory agents should be intensively studied. They may provide valuable models for new classes of anti-inflammatory drugs: there are historical precedents for this approach, for example salicin, aspirin and cortisone and the synthetic corticosteroids. Furthermore, the essentially pragmatic nature of current screening programmes militates against the discovery of 'new' anti-inflammatory compounds. Thus, one of the difficulties of searching for new anti-inflammatory agents is that it is tempting to select the present inadequate design tests that give positive results and then, with the aid of these tests, to search for further compounds giving positive results. Such methodology may lead to 'old' anti-inflammatory agents instead of 'new' (SPECTOR and WILLOUGHBY, 1968).

The natural regulation or remission of inflammatory processes is a neglected subject and it is in this area that a study of anti-inflammatory agents of animal origin might be expected to throw some much needed light. There exists a paradoxical situation that inflammation is a natural defence mechanism which, in normal situations, should be left alone but during the course of various diseases may need careful control (SKIDMORE, 1974). It seems likely that there are certain key areas in which such control can be exercised and a search for natural regulators may be more rewarding than the present empirical manufacture of chemical congeners of the unsatisfactory synthetic drugs.

B. Definition and Evaluation of Anti-Inflammatory Activity

'Anti-inflammatory' is a very broad description which may be applied to drugs which inhibit any of the facets of inflammation, whether observed as part of an experimentally induced system or as a clinical manifestation in man. This definition embraces the term 'anti-rheumatic', which should be reserved for substances which suppress the inflammation occurring in the human connective tissue and arthritic disorders (SMITH, 1975).

This is not merely a semantic difficulty since it is abundantly clear that current research is largely concerned with developing anti-inflammatory rather than anti-

Table 1. Laboratory evaluation of anti-inflammatory action

Inhibition of carrageenin-induced paw oedema	(rat)
Inhibition of UV-induced erythema	(guinea pig)
Adjuvant-induced arthritis	(rat)
Cotton pellet granuloma	(rat)

rheumatic drugs. Classical anti-inflammatory agents do not really pretend to cure the underlying disease or even to prevent completely tissue injury or progressive loss of function (Paulus, 1974). It is loss of function that is the major clinical problem in the chronic rheumatoid diseases rather than the suppression of a phase of acute inflammation and the consequent amelioration of the discomfort caused by one or more of the cardinal signs of inflammation. The acid test of any new anti-rheumatic remedy is the results of observations in the relevant human diseases. In the absence of acceptable animal models for rheumatoid arthritis and allied conditions, however, a preliminary evaluation of anti-inflammatory agents of animal origin must be conducted within the framework of existing screening programmes.

The most popular methods for the evaluation of anti-inflammatory activity in the laboratory have been comprehensively and lucidly reviewed by Swingle (1974). Most workers elect to use a battery of tests based on a modification either of one of the cardinal signs of inflammation or one of the events occurring during the inflammatory process. Thus, one of the most widely used assays is the measurement of swelling induced in the rat's paw by the subplantar injection of carrageenin. There are many variants, in that a number of different irritants may be used and the inflammatory exudate may be induced in sites other than the paw. The emigration of leucocytes into the inflammatory exudates may be studied separately, as can the erythrematous response to uv light, X-rays and chemical irritants in depilated skin. All these inflammatory reactions tend to be relatively short-lived and it is usual to proceed to other assays with some element of chronicity. A well-known procedure is adjuvant-induced arthritis in the rat and a further group of tests which reflect some of the more chronic aspects of inflammation are the various granuloma reactions.

Thus, the initial investigation of the anti-inflammatory spectrum of a new drug or natural substance could comprise the battery of tests given in Table 1.

The information gained from this preliminary screening programme may be supplemented in one or more of several ways. It is conventional to investigate the analgesic and antipyretic activities of the test substance. Both pain and heat are cardinal signs of inflammation and the relevant procedures should be concerned with the suppression of the pain and hyperpyrexia occurring at locally defined areas of inflammation. In most instances, however, the chosen methods preferentially detect centrally acting analgesics and antipyretics.

A second group of assays may be used to assess anti-allergic and immunosuppressive properties. They comprise not only the well-known and widely used procedures for the production of local hypersensitivity reactions, such as passive cutaneous anaphylaxis and the Arthus and Shwartzman reactions, but also tests based on suppression of homograft responses and on experimental auto-immune diseases, including adjuvant-induced arthritis. This group has recently been reviewed in detail by Rosenthale (1974).

A further and rather large category are the many and varied in vitro reactions. These are of two main types. They may be based on some property peculiar to a section of known anti-inflammatory drugs and include uncoupling of oxidative phosphorylation, inhibition of denaturation of proteins, stabilisation of erthrocytic membranes, or the acceleration of an interchange reaction between the sulphhydryl group of serum proteins and a synthetic disulphide. There is little, if any evidence that these reactions are relevant to inflammation in vivo and they are used empirically as screening tests to develop further drugs of the same type. Alternatively, the in vitro tests are considered to represent one or more aspects of inflammation thought to be concerned in supporting inflammatory processes. In this category are procedures based on stabilisation of lysosomal membranes, platelet aggregation, chemotaxis of leucocytes and interference with the biosynthesis, release and action of putative chemical mediators of inflammation. It should be recognised that these reactions only purport to reflect one of the many components which are assumed to contribute to the vicious circle which supports chronic inflammation. No information is available about the relative importance of these different components with respect either to the initiation or to the maintenance of the inflammatory process in clinical situations. It is not even known if they are essential, or if more important components remain undiscovered. Their role as screening tests for anti-inflammatory and anti-rheumatic substances must be viewed with extreme caution, although they may provide some useful clues about modes and sites of action.

The final source of extra data is man, i.e. from patients suffering from either hypersensitivity reactions or the rheumatic diseases. The quality and quantity of the clinical information is variable. At worst it may comprise a random report based on purely subjective criteria that some patients appear to do rather well on a new drug. The other end of the spectrum is represented by the double-blind crossover clinical trial conducted with the proper safeguards of large numbers of matched patients, the use of placebos and reference drugs, and proper statistical design and evaluation. There are, however, many problems inherent in the clinical trials of anti-arthritic drugs, for example a disease such as rheumatoid arthritis is subject to spontaneous remission and relapses. It may not even be a single entity so that a subsection of the chosen patients who respond to a given drug might have a disease of distinctive aetiology. Patients selected for such trials are often refractory to standard therapy and this bias may preclude a fair trial. Thus, the information from man is rarely as controlled or complete as should be available from animal testing but at least it has been obtained in the relevant species.

C. Mechanisms of Action

It is often said, albeit somewhat cynically, that the most effective anti-inflammatory agent is death. In less extreme circumstances, toxicity of many kinds are associated with a depression of the inflammatory responses in an organism. Thus, it is incumbent on an investigator to show that the agent under test is not producing a spurious anti-inflammatory effect merely by poisoning the experimental animal model. One example is adjuvant-induced arthritis in the rat. Not only is the natural reaction to the adjuvant a severe one, the swelling of the injected paw being relatively enormous and frequently accompanied by an abrupt decrease in body weight, but the subsequent programme involves the chronic administration of the test substance over several days. The general condition of the animals may be of more significance than the size of the paws in distinguishing between generalised toxicity and a true anti-inflammatory activity. The development of carrageenin-induced paw oedema in the rat may be inhibited by several compounds which are not usually classified as anti-inflammatory agents but it has been pointed out that many of these have been administered in doses that would be expected to produce behavioural or autonomic effects (SWINGLE, 1974). Even some of the well-known non-steroid anti-inflammatory drugs, aspirin, phenylbutazone and indomethacin, cause gastric haemorrhages at doses required for inhibition of the oedema. Thus, the test is incapable of distinguishing between toxic and anti-inflammatory properties of these substances.

The measurement of local oedema, as in irritant-induced paw oedema tests, is the most common method of assessing experimental anti-inflammatory activity. In these acute inflammatory reactions haemodynamic changes predominate in the initial phases. Any substance which effects plasma volume, blood pressure, or even diuresis, is potentially capable of reducing the formation of local oedema. It is known (GARATTINI et al., 1965) that drugs effective in changing vascular calibre, such as noradrenaline, or in producing hypotension, e.g. ganglion-blocking agents, cause non-specific inhibition in paw oedema tests. Thus, the investigation of a new anti-inflammatory agent should not neglect its possible effects on cardiovascular function and vascular tone.

The further study of possible mechanisms of action should include two main areas. These comprise possible interactions, either with endogenous anti-inflammatory systems, or with the biosynthesis, release and action of mediators that either increase vascular permeability or cause the emigration of peripheral leucocytes into inflammatory exudates. In the first category are stimulation of neuro-endocrine systems and counter-irritation.

The most important neuro-endocrine system is the so-called anterior pituitary-adrenal cortex axis. Natural adrenocorticosteroids are anti-inflammatory agents and the increased endogenous release of these substances after the injection of ACTH is effective in preventing the formation of local oedema. Many drugs and foreign chemicals cause a non-specific stimulation of the pituitary-adrenal axis and this may be dose-dependent. One example is the salicylates (SMITH, 1966). Aspirin and sodium salicylate, in relatively large amounts cause responses, both direct and indirect, which are typical of adrenocortical stimulation. These responses, observed in intact animals, are abolished by adrenalectomy or hypophysectomy. If smaller doses of the drugs, comparable to those used in the therapy of the human rheumatic diseases, are administered, the adreno-cortical stimulation does not occur but the anti-inflammatory activity persists even in adrenalectomized animals. Thus, the experimental anti-inflammatory activity of large doses of aspirin has at least two components, one of which, involving stimulation of the pituitary-adrenal axis, may be considered to be a toxic action of the drug. Other substances, however, may cause experimental anti-inflammatory effects solely through stimulation of the neuro-endocrine system, possible examples being tetrahydrocannabinol (SOFIA et al., 1973), carnosine (NAGAI et al., 1970) and glucagon (GARCIA LEME et al., 1975).

Counter-irritation may be defined as the ability of a localised irritation to produce a systemic anti-inflammatory effect. Thus the intraperitoneal injection of acetic acid will block the paw oedema induced by the subsequent subplantar injection of carrageenin. Any material producing local irritation, i.e. an inflammatory response, is capable of counteracting a second inflammatory reaction elicited by the same or a different irritant at a remote site in an organism. The suggested mechanisms are many and varied ranging from adrenocortical stimulation to depletion of stores of mediator precursors. The most interesting is the production of anti-inflammatory proteins in response to the initial irritation and this aspect will be described later in the present chapter (Sect. D.VI.3.). Whatever is the mechanism or combination of mechanisms of counter-irritation, it is of practical importance to determine if any material showing positive results in an anti-inflammatory screening programme possesses local irritant activity. If so then either an effort should be made to prepare it in a form devoid of local irritant activity or its status as an anti-inflammatory agent must be open to question.

The various mediators of inflammation can be generally divided into those agents involving vascular permeability and those with leucotactic properties (WARD, 1974a). As a general rule, each mediator has one or the other biological activity, but not both, and are best considered as separate groups. The main mediators of vascular permeability are the vasoactive amines, histamine, and 5-hydroxytryptamine (5-HT), the polypeptide kinins and the prostaglandins. Others include the slow reacting substance of anaphylaxis (SRS-A), the leucokinins, lymph node permeability factor and the anaphylatoxins derived from complement. The relative importance of these mediators in various types of inflammation is still a matter for speculation. In general, it appears that they may play an important part in the earlier phases of inflammatory responses and it has been suggested that they may act in a serial and sequential manner (WILLOUGHBY and DI ROSA, 1971). Despite the lack of detailed knowledge about the roles of the mediators it is necessary that any interactions between them and anti-inflammatory substances are investigated. Some evidence may become available during the initial screening programme if a battery of paw oedema tests has been used. Some of these reactions, the so-called 'anaphylactoid' oedemas, are thought to be mediated to a large extent by the release of the vasoactive amines. Thus, a compound active against dextran and ovalbumin-induced paw swellings can be suspected of some inherent antihistamine and anti-5-HT activity (SWINGLE, 1974).

The second class of inflammatory mediators comprise the leucotactic factors. With the exception of eosinophil chemotactic factors either released during anaphylaxis or produced from lymphocytes, the most important are peptides derived from complement proteins. Enzymes intrinsic to the complement system are capable of generating leucotactically active cleavage products from C3 and C5 after activation of the system by either the classical or alternate pathway (VOGT, 1974). Enzymes extrinsic to complement are also able to release leucotactic peptides and such enzymes may be derived from bacteria, viruses and from normal mammalian tissues, including leucocytes (JANOFF, 1972). The methods for the study of cellular exudation in vivo are limited. The most widely used include counting the emigration of polymorphonuclear and mononuclear leucocytes into inflammatory exudates, such as those found after the intrapleural or intraperitoneal injection of irritants, or after the implantation of inert porous sponges. Modifications of the Boyden chamber technique (BOYDEN, 1962) are preferred by most workers to assay chemotaxis in vitro.

The method enables the possible action of an anti-inflammatory substance on either the release or the action of chemotactic agents to be studied. Further experiments on the effects of the test substance on circulating complement titres in vivo and on the activation of the complement system in vitro may be performed with standard methods.

D. Individual Agents

In the present chapter no-attempt has been made to provide a comprehensive account of every agent. Thus, although the polypeptide ACTHs, the adrenocortical hormones and catecholamines are anti-inflammatory agents of animal origin we have not provided separate detailed accounts of their chemistry and biological activities. Steroids are described in Chapter 37 and excellent contemporary accounts of the others are readily available. No attempt has been made to classify the remainder in a logical manner. In many instances all the literature has to offer is an amorphous mass of data varying in both quality and quantity. We have, therefore, made a personal selection on the grounds of what appears to be interesting and reasonably documented. Few aspects of the anti-inflammatory field are free from controversy and it is hoped that the present topic will be no exception.

I. Alkoxyglycerols

Fatty acid esters of the α-hydroxyl group of glycerol are found in a variety of animal tissues such as fish liver oils, bone marrow and egg yolk (PRELOG and BEYERMANN, 1945; HALLGREN and LARSSON, 1962). The hexadecyl derivative is known as chimyl, the octadecyl as batyl and the octadecenyl as selachyl alcohol.

$CH_2O\ CH_2(CH_2)_7CH = CH(CH_2)_7CH_3$

$CHOH$ Selachyl alcohol
                                                    3-(9-octadecenyloxy)-1,2-propanediol
CH_2OH

The topical application of batyl and selachyl alcohols accelerated the rate of wound healing (BODMAN and MAISIN, 1958) and their oral administration reduced the volume of exudate formed in croton oil-induced granuloma pouches in the rat (BURFORD and GOWDEY, 1968). The lack of activity after parenteral injection suggested that the 'active' forms were the liberated fatty acids. No information appears to be available about the octadecenyl acid, but polyunsaturated fatty acids, such as linoleic, have been studied as anti-inflammatory agents. In one set of experiments it was found that linoleic acid inhibited the early stages of adjuvant-induced arthritis in the rat (STUYVESANT and JOLLEY, 1968). Other workers (MERTIN et al., 1973; FIELD et al., 1974) provided evidence that the fatty acid suppressed cellular immunity in vitro. Attempts to extend this finding to in vivo situations have not yielded definite results. Although RING et al. (1974) claimed that the oral and intraperitoneal administration of linoleic acid caused a prolongation of skin allografts in the rat, this could have been due to a non-specific toxic effect. Furthermore, BROCK and FIELD (1975) found no increase in the survival time of tail grafts in mice after the subcutaneous injection of the relatively non-toxic triglyceride esters of the acid. Linoleic acid has also been used in the treatment of multiple sclerosis. MILLAR et al. (1973) carried out a controlled study in which the fatty acid was given for two years in a dose of about 8 g twice daily. There was a rise in the serum linoleate fraction and clinical relapses in the treated patients were less severe and of shorter duration. No conclusion, however, could be drawn concerning the overall progress of the disease.

II. N(2-hydroxyethyl) Palmitamide

During an investigation into the possible role of environmental factors which increased susceptibility to rheumatic fever in the underprivileged, COBURN and MOORE (1943) found that reinforcing poor diets with egg yolk appeared to prevent the recurrence of rheumatic fever in spite of repeated attacks of haemolytic streptococcal infection.

The phospholipid fraction from egg yolk showed experimental anti-inflammatory activity in a passive Arthus reaction in the guinea pig (COBURN et al., 1954). The active substance was further purified by LONG and MARTIN (1956) and subsequently identified as N(2-hydroxy-ethyl) palmitamide (KUEHL et al., 1957). It is present in high concentrations in brain tissue of rats and guinea pigs (BACHUR et al., 1965).

$$CH_3(CH_2)_{14}\,CONHCH_2CH_2OH \quad N(2\text{-hydroxyethyl) palmitamide}$$

The synthetic substance was found to be active at very low concentrations (0.3 μg/kg) in a local joint anaphylaxis test in the guinea pig (GANLEY et al., 1958). In contrast to the alkoxyglycerols, this activity appeared to be associated with the ethanolamine moiety and not with the fatty acid. There was some structural specificity in that although ethanolamine was active, the corresponding amino-propanols were not. Furthermore, some of the in vivo metabolites of ethanolamine, such as the N-monomethyl and dimethyl compounds and choline, showed activity, whereas serine and betaine were inactive. On the other hand, GANLEY et al. (1959) reported that N(2-hydroxyethyl) palmitamide, ethanolamine, and palmitic acid were active against passive anaphylaxis and 5-HT toxicity in the mouse, and provided data that other fatty acids were effective in the latter test.

Although N(2-hydroxyethyl) palmitamide depressed the sensitivity of BCG infected guinea pigs to tuberculin, its anti-inflammatory activity in other animal models is not impressive. Thus, it is reported to be inactive in the cotton pellet granuloma assay (GANLEY et al., 1958), either inactive (PERLIK and MASEK, 1974) or less active than indomethacin in the carrageenin-induced rat paw oedema test (BENEVUTI et al., 1968), and to have no effect on 5-HT-induced oedema in the rat or on the primary lesions of adjuvant-induced arthritis in the same species, although daily dosage of the substance over a 6-week period decreased the severity of the secondary lesions (PERLIK et al., 1971). A limited clinical trial of its possible prophylactic effects in preventing recurrences of rheumatic fever in children did not produce a statistically significant effect (COBURN and RICH, 1960). A controlled clinical trial of N(2-hydroxy-ethyl) palmitamide at an oral dose of 1.8 g per day for 6 weeks conducted under double blind conditions on patients with rheumatoid arthritis revealed that the substance, although showing some anti-rheumatic activity on grip strength and joint size, was less effective than a daily dose of 3 g of aspirin (PERLIK and MASEK, 1974).

The later history of the substance is somewhat mysterious. It has been reported to lower blood alcohol concentrations in man (KRSIAK et al., 1972), change the distribution of barbiturates between the blood and tissues of the mouse (Buchar et al., 1973) and alter sexual behaviour in the rat (Tikal et al., 1973). The initial promise of the substance as a powerful anti-inflammatory agent in delayed sensitivity reactions has not been fulfilled. It does not appear to have been tested in serum sickness. The emphasis of the animal work has been concerned with its analgesic activity, its possible effects in augmenting resistance to microbial toxins and traumatic shock and with miscellaneous and apparently unrelated actions (Raskova and Masek, 1967; Masek and Raskova, 1967).

III. Vitamins

There is a fragmentary literature on the anti-rheumatic and anti-inflammatory activities of members of this group. There is no evidence that one or more of the human diseases of connective tissue are associated with a specific deficiency of any of the vitamins. Obviously, adequate intake of the various factors is an important consideration in the treatment of patients with chronic disabling diseases and any associated dietary deficiency could impair the effectiveness of therapy with anti-rheumatic drugs. There is no convincing evidence that the administration of extra amounts of the vitamins is of any benefit (Traeger, 1946). An illustrative example is cyanocobalamin. Beneficial results were reported in 30 of 33 patients with osteoarthritis treated with the vitamin (Hallahan, 1952) but Zuckner (1954) found that 16 similar patients failed to respond to intramuscular doses, of up to 1mg, of B_{12}. The explanation for the discrepant results appeared to be the failure to use placebos in the earlier study. A further instance is calciferol and related substances. These were widely used at one period to treat arthritic conditions (Horwitz and Joseph, 1946) but studies of large numbers of patients over long periods of time suggested that they were of very limited value and the incidence of undesirable side-effects led to their abandonment (Rawls, 1947).

The second type of observation is the finding that some vitamins possess experimental anti-inflammatory activity. Ascorbic acid inhibits β-glucuronidase in vitro (Dolbeare, 1971), and since the activity of this enzyme increases in the synovial fluid of patients with rheumatoid arthritis and in the serum of rats during the development of polyarthritis, the vitamin was tested in several animal models. It was active at a dose of 20 mg/kg against the sterile peritonitis-polyarthritis induced by injecting heat-killed mycobacterium, moderately effective against adjuvant-induced arthritis, almost inactive against carrageenin-induced paw oedema and totally inactive against ultraviolet light-induced erythema (Dolbeare and Martlage, 1972). A similar situation has occurred with tocopherol which was found both to stabilize rat liver lysosomes (Brown and Pollock, 1972) erythrocyte and leucocyte membranes (Brown and Mackey, 1968; Mizushima et al., 1970) and to prevent the heat-induced aggregation of human and rat globulins in vitro (Taylor and Brown, 1974). Despite these in vitro effects (see Section D.II.) the daily administration of the vitamin had no action on the development of adjuvant-induced polyarthritis in the rat (Taylor and Brown, 1974). In other studies large systemic doses of the vitamin, up to 20 mg, have been claimed to be slightly active against dextran-induced paw oedema in the rabbit and topical administration has been reported to reduce the cutaneous inflammation caused by the application of such materials as croton oil and plasters (Kamimura, 1972). Vitamin K_1 and K_3 have been examined in a number of animal models by GÖRÖG et al. (1968). They were reported to be active in cotton pellet granuloma, croton oil-induced granuloma pouch and kaolin-induced paw oedema tests in the rat but inactive in other types of rat pedal oedemas and against uv light-induced erythema in the guinea pig.

IV. Amino Acids

Interest in the amino acids has been stimulated by several different types of observations. Firstly, there are reports of low concentrations of histidine in the serum of patients with rheumatoid arthritis (BORDEN et al., 1950; GERBER and TANENBAUM, 1969; GERBER, 1975). The results of an initial study suggested that the oral administration of histidine to such patients yielded some degree of clinical improvement (GERBER, 1969) but no statistically significant changes were observed using larger numbers of patients in a double blind controlled clinical trial (PINALS and GERBER, 1973). The amino acid in doses of 500 (oral) and 100 (intravenous) mg/kg body weight does not inhibit the development of carrageenin-induced paw oedema in the rat (HIRSCHELMANN and BEKEMEIER, 1973).

A second reason appears to be the finding that conventional anti-rheumatic drugs share a common action in displacing L-tryptophan from its binding site to circulating proteins (MCARTHUR et al., 1971). L-tryptophan exerts weak experimental anti-inflammatory effects in carrageenin-induced paw oedema (HIRSHELMANN and BEKEMEIER, 1973) and as a local and systemic antileucotactic agent in peritoneal irritation induced by gelatin in the rat (DAVIS et al., 1968; DAVIS, 1972) L-phenylalanine was inactive in paw swelling but approximately as active as tryptophan in the peritoneal irritation test.

The possible interactions of anti-rheumatic drugs with sulphydryl groups, coupled with the use of D-penicillamine in the treatment of the human rheumatic diseases, has stimulated interest in the sulphur containing amino acids. Cysteine is the most impressive, being active in skin tests (BAILEY and SHEFFNER, 1967), in dextran and carrageenin-induced paw oedema (THOMAS and WEST, 1973) and in adjuvant-induced arthritis in the rat (RYZEWSKI, 1966). Its efficacy in the treatment of rheumatoid arthritis has been stated to be modest (SHEN, 1967). There have also been attempts to investigate either natural or synthetic derivatives of the amino acids. Thus, small peptides such as glutathione and carnosine have been reported to exert some experimental anti-inflammatory actions (NAGAI et al., 1970; NAGAI, 1971; THOMAS and WEST, 1973) and a limited series of esters of amino acids and a dipeptide have been prepared and tested without much success by GECSE et al. (1971) and HIRSCHELMANN and BEKEMEIER (1973). It is possible that synthetic anti-inflammatory drugs based on natural amino acids as model compounds may be developed. However, the published work on the anti-inflammatory and anti-rheumatic activities of the natural amino acids is both sparse and unconvincing.

V. Peptides

1. Peptide 401

It is a traditional belief in folklore that beekeepers are immune to rheumatism and the sting of bees has been used since ancient times as a popular remedy for the treatment of various arthritic and rheumatoid conditions (BECK, 1935). The venom of the honey bee, *Apis mellifera*, contains a complex mixture of constituents ranging from macromolecules (including phospholipase A, hyaluronidase and non-enzymic antigenic proteins) through polypeptides and lipids to small molecules such as amino acids, histamine, sugars, and inorganic salts (DINIZ and CORRADO, 1971). At least 11 unidentified compounds are present.

The minimum lethal dose of the venom in man is estimated as 7 mg/kg which represents about 200–500 simultaneous bee stings in a non-sensitized individual. One sting, however, can be fatal in a sensitized person. The general toxicity is not surprising since the most abundant polypeptide component, mellitin, is a potent haemolysin and a mast cell degranulator, another polypeptide, apamin, is a neuro-toxin and the enzyme phospholipase A possesses multiple pharmacological actions. The serious use of such a mixture as a therapeutic agent is scarcely credible despite the enthusiasm of its practitioners (see BECK, 1935). Many of the published reports are impossible to evaluate because of the unscientific way in which the work was carried out. Patients who appeared to respond to venom therapy were receiving other treatments such as enriched diets, heat to the joints, etc., and no controls were used (ANON, 1938). A recent clinical opinion (ANON, 1975) is that it has not been established if bee venom therapy is of any value in treating non-articular rheuma-tism. Any beneficial effect which might occur would appear to result through a counter-irritant mechanism and there is some evidence that stimulation of the adre-nal cortex and the release of natural corticosteroids may be involved (HAMMERAL and PITCHLER, 1960; VICK and BROOKS, 1972).

An unexpected twist to the story has occurred in the last few years. Amongst the basic peptides in bee venom is a relatively minor component containing 22 amino acid residues, which was originally described as a mast cell degranulating peptide MCDP (BREITHAUPT and HABERMANN, 1968). The primary sequence of amino acids was elucidated by HAUX (1969) and subsequently VERNON et al. (1969) determined the position of the two disulphide bridges in the peptide, subsequently designated 401. In earlier studies they had fractionated freeze-dried bee venom, tested all the fractions for anti-inflammatory activity and found such activity to be associated only with the basic peptide fraction (SHIPOLINI et al., 1971 a, b). Using the carrageenin-induced rat paw oedema test, BILLINGHAM et al. (1973) found peptide 401, but not the other basic peptides mellitin and apamin, to possess anti-inflammatory activity. The spectrum of activity was extended to include the accumulation of protein in the synovial cavity of rat knee joints after the intra-articular injection of turpentine, the developing and established adjuvant-induced arthritis in the rat and tests involving the extravasation of protein-bound dye produced by the intradermal injection of a number of inflammatory mediators. The anti-inflammatory activity was found to be produced independently of the local irritant effect of the peptide and was not due to its ability to lyse mast cells. The investigation was taken a stage further by HANSON et al. (1974), who produced evidence that the anti-inflammatory activity was not primarily due to alteration in either vasomotor activity or the release of endogenous cortico-steroids. They concluded that the peptide acted by rendering vascular en-dothelium anergic to inflammatory stimuli.

There are some reservations concerning the possible usefulness of peptide 401 as an anti-inflammatory agent. Firstly, the published work refers only to activity in the rat and the substance appears to be devoid of anti-inflammatory activity in another species, the guinea pig. More importantly, it possesses toxic effects on the central nervous system. Thus, animals given non-lethal doses exhibited a pattern of activity characterised by hyperactivity, continuous tremors and intermittent convulsions (VERNON et al., 1969). Unless the undesirable pharmacological properties can be separated from the anti-inflammatory activity by modifying the chemical structure of the peptide then the therapeutic future does not appear to be rosy. The two disulphide bridges appear to be essential for anti-inflammatory activity since reduction followed by carboxymethylation destroyed such activity (BILLINGHAM et al., 1973) but reduction followed by reoxidation of the corresponding tetrathiol to a mixture of isomeric docasopeptides containing the disulphide bridges, did not (VERNON et al., 1969).

2. Rabbit Skin Protease Inhibitor

Cutaneous Arthus reactions reach a maximum between approximately 4 and 8 h and begin to decline in intensity about 24 h after the injection of the immune reactants (COCHRANE and JANOFF, 1974). One mechanism to explain this reduction in the inflammatory response is destruction of the offending antigen, but an alternative is the presence of inhibitory substances. It has been shown by HAYASHI and his co-workers (HAYASHI, 1975) that SH-dependent proteases are released into the injured sites in cutaneous Arthus reactions and thermal injury in rodents and act as permeability factors. The local concentration of the proteases parallels the increasing intensity of the skin reactions but they become inactivated due to the production of inhibitors. One of these inhibitors has been isolated from bovine, guinea pig and rabbit sera (TOKAJI, 1971) and appears to be a glycoprotein (see Sect. D.VI, 3). The second inhibitor is synthesized locally and was isolated both from the euglobin fraction of burned and active Arthus skin sites (MATSUBA, 1960; HAYASHI et al., 1965) and from cultures of peritoneal mononuclear cells (TOKUDA et al., 1960). It behaved as a homogenous substance on electrophoresis and ultracentrifugation (UDAKA and HAYASHI, 1965a,b) and yielded a mixture of 17 different amino acids on hydrolysis (KAMBARA et al., 1968). No further information about its structure has been published except that it is reported to have a molecular weight of 12000 daltons (TOKAJI, 1971) and to be a peptide (HAYASHI et al., 1969; HAYASHI, 1975).

The potential interest of these observations is that a polypeptide material produced locally in the skin of rodents may limit the development of inflammatory responses by an apparently specific mechanism of action. However, the restricted information available about the characterisation of the protease inhibitor does not allow further conclusions to be drawn.

3. Aprotinin (Trasylol)

The history of aprotinin begins in the late 1920s with the discovery of kallikrein, the enzyme producing kinins from globulin precursors. Shortly after, an inactivator of kallikrein was found in serum and subsequently isolated in a pure form from bovine parotid glands and lung (AUHAGEN, 1967). The inactivator proved to be a basic polypeptide, with a primary sequence of 58 amino acids and 3 disulphide bridges (ANDERER and HÖRNLE, 1965, 1966), which inhibited a variety of proteases including trypsin, chymotrypsin, plasmin and leucocytic proteases (SPILBERG and OSTERLAND, 1970).

The substance was marketed as Trasylol and became a popular form of treatment for acute pancreatitis. The basis for this was a combination of the effectiveness of aprotinin in experimentally induced pancreatitis in the laboratory and the belief that many of the acute manifestations of the human disease are due to the formation of vasoactive peptides by the proteolytic enzymes released from the inflamed pancreas (TRAPNELL, 1972). A number of the earlier reports were favourable but later clinical trials of aprotinin in the treatment of acute pancreatitis showed no benefit from the drug (ANON, 1974). The reputation of the drug was eroded and gradually it fell out of fashion. Interest in the topic has now been reawakened by the results of a prospective randomized double-blind trial of aprotinin in over 100 patients with acute pancreatitis over a 5-year period (TRAPNELL et al., 1974). Statistically significant improvements in the mortality rate and in the course of the disease in the treated patients were reported. A second clinical application of the polypeptide is the treatment for burns (BERTELLI et al., 1969).

Aprotinin has also been studied in irritant-induced paw oedema reactions in the rat. Some workers (DI ROSA and SORRENTINO, 1968; BOLAM et al., 1973) have used it as an investigative substance to assess either the relative importance of kinins in these acute inflammatory reactions or whether other anti-inflammatory drugs interact with the kinin system. FORSTER (1969) investigated the spectrum of activity of aprotinin in various types of rat paw oedemas and concluded that inhibition of plasmin was an important factor in the mode of action of the polypeptide. Other animal studies have been reported by MARTELLI et al. (1969) who found that the intraperitoneal injection of 10000 units of aprotinin/kg in the rat reduced the release of bradykinin by 80% but did not inhibit the development of carrageenin-induced oedema. The injection of 25000 units/kg caused a reduction of 35% in the carrageenin oedema and of 93% in the bradykinin output. MARCY (1972) observed that the anti-carrageenin activity of the polypeptide was enhanced if it was administered locally with the carrageenin. A clinical trial of aprotinin in patients with various joint conditions was carried out by MARCY et al. (1972). The results were variable except that the treatment appeared to be more successful in the patients with inflammatory rather than degenerative conditions.

The obvious disadvantage of aprotinin as a potential anti-rheumatic drug is that it has to be administered by injection. Nevertheless, it is surprising that more controlled clinical trials have not been performed unless its controversial history in acute pancreatitis militated against its use. A further reason may be that it is merely an inhibitor of kinin formation and could only have a limited role to play as an anti-inflammatory agent as shown by its relatively modest performance in animal models.

Other polypeptide substances or mixtures with anti-inflammatory properties are the adrenocorticotrophic hormones and Lysoartrosi (Sect. D.VII.3).

VI. Proteins

1. Exogenous Enzymes

In recent editions of the British "Monthly Index of Medical Specialities" and the American "Physicians Desk Reference", a substantial number of therapeutic preparations, listed as having clinical anti-inflammatory activity, are enzymes. They are obtained from a variety of sources but many, such as trypsin and chymotrypsin, are of animal origin. Their chief clinical usefulness seems to be as prophylactic agents to shorten the course of inflammatory responses which are part of the post-operative trauma after plastic and dental surgery or which follow athletic injuries.

The main reservations about the use of these materials have been admirably summarised (FISHER, 1974) as follows: incredulity that such macromolecules could be absorbed after oral administration, the small number of well-controlled clinical studies compared to the much larger number of testimonials, the inflammagenic (irritant) nature of many of the enzyme preparations and the general ignorance of how they might act.

Some investigators (AMBRUS et al., 1967) have concluded that trypsin and chymotrypsin are absorbed from the gastrointestinal tract into the circulation because of the increased serum concentrations, either of the enzyme activities or of incorporated radioactive tracers, found after the oral administration of the enzyme preparations. There is animal evidence (FISHER, 1974) that orally administered pancreatic enzymes reduce the swelling in a number of paw oedemas.

The clinical data ranges from opinions based on the average recovery time of professional association footballers from soft-tissue and ligamentous injuries to double-blind clinical trials. The following articles comprise a representative cross-section (MOORE, 1963; BERN, 1964; BLONSTEIN, 1967; BOYNE and MEDHURST, 1967; BUCK and PHILLIPS, 1970; DE FIEBRE et al., 1967; BAZERQUE et al., 1972).

The irritancy of the enzyme preparations is of less relevance in oral administration than when the preparations are administered parenterally. Here there is a large body of evidence not only that endogenous proteases may participate in the development of inflammatory reactions but also that exogenous enzymes can act as inflammagenic stimuli (FISHER, 1974). The general consensus of opinion seems to be that the anti-inflammatory effects observed following the injection of a proteolytic enzyme are due to a non-specific counter-irritation mechanism (see Sect. D.VI.3).

The empirical use of many classes of natural drugs in man has never been jeopardised by a lack of knowledge of their modes of action. Whether oral enzymes have a place in therapy will probably depend on purely pragmatic observations that they produce more benefit than alternative available treatments. Despite the earlier controversies about the rationale for their use and their clinical effectiveness (COUNCIL ON DRUGS, 1964) they are still available and widely prescribed.

2. Orgotein

A preparation which has emerged from the patent literature is orgotein. This is the non-proprietory name assigned by the UNITED STATES ADOPTED NAMES COUNCIL (1971) for a group of water-soluble protein congeners containing chelated divalent metals isolatable from liver, red blood cells and other animal tissues. It is available under the trade names Palosein for veterinary treatment and Ontosein for investigational use in human disease.

The history of the preparation is said to have started with some clinical observations on the apparent usefulness of a number of crude preparations of animal organs in ameliorating the inflammatory manifestations of various acute and chronic urological conditions. A search was made for a common constituent of these preparations with anti-inflammatory activity and a series of patents were produced describing the isolation and characterisation of more and more highly purified fractions from sources such as bovine red blood cells and liver (British Patent, 1966; U.S. Patent, 1972).

The preparation isolated from bovine liver behaves as a single component on ultracentrifugation and electrophoresis, has a molecular weight of about 33 000 daltons and its content of Cu and Zn is stated to be particularly important for physiological activity. Similar proteins can be isolated from several tissues of many species and have been described in the literature since 1939 (Mann and Keilin, 1939; Carrico and Deutsch, 1970; Wood et al., 1971).

The only enzymic function discovered for these metalloproteins is as superperoxide dismutases (McCord and Fridovich, 1969). Super-peroxide free radicals have a fleeting existence in aqueous media and their production in biological systems is uncertain. They may be produced by enzymes such as xanthine oxidase and it has been suggested that the possible role of super-peroxide dismutases is to protect organisms against the damaging effects of the free radicals (McCord et al., 1971).

There is very little published information about the anti-inflammatory activity of orgotein. An abstract (Huber et al., 1968) of a paper read at a meeting states that the material is active in several test procedures in rats, guinea pigs and rabbits and that it has been found to be equal to or more potent than prednisone and phenylbutazone on a weight for weight basis. The patents make a number of claims, a typical one (U.S. Patent, 1972) being that it is an effective anti-inflammatory agent in carrageenin-induced rat paw oedema, cotton-pellet-induced rat granuloma, adjuvant-induced rat paw arthritis and antigen-induced guinea pig skin oedema. It is stated to be effective in adrenalectomised animals. A booklet described as providing background data (Fisons, 1973), provides more detail on the material including the results of experiments showing that it possesses significant activity in a number of anti-inflammatory tests in which the inflammatory insult is immunological in nature. Orgotein itself is only a very weak immunogen and does not produce sensitization in either the guinea pig or the horse (Carson et al., 1973). No evidence of any toxic effects in conventional toxicity studies, including reproductive and teratological tests, in mice, rats, rabbits, guinea pigs and monkeys were observed.

The remaining publications on the substance comprise some papers on its use in the treatment of experimental and pathological inflammatory conditions in animals and man. Cushing et al. (1973) described a model of induced inflammation in the horse involving the injection of a counter-irritant, containing iodine, ether, and soybean oil, which achieved a reproducible swelling between the fetlock and carpal joints. The intramuscular injection of 5 mg doses of orgotein for several days after the injection of the irritant caused a significant reduction of the swelling. In another study, Decker et al. (1974) reported that the administration of up to three doses, of between 5 and 15 mg, of orgotein by either local or intra-articular injection caused a rapid response in seventy horses with various joint and limb conditions. The patents also contain a number of claims that racehorses, police horses etc., with conditions described as traumatic arthritis, azoturia and respiratory tract viral infections responded to very small amounts of the material, of the order of several milligrams. A double blind study in which dogs were given a total of 25 mg of orgotein over a period of a week reported that gait impairment associated with pain, due mainly to what is described as a disc syndrome, was markedly improved (Breshears et al.,

1974). Finally, there is a clinical report (MARBERGER et al., 1974) on the treatment of patients with a variety of inflammatory conditions of the urinary tract. It was stated that the drug was not only well tolerated upon systemic administration but gave no side-effects when administered by special routes such as intra-murally by catheter into the bladder wall and locally in the plaques of induration penis plastica. Excellent results were claimed in chronic interstitial cystitis with a particularly good result in the treatment of radiation cystitis in the female.

It is extremely difficult to assess the potential of orgotein as an anti-inflammatory agent, particularly for therapy. There is a paucity of detailed information in the literature about its testing and comparison with other drugs in animal models, the available data being restricted either to claims in patents or statements in abstracts. Nevertheless, it represents a new class of anti-inflammatory agents of animal origin in that it is a metallo-protein material with very weak immunogenic activity which appears to be well tolerated when given by a variety of routes to many species. The veterinary reports, especially those concerned with the horse, are surprising in the small amount of material required for a beneficial effect to be expected. In this species, at least, it appears to act as a homeopathic remedy. It will be of some interest to see if the claims made for the substance in the patent literature are substantiated in carefully controlled animal studies and clinical trials in diseases such as rheumatoid arthritis.

3. Inflamed Tissue Factors

The use of counter-irritants for the relief of inflammation and pain dates back to antiquity. Two thousand years ago the Romans were using stinging nettles to relieve their rheumatism. The term 'counter-irritant' was introduced at the end of the last century (GILLIES, 1895). It was coined to define the phenomenon that irritation leading to inflammation at one site in an organism would counteract subsequent inflammatory responses at remote sites of the same organism (BONTA and NOORDHOEK, 1973). Many mechanisms have been advanced to explain counter-irritation (ATKINSON and HICKS, 1975a). One of the more interesting is that the initial inflammatory reaction may cause the production of endogenous anti-inflammatory substances which enter the circulation and are transported to other parts of the body.

The first report that anti-inflammatory activity could be detected in inflammatory exudates appears to be that of RINDANI (1956). This observation was followed by a minor flood of papers (DI PASQUALE and GIRERD, 1961; DI PASQUALE et al., 1963; ROBINSON and ROBSON, 1964, 1966; BONTA et al., 1970; NOORDHOEK and BONTA, 1974; GARCIA LEME and SCHAPORAL, 1975) showing that inflammatory exudates and perfusates inhibited a variety of inflammatory models including carrageenin-induced paw oedema, adjuvant arthritis, granuloma formation and delayed hypersensitivity.

In a series of publications from a single laboratory (ROBINSON and ROBSON, 1966; BILLINGHAM et al., 1969a, 1969b; BILLINGHAM and ROBINSON, 1972) it has been reported that the anti-inflammatory activity found in inflammatory exudates could be destroyed either by heating above 70° C or by exposure to pronase and that it behaved as a protein on gel chromatography. Furthermore, the anti-inflammatory fraction could be separated by polyacrylamide electrophoresis as a single peak which is virtually devoid of local irritancy. The last finding is of some importance, since a second group of workers (ATKINSON et al., 1969, 1971; ATKINSON and HICKS, 1971, 1975a) have maintained that the anti-inflammatory activity of inflammatory exudates is due to the irritant properties of one or more constituents present. The evidence presented in favour of this contention is the correlation found between the irritant and systemic anti-inflammatory activities of a number of inflammatory exudates. It seems to be suggested that any anti-inflammatory activity occurring in inflammatory exudates produced by the local injection of so-called counter-irritants is itself mediated by a further counter-irritant mechanism. This may lead to semantic confusion unless a more precise and acceptable definition of exactly what is meant by counter-irritation is forthcoming.

A second area of disagreement is whether anti-inflammatory activity can be detected in the blood of animals which have received an inflammatory stimulus. It was first suggested by LADEN et al. (1958) that anti-inflammatory factors are produced at an inflammatory site, enter the bloodstream and exert inhibitory effects on inflammation at distant parts of the body. They reported some preliminary results which indicated that blood taken from silver nitrate–treated rats could produce anti-inflammatory effects when injected into the other rats with pleural inflammation but no details of the work were given. Subsequently, GOLDSTEIN et al. (1967) claimed that in parabiotic rats the systemic anti-inflammatory activity of intraperitoneally administered kaolin was effected by the blood.

ROBINSON and ROBSON (1964) reported that the plasma from adrenalectomized animals implanted with plastic sponges caused a significant reduction in the deposition of granulation tissue around cotton wool pellets in adrenalectomized but not in intact recipient animals. The comparison was made with corresponding saline-treated controls, but when the comparison was made with plasma from animals not implanted with sponges the effect was no longer statistically significant. Thus, the evidence for the presence of the anti-inflammatory factor in plasma was not conclusive. In a later paper (BILLINGHAM et al., 1969a) more acceptable data was produced that serum from adrenalectomized animals, bearing polyester sponges, possessed significant anti-inflammatory activity. The negative findings obtained by DI PASQUALE et al. (1963) were explained as being due to the latter workers using a croton oil pouch technique because the capsule which formed around the pouch may have prevented the passage of the anti-inflammatory substance into the blood. The results have been challenged by ATKINSON and HICKS (1975b) who, in a careful series of experiments, failed to find any anti-inflammatory activity in adrenalectomized rats in which sponges had been implanted, even when the irritancy of the sponge implants had been augmented with croton oil. In additional work they found that no anti-inflammatory activity could be detected in plasma samples obtained from rats treated with doses of acetic acid capable of producing pronounced systemic anti-inflammatory effects. They concluded that the induction of such inflammatory lesions in rats does not appear to lead to detectable release of endogenous anti-inflammatory substances into the circulation.

The resolution of this dispute must await the results of further work but it is of some interest to note that ATKINSON and HICKS (1975b) found a qualitative difference between two strains of rats in their ability to produce anti-inflammatory activity in inflammatory exudates. If there are strain differences then it is more than likely that there are species differences and it will be of some importance to determine whether other and larger mammalian species are able to produce greater quantities of endogenous anti-inflammatory proteins in local inflammatory exudates and whether these may be detected in the circulation. The only available evidence is that inflammatory exudates collected from partial gastrectomy sites in man possess anti-inflammatory activity in the carrageenin-induced rat paw oedema reaction (BILLINGHAM et al., 1969b), that at least one of the proteins in antilymphocytic serum has anti-inflammatory effects in several animal tests (BILLINGHAM et al., 1970) and, less relevantly, that injections of relatively large quantities (2–10 ml) of serum from patients with either active rheumatoid arthritis (HIGHTON, 1963) or from pregnant women (PERSELLIN et al., 1974) have been reported to cause anti-inflammatory effects in animal models.

The anti-inflammatory protein described by ROBINSON and his co-workers is thought to be of hepatic origin on the basis of perfusion experiment using livers from rats in which polyester sponges had been implanted. Considerable anti-inflammatory activity was found in the perfusion plasma of these animals whereas plasma from perfusions of control rat livers did not inhibit the carrageenin-induced rat paw oedema (BILLINGHAM et al., 1971). When the animals were pretreated with actinomycin D, before the removal of the liver for the perfusion studies, the appearance of the anti-inflammatory activity was blocked. A similar observation has been reported by VAN GOOL and LADIGES (1969) except that the anti-inflammatory protein was identified as foetal α_2-globulin. In later work, VAN GOOL et al. (1974) presented evidence that this acute phase protein is present in both inflammatory exudates and the circulation of rats after different types of injury but is absent in the plasma of normal rats. Furthermore, the purified protein inhibited the development of carrageenin-induced rat paw oedema when administered by intravenous injection.

These findings prompt some interesting speculations. Firstly, is the anti-inflammatory protein, described by BILLINGHAM and his co-workers, identical with foetal α_2-globulin or with another acute phase protein? Secondly, are acute phase proteins part of an autoregulatory mechanism in inflammation? Finally, is the liver concerned in the overall control of inflammation? It is possible that an inflammatory insult may cause the local production of a 'triggering' factor, akin to the humoral initiator substance described by BOGDEN et al. (1966). This factor enters the circulation and stimulates the liver to produce acute phase proteins. One or more of these may act as anti-inflammatory substances to limit the further development both of the original reaction and of subsequent inflammatory responses at remote sites. Other proteins with anti-protease activities, including α_2-macroglobulin (BARRET, 1974) and α_1-antitrypsin, have been detected in the synovial fluid of patients with rheumatoid arthritis (CAPSTICK et al., 1975; BRACKERTZ et al., 1975). It has been suggested that these proteins might also exert anti-inflammatory effects in vivo either by limiting tissue damage due to released leucocytic proteases or by stabilizing intralysosomal membranes (see ALLISON and DAVIES, 1974).

4. Antileucotactic Agents

A major aspect of acute and chronic inflammatory reactions is the appearance in the inflammatory exudates of large numbers of leucocytes from the blood. Anti-leucotactic agents could interfere with this phenomenon either by inhibiting chemotaxis, i.e., the directed migration of the white cells, or by affecting the random, i.e. non-directional, migration (GOETZL, 1975). Chemotaxis is a very difficult phenomenon to prove by direct observation in vivo but the circumstantial evidence for the involvement of chemotactic mediators in leucocyte accumulation appears to be overwhelming (GRANT, 1973). A number of such mediators have been identified and the most widely studied are certain peptides, C3a and C5a, derived from the complement cascade (WARD, 1974 b, 1975).

Leucotaxis could be modified by an interference with the production of complement derived chemotactic mediators, either by complete inhibition of the activation of haemolytic complement or by a selective inhibition of the release of the chemotactic peptides. Secondly, the released chemotactic factors could be destroyed, e.g. by enzymatic attack. Finally, an anti-leucotactic agent could antagonise the action of the chemotactic factors on leucocyte cell surfaces. Proteins have been isolated from animal tissues which act by each of these mechanisms.

Natural complement inhibitors include C1 esterase inhibitor C4 inactivator and C6 inactivator (MÜLLER-EBERHARD, 1969; FEARON and AUSTEN, 1975). One of the most interesting regulatory proteins for complement activation is C3b inactivator (KAF). The alternative pathway of complement is activated by its end product, C3b, which interacts with other components of the pathway to produce the enzyme C3 convertase which then acts on more C3. The system is modulated in serum by the presence of C3bI inactivator which enzymically changes C3bI, thus preventing further activation of the pathway. Activation of the alternate pathway of complement is thought to be of some importance in inflammation (ALLISON and DAVIES, 1974; GOLDSTEIN and WEISSMANN, 1974; RUDDY and AUSTEN, 1975). It has recently been suggested (LACHMANN and HALBWACHS, 1975) that C3bI inactivator could be injected locally, e.g. into an inflamed joint, in order to suppress the activation of local complement thus reduce the release of leucotactic peptides. A further potential regulatory substance, which is not a protein, has been isolated from normal human plasma (WALKER et al., 1975 b). This material, termed the human plasma factor, is described in Section D. VIII of the present chapter. It merits mention at this point since its mechanism of action appears to be a selective inhibition of the release of chemotactic factors when complement is activated by the alternative but not by the classical pathway.

Chemotactic factor inactivator is found in small quantities in normal human serum, which, after concentration and partial purification (BERENBERG and WARD, 1973), blocks the actions of a number of chemotactic factors, derived from complement, lymphocytes etc., for both polymorphonuclear and mononuclear phagocytes (WARD and BERENBERG, 1974). Further purification of the active material showed that it contained at least two proteins, one being a 7S β-globulin and the other a 4S α-globulin (TILL and WARD, 1975). Both proteins inactivated chemotactic factors derived from bacteria and also kallikrein but for the complement derived peptides the β-globulin is specific for C3 fragments whereas the α-globulin is specific for C5 chemotactic peptides. These antagonistic activities are heat labile and time, temperature and pH-dependent and it has been suggested that chemotactic factor inactivator is an enzyme. It has the ability to hydrolyse bradykinin but not angiotensin I or angiotensin II (WARD et al., 1974). Both the α- and β-globulin components inactivate the lymphokine macrophage inhibitory factor (WARD and ROCKLIN, 1975) and thus could regulate lymphokine production (see Sect. D.VI.5) not only directly but also indirectly by inactivating C3b. A tryptic digest of C3b, which has similar physical and chemical properties to C3b but has only weak leucotactic properties has been shown to stimulate B lymphocytes to produce the lymphokine, monocyte chemotactic factor. This process occurs with non-transformed cells, in the absence of antigen and without concomitant cellular proliferation, and is evidence that lymphokines may be produced by non-immunological stimuli (SANDBERG et al., 1975).

Elevated levels of chemotactic factor inactivator are found in Hodgkin's disease and cirrhosis (WARD and BERENBERG, 1974; MADERAZO et al., 1975). These clinical states appear to be associated with a decreased ability to produce inflammatory skin reactions and with an increased susceptibility to infections. Similar findings have been described in patients with skin test anergy occurring during acute illness (VAN EPPS et al., 1974). The presence of chemotactic inhibitory activity directly paralleled the skin test anergy. Three separate inhibitors were isolated and some of the published properties suggest that at least one of them is identical to the chemotactic factor inactivator. Although there are raised activities of chemotactic factor inactivator in some disease states there is no apparent correlation with increased quantities of the actual proteins. It has been suggested that this is due to the absence of an antagonist to the inactivator, rather than to increased concentrations of the inactivator protein (SORIANO et al., 1973; HUGHES et al., 1974). Thus, it appears that there may be a complex system of inactivators and inactivator antagonists which may function as a natural anti-inflammatory mechanism, causing the production of antileucotactic, anti-lymphokine and other effects.

The third point of attack for anti-chemotactic factors is to prevent the chemotactic peptides acting on the appropriate receptor sites on leucocyte cell surfaces (SNYDERMAN et al., 1975). An impaired leucotactic responsiveness has been demonstrated in children with recurrent infections but no intrinsic neutrophil defect (WARD and SCHLEGEL, 1969; SMITH et al., 1972). There was evidence of a neutrophil immobilising factor in the serum of the children which was inactivated by normal serum. A second factor, described by GOETZL and AUSTEN (1972) acts directly on leucocytes rendering them unresponsive to chemotactic stimuli. The substance appears to be a small protein, of molecular weight 5000 daltons, which was released by leucocytes during phagocytosis or after exposure to endotoxin and has a much greater effect on polymorphonuclear than on mononuclear phagocytes (GOETZL et al., 1973). The authors suggest that at low concentrations the factor may immobilise neutrophils in inflammatory exudates without affecting phagocytic and other activities but as its concentration increases with time, the factor may preferentially limit the migration of polymorphonuclear leucocytes and thus cause the transition from a predominantly polymorphonuclear cell population to a mononuclear cell population.

Cellular migration could also be affected by modifying the random, i.e. non-directional, migration of leucocytes. Macrophage migration is inhibited by migration-inhibiting factors produced by cultured polymorphonuclear leucocytes (STASTNY and ZIFF, 1970) and by antigen-stimulated lymphocytes (ROCKLIN et al., 1972). The latter cells are also able to produce a leucocyte migration-inhibiting factor (ROCKLIN, 1975). The possible roles and importance of both the above factors and of other lymphokines in inflammatory reactions remains to be elucidated and whether the substances should be considered as either anti-inflammatory or pro-inflammatory remains problematic. It seems highly likely that more controlling mechanisms of chemotaxis will be discovered. Their potential use in therapeutics is uncertain, since the systemic administration of the more general type of inhibitor, such as crude chemotactic factor inactivator preparations, would seem to be undesirable if only on the basis that an increased susceptibility to infection would be expected to occur. Nevertheless, they may have a useful role when injected locally into inflamed sites. More specific anti-chemotactic activities are required and it may well be that subfractionation of the present crude preparations could produce useful and specific antagonists of leucotaxis.

5. Antiproliferative Agents

Chronic inflammatory reactions are characterised by their persistence and tissue responses, i.e. the infiltration of cells of many kinds (SPECTOR, 1974). The basic cell type is the macrophage, derived from circulating monocytes, which may give rise to epithelioid and giant cells but lymphocytes and fibroblasts are prominent constituents of granulomatous deposits. Several mechanisms, including the sustained emigration of mononuclear leucocytes and the proliferation of macrophages, are responsible for the maintenance of chronic inflammation. Anti-leucotactic agents (Sect. D.VI.4) which inhibit the chemotaxis of mononuclear leucocytes, would be expected to interfere with chronic inflammatory reactions but another point of attack is on the mitotic division of macrophages in the lesions. Any cytostatic or cytotoxic agent could affect the development of chronic granulomata and the natural adrenal corticosteroids may affect the mitotic rate (FISHER, 1974). Conventional anti-rheumatic drugs have been reported to suppress the proliferation of granulation tissue (KULONEN and POTILA, 1975).

A group of natural substances which may be relevant to this area are the chalones (FISHER, 1974). These have been defined as substances produced by a tissue which inhibits the rate of cell production in that tissue. Theoretically there are as many chalones as there are cell types and each is specific for its own type. Furthermore, those chalones which have been isolated although tissue specific are not species specific suggesting that they may be potential therapeutic agents. Thus, it is possible to envisage a chalone produced from macrophages in one species that might inhibit the proliferation of macrophages in chronic granulomatous lesions in another species. One lymphoid chalone from the spleen of various species has been isolated by HOUCK et al. (1971) and characterised as a protein with a molecular weight between 30000 and 50000 daltons and a second, described as a protein-fraction, has been extracted from bovine spleen (GARCIA-GIRALT et al., 1970).

Lymphocytes, when exposed to mitogens and antigens, undergo a transformation and liberate a group of biologically active substances termed lymphokines. Their effects on cell proliferation range from stimulation to cytotoxicity. Antiproliferative activities which have been distinguished include cloning inhibition factor, lymphotoxin and proliferation inhibition factor (JEFFES and GRANGER, 1975), although it is not yet clear if these are separate substances. The presence of macrophages as well as lymphocytes is required to produce other lymphokines such as monocyte chemotactic factor, macrophage activating factor, migration inhibitory factor (MIF) and lymphocyte proliferation factor (NELSON and LEU, 1975; WAHL et al., 1975).

Macrophages alone are capable of producing substances affecting their proliferation when cultured in vitro. One of particular interest is a factor of molecular weight less than 1400 daltons which is not a peptide and is capable of reversibly inhibiting thymidine incorporation and proliferation in a number of cell lines (WALDMAN and GOTTLIEB, 1973; CALDERON et al., 1974; CALDERON and UNANAE, 1975). It is proposed that the substance acts as a neutral anti-proliferative agent in situations where macrophages conglomerate around target cells as in granulomata. A second factor, which may be a small peptide is released by macrophages, lymphocytes or HeLa cells in culture and acts as an inhibitor of protein biosynthesis in vitro (ULRICH, 1974). Macrophages also release immunoregulatory globulins (COOPERBAND et al., 1972) and another factor (NELSON, 1973) which inhibits lymphocyte transformation and hence would lead to a decrease in the production of lymphokines in mixed populations of the cell types.

The major difficulties with antiproliferative factors from animal cells are their multiplicity, interrelationships, and relative lack of characterisation. This aspect of inflammation is a virtually unexplored topic and could yield some extremely interesting anti-inflammatory agents. The concept that some of the more important cell types involved in chronic inflammation produce factors which may limit their own proliferation and that of other cells is most attractive. Factors of low molecular weight rather than macromolecules are of particular interest since they could both be synthesized and act as models for new classes of anti-inflammatory drugs.

6. Antilymphocytic Serum

A marked feature of the various antilymphocytic sera is their mulitplicity of actions (TURK and WILLOUGHBY, 1969). The materials, generically termed ALS, are widely known for their ability to impair immunological responsiveness especially of cell-mediated immunity. They have been used as adjuncts in immunosuppressive therapy after renal and liver transplantation in man and one of the experimental indices to assess their immunosuppressive potency is the survival of homografts in animals. The main immunosuppressive component of ALS in vivo is an IgG immunoglobulin (ALG) and it is of great interest to determine whether this constituent is solely responsible for the various anti-inflammatory activities of ALS preparations. The effectiveness of ALS in Arthus reactions and adjuvant-induced arthritis in the rat (CURREY and ZIFF, 1966) is explicable on this basis, since immune disturbances are prominent in these experimental models. The anti-inflammatory activity against carrageenin-induced paw oedema is less straightforward, particularly as there is evidence (PERPER et al., 1969) that the immunosuppressive and anti-carrageenin activities of ALS preparations, collected at different time intervals after the immunisation of horses with rat spleen lymphocytes, did not run parallel.

Antilyphocytic sera, produced by immunising rabbits with either rat or guinea pig thymocytes, were tested by BILLINGHAM et al. (1970) against skin homograft survival and carrageenin-induced oedema anti-inflammatory reactions in the rat. The anti-rat preparation was active in both tests and when it was fractionated on a Sephadex column the IgG fraction was again active in the two tests, but a second protein fraction possessed anti-inflammatory but not immunosuppressive activity. The anti-guinea pig preparation was inactive in the immunosuppressive reaction but active in the anti-inflammatory test. Fractionation as before showed that the IgG compound was inactive whereas the second protein fraction contained the anti-inflammatory activity. It was concluded that there are two anti-inflammatory components in ALS but only one of them, the IgG immunoglobulin, had species specificity. Further studies on the anti-inflammatory spectrum of antithymocytic serum have been carried out by Teodorczyk et al. (1975). It was found that the preparation possesses a non-specific anti-inflammatory activity besides the specific action on lymphocytes, that the mechanism of this action did not involve an antagonism of chemical mediators of inflammation, including histamine, 5-HT bradykinin and prostaglandin E_2, but that it may be concerned with depletion of circulating complement. Similar observations were reported in earlier work by Turk et al. (1968) except that conflicting results on the antiproliferative activity of the ALS preparation were observed. It therefore appears that ALS preparations contain not only antibodies directed against lymphocytes but also one or more proteins with non-specific anti-inflammatory activities. It has been suggested that this second group of proteins may be identical to inflamed tissue factors (Sect. D.VI.3). Theoretically, the production of specific antisera against components of inflammatory reactions should not only provide information about the relative importance, if any, of these components in acute and chronic inflammation but also yield potential therapeutic agents. While ALS and ALG preparations have been used therapeutically as immunosuppressive preparations there are difficulties, such as foreign protein reactions and the risk of enhancing malignant conditions, which militate against their widespread employment in the more chronic rheumatic diseases. A recent account of the therapeutic uses of ALG in autoimmune diseases including polyarthritis, states that the results of clinical trials are mostly still inconclusive although occasional positive results have been reported (Balnec and Brendel, 1974).

VII. Tissue Hydrolysates

1. Catrix

The topical application of powdered cartilage to sutured abdominal incisions in the rat has been found to cause an increase of 20% in the tensile strength of the wounds (Prudden et al., 1957). This observation was followed by a number of papers in which the local and parenteral use of preparations of cartilage, from a variety of animal sources, was reported to accelerate the rate of healing both of closed incised and open granulating wounds (Houck et al., 1962; Prudden et al., 1963; Sabo et al., 1965). The preparation which has been most widely used in recent years is catrix, defined as an activated acid pepsin-digested tracheal cartilage of calf origin. In addition to its wound-healing properties it has been stated to possess both experimental anti-inflammatory and clinical anti-rheumatic actions. It is claimed that catrix is equivalent to indomethacin as an anti-inflammatory agent in both carrageenin-induced paw oedema and adjuvant-induced arthritis tests in the rat (Prudden, 1975). Furthermore it has been reported to produce clinical improvement in patients with rheumatoid arthritis, psoriasis and progressive systemic sclerosis (Prudden and Balassa, 1974).

The active material in the hydrolysed cartilage extract with respect to its wound-healing properties was stated to be a protein, perhaps associated with an acid mucopolysaccharide (PRUDDEN et al., 1963). Similar properties were found with various kinds of animal chitins, which are polymers of N-acetylglucosamine (PRUDDEN et al., 1970). However, the polymeric forms of N-acetylglycosamine are only weakly anti-inflammatory according to PRUDDEN and BALASSA (1974), and these authors suggest that catrix, being composed of polysaccharides and glycoproteins, acts by coating cellular membranes and preventing auto-immune reactions.

2. Livingston Lysate

Filtrates of fresh mammalian tissues, including human placenta, incubated under pressure in the presence of unknown populations of micro-organisms were reported by LIVINGSTON (1958) to cause the regression of spontaneous tumours in dogs and cats. In a later paper (LIVINGSTON et al., 1959), the preparation was modified by the addition of antibiotics to yield a sterile autolysate of human placental tissue which possessed anti-tumour activity in mice with transplanted lymphosarcomas. This preparation, which is apparently devoid of any experimental anti-inflammatory properties either in vitro or in vivo, was used by MAXSON and COMPTON (1969) in a double-blind study, versus a placebo composed of an amino acid mixture, in patients with rheumatoid arthritis and osteoarthritis. Their reason for the investigation appears to be based on the non sequitur that, since pregnant women suffering from one of the systemic rheumatic diseases sometimes have remissions during gestation, a lysate of human placental tissue was worthy of trial as a possible anti-arthritic agent. Nevertheless, they found a statistically significant improvement in pain symptoms and functional disabilities and emphasised the lack of adverse reactions to the lysate. The chemical complexity of the material renders any evaluation of a possible active constituent to pure speculation although it is stated by MAXSON and COMPTON (1969) that it may be either a nucleotide or polynucleotide.

3. Lysoartrosi

This preparation is a commercially available hydrolysate of bovine spleen which contains a mixture of amino acids and polypeptides. The material has been separated on DEAE cellulose as the copper complexes into five main fractions, (CORNET et al., 1971). Some of the fractions containing polypeptides have been reported to exert a variety of experimental anti-inflammatory activities both in vivo and in vitro. Thus, they may act either independently or synergystically on carrageenin- and 5-HT-induced paw oedema in the rat and on the extravasation of protein-bound dye after the intradermal injection of 5-HT (PACINI and GOMARASCA, 1971; D'ATRI and GOMARASCA, 1971). As well as anti-5-HT effects, the polypeptide fractions exert antihistamine, anti-bradykinin and anti-prostaglandin activities in organ bath experiments (GOMARASCA and D'ATRI, 1971; GOMARASCA et al., 1971; D'ATRI et al., 1972). The material has also been reported to interact with circulating complement in the rat in vivo causing a decreased haemolysis (CERUTTI and FORLANI, 1974). Finally, there are claims that lysoartrosi is useful in the management of symptoms in patients with recurrent arthrosis (MANCA and BERTINI, 1971; ZANASI et al., 1971).

The available information on lysoartrosi is too limited for any precise opinion on its anti-inflammatory or anti-rheumatic potential to be formulated. The polypeptide components appear to be responsible for its biological activities but considerable work needs to be done on their separation and characterisation. The published material shows that there is a wide range of interactions with the effects of the common mediators of inflammation suggesting that these may be produced at receptor sites rather than on either biosynthetic or release mechanisms.

VIII. Human Plasma Factor

A substance of low molecular weight, below 1000 daltons, has been reproducibly separated from pooled human plasma by a stepwise process involving ultrafiltration followed by column chromatography using Sephadex G25·and ion exchange resins (Ford-Hutchinson et al., 1973; Walker et al., 1975a). Little has been published on the chemical characterisation of the material, termed human plasma factor (HPF), except that it is not a linear peptide or similar molecule. However, it has an interesting range of experimental anti-inflammatory activity (Smith and Ford-Hutchinson, 1975) as shown in Table 2.

Thus it shows anti-inflammatory activity against the carrageenin-induced paw swelling in several species. The intravenous injection of single doses 30 min before the subplantar administration of the irritant causes an inhibition of the paw oedema up to 80% and the effect may be considerably prolonged by giving spaced injections (Ford-Hutchinson et al., 1974). Although it shows activity in an acceptable range of animal tests (see Table 1) it possesses neither analgesic nor antipyretic properties (Smith et al., 1974a) and did not affect either the persistence or the proliferation of mononuclear cells in chronic granulomatous deposits after the implantation of either cotton wool pellets or polyvinyl sponges (Elliott et al., 1974a).

The possible mechanisms of action of the plasma factor have also received some attention. Intravenous injection of HPF inhibited carrageenin-induced paw oedema in adrenalectomized as well as intact rats, did not affect blood pressure of anaesthetised animals and only caused a very minor degree of local irritation (Elliott et al., 1974b). Its lack of activity in the dextran anaphylactoid reaction, in passive cutaneous anaphylaxis and in the cutaneous responses to the intradermal injection of histamine, 5-HT, bradykinin and prostaglandins, suggested that it did not act primarily by interfering with chemical mediators of inflammation. This conclusion was confirmed by the results of further work; groups of rats were either pretreated with substances which depleted preformed stores of mediators or inhibited their formation or release, or treated with antagonists which blocked the actions of the released mediators during the experiments (Bolam et al., 1973; Smith et al., 1974b). No evidence of a primary interference with either the biosynthesis, release or action of either vasoactive amines, kinins or prostaglandins was obtained.

A significant observation in the experiments with cutaneous reactions was the contrast between the activity of HPF in the Arthus test and its lack of effect in passive cutaneous anaphylaxis. The former reaction is dependent on leucocyte migration (Cochrane and Janoff, 1974) and HPF significantly reduced the infiltration of polymorphonuclear and mononuclear leucocytes into the inflammatory exudates produced by the intrapleural,injection of turpentine and carrageenin in the rat. A sizeable inhibition, amounting to 90%, occurred with the emigration of both cell types into the exudates found in porous inert sponges implanted subdermally (Ford-Hutchinson et al., 1975).

Table 2. Spectrum of anti-inflammatory activity of HPF active against

Test system	Species
Active against:	
Acute paw oedemas	
Carrageenin	Rat, Mouse Guinea pig
Dextran	Rat
Kaolin	Rat
Yeast	Rat
Zymosan	Rat
Adjuvant arthritis	Rat
Ultraviolet erythema	Guinea pig
Reversed passive Arthus	Rat, Rabbit
Extravasation of protein-bound dye after intradermal injection of irritants	Rat
Turpentine- and carrageenin-induced pleurisy	Rat
Leucocyte emigration in implanted sponge	Rat, Mouse
Chemotaxis of leucocytes (Boyden chamber)	Rat, Man
Inactive against:	
Systemic dextran anaphylactoid reaction	Rat
Passive cutaneous anaphylaxis	Rat
Extravasation of protein-bound dye after intradermal injection of mediators	Rat
Xylene ear test	Mouse
Granuloma formation	Rat, Mouse
Analgesic tests:	
Hot plate	Mouse
Phenylquinone writhing	Mouse
Endotoxin-induced pyrexia	Rabbit

The next step was an exploration of possible interactions of HPF with leucotactic mediators. Those derived from the complement cascade are thought to be of particular importance (WARD, 1974a), HPF interfered with the release of the complement-derived chemotactic peptides rather than with their effects on the leucocyte cell surfaces (WALKER et al., 1975a, b). Furthermore, this inhibition occurred only when complement was activated by endotoxin and zymosan (alternative or properdin pathway) and not by antigen-antibody complexes (classical pathway) and was more pronounced for the human complement-leucocyte system than in corresponding animal systems (WALKER et al., 1975a). The experiments were performed using in vitro Boyden chamber technique and the findings were confirmed by independent measurement of the release of anaphylatoxin activity from human and guinea pig serum (WALKER et al., 1975). It was suggested that the mechanism of the anti-inflammatory action in vivo of HPF involves a local and selective inhibition of the release of complement-derived chemotactic factors possibly due to an interference with the C3 activator system thus checking the invasion of developing inflammatory exudates by leucocytes (WALKER et al., 1975).

The existence of a substance in normal human plasma with a wide range of experimental anti-inflammatory activity in animal models and an apparently specific mode of action raises some interesting questions. Is it one of the naturally occurring control mechanisms in inflammation and what is its relevance to the human rheumatic diseases? However, more information must be obtained about its chemistry and biological activity in man before its therapeutic potential can be assessed.

IX. Prostaglandins

The possible roles of the prostaglandins as either mediators or modulators of inflammatory reactions is described elsewhere (Chaps. 17 and 31). An aspect of these substances which merits attention in the present account is the anti-inflammatory activities of this class of mediators.

It was first reported by ASPINALL and CAMMARATA (1969) that PGE_2 in a dose of 500 µg given twice daily inhibited the development of adjuvant-induced arthritis in the rat but did not affect either carrageenin-induced paw oedema or the granuloma pellet reaction in the same species. A number of authors (ZURIER and QUAGLIATA, 1971; GLENN and ROHLOFF, 1972; ASPINALL et al., 1974; ZURIER and WEISSMANN, 1972; DI PASQUALE et al., 1973) have confirmed and extended these observations. Prostaglandins other than PGE_2 were found to exert anti-inflammatory effects by some but not by all workers and the spectrum of anti-inflammatory activity was extended to include mycoplasma-induced arthritis and further types of rat pedal oedema.

The common factor in all the published work is the high doses of prostaglandins employed. Indeed the term 'heroic' is not inappropriate since amounts ranging from 0.5 to 10 mg were administered either as single or repeated injections. It is therefore not surprising to discover that the mechanism of the anti-inflammatory effects has been ascribed to non-specific actions. One of these is prostration due to salt deficiency (GLENN and ROHLOFF, 1972) since diarrhoea is a manifestation occurring in the rat (ZURIER and QUAGLIATA, 1971). Another is adrenocortical stimulation because such doses of prostaglandins cause adrenal hyperplasia (GLENN et al., 1972) and the release of pituitary ACTH (DEWIED et al., 1969). A third is vascular disturbances, particularly as other unrelated vasoactive drugs, such as isoprenaline, digitonin and ethyl alcohol, are capable of inducing similar experimental anti-inflammatory effects (GLENN and ROHLOFF, 1972). Nevertheless, some more specific modes of action have been suggested including inhibition of macrophage migration factor (ASPINALL et al., 1974), an interference with the release of lysosomal enzymes (ZURIER and WEISSMANN, 1972) and an effect on lymphocyte transformation (ZURIER and QUAGLIATA, 1971).

There are a few other points of interest with respect to the possible involvement of the prostaglandins as controlling agents in inflammatory reactions. One is the distribution of the various members, in particular those of the E and F series in various inflammatory exudates. The results of VELO et al. (1973) and GIROUD et al. (1974) have revealed that in carrageenin-induced pleurisy and peritonitis the initial rise in E-type prostaglandins is succeeded at later time intervals by a rise in the relative content of F-type prostaglandins. It was tentatively suggested that these are antagonistic activities of the two types of prostaglandins and that they may balance the effects of each other. Also there is evidence that the prostaglandins may stimulate the production of cyclic nucleotides, that these are opposing activities of cAMP and cGMP and that while PGE_2 affects cAMP, $PGF_{2\alpha}$ perferentially affects cGMP (PAOLETTI et al., 1974; KUEHL, 1974). Thus, attention is now being directed to the possible roles of cyclic nucleotide concentrations and ratios in the control of inflammation.

E. Summary and Conclusions

The impression gained after reviewing anti-inflammatory agents of animal origin is one of disappointment. Many substances have been studied with high hopes that have not been realised either because of ineradicable and unacceptable toxicity or because the experimental and clinical activities have not compared favourably with the conventional and unsatisfactory anti-rheumatic drugs in current use.

In the introduction two main reasons were given why natural anti-inflammatory substances should be taken seriously. The first is that they could serve as models for novel anti-inflammatory drugs. It is materials of low molecular weight which are of immediate interest in this context since they are more likely to be identified and serve as the basis of synthetic programmes. Very few substances of low molecular weight from animal tissues possess both a high and useful spectrum of anti-inflammatory activity either in the laboratory or the clinic. Neither the alkoxyglycerols nor N(2-ethoxy)palmitamide have fulfilled their early promise and the pilot studies on small peptides do not appear promising. Substances of potential interest comprise the antiproliferative factor of CALDERON et al. (1974) and the human plasma factor (Sect. D.VIII), but too little is known about either their chemical nature or possible effectiveness in man for useful conclusions to be drawn at this stage.

The polypeptides have not been rewarding. Lysoartrosi is still an undefined mixture, the polypeptide fraction described by HAYASHI as a protease inhibitor in rabbit skin has not been characterised and aprotinin is a curiously vague material with respect to inflammatory reactions. The most promising is peptide 401 but the inherent toxicity of the intact molecule militates against its therapeutic use. There has been no indication either that anti-inflammatory activity is associated with part of the structure or that minor chemical modifications could dissociate toxicity from anti-inflammatory activity. Systematic synthesis of related structures would be an awesome task since the number of structural variants of a peptide with 22 residues is 10^{28}.

It is even less likely that macromolecules, such as proteins, could be considered as models for synthetic programmes. Nevertheless it is this class of anti-inflammatory agents of animal origin which is of greater interest biologically. Some of the antileucotactic and antiproliferative proteins and also the acute phase proteins are of particular importance since they may act as autoregulatory factors in inflammation. Their interrelationships, functions and activities in vivo merit special attention in the near future. It is in this area that useful information about natural regulatory mechanisms in acute and chronic inflammatory processes might accrue and lead to the development of suitable methodology for detecting types of anti-inflammatory activity more relevant to human disease. The era of screening programmes designed to produce drugs which only mimic the existing unsatisfactory drugs should then die a natural and unlamented death.

References

Allison, A. C., Davies, P.: Mechanisms underlying chronic inflammation. In: Velo, G. P., Willoughby, D. A., Giroud, J. P. (Eds.): Future Trends in Inflammation, pp. 449—480. Padua: Piccin Medical Books 1974

Ambrus, J. L., Lassmann, H. B., De Marchi, J. J.: Absorption of exogenous and endogenous proteolytic enzymes. Clin. Pharmacol. Ther. **8**, 362—368 (1967)

Anderer, F. A., Hörnle, S.: Strukturuntersuchungen am Kallikrein-Inaktivator aus Rinderlunge: I. Molekulargewicht, Endgruppenanalyse und Aminosäure-Zusammensetzung. Z. Naturforsch. **20**, 457 (1965)

Anderer, F. A., Hörnle, S.: The disulfide linkages in kallikrein inactivator of bovine lung. J. biol. Chem. **241**, 1568—1572 (1966)

Anon.: Bee venom for arthritis. Brit. med. J. (1938) **I**, 858

Anon.: Bee venom therapy for rheumatism. Brit. med. J. (1975) **II**, 440

Anon.: Trasylol for pancreatitis. Brit. med. J. (1974) **III**, 133—134

Aspinall, R. L., Cammarata, P. S.: Effect of prostaglandin E_2 on adjuvant arthritis. Nature **224**, 1320—1321 (1969)

Aspinall, R. L., Cammarata, P. S., Nukao, A., Jiu, J., Miyano, M., Baker, D. E., Pautsch, W. F.: Effects of various prostaglandins on two laboratory models of chronic arthritic inflammation. Advanc. Biosci. **9**, 419—425 (1974)

Atkinson, D. C., Boura, A. L., Hicks, R.: Observations on the pharmacological properties of inflammatory exudate. Europ. J. Pharmacol. **8**, 348—354 (1969)

Atkinson, D. C., Hicks, R.: Relationship between the anti-inflammatory and irritant properties of inflammatory exudate. Brit. J. Pharmacol. **41**, 480—487 (1971)

Atkinson, D. C., Hicks, R.: The anti-inflammatory activity of irritants. Agents Actions **5**, 239—249 (1975a)

Atkinson, D. C., Hicks, R.: The possible occurrence of endogenous anti-inflammatory substances in the blood of injured rats. Brit. J. Pharmacol. **53**, 85—91 (1975b)

Atkinson, D. C., Whittle, B. A., Hicks, R.: A further observation on the anti-inflammatory activity of inflammatory exudate. Europ. J. Pharmacol. **16**, 254—256 (1971)

Auhagen, E.: Chemistry and biochemistry of trasylol. In: Leonardi, A., Walsh, J. (Eds.): Drugs of Animal Origin, pp. 69—79. Proceedings of the First International Symposium, Milan: Ferro Edizioni 1967

Bachur, N. R., Masek, K., Melmon, K. L., Udenfriend, S.: Fatty acid amides of ethanolamine in mammalian tissues. J. biol. Chem. **240**, 1019—1024 (1965)

Bailey, K. R., Sheffner, A. L.: The reduction of experimentally induced inflammation by sulfhydryl compounds. Biochem. Pharmacol. **16**, 1175—1182 (1967)

Balnec, H., Brendel, W.: The use of antilymphocyte serum in clinical practice. In: Brent, L., Holborrow, I. (Eds.): Progress in Immunology, Vol. II, Vol. V, pp. 401—403. New York: American Elsevier Publishing Co. 1974

Barret, A. J.: The function of α_2 macroglobulin: control of extracellular proteolytic activity. In: Velo, G. P., Willoughby, D. A., Giroud, J. P. (Eds.): Future Trends in Inflammation, pp. 429—432. Padua: Piccin Medical Books 1974

Bazerque, P. M., Galmarini, J. C., Evangelista, J. C.: Prueva Ciega Doble Sobre el Efecto Anti-Inflamatorio de Enzimas Proteoliticas. Medicina (B. Aires) **32**, 357—362 (1972)

Beck, B.: Bee Venom Therapy: Bee Venom, Its Nature, and Its Effect on Arthritic and Rheumatoid Conditions. New York: Appleton-Century 1935

Benevuti, F., Lattanzi, F., De Gori, A., Tarli, P.: Effects of some palmitoyl ethanolamide derivatives on carrageenan-induced rat paw oedema. Boll. Soc. ital. Biol. sper. **44**, 809—813 (1968)

Berenberg,J.L., Ward,P.A.: Chemotactic inactivator in normal human serum. J. clin. Invest. **52**, 1200—1206 (1973)

Bern,G.: Clinical trial of an oedema-reducing preparation, α-chymotrypsin. Acta chir. scand. **127**, 35—38 (1964)

Bertelli,A., Donati,L., Marek,J.: Pharmacological treatment in burns. In: Bertelli,A., Houck,J.C. (Eds.): Inflammatory Biochemistry and Drug Interactions. International Symposium, Como, p.66. Amsterdam: Excerpta Medica 1969

Billingham,M.E.J., Gordon,A.H., Robinson,B.V.: Role of the liver in inflammation. Nature (New Biol.) **231**, 26—27 (1971)

Billingham,M.E.J., Morley,J., Hanson,J.M., Shipolini,R.A., Vernon,C.A.: An anti-inflammatory peptide from bee venom. Nature (New Biol.) **245**, 163—164 (1973)

Billingham,M.E.J., Robinson,B.V.: Separation of irritancy from the anti-inflammatory component of inflammation exudate. Brit. J. Pharmacol. **44**, 317—320 (1972)

Billingham,M.E.J., Robinson,B.V., Gaugas,J.M.: Two anti-inflammatory components in anti-lymphocytic serum. Nature (Lond.) **227**, 276—277 (1970)

Billingham,M.E.J., Robinson,B.V., Robson,J.M.: Partial purification of the anti-inflammatory factor(s) in inflammatory exudate. Brit. J. Pharmacol. **35**, 543—557 (1969a)

Billingham,M.E.J., Robinson,B.V., Robson,J.M.: Anti-inflammatory properties of human inflammatory exudate. Brit. med. J. **(1969c)** II, 93—96

Billingham,M.E.J., Robinson,B.V., Robson,J.M.: The partial purification of anti-inflammatory factor(s) found during experimental and clinical inflammation. In: Bertelli,A., Houck,J.C. (Eds.): Inflammation Biochemistry and Drug Interaction, pp.204—209. Amsterdam: Excerpta Medica Foundation 1969b

Blonstein,J.L.: Oral enzyme tablets in the treatment of boxing injuries. Practitioner **198**, 547—548 (1967)

Bodman,J., Maisin,J.H.: The α glyceryl ethers. Clin. chim. Acta **3**, 253—274 (1958)

Bogden,A.E., Gray,J.H., Fuss,F.R.: Initiation of alpha-2-glycoprotein synthesis by a trauma-associated humoral factor. Proc. Amer. Ass. cancer Res. **7**, 8A (1966)

Bolam,J.P., Elliott,P.N.C., Ford-Hutchinson,A.W., Smith,M.J.H.: Histamine, 5-hydroxytryptamine, kinins and the anti-inflammatory activity of human plasma fraction in carrageenin-induced paw oedema in the rat. J. Pharm. (Lond.) **26**, 434—440 (1973)

Bonta,I.L., Bhargava,N., De Vos,C.J.: Specific oedema-inhibiting property of a natural anti-inflammatory factor collected from inflamed tissue. Experentia (Basel) **26**, 759—760 (1970)

Bonta,I.L., Noordhoek,J.: Anti-inflammatory mechanism of inflamed-tissue factor. Agents Actions **3**, 348—356 (1973)

Borden,A.L., Wallraff,E.B., Brodie,E.C., Holbrook,W.P., Hill,D.F., Stephens,C.A.L., Kent,L.J., Kammerer,J.R.: Plasma levels of free amino acids in normal subjects compared with patients with rheumatoid arthritis. Proc. Soc. exp. Biol. (N.Y.) **75**, 28—30 (1950)

Boyden,S.: The chemotactic effect of mixtures of antibody and antigen on polymorphonuclear leucocytes. J. exp. Med. **115**, 453—466 (1962)

Boyne,P.S., Medhurst,H.: Oral anti-inflammatory enzyme therapy in injuries to professional footballers. Practitioner **198**, 543—546 (1967)

Brackertz,D., Hagmann,J., Kueppers,F.: Proteinase inhibitors in rheumatoid arthritis. Ann. rheum. Dis. **34**, 225—230 (1975)

Breithaupt,H., Habermann,E.: Mastzelldegranulierendes Peptid (MCD-peptid) aus Bienengift: Isolierung biochemische und pharmakologische Eigenschaften. Naunyn-Schmiedeberg's Arch. exp. Path. Pharmak. **261**, 252—270 (1968)

Breshears,D.E., Brown,C.D., Riffel,D.M., Cobble,R.J., Chessman,S.F.: Evaluation of orgotein in treatment of locomotor dysfunction in dogs. Mod. vet. Pract. **55**, 85—93 (1974)

British Patent: Therapeutically active metal chelates of proteins. No.1, 160, 151 (1966)

Brock,J., Field,E.J.: Unsaturated fatty acids and transplantation. Lancet **(1975)** I, 1382—1383

Brown,J.H., Mackey,H.K.: Further studies on erythrocyte anti-inflammatory assay. Proc. Soc. exp. Biol. (N.Y.) **128**, 504—509 (1968)

Brown,J.H., Pollock,S.H.: Stabilization of hepatic lysosomes of rats by vitamin E and selenium in vivo as indicated by thermal labilization of isolated lysosomes. J. Nutr. **102**, 1413—1419 (1972)

Buchar,E., Masek,K., Obermajerova,H., Seifert,J., Havlik,I.: Lipid-induced changes of pentobarbital distribution and metabolism. Pharmacology (Basel) **10**, 152—160 (1973)

Buck, J. E., Phillips, N.: Trial of chymoral in professional footballers. Brit. J. clin. Prac. **24**, 375—377 (1970)

Burford, R. G., Gowdey, C. W.: Anti-inflammatory activity of alkoxyglycerols in rats. Arch. int. Pharmacodyn. **173**, 56—70 (1968)

Calderon, J., Unanue, E. R.: Two biological activites regulating cell proliferation found in cultures of peritoneal exudate cells. Nature (Lond.) **253**, 359—361 (1975)

Calderon, J., Williams, R. T., Unanue, E. R.: An inhibitor of cell proliferation released by cultures of macrophages. Proc. nat. Acad. Sci. (Wash.) **71**, 4273—4277 (1974)

Capstick, R. B., Lewis, D. A., Cosh, J. A.: Naturally occurring anti-inflammatory factors in the synovial fluid of patients with rheumatic disease and their possible mode of action. Ann. rheum. Dis. **34**, 213—218 (1975)

Carrico, R. J., Deutsch, H. F.: The presence of zinc in human cytocuprein and some properties of the apoprotein. J. biol. Chem. **245**, 723—727 (1970)

Carson, S., Vogin, E. E., Huber, W., Schulte, T. L.: Safety test of orgotein, an anti-inflammatory protein. Toxicol. appl. Pharmacol. **26**, 184—202 (1973)

Cerutti, S., Forlani, A.: Interzione in vivo di una Preparazione Biologica ad Attivata Antinflammatoria verso il Complemento. Gazz. med. ital. **133**, 537—546 (1974)

Coburn, A. F., Graham, C. E., Haninger, J.: The effect of egg yolk in diets on anaphylactic arthritis (passive Arthus phenomenon) in the guinea-pig. J. exp. Med. **100**, 425—435 (1954)

Coburn, A. F., Moore, L. V.: Nutrition as a conditioning factor in the rheumatic state. Amer. J. Dis. Child. **65**, 744—756 (1943)

Coburn, A. F., Rich, H.: A limited clinical evaluation of an egg yolk fraction in the prevention of Rheumatic recurrences. A. I. R. Arch. interamer. Rheum. (Rio de J.) **4**, 498—515 (1960)

Cochrane, G. G., Janoff, A.: The Arthus reaction: a model of neutrophil and complement-mediated injury. In: Zweifach, B. W., Grant, L., McCluskey, R. T. (Eds.): The Inflammatory Process, 2nd Ed., Vol. III, pp. 85—162. New York: Academic Press 1974

Cooperband, S. R., Badger, A. M., Davis, R. C., Schmidt, K., Mannick, J. A.: The effect of immunoregulation α globulin (IRA) upon lymphocytes in vitro. J. Immunol. **109**, 154—163 (1972)

Cornet, F., De Marchi, G., Scolastico, C.: Isolamento e Carraterizzazione dei Polipeptidi ottenuti da Lysoartrosi. Minerva med. (Torino) **62**, 65—70 (1971)

Council of Drugs: Enzymes proposed as systemic anti-inflammatory agents. J. Amer. med. Ass. **188**, 875—876 (1964)

Currey, H. F. L., Ziff, M.: Suppression of experimentally induced polyarthritis in the rat by heterologous anti-lymphocyte serum. Lancet **(1966)**II, 889—891

Cushing, L. S., Decker, W. E., Santos, F. K., Schulte, T. L., Huber, W.: Orgotein therapy for inflammation in horses. Mod. vet. Pract. **54**, 17—21 (1973)

D'Atri, G., Galimberti, E., Mascaretti, L.: Attivata di una Preparazione Bioligica e di Frazioni Polipeptidi in essa contenute verso L'azione contratterante delle Prostaglandine. Boll. chim.-farm. **111**, 616—625 (1972)

D'Atri, G., Gomarasca, M.: Attivita del Lysoartrosi o dei Polipeptidi in esso contenuti Sull'inflammazione Indotta da Serotina. Minerva med. (Torino) **62**, 71—87 (1971)

Davis, R. H.: Antiphlogistic activity of L-phenylalanine and L-tryptophane within the mouse peritoneal cavity. Experentia (Basel) **28**, 1230—1231 (1972)

Davis, R. H., Fisher, J. S., McGowan, L.: Local antiphlogistic activity of L-phenylalanine and L-tryptophane. J. Endocr. **41**, 603—604 (1968)

Decker, W. E., Edmonson, A. H., Hill, H. E., Holmes, R. A., Padmore, C. L., Warren, H. H., Wood, W. C.: Local administration of orgotein in horses. Mod. vet. Pract. **55**, 773—774 (1974)

De Fiebre, C. W., Ramsay, A. G., Golberg, R. I., Shuman, F. I.: Statistical analysis of oral enzyme therapy. In: Leonardi, A., Walsh, J. (Eds.): Drugs of Animal Origin, pp. 103—110. Milan: Ferro Edizioni 1967

deWied, D., Witter, A., Versteeg, D. H. G., Mulder, A. H.: Release of ACTH by substances of central nervous system origin. Endocrinology **85**, 561—569 (1969)

Diniz, C. R., Corrado, A. P.: Venoms of insects and arachnids. In: International Encyclopedia of Pharmacology and Therapeutics, Section 71. Oxford: Pergamon Press 1971, Vol. II, Part IV, pp. 117—140

Di Pasquale, G., Girerd, R. J.: Anti-inflammatory properties of lyophilized inflammatory exudates. Amer. J. Physiol. **201**, 1155—1158 (1961)

Di Pasquale, G., Girerd, R. J., Beach, V. L., Steinetz, B. G.: Antiphlogistic properties of lyophilised granuloma pouch exudates in intact or adrenalectomised rat. Amer. J. Physiol. **205**, 1080—1082 (1963)

Di Pasquale, G., Rassaert, C., Richter, R., Welaj, P., Tripp, L.: Influence of prostaglandins (PG) E_2 and $F_{2\alpha}$ on the inflammatory process. Prostaglandins **3**, 741—757 (1973)

Di Rosa, M., Sorrentino, L.: The mechanism of the inflammatory effect of carrageenin. Europ. J. Pharmacol. **4**, 340—342 (1968)

Dolbeare, F. A.: Lipid oxidation-linked stabilization of lysosomes by ascorbate. Fed. Proc. **30**, 1092A (1971)

Dolbeare, F. A., Martlage, K. A.: Some anti-inflammatory properties of ascorbic acid. Proc. Soc. exp. Biol. (N.Y.) **139**, 540—543 (1972)

Elliott, P. N. C., Bolam, J. P., Ford-Hutchinson, A. W., Smith, M. J. H.: The effects of a human plasma fraction on adjuvant arthritis and granuloma pellet reactions in the rat. J. Pharm. (Lond.) **26**, 751—752 (1974 a)

Elliott, P. N. C., Ford-Hutchinson, A. W., Smith, M. J. H.: Anti-inflammatory and irritant effects of a fraction from normal human plasma. Brit. J. Pharmacol. **50**, 253—257 (1974 b)

Fearon, D. T., Austen, K. F.: Inhibition of complement-derived enzymes. Ann. N.Y. Acad. Sci. **256**, 441—450 (1975)

Field, E. J., Shenton, B. K., Joyce, G.: Specific laboratory test for diagnosis of multiple sclerosis. Brit. med. J. I, 412—414 (1974)

Fisher, J. D.: Anti-inflammatory proteins and peptides. In: Scherrer, R. A., Whitehouse, M. W., (Eds.): Anti-inflammatory Agents, Vol. 1, pp. 363—384. New York: Academic Press 1974

Fisons Limited: Orgotein: Background Data for Clinical Investigators, 1st Edit. 1973

Ford-Hutchinson, A. W., Elliott, P. N. C., Bolam, J. P., Smith, M. J. H.: The effects of a human plasma fraction on carrageenan-induced paw oedema in the rat. J. Pharm. (Lond.) **26**, 878—881 (1974)

Ford-Hutchinson, A. W., Insley, M. Y., Elliott, P. N. C., Sturgess, E. A., Smith, M. J. H.: Anti-inflammatory activity in human plasma. J. Pharm. (Lond.) **25**, 881—886 (1973)

Ford-Hutchinson, A. W., Smith, M. J. H., Elliott, P. N. C., Bolam, J. P., Walker, J. R., Lobo, A. A., Badcock, J. K., Colledge, A. J., Billimoria, F. J.: Effects of a human plasma fraction on leucocyte migration into inflammatory exudates. J. Pharm. (Lond.) **27**, 106—112 (1975)

Forster, G.: Proteases in inflammation: on the possible mode of action of the protease inhibitor, Trasylol. In: Bertelli, A., Houck, J. C. (Eds.): Inflammation Biochemistry and Drug Interaction, pp. 53—75. Amsterdam: Excerpta Medica Foundation 1969

Ganley, O. H., Graessle, D. E., Robinson, H. J., Rahway, N. J.: Anti-inflammatory activity of compounds obtained from egg yolks, peanut oil and soybean lecithin. J. Lab. clin. Med. **51**, 709—714 (1958)

Ganley, O. H., Robinson, H. J., Rahway, N. J.: Antianaphylactic and antiserotonin activity of a compound obtained from egg yolk, peanut oil and soybean lecithin. J. Allergy **30**, 415—419 (1959)

Garattini, S., Jori, A., Bernardi, D., Carrara, C., Paglalunga, S., Segre, D.: Sensitivity of local oedemas to systemic pharmacological effects. In: Non-Steroidal Anti-inflammatory Drugs. Garattini, S., Dukes, M. N. G., (eds.). Amsterdam: Excerpta Medica Foundation 1965

Garcia-Giralt, E., Lasalvia, E., Florentine, I., Mathé, G.: Evidence for a lymphocyte chalone. Rev. Europ. Et. clin. biol. **15**, 1012—1015 (1970)

Garcia Leme, J., Morato, M., Souza, M. Z. A.: Anti-inflammatory action of glucagon in rats. Brit. J. Pharmacol. **55**, 65—68 (1975)

Garcia Leme, J., Schaporal, E. E. S.: Stimulation of the hypothalama-pituitary-adrenal axis by compounds formed in inflamed tissue. Brit. J. Pharmacol. **53**, 75—83 (1975)

Gecse, A., Zsilinszky, E., Lonovics, J., West, G. B.: C-Phenylglycine-n-heptyl ester as an inhibitor of mediators of allergic reactions. Int. Arch. Allergy **41**, 174—179 (1971)

Gerber, D. A.: Treatment of rheumatoid arthritis with histidine. Arthr. Rheum. **12**, 295 (1969)

Gerber, D. A.: Low free serum histidine concentrations in rheumatoid arthritis. J. clin. Invest. **55**, 1164—1173 (1975)

Gerber, D. A., Tanenbaum, L.: Abnormal oral histidine tolerance test in rheumatoid arthritis. Arthr. Rheum. **12**, 296 (1969)

Gillies, C. H.: The Theory and Practice of Counter-irritation. London: MacMillan 1895

Giroud, J. P., Velo, G. P., Dunn, C. J., Timsit, J., Willoughby, D. A.: Distribution of prostaglandins in inflammatory exudates. In: Velo, G. P., Willoughby, D. A., Giroud, J. P. (Eds.): Future Trends in Inflammation, pp. 19—36. Padua: Piccin Medical Books 1974

Glenn, E. M., Rohloff, N.: Antiarthritic and anti-inflammatory effects of certain prostaglandins. Proc. Soc. exp. Biol. (N.Y.) **138**, 290—294 (1972)

Glenn, E. M., Rohloff, N., Bowmann, B., Lyster, S.: Anti-inflammatory and pro-inflammatory effects of certain prostaglandins. Arthr. Rheum. **15**, 110 (1972)

Goetzl, E. J.: Plasma and cell-derived inhibitors of human neutrophil chemotaxis. Ann. N.Y. Acad. Sci. **256**, 210—221 (1975)

Goetzl, E. J., Austen, K. F.: A neutrophil-immobilizing factor derived from human leucocytes. J. exp. Med. **136**, 1564—1580 (1972)

Goetzl, E. J., Gigli, I., Wasserman, S. I., Austen, K. F.: A neutrophil immobilizing factor derived from human leukocytes. II. Specificity of action of polymorphonuclear leukocyte mobility. J. Immunol. **111**, 938—945 (1973)

Goldstein, I. R., Weissman, G.: Generation of C5-derived lysosomal enzyme-releasing activity (C5a) by lysates of leucocyte lysosomes. J. Immunol. **113**, 1583—1588 (1974)

Goldstein, S., Shemano, I., Demeo, R., Beiler, J. M.: Anti-inflammatory activity of several irritants in three models of experimental inflammation in rats. Arch. int. Pharmacodyn. **167**, 39—53 (1967)

Gomarasca, P., D'Atri, G.: Interazione tra Lysoartrosi ed Istamina. Minerva med. (Torino) **62**, 142—160 (1971)

Gomarasca, P., D'Atri, G., Titobello, A.: Attivata Antibradikininica del Lysoartrosi. Minerva med. **62**, 133—141 (1971)

Görög, P., Kovács, I. B., Szporny, L., Fekete, G.: Antiinflammatory and antianaphylactic actions of vitamins K_1 and K_3. Arzneimittel-Forsch. **18**, 227—230 (1968)

Grant, L.: The sticking and emigration of white blood cells in inflammation. In: Zweifach, B. W., Grant, L., McCluskey, R. T. (Eds.): The Inflammatory Process, Vol. II, pp. 205—249. New York: Academic Press 1973

Hallahan, J. D.: Relief of osteo-arthritis and osteoporosis with vitamin B_{12}. Amer. Pract. **3**, 27—32 (1952)

Hallgren, B., Larsson, S.: Glyceryl ethers in man and cow. J. Lipid Res. **3**, 39—43 (1962)

Hammeral, A. M., Pitchler, O.: On therapy with apiforty. Med. Clin. N. Amer. **55**, 2015—2021 (1960)

Hanson, J. M., Morley, J., Soria-Herrera, C.: Anti-inflammatory property of 401 (MCD-peptide), a peptide from the venom of the bee Apis mellifera (L). Brit. J. Pharmacol. **50**, 383—392 (1974)

Haux, P.: Die Aminosäurensequenz von MCD-Peptid, einem spezifisch Mastzelldegranulierenden Peptid aus Bienengift. Hoppe-Seyler's Z. physiol. Chem. **350**, 536—546 (1969)

Hayashi, H.: The intracellular neutral SH-dependent protease associated with inflammatory reactions. Int. Rev. Cytol. **40**, 101—151 (1975)

Hayashi, H., Udaka, K., Miyoshi, H., Kudo, S.: Further study of correlative behaviour between specific protease and inhibitor in cutaneous Arthus reactions. Lab. Invest. **14**, 665—673 (1965)

Hayashi, M., Koono, M., Yoshinaga, M., Muto, M.: The role of an SH-dependent protease and its inhibitors in the Arthus-type hypersensitivity reaction. In: Bertelli, A., Houck, J. C. (Eds.): Inflammation Biochemistry and Drug Action, pp. 34—52. Amsterdam: Excerpta Medica Foundation 1969

Highton, T. C.: The effect of sera from patients with rheumatoid arthritis in carrageenan granuloma pouches, skin wounds and weight gain in rats. Brit. J. exp. Path. **44**, 137—144 (1963)

Hirschelmann, R., Bekemeier, H.: Examination of dipeptides, amino-acids and substituted amino acids for anti-inflammatory activity in carrageenan oedema. Acta biol. med. germ. **31**, 899—901 (1973)

Horwitz, H., Joseph, N. R.: Prolonged observation in a group of arthritic patients. Industr. Med. **15**, 100—105 (1946)

Houck, J. C., Irausquin, H., Leikin, S.: Lymphocyte DNA synthesis inhibition. Science **173**, 1139—1141 (1971)

Houck, J. C., Jacob, R. A., DeAngelo, L., Vickers, K.: The inhibition of inflammation and the acceleration of tissue repair by cartilage powder. Surgery **51**, 632—638 (1962)

Huber, W., Schulte, T. L.: Method of Treating Post-Traumatic Arthritis. U.S. Patent No. 3,637,641 (1972)

Huber, W., Schulte, T. L., Carson, S., Goldhamer, R. E., Vogin, E. E.: Some chemical and pharmacological properties of a novel anti-inflammatory protein. Toxicol. appl. Pharmacol. 12, 208 (1968)

Hughes, W., Armendariz, M., Goldman, A.: Deficiency of an antagonist to a serum inhibitor of leukotaxis in cirrhotic patients. Gastroenterology 66, 846 (1974)

Janoff, A.: Neutrophil proteases in inflammation. Ann. Rev. Med. 23, 177—190 (1972)

Jeffes, E. W. B., Granger, G. A.: Relationship of cloning inhibition factor, "Lymphotoxin" factor and proliferation inhibition factor release in vitro by mitogen-activated human lymphocytes. J. Immunol. 114, 64—69 (1975)

Kambara, T., Aimoto, T., Hayashi, H.: Incorporation of ^{35}S-methionine or ^{35}S-cystine into polypeptide protease inhibitor in the rabbit skin with healing inflammation. Tohoku J. exp. Med. 94, 237—240 (1968)

Kamimura, M.: Antiinflammatory activity of vitamin E. J. Vitaminol. 18, 201—209 (1972)

Krsiak, M., Sechserova, M., Perlik, F., Elis, J.: Effect of palmitoyl ethanolamide on alcohol intoxication in man. Activ. nerv. sup. (Praha) 14, 187 (1972)

Kuehl, F. A.: Prostaglandins, cyclic nucleotides and cell function. Prostaglandins 5, 325—340 (1974)

Kuehl, F. A., Jacob, T. A., Ganley, O. H., Ormond, R. E., Meisinger, M. A. P.: The identification of N(2-hydroxyethyl) palmitamide as a naturally occurring anti-inflammatory agent. J. Amer. chem. Soc. 79, 5577—5578 (1957)

Kulonen, E., Potila, M.: Effect of the administration of anti-rheumatic drugs on experimental granuloma in rat. Biochem. Pharmacol. 24, 219—225 (1975)

Lachmann, P. J., Halbwachs, L.: The influence of C3b inactivator (KAF) concentration on the ability of serum to support complement activation. Clin. exp. Immunol. 21, 109—114 (1975)

Laden, C., Blackwell, R. Q., Fosdick, L. S.: Anti-inflammatory effects of counterirritants. Amer. J. Physiol. 195, 712—718 (1958)

Livingston, W. S.: The treatment of spontaneous tumors of the dog and cat with a filtrate from a tissue lysate. J. nat. Cancer. Inst. 20, 245—271 (1958)

Livingston, W. S., Bennett, L. R., Lamson, B. G.: Growth inhibition of transplantable mouse lymphosarcoma by a filtrate from placental lysates. J. nat. Cancer. Inst. 23, 587—602 (1959)

Long, D. A., Martin, A. J. P.: Factors in arachis oil depressing sensitivity to tuberculin in BCG infected guinea-pigs. Lancet (1956)I, 464

McArthur, J. N., Dawkins, P. D., Smith, M. J. H., Hamilton, E. B. D.: Mode of action of antirheumatic drugs. Brit. med. J. (1971)II, 677—679

McCord, J. M., Fridovich, I.: Superoxide dismutase. An enzymic function for erythrocuprein (hemocuprein). J. biol. Chem. 244, 6049—6053 (1969)

McCord, J. M., Keele, B. B., Fridovich, I.: An enzyme-based theory of obligate anaerobrosis: the physiological function of superoxide dismutase. Proc. nat. Acad. Sci. (Wash.) 68, 1024—1027 (1971)

Maderazo, E. F., Ward, P. A., Quintiliami, R.: Defective regulation of chemotaxis in cirrhosis. J. Lab. clin. Med. 85, 621—630 (1975)

Manca, M., Bertini, G.: La nostra Esperienza sull'impiego di Lisati Proteici die Organo nel Trattamento delle Atropatie Croniche. Minerva med. (Torino) 62, 168—173 (1971)

Mann, T., Keilin, D.: Haemocuprein and hepatocuprein, copper protein compounds of blood and liver in mammals. Proc. roy. Soc. B. 126, 303—315 (1939)

Marberger, H., Huber, W., Bartsch, G., Schulte, T., Swoboda, P.: Orgotein: a new anti-inflammatory metalloprotein. Drug evaluation of clinical efficacy and safety in inflammatory conditions of the urinary tracts. Int. Urol. Nephrol. 6, 61—74 (1974)

Marcy, R.: Etude des Effets de l'Aprotinine administrée par voie para et intra-articulaire. I. Et. exp. Thérapie 27, 1021—1030 (1972)

Marcy, R., Loyau, G., Dumas, M.: Étude des Effets de l'Aprotinine administrée par voie para et intra-articulaire. II. Etude Clinique. Thérapie 27, 1031—1041 (1972)

Martelli, E. A., Corsico, N., Fogagnolo, E.: Significance of the release of bradykinin in local inflammatory reactions and related effect of antiphlogistic drugs. In: Bertelli, A., Houck, J. C. (Eds.): Inflammation Biochemistry and Drug Interaction, pp. 185—196. Amsterdam: Excerpta Medica Foundation 1969

Masek, K., Raskova, H.: Pharmacology of palmitoyl ethanolanide. In: Leonardi, A., Walsh, J. (Eds.): Drugs of Animal Origin, pp. 199—209. Milan: Ferro Edizioni 1967

Matsuba, K.: Studies of the certain protease-inhibitor system in the mechanism of Arthus-type hypersensitivity reaction. I. Inhibition of the reaction by euglobulin inhibitor. Mie med. J. **10**, 21—25 (1960)

Maxson, T. R., Compton, E. L.: Controlled study of a new anti-arthritic substance. Ann. Allergy **27**, 54—64 (1969)

Mertin, J., Shenton, B. K., Field, E. J.: Unsaturated fatty acids in multiple sclerosis. Brit. med. J. **(1973)**II, 777—778

Millar, J. H. D., Zilka, K. J., Langman, M. J. S., Wright, H. P., Smith, A. D., Bellin, J., Thompson, R. H. S.: Double blind trial of linoleate supplementation of the diet in multiple sclerosis. Brit. med. J. **(1973)**II, 765—768

Mizushima, Y., Sakai, S., Yamaura, M.: Mode of stabilizing action of non-steroid anti-inflammatory drugs on erythrocyte membrane. Biochem. Pharmacol. **19**, 227—234 (1970)

Moore, F. T.: Some further views of alpha-chymotrypsin in facial surgery. Brit. J. plast. Surg. **16**, 387—390 (1963)

Müller-Eberhard, H. J.: Complement. Ann. Rev. Biochem. **38**, 389—465 (1969)

Nagai, K.: Physiological implications of carnosine on the inflammation. J. Nihon. Univ. Sch. Dent. **13**, 1—11 (1971)

Nagai, K., Murakami, H., Sano, A., Kabutake, H.: Die physiologische Bedeutung von Carnosin und Homocarnosin bei der Inflammation. Arzneimittel-Forsch. **20**, 1876—1878 (1970)

Nelson, D. S.: Production by stimulated macrophages of factors depressing lymphocyte transformation. Nature (Lond.) **246**, 306—307 (1973)

Nelson, R. D., Leu, R. D.: Macrophage requirement for production of guinea-pig migration inhibitory factor (MIF) in vitro. J. Immunol. **114**, 606—609 (1975)

Noordhoek, J., Bonta, I. L.: Mechanism of the anti-inflammatory effect of carrageenin pouch exudate. In: Velo, G. P., Willoughby, D. A., Giroud, J. P. (Eds.): Future Trends in Inflammation, pp. 249—258. Padua: Piccin Medical Books 1974

Pacini, N., Gomarasca, M.: Azione antiedemigena del Lysoartrosi e delle frazioni Polipeptidiche in esso contenute. Minerva med. (Torino) **62**, 125—132 (1971)

Paoletti, R., Berti, F., Fumagalli, R., Folco, G. C.: Some interrelations between prostaglandins and cyclic nucleotides. In: Future Trends in Inflammation. Velo, G. P., Willoughby, D. A., Giroud, J. P. (Eds.). Padua: Piccin Medical Books 1974, pp. 11—18

Paulus, H. E.: Evaluation for clinical efficacy. In: Scherrer, R. A., Whitehouse, M. W. (Eds.): Anti-Inflammatory Agents, Vol. II, pp. 217—233. New York: Academic Press 1974

Perlik, F., Elis, J., Raskova, H.: Anti-inflammatory properties of N(2-hydroxyethyl) palmitamide. Acta physiol. Acad. Sci. hung. **39**, 395—400 (1971)

Perlik, F., Masek, K.: The effect of N(2-hydroxyethyl) palmitamide on inflammatory processes in animal and man. In: Velo, G. P., Willoughby, D. A., Giroud, J. P. (Eds.): Future Trends in Inflammation, pp. 301—305. Padua: Piccin Medical Books 1974

Perper, R. J., Glenn, E. M., Monovich, R. E.: Separation of anti-inflammatory and immunosuppressive activities in heterologous anti-lymphocyte serum. Nature (Lond.) **223**, 86—87 (1969)

Persellin, R. H., Vance, S. E., Peery, A.: Effect of pregnancy serum on experimental inflammation. Brit. J. exp. Path. **55**, 26—32 (1974)

Pinals, R. S., Gerber, D. A.: Treatment of rheumatoid arthritis with histidine: a double-blind trial. Arthr. Rheum. **16**, 126—127 (1973)

Prelog, V., Beyermann, H. C.: Untersuchungen über Organextrakte. Über die Isolierung von Chimyl-alkohol (d-α-Hexadecyl-glyceryläther) aus Schweinemilz. Helv. chim. Acta **28**, 350—351 (1945)

Prudden, J. F.: Personal communication (1975)

Prudden, J. F., Balassa, L. L.: The biological activity of bovine cartilage preparations. Semin. Arthr. Rheum. **3**, 287—321 (1974)

Prudden, J. F., Gabriel, O., Allen, B.: The acceleration of wound healing. Arch. Surg. (Chicago) **86**, 157—161 (1963)

Prudden, J. F., Migel, P., Hanson, P., Friedrich, L., Balassa, L.: The discovery of a potent pure chemical wound-healing accelerator. Amer. J. Surg. **119**, 560—564 (1970)

Prudden, J. F., Nishihara, G., Baker, L.: The acceleration of wound-healing with cartilage. I. Surg. Gynec. Obstet. **105**, 283—286 (1957)

Raskova, H., Masek, K.: Nouvelles possibilités d'augmentation de la résistance non-spécifique. Thérapie 22, 1241—1246 (1967)

Rawls, W. B.: Evaluation of present day therapy in rheumatoid arthritis, N.Y. Med. 3, 19—22 (1947)

Rindani, T. H.: Recovery of an anti-inflammatory fraction from inflammatory exudates. Indian J. med. Res. 44, 673—676 (1956)

Ring, J., Siefert, J., Mertin, J., Brendel, W.: Prolongation of skin allografts in rats by treatment with linoleic acid. Lancet (1974)II, 1331

Robinson, B. V., Robson, J. M.: Production of an anti-inflammatory substance at a site of inflammation. Brit. J. Pharmacol. 23, 420—432 (1964)

Robinson, B. V., Robson, J. M.: Further studies on the anti-inflammatory factor found at a site of inflammation. Brit. J. Pharmacol. 26, 372—384 (1966)

Rocklin, R. E.: Partial characterization of leukocyte inhibitory factor by concanavalin A-stimulated human lymphocytes. J. Immunol. 114, 1161—1165 (1975)

Rocklin, R. E., Remold, H. G., David, J. R.: Characterization of human migration inhibiting factor (MIF) from antigen-stimulated lymphocytes. Cell. Immunol. 5, 436—445 (1972)

Rosenthale, M. E.: Evaluation for immunosuppressive and antiallergic activity. In: Scherrer, R. A., Whitehouse, M. W. (Eds.): Anti-Inflammatory Agents, Vol. II, pp. 123—192. New York: Academic Press 1974

Ruddy, S., Austen, K. F.: Activation of the complement and properdin systems in rheumatoid arthritis. Ann. N.Y. Acad. Sci. 256, 96—104 (1975)

Ryzewski, J.: Wplys Cysteiny na Powstawanie i Przebieg Poadjuwansowego Wielostawowego Sapalenia u Szczurow. Reum. pol. 4, 227—234 (1966)

Sabo, J. C., Oberlander, L., Enquist, I. F.: Acceleration of open wound healing by cartilage. Arch. Surg. (Chicago) 90, 414—417 (1965)

Sandberg, A. L., Wahl, S. M., Mergenhagen, S. E.: Lymphokine production of C3b-stimulated B cells. J. Immunol. 115, 139—144 (1975)

Shen, T. Y.: Non-steroidal anti-inflammatory agents. Ann. Rep. med. Chem., Section 21, 215—226 (1967)

Shipolini, R. A., Callewaert, G. L., Cottrell, R. C., Doonan, S., Vernon, C. A.: Phospholipase A from bee venoms. Europ. J. Biochem. 20, 459—468 (1971 a)

Shipolini, R. A., Callewaert, G. L., Cottrell, R. C., Vernon, C. A.: The primary sequence of phospholipase A from bee venom. FEBS Lett. 1, 39 (1971 b)

Skidmore, I. F.: Targets in inflammation therapy. In: Scherrer, R. A., Whitehouse, M. W. (Eds.): Anti-Inflammatory Agents, Vol. II, pp. 23—25. New York: Academic Press 1974

Smith, C. W., Hollers, J. C., Dupree, E., Goldman, A. S., Lord, R. A.: A serum inhibitor of leukotaxis in a child with recurrent infections. J. Lab. clin. Med. 79, 878—885 (1972)

Smith, M. J. H.: Interactions with endocrine systems In: Smith, M. J. H., Smith, P. K. (Eds.): The Salicylates, pp. 107—153. New York: Interscience Publications 1966

Smith, M. J. H.: Mode of action of antirheumatic drugs. In: Holt, P. J. L. (Ed.): Current Topics in Connective Tissue Diseases. London: Churchill Livingstone 1975

Smith, M. J. H., Colledge, A. J., Elliott, P. N. C., Bolam, J. P., Ford-Hutchinson, A. W.: A human plasma fraction with anti-inflammatory but without either analgesic or antipyretic properties. J. Pharm. (Lond.) 26, 836—837 (1974 a)

Smith, M. J. H., Ford-Hutchinson, A. W.: An anti-inflammatory substance in normal human plasma. Agents Actions 5, 318—321 (1975)

Smith, M. J. H., Ford-Hutchinson, A. W., Elliott, P. N. C., Bolam, J. P.: Prostaglandins and the anti-inflammatory activity of a human plasma fraction in carrageenan-induced paw oedema in the rat. J. Pharm. (Lond.) 26, 692—698 (1974 b)

Snyderman, R., Pike, M. C., Altman, L. C.: Abnormalities of leukocyte chemotaxis in human disease. Ann. N.Y. Acad. Sci. 256, 386—401 (1975)

Sofia, R. D., Nalepa, S. D., Herakal, J. J., Vassar, H. B.: Anti-oedema and analgesic properties of D-9-tetrahydrocannabinol (THC): J. Pharmacol. exp. Ther. 186, 646—655 (1973)

Soriano, R. B., South, M. A., Goldman, A. S., Smith, C. W.: Defect of neutrophil motility in a child with recurrent bacterial infections and disseminated cytomegalovirus infection. J. Pediat. 83, 951—958 (1973)

Spector, W. G., Chronic inflammation. In: Zweifach, B. W., Grant, L., McCluskey, R. T. (Eds.): The Inflammatory Process 2nd Ed., Vol. III, pp. 277—280. New York: Academic Press 1974

Spector, W. G., Willoughby, D. A.: The Pharmacology of Inflammation. London: The English Universities Press 1968

Spilberg, I., Osterland, C. K.: Anti-inflammatory effect of the trypsin-kallikrein inhibitor in acute arthritis induced by urate crystals in rabbits. J. Lab. clin. Med. **76**, 472—479 (1970)

Stastny, P., Ziff, M.: Inhibitor of macrophage migration produced by polymorphonuclear leucocytes. J. reticuloendoth. Soc. **7**, 140—145 (1970)

Stuyvesant, V. W., Jolley, W. B.: Composition of the oily phase of adjuvant in the induction of arthritis. Fed. Proc. **27**, 474 (1968)

Swingle, K. F.: Evaluation for anti-inflammatory Activity. In: Scherrer, R. A., Whitehouse, M. W. (Eds.): Anti-Inflammatory Agents, Vol. II, pp. 33—122. New York: Academic Press 1974

Taylor, J. L., Brown, J. H.: Inhibition of Protein Aggregation by vitamin E and selenium. Proc. Soc. exp. Biol. (N.Y.) **145**, 32—36 (1974)

Teodorczyk, J., Szymaniec, S., Blaszczyk, B., Ludwikowska, A., Gieldanowski, J.: Studies on anti-inflammatory activity of anti-thymocytic serum. Arch. Immunol. Ther. exp. **23**, 83—89 (1975)

Thomas, G., West, G. B.: Amino acids and inflammation. Brit. J. Pharmacol. **47**, 662 P (1973)

Tikal, K., Benesova, D., Frankova, S.: Effects of centrophenoxine and palmityl ethanolomine on the social behaviour of rats malnourished in early postnatal life. Activ. nerv. sup. (Praha) **15**, 150—151 (1973)

Till, G., Ward, P. A.: Two distinct chemotactic factor inactivators in human serum. J. Immunol. **114**, 843—847 (1975)

Tokaji, G.: The chemical pathology of thermal injury, with special reference to burns SH-dependent protease and its inhibitor. Kumamoto med. J. **24**, 68—86 (1971)

Tokuda, A., Hayashi, H., Matsuda, K.: Biochemical study of cellular antigen-antibody reaction in tissue culture. II. Release of a protease inhibitor. J. exp. Med. **112**, 249—255 (1960)

Traeger, C. H.: Use of vitamins in treatment of chronic arthritis. Med. Clin. N. Amer. **30**, 616—622 (1946)

Trapnell, J. E.: The natural history and management of acute pancreatitis. In: Howat, H. T. (Ed.): Clinics in Gastroenterology; The Exocrine Pancreas, Volume I, pp. 147—166. London: W. B. Saunders 1972

Trapnell, J., Rigby, C. C., Talbot, C. H., Duncan, E. H. L.: A controlled trial of trasylol in the treatment of acute pancreatitis. Brit. J. Surg. **61**, 177—182 (1974)

Turk, J. L., Willoughby, D. A.: An analysis of the multiplicity of the effects of antilymphocytic serum. Antibiot. et Chemother. (Basel) **15**, 267—284 (1969)

Turk, J. L., Willoughby, D. A., Stevens, J. E.: An analysis of the effects of some types of anti-lymphocyte sera on contact hypersensitivity and certain models of inflammation. Immunology **14**, 683—695 (1968)

Udaka, K., Hayashi, H.: Further purification of a protease inhibitor from rabbit skin with healing inflammation. Biochim. biophys. Acta. **97**, 251—261 (1965 a)

Udaka, K., Hayashi, H.: Molecular-weight determination of a protease inhibitor from rabbit skin with healing inflammation. Biochim. biophys. Acta **104**, 600—603 (1965 b)

Ulrich, F.: A dialysable protein synthesis inhibitor release by mammalian cells in vitro. Biochem. biophys. Res. Commun. **60**, 1453—1459 (1974)

United States Adopted Names Council: New Names, List No. 106, J. Amer. Med. Ass. **218**, 1936 (1971)

Van Epps, D. E., Palmer, D. L., Williams, R. C.: Characterisation of serum inhibitors of neutrophil chemotaxis associated with anergy. J. Immunol. **113**, 189—199 (1974)

Van Gool, J., Ladiges, N. C. J. J.: Production of foetal globulin after injury in rat and man. J. Path. **97**, 115—126 (1969)

Van Gool, J., Schreuder, J., Ladiges, N. C. J. J.: Inhibitory effect of foetal α_2 globulin, an acute phase protein, on carrageenin oedema in the rat. J. Path. **112**, 245—261 (1974)

Velo, G. P., Dunn, C. J., Giroud, J. P., Timsit, J., Willoughby, D. A.: Distribution of prostaglandins in inflammatory exudates. J. Path. **111**, 149—158 (1973)

Vernon, C. A., Hanson, J. M., Brimblecombe, R. W.: Peptides. British Patent No. 1, 314, 823 (1969)

Vick, J. A., Brooks, R. B.: Pharmacological studies of major fractions of bee venom. Amer. Bee J. **112**, 288—289 (1972)

Vogt, W.: Activation, activities and pharmacologically active products of complement. Pharmacol. Rev. **26**, 125—169 (1974)

Wahl, S. M., Wilton, J. M., Rosentreich, D. L., Oppenheim, J. J.: The role of macrophages in the production of lymphokines by T and B lymphocytes. J. Immunol. **114**, 1296—1301 (1975)

Waldman, S. R., Gottlieb, A. A.: Macrophage regulation of DNA synthesis in lymphoid cells: effects of a soluble factor from macrophages. Cell. Immunol. **9**, 142—156 (1973)

Walker, J. R., Badcock, J. K., Ford-Hutchinson, A. W., Smith, M. J. H., Billimoria, F. J.: Effects of a human plasma fraction on the release of chemotactic factors and anaphylotoxin from complement. J. Pharm. (Lond.) **27**, 747—753 (1975 a)

Walker, J. R., Smith, M. J. H., Ford-Hutchinson, A. W., Billimoria, F. J.: Mode of action of an anti-inflammatory fraction from normal human plasma. Nature (Lond.) **254**, 444—446 (1975 b)

Ward, P. A.: The inflammatory mediators. Ann. N. Y. Acad. Sci. **221**, 290—298 (1974 a)

Ward, P. A.: Leukotaxis and leukotactic disorders. Amer. J. Path. **77**, 520—538 (1974 b)

Ward, P. A.: Complement-dependent phlogistic factors in rheumatoid synovial fluids. Ann. N. Y. Acad. Sci. **256**, 169—176 (1975)

Ward, P. A., Berenberg, J. L.: Defective regulation of inflammatory mediators in Hodgkin's disease. New Engl. J. Med. **290**, 76—80 (1974)

Ward, P. A., Data, R., Till, G.: Regulatory control of complement-derived chemotactic and anaphylatoxin mediators. In: Brent, L., Holborrow, J. (Eds.): Progress in Immunology, Vol. I, pp. 209—215. North-Holland Publishing Co. 1974

Ward, P. A., Rocklin, R. E.: Regulation of MIF by a factor in human serum. J. Immunol. **115**, 309—311 (1975)

Ward, P. A., Schlegel, R. J.: Impaired leucotactic responsiveness in a child with recurrent infections. Lancet **(1969)**II, 344—347

Willoughby, D. A., Di Rosa, M.: A unifying concept for inflammation: a new appraisal of some old mediators. In: Immunopathology of Inflammation, pp. 28—38. Amsterdam: Excerpta Medica 1971

Wood, E., Dalgliesh, D., Bannister, W.: Bovine erythrocyte cuprozinc protein. Europ. J. Biochem. **18**, 187—193 (1971)

Zanasi, R., Volonteri, G., Castaldi, D.: Valutazione Clinica dell'impiego nell 'artrosi di un Farmaco ad Azione Antirheumatica e Antiflogistica. Minerva med. (Torino) **62**, 174—178 (1971)

Zuckner, J.: Vitamin B_{12} therapy in osteoarthritis. Missouri Med. **51**, 450—451 (1954)

Zurier, R. B., Quagliata, F.: Effect of prostaglandin E_1 on adjuvant arthritis. Nature (Lond.) **234**, 304—305 (1971)

Zurier, R. B., Weissman, G.: Effect of prostaglandins upon enzyme release from lysosomes and experimental arthritis. In: Ramwell, P. W., Pharriss, B. B. (Eds.): Prostaglandins in Cellular Biology, Vol. I, pp. 151—168. New York: Plenum Press 1972

CHAPTER 39

Anti-Inflammatory Substances of Plant Origin

M. GÁBOR

A. Introduction

Until recently, information on anti-inflammatory agents of plant origin was sparse. The first reviews dealt primarily with the phenylbenzo-γ-pyrones (flavonoids) (GÁBOR, 1972a, 1975); however, there are other substances of plant origin with anti-inflammatory action. Although these are not as potent as the non-steroid anti-inflammatory agents knowledge of the structure activity relationships may lead to newer and more effective preparations.

The aim of the present chapter is to report on the anti-inflammatory agents of plant origin and on the data and conceptions to date regarding their mechanisms of action. It appears logical to include a discussion of the anti-inflammatory action of some synthetic and semi-synthetic derivatives of naturally occurring materials.

B. Anti-Inflammatory Action of Phenylbenzo-γ-Pyrone (Flavone) Derivatives

I. The Occurrence of Flavonoid Compounds in Nature

The phenylbenzo-γ-pyrones (flavonoids) are very widespread pigments in the plant kingdom. The monograph by HARBORNE (1967) presents a detailed account of the general distribution of flavonoids in both higher and lower plants (algae, fungi, mosses, ferns). It discusses the flavonoids of the gymnosperms (Cycadaceae, Ginkgoaceae, Taxaceae, Podocarpaceae, Pinaceae, Taxodiaceae, Cupresseaceae). A detailed study is made of the flavonoids of the dicotyledons, the Archichlamydeae (flavonoids of Ranunculaceae, Paeoniaceae, Papaveraceae, Cruciferae, Rosaceae, Leguminosae, Vitaceae, Theaceae, Rutaceae, Umbelliferae). *The Flavonoids* (HARBORNE et al., 1975) is the most up-to-date account of the occurrence and distribution of the various flavone compounds.

II. The Chemistry of Flavonoid Compounds

The first comprehensive monographs on the chemistry of the flavonoid compounds were published by GEISSMAN (1962) and DEAN (1963). Of the more recent works, mention may be made of the review by COURBAT (1972); *The Flavonoids*, edited by HARBORNE et al. (1975); and *Topics in Flavonoid Chemistry and Biochemistry*, edited by FARKAS et al. (1975).

Prior to the discussion of the anti-inflammatory action of the flavonoids, it is convenient to tabulate the flavone compound types occurring in this chapter

Table 1. Naturally occuring flavonoids and some related compounds (basic skeletons)

I γ–Pyrone

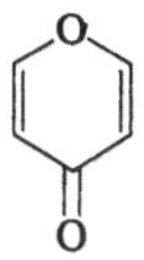

II Chromone
(benzo–γ–pyrone)

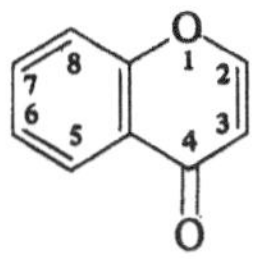

III Flavone
(2–phenylbenzo–γ–pyrone)

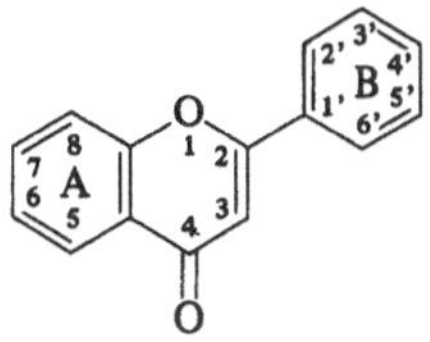

IV Isoflavone
(3–phenylbenzo–γ–pyrone)

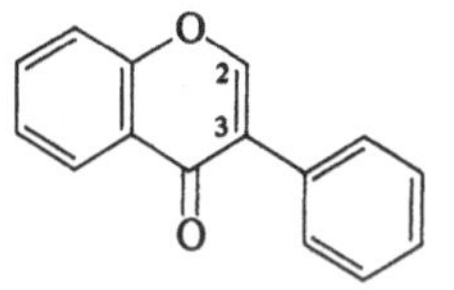

V Flavonol
(3–hydroxyflavone)

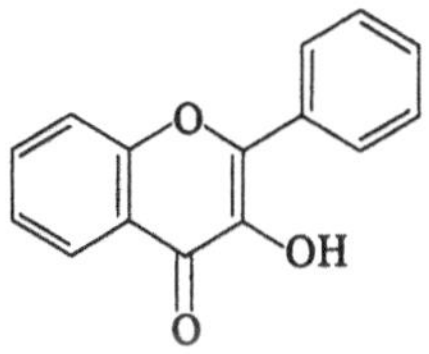

VI Flavanone
(2,3–dihydroflavone)

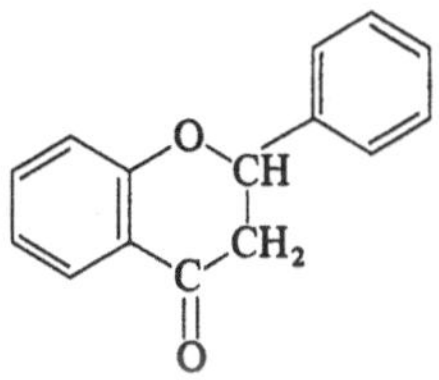

VII Flavanonol
(3–hydroxyflavanone)

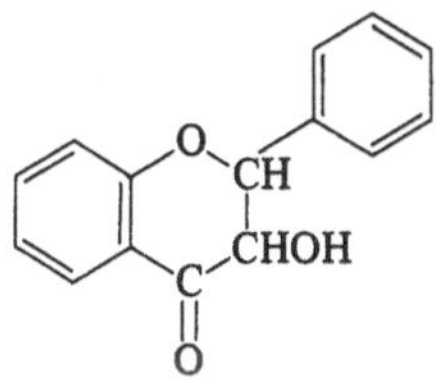

VIII Chalcone
(benzalacetophenone)

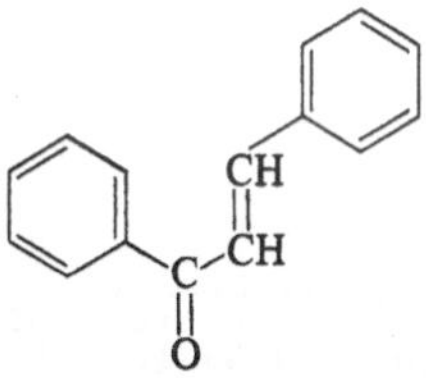

IX R = H Flavan
R = OH Catechin

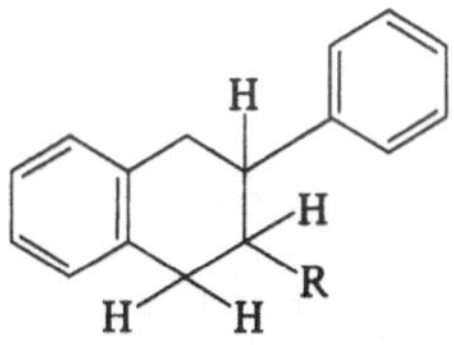

X Anthocyanidin
(flavylium salt)

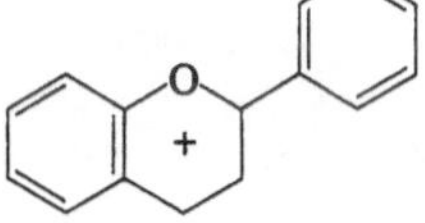

XI Aurone
(2–benzalcoumaranone–3)

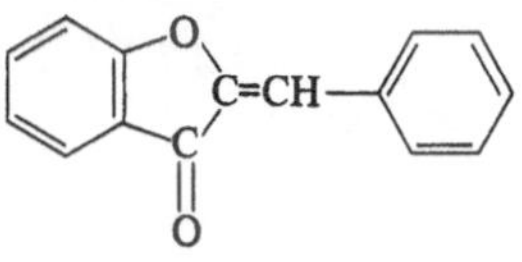

(Table 1) and some of their derivatives (Table 2). The flavone skeleton is 2-phenyl-benzo-γ-pyrone, a γ-pyrone derivative.

It should be noted here that O-(β-hydroxyethyl)rutin (Venoruton, Zyma S.A., Nyon), which will be mentioned frequently below, contains a mixture of hydroxyethylrutins in fixed proportions prepared by the hydroxyethylation of rutin. The five

Table 2. Chemical structures of some flavonoids

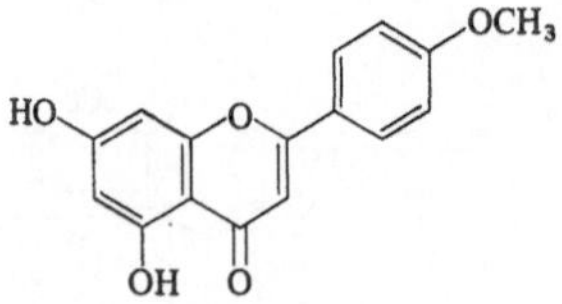

Acacetin

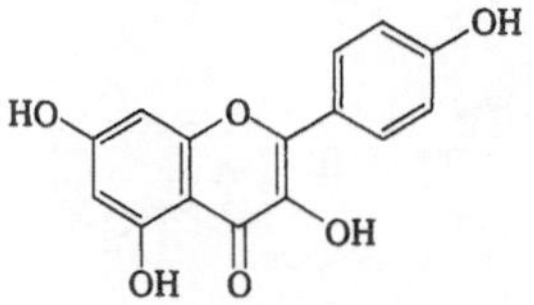

Kaempferol

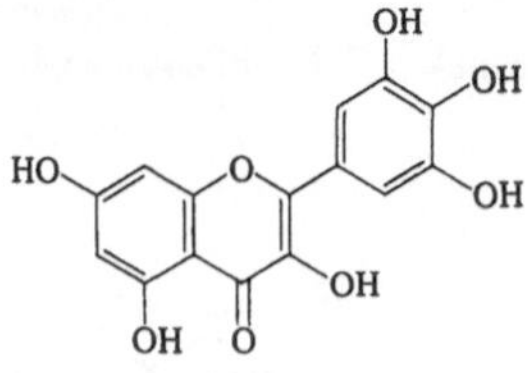

Myricetin

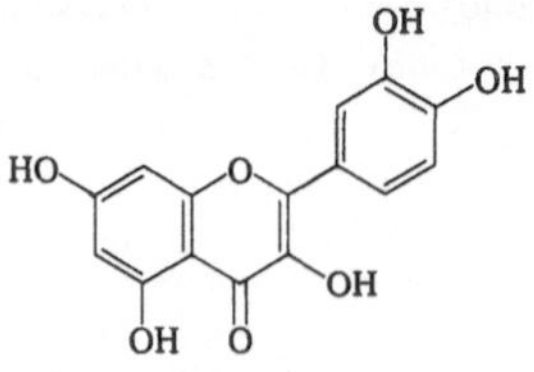

Quercetin

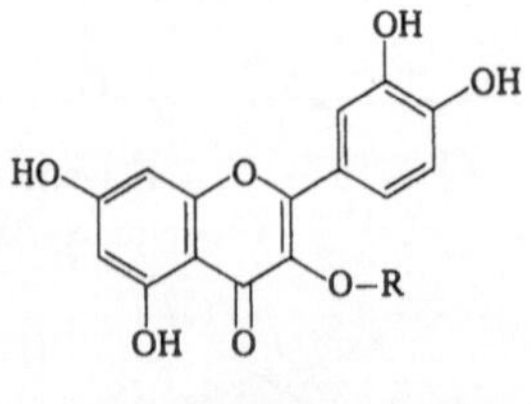

Rutin
R = Rhamnosido–glucose

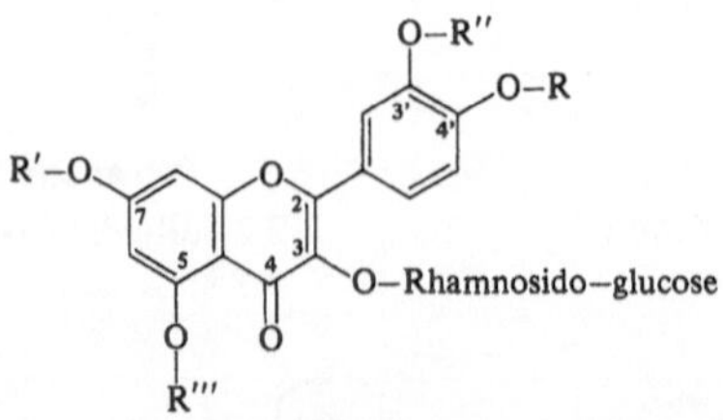

Hydroxyethylrutin

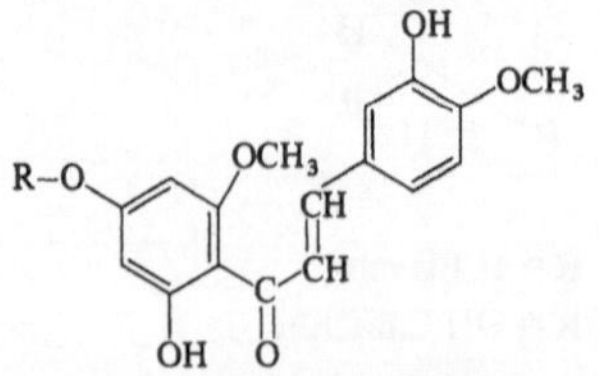

Hesperidin methylchalcone

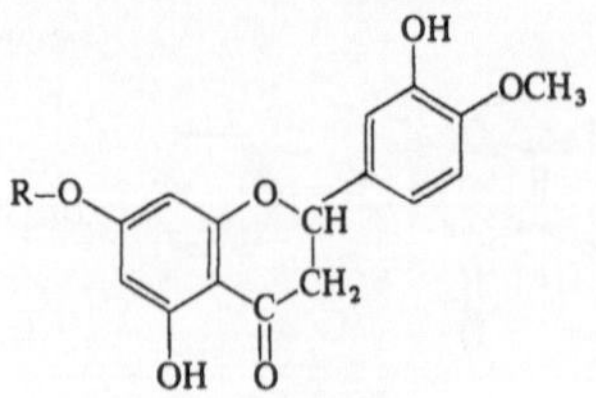

	R	R'	R''	R'''
5, 7, 3'4' – Tetrahydroxyethylrutoside	HE	HE	HE	HE
5, 7'4' – Trihydroxyethylrutoside	HE	HE	H	HE
7, 3'4' – Trihydroxyethylrutoside	HE	HE	HE	H
7,4' – Dihydroxyethylrutoside	HE	HE	H	H
4' – Monohydroxyethylrutoside	HE	H	H	H

$$HE = -CH_2CH_2OH$$

Hesperidin
R = Rhamnosido–glucose

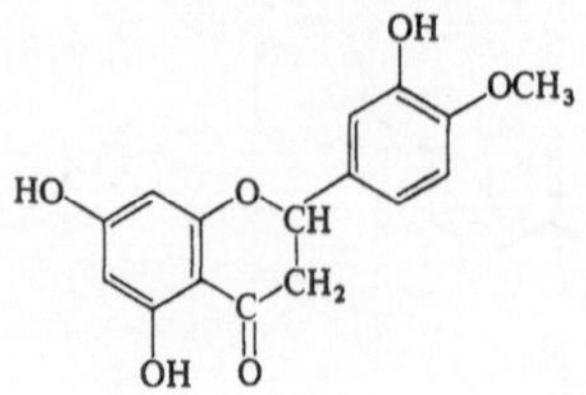

Hesperetin

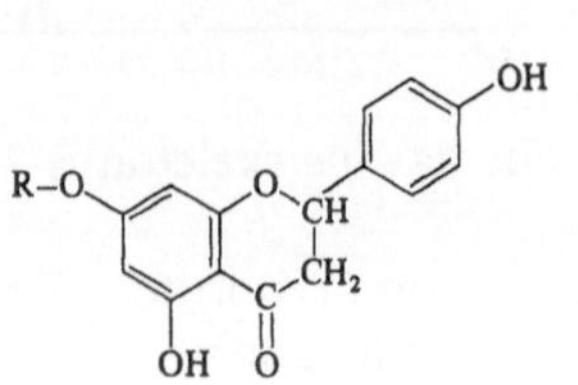

Naringin

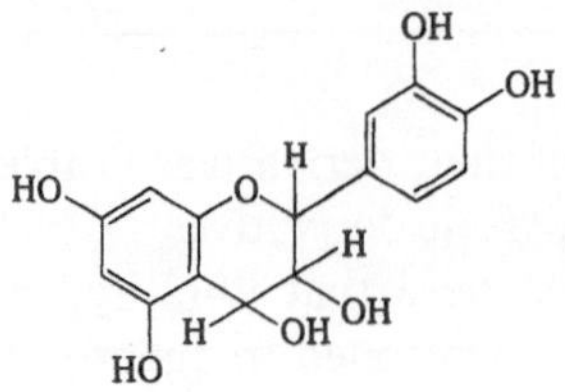

Leucocyanidin

major components of the mixture have been identified by UV spectrophotometry (COURBAT et al., 1966a, b); they are: 5,7,3',4'-tetrahydroxyethylrutin, 5,7,4'-trihydroxyethylrutin, 7,3',4'-trihydroxyethylrutin, 7,4'-dihydroxyethylrutin, and 4'-monohydroxyethylrutin.

III. The Anti-Inflammatory Action of Flavonoids

Great interest has been shown in the flavonoids in recent years. More than a dozen reviews have appeared; however, if the largest reviews (BÖHM, 1968; SHILS-GOODHART, 1956; GRIFFITH et al., 1955) are examined, it is found that the anti-inflammatory action of flavonoids is dealt with in a few lines or is not mentioned at all, although this question has already been treated in numerous publications. Widespread studies over about 20 years required that a comprehensive picture be obtained of this field (GÁBOR, 1972a, 1975). In the following, the anti-inflammatory action of the bioflavonoids is discussed.

1. Influence on Mouse and Rat Paw Oedema

GROSS(1950a, b) reported that when rutin was administered subcutaneously (s.c.) (100 mg/kg in propylene glycol) 2 h before the local application of egg white, oedema formation in rats was inhibited. The solvent, propylene glycol, itself (100 mg/kg s.c.) had a smaller, but pronounced inhibiting action.

KÜCHLE and WEGENER (1951) attempted to influence rat paw oedema induced by a subplantar injection of 0.1 ml egg white or of egg white diluted in a ratio 1:10 with physiological salt solution, by treatment with rutin (Birutan, Merck), citrin (Citrin, Hoechst), and epicatechin (Citrin "E", Hoechst). The rats received the flavonoids in 100 mg/kg doses s.c. 1 h before the local application. Oedema formation was moderately retarded by rutin and inhibited by 20% by citrin. The effect of epicatechin on oedema caused by undiluted egg white was not pronounced, but the oedema caused by the diluted egg white was inhibited by 19%.

VOGEL and MAREK (1961) were able to significantly decrease rat paw oedema induced by subplantar polyvinylpyrrolidone (0.2 ml of 24% w/v solution) by the intravenous (i.v.) injection of rutin (100 mg/kg).

Hesperidin, neohesperidin, and naringin in doses of 100 mg/kg intraperitoneally (i.p.) led to a considerable reduction of formaldehyde-induced inflammation in mouse paw, but rutin was inactive (NORTHOVER and SUBRAMANIAN, 1962). The experimental animals were treated with the flavanone glycosides on two occasions (24 h and 30 min) before oedema was induced. None of the flavone and flavanone glycosides were active against inflammation induced by 5-hydroxytryptamine (5-HT).

TEXL (1963) found that rat oedema caused by formalin or hyaluronidase was significantly inhibited by the combined administration of vitamin C (100 mg/kg) and tea leaf catechin complex (tea tannin: 100 mg/kg s.c.). This effect was not observed in adrenalectomized rats. It is interesting to note that the application of tea tannin or vitamin C alone does not significantly affect the experimentally produced inflammation.

Likewise, in the mouse experiments of VOGIN and ROSSI (1963), paw oedema produced by 5-HT was not affected by orally applied doses of ascorbic acid of 150,

300, 600, and 1200 mg/kg. Pretreatment with hesperidin methylchalcone was similarly without effect. Paw oedema caused by 5-HT was also not decreased to a significant extent by the combined application of ascorbic acid (150 mg/kg) and hesperidin-methylchalcone (150 and 600 mg/kg).

MARTIN et al. (1953) found that paw oedema induced in rats by ovalbumin can be moderated to an appreciable extent with phosphorylated hesperidin (200 mg/kg or 2 × 200 mg/kg, administered orally or s.c.). Also worthy of mention is the synergistic effect of phosphorylated hesperidin administered with trypsin.

According to the studies of FORMANEK and HÖLLER (1960), orally administered O-(β-hydroxyethyl)rutin (Venoruton or Paroven, Zyma S.A., Nyon: 2 g/kg) inhibits rat paw oedema induced by the application of dextran or hyaluronidase, whereas formalin oedema and serum oedema are not affected. However, it was found by GROSS (1950a) that if rutin is administered (100 mg/kg s.c.) 2 h before the formalin injection, the acute formalin inflammation is inhibited.

VAN CAUWENBERGE and FRANCHIMONT (1967) were able to inhibit oedema induced by formalin, dextran, 5-HT, and bradykinin with an O-(β-hydroxyethyl) rutin (Z 6000, Labor. Zyma) treatment, but they could not affect the extent of oedema caused by histamine. This rutin derivative was administered (30 mg/kg i.p.) to rats 48, 24, 6, and 1 h before the oedema-inducing injection. The intensity of the oedema in adrenalectomized rats did not decrease after the application of trihydroxyethylrutin.

According to the investigations of LECOMTE and VAN CAUWENBERGE (1974), a new hydroxyethylated rutin derivative, 7-monohydroxyethylrutoside (Z 12007, Zyma S.A., Nyon) in a dose of 30–50 mg/kg i.p. decreases or delays the extent or the development of rat paw oedema induced by histamine (50 µg), bradykinin (0.5 µg), or carrageenin (1 mg). It proved ineffective, however, against oedema induced by 5-HT, formalin, or dextran.

KHADZHAI et al. (1969) found that mouse paw oedema induced by formalin decreases by 34–72% as a result of preliminary treatment with acacetin (25, 50, 100 mg/kg p.o.). The experimental animals received the acacetin in a 1% starch mucilage suspension 2 h before the oedema was induced.

In the experiments of BONTA (1969), injection of a large dose of rutin (500 mg/kg i.p.) led to a pronounced inhibition (ca. 50% or more) of rat paw oedema induced by histamine and to moderate inhibition (25–30%) of oedema induced by 5-HT, compound 48/80, egg white, snake venom, kaolin, or polyvinylpyrrolidone.

According to RIESTERER and JAQUES (1970), the extent of traumatic oedema in rats can be significantly reduced by the application of rutin (300 mg/kg p.o.). LEUSCHNER (1970) and LEUSCHNER and LEUSCHNER (1971) have also reported on the similar effect of O-(β-hydroxyethyl)rutin used in gel form.

The studies of VAN CAUWENBERGE et al. (1971) indicated that (+)-catechin (4 mg/100 g s.c.) moderately inhibits rat paw oedema induced by 5-HT, dextran, and formalin, but does not affect that induced by histamine and bradykinin.

The anti-inflammatory effect of taxifolin (dihydroquercetin) was examined by GUPTA et al. (1971). Administered i.p. in a dose of 40 mg/kg, taxifolin (similarly to hydrocortisone) significantly inhibited oedema induced by carrageenin in the hind paw of rats.

It is interesting to note that DHAWAN and SRIMAL (1973) reported on the anti-inflammatory action of a chroman derivative (3,4-trans-2,2-dimethyl-3-phenyl-4-

[-(β-pyrrolidinoethoxy)-phenyl]-7-methoxychroman; Centchroman). When given orally, Centchroman inhibited carrageenin-induced paw oedema in both mice (20–160 mg/kg) and rats (20–80 mg/kg). It should be noted here that a marked anti-inflammatory action was observed in the granuloma body of rats, in formaldehyde-induced arthritis, and in adjuvant arthritis.

The anti-inflammatory activity of *Vaccinium myrtillus* anthocyanosides has recently been described by LIETTI et al. (1976). The anthocyanoside preparation employed (equivalent to 25% of anthocyanidins) demonstrated significant anti-oedema properties. Carrageenin oedema was induced in male Sprague-Dawley rats (A 1% carrageenin suspension in saline (0.1 ml/rat) was injected into the subplantar region of the right hind paw). *Vaccinium myrtillus* anthocyanosides were given 15 min (i.v.) or 60 min (orally) before carrageenin injection. Use of three doses of the product (50, 100, and 200 mg/kg p.o.) revealed a dose-response relationship. The dose of 200 mg/kg p.o. reduced the oedema by 45%.

The anti-inflammatory principles of *Caesalpinia sappan* L. wood and of *Haematoxylon campechianum* L. wood have recently been reported by HIKINO et al. (1977). The active substances isolated (brazilin and haematoxylin) are indenochromen derivatives and are related to flavonoids. Their investigations showed that administration of brazilin to rats in a dose of 10 mg/kg p.o. before the induction of carrageenin oedema suppressed the foot swelling, the effect being larger than that of 100 mg/kg p.o. berberine chloride, a reference. (Berberine is an alkaloid from the plant *Berberis aristata*.) Haematoxylin exerted a dose-dependent activity; application of 100 mg/kg p.o. was superior to that of berberine chloride in the same dose.

Gossypin and O-(β-hydroxyethyl)rutin inhibited carrageenin-induced rat paw oedema (PARMAR and GHOSH, 1974). Gossypin, which was isolated from *Hibiscus vitifolius* flowers, showed a graded inhibition following three different doses $(1 \times 10^{-4}, 2 \times 10^{-4},$ and 4×10^{-4} M/kg i.p.). After O-(β-hydroxyethyl)rutin $(4 \times 10^{-4}$ M/kg i.p.), paw swelling was inhibited to 59%.

Cherry stalk extract (inventor: KRÁLIK; German patent No.: 1117822, 1962) effectively inhibited oedema induced by carrageenin, dextran, 5-HT, and hyaluronidase in the hind paw of rats (GÁBOR and BLAZSÓ, 1974). In an earlier study GÁBOR and IVÁN (1972) measured the influence of the water-soluble O-(β-hydroxyethyl) rutin (Venoruton, Zyma S.A., Nyon: 100 mg/kg i.p.) on the rat paw oedema-inhibiting effect of butazolidin (50 or 100 mg/kg i.p.) (GÁBOR and IVÁN,, 1972). Compared with the oedema of rats pretreated only with butazolidin, the combined administration of these two drugs significantly decreased rat paw oedema induced by 5-HT or hyaluronidase. A moderate difference was observed in the case of formaldehyde-oedema. For paw oedema provoked by dextran no difference was observed when butazolidin was administered alone or in combination with the rutin derivative.

Rat paw oedema induced by dextran or carrageenin is decreased by large doses of the drug combination used by TARAYRE and LAURESSERGUES (1976), which contains among others flavonoids (hesperidin methylchalcone, methyl-4-esculetol sodium monoethanoate, *Ruscus aculeatus* sterol, and ascorbic acid, Cyclo 3: P. Fabre Centre, Castres, France).

A similarly significant decrease of dextran and carrageenin oedemas was recently reported by TARAYRE and LAURESSERGUES (1977); proteolytic enzymes were included in the combination: chymotrypsin—trypsin complex (Zymolean), hesperidin meth-

Table 3. Inhibition of different rat and mouse paw oedemas by flavonoids

Reference	Flavonoid	Dose (mg/kg)	Oedema inducer													
			5-Hydroxytryptamine	Histamine	Bradykinin	Compound 48/80	Hyaluronidase	Egg white	Formaldehyde	Cobra venom (early phase)	Cobra venom (delayed phase)	PVP	Dextran	Kaolin	Trauma	Carrageenin
GROSS (1950b)	Rutin	s.c. 100						+								
KÜCHLE and WEGENER (1951)	Rutin	s.c. 100						+								
MARTIN et al. (1953)	Epicatechin	s.c. 100						+								
	Phosphorylated hesperidin	p.o. 200 or s.c. 2 × 20														
FORMANEK and HÖLLER (1960)	HR+	p.o. 2000					+		−							
VOGEL and MAREK (1961)	Trimethylolrutin	i.v. 100										+	+			
TEXL (1963)	Vitamin C	s.c. 100					+		+							
	Tea leaf catechol complex															
VOGIN and ROSSI (1963)	Vitamin C + HMC++	p.o. 150–1200 +150 and 600	−													
CAUWENBERGE and FRANCHIMONT (1967, 1968)	HR+	i.p. 30	+	−	+				+							
BONTA (1969)	Rutin	i.p. 500	+	+										+		
KHADZHAI et al. (1969)	Acacetin	p.o. 25–100		++				++								
RIESTERER and JAQUES (1970)	Rutin	p.o. 300	+	+		+				+	+		+	+		+
LEUSCHNER (1970)	HR+	gel form														
GUPTA et al. (1971)	Taxifolin	i.p. 40														
CAUWENBERGE et al. (1971)	[+]-Catechin	s.c. 40	+	−	−			+								
DHAWAN and SRIMAL (1973)	Centchroman	p.o. 20–60													+	
PARMAR and GHOSH (1974)	Gossypin	i.p. 4×10^{-4} M													+	++
	HR+															
GÁBOR and BLAZSÓ (1974)	Cherry stalk extract	i.p. 60, 120, 250	+				+						+			+
LIETTI et al. (1976)	Anthocyanosides	p.o. 50, 100, 200														
TARAYRE and LAURESSERGUES (1976)	HMC + Methyl-4-esculetol	p.o. 40, 5														
HIKINO et al. (1977)	Brazilin, Haematoxylin	p.o. 10, 50, 100														

+ HR = 0-(β-hydroxyethyl)rutin. + +HMC = hesperidin methylchalcone. PVP = polyvinylpyrrolidone.

ylchalcone, methyl-4-esculetol sodium monoethanoate, and ascorbic acid. The combination showed a more complete spectrum of action than non-steroid anti-inflammatory substances against initial symptoms of inflammation.

For the convenience of the reader, the results of the various studies listed above are given in Table 3.

2. Generalized Dextran Oedema in Rats

It is well known that the i.p. injection of dextran into experimental animals leads to the development of oedema localized to the limbs, the cheeks, and the scrotum. The influence of flavonoids on generalized dextran oedema in rats was reported by HAMMERSEN and MÖHRING (1968, 1970) and HAMMERSEN (1972).

According to histologic studies of the subcutaneous connective tissue at the back of the paws of dextran-treated experimental animals, the endothelia of the blood vessels show the same changes, the button-like and wart-like protrusions being the most striking. In addition, the larger intracytoplasmatic vacuoles and vesicles multiply; this can lead to the formation of transendothelial ducts.

When O-(β-hydroxyethyl)rutin is injected (10 mg/100 g i.v.) 1 h before the induction of dextran oedema or is administered for 7 days (30 mg/100 g orally daily), the normally occurring endothelial changes are appreciably decreased. Most conspicuous is the regression of the endothelial protrusions tending towards the lumen. Apart from this, the cytoplasmatic cell changes largely disappear and the larger intraendothelial vacuoles decrease significantly. This can be attributed to the absence of transendothelial dehiscence. In contrast, the intercellular openings do not disappear, but their number and extent decrease.

3. Generalized Phospholipase Oedema in Rats

To induce phospholipase oedema, HAMMERSEN and MÖHRING (1972) and HAMMERSEN (1972) injected 0.1 mg phospholipase A dissolved in 0.1 ml saline into the scrotum of anaesthetized rats. Specimens (m. cremaster and subcutaneous tissue) were taken 10, 20, 30, and 60 min after enzyme injection. As a marker, carbon suspension (0.1 mg/100 g i.v.: C 11/1431a G. Wagner, Hanover) was given 5 min before the enzyme. In the course of the histologic processing, partly specific alterations of the venous vessels and a rather characteristic deformation of the red blood cells were demonstrated: "They exhibited numerous spinous processes that very often due to the plane of section give the impression of isolated profiles lying free in the vascular lumen. These phenomena probably represent the early phase in the development of the so-called thorn-apple form of erythrocytes as a result of enzyme-induced damage of the cell membrane".

Pretreatment of the rats with O-(β-hydroxyethyl)rutin at a dose level of 100 mg/kg body weight i.v. 1 h prior to the oedema challenge, reduced or prevented some of the rather severe damage of the endothelial and red blood cells. The most obvious effect was the absence of the striking alterations of the erythrocytes. The carbon suspension leaked out of the venous vessels only in very rare cases; whereas in the untreated animals most of the larger venules leaked, and quite often more than one interendothelial gap was found in a vascular cross-section. The endothelial processes were more or less completely reduced in the pretreated animals, so that most of the venous vessels gave a normal appearance of their inner outlines.

4. Effect on the Development of the Granuloma Pouch

Using the Selye granuloma pouch method (1953), Salgado and Green (1955) investigated the anti-inflammatory actions of calcium flavone glycoside, lemon bio-flavonoid complex, hesperidin complex, hesperidin, hesperidin methylchalcone, hesperetin, naringin, and naringenin. The granuloma pouch was induced in rats by the injection of croton oil; directly afterwards, and daily for 10–12 days, the animals received a bioflavonoid treatment (once daily in the case of s.c. administration, twice daily in the case of oral application). The parenteral injection produced a significant reduction in the volume of the inflammatory exudate, whereas the oral doses (200, 800, or 1600 mg/kg) were ineffective.

The greatest anti-inflammatory effect was observed after treatment with naringin (100 mg/kg), naringenin (43 mg/kg), and purified hesperidin (100 mg/kg); the smallest effect after treatment with the hesperidin complex (100 mg/kg). With hesperidin methylchalcone (100 mg/kg), a very small effect or none at all was observed. Experiments on adrenalectomized rats showed that the anti-inflammatory effect is independent of the hypophysis-adrenal gland system.

The anti-inflammatory action of O-(β-hydroxyethyl)rutin was also examined by Radouco-Thomas et al. (1964) using the Selye granuloma pouch technique. They compared the effects on rats of daily oral treatments for 10 days of rutin derivative (1, 2, and 4 g/kg), phenylbutazone (0.1 g/kg), and acetylsalicylic acid (0.2 g/kg). Treatment was begun 3 days before the granuloma pouch was induced, and the weight of the 8-day granulomatous wall and the volume of the exudate were measured. The study showed that the weight of the wall was decreased on average by 26% by the phenylbutazone, by 24% by the highest dose of the rutin derivative, and by 18% by the acetylsalicylic acid. The decrease of the volume of exudate after phenylbutazone and acetylsalicylic acid treatments was 52% and 35% respectively. O-(β-hydroxyethyl)rutin (4 g/kg) reduced the formation of exudate by 36%. The effect of smaller doses of the rutin derivative was less pronounced. It is also worth mentioning that in experiments on rats, Radouco-Thomas et al. did not observe mortalities after the oral administration of the rutin derivative in doses of 40 g/kg. (After i.p. injection of this compound the LD_{50} was 27 g/kg).

Van Cauwenberge and Franchimont (1968) treated rats with small doses of O-(β-hydroxyethyl)rutin (3 mg/100 g i.p.) for 9 days following injection of croton oil to induce granuloma pouch. In contrast to the previous experiments, these small doses did not affect the extent of inflammation: neither the weight of the granuloma pouch nor the volume of exudate decreased. In more recent experiments, the application of larger doses (10, 25, 50, 100, and 200 mg/kg) also proved ineffective (Van Cauwenberge et al., 1969).

5. Inflammation Caused by Cotton Pellet

Little has been published on the influence of flavonoids on cotton pellet-induced inflammation. Texl (1963) implanted sterile cotton wool under the skin of rats using the method of MEIER et al. (1950). At the same time as the implantation, tea tannin was administered in 100 mg/kg doses s.c. or orally, either alone or with vitamin C in 100 mg/kg doses. In some cases, vitamin C was administered alone in 100 mg/kg. The controls were injected with physiological salt solution. The treatment was repeated on the 2nd, 4th, and 6th days. In certain experimental groups, the granuloma was removed on the 7th day and weighed after drying. When tea tannin was administered s.c. with vitamin C, the weight of the granuloma decreased by 31% compared with the control. With oral administration, the effect was not significant. Treatment with vitamin C alone also proved ineffective.

According to the studies of VAN CAUWENBERGE and FRANCHIMONT (1968), O-(β-hydroxyethyl)rutin (Z 6000, Labor. Zyma) treatment with 3, 10, and 200 mg/100 g caused no significant change, either in the total weight of the inflamed tissue in the vicinity of the implanted cotton wool or in the weight of the isolated "foreign body" wall. In contrast, 50 mg/100 g produced a significant weight decrease of both the abscess formed near the cotton pellet and the granulomatous wall. Doses of 25 and 100 mg/100 g decreased only the weight of the granulomatous wall.

In experiments with foreign body implantation, MAKAROV and KHADZHAI (1969) demonstrated the anti-inflammatory effect of quercetin, kaempferol, kaempferol-7-rhamnoside, and kaempferol-3,7-dirhamnoside. The rats received the flavonoids for 7 days in a daily oral dose of 50 mg/kg in a 1% starch suspension.

The anti-inflammatory activities of two indenochromen derivatives (brazilin and hematoxylin, from the heart-wood of *Caesalpinia sappan* L. and *Haematoxylon campechianum* L., respectively), with berberine chloride as reference, have recently been determined by the cotton pellet method in rats (HIKINO et al., 1977). Although haematoxylin in doses of 10 and 50 mg/kg/day did not exert an anti-inflammatory effect, the activity of brazilin in doses of 10 and 50 mg/kg/day was found about equivalent to the same doses of berberine chloride in the experimental inflammation model. However, a side-effect leading to a decrease in body weight gain was also observed. On the basis of the above results, it is expected that brazilin is of higher potency than berberine chloride in the treatment of both acute and chronic inflammatory conditions, while hematoxylin shows a considerable effectiveness for acute inflammation, though it possesses little activity for chronic inflammation. According to HIKINO et al. (1977), "these properties of brazilin support the clinical application of the crude drug sappan wood in certain inflammatory disorders."

6. Erythema Produced by UV Radiation

We recently reported a procedure for the evaluation of UV-induced erythema and of experiments with a flavone derivative using this method (ANTAL and GÁBOR, 1971; GÁBOR and ANTAL, 1972). Two circular regions of 20-mm diameter and 10 mm apart of the depilated skin on one side of the spinal column on the backs of albino guinea pigs were irradiated for 20 min with a 350 W analytical quartz lamp. The development of the erythema was followed by a photo cell method. The photo cell current was led into a Hellige D.C. amplifier and the amplified current recorded with a Hellige multiscriptor. The time of appearance of the erythema was also noted. On the following day these experimental animals were treated with O-(β-hydroxyethyl)-rutin (Venoruton, Zyma, Nyon: 250 mg/kg s.c.). Eighty minutes after the administration of the rutin derivative, the guinea pigs were irradiated in the symmetrical regions on the other side of the spinal column in the same way and for the same time as previously. The intensity of the erythema was recorded every 30 min. The results showed that the flavonoid treatment does not prevent the occurrence of the erythema, but it does lead to a pronounced decrease in its intensity (GÁBOR and ANTAL, 1972).

Only one paper had previously been written on the influence of flavonoids on UV erythema: the erythema-inhibiting action of hesperidin was described by WINDER et al. (1958).

It should be mentioned that in guinea pig experiments some synthetic chalcone and dihydrochalcone derivatives of salicylic acid (the chalcones belong structurally among the flavonoids) inhibited UV erythema to the same extent as aspirin. The dose applied was 300 mg/kg orally (LESPAGNOL et al., 1972).

TARAYRE and LAURESSERGUES (1975) recently described the erythema-inhibiting effect of hesperidin methylchalcone (HMC). In experiments on guinea pigs, significant effects were observed 5 and 7 h after irradiation following oral administration of HMC (750 mg/kg) or local application of an ointment containing 10% HMC. In the case of i.p. administration (300 mg/kg), the degree of the UV erythema decreased to a significant extent 2 h after irradiation.

TARAYRE and LAURESSERGUES (1976) also observed that large oral doses of HMC employed in a combination (*Ruscus aculeatus* sterol, methyl-4-esculetol sodium methanoate, hesperidin methylchalcone, and ascorbic acid, Cyclo 3: P. Fabre Centre, Castres, France) similarly decrease the UV erythema of guinea pigs to a significant extent.

7. Inflammation Produced by Mustard Oil

GROSS and MEIER (1948) reported that the development of chemosis induced by drops of 10% mustard oil in the sac of the conjunctiva of rabbits was affected to only a small extent by rutin (25–100 mg/kg i.v. or s.c.) in propylene glycol solution. (The time of administration of the rutin was not apparent.) A good protecting action was attained, however, if the rabbits were treated with rutin (50–100 mg/kg s.c.) in propylene glycol 2 h before the mustard oil drops were applied to induce the inflammation (GROSS, 1950b).

GÁBOR and SZÓRÁDY (1952) succeeded in decreasing the inflammation induced by mustard oil on the depilated skin of the backs of rabbits with haematoxylin one of the indenochromene derivatives included as bioflavonoids. (Haematoxylin occurs in logwood, *Haematoxylon campechianum*.) As a result of the haematoxylin treatment (200 mg/kg i.p.), the skin reaction decreased in every experimental animal. Those rabbits which reacted to the mustard oil plaster with very strong skin inflammation and with scale and scab formation on the control side, displayed at most a strong reddening of the skin after the haematoxylin treatment (The extent of the skin reaction was decided 24 h after removal of the plaster.).

8. Influence on the Permeability-Increasing Action of Inflammatory Exudate

SOKOLOFF et al. (1951) found that the permeability increase induced in rabbits by the leucotaxin isolated from the inflammatory exudate (3 mg per animal s.c.) was inhibited by a bioflavonoid ("Citrus Vitamin P": 10 mg/kg s.c. administered 20 min before the leucotaxin injection). The study was made using the technique of MENKIN (1940).

MENKIN (1959) later studied the effect of "Citrus Vitamin P" (CVP) on the increase of capillary permeability induced in rabbits by the exudate, using another method. (The exudate was produced by the intrapleural injection of turpentine oil.) CVP (5–10 mg) was mixed with 0.25 ml of alkaline or acidic exudate: the mixture was allowed to stand for 10–15 min and was then injected intracutaneously into the abdominal skin of the rabbits.

For comparison, 10 mg exudate mixed with cortisone acetate was injected into another region of the abdominal skin. After this, a 1% trypan blue solution was injected into the ear vein of the animals. A trypan blue spot appeared on the site of injection of the exudate alone, while merely a brown discoloration was observed on the site of the injection of exudate mixed with CVP. The CVP also inhibited migration of leucocytes. Cortisone acetate also impeded and decreased the outflow of the dye and of the leucocytes. On the basis of these results, MENKIN (1959) noted that CVP deserves further attention as an anti-inflammatory agent.

9. Influence on the Inflammation Produced by Red Paprika (Capsicum annuum L. Solanaceae)

According to the experiments of JANCSÓ (1965), a small piece of strongly pungent paprika attached to the inside surface of the arm induces an acute inflammatory reaction. We have studied (GÁBOR, 1972a) the change of capillary resistance (CR) and the effectiveness of flavonoids on this in albino guinea pigs. The CR was determined with the LAVOLLAY and NEUMANN (1949) apparatus. The diameter of the suction bell was 8.5 mm, and suction was applied for 30 s.

Paprika discs (1.5 cm diameter) were applied to the depilated backs of 30 guinea pigs of both sexes weighing 270–360 g. The CR decreased significantly at the site of the paprika disc in every animal, on average by 5.4 cm Hg. As is well known, the compound responsible for the hot taste of paprika is capsaicin. In another experimental series on 15 different guinea pigs, we showed that the result of an exactly similar treatment with Capsoderma ointment (Biogal, Debrecen) containing capsaicin was a decrease of CR in every animal, on average by 4.8 cm Hg.

In another series of experiments, 30 guinea pigs were treated with hesperidin methylchalcone (250 mg/kg i.p.); paprika discs were then applied to half of these animals and the Capsoderma ointment to the other half. Determination of the CR 45 min after the injections showed that it had not decreased. (In these latter two series the CR before the application of the paprika discs and the Capsoderma ointment was 24.46 and 24.80 cm Hg respectively, and after the hesperidin methylchalcone treatment 24.33 and 24.66 cm Hg respectively.) Thus, the decrease of capillary resistance can be completely avoided by previous treatment with hesperidin methylchalcone.

10. Effect of Citrus Flavonoid Complex on Experimentally Induced Mucous Membrane Inflammation

The mucous membrane method for the study of anti-inflammatory substances was developed by KÁTÓ and GÖZSY (1969). One milliliter of diluted formaldehyde solution (1 ml formaldehyde + 14 ml distilled water) was injected by tube into the recta (washed to a depth of 5 cm with physiological salt solution) of rats. Four hours later, a colloidal carbon suspension was injected into the tail vein (1 ml/100 g). (Preparation of the suspension: 30 ml "Günther" Indian ink was suspended in 70 ml of a 3% gelatin solution prepared with distilled water.) One hour after the injection of the carbon suspension, the animals were killed by decapitation and the recta taken out, cut open longitudinally, washed in running water, and spread out on white paper. Determination of the intensity of the carbon deposition in the rectum was made using an empirically prepared scale. The rectal application of diluted formalin led to vasodilatation and an increase of vascular permeability in the mucous membrane. Using this method, KÁTÓ and GÖZSY (1969) showed that the application of citrus flavonoid complex (CFC) inhibits blood vessel damage caused by formaldehyde in the mucous membrane. Rats received 0.5 ml of a CFC solution i.v. on two occasions: 30 or 60 min before or after the formaldehyde injection.

11. Influence on Experimentally Induced Thrombophlebitis

A method for developing thrombophlebitis experimentally has been evolved by FÖLDI and ZOLTÁN (1965). The hind legs of dogs were depilated and the circumference measured at the height of the patella. The animals were anaesthetized and the homolateral external iliac vein was ligated. Turpentine oil (0.2 ml) was injected into the lymphatic lumen along the saphenous vein in the lower leg. In this way a strong oedematous inflammation was induced, and the extent of the inflammation was recorded by daily measurement of the circumference of the limb at the patella. A Melilotus preparation, Esberiven [Schaper-Brümmer, Salzgitter-Ringelheim; composition: sodium salt of the sulphuric acid ester of rutin (50 mg) and cumarin (1 mg) to 2 ml], was administered twice daily to examine its effect on the experimentally produced thrombophlebitis. An average of 17 days was necessary for the circumference of the limbs of the untreated animals to decrease to the original value, while in the treated animals only 7.5 days was necessary. The increase in the limb circumference of the untreated dogs was 158% relative to the starting value, in the treated animals only 120%. The difference was statistically significant.

Recent studies by FÖLDI et al. (1970) show that the daily application (i.m.) of rutin (25 mg/kg) and of cumarin (4 mg/kg) (the essential components of Esberiven) exerts a statistically significant effect on experimental thrombophlebitis. A potentiation of the effect was observed with simultaneous administration of the two substances.

The formation of oedemas following osteotomy of the femur and osteosynthesis in dogs was largely suppressed by the coumarin preparation Esberiven. The swelling was significantly less and subsided more quickly (HOPF et al., 1971).

It may be mentioned here that MIRKOVITCH et al. (1972) showed that the development of experimentally induced thrombosis in dogs can be averted by the administration of large doses of O-(β-hydroxyethyl)rutin (500 mg/kg i.v., daily). A difference was found in the histologic pictures between treated and control animals. As a result of therapy with rutin derivatives, haematomas were much rarer and less extensive, and the oedemas too were smaller. The majority of the capillaries were open and permeable, and the endothelium showed no change. According to later studies, (+)-catechin in a daily dose of 250 mg/kg proved similarly effective in preventing the development of experimentally-induced thrombosis (NIEBES, 1972).

12. Allergic and Hyperimmune Inflammation of the Skin and Joints

FASSBENDER and PIPPERT (1954) produced allergic and hyperimmune inflammation and Arthus phenomenon in the thighs and hind legs of rabbits sensitized with equine serum by re-injection of the serum s.c. For 3 days before the re-injection and for 36 h after it, the animals received a 12-hourly treatment of rutin (Birutan, Merck) (i.v., 500 mg rutin per animal in all). The animals were killed and the appropriate skin area and knee-joints processed histologically. The inflammatory change was classified into one of four grades of severity. In the lighter cases of Arthus phenomenon, merely moderate oedema and slight granulocytosis were observed in the control animals; in the more serious cases, pronounced granulocytic infiltration and necrosis. Study of the joints showed that in the mildest cases, slight oedema of the articular villi and a small amount of proliferation in the joint membrane could be observed. In the most serious changes, large-scale granulocyte infiltration, fibrinoid necrosis, and granuloma could be seen in the articular capsule and fibrin and pus cells in the articular cavity, while the surroundings of the joint were infiltrated by granulocytes and lymphocytes.

The i.v. rutin treatment of the rabbits clearly and strongly inhibited the inflammation both in the skin and in the joint. The phenomenon is explained by the capillary sealing and exudation inhibiting actions of the rutin and by its protective effect on the capillary wall and anaphylactic shock.

13. Data on the Mechanism of the Anti-Inflammatory Effect of Flavonoids

Previous chapters of this volume have already dealt in detail with the inflammatory mediators histamine, 5-HT bradykinin, prostaglandin, and lysosomal enzymes (see Chap. 9, 11, 12, 14, and 16).

A number of reviews have appeared on the chemical mediators of inflammation (SPECTOR and WILLOUGHBY, 1965, 1968; FRIMMER, 1971; ROCHA E SILVA and GARCIA LEME, 1972; WILHELM, 1965, 1973). In the following we shall deal with the mechanism of the anti-inflammatory action of flavonoids, with particular regard to our knowledge of the flavonoids relating to mediators, and shall also touch briefly on the effects of the flavonoids on vascular permeability.

a) Histamine, 5-hydroxytryptamine

Even though several decades have passed since the investigations by DALE and LAIDLAW (1910), research on histamine remains unchangingly in the foreground of attention. Several handbooks and the proceedings of symposia and congresses are of assistance in providing an overall picture of the results and in illustrating the pharmacologic effects (ROCHA E SILVA, 1955; WOLSTENHOLME and O'CONNOR, 1956; ROCHA E SILVA, 1966; MASLINSKY, 1973). Investigations into 5-HT are accompanied by similar interest (GARATTINI and VALZELLI, 1965; ERSPAMER, 1966; SPECTOR and WILLOUGHBY, 1965, 1968; GÖZSY and KÁTÓ, 1970). The roles of these two mediators in inflammation have been dealt with in numerous publications and are also discussed in several chapters of the present volume.

Effect on oedema induced by histamine and 5-HT. As described in an earlier section, O-(β-hydroxyethyl)rutin administered i.p. in a dose of 30 mg/kg could not avert paw oedema induced in rats with histamine, whereas a significant inhibition was observed in the case of 5-HT-induced oedema (VAN CAUWENBERGE and FRAN-CHIMONT, 1967; VAN CAUWENBERGE et al., 1969). After the injection of a large dose of rutin (500 mg/kg i.p.), BONTA (1969) observed a marked inhibition (approximately 50% or more) in rat paw oedema induced by histamine and moderate inhibition (25–30%, $P < 0.05$) in that induced by 5-HT. According to LECOMTE and VAN CAUWEN-BERGE (1974), mono-(O-β-hydroxyethyl)-7-rutin has a small anti-oedematous effect in rats; it inhibits the action of histamine.

It is worth mentioning that a very large dose of O-(β-hydroxyethyl)rutin, its components, or mono-(O-β-hydroxyethyl)-7-rutin release histamine and 5-HT in rats, as shown by hypotension and oedema. The rutin derivatives do not release histamine in either rabbit or man (LECOMTE and VAN CAUWENBERGE, 1972, 1974). LECOMTE (1971) observed release of endogenous histamine and 5-HT in rats after large doses of other flavonoids (esculin, methylesculin, and anthocyanin). In in vitro experiments, BAECKELAND and LECOMTE (1969) demonstrated that degranulation of isolated peritoneal mastocytes of rat is not brought about by the aminoliberator O-(β-hydroxyethyl)rutin, even in a concentration of 10 mg/ml.

Influence on the vascular permeability-increasing effect of histamine and 5-HT. Leakage of protein-bound dye into the skin is one of the most widely used techniques in the study of vascular permeability. The general principle is to inject an experimental animal i.v. with a vital dye, usually trypan blue, pontamine blue, or Evans blue. The dye forms a stable complex with circulating plasma albumin. A small volume of the test substance is then injected into the shaved or depilated skin. If the substance under test increases the vascular permeability, the injection site soon becomes colored with the protein-bound dye. Varying degrees of accuracy have been claimed for the quantitative assay of this change by measuring the diameter of the area of dye leakage or assessing by naked eye on an arbitrary unitary scale. However, the most accurate method is to extract the protein-bound dye from the injection site and measure the resultant color (SPECTOR and WILLOUGHBY, 1968).

Utilizing this method in rats, VAN CAUWENBERGE et al. (1969) showed that after the administration of O-(β-hydroxyethyl)-rutin (100 mg/kg i.p.), the time for appearance of the blue stain at the site of intradermally injected histamine (50 µg) or 5-HT (2.5 µg) was significantly longer than in the control animals. The vascular permeability effect of intradermal histamine is blocked by an antihistamine (pyribenzamine); the action of CFC is much less pronounced (KÁTÓ and GÖZSY, 1969).

Isolated organs. In connection with the effects of flavonoids on the actions of histamine and 5-HT FELIX (1970) showed that O-(β-hydroxyethyl)rutin (0.06 mmole/liter) inhibits the contraction induced by histamine (0.02 mmole/liter) in the isolated ileum of guinea pigs. Our studies on the isolated uterus of rats show that the application of O-(β-hydroxyethyl)rutin in a concentration of 10^{-4} g/ml significantly inhibits smooth muscle contraction induced by 5-HT (GECSE et al., 1972).

Effects of flavonoids in allergy and anaphylactic shock. Histamine plays an important role in allergic reactions and anaphylactic shock. The recognition of this fact led to the development of anti-histaminic substances. These possess a characteristic inhibitory effect on histamine, affecting capillary permeability and resistance. Numerous publications are known on the study of the influence of the flavonoids on the effects produced by histamine (BÖHM, 1968). Opinions differ with respect to the efficacy of the flavonoids in allergic conditions, particularly in anaphylactic shock. It can be stated that according to their mode of action, flavonoids are not anti-histaminic; their efficacy is much less pronounced. As reported by SHILS and GOODHART (1956), it may be concluded that, as regards histamine shock, a few of the flavonoids (quercetin sodium sulphonate and rutin) have at most only a slight protective action, and then only with histamine levels below LD_{100}.

Inhibition of histidine decarboxylase. The flavonoids inhibit many enzymes (BÖHM, 1968; GÁBOR, 1972a, 1975), among them histidine decarboxylase. MARTIN et al. (1949) showed that the most effective was d-catechin (100 µg/ml); quercetin had a lower activity (1000 µg/ml). Rutin, homoeriodictyol, hesperidin and its derivatives, esculin, and esculetin were ineffective. Ascorbic acid alone exhibited a minimal effect, but if rutin or hesperidin methylchalcone was added, then an inhibitory effect was observed. Since the inhibitors act only in concentrations of 1:1000 to 1:10000, MARTIN et al. consider the inhibition probably nonspecific. BARTLETT's theory (1948) of the mechanism of action of flavonoids is that it is due to the formation of quinones, which then react either with the sulfhydryl or with the amino groups of proteins.

Our own examinations indicate that the indenochromene derivatives (haematoxylin, haematein, brasilin, and brasilein), which can be classified among the flavonoids, markedly inhibit histidine decarboxylase (GÁBOR et al., 1952). Most effective were haematein and brasilein, which possess an already-developed quinoidal structure. The inhibitory effect was additive between the members of the ascorbic acid and haematoxylin group.

LORENZ et al. (1973) mentioned that in an investigation with several flavonoids, some of them inhibited histidine decarboxylase of different sources. Especially effective was (+)-catechin. This substance was a potent inhibitor of the specific "acid histidine decarboxylase" from rat stomach. In a final concentration of 10^{-6} M, the flavonoid lowered the enzyme activity by more than 50%. Also, the unspecific or alkaline histidine decarboxylase from guinea pig kidney was inhibited by (+)-catechin to a considerable extent (58% at 10^{-5} M).

LORENZ et al. (1973) studied the effect of another flavonoid, tri-O-(β-hydroxyethyl)rutin, on gastric histidine decarboxylase only in rats. In a 10^{-3} M concentration it inhibited the "acid histidine decarboxylase" of rat stomach by about 80%, whereas the mixture of hydroxyethylrutins (Venoruton, Paroven, Zyma S.A., Nyon) in 10^{-3} M concentration lowered the enzyme activity by 60%.

Action on enzymes of histamine metabolism. A study was made of the effects of flavonoids on histamine methyltransferase from pig antrum mucosa and on diamine oxidases from pig kidney and from pea seedlings (LORENZ et al., 1973). No inhibition of histamine methyltransferase was observed with (+)-catechin (10^{-3} M) and tri-O-(β-hydroxyethyl)rutin (10^{-4} M). A marked inhibitory effect was measured on glutamate dehydrogenase (50% at a (+)-catechin concentration of 10^{-3} M and 10% at 10^{-4} M). Tri-O-(β-hydroxyethyl)rutin did not inhibit glutamate dehydrogenase.

b) Noradrenaline

As reported by SPECTOR and WILLOUGHBY (1965), considerable evidence exists today that during inflammation vasoactive hormones are released and immediately destroyed, and that the active form of these hormones can restore vascular permeability to normal. The most likely substances to act as local anti-inflammatory hormones are adrenaline and noradrenaline. According to Gözsy and Kátó (1970): "among the many factors proposed, only noradrenaline, histamine (and 5-HT) fulfil the criteria of a chemical mediator of the inflammatory process."

Especially worthy of attention are the studies of Kátó and Gözsy (1969) relating to the role and effect of noradrenaline. Kátó and Gözsy emphasized that the catecholamines are natural anti-inflammatory hormones in the early stage of inflammation. As is well known, when histamine is injected into the abdominal skin of rats immediately after intradermal injection of noradrenaline in the same spot, it no longer causes vasodilatation and the increase of capillary permeability. When, however, the administration of histamine follows 4 h after the injection of noradrenaline, very considerable local vasodilatation, rupture of the capillaries and total destruction and degranulation of the mastocytes ensue. This early blood vessel reaction is inhibited in rats treated with CFC.

In further experiments they demonstrated the potentiality of subeffective doses of noradrenaline opposing the effect of histamine. Noradrenaline (20–150 ng) does not affect the vasodilatation induced by histamine. In rats pretreated with CFC, however, the vascular effects of histamine were inhibited by the same doses of noradrenaline. This latter resulted Kátó and Gözsy (1969) to believe that the physical or enzym (catechol-O-methyltransferase or monoamine oxidase) inactivation of noradrenaline is inhibited by CFC. More recent researches have led to the recognition of exact correlations between the chemical structures of the various flavone derivatives and the inhibiting effect of catechol-O-methyltransferase (SCHWABE and FLOHÉ, 1972; GUGLER and DENGLER, 1973).

Kátó and Gözsy (1969) concluded that the essential pharmacologic action of the water-soluble flavonoids is the protection of the mastocytes from disintegration and degranulation during stress. As a result, the liberation of the preinflammatory amines is inhibited. On the other hand, the flavonoids obstruct the physical inactivation of noradrenaline. The protection of the vascular integrity is the cumulative effect of these two factors: the prevention of liberation of the preinflammatory amines and the inhibition of inactivation of the anti-inflammatory amines.

c) Bradykinin

The anti-bradykinin effects of anti-inflammatory drugs were first summarized by ERDÖS (1968). The role of the kinins in inflammation was described in detail by LEWIS (1970). Study of the vasopeptides remains unchangingly in the foreground of research (BACK and SICUTERI, 1972; Kinin 75, International Symposium on Vasopeptides, Fiesole, July 15–17, 1975).

GASCON and WALASZEK (1966) showed that an isoflavone derivative, osajin, isolated from the fruit of *Maclura pomifera* (hedge apples or osages oranges), applied to isolated segments of the ileum of guinea pigs antagonized the musculotropic activity of valyl[5] angiotensin II amide but not that of bradykinin. Later, GARCIA LEME, and WALASZEK (1967) reported on flavonoids with other chemical structures (apiin and hesperidin) as antagonists of bradykinin. Similarly, in experiments on segments of guinea pig ileum, CHAU and HALEY (1969) found that flavonoids inhibited the action of bradykinin in the following order of descending potency: quercetin, rhamnetin, and homoeriodictyol. Morin and esculin showed some activity. All of the other compounds (catechin, xanthorhamnin, rottlerin, quercitrin, esculetin, 4-methylesculetin, and phlorizin) were ineffective within the dose range used. The experimental results permit some conclusions as to the correlation of chemical structure and effect. Antagonism of the spasmogenic activity of bradykinin by flavonoid compounds appears to involve the presence of free phenolic hydroxy groups in the 5,7-positions of the benzo-γ-pyrone nucleus of the aglycone, because methoxylation in position 7 decreases the activity ten times (quercetin vs. rhamnetin). Shifting of one hydroxy from the 3'- to the 2'-position decreases the activity (quercetin vs. morin). In general, the aglycones have greater activity than the glycosides (quercetin vs. quercitrin, and rhamnetin vs. xanthorhamnin).

GARCIA LEME and WALASZEK (1973) recently reported that khellin, furochromon, apiin, and hesperetin produce an inhibition of the responses of the isolated guinea pig ileum to bradykinin. The antagonism between khellin and bradykinin seemed to be competitive, while hesperetin and apiin blocked bradykinin in a noncompetitive manner. In the experiments of GARCIA LEME and WALASZEK (1973) to combat the development of rat paw oedema induced by local injection of bradykinin, highly significant differences were found between the values obtained at the observation times of 30 min, 2 h, and 4 h for the groups receiving khellin and apiin and the control group.

Mention may also be made of the anti-bradykinin effects of two biflavonoids, amentoflavone and cupressuflavone, obtained from *Gingko biloba* and *Cupressus torulosa* respectively, as exhibited on the isolated ileum of guinea pig (RAMASWAMY, 1970). One of the biflavone constituents, apigenin, exerted only a weak effect.

Our own investigations on the isolated uterus of rats indicate that O-(β-hydroxy-ethyl)rutin administered in a concentration of 10^{-4} g/ml considerably inhibits the smooth muscle contraction induced by bradykinin (GECSE et al., 1972). The effect can be enhanced by increasing the quantity of the rutin derivative. The permeability increase induced in rats by bradykinin administered i.c. can be reduced to a significant extent by the preliminary treatment of the experimental animals with the rutin derivative (100–500 mg/kg i.p.) or hesperidin methylchalcone (250–500 mg/kg i.p.).

d) Lysosomes

The biologic and pathologic importance of the lysosomes is well known (DINGLE and FELL, 1969). The possible relationships of lysosomes and their enzymes to inflammation have been reviewed by WEISSMANN (1967) and CHAYEN and BITTENSKY (1971). Lysosomes secrete their enzyme content into the extracellular space following inflammation or other effects. Compounds stabilizing the lysosome membrane inhibit the release of the enzyme content and the occurrence of inflammation.

The flavonoids [rutin, tri(hydroxyethyl)rutin, magnesium flavonic chelates] exert a stabilizing influence on the lysosomes in vitro (VAN CANEGHEM, 1972). The three drugs seem to be about equally active. VAN CANEGHEM found no stabilizing action of the anthocyanosides of *Vaccinium myrtillus*.

According to NIEBES and PONARD (1975), (+)-cyanidanol-3 ((+)-catechin), administered by subcutaneous injection at a dose of 100–200 mg/kg/day for 6–20 days, exerts in vivo a stabilizing effect on lysosomal membranes in rat liver. The same was also demonstrated in animals whose lysosomes had been rendered fragile by intoxication with galactosamine and ethanol.

e) Prostaglandins

The prostaglandins (PGs) and related compounds are discussed in detail in Chapter 12. Their chemistry, biosyntheses, and biological effects have been dealt with in numerous publications (RAMWELL and SHAW, 1971; KARIM, 1972; SOUTHERN, 1972; HORTON, 1972; VANE, 1972; RAMWELL, 1973; ANDERSEN and RAMWELL, 1974; FLOWER, 1974; KÖNIG, 1975; SAMUELSSON and PAOLETTI, 1976).

PGs are known to be mediators in the inflammatory response (ARORA et al., 1970; KALEY and WEINER, 1970; WILLIAMS and MORLEY, 1973), but they do not appear to be the initial mediators (GOLDYNE, 1975).

A number of substances are now known which antagonize the effects of the PGs (EAKINS and SANNER, 1972). Among these is a phosphorylated derivative of phloretin, polyphloretin phosphate (PPP), which can be classified chemically among the flavonoids. Phloretin is the aglycone of phlorizin. (The latter can be obtained from the bark or root-bark of apple, pear, cherry, and plum, and also from *Kalmia augustifolia*.)

Phloretin

According to DICZFALUSI et al. (1953), PPP possesses a very high inhibitory effect on several enzymes, above all alkaline phosphatase, urease, and hyaluronidase.

In vivo experiments. Many data are already available concerning the effect and mechanism of action of PPP. Rat paw oedema induced by egg white (1.5 ml/100 g i.p.) or dextran (Macrodex: 2 ml/100 g i.p.), and lung oedema induced by adrenaline (0.25 mg/kg i.v.) in guinea pigs, can be reduced to a significant extent with PPP (10 mg/100 g i.v.). PPP has a general permeability-reducing effect on capillaries (FRIES, 1960).

PPP (10 mg/ml) infused (at a rate of 0.5 mg/min) into the lingual artery of rabbits inhibits or markedly antagonizes the rise in intraocular pressure normally seen after the intracameral injection of 1 µg PGE_2 (BEITCH and EAKINS, 1969).

In anaesthetized rabbits, injection of PPP (25–200 mg/kg i.v.) results in a variable antagonism to the fall in blood pressure produced by intravenous injections of $PGF_{2\alpha}$; vasodepressor responses produced by PGE_2 and acetylcholine are not antagonized (EAKINS et al., 1970).

In cat experiments, it was demonstrated that PPP antagonizes some smooth muscle actions of prostaglandins: the effects of $PGF_{2\alpha}$ on tracheobronchial tree, ileum, and blood pressure. However, PPP antagonizes the action of PGE_2 only on the ileum and does not inhibit its effects on the tracheobronchial tree and on blood pressure (VILLANUEVA et al., 1972).

In vitro experiments. PPP (2.5–20 µg/ml) reversibly inhibited contractions of the jird colon (*Meriones libycus*; the species is now known as *Meriones shawi*) produced by PGE_2 or $PGF_{2\alpha}$. $PGF_{2\alpha}$ was more readily antagonized than PGE_2 (EAKINS et al., 1970; EAKINS and KARIM, 1970).

PPP (2.5–30 µg/ml) reversibly antagonized contractions produced by PGE_2 and $PGF_{2\alpha}$ on the isolated rabbit jejunum and uterus as well. It was concluded from the

Table 4. Effect of polyphloretin phosphate (PPP) on some responses to prostaglandins in vivo (EAKINS, 1971)

Species	Measurement	Prostaglandin	Response	Antagonism by PPP	Route & dose of PPP
Rabbit	Blood pressure	$PGF_{2\alpha}$ (i.v.)	Fall in blood pressure	+	
		PGE_2 (i.v.)	Fall in blood pressure	−	25—200 mg/kg i.v.
Rabbit	Intraocular pressure (IOP)	$PGF_{2\alpha}$ (i.c.)	Rise in IOP	+	Topical 1%—10%
		PGE_2 (i.c.)	Rise in IOP	+	i.a. infusion (0.5 mg/min)
Rabbit	Protein concentration in aqueous humor	$PGF_{2\alpha}$ (i.c.)	Increase	+	Topical 1%—10%
		PGE_2 (i.c.)	Increase	+	i.a. infusion (0.5 mg/min)
Mouse	Gastrointestinal activity	PGE_2 (i.p.; j.v.)	Diarrhea	+ i.p.	50–200 mg/kg

results that PPP is a selective antagonist to the PGs on these tissues, for contractions produced by other agonists, such as acetylcholine, angiotensin, 5-HT, and bradykinin, were not reduced by concentrations of PPP that markedly antagonized responses to the PGs (EAKINS et al., 1970).

EAKINS et al. (1971) later examined the PG-blocking activity of compounds structurally and functionally related to PPP, including the parent dihydrochalcone, phloretin, and the corresponding glucoside, phlorizin. PPP was a specific reversible, surmountable antagonist of the smooth-muscle-stimulating actions of prostaglandins E_2 and $F_{2\alpha}$. Phloretin and phlorizin were 20–40 times less active and nonspecific antagonists of PG action. From this it can be concluded that the PG-blocking activity of PPP is not a property of the parent dihydrochalcone moiety itself. It is nevertheless assumed that "the possibility exists that shorter-chain phosphorylated esters of phloretin, including the monomer, may possess prostaglandin-blocking activity" (EAKINS et al., 1971). The mechanism of action involved in the interactions observed between PPP and the PGs in their experiments may also be explained by the concept of allosteric interaction proposed by KOSHLAND (1964).

The effect of PPP on some smooth muscle actions of PGs in vitro was well summarized by EAKINS (1971).

CRUTCHLEY and PIPER (1973) later reported that in isolated guinea pig lung experiments PPP inhibited the inactivation of PGE_2, $PGF_{2\alpha}$, and $PGF_{2\beta}$ (ED_{50}: 1.4 µg/ml, 10^{-7} M for each). On the other hand, they mentioned that diphloretin phosphate (DPP) also prevented the inactivation of PGE_2 and $PGF_{2\alpha}$ (ED_{50}: 0.45 µg/ml, 6 × 10^{-7} M); at concentrations greater than 5 µg/ml, DPP antagonized contractions of the assay tissues induced by $PGF_{2\beta}$.

The experiments of GANESAN and KARIM (1973) showed that at low dose levels PPP (50–800 ng/ml) potentiates the effect of prostaglandin E_2 on the isolated rat stomach fundus preparation. No such potentiation could be demonstrated for PG 15 (S) 15 methyl E_2 methyl ester, a synthetic analogue of PGE_2. It is worth mentioning that with higher doses (up to 640 µg/ml), PPP completely abolishes the stimulant

Table 5. Effect of polyphloretin phosphate (PPP) on some smooth muscle actions of prostaglandins in vitro. (Eakins, 1971)

Preparation	Prostaglandin	Response	Antagonism by PPP
Colon, Jird	$PGF_{2\alpha}$; PGE_2	Contraction	+
Jejunum, Rabbit	$PGF_{2\alpha}$; PGE_2	Contraction	+
Uterus, Rabbit (N.P.)	$PGF_{2\alpha}$; PGE_2	Contraction	+
Uterus, G. pig (N.P. & P.)	$PGF_{2\alpha}$; PGE_2	Contraction	+
Uterus, Rat (N.P. & P.)	$PGF_{2\alpha}$; PGE_2	Contraction	+
Uterus, Monkey (N.P.)	$PGF_{2\alpha}$; PGE_2	Contraction	+
Trachea, Rabbit	PGE_2	Relaxation	−
Umbilical cord, human	PGE_1	Relaxation	−
	PGE_2; $PGF_{2\alpha}$	Contraction	−

N.P. = Nonpregnant.
P.   = Pregnant.

effect of PGE_2. PPP also stimulates the longitudinal muscle of isolated human jejunum.

Taking into consideration the fact that in the investigations of MARRAZZI and MATSCHINSKY (1972) PPP was a potent inhibitor of PG 15-OH dehydrogenase, whereas PG 15 (S) 15 methyl E_2 methyl ester is not a substrate for the dehydrogenase (BUNDY et al., 1971), GANESAN and KARIM (1973) produced evidence to show that the potentiation of PGE_2 and the direct stimulant action of PPP are due to inhibition of PG 15-OH dehydrogenase. PARK and DYER (1973) and STRANDBERG and TUVEMO (1975) found that PPP inhibits contractions of the isolated human umbilical artery induced by PGE_2 and $PGF_{2\alpha}$ respectively.

f) The Effect of Flavonoids on Vascular Permeability

Increased vascular permeability is considered to be the most characteristic sign of the early inflammatory reaction. Current knowledge relating to the capillary permeability (structural and physiologic considerations, connective tissue mediation of increased vascular permeability in inflammation) is treated in detail by ZWEIFACH et al. (1973).

Attention was directed to the effects of flavonoids on capillary permeability by ARMENTANO et al. (1936). They were the first to show that pathologically increased capillary permeability is normalized by flavone derivatives (hesperidin, eriodictyol) isolated from lemon juice. A number of monographs later dealt with the effect of flavonoids on vascular permeability (GRIFFITH et al., 1955; SHILS and GOODHART, 1956; BÖHM, 1968). Many studies have been made on the effects of flavonoids on permeability changes induced by chloroform, histamine, 5-HT, and bradykinin. The effects of flavonoids on the permeability increase caused by heat, X-rays, etc. are also known (reviewed by GÁBOR, 1972 b).

14. Discussion

If the results of the studies of the anti-inflammatory action of flavonoids are considered, the following findings emerge:

1. According to the overwhelming majority of authors (GROSS, 1950b; KÜCHLE and WEGENER, 1951; MARTIN et al., 1953; VOGEL and MAREK, 1961; NORTHOVER and SUBRAMANIAN, 1962; TEXL, 1963; FORMANEK and HÖLLER, 1960; VAN CAUWENBERGE and FRANCHIMONT, 1967, 1968; VAN CAUWENBERGE et al., 1969, 1971; BONTA, 1969; KHADZHAI et al., 1969; RIESTERER and JAQUES, 1970; LEUSCHNER, 1970; LEUSCHNER and LEUSCHNER, 1971; GUPTA et al., 1971; DHAWAN and SRIMAL, 1973; PARMAR and GHOSH, 1974; GÁBOR and BLAZSÓ, 1974; LIETTI et al., 1976; TARAYRE and LAURESSERGUES, 1976; HIKINO et al., 1977), prior treatment with flavonoids decreases the extent of oedema induced in mouse and rat paw by different methods.

2. The blood vessel endothelial changes usually appearing in generalized dextran oedema are significantly decreased by treatment with a rutin derivative (HAMMERSEN and MÖHRING, 1968, 1970; HAMMERSEN, 1972).

3. The pretreatment of rats with 0-(β-hydroxyethyl)rutin is able to reduce or prevent some rather severe damage of the endothelial and red blood cells caused by the injection of phospholipase A (HAMMERSEN and MÖHRING, 1972; HAMMERSEN, 1972).

4. According to SALGADO and GREEN (1955), the volume of inflammatory exudate in the granuloma pouch can be significantly decreased by a parenteral flavonoid treatment. As a result of the oral administration of large doses of trihydroxyethylrutoside, RADOUCO-THOMAS et al. (1964) observed a decrease of both the weight of the granuloma pouch wall and the volume of the exudate. In contrast to the above-mentioned experiments, 0-(β-hydroxyethyl)rutin treatment did not decrease either the weight of the granuloma pouch or the exudate volume in the studies by VAN CAUWENBERGE and FRANCHIMONT (1968), and VAN CAUWENBERGE et al. (1969).

5. According to TEXL (1963), VAN CAUWENBERGE and FRANCHIMONT (1968), MAKAROV and KHADZHAI (1969), and HIKINO et al. (1977), inflammation induced by foreign body implantation can be reduced considerably by a prior treatment with flavonoids.

6. The intensity of the erythema produced by UV irradiation can be markedly reduced by the use of hesperidin, hesperidin methylchalcone or 0-(β-hydroxyethyl)-rutin (WINDER et al., 1958; GÁBOR and ANTAL, 1972; LESPAGNOL et al., 1972; TARAYRE and LAURESSERGUES, 1975, 1976).

7. Inflammation induced by the application of mustard oil to the eye or the skin is moderated by flavonoid treatment, rutin, or indenochromene derivatives (GROSS and MEIER, 1948; GROSS, 1950a; GÁBOR and SZÓRÁDY, 1952).

8. The capillary permeability increase induced by inflammatory exudate can be inhibited by a CVP treatment (SOKOLOFF et al., 1951; MENKIN, 1959).

9. The decrease of skin capillary resistance during inflammation caused by the application of red paprika can be avoided by the prior treatment of the animals with hesperidin methylchalcone (GÁBOR, 1972a).

10. CFC treatment inhibits the capillary permeability increase and the vasodilatation brought about in the rectal mucosa of the rat by a formaldehyde solution (KÁTÓ and GÖZSY, 1969).

11. The recovery time from thrombophlebitis experimentally induced in the hind legs of dogs is substantially shortened as a result of treatment with Esberiven preparation containing rutin and cumarin, and the degree of tumescence is significantly

less compared with the controls (FÖLDI and ZOLTÁN, 1965; FÖLDI et al., 1970; HOPF et al., 1971).

Experimental thrombosis in dogs can be prevented and the damage to the venous wall can be inhibited by the administration of O-(β-hydroxyethyl)rutin (MIRKO-VITCH et al., 1972).

12. FASSBENDER and PIPPERT (1954) found that allergic-hyperimmune inflammation in rabbits can be strongly inhibited by rutin treatment.

The above-mentioned model studies have demonstrated the anti-inflammatory action of the flavonoids. The experimental results point to the likely anti-inflammatory effect of certain flavone derivatives. In Section B.III.13 we dealt with the mechanism of the anti-inflammatory effect of flavonoids, with particular regard to the mediator substances. In the future it appears worthwhile to carry out studies on the antagonistic effects of prostaglandins and on the possible inhibition of prostaglandin biosynthesis with various flavonoids. (We are at present performing such experiments.)

With regard to the mechanism of action, mention may be made here of the studies of VAN CAUWENBERGE and FRANCHIMONT (1968). According to their experiments, 1 or 2 h after the injection of O-(β-hydroxyethyl)rutin (3 mg/100 g i.p.) the ascorbic acid and cholesterol contents of the adrenal glands decrease significantly, while the fluorescing steroid level of the blood plasma significantly increases. The increase of the plasma steroid level follows 2–4 h after the intramuscular (i.m.) administration of the chemical and 4 h after its oral administration. Hence, the mode of action of the rutin derivative is probably based on the stimulation of the adrenal cortex.

Our knowledge relating to the anti-inflammatory action of bioflavonoids has increased to a significant extent during the past 20 years, and we have come nearer to an understanding their mechanism of action. It must be noted, however, that with very few exceptions, researchers have carried out only one model study for the demonstration of anti-inflammatory action, although, as WINTER (1966a, b) and others have emphasized, numerous tests must be made to check the effect.

Even today, the relation between the anti-inflammatory effect of the bioflavonoids and their biochemical effects has not been elucidated. As is well known, the flavone compounds are polyvalent, that is, they affect several enzymes (hyaluronidase, histidine decarboxylase, xanthinoxidase, succinoxidase, etc.). The effects of the flavonoids on the enzymes are attributed to SH-blocking and the complexing of certain essential metal ions.

In the future it seems very important to carry out further biochemical studies: demonstrating the effect on interrupting oxidative phosphorylation, on proteolytic enzymes [e.g., chymotrypsin, to which the degranulation of mast cells and the liberation of histamine are attributed (PASTAN and ALMQUIST, 1966)], etc.

C. Anti-Inflammatory Activity of Natural Plant Coumarins (Benzo-α-Pyrones)

The occurrence and the chemistry of the coumarins have been reported, among others, by DEAN (1963) and KUZNECOVA (1967), and their biological effects by KHADZHAI (1965) and FEUER (1974).

The contents of *Melilotus officinalis* (L.) (common melilotus) include coumarin and flavones. The effect of the standardized extract (Esberiven, Schaper and Brümmer, Salzgitter-Ringelheim) on experimentally induced thrombophlebitis is described above, and its other anti-inflammatory effects have been reported in a number of publications. In rat experiments with the SELYE (1953) granuloma method, groups of animals were treated for 10 days with 0.5 ml Esberiven daily, 0.5 ml Melilotus extract daily, or 10 mg rutin i.m. daily, while the controls received 0.5 ml physiological salt solution (KELLNER, et al., 1961). As a result of the treatments with Esberiven or Melilotus extract, the weight of the granuloma pouch and the volume of exudate decreased significanctly compared with the controls. Rutin treatment per se did not exhibit a significant anti-inflammatory effect.

Oedema induced by egg white in the hind paw of rat was inhibited by 40–50% by Esberiven (Melilotus extract standardized to 0.05% coumarin and with 2.5% vitamin P factor) administered in a dose of 1 ml/kg 15 min before and 24 h after inducement of the oedema (SHIMAMOTO and TAKAORI, 1965).

In the later studies of FÖLDI-BÖRCSÖK et al. (1971) and FÖLDI-BÖRCSÖK (1972), coumarin given i.p. in a dose of 50 mg/kg significantly inhibited rat paw oedema produced by carrageenin or by thermal injury (52 or 55° C). However, coumarin did not inhibit egg-white-induced oedema and kaolin arthritis. A dose-dependent coumarin effect was observed in the case of oedema due to lymphatic obstruction. Histologic examinations showed the oedema to be appreciably less marked in coumarin-treated animals.

CASLEY-SMITH and PILLER (1974) consider that coumarins substantially reduce the amount of high-protein oedemas.

They do this not by increasing lymph flow (although they can do this), not by reducing protein leakage from the blood vessels, nor by causing increased endocytosis of proteins per se, but by causing increased lysis of the accumulated proteins in the tissue. The resulting fragments can then rapidly enter the blood vessels, because they are small enough to pass down the intercellular junctions, their concentration gradients are directed from the tissues to the blood, and their diffusion coefficients are high. Thus, the excessive amounts of protein are removed, and the oedema fluid is released.

PILLER (1975) recently reported that coumarin has two main effects: one is to cause vascular injury, thus allowing extra protein and fluid into the tissue; the other is to stimulate phagocytosis, enzyme production and thus proteolysis, and a subsequent removal of protein and fluid from the injured tissues. PILLER makes the interesting observation that a medium-range temperatures the proteolytic actions of coumarin outweigh its injurious nature.

In the most recent reviews, CASLEY-SMITH (1976) discussed the actions of the benzopyrones on the blood—tissue—lymph system, while PILLER (1977a) provided a comprehensive picture of the mechanism of action of coumarin. In possession of the numerous data, he gives an explanation of its effectiveness as a therapy for thermally injured tissue:

"Coumarin binds rapidly to the serum albumins, and the protein binding capacity of a substance provides insight into its interaction with sites of biological activity. Together with proteins, flowing in through the damaged capillary endothelium after thermal injury, it is taken up by the monocytes in the inflamed tissues and by the resident macrophages. Coumarin can stimulate these cells to enhanced proteolysis of the engulfed protein, which is digested to debris of molecular weight < 1000. This is, on the other hand, readily utilizable protein for the large number of monocytes to mature and differentiate into macrophages. Coumarin may dissociate from protein in the tissue and cause local site activation or even activate all cell sites, increasing cell numbers, or may rejuvenate older phagocytic cells and stimulate the reticulo-endothelial system (RES). A passing histamine-like effect of coumarin and other benzopyrones is an indirect stimulant for the RES. The released injurious amines open additional numbers of endothelial intercellular junctions, allowing extra protein and fluid into the interstitial tissues. A reinforced phagocytosis follows and results in more rapid and complete digestion. The action of the drug in causing the opening of intercellular junctions is very beneficial. The extra protein is of little consequence, since its inflow is more than compensated for by the other actions of the drug, which results in its lysis.

Coumarin has also a number of other important actions on the vascular system. It causes constriction of the precapillary sphincters and a dilatation of the arterio-venous anastomosis. The result is an increased blood pressure and flow and a better oxygen supply of the area.

It is able to restore the deformability of the red blood cell to near normal levels and to protect the thrombocyte by membrane stabilizing. The result is a reduced likelihood of thrombosis and embolism. By increasing the glucose uptake and transport, the benzopyrones can improve the chance of survival of those cells in stagnant areas of the circulation."

In another very recent paper PILLER (1977b) provides data on the most effective doses of benzopyrone in treatment of mild thermal oedema.

In a discussion of the anti-inflammatory action of coumarin, it should be mentioned that, in contrast to the earlier-reported results, FONTAINE et al. (1967) found that coumarin itself and 19 of its derivatives did not exhibit a significant anti-inflammatory effect compared with aspirin (guinea pig UV erythema test) or phenyl-butazone (carrageenin-induced rat paw oedema test): not even 50% of the aspirin or phenylbutazone activity could be observed. The differences between the results can probably be explained by the different modes of administration. In contrast to the previous experiments, FONTAINE et al. (1967) gave the coumarin in an oral dose of 50 mg/kg.

The carrageenin-induced rat paw oedema method was recently utilized to study the anti-inflammatory effects of some natural plant coumarins (apetalolide, calophyllolide, calophyllic acid, inophyllolide, tomentolide-A, and tomentolide-B) (CHATUR-

Apetalolide   Calophyllolide   Calophyllic acid

Inophyllolide   Tomentolide—A   Tomentolide—B

VEDI et al., 1974). Of these coumarin derivatives, calophyllolide, inophyllolide, to-mentolide-A, and tomentolide-B caused decreased of 24.5–60.7% in the volume of oedema. The doses applied were 40 mg/kg i.p. Calophyllolide possessed the maximum anti-inflammatory activity of 60.7%. Hydrocortisone, at a dose of 10 mg/kg, exhibited an anti-inflammatory activity of 44%.

D. Anti-Inflammatory Activity of Natural Plant Triterpenoids

I. Escin

The therapeutically active principle of horse-chestnut *(Aesculus hippocastanum)*, escin, has been described and studied pharmacologically by LORENZ and MAREK (1960). Its site and mechanism of action have been described by VOGEL and UEBEL (1960) as well as by VOGEL et al. (1963) and PREZIOSI and MANCA (1965). Experimental and clinical studies with tritium-labelled escin have shown it capable of normalizing abnormal conditions of permeability (ASHER, 1968). Its capillary resistance-increasing effect has been reviewed by Gábor (1974). Chemical analysis has been carried out by PATT and WINKLER (1960). According to these examinations, the active principle of horse-chestnut saponin escin is escigenin, which contains a pentacyclic triterpene skeleton with an oxide ring.

Escigenin $C_{30}H_{48}O_5$

LORENZ and MAREK (1960) observed that ovalbumin-induced rat paw oedema could be inhibited by saponin escin and esculus extracts. It was later also demonstrated that a gel containing 1% micronized escin and 1% buphenine, applied to the backs of rats, strongly inhibited kaolin-oedema of the paw. Both active ingredients are involved in the anti-oedemic effect (LORENZ and REIFFER, 1967).

The mechanism of action of horse-chestnut saponin escin was extensively studied by VOGEL et al. (1970). The drug was tested on rat paw oedema following local application of ovalbumin, dextran, carrageenin, hyaluronidase, bradykinin, compound 48/80, 5-HT, histamine, aerosol, kaolin, bee poison, and formalin, and oedema in local Arthus phenomenon. Escin inhibited inflammation, e.g., the paw oedemas induced by ovalbumin, dextran, carrageenin, bradykinin and compound 48/80, and the local Arthus oedema. Its inhibitory effect was mostly restricted to the initial phase of the other oedemas. The exudation caused by the subcutaneous (s.c.) implantation of an adsorbent foreign body and the exudation occurring in a mycobacterial granuloma pouch were also inhibited. On the other hand, escin was ineffective in the late reparative phase; in the neoplastic connective tissue of the croton oil granuloma

pouch test and cotton pellet test, as well as in the immunologically induced polyarthritis of rats, it had no effect. Since the initial phase of inflammation is characterized
by disturbed permeability of the vascular walls, the authors advanced the hypothesis
that escin seals the capillaries by reducing the number and/or diameter of the small
pores of the capillary wall through which the exchange of water occurs. This conclusion is supported by the observation that escin is able to shift back to normal the
permeability of the plasma-lymph barrier enhanced by bradykinin injection.

Recently ROTHKOPF and VOGEL (1976) tested the efficacy of the horse-chestnut
saponin escin on two further models of inflammation: the rat serous peritonitis
provoked by i.p. injection of formalin solution and the rat serous pleurisy provoked
by intrapleural injection of Evans blue/carrageenin. The results showed "escin to be
an antiexudative substance with regard to its exudation inhibitory effect determined
by the reduction of exudative fluid."

II. Glycyrrhetinic Acid

The anti-inflammatory effect of one of the constituents of liquorice (Glycyrrhiza
glabra), glycyrrhetinic acid, has been reported by several authors (SOMERS, 1957;
D'ARCY and KELLETT, 1957; LOGEMAN et al., 1957).

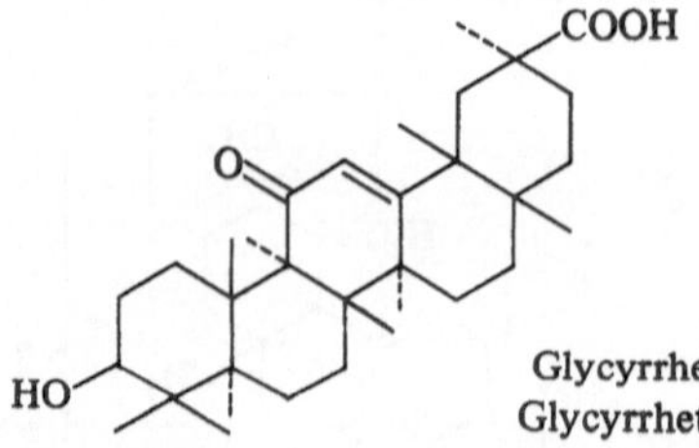

Glycyrrhetic acid
Glycyrrhetinic acid

Although the structure shows a resemblance to that of hydrocortisone, the acid
has no glucocorticoid action.

The anti-inflammatory activity of glycyrrhetinic acid has been determined by the
following methods: cotton pellet- and formaldehyde-induced rat paw oedema, the
granuloma pouch method, and the tuberculin reaction in BCG-sensitized guinea
pigs. The results obtained in the four different kinds of tests show that glycyrrhetinic
acid is an active anti-inflammatory agent (FINNEY and SOMERS, 1958). It was later
reported that glycyrrhetinic acid hydrogen succinate, as the disodium salt, has a
powerful anti-inflammatory action in rats. As assessed by the cotton pellet method, it
had 0.23 times the activity of hydrocortisone hemisuccinate (FINNEY and TÁRNOKY,
1960). The anti-inflammatory actions of β-glycyrrhetinic acid and glycyrrhetinic acid
were measured by depression of granuloma tissue formation by the cotton pellet
technique in adrenalectomized rats as well (KRAUS, 1960). The two preparations
significantly depressed the granulation tissue formation.

In the review by WHITEHOUSE (1965), it is mentioned that "the 18β-glycyrrhe-
t(in)ic acid did at one time enjoy some popularity as an anti-rheumatic drug. Small
clinical trials have not really substantiated its anti-rheumatic efficacy, although the
3-hemisuccinate ester of this acid ("Biogastrone") does have a beneficial action on
and promotes the healing of gastric ulcers (DOLL et al., 1962), perhaps through a
local anti-inflammatory effect."

III. Other Triterpenoids

Anti-inflammatory properties of two plant triterpenoids, α- and β-amyrin acetates, as exhibited by the protection of carrageenin-induced oedema and formaldehyde-induced arthritis and by the decrease in the formation of tissue induced by "cotton wool" implantation, have been reported by GUPTA et al. (1969, 1971).

Recently, newer triterpenoids were investigated for anti-inflammatory activity by CHATURVEDI et al. (1974): friedelin and friedelan-3β-ol decreased the volume of carrageenin-induced oedema in rats and exhibited 17% and 51% anti-inflammatory activity respectively when used in a dose of 30 mg/kg i.p. Hydrocortisone in a dose of 10 mg/kg i.p. exhibited 44% anti-inflammatory activity.

Still more recently, some other plant triterpenoids (hederagenin methyl ester acetate, hederagenin, α- and β-amyrin caprylates, erythrodiol caprylate, dihydrobetulic acid, friedelinoxime, and acetyl methyl ursolate) were evaluated for anti-inflammatory activity by CHATURVEDI et al. (1976). The substances exhibited anti-inflammatory activity against carrageenin-induced oedema, except for α-amyrin caprylate and friedelinoxime. The compounds were tested in a dose of 40 mg/kg i.p., while sodium salicylate, as a reference drug, was used in a dose of 100 mg/kg (anti-inflammatory activity, 33.3%). The maximum inhibition of 48% was observed with hederagenin.

E. Colchicine

As is well known, colchicine, an alkaloid from *Colchicum autumnale* (autumn crocus), is used in the treatment of acute gout. A common mechanism for its anti-inflammatory effect was reported by MALAWISTA (1968).

An acute attack of gout apparently occurs as a result of an inflammatory reaction to crystals of monosodium urate that are deposited in the joint tissue from hyperuric body fluids; the reaction is aggravated as more urate crystals accumulate (GOODMAN and GILMAN, 1971). From this starting-point, several attempts have been made to use colchicine to influence sodium-urate-induced paw swelling in rats and mice. Experimental data on colchicine (DENKO and WHITEHOUSE, 1970) and on colchicine and 17 of its derivatives (ZWEIG et al., 1972) showed that demecolchicine, colchiceinamide, trimethylcolchicinic acid methyl ether, and trimethylcolchinic acid ethyl ether were almost as effective as colchicine in inhibiting the oedema induced in the rat hind paw by subplantar injection of sodium urate crystals. From a study of various colchicine derivatives with regard to the correlation of chemical structure and effect, FITZGERALD et al. (1971) found that the methoxytropone moiety and the nitrogen function of colchicine are essential for anti-inflammatory activity. (The experimental model of inflammation consisted of mouse paw swelling induced by a subplantar injection of a suspension of microcrystalline sodium urate.)

Most recently, the effects of colchicine and its analogs (trimethylcolchicinic acid, colchiceine, N-desacetyl-N-methylcolchicine, 2-desmethylcolchicine glucoside) on carrageenin-induced rat paw oedema have been studied by CHANG (1975a). The drugs were administered as solutions in saline, either orally (33 mg/kg) 1 h prior to the injection of carrageenin, or intravenously (1 mg/kg) 15 min before the injection of carrageenin. Of the compounds used, colchicine and N-desacetyl-N-methylcolchicine suppressed the development of the inflammation by about 50–60%. The other substances had no significant effect. Colchicine (2 mg/kg i.p.) and N-desacetyl-N-methylcolchicine (2 mg/kg i.p.) also suppressed the reversed passive Arthus reaction in the rat. In the latter experiments, the inflammatory response was measured by using radioiodinated (^{131}I) human serum albumin and Evans blue.

Further investigations by CHANG (1975b) showed that colchicine, desacetylmethylcolchicine, and colchiceine suppress the phagocytosis of starch granules by rabbit peritoneal polymorphonuclear leucocytes in vitro. Colchicine at concentrations as high as 10^{-4} M has no effect on the chemotaxis of polymorphonuclear leucocytes in response to immune-complex-activated chemotactic factors. According to CHANG: "these results do not support the contention that the suppression of phagocytosis or chemotaxis plays a significant role in the anti-inflammatory activity of colchicine." [The reader is referred to the publication by CHANG (1975b) for the details.]

The anti-inflammatory effect of colchicine has also been compared with those of phenylbutazone and indomethacin by CHANG (1975c). Colchicine suppresses the development of carrageenin-induced oedema in the rat with a minimum effective oral dose of 6.0 mg/kg. The slope of the dose-response regression line for colchicine differs significantly from those for indomethacin and phenylbutazone. Based on the dosages required to achieve a 50% suppression of this inflammation, colchicine is 0.6 and 1.5 times as potent as indomethacin and phenylbutazone respectively.

F. Essential Components of Camomile

The phytochemical examination and pharmacological effects of extracts and volatiles of the camomile flower (*Matricaria chamomilla* L.) have been described in numerous reviews and publications (KRISTEN and SCHMIDT, 1957; ISAAC and SCHIMPKE, 1965; POETHKE and BULIN, 1969a, b; LINDE and CRAMER, 1972; SCHILCHER, 1972, 1973; THIEMER et al., 1973; ISAAC, 1974).

According to our present knowledge, the components responsible for the anti-inflammatory effect of camomile are: I. the azulenes; II. (-)-α-bisabolol; III. cis-2[hexadiine-(2,4)-yilidine]-1,6-dioxaspiro-(4,4)-nonene-(3) (EN-IN-dicycloether); and IV. the flavonoids.

I. The Azulenes

The chemistry of the azulenes has been reviewed by HAGEN-SMIT (1948). The camomile flower contains matricin (prochamazulene), which on steam distillation is converted via chamazulene-carboxylic acid to chamazulene (1,4-dimethyl-7-ethylazulene).

| Matricin (Prochamazulene) | Chamazulene—carboxylic acid | Chamazulene |

ARNOLD (1927), HEUBNER and GRABE (1933), and HEUBNER and ALBATH (1939) demonstrated the anti-inflammatory action of an infusion prepared from the camomile flower and of the azulene-containing fraction of camomile oil. Although doubt was cast on these results (BROCK et al., 1954; OETTEL and WILHELM-KOLLMANS-PERGER, 1955, 1956; BOGS and MEINHARD, 1955), attention turned to research on the anti-inflammatory effects of camomile oil and the azulenes.

The investigations by JANCSÓ (1947a, 1947b) showed that one of the components of camomile oil, chamazulene, is a "special histamine-releasing substance." If the skin of mouse, rat, or guinea pig were smeared with chamazulene, and Indian ink was administered 0.5–3 h later i.v., then deep-extending, strong, regular pictures of angioendothelial phagocytic activity could be observed at the treated site. Azulene exerts a long-lasting histamine-releasing effect in the tissues. In the view of JANCSÓ, "chamazulene or the blue oil of the camomile does not have an anti-inflammatory effect; on the contrary, it can be utilized in therapy to enhance sluggish inflammatory reactions and make them more intensive."

The basis of the theory developed by STERN, however, is that azulene inhibits histamine release in both allergic (STERN, 1951) and inflammatory (STERN and MI-LIN, 1956) processes and antagonizes the effect of the histamine liberator (compound 48/80). After injection of compound 48/80 (5 µg) into cats (2.5 kg) treated with the water-soluble guaiazulene (1,4-dimethyl-7-isopropylazulenesulphonic acid sodium salt (Azulene SN) (20 mg), the blood pressure no longer decreased. In rats, guaiazulene (10 mg) inhibited the cheek and paw oedema-inducing effects of egg white (i.p.) and the histamine liberator compound 48/80 (100 µg). Later studies showed that guaiazulene significantly inhibits the reduction of histamine induced in the skin of rats by compound 48/80 (STERN, 1959).

Hind paw oedema induced by the subplantar (s.p.) injection of kaolin in rats can be significantly inhibited by treatment s.c. as orally with natural azulenes (total extract of *Flores chamomillae*, etheric camomile oil) and synthetic azulene (S-guaiazulene = 1,4-dimethyl-7-isopropylazulene) (ZIERZ et al., 1957). These results were confirmed in essence by the further studies of SEIKEL (cited in KRISTEN and SCHMIDT, 1957). Guaiazulene inhibited dextran oedema markedly, and hyaluronidase and formaldehyde and histamine oedemas moderately. It was suggested that the oedema-inhibiting effect of guaiazulene was based on histamine-releasing action, antihistamine action, 5-HT-release-inhibiting action, antihyaluronidase action and, probably, capillary permeability decreasing action (UDA, 1960).

Mention must also be made of the work of YAMASAKI et al. (1958), according to which guaiazulene inhibits the passive cutaneous anaphylaxis (PCA) of rats by i.p. injection or external application to the local skin. It inhibited the depletion of the skin histamine after a large dose of dextran given i.p. It lessened the increase of urinary excretion of histamine after i.p. injection of various classes of histamine liberators such as sinomenine, decylamine, Na cholate, Tween 20, dextran, and egg white. The drug suppressed local staining or granulopexy after dermal inoculation of sinomenine solution manifested by vascular injection of trypan blue or Indian ink in the rat. In vitro anaphylactic histamine release from the minced lung of the sensitized guinea pig was inhibited by 10^{-5}–10^{-6} M guaiazulene. These results suggest that the anti-inflammatory as well as anti-allergic effects of guaiazulene may be due to interference with the release of inflammatory substances including histamine from the tissue cells by a mechanism, the nature of which is direct on cells rather than mediatory via pituitary-adrenal activation. Guaiazulene was found to have slightly antipyretic, analgesic, local anaesthetic, and antihistaminic properties. These will favor the clinical anti-inflammatory effect.

Jeličić-Hadžović and Stern (1972) recently reported that guaiazulene (Azulon liquidum: Chemiewerk, Homburg, Frankfurt) in a concentration of 0.045 µg/ml blocks contractions produced by histamine, 5-HT, or bradykinin in the isolated intestinal loop of guinea pigs.

According to more recent data, an increasing influence on the oxidative phosphorylation was seen in rat liver mitochondria after application of camomile extract. Only the phosphorylation/oxidation ratio changed slightly (Thiemer et al., 1973).

II. (-)-α-Bisabolol

The anti-inflammatory action of the sesquiterpene alcohol, (-)-α-bisabolol, has been examined only in recent years.

α−Bisabolol

Jakovlev and Schlichtegroll (1969) used the carrageenin oedema and the cotton pellet granuloma methods to study the anti-inflammatory effect of bisabolol in comparison with guaiazulene, azulene SN, phenylbutazone, and indomethacin (Table 6). It can be seen that bisabolol exhibited only a slight activity in this test, in contrast to the cotton pellet test (Table 7).

The experimental results of Jakovlev and Schlichtegroll (1969) may give an explanation as to why the total extract of camomile is more effective than would correspond to the azulene content.

Further experiments proved that new derivatives of (-)-α-bisabolol exhibit considerably larger oedema-inhibiting effects than (-)-α-bisabolol itself (Thiele et al., 1969). For instance, the paw oedema induced in rats by egg white can be moderated to an appreciable extent (47%) with cyclopentanecarboxylic acid bisabolol ester (300 mg/kg orally), whereas (-)-α-bisabolol (500 mg/kg orally) has a corresponding effect of only 18%.

Table 6. Carragenin-induced rat paw oedema

	ED_{50} mg/kg orally
Bisabolol	850
Guaiazulene	1100
Azulene SN	2200
Phenylbutazone	16
Indomethacin	4,5

Table 7. Cotton pellet granuloma (rat experiments)

	ED_{50} mg/kg orally
Bisabolol	30
Guaiazulene	32
Azulene SN	34
Camomile oil	35
Phenylbutazone	33
Indomethacin	4,5

III. EN-IN-Dicycloether

The exact chemical name of this compound is cis-2-[hexadiin(2,4)-ylidine]-1,6-diox-aspiro-(4,4)-nonene-3; it is a spirocyclic polyin derivative.

cis—Spiroether

Its anti-inflammatory effect was demonstrated by BREINLICH and SCHARNAGEL (1968). EN-IN-dicycloether (80 or 40 mg/kg i.p.) given 30 min before the induction of generalized dextran oedema in rats significantly inhibited the dextran oedema. Guaiazulene (25–50 mg/kg i.p.) proved substantially less effective. EN-IN-dicycloether also inhibited the decrease of the plasma kininogen, but it did not affect rat paw oedema induced by histamine, 5-HT, or bradykinin. It may be mentioned that s.p. injection of the dicycloether into the hind paw of rats caused an oedematous inflammation, even in a dose of 0.25 µg.

IV. Flavonoids

A detailed account of the anti-inflammatory effects of the flavonoids has already been given above. Here it is desired simply to deal briefly with the flavones of camomile. Of the numerous relevant data, reference will be made to the work of HÖRHAMMER et al. (1963). They used thin-layer chromatography to detect a total of 11 flavones in a methanolic camomile extract: among others, apigenin, apigenin-7-glycoside (apigetrin), quercetin-7-glycoside (quercimeritrin), patulitrin, and luteolin-7-glycoside. HÄNSEL et al. (1966) also reported the presence of a lipophilic flavone (5,4'-dihydroxy-3,6,7,3'-tetramethoxyflavone). As regards the flavonoids listed, JANKU (cited in HAVA and JANKU, 1957; ISAAC and SCHIMPKE, 1965) described the anti-phlogistic effect of apigenin.

H. Miscellaneous

The anti-inflammatory effect of extracts of a shrub, *Ruscus aculeatus* L., administered i.p. or as a suppository, was demonstrated by CHEVILLARD et al. (1965) on kaolin-induced rat paw oedema.

CHATURVEDI and SINGH (1965) screened fifteen indigenous drugs for their action in experimental arthritis produced by s.p. formaldehyde injection in rats. The most effective proved to be decoctions of *Dalbergia lanceolaria, Sida humilis, Pluchea lanceolata, Vitex negundo,* and *Paederia foetida.*

GUJRAL et al. (1960) similarly examined the effect of gum guggul in formalde-hyde-induced arthritis in rats. This substance is an exudate obtained by incision of the bark of the shrub *Balsamodendron mukul Hook.* All the fractions obtained by direct extraction of the crude drug possessed a highly significant activity as compared with hydrocortisone and butazolidin as reference standards.

SHARMA and SHARMA (1977) have recently made a comparison of the anti-inflammatory activity of Commiphora mukul with those of phenylbutazone and ibuprofen in mycobacterium-induced adjuvant arthritis in rabbits. (Inflammatory syndrome was induced in the right hock joint of rabbits by intra-articular injection of the killed mycobacterial adjuvant in liquid paraffin.) Development of this arthritic syndrome was studied for five months with and without drugs. The three drugs [phenylbutazone, ibuprofen, and the petroleum ether extract (fraction "A") of the gum exudate (gum guggul) from the trunk of the plant Commiphora mukul] were administered orally in a daily dose of 100, 100, and 500 mg/kg, respectively, for a period of five months. All three anti-inflammatory agents decreased the thickness of the joint swelling during the course of drug treatment.

Curcuma longa (Linn.), known as "Haldi", has been reported to possess anti-inflammatory activity. A comparison of the anti-inflammatory activities of various extracts of *Curcuma longa* was recently made by YEGNANARAYAN et al. (1976). In the cotton pellet test, the petroleum ether extract was most potent, its activity being similar to that of indomethacin. In carrageenin-induced paw oedema, 80 mg/kg of the water extract almost completely suppressed inflammation; 40 mg/kg of the water extract had as much anti-inflammatory activity as that of 5 mg/kg indomethacin. In the granuloma pouch method, the water extract was the most potent, its activity being similar to that of hydrocortisone.

The anti-inflammatory effect of berberine in rats injected locally with cholera toxin has been studied by AKHTER et al. (1977). As already mentioned, berberine is an alkaloid from the plant *Berberis aristata*. Berberine (30 mg/kg i.p.) was found to be an effective inhibitor of the local rat neck inflammation induced by cholera toxin. Cholera toxin was injected subcutaneously in the dorsum of the neck region. To judge the severity of inflammation, the neck circumference was measured in mm at frequent intervals up to 96 h, and the percentage increase over the preinjection value was calculated for each rat. The effect of berberine (10 mg/kg i.p.) was also studied on rat neck inflammation induced by carrageenin. The neck circumference was measured over a 24-h period. Carrageenin injection produced neck swelling, which reached a maximum after about 6 h. In this dose, berberine proved entirely ineffective (a dose of 30 mg/kg was not examined), whereas indomethacin (2 mg/kg i.p.) was very effective. In further experiments, a study was made of the effect of i.p.-injected berberine on chronic inflammation induced by cotton pellet in rats. In a dose of 10 mg/kg, berberine did not inhibit the growth of the granuloma at all, but in a dose of 30 mg/kg it did reduce it significantly. [Hydrocortisone (3 mg/kg i.p.) impressively reduced the weight of the granuloma.] According to AKHTER et al. (1977), these data suggest that berberine is not a classic anti-inflammatory agent.

References

Akhter, M. H., Sabir, M., Bhide, N. K.: Anti-inflammatory effect of berberine in rats injected locally with cholera toxin. Indian J. Med. Res. **65**, 133—141 (1977)

Andersen, N. H., Ramwell, P. W.: Biological aspects of prostaglandins. Arch. intern. Med. **133**, 30—50 (1974)

Antal, A., Gábor, M.: UV erythema értékelésére szolgáló készülék (Apparat für die Bewertung des UV-Erythems). Kisérl. Orvostud. **23**, 478—481 (1971). Cited in: Gábor, M.: The Anti-Inflammatory Action of Flavonoids. Budapest: Akadémiai Kiadó 1972

Armentano, L., Bentsáth, A., Béres, T., Rusznyák, St., Szent-Györgyi, A.: Über den Einfluß von Substanzen der Flavongruppe auf die Permeabilität der Kapillaren. Vitamin P. Dtsch. med. Wschr. **62**, 1325—1328 (1936)

Arnold, W.: Über Kamille, Pfefferminze und Fenchel. Naunyn-Schmiedeberg's Arch. exp. Path. Pharmak. **123**, 129—159 (1927)

Arora, S., Lahiri, P. K., Sanyal, R. K.: The role of Prostaglandin E_1 in inflammatory process in the rat. Int. Arch. Allergy **39**, 186—191 (1970)

Ascher, P. W.: Untersuchung der Pharmakodynamik und Pharmakokinetik des Aescins am Beispiel des Hirnödems. Wien. med. Wschr. **118**, 1050—1051 (1968)

Back, N., Sicuteri, F. (Eds.): Vasopeptides: Chemistry, Pharmacology, and pathophysiology. Proceedings of the Symposium on Vasopeptides. Florence, Italy, 1971. New York-London: Plenum Press 1972

Baeckeland, E., Lecomte, J.: Dérivés hydroxyétilés du rutoside isolés du rat. C.R. Soc. Biol. (Paris) **163**, 2226—2229 (1969)

Bartlett, G. R.: Inhibition of succinoxydase by the vitamin P-like flavonoid 2′,3,4-trihydroxy chalcone. J. Pharmacol. exp. Ther. **93**, 329—337 (1948)

Beitch, B. R., Eakins, K. E.: The effects of prostaglandins on the intraocular pressure of the rabbit. Brit. J. Pharmacol. **37**, 158—167 (1969)

Bogs, U., Meinhard, J.: Zur Herstellung von Kamillen-Fluidextrakt. Pharmazie **10**, 653—658 (1955)

Böhm, K.: The Flavonoids. A Review of Their Physiology, Pharmacodynamics and Therapeutic Uses. Aulendorf, Württ.: Editio Cantor KG. 1968

Bonta, I. L.: Microvascular lesions as a target of anti-inflammatory and certain other drugs. Acta physiol. pharmacol. neerl. **15**, 188—222 (1969)

Breinlich, J., Scharnagel, K.: Pharmakologische Eigenschaften des EN-IN-Dizykloäthers aus *Matricaria chamomilla*. Arzneimittel-Forsch. **18**, 429—431 (1968)

Brock, N., Kottmeier, J., Lorenz, D., Veigel, H.: Zur Frage der antiphlogistischen Wirkung von Azulenen im Tierversuch. Ein Beitrag zur Prüfungsmethodik entzündungswidriger Substanzen. Naunyn-Schmiedeberg's Arch. exp. Path. Pharmak. **223**, 450—464 (1954)

Bundy, G., Lincoln, F., Nelson, N., Pike, J., Schneider, W.: Novel prostaglandin syntheses. Ann. N.Y. Acad. Sci. **180**, 76—90 (1971)

Casley-Smith, J. R.: The actions of the benzo-pyrones on the blood-tissue-lymph-system. Folia Angiol. **24**, 7—22 (1976)

Casley-Smith, J., Piller, N. B.: The pathogenesis of oedemas, and the therapeutic action of coumarin and related compounds. In: Földi, M. (Ed.): Folia angiologica Supplementa, Basic Lymphology, Second Ringelheim Symposion, Vol. III, pp. 33—59. Berlin-Wien: Haupt & Koska HG. 1974

Chang, Y.-H.: Mechanism of action of colchicine. I. Effects of colchicine and its analogs on the reversed passive Arthus reaction and the carragenan-induced hindpaw edema in the rat. J. Pharmacol. exp. Ther. **194**, 154—158 (1975a)

Chang, Y.-H.: Mechanism of action of colchicine. II. Effect of colchicine and its analogs on phagocytosis and chemotaxis in vitro. J. Pharmacol. exp. Ther. **194**, 159—164 (1975b)

Chang, Y.-H.: III. Anti-inflammatory effects of colchicine compared with phenylbutazone and indomethacin. Arthritis Rheum. **18**, 493—496 (1975c)

Chaturvedi, G. N., Singh, R. H.: Experimental studies on the anti-arthritic effect of certain indigenous drugs. Indian J. med. Res. **53**, 71—80 (1965)

Chaturvedi, A. K., Parmar, S. S., Bhatnagar, S. C., Misra, G., Nikam, S. K.: Anticonvulsant and anti-inflammatory activity of natural plant coumarins and triterpenoids. Res. Commun. chem. path. Pharmacol. **9**, 11—22 (1974)

Chaturvedi, A. K., Parmar, S. S., Nigam, S. K., Bhatnagar, S. C., Misra, G., Sastry, B. V. R.: Anti-inflammatory and anticonvulsant properties of some natural plant triterpenoids. Pharmacol. Res. Commun. **8**, 199—210 (1976)

Chau, T. T., Haley, T. J.: Flavonoid antagonism of the spasmogenic effect of angiotensin, bradykinin and eledoisin of guinea pig ileum. J. pharm. Sci. **58**, 621—623 (1969)

Chayen, J., Bitensky, L.: Lysosomal enzymes and inflammation with particular reference to rheumatoid diseases. Ann. rheum. Dis. **30**, 333—405 (1969)

Chevillard, L., Ranson, M., Senault, B.: Activité anti-inflammatoire d'extraits de fragon épineux (*Ruscus aculeatus* L.). Méd. Pharmacol. exp. **12**, 109—114 (1965)

Courbat, P.: Quelques généralités sur les composés flavonoïdes. In: Clinical Pharmacology: Flavonoids and vascular wall. Symposia angiologica Santoriana, 4th International Symposium, Fribourg-Nyon, 1972, pp. 3—29. Basel-München-Paris-London-New York-Sydney: S. Karger 1972

Courbat, P., Favre, J., Guerne, R., Uhlmann, G.: Contribution à l'étude d'un produit de β-hydroxyéthylation du rutoside. Partie 1. Isolement et identification des constituants majeurs par chromatographie sur papier. Helv. chim. Acta **49**, 1203—1211 (1966a)

Courbat, P., Uhlmann, G., Guerne, R.: Contribution à l'étude d'un produit de β-hydroxyéthylation du rutoside. Identification des constituants majeurs par spectrophotométrie ultraviolette. Helv. chim. Acta **49**, 1420—1424 (1966b)

Crutchley, D. J., Piper, P. J.: Inhibition of the inactivation of prostaglandins in guinea pig lungs. Naunyn-Schmiedebergs Arch. Pharmacol. **279**, 27 (1973)

Dale, H. H., Laidlaw, P. P.: The physiological action of β-iminazolylethylamine. J. Physiol. (Lond.) **41**, 318—344 (1910)

D'Arcy, P. F., Kellett, D. N.: Glycyrrhetinic acid. Brit. med. J. **1**, 647 (1957)

Dean, F. M.: Naturally occuring oxygen ring compounds. London: Butterworths 1963

Denko, C. W., Whitehouse, M. W.: Effects of colchicine in rats with urate crystal-induced inflammation. Pharmacology (Basel) **3**, 229—242 (1970)

Dhawan, B. N., Srimal, R. C.: Anti-inflammatory and some other pharmacological effects of 3,4-*trans*-2,2-dimethyl-3-phenyl-4-[p-(β-pyrrolidinoethoxy)-phenyl]-7-methoxy-chroman (Centchroman) Brit. J. Pharmacol. **49**, 64—73 (1973)

Diczfalusy, E., Fernö, O., Fex, H., Högberg, B., Linderot, T., Rosenberg, Th.: Synthetic high molecular weight enzyme inhibitors. I. Polymeric phosphates of phloretin and related compounds. Acta chem. scand. **7**, 913—920 (1953)

Dingle, J. T., Fell, H. B. (Eds.): Lysosomes in Biology and Pathology. Amsterdam: North-Holland 1969

Doll, R., Hill, I. D., Hutton, C., Underwood, D. J.: Clinical trial of a triterpenoid liquorice compound in gastric and duodenal ulcer. Lancet **II**, 793 (1962)

Eakins, K. E.: Prostaglandin antagonism by polymeric phosphates of phloretin and related compounds. Ann. N.Y. Acad. Sci. **180**, 386—395 (1971)

Eakins, K. E., Karim, S. M. M.: Polyphloretinphosphate—a selective antagonist for prostaglandin $F_{1\alpha}$ and $F_{2\alpha}$. Life Sci. **9**, 1—5 (1970)

Eakins, K. E., Karim, S. M. M., Miller, J. D.: Antagonism of some smooth muscle reactions of prostaglandins by polyphloretin phosphate—a selective antagonist for prostaglandins $F_{1\alpha}$ and $F_{2\alpha}$. Life Sci. **9**, 1—5 (1970)

Eakins, K. E., Miller, J. D., Karim, M. M.: The nature of the prostaglandin-blocking activity of polyphloretin phosphate. J. Pharmacol. exp. Ther. **176**, 441—447 (1971)

Eakins, K. E., Sanner, J. H.: Prostaglandin antagonists. In: Karim, S. M. M. (Ed.): The Prostaglandins, pp. 263—292. New York: Wiley-Interscience 1972

Erdös, E. G.: Effect of nonsteroidal anti-inflammatory drugs in endotoxin shock. Biochem. Pharmacol. Suppl., 283—291 (1968)

Erspamer, V. (Ed.): 5-Hydroxytryptamine and Related Indolealkylamines. Handbook experimental Pharmakology. Berlin-Heidelberg-New York: Springer 1966

Farkas, L., Gábor, M., Kállay, F. (Eds.): Topics in Flavonoid Chemistry and Biochemistry. Proceedings of the Fourth Hungarian Bioflavonoid Symposium Keszthely, 1973. Budapest: Akadémiai Kiadó 1975

Fassbender, H. G., Pippert, H. K.: Die allergisch-hyperergische Entzündung von Haut und Gelenken unter dem Einfluß von Hyaluronidase und Rutin. Z. ges. exp. Med. **123**, 210—218 (1954)

Felix, W.: Wirkungsmechanismus der internen Therapie mit „Venopharmaka". Dtsch. med. Wschr. **21**, 456—466 (1970)

Feuer, G.: The metabolism and biological actions of Coumarins. In: Ellis, G. P., West, G. B. (Eds.): Progress in Medicinal Chemistry, Vol. 10, pp. 85—158. Amsterdam-London: North-Holland 1974

Finney, R. S. H., Somers, G. F.: The anti-inflammatory activity of glycyrrhetinic acid and derivatives. J. Pharm. (Lond.) **10**, 613—620 (1958)

Finney, R. S. H., Tárnoky, A. L.: The pharmacological properties of glycyrrhetinic acid hydrogen succinate (disodium salt). J. Pharm. (Lond.) **12**, 49—58 (1960)

Fitzgerald, T. J., Williams, B., Uyeki, E. H.: Colchicine on sodium urate-induced paw swelling in mice: structure-activity relationships of colchicine derivatives. Proc. Soc. exp. Biol. (N.Y.) **136**, 115—120 (1971)

Flower, R. J.: Drugs which inhibit prostaglandin biosynthesis. Pharmacol. Rev. **26**, 33—67 (1974)

Földi, M., Zoltán, Ö. T.: Experimentelle Thrombophlebitis und deren therapeutische Beeinflussung. Arzneimittel-Forsch. **15**, 901—903 (1965)

Földi, M., Zoltán, Ö. T., Piukovich, I.: Die Wirkung von Rutin und Cumarin auf den Verlauf einer experimentellen Thrombophlebitis. Arzneimittel-Forsch. **20**, 1629—1635 (1970)

Földi-Börcsök, E.: Effect of external lymph drainage and of coumarin treatment injury in the rat hind leg. Brit. J. Pharmacol. **46**, 254—259 (1972)

Földi-Börcsök, E., Bedall, F. K., Rahlfs, V. W.: Die antiphlogistische und ödemhemmende Wirkung von Cumarin aus *Melilotus officinalis*. Arzneimittel-Forsch. **21**, 2025—2030 (1971)

Fontaine, L., Grand, M., Molho, D., Boschetti, E.: Activité anti-inflammatoire expérimentale de coumarins, indane-diones et acyl-indan-diones apparentées aux anticoagulants oraux. Méd. Pharmacol. exp. **17**, 497—507 (1967)

Formanek, K., Höller, H.: Über den Einfluß von Trioxyäthylrutin auf das experimentell erzeugte Ödem der Rattenpfote. Wien. med. Wschr. **110**, 697—699 (1960)

Fries, B.: The edema-inhibiting action of polyphloretin-phosphate (PPP) in some types of capillary damage. An experimental investigation. Acta chir. scand. **119**, 1—7 (1960)

Frimmer, M.: Biochemie und Pathophysiologie von Entzündungsmediatoren. Int. Z. klin. Pharmakol. Ther. Toxikol. **2**, 144—151 (1971)

Gábor, M.: The Anti-Inflammatory Action of Flavonoids. Budapest: Akadémiai Kiadó 1972a

Gábor, M.: Pharmacologic effects of flavonoids on blood vessels. In: Comèl, M., Laszt, L. (Eds.): Clinical Pharmacology: Flavonoids and Vascular Wall. Symposia angiologica santoriana. 4th International Symposium, Fribourg-Nyon 1972. Basel-München-Paris-London-New York-Sydney: Karger 1972b

Gábor, M.: Influence of flavonoids on decrease of capillary resistance in inflammation caused by red paprika (*Capsicum annuum* L. *Solanaceae*). In: Gábor, M.: The Anti-Inflammatory Action of Flavonoids, pp. 78—83. Budapest: Akadémiai Kiadó 1972c

Gábor, M.: Pathophysiology and Pharmacology of Capillary Resistance. Budapest: Akadémiai Kiadó 1974

Gábor, M.: Abriß der Pharmakologie von Flavonoiden unter besonderer Berücksichtigung der antiödematösen und antiphlogistischen Effekte. Budapest: Akadémiai Kiadó 1975

Gábor, M., Antal, A.: Influence of O-(β-hydroxyethyl)rutin on erythema induced by UV radiation. In: Gábor, M.: The Anti-Inflammatory Action of Flavonoids, pp. 84—93. Akadémiai Kiadó 1972

Gábor, M., Blazsó, G.: In: Gábor, M.: Abriß der Pharmakologie von Flavonoiden, unter besonderer Berücksichtigung der antiödematösen und antiphlogistischen Effekte. Budapest: Akadémiai Kiadó 1975

Gábor, M., Iván, J.: Effect of O-(β-hydroxyethyl)rutin on the oedema-preventing action of butazolidin. In: Gábor, M.: The Anti-Inflammatory Action of Flavonoids, pp. 94—100. Budapest: Akadémiai Kiadó 1972

Gábor, M., Szórády, I.: Die Beeinflussung der experimentellen Senfölentzündungen mit Hämatoxylin. Acta physiol. Acad. Sci. hung. **3**, 405—407 (1952)

Gábor, M., Szórády, I., Dirner, Z.: The inhibiting effect of the members of the haematoxylin group on the action of histidin-decarboxylase. Acta physiol. Acad. Sci. hung. **3**, 595—600 (1952)

Ganesan, P. A., Karim, S. M. M.: Polyphloretin phosphate temporarily potentiates prostaglandin E_2 on the rat fundus, probably by inhibiting PG-15-hydroxyde-hydrogenase. J. Pharm. (Lond.) **25**, 229—233 (1973)

Garcia Leme, J., Walaszek, E. J.: Antagonists of pharmacologically active peptides: effect on guinea pig ileum and inflammation. Pharmacologist **9**, 242 (1967)

Garcia Leme, J., Walaszek, E. J.: Antagonists of pharmacologically active peptides. Effect on guinea pig ileum and inflammation. Pharmacology and the Future of Man, Proceedings 5th International Congr. Pharmacology, San Francisco 1972. Basel: Karger 1973, Vol. V, pp. 328—335

Garattini, S., Valzelli, L.: Serotonin. Amsterdam-London-New York: Elsevier 1965

Gascon, A. L., Walaszek, E. J.: Inhibition of valyl[5] angiotensinamide II by osajin. J. Pharm. (Lond.) **18**, 478—479 (1966)

Gecse, Á., Zsilinszky, N., Horpácsy, G., Gábor, M.: Data on the mechanism of the anti-inflammatory effect of flavonoids. In: Gábor, M.: The Anti-Inflammatory Action of Flavonoids. Budapest: Akadémiai Kiadó 1972

Geissman, T. A.: The Chemistry of Flavonoid Compounds. Oxford-London-New York-Paris: Pergamon Press 1962

Goldyne, M. E.: Prostaglandins and cutaneous inflammation. J. invest. Derm. **64**, 377—385 (1975)

Goodman, L. S., Gilman, A.: The pharmacological basis of therapeutics, 4th ed. London: McMillan 1971

Gözsi, B., Kátó, L.: Balancing Mechanisms in Acute Inflammation. Montreal: Thérien Frères 1970

Griffith, J. G. Jr., Krewson, Ch. F., Naghski, J.: Rutin and Related Flavonoids. Chemistry—Pharmacology-Clinical applications. Easton, Pa.: Mack Publ. Co. 1955

Gross, F.: Unspezifische Beeinflussung entzündlicher Reaktionen. Schweiz. med. Wschr. **80**, 697—701 (1950a)

Gross, F.: Zur Auslösung und Beeinflussung der Oedembildung nach Injektion von Hühnereiweiß an der Ratte. Naunyn-Schmiedebergs Arch. exp. Path. Pharmak. **211**, 421—426 (1950b)

Gross, F., Meier, R.: Die Wirkung von synthetischen Antihistaminkörpern auf die Senfölchemosis am Kaninchenauge. Experientia (Basel) **4**, 400—402 (1948)

Gugler, R., Dengler, H. J.: Inhibition of human liver catechol-O-methyltransferase. Naunyn-Schmiedebergs Arch. Pharmakol. **276**, 223—233 (1973)

Gujral, M. L., Sareen, K., Tangri, K. K., Amma, M. K. P., Roy, A. K.: Anti-arthritic and anti-inflammatory activity of gum guggul (Balsamodendron mukul Hook). Ind. J. Physiol. Pharmacol. **4**, 267—273 (1960)

Gupta, M. B., Bhalla, T. N., Gupta, G. P., Mitra, C. R., Bhargava, K. P.: Anti-inflammatory activity of natural products. I. Triterpenoids. Eur. J. Pharmacol. **6**, 67—70 (1969)

Gupta, M. B., Bhalla, T. N., Gupta, G. P., Mitra, C. R., Bhargava, K. P.: Anti-inflammatory activity of taxifolin. Jap. J. Pharmacol. **21**, 377—382 (1971)

Gupta, M. B., Bhalla, T. N., Tangri, K. K., Bhargava, K. P.: Biochemical study of the anti-inflammatory activity of α- and β-amyrin acetate. Biochem. Pharmacol. **20**, 401—405 (1971)

Haagen-Smit, A. J.: Azulenes. In: Progress in the Chemistry of Organic Natural Products. Zechmeister, L. (Ed.). Wien: Springer-Verlag 1948, pp. 40—71

Hammersen, F.: The fine structure of different types of experimental edemas for testing the effect of vasoactive drugs demonstrated with a flavonoid. In: Comèl, M., Laszt, L. (Eds.): Clinical Pharmacology: Flavonoids and Vascular wall. Symposia angiologica santoriana. 4th. International Symposium, Fribourg-Nyon 1972, pp. 194—222. Basel-München-Paris-London-New York-Sydney: Karger 1972

Hammersen, F., Möhring, E.: Der Feinbau der Endstrombahn beim Dextran-Ödem und deren Beeinflussung durch HR. Fortschr. Med. **86**, 925—927 (1968)

Hammersen, F., Möhring, E.: Das Dextran-Ödem der Ratte als morphologisches Modell zur Prüfung gefäßaktiver Pharmaka. Dtsch. med. Wschr. **21**, 472—478 (1970)

Hammersen, F., Möhring, E.: Zum Feinbau enzymatisch bedingter Endothel- und Erythrozytenveränderungen (Phospholipase-Ödem) und deren Beeinflussung durch HR. Dtsch. med. Wschr. **23**, 406—409 (1972)

Hänsel, R., Rimpler, H., Walther, K.: Ein lipophiles Flavon aus der Kamille (Matricaria chamomilla L.). Naturwissenschaften **53**, 19 (1966)

Harborne, J. B.: Comparative Biochemistry of the Flavonoids. London-New York: Academic Press 1967

Harborne, J. B., Mabry, T. J., Mabry, Y. H., Eds.: The Flavonoids. London: Chapman & Hall 1975

Hava, M., Janku, I.: The pharmacology of camomile and juniper. Rev. Czech. Med. **3**, 1—9 (1957)

Heubner, W., Albath, W.: Über die entzündungswidrige Wirkung des Rein-Azulens aus *Matricaria chamomilla L*. Naunyn-Schmiedebergs Arch. exp. Path. Pharmak. **192**, 383—388 (1939)

Heubner, W., Grabe, F.: Über die entzündungswidrige Wirkung des Kamillenöls. Naunyn-Schmiedebergs Arch. exp. Path. Pharmak. **171**, 329—339 (1933)

Hikino, H., Taguchi, T., Fujimura, H., Hiramatsu, Y.: Antiinflammatory principles of *Caesalpinia sappan* wood and of *Haematoxylon* Campechianum wood. Planta Med. **31**, 214—220 (1977)

Hopf, G., Kaessmann, H. J., Pekker, I., Schäfer, E. A., Weber, H. G.: Experimentelle Untersuchungen der Beeinflussung des postoperativen Extremitätenödems am Hunde mit einem Cumarin-Präparat. Arzneimittel-Forsch. **21**, 854—855 (1971)

Hörhammer, L., Wagner, H., Salfner, B.: Neue Flavonglykoside aus der Kamille *(Matricaria chamomilla L.)*. 3. Mitteilung über Compositen- und Papilionaceenflavone. Arzneimittel-Forsch. **13**, 33—36 (1963)

Horton, E. W.: Prostaglandins. Berlin-Heidelberg-New York: Springer Verlag 1972

Isaac, O.: Fortschritte in der Kamillenforschung. Dtsch. Apoth.-Ztg. **114**, 255—260 (1974)

Isaac, O., Schimpke, H.: Alte und neue Erkenntnisse der Kamillenforschung. Mitt. dtsch. pharm. Ges. **35**, 133—147, 157—170 (1965)

Jakovlev, V., Schlichtegroll, A.: Zur entzündungshemmenden Wirkung von (-)-α-Bisabolol, einem wesentlichen Bestandteil des Kamillenöls. Arzneimittel-Forsch. **19**, 615—616 (1969)

Jancsó, M.: Histamin: A reticulo-endotheliális sejtrendszer élettani aktivátora (Histamine, the biological activator of the reticuloendothelial cell system). Orv. Lapja **3**, 1025—1030 (1947a)

Jancsó, N.: Histamine as a physiological activator of the reticuloendothelial system. Nature (Lond.) **160**, 227—228 (1947b)

Jancsó, M.: Idegi mechanizmusok szerepe a gyulladá sban. Orv. Hetil. **106**, 289—296 (1965)

Jeličić-Hadžović, J., Stern, P.: Azulene und Bradykinin. Arzneimittel-Forsch. **22**, 1210—1211 (1972)

Kaley, G., Weiner, R.: Prostaglandin E_1: a potential mediator. Ann. N.Y. Acad. Sci. **180**, 338—350 (1970)

Karim, S. M. M., Ed.: The Prostaglandins. New York: Wiley — Interscience 1972

Kátó, L., Gözsy, L.: Effets vasculaires des bioflavonoïdes chez le rat. Vie méd. **50**, 33—42 (1969)

Kellner, M., Kovách, A. G. B., Földi, M.: Über die antiphlogistische Wirkung des Melilotusextraktes Esberiven. Arzneimittel-Forsch. **15**, 326—328 (1961)

Khadzay, Ya. I.: Biological properties and pharmacological activity of coumarins and furocumarins. Akad. Nauk SSSR, Ser. 5, Rast. Syr'e **12**, 25—30 (1965). See Chem. Abst. **64**, 1185d

Khadzay, Ya. I., Obolentseva, G. V., Serdyuk, A. D.: On the pharmacology of acacetine. Farmakol. i Toksikol. **32**, 451—453 (1969)

König, H.: Zur Chemie der Prostaglandine-Biogenese, Stoffwechsel, Totalsynthese. Klin. Wschr. **53**, 1041—1048 (1975)

Koshland, D. E. Jr.: Conformation changes at the active site during enzyme action. Fed. Proc. **23**, 719—726 (1964)

Kraus, S. D.: Glycyrrhetinic acid—a triterpene with antioestrogenic and anti-inflammatory activity. J. Pharm. (Lond.) **12**, 300—306 (1960)

Kristen, G., Schmidt, W.: Kamille und Azulene. Pharmakologie — Therapie — Galenik. Mitt. dtsch. pharm. Ges. **27**, 105—114 (1957)

Küchle, H. J., Wegener, H.: Quantitative Untersuchungen über Wirksamkeit und Wirkungsstärke entzündungshemmender Substanzen. Z. ges. exp. Med. **118**, 136—142 (1951)

Kuznecova, G. A.: Naturally occuring coumarins and furocoumarins. Nauka 1967

Lavollay, J., Neumann, J.: Les substances actives contre la fragilité vasculaire. Expos. ann. Biochim. méd. **10**, 59 (1949)

Lecomte, J.: Pouvoir amino-libérateur des bioflavonoïdes chez le rat. C.R. Soc. Biol. (Paris) **165**, 433—435 (1971)

Lecomte, J., Van Cauwenberge, H.: Le pouvoir amino-libérateur du quelques bioflavonoïdes chez le rat. In: Comèl, M., Laszt, L. (Eds.): Clinical Pharmacology: Flavonoids and Vascular Wall. Symposia angiologica santoriana, 4th International Symposium, pp. 179—193. Fribourg-Nyon 1972, Basel-München-Paris-London-New York-Sydney: Karger 1972

Lecomte, J., Van Cauwenberge, H.: Sur quelques propriétés pharmacologiques du mono (O.β.hydroxy éthyl) 7 rutoside chez le rat. Arch. int. Pharmacodyn. **208**, 317—327 (1974)

Lespagnol, A., Lespagnol, Ch., Lesieur, D., Cazin, J. Cl., Cazin, M., Beerens, H., Romond, Ch.: Activités analgésique, antiinflammatoire et antimicrobienne des chalcones et dihydrochalcones dérivées de l'acide salicylique. Bull. Chim. thér. 365—369 (1972)

Leuschner, F.: Über die perkutane Beeinflussung von experimentellen Ödemen und Gewebsschäden bei Ratten. 2nd Czechoslovak Congress of Internal Medicine; Pathogenesis and Therapy in Edema, Bratislava 1970

Leuschner, F., Leuschner, A.: Über die perkutane Beeinflussung von experimentellen Ödemen und Gewebeschäden bei Ratten. **56**, 612—618 (1972)

Lewis, G. P.: Kinins in inflammation and tissue injury. In: Bradykinin, Kallidin and Kallikrein. In: Erdös, E. G. (Ed.): Handbook of Experimental Pharmacology. Berlin-Heidelberg-New York: Springer Verlag 1970, Vol. XXV, pp. 516—530

Lietti, A., Cristoni, A., Picci, M.: Studies on Vaccinium myrtillus anthocyanosides. I. Vasoprotective and antiinflammatory activity. Arzneimittel-Forsch. Drug Res. **26**, 829—832 (1976)

Linde, H., Cramer, G.: (-)-α-Bisabolol and cis-2-[Hexadiin-(2,4)-yliden]-1,6-dioxaspiro-[4,4]-nonen-(3) in handelsüblichen Kamillen-Extrakten. Arzneimittel-Forsch. **22**, 583—585 (1972)

Logeman, W., Lauria, F., Tosolini, G.: Über Ketole der 18α- und 18β-Glycyrrhetinsäure. Chem. Ber. **90**, 601—604 (1957)

Lorenz, W., Kusche, J., Barth, H., Mathias, Ch.: Action of several flavonoids on enzymes of histamine metabolism in vitro. In: Histamine. Mechanisms of Regulation of the Biogenic Amines Level in the Tissues With Special Reference to Histamine, Proceedings of Satellite Symposium of the XXVth International Congress of Physiological Sciences, Łódź, Poland 1971, Maślinski, C. (Ed.)., pp. 265—269, Stroudsburg, Penn.: Dowden, Hutchinson & Ross Inc. 1973

Lorenz, D., Marek, M. L.: Das therapeutisch wirksame Prinzip der Roßkastanie *(Aesculus hippocastanum)*. 1. Mitt.: Aufklärung des Wirkstoffes. Arzneimittel-Forsch. **10**, 263—272 (1960)

Lorenz, D., Reiffer, F.: Die oedemhemmende Wirksamkeit von Aescin und Buphenin bei cutaner Anwendung am Kaolin-Oedem der Rattenpfote. Arzneimittel-Forsch. **17**, 1083—1084 (1967)

Makarov, V. A., Khadzai, Ya. I.: Antiphlogistic and P-vitaminogenic activity of blackthorn flavonols. Farmakol. i Toksikol. **32**, 438—441 (1969)

Malawista, S. E.: Colchicine: a common mechanism for its anti-inflammatory and anti-mitotic effects. Arthr. Rheum. **11**, 191—197 (1968)

Marrazzi, M. A., Matschinsky, F. M.: Properties of 15-hydroxyprostaglandin dehydrogenase: structural requirements for substrate binding. Prostaglandins **1**, 373—388 (1972)

Martin, G. J., Brendel, R., Beiler, J. M.: Effects of parenterally administered trypsin and phosphorylated hesperidin. Arch. int. Pharmacodyn. **96**, 124—129 (1953)

Martin, G. J., Graff, M., Brendel, R., Beiler, J. M.: Effect of vitamin P compounds on the action of histidine decarboxylase. Arch. Biochem. **21**, 177—180 (1949)

Maslinsky, C., Ed.: Histamine. Mechanisms of Regulation of the Biogenic Amines Level in the Tissues With Special Reference to Histamine, Proceedings Satellite Symposium of the XXVth International Congress of Physiological Sciences, Łódź, Poland 1971. Stroudsburg, Penn.: Dowden, Hutchinson & Ross Inc. 1973

Menkin, V.: Effect of adrenal cortex extract on capillary permeability. Amer. J. Physiol. **129**, 691—697 (1940)

Menkin, V.: Anti-inflammatory activity of some water-soluble bioflavonoids. Amer. J. Physiol. **196**, 1205—1210 (1959)

Meyer, R., Schuler, W., Desaulles, P.: Zur Frage des Mechanismus der Hemmung des Bindegewebswachstums durch Cortisone. Experientia (Basel) **6**, 469—471 (1950)

Mirkovitch, V., Borgeaud, J., Meyer, S., Niebes, P.: Prévention de thrombose expérimentale par O-(β-hydroxyéthyl)-rutosides. Helv. chir. Acta **39**, 379—382 (1972)

Niebes, P.: Influence des flavonoïdes sur la métabolisme des mucopolysaccharides dans la paroi veineuse. In: Comèl, M., Laszt, L. (Eds.): Symposia Angiologica Santoriana, 4th International Symposium, Fribourg-Nyon, Clinical Pharmacology: Flavonoids and Vascular Wall, pp. 94—102. Basel-München-Paris-New York-Sydney: Karger 1972

Niebes, P., Ponard, G.: Stabilization of rat liver lysosomes by (+)-cyanidanol-3 in vivo. Biochem. Pharmacol. **24**, 905—909 (1975)

Northover, B. J., Subramanian, G.: A study of possible mediators of inflammatory reactions in the mouse foot. Brit. J. Pharmacol. **18**, 346—355 (1962)

Oettel, H., Wilhelm-Kollmansperger, G.: Zur Frage der antiphlogistischen Wirkung von Azulenen. I. Mitteilung. Naunyn-Schmiedebergs Arch. exp. Path. Pharmak. **226**, 473—485 (1955)

Oettel, H., Wilhelm-Kollmansperger, G.: Zur Frage der antiphlogistischen Wirkung von Azulenen. II. Mitteilung. Naunyn-Schmiedebergs Arch. exp. Path. Pharmak. **228**, 331—339 (1956)

Park, M. K., Dyer, D. C.: Effect of polyphloretinphosphate and 7-oxa-13 prostynoic acid on the vasoactive actions of prostaglandin E_2 and 5-hydroxytryptamine on isolated human umbilical arteries. Prostaglandins **3**, 913—920 (1973)

Parmar, N. S., Ghosh, M. N.: Some pharmacological studies of bioflavonoids in rats. Bull. Jipmer clin. Soc. **10**, 183—190 (1974)

Pastan, J., Almqvist, S.: Purification and properties of mast cell protease. J. biol. Chem. **241**, 5090—5094 (1966)

Patt,P., Winkler,W.: Das therapeutisch wirksame Prinzip der Roßkastanie *(Aesculus hippocasta-num)*. 2. Mitt.: Zur Chemie des Wirkstoffes. Arzneimittel-Forsch. **10**, 273—275 (1960)

Piller,N.B.: The resolution of thermal oedema at various temperatures under coumarin treatment. Brit. J. exp. Path. **56**, 83—91 (1975)

Piller,N.B.: An integration of the modes of action of coumarin. An explanation of its effectiveness as a therapy for thermally injured tissue. Arzneimittel-Forsch. (Drug Res.) **27**, 1135—1138 (1977a)

Piller,N.B.: Benzopyrone treatment of mild thermal oedema: determination of the most effective doses. Arzneimittel-Forsch. (Drug Res.) **27**, 1138—1141 (1977b)

Poethke,W., Bulin,P.: Phytochemische Untersuchung einer neue gezüchteten Kamillensorte. 1. Mitt.: Flavonglykoside und Cumarinderivate. Pharm. Zentralh. **108**, 733—746 (1969a)

Poethke,W., Bulin,P.: Phytochemische Untersuchung einer neu gezüchteten Kamillensorte. 2. Mitt.: Ätherisches Öl. Pharm. Zentralh. **108**, 813—823 (1969b)

Preziosi,P., Manca,P.: Die Antiödem- und die antiinflammatorische Wirkung von Aescin und ihre Beziehung zur Hypophysen-Nebennieren-Achse. Arzneimittel-Forsch. **15**, 404—413 (1965)

Radouco-Thomas,S., Grumbach,P., Nosal, Gl., Radouco-Thomas,C.: Anti-inflammatory effect of trihydroxyethylrutoside assessed in the granuloma pouch. Life Sci. **3**, 459—464 (1964)

Ramaswamy,A.S.: Pharmacological action of the biflavonoids from the Gymnosperms with special reference to *Ginkgo biloba* L. J. med. Ass. **55**, 163—165 (1970)

Ramwell,P.W., (Ed.): The Prostaglandins. New York-London: Plenum Press 1973

Ramwell,P., Shaw,J.E., (Eds.): Prostaglandins. Ann. N.Y. Acad. Sci. **180**, 1971

Riesterer,L., Jaques,R.: The influence of anti-inflammatory drugs on the development of an experimental traumatic paw oedema in the rat. Pharmacology (Basel) **3**, 243—251 (1970)

Rocha e Silva,M.: Histamine. Its Role in Anaphylaxis and Allergy. Springfield, Illinois: Charles C. Thomas 1955

Rocha e Silva,M. (Ed.): Histamine and Anti-Histaminics, Handbook of Experimental Pharmacology. Berlin-Heidelberg-New York: Springer 1966, Vol. XVIII/1

Rocha e Silva,M., Garcia Leme,J.: Chemical Mediators of the Acute Inflammatory Reaction. Oxford-New York: Pergamon Press 1972

Rothkopf,M., Vogel,G.: Neue Befunde zur Wirksamkeit und zum Wirkungsmechanismus des Roßkastaniensaponins Aescin. Arzneimittel-Forsch. (Drug Res.) **26**, 225—235 (1976)

Salgado,E., Green,D.M.: Action of bioflavonoids on inflammation. J. appl. Physiol. **8**, 647—650 (1955)

Samuelsson,B., Paoletti,R. (Eds.): Advances in Prostaglandin and Thromboxane Research. New York: Raven Press 1976

Schilcher,H.: Neuere Erkenntnisse bei der Qualitätsbeurteilung von Kamillenblüten bzw. Kamillenöl. Teil 1: Quantitative Gehaltsbestimmung des ätherischen Öles in Flores Chamomillae. Dtsch. Apoth.-Ztg. **112**, 1497—1500 (1972)

Schilcher,H.: Neuere Erkenntnisse bei der Qualitätsbeurteilung von Kamillenblüten bzw. Kamillenöl. Teil 2: Qualitative Beurteilung des ätherischen Öles in Flores Chamomillae. Planta med. **23**, 132—144 (1973)

Schwabe,K.-P., Flohé,L.: Catechol-O-Methyltransferase, III. Beziehungen zwischen der Struktur von Flavonoiden und deren Eignung als Inhibitoren der Catechol-O-Methyltransferase. Hoppe-Seylers Z. physiol. Chem. **353**, 476—482 (1972)

Selye,H.: Use of "Granuloma Pouch" technique in the study of antiphlogistic corticosteroids. Proc. Soc. exp. Biol. (N.Y.) **82**, 328—333 (1953)

Sharma,J.N., Sharma,J.N.: Comparison of the anti-inflammatory activity of *Commiphora* mukul, an indigenous drug, with those of phenylbutazone and ibuprofen in experimental arthritis induced by mycobacterial adjuvant. Arzneimittel-Forsch. (Drug Res.) **27**, 1455—1457 (1977)

Shils,M.E., Goodhart,R.S.: The Flavonoids in Biology and Medicine. A Critical Review. New York: The National Vitamin Foundation 1956

Shimamoto,K., Takaori,S.: Pharmakologische Untersuchungen mit einem *Melilotus*-Extrakt. Arzneimittel-Forsch. **15**, 897—899 (1965)

Sokoloff,B., Eddy,W.H., Redd,J.B.: The biological activity of a flavonoid (Vitamin "P") compound. J. clin. Invest. **30**, 395—400 (1951)

Somers, G. F.: Glycyrrhetinic acid. Brit. med. J. I, 463 (1957)

Southern, E. M., Ed.: The Prostaglandins. Clinical Applications in Human Reproduction. Mount Kisco, New York: Futura Publ. Co. Inc. 1972

Spector, W. G., Willoughby, D. A.: Chemical mediators. In: The Inflammatory Process, Zweifach, B. W., Grant, L., McCluskey, R. T. (Eds.). New York-London: Academic Press 1965, pp. 427—448

Spector, W. G., Willoughby, D. A.: The Pharmacology of Inflammation. London: English Universities Press 1968

Stern, P.: Antiallergische Wirkung der Azulene. In: Premier Congrês International d'Allergie, Zürich-Basel-New York: Karger 1951, pp. 542—545

Stern, P.: Beitrag zur Wirkungsweise der Azulene. Arzneimittel-Forsch. 9, 551—553 (1959)

Stern, P., Milin, R.: Die antiallergische und antiphlogistische Wirkung der Azulene. Arzneimittel-Forsch. 6, 445—450 (1956)

Strandberg, K., Tuvemo, T.: Reduction of the tone of the isolated human umbilical artery by Indomethacin, Eicosa-5,8,11,14-tetraynoic acid and polyphloretin phosphate. Acta physiol. scand. 94, 319—326 (1975)

Tarayre, J. P., Lauressergues, H.: Preuve pharmacologiques de l'activité de l'hespéridine méthyl chalcone. Angéiologie 27, 197—203 (1975)

Tarayre, J. P., Lauressergues, H.: Etude de quelques propriétés pharmacologiques d'une association vasculotrope. Ann. Pharm. Fr. 34, 375—382 (1976)

Tarayre, J. P., Lauressergues, H.: Advantages of a combination of proteolytic enzymes, flavonoids and ascorbic acid in comparison with non-steroid anti-inflammatory agents. Arzneimittel-Forsch. (Drug Res.) 27, 1144—1149 (1977)

Texl, A.: The Effect of Catechol Complexes from Tea Leafs on Experimental Inflammation 19, 515—519 (1963)

Thiele, K., Jakovlev, V., Isaac, O., Schuler, W. A.: Äther und von (-)-α-Bisabolol und analogen Mono- und Sesquiterpenoiden mit antiphlogistischer Wirkung. Arzneimittel-Forsch. 19, 1878—1882 (1969)

Thiemer, K., Stadler, R., Isaac, O.: Biochemische Untersuchungen von Kamillen-Inhaltstoffen. II. Einfluß von Kamillenextrakt auf die oxydative Phosphorylierung und den Hautstoffwechsel des Meerschweinchens. Arzneimittel-Forsch. 23, 756—759 (1973)

Uda, T.: The mode of inhibiting action of guaiazulene and some other antiinflammatory agents on anaphylactoid edemas. Nippon Yakurigaku Zasshi 56, 1151—1163 (1960). See Chem. Abst. 56, 4058h (1962)

Van Caneghem, P.: Influence of some hydrosoluble substances with vitamin P activity on the fragility of lysosomes in vitro. Biochem. Pharmacol. 21, 1543—1548 (1972)

Van Cauwenberge, H., Franchimont, P.: Action du Z 6000 (trihydroxyethylrutoside) sur divers tests d'inflammation expérimentale réalisés chez le rat. Arch. int. Pharmacodyn. 170, 74—80 (1967)

Van Cauwenberge, H., Franchimont, P.: Untersuchung der antiphlogistischen Eigenschaften von Trihydroxyäthylrutosid. Zbl. Phlebol. 7, 110—121 (1968)

Van Cauwenberge, H., Lecomte, J., Cession-Fossion, A.: Sur quelques activités pharmacologiques de la (+)-catechine chez le rat. C.R. Soc. Biol. (Paris) 165, 1195—1198 (1971)

Van Cauwenberge, H., Lecomte, J., Franchimont, P.: De la recherche expérimentale à la recherche clinique dans le domaine des affections capillaro-veineuses. Vie méd. 50, 108—116 (1969)

Vane, J. R.: Prostaglandins in the inflammatory response. In: Lepow, J.-H., Ward, P. A. (Eds.): Inflammation Mechanisms and Control, pp. 261—279. London: Academic Press 1972

Vane, J. R.: Prostaglandins as mediators of inflammation. In: Samuelsson, B., Paoletti, R. (Eds.): Advances in Prostaglandin and Thromboxane Research, pp. 791—801. New York: Raven Press 1976

Villanueva, R., Hinds, L., Katz, R. L., Eakins, K. E.: The effect of polyphloretin phosphate on smooth muscle actions of prostaglandins in the cat. J. Pharmacol. exp. Ther. 180, 78—85 (1972)

Vogel, G., Marek, M. L.: Rattenpfoten-Ödem durch Polyvinylpyrrolidon und seine pharmakologische Beeinflußbarkeit. Eine einfache Methode zur Beurteilung der Kapillarpermeabilität für Flüssigkeit und definierte Makromoleküle. Arzneimittel-Forsch. 11, 356—362 (1961)

Vogel, G., Marek, M. L., Oertner, R.: Untersuchungen zum Mechanismus der therapeutischen und toxischen Wirkung des Roßkastanien-Saponins Aescin. Arzneimittel-Forsch. **20**, 699—703 (1970)

Vogel, G., Marek, M. L., Stoeckert, I.: Weitere Untersuchungen zum Wirkungsmechanismus des Roßkastanien-Saponins Aescin. Arzneimittel-Forsch. **13**, 59—64 (1963)

Vogel, G., Uebel, H.: Das therapeutisch wirksame Prinzip der Roßkastanie *(Aesculus hippocastanum)*. 3. Mitt.: Zur Frage von Angriffspunkt und Wirkungsmechanismus. Arzneimittel-Forsch. **10**, 275—280 (1960)

Vogin, E. E., Rossi, G. V.: Radiometric quantitation of the inhibition of 5-hydroxytryptamine-induced edema in mice. Arch. int. Pharmacodyn. **144**, 151—160 (1963)

Weissmann, G.: The role of lysosomes in inflammation and disease. Ann. Rev. Med. **18**, 97—112 (1967)

Whitehouse, M. W.: Some biochemical and pharmacological properties of anti-inflammatory drugs. In: Jucker, E. (Ed.): Progress in Drug Research, Vol. VIII, pp. 321—429. Basel-Stuttgart: Birkhäuser 1965

Wilhelm, D. L.: Chemical Mediators. In: Zweifach, B. W., Grant, L., McCluskey, R. T. (Eds.): The Inflammatory Process, pp. 389—425. New York-London: Academic Press 1965

Wilhelm, D. L.: Chemical Mediators, 2nd ed. In: Zweifach, B. W., Grant, L., McCluskey, R. T. (Eds.): The Inflammatory Process, Vol. II, pp. 251—301. New York-London: Academic Press 1973

Williams, T. J., Morley, J.: Prostaglandins as potentiators of increased vascular permeability in inflammation. Nature (Lond.) **246**, 215—217 (1973)

Winder, C. V., Wax, J., Burr, V., Been, M., Rosière, C. E.: A study of pharmacological influences on ultraviolet erythema in guinea pigs. Arch. int. Pharmacodyn. **116**, 261—292 (1958)

Winter, C. A.: Nonsteroid antiinflammatory agents. In: Jucker, E. (Ed.): Progress in Drug Research, Vol. 10, pp. 139—203. Basel-Stuttgart: Birkhäuser 1966a

Winter, C. A.: Nonsteroid anti-inflammatory agents. Ann. Rev. Pharmacol. **6**, 157—174 (1966b)

Wolstenholme, G. E. W., O'Connor, C. M., (Eds.): Histamine. CIBA Foundation Symposium. London: J. & A. Churchill Ltd 1956

Yamasaki, H., Irino, S., Saito, N., Kondo, K., Jinzenji, K., Yamamoto, T.: Pharmacology of guaiazulene with special reference to anti-inflammatory effect due to inhibition of histamine release. Nippon Yakurigaku Zasshi **54**, 362—377 (1958). See Chem. Abst. **53**, 10525d (1959)

Yegnanarayan, R., Saraf, A. P., Balwani, J. H.: Comparison of anti-inflammatory activity of various extracts of *Curcuma longa*. Linn. Indian J. Med. Res. **64**, 601—608 (1976)

Zierz, P., Lehmann, A., Craemer, R.: Die Beeinflußbarkeit akuter Entzündungsvorgänge durch Azulene. Hautarzt **8**, 552—556 (1957)

Zweifach, B. W., Grant, L., McCluskey, R. T.: The Inflammatory Process, 2nd Ed., New York-London: Academic Press 1973, Vol. II

Zweig, M. H., Maling, H. M., Webster, M. E.: Inhibition of sodium urate-induced rat hindpaw edema by colchicine derivatives: correlation with antimitotic activity. J. Pharmacol. exp. Ther. **182**, 344—350 (1972)

CHAPTER 40

A Critical Comparison of the Evaluation
of Anti-Inflammatory Therapy
in Animal Models and Man

P. J. L. HOLT

A. Introduction

This chapter is purposely written from the point of view of the practising clinician in
the hope that it may illustrate some of the difficulties in moving from in vitro or
animal models of inflammation to the human organism and of assessing the clinical
action of anti-inflammatory agents. It is primarily concerned only with the inflammation of arthritis and associated conditions which invariably form the major indication for this form of therapy.

Inflammation is a normal and necessary defence and repair response best left
unmodified unless it becomes uncontrolled and *detrimental*. The clinician is faced
with various forms of inflammation. The inflammation of arthritis is fundamentally
distinct from that of acute infection, for example pneumonia, principally because of
the element of chronicity that has appeared and the frequent absence of obvious
aetiology. Consequently, the ability to influence the inflammation significantly is
often much reduced. In certain cases, the provocative agent is known, for example in
microcystalline disease, in others infection is likely but its nature is unknown. In
both examples it is possible to use anti-inflammatory and analgesic therapy, but in
the first a specific therapy against the known provoking agent is much more effective.
This approach has the advantage of not interfering with the useful components of the
normal inflammatory responses at other sites in the body. Where the aetiological
agent is unknown, the clinician is left with the alternative of treating the results of
this agent and the receptive host, often at a time when the initial picture of agent
versus host has changed to more of an antoimmune i.e. host versus host situation,
where the initiating agent has become largely irrelevant. At this later stage, and
presuming the causative agent is not still influencing the disease, the problem of
treatment resolves itself into that of regulation of the autoimmune process and in
particular trying to re-set the regulatory mechanisms to control unwanted responses
while retaining beneficial responses, i.e. selective regulation. This field is still in its
infancy.

The aetiology of most of the rheumatic diseases is completely unknown, as are
the factors governing the host responses. The diversity of initiating agents and responses leads to great difficulty in defining the disease type. Thus, the concept of a
spectrum of diseases due either to a variety of similar insults or a variety of similar,
but not identical, host responses has arisen.

The permutation of these variables will produce many different disease pictures,
some of which may in fact be different diseases. Moreover, rheumatoid *disease* and
similar inflammatory syndromes can manifest as inflammation in joints, or in organs
and tissues with little joint change but severe ill-health.

If inflammatory disease cannot be subdivided into different types, is it possible to classify according to severity or stage? This is difficult though not impossible and will be discussed later.

It follows that if a disease syndrome can be the common expression of several different aetiological agents or host responses, an agent highly effective against only one variable will show up relatively badly in a formal trial where many variables may be present. Even so, the benefit in individual cases may be excellent. Conversely, a drug effective at a single site in the inflammatory reaction may be brilliantly successful in a number of cases of disease of different pathogenesis while overall results may be decreed poor: hence the clinical practice of trial and error with drug therapy.

In planning therapy, several concepts are possible but are not usually individually analysed in the clinical situation. One can treat the causative agent, treat the inflammatory reaction at several rate-limiting steps—either singly or together—to slow down the overall inflammatory response, influence the normal responses of the host to prevent acute inflammation becoming chronic, or give therapy known to work but whose mode of action is unknown. Thus, where the cause of the inflammation is clear, its assessment is relatively simple because the variables are measurable. These are the presence of organism (or chemical), the inflammation provoked (both local and general) and the resulting specific and non-specific immunological and biochemical changes.

A relatively stable situation is found in animal models where a standard insult is provided to a relatively uniform (standard) animal population. Here, either variable (insult or animal population) may be altered. In most inflammatory diseases in man the conditions are more complex: a third variable is present. Man is in essence an outbred population subject to genetic and environmental variations some of which the individual may himself influence. He certainly influences his own reactions and the interpretation of the tests applied.

A different type of problem arises where the pathogenesis of the disease is not clear. In osteoarthrosis (osteoarthritis in U.S.A.) opinions vary as to the inflammatory component, some authorities using analgesics only and others anti-inflammatory agents. In some diseases, and scleroderma is an example, inflammation may be present at certain stages of the disease only. This raises the question whether the differentiation between analgesics and analgesic/anti-inflammatory compounds has any importance apart from that of defining clinical objectives. Certainly, the side effects of analgesic/anti-inflammatory compounds are considerably more than those of the pure analgesics.

The variety of active chemicals—from gold to basic or acidic, alicyclic, aromatic or even more complicated compounds—implies a variety of sites of actions and a variety of toxic reactions. The suggestion follows, therefore, that more than one drug could summate therapeutically. This might occur if several steps in the inflammatory process were being suppressed more or less equally but not if the suppression depended on a single rate-limiting step. Further, since gold, penicillamine and chloroquine are not demonstrably anti-inflammatory compounds in animal screening tests, we return to the practical solution of testing the effect of drugs in patients and of identifying the chance benefit of therapy given for other conditions in order to detect potential anti-inflammatory compounds.

B. Comparison of Models of Inflammation With the Human Situation

The clinical situation has many differences from the laboratory experiment, principally because the latter is an artificial situation in which the conditions can, at least in part, be controlled (this may or may not be an advantage in assessing drug efficiency which depends on whole body responses). This type of work may represent the purest type of experiment but is only of interest in terms of a 'single step' or circumscribed approach to anti-inflammatory treatment in which one variable at a time is examined. Thus, it is difficult to extend the relevance of in vitro work, even when whole tissues are used, to the clinical situation where multiple factors are present. The isolation of cells or tissues from their normal homeostatic mechanisms, while facilitating evaluation, greatly reduces the significance of the changes produced by drugs. Although in vitro models must have biological significance, the practising clinician can find little interest in events happening outside the physiological and pathological limits.

Experiments in animals or humans, while having more meaning, do represent 'pure diseases' rather than the *spectrum* of diseases found clinically and presumably resulting from an admixture of genetic, environmental and aetiological agents. Some of the differences between models of inflammation and the human diseases may be summarized as follows:

1. The aetiological agent is apparent in many of these laboratory models, though its relevance for the pathogenesis is not clear and indeed the same clinical picture may be produced by different agents. The time of challenge, and thus the time course of the experimental syndrome, are known. Only in Reiter's syndrome, rheumatic fever and the infective arthritides, can the date of onset of the challenge be estimated in humans: in none of the other rheumatic diseases is this known. Thus, the clinician might be dealing with a fresh infection, activation of a latent process, or the end result of some slowly developing aberration of metabolism or immunity. These different situations have different pathogenetic postulates and therapeutic concepts. In those due to infection, removal of the infection should be definitive; in those due to activation of a latent process or the evolution of a prolonged process, presumably some homeostatic mechanism has failed and needs correction.

In none of the human rheumatic or connective tissue diseases is the pathogenesis understood, although parts of the process may be suspected and indeed copied.

The ability to determine the initiation of the inflammatory model allows a 'before and after' comparison to be made. This, together with the use of uniform animals, provides a more clearly defined baseline to the experiments.

2. By selective breeding, animal strains of greater or lesser susceptibility and even with different spectra of response can be obtained. The realism of many of these animal models is doubtful; they tend to run a self-limiting course or there is a very strong inherited component to the disease. Some of these genetic factors have been partly worked out. This concept of selective breeding to obtain specific susceptibility and reproducibility is completely opposed to the human situation where, by natural selection, the numbers of susceptible people should decrease. Heredity is a factor in the rheumatic diseases, but perhaps of less importance than previously thought and its influence is difficult to separate from the associated effects of co-habitation and environment—factors that the human is able to alter. Ethnic and geographical variations in rheumatic diseases are well recognised.

3. Preconditioning of animals can influence the onset of the subsequent disease and its character. Similar mechanisms may exist in humans, but have not been demonstrated. However, alteration of immune reactions by collateral infection or disease is recognised and treatment may influence the immune response, not always beneficially. The ability to monitor and detect potentially harmful alterations in these responses is very limited. During the course of therapeutic studies in the human, environmental conditions are very liable to change. Thus, exposure to UV light, increased exercise during the summer, and cold and damp during the winter, will affect either the true incidence of the disease or the character and severity of the symptoms arising. Most human trials are performed on outpatients where the daily activities, and in particular the activity in the clinic just before being tested, are not supervised. The conditions under which animals are tested are quite different. The animal has standard and unvarying surroundings usually within a restricted area and is commonly examined at the same time each day.

4. The actual inflammation produced in animals is unlike the clinical situation. Thus, either local inflammation is used, as in the UV light-induced inflammation, or inflammation is localised to selected areas of skin or joints by direct injury or injection; multiple joint involvement is rare. Alternatively, when a generalised response is produced, as in the rat adjuvant disease model, the disease bears more resemblance to a septicaemia or embolic phenomena and the joint inflammation is incidental. These models are seldom chronic but have definite patterns and phases which are not simulated in the human. The concept of inflammation as held by the clinician is rather broader than that of the laboratory biologist. The clinical picture embraces general ill-health and psychological alterations, some as part of the disease and some in response to the disease. Human disease is usually multisystem, while animal models are often localised either to a single joint or organ such as the skin. Thus the multisystem clinical pattern of rheumatoid arthritis, ankylosing spondylitis and scleroderma have not been mimicked. The associated ill-health of the animal may be of greater or lesser importance than in the corresponding human situation but is much more difficult to evaluate. It is an amalgamation of many different factors and, although several features are measured, it is usually the average or total that is used in assessment. In the animal models, however, a single feature is usually selected for measurement. Of the many models proposed, that most closely resembling a human disease is probably the New Zealand cross mouse model for immune complex disease and systemic lupus erythematosus (TALAL, 1970).

5. The differential sex incidence found in rheumatoid arthritis (1:2, M:F) or ankylosing spondylitis (3:1, M:F) does not occur in animal models of inflammation. Furthermore, because few of these animal models are age dependent, the varying clinical pictures produced at different ages in the human are not reproduced.

6. The metabolism or side-effects of the drugs given to animals often bear little relationship to that found when subsequently used in humans. The dose administered in the animal is adjusted according to serum levels or some measurement of inflammation. In the human, adjustments are more usually varied according to the patient's estimate of benefit and side-effects of the treatment. Different drugs may affect different aspects of inflammation in animal models. Thus, indomethacin is a powerful inhibitor of carregeenin inflammation but not of that produced by other irritants. This has certain similarities to the human situation where the clinician may feel that one drug may be more efficient in one type of inflammation than another.

The benefit obtained with indomethacin and phenylbutazone in ankylosing spondylitis is thought to be better than that obtained with salicylate. BECK and WHITEHOUSE (1973) have demonstrated that the induction of disease (adjuvant arthritis in the rat) may itself alter hepatic drug metabolism and the effectiveness of the administered drug. Altered hepatic enzyme activity is known to exist in inflammatory diseases in the human.

7. The therapeutic possibilities of rest in inflammatory arthritis cannot be tested in animal models of disease and since this is often used in humans in combination with non-steroid anti-inflammatory drugs, the conditions of trials are not comparable.

8. Perhaps the greatest imponderable is that of psychological effects on the natural history. It is well known that animals respond to stress and, although this variable can be mitigated by use of suitable controls, it may well have an effect on any trial of therapy. Vocalisation or other types of response are conditioned in the human by the possibility of communication and the results of tribal experience; this communication is impossible certainly between the lower animals. On the other hand, faith—a feeling few of the laboratory animals can have developed—may well be very effective in the human, producing the well-known placebo response.

9. Where the stimulus and response (e.g. pain, swelling) can be measured, then a correlation between the two can be constructed. Where different stimuli are used, the correlation curves obtained differ. This rather pure type of experiment is possible only with certain models.

10. The ability to alter the internal homeostatic mechanisms of the animal, e.g. by adrenalectomy, may allow better definition of the pathway of action of drugs and also whether the drug is acting directly or indirectly on the inflammation. Only indirect information is available in the human.

If these animal models are of any value they may simply point the way to drugs likely to be useful in man. Equally, they may well completely miss other drugs of value. For some of the most effective drugs, such as gold, penicillamine and chloroquine, there are no animal models available. Models developed to detect the antirheumatic potential of these latter drugs might be of far more value as screening methods for new anti-rheumatic drugs.

C. Analysis of Parameters of Inflammation in Man

In the evaluation of inflammation in the human, two facets are available which are not present with animal models: subjective and emotive evaluation, and functional testing. Although an animal may grimace or writhe, it cannot express itself more clearly, and functional testing in animals is limited to running (treadmill), random mobility or clinging tests. In general, clinical tests of inflammation can be subdivided into the completely subjective, the completely objective or a combination of the two in which the degrees of subjectivity and objectivity depend on the patient's or doctor's ability to alter the results by their own interpretation. Hence the use of varying degrees of 'blindness.'

The classical features of inflammation are pain, swelling, heat, redness, tenderness and loss of function. Of these, pain is subjective but can be compared by the analogue principle, swelling is objective and measurable, heat and redness reflect vascularity and can be measured as blood flow or temperature, although it is technically difficult to obtain reproducible results. Tenderness is directly measurable but subject to individual and periodic variation due to psychological and external influences. Loss of function, a reflection among other things of pain, tenderness, swelling, stiffness and muscle weakness, is measurable by tests of strength and timed function tests such as climbing stairs or walking on the flat, or tests of dexterity as in 'activities of daily living' studies. Stiffness after rest is characteristic of inflammation and, together with the well-being of the patient, represents sensitive early symptoms of improvement or deterioration, but neither feature is quantifiable. It is quantitation that is important and difficult since, theoretically at least, if the improvement was obvious accurate assessment would be unnecessary. Usually, relatively small changes in clinical status occur during drug studies and since the majority of the patients used are of only moderate to medium severity, i.e. neither minimal nor very severe, the possibility of clear-cut change, i.e. from minimal to normal or from very severe to moderate or minimal, is lost

The more effective the drug, the less discriminating the test needs to be. However, when comparing increasingly effective drugs, the possible difference in clinical benefit obtained becomes progressively smaller so that the discriminatory value of the test must progressively increase.

Tests must be chosen which measure potentially reversible features with accuracy and with little chance for random error. These features vary in individual patients and different diseases so that when a group is examined, a compromise in the selected tests may be necessary. This is of some importance since many patients with arthritis may not be affected both in their hands and in their feet; in these cases demonstration of changes will only be possible in either hands or feet. It is scientifically impossible to compare changes in the hands of one patient with those in the feet of another patient, although this type of information forms the basis of most trials. Furthermore, all types of dysfunction do not respond equally; thus, weakness of grip due to tenosynovitis may respond to anti-rheumatic treatment much less satisfactorily than that due to articular synovitis. A series of tests on a varied group of patients will show changes in some parameters in some patients and in different parameters in others. However, the magnitude of these changes will be reduced by the absence of any change in those tests where there was no possibility of change from the start.

Since the baseline, i.e. normal, value of most of these parameters in a patient is not usually known, it is more convenient to record change in a value by difference rather than percentage. Further, since the degree of change may vary between different joints, either change in an index joint or a summation of the change in several joints can be measured. Certain tests are only applicable to certain joints, e.g. grip to hands and walking time to legs.

Laboratory tests are largely concerned with acute phase reactants and immune processes. While the normal values of these are known and hence the *potential* goal in biochemical terms, in practice the changes are usually not completely sensitive or reversible and thus the practical end point is often unknown. Nor is the clinical significance of improving these parameters known, for their correlation with disease activity and more importantly disease progression or regression is not clear and may vary from individual to individual.

I. Stiffness

Stiffness experienced in either joints or muscle is very suggestive of inflammation and is almost universal in rheumatoid arthritis and common in all forms of inflammatory arthritis. Thus, it is a very useful determinant in epidemiological surveys. It is characteristically worsened by inactivity and improved by activity. The symptom of stiffness is not one that is normally experienced and thus the interviewer may have some difficulty in interpreting the patient's symptoms. Nor is the patient always clear of what is implied; thus, 'stiffness' of a few minutes' duration is best ignored and *pain* on first moving a joint rather different in its significance. Although difficult to quantify, it is easier for the patient to give an approximate duration than to express a degree of severity of stiffness. It is a reduction in duration rather than severity that heralds improvement. With cortisone, stiffness eventually disappears completely, often in a matter of days, but with non-steroid anti-inflammatory drugs the disappearance is incomplete. Most rheumatoid patients find the symptoms worse first thing in the morning ('morning stiffness'), when stiffness may persist for 4 h. Other patients with polymyalgia rheumatica (an inflammatory disease of unknown pathogenesis) have stiffness all day with only mild relief from exercise. Quite different from the stiffness experienced by the rheumatoid patient is the pain and stiffness associated with other inflammatory diseases such as ankylosing spondylitis, where the capsules, ligaments and tendon insertions may be painful and lead to 'stiffness.' In these cases, the symptoms are often more widespread, involve central areas of the body, have a prominent pain and tenderness component and move from place to place. The stiffness and more prominent tenderness found in inflammation of muscles (myositis) are again different in character.

Attempts to measure joint stiffness objectively have not been completely successful (WRIGHT and JOHNS, 1961; BACKLUND and TISELIUS, 1967) nor is it known what causes joint stiffness, although the periarticular tissue seems to be predominantly responsible (WRIGHT et al., 1969).

II. Pain

The symptom of pain is purely subjective and without definition. Its interpretation varies between individuals, and is dependent on factors such as age, physical and psychological status, the menstrual cycle and climatic conditions and previous experience. Natural variation in pain threshold probably explains the gross joint destruction found in individuals with high pain thresholds. This feature of inflammation is perhaps the most difficult of all to evaluate. It depends on personal appraisal of the quality and severity of a symptom, translation of which to a common scale of experience is difficult. Since it often produces psychological changes, these may in turn influence the patient's response. Thus, alteration in the character and severity of the pain may be more meaningful than trying to assign a value to it. Assessment is by the analogue method which allows a patient to make his own assessment of pain severity and changes in it (HUSKISSON, 1974). This technique is more useful and easier for the patient to answer than the use of a series of standard questions such as "pain absent?," "mild?" "severe?" or "very severe?" The patient finds the choice of one of these values hard.

III. Joint Tenderness

This is a useful sign of inflammation and is particularly helpful in demarcating clinically the sites of active inflammation. Its measurement is not easy and wide variations in the results are obtained. However, it has a useful stimulus-response relation. Very tender joints need little pressure to elicit pain; as inflammation resolves, the pressure needed to elicit the same response increases rapidly until in the normal joint considerable pressure is necessary. Various methods have been proposed for measuring this tenderness usually based on linear compression (McCARTY et al., 1968; RITCHIE et al., 1968). In these methods, pressure or alternatively pressure and/or movement is used in joints to elicit pain, and the pain (not strictly tenderness) elicited by either method is given a simple value according to its severity, so that the sum total of all painful joints at that time is obtained. Tenderness may be measured by circumferential pressure (HAWKINS and HOLT, 1966) and the results are reproducible. More complex systems, which take into account the relative joint size (LANSBURY, 1958) or the presence of soft tissue swelling (Co-operating Clinics, Committee of American Rheumatism Association, 1970), tend to be impractical. Accurate localisation of tenderness is important, for it may be very localised and may differ in distribution from the associated pain which can be referred to a distance. Occasionally, there may be little pain but marked tenderness as in localised tenosynovitis. Conversely, deep pain such as that arising in bones may not be associated with tenderness. Nor are dysfunction and tenderness directly related, although pressure induced tenderness may inhibit grip and be felt as pain. With any method of assessment, experience of both observer and patient will improve the reproducibility of results and repeated estimations will indicate the reliability of the observations and their correlation with disease activity. Initially, wide variations occur particularly between observers, but these become much less with practice.

IV. Grip Strength

Grip strength depends on the stability of the joints and tendons, the integrity of the muscles and nerves of the hand and forearm and the degree of painful inhibition of the muscles. Careful assessment of the test situation is necessary; a solitary painful joint or tendon may result in marked weakness of the total hand. Rapid deterioration which is partly due to associated muscle weakness, is much more clearly monitored than changes produced by improvement. Because of the multiple factors involved and since many of the above causes of weakness may take a considerable time to recover, this test is not suitable for short-term trials.

Grip strength compared either by the squeezing of two of the physician's fingers or more accurately by squeezing various mechanical devices, is a useful guide to progress. It is a relatively easy test to perform and, provided the patient co-operates fully, is reproducible with a wide range of response between active and inactive states. The simplest method is to inflate a folded sphygmomanometer cuff or Davis bag to 30 mm Hg (some authorities use 20 mm and different results are obtained), and attach it to a sphygmomanometer, the mercury column of which is shielded from the view of the patient (SAVAGE, 1966). Values in consecutive inflations should lie within 20 mm of each other and an average of these values is taken. Normal man should exceed 300 mm Hg and woman 250 mm Hg; rheumatoid patients may lie in the 50–100 mm Hg range. This method is useful to detect patients who are not fully trying or are frankly malingering because the inability to reproduce the same degree of pressure—unless maximal exertion is used—leads to wide fluctuations in the apparent strength of the patient. It has been suggested that there may be a diurnal variation in grip strength (WRIGHT, 1959) but LEE et al. (1974a) could not confirm this. They found an observer error of up to 20 mm Hg in this method; this is less than the range of change to be expected from an effective anti-rheumatic drug.

Preliminary exercising of the hand may reduce some of the stiffness and lead to more uniform results. Splinting of the wrist or supporting the forearm can considerably increase the apparent grip strength, whilst repeated testing leads to early fatigue in the rheumatoid patient and spuriously low readings.

Arthritis is often assymmetrical and may only affect a part of the hand, although the local problem may be reflected in total hand dysfunction. It may, therefore, be more advantageous to measure either pressure between the first and second fingers (pinch) or the power of flexion of an individual finger. Special machines have been designed to do this (reviewed by DICKSON and NICOLLE, 1975).

V. Joint Size

Enlargement of joints is characteristic of most types of arthritis, although a relatively minor enlargement may be associated with severe disability when the capsule is mainly involved, as in rheumatic fever and ankylosing spondylitis. Enlargement is made up of several components; bone overgrowth, which is irreversible, soft tissue thickening which is slowly reversible unless it is of long duration and organised, and fluid swelling which is potentially rapidly and completely reversible. However, reversibility of fluid swelling is only a reliable index when due to inflammation; non-inflammatory fluid swelling responds poorly to anti-inflammatory drugs. Although swelling can be appreciated by palpation, as the changes in size tend to be small and slow, instruments have been developed to measure the swelling. The use of circumferential measurement allows a more accurate measure than linear width; not only are the differences greater but the correct alignment is less critical. For this reason, the interphalangeal joints of the fingers are usually chosen since they are accessible, reasonably uniform and allow reproducible results to be obtained; other joints such as the knee are less configerationally suitable. Originally estimated by jeweller's rings, measurement of the finger joints using the standard strain gauge type apparatus issued by Geigy is now almost universal and gives highly reproducible results. Measurement of several joints avoids sampling errors but recordings of individual joints may show greater changes. The same gauge should be used throughout and occasionally calibrated. Both aspirin and cortisone have demonstrable anti-inflammatory effects using these tests, (BOARDMAN and HART, 1967). Estimations of foot swelling by water displacement have now been largely abandoned.

VI. Blood Flow and Vascular Permeability

Increased blood flow and vascular permeability are prominent aspects of inflammation. They can be measured in several ways. Increased blood flow leads to an increase in temperature in the limbs, which are normally a few degrees colder than the rest of the body. Early workers (e.g. HORVATH and HOLLANDER, 1949) showed that the intra-articular temperature rose with inflammation but the techniques necessary to measure this directly are not in general practical and can be used only in large joints such as the knee. An indirect index of this increased temperature may be obtained by the use of external thermography (COLLINS et al., 1974). This measures the infrared radiation given off by the body, which is dependent on local temperature, and can be used to scan for hot inflamed areas. Although these techniques are improving and may well become rapid non-invasive methods of analysis, they are at present research tools only, requiring experience and elaborate facilities to obtain reproducible results.

Radioactive traces can be used to study the synovial blood flow. Following intra-articular injection, xenon (133 Xe) is cleared from the joint at a rate proportional to the synovial vascularity and is promptly excreted by the lungs so that there is no recirculation to produce a raised background (DICK, 1972). Conversely, radioactive technetium (98 m TC), after intravenous injection, slowly leaks into the synovial cavity from capillaries and is then sequestrated, leading to an increasing radioactivity over the inflamed joints. Thus, soon after injection, radioactivity registers capillary blood flow and at a later stage capillary permeability (DICK, 1972). These tests are less useful than their initial results indicated.

VII. Radiographic Changes

Basically, two types of change may be seen; alteration in the soft tissues—synovial fluid, synovium or capsule—or of bone, either as regional osteoporosis or local erosions of the bone in the form of joint erosions or bone cysts. These latter are usually slow in evolution and even slower in resolution. Further, they are hard to quantify, due to variations in radiological technique and the difficulty of measuring the resulting radiological density. Resolution of inflammatory erosions or osteoporosis, changes which greatly impress clinicians, is *very* slow. Methods of measuring bone density have been evaluated but at present are time consuming, expensive and still too insensitive for short-term assessment. There are strong possibilities of improvement in these techniques, particularly with computerised bone scanning, but they will probably remain expensive. Of equal interest and as yet incompletely evaluated, are methods of measuring the bone density distribution. This allows very small (mm^3) local changes to be compared and is of theoretical as well as practical interest in demonstrating the serial changes in bone density around sites of inflammation, (DICKSON and NICOLLE, 1975). They do not allow changes in bone architecture to be differentiated.

Radiological changes in bone reflect many local and systemic variables. Alteration may be due to factors such as malnutrition, local and general inactivity, the therapy employed or, more specifically, the local inflammation. The inflammation produces decreased mobility, increased local bone destruction and regional osteoporosis (occasionally anabolism in the form of boney outgrowths), or periostitis. When the inflammation is mild and intermittant there will be precocious epiphyseal development.

Progressive radiological joint deformity is a poor indicator of inflammation, since it may progress in spite of healing, the changes occurring over months and are thus impractical for short-term studies. Regression is even slower. Over longer periods, the radiological appearances must be interpreted against the natural changes in bone density occurring with age.

VIII. Tests of Functional Ability

These are either tests of physical activity, such as walking time or the time taken to ascend or descend stairs, or of tests of dexterity. They are thus composite tests involving several joints and a number of features such as stiffness, pain, strength and stability. They are crude but practical tests, useful in assessing a patient's problems in relationship to daily living. When they are repeated too often, learning or boredom may alter their value. Composites of various tests have been proposed but add little to their value and moreover the techniques become progressively more time consuming for the clinician and irksome for the patients. Formal estimates of functional status of disease index have been proposed. They measure slightly different aspects of the patient's overall condition. The simplest functional estimates are those suggested by STEINBROCKER et al. (1949) which list four grades and that of the MEDICAL RESEARCH COUNCIL (1954) which lists five scale points.

IX. Laboratory Assessment of Disease Activity

These tests, since they are objective, might theoretically be of more value than clinical assessment. However, there are several defects, other than the purely technical aspects.

1. In spite of clinically severe disease, little change from normal may be found in the laboratory tests and in particular the erythrocyte sedimentation rate (ESR) may be normal, while severe systemic disease with little arthritis may be associated with a markedly elevated ESR and acute phase reactants.

2. Conversely, although showing some fall with the initial clinical improvement, acute phase reactants may remain elevated in spite of apparently complete clinical remission (McCONKEY et al., 1973).

3. Biochemical and immunological changes in the serum seem to reflect in part the extent as well as the severity of the process. Thus, severe inflammation of a single joint may be associated with normal biological tests.

4. Different diseases are associated with different responses; thus, the acute phase reactants may not be equally elevated in spite of clinically equivalent inflammation. In some diseases, acute phase reactants may be decreased such as complement (C_3) in systemic lupus erythematosus, and in others raised as in rheumatoid arthritis (VERSEY et al., 1973), characteristically C-reactive protein is *not* raised in systemic lupus erythematosus, unless infection is present, but is raised in rheumatoid arthritis.

The laboratory correlates of inflammation fall into various categories: the nonspecific, such as ESR in which increased sedimentation of the red blood cells occurs due to the effect of fibrinogen and macroglobulins, producing rouleaux formation and thus increasing sedimentation; the acute phase reactants such as C-reactive protein, haptoglobin, complement, fibrinogen etc., which reflect alteration of inflammation much more rapidly and to a greater degree than the immunoglobulins. Little change in any of these parameters has been found with most of the non-steroid anti-inflammatory drugs, but chloroquine, gold and penicillamine have shown a tendency of reduce these titres in association with clinical improvement.

Biochemical changes specific for the inflammatory disease are few. Immunoglobulins, mainly of the IgM type, are responsible for the positive sheep cell and latex fixation test found in rheumatoid diseases. High titres of IgM broadly correlate with the presence of chronicity and complications in rheumatoid disease. Although fluctuations of the titres occur, persistent lowering suggests improvement in the patient's condition. Increased antibodies to double-stranded deoxyribonucleic acid (DNA) are very characteristic of active systemic lupus erythematosus and are not found in inactive disease. When elevated they are a useful means of monitoring treatment, a reduction of elevated levels indicating clinical improvement (HUGHES, 1971). Various other antibodies are found whose presence correlate fairly well with disease states but alteration of their titres with treatment is not well documented.

Anaemia and lowered serum iron, often with normal bone marrow iron stores, are common in active inflammation particularly when it is generalised. Slow recovery of both may follow successful treatment.

Since immunosuppression is the objective of some of the therapies used, assessment of immunosuppression either by lymphocyte function in vitro or by skin tests has been tried but not very successfully. These tests may be influenced in different ways both by anti-inflammatory therapy and cytotoxic therapy. In particular, many of the tests take too long to be useful in adjusting the treatment of the patient.

The serum levels of a variety of enzymes are elevated in severe disease, probably as a non-specific association of the inflammation. These regress with treatment. Although many of these enzymes are also elevated in liver disease, it is debatable whether they represent liver disease in this context. However, they do present difficulties when assembling patients for studies of drug treatment since they tend to be raised in those patients who have the most active inflammation and who are therefore most likely to show benefit with treatment. Trialists are unhappy to use these patients because of the difficulty in distinguishing the raised enzyme levels of liver disease from those provoked by drug toxicity.

Other techniques of assessment such as following the joint pathology by serial synovial biopsy and arthroscopy are probably unjustified and are associated with too many variables. Repeated synovial fluid aspirations are feasible and ethical under certain circumstances. The changes represent those of an inflammatory situation with increased leucocytes, fibrinogen, protein and enzymes of various types including peptidases and collagenases which result in a partial degradation of hyaluronic acid (HOLT et al., 1968). The result is an opalescent fluid of low viscosity which forms a poor clot with acetic acid. Alteration of these findings, which represent the end result of many factors, is a useful non-specific parameter of effective therapy.

D. Clinical Trials

It is first important to consider why clinical trials are undertaken. Fundamentally, they represent a dissatisfaction with present treatment either pharmacological, surgical, physical or psychological. However, certain additional benefits accrue. The following discussion is limited to some aspects of drug trials since many comprehensive reviews are available. FEINSTEIN (1972, 1973) has pointed out some of the fallacies of 'control' in the design of clinical experiments and should be read in full.

I. Objectives

The objectives or benefits of clinical trials and assessment may be itemised as follows.

1. Improvement of Therapeutic Methods at Present Available

Initial treatment schedules are seldom permanently adhered to in clinical practise. Changes in timing and dosage are common, either because of the realisation of increasing benefit with no increase in toxicity or because side-effects may be reduced by an altered treatment regime. Ibuprofen represents a good example of different therapeutic approaches; it was introduced into the U.S.A. in a daily dose of 8– 16×200 mg tablets, but in England at 3×200 mg tablets daily. The question arises that if a drug is effective at 600 mg, is the added advantage of using 3200 mg worthwhile? Obviously, without controlled clinical trials, the correct dosage would not be evaluated. With indomethacin a high incidence of side-effects was found with the early formulation when approximately 300 mg/day was administered. With the new formulation which resulted in more even absorption, the daily dosage has been reduced to 100 mg/day with more benefit because of the reduced side-effects. Unfortunately, this change has not been fully appreciated and the results obtained with the earlier formulation are persistently quoted. The use of prednisone in children can be valuable but is associated with growth retardation. By giving the prednisone as a single daily dose in the morning, the normal circadian rhythm is mimicked. The suppression of the hypothalmic-pituitary-adrenal axis is even further reduced by giving twice the daily dose of prednisone as a single morning dose on alternate days, when growth can often be shown to recommence (ANSELL and BYWATERS, 1974).

2. Optimum Benefit in a Patient

Although all patients are obviously not included in formal trials, a beneficial association of some varieties of disease and different therapeutic regimes may be established and lead to a more rational treatment of the individual patient. It is the identification of subgroups of patients that allows the use of more rational therapy.

3. Improvement of Methods of Monitoring Inflammation in Patients

The present methods of measuring facets of inflammation are barely adequate and need improvement to detect smaller degrees of alteration in disease activity as the margin of therapeutic advance gets progressively less. The assessment techniques are blunderbuss and do not measure isolated pathways of inflammation; thus, different types of therapeutic effect ar not distinguished. The part played by other factors such as psychological response should also be defined.

4. Development of New Human Models for the Evaluation of Drugs

The clinical impression that not all drugs are equally effective in all inflammatory diseases implies multiple pathological and biological systems. Analysis of this situation by defining different models such as isolated osteoarthrosis of the hip instead of osteoarthrosis in general, neoplastic bone pain, the recording of pain threshold in different types of disease and the development of new models of skin or other inflammation, are all examples of this approach.

5. Discovery of New Therapeutic Agents

This is the more immediately obvious virtue of clinical trials and will be discussed further later

6. Promotion of More Scientific Management of Disease

Much of clinical management is based on clinical judgement, with little scientific basis. Attempts at scientific analysis of clinical material, i.e. patients, are increasingly being undertaken but until they are routinely practical there is unlikely to be any major advance in the management of patients. The practical (pragmatic) approach is relatively easy, but ensures a static standard. The assessment for trial purposes presupposes that the relative possibilities for treatment of each clinical problem are evaluated and recorded. This in both the short and long term must improve the practitioner's knowledge and care of the disease, and in particular the long-term evaluation of disease.

It is often difficult to define the therapeutic objectives in treating arthritis. It is, perhaps, most easily summarised as improvement of function. Thus, anything which impairs function must be treated. This might include pain, weakness, limited range of motion, instability of the joint or sensory deficits. Each of these facets may have several causes. Thus, the therapeutic possibilities are manifold. Improved function also implies rehabilitation both psychologically and physically.

In conducting a clinical trial three aspects, each of which may have many subsidiary features are considered: the dose of drug given and its metabolism, the response of the patient and the side-effects. Some limitation of the problems or the extent of their analysis is usually made to allow groups of patients to be compared. Since the individual patients may have only some of the total abnormalities of the whole group and it is impossible to equate different parameters, e.g. stiffness in one patient with joint swelling in another, the margin of change between treated and untreated groups tend to be blurred. The alternative is to take single patients and assess one or two features capable of improvement before and after treatment and then compare the number of patients who have improved (using different parameters as criteria) with those who have not improved.

Attempts should be made to reduce the many variables. There has been some success with careful selection of assessment methods and patients and with clear and usually circumscribed objectives being outlined for each trial. The duration of a trial is important. Initially short periods of drug treatment are employed. But short-term trial results can only be used to infer changes over the short term and not those following long-term therapy.

When the objective has been defined, and this will depend in part on the supposed action of the drug, e.g. analgesic or anti-inflammatory, the technique of measuring the patient's response must also be considered.

It will be obvious that a trial implies a comparison either with currently accepted therapy or with a projected normality for that patient. The latter concept is difficult and can only be fully approached in biochemical terms where the range of normality is known. It is also obvious that the problems likely to be involved in the trial treatment should be considered. These must be balanced against the need for new therapies and the severity of the disease, i.e. what risks can legitimately be taken. Once started, provided serious toxicity does not occur, the trial must continue until a statistical answer is obtained; early results may be misleading.

II. Assessment

Any method that relies on the patient's response to the clinician's stimulus, whether as a question or a physical function such as squeezing a tender joint, has two poorly controlled variables. It is likely to give the most reproducible results when applied by one observer and that after much continuous practise. Thus, an estimate of both intra- and inter-observer error of a particular test is important in assessing the significance of the results obtained. The fact that different observers may grade responses differently and thus confuse results, illustrates the point that clinicians often have difficulty in defining what constitutes improvement and also in defining functional states. Improvement in one area is often accompanied by deterioration elsewhere. Perhaps the greatest difficulty lies in the assessment of the significance of side-effects, and the reports of the incidence of toxicity of drug therapy are often unreliable. Thus, these evaluations are the sum total or average of many different forms of therapy and in particular, different standards of patient monitoring. What one physician may regard as a relatively safe drug may be disastrous in the hands of another. Furthermore, the patient may not agree with his physician's assessment.

Any test of inflammation is subject to non-standard conditions because of the alteration in general status of the patient. Inflammatory diseases have a large systemic component which, apart from organic changes, manifests itself as general ill-health, weight loss and a lowering of morale. Thus, changes of morale and psychological mood associated with the systemic component may be important in altering the patient's reaction to test procedures, increased physical activity may result in increased joint symptoms. Improvement in one joint of the leg (for instance by local injection) may throw an increased strain on another joint.

The concept of base-line in the sense of maximum achievement of function or complete relief of symptoms is important because it determines the type of test employed. Thus, if a partially effective drug such as aspirin is already being given (perhaps because it is not felt possible to take the patient off all therapy), and it is desired to test the effectiveness of a second drug, then the margin for potential improvement is reduced, the first drug (e.g. aspirin) having already produced some benefit. Evaluation of the second drug is harder and probably needs more patients to obtain statistical significance. The technique of replacing the background drug (aspirin), once a plateau response has been achieved, by a placebo and seeing whether there is a marked change in inflammatory indices, is useful. Moreover, it is found that the withdrawal of an effective drug produces more dramatic clinical change than the change produced during the institution of the same therapy. Thus, replacement of an effective background drug (aspirin), or of a trial drug being used alone, by a placebo may be a most useful method of demonstrating anti-inflammatory activity. There are problems of interpretation with this method which are being increasingly recognised as the effects of both competitive and non-competitive binding (KOCH-WESER and SELLERS, 1976) and enzyme induction (GELEHRTER, 1976) are more fully appreciated. This technique works well only with rapidly acting drugs.

In drug trials, little attention is usually paid to the optimum timing of methods of therapy and rather rigid schedules are laid down. More recently, either freedom of therapeutic adjustment has been used, or estimations of serum drug levels have allowed dosage to be adjusted and the serum levels obtained to be compared with the effectiveness of treatment. This is valuable for two reasons. First very different serum levels may be obtained in different patients: salicylates are a good example and since many of these drugs are protein bound (principally to albumin), their concentrations may vary with the varying albumin levels found in these diseases. Secondly, it also ensures that treatment is being taken, a factor often overlooked.

With some drugs there is a good correlation between serum levels of the drug and clinical benefit but with others there is none. Aspirin and indomethacin are good examples of the first and gold a good example of the second type of response. When the drugs are avidly retained in the tissues, serum levels seem to be of less importance than when the drugs have a short half-life such as occurs with salicylate. These forms of therapeutic adjustment can be undertaken without destroying the 'blindness' of the investigation.

The initial stages of the introduction of a drug involve an extrapolation of the findings with drugs used in animals and these are notoriously unreliable. They will, however, give some indication of the likely length of the trial.

III. Patient Selection

The problem of the selection of suitable patients has already been mentioned. The inflammatory arthritides are a mixed group of conditions. Several criteria have been proposed to allow some coherent subdivision. In order to illustrate the variable clinical pictures that are considered relatively homogenous, the commonly used American Rheumatism Association criteria for rheumatoid arthritis (AMERICAN RHEUMATISM ASSOCIATION, 1959) are appended in abbreviated form. These criteria are intended primarily for surveys of an epidemiological nature but have been used widely in the clinical trial field. For a full discussion the original should be consulted.

1. Morning stiffness (1 h or more)
2. Pain on motion or tenderness of a joint
3. Swelling—soft tissue or fluid of a joint
4. Swelling—of at least one other joint
5. Symmetrical joint involvement of both sides of the body
6. Subcutaneous nodules over bony prominences
7. X-ray changes typical of rheumatoid arthritis
8. Positive sheep cell agglutination test
9. Poor mucin clot from synovial fluid
10. Characteristic synovial histology
11. Characteristic nodule histology

A similar list of 20 exclusions, i.e. features nullifying the diagnosis, must also be considered. Any seven of the above criteria are sufficient to make a diagnosis of *classical* rheumatoid arthritis, any five of *definite* rheumatoid arthritis and any three of *probable* rheumatoid arthritis. This method uses no weighting for the relative importance of each criteria. Thus, many clinicians would consider a characteristic nodule is far more useful in diagnosis than any of the other features. For systemic lupus erythematosus sixteen features have been suggested any four of which are sufficient to make the diagnosis (COHEN et al., 1971). Similar criteria exist for other conditions and all are under continued review as different diseases are discovered within the present umbrella of diagnosis.

Although there are few facts to refer to, clinically it seems that social and family background may influence the patient's reaction to disease and to clinical trials. Further, outside factors such as chronic infection may influence the disease incidence in some countries.

A more important variable is that of ethnic background. Thus, negroes seem to be much more susceptible to systemic lupus erythematosus than caucasians and the clinical features may be rather different in the two groups, for which a genetic basis seems to be emerging (GOLDBERG et al., 1976) suggesting genetic influences in the pathogenesis and expression of systemic lupus erythematosus.

These variables can, where appropriate, be allowed for by stratification of the cases. However, the more stratification necessary, the more complicated the trial becomes and the more patients are required to give adequate group numbers.

The coincidental use of other non-anti-inflammatory drugs may have a serious effect on the interpretation of drug trials. Phenobarbitone, a strong hepatic enzyme inducer markedly reduces the clinical effectiveness of phenylbutazone (CHEN et al., 1962; LEVI et al., 1968), this simple fact greatly reduces the significance of many of the early trials of phenylbutazone where the use of phenobarbitone was not specifically mentioned. The opposite effect, inhibition, has been shown with flurbiprofen (CHALMERS et al., 1973). Other unsuspected changes may occur; antidepressants are often used in the treatment of the arthritic. HAYDU et al. (1974) have shown that one of these, imipramine, may reduce the titre of rheumatoid factor often found in the depressed patient. Their preliminary results suggested a similar benefit in rheumatoid arthritis. However, HAYDU et al. (1974) used 150 mg per day; other work using 75 mg day in rheumatoid arthritis has shown no benefit (DICK and FOWLER, 1976).

Raised serum enzyme levels suggesting liver damage but without other evidence of liver disease, have been found following aspirin treatment in children with rheumatoid arthritis and dermatomyositis (RUSSELL et al., 1971) and in systemic lupus erythematosus (SEAMAN et al., 1974). This is obviously of importance when formulations containing aspirin are used in association with drugs under trial.

To obtain a certain uniformity amongst the patients they can be assessed in three further ways, all of which have their special advantages. The original criteria of anatomical stage of disease, functional class and therapeutic criteria for responses (STEINBROCKER et al., 1949), although modified by subsequent workers, still represent valid and instructive concepts which should be consulted to obtain a background to the difficulties likely to be encountered. In summary, the anatomical stage tries to define the clinical and radiological changes present. These will obviously vary for different parts of the body but either an average (subjective) for all the joints can be obtained or changes in a single joint can be measured. This type of assessment can be used for charting progression of the disease and is now mainly confined to the radiological changes, other factors being measured as under 'parameters of inflammation' or as a functional capacity.

Functional capacity is an overall measure of the patient's ability to lead a normal life or to continue his work, and his ability to look after himself in the activities of daily living. Two slightly different systems of functional assessment have been used, that of STEINBROCKER et al. (1949) and that of the MEDICAL RESEARCH COUNCIL (1954).

In assessing disease activity for formal trials, complicated systems as described in the section 'parameters of inflammation' are used or the original STEINBROCKER criteria which are purely clinical except for the addition of an ESR. DUTHIE et al. (1955) proposed a simple system which included, in addition to the ESR, the degree of anaemia. More recently, there has been a tendency to return to a clinically based system (RITCHIE et al., 1968) which combines assessment of inflammation (or tenderness) and a record of the distribution of joints involved.

It will be obvious that all these forms of assessment are highly subjective: hence the importance of using controls in the form of placebos, crossover studies and most important of all, 'blindness'.

IV. Placebo Response

This important feature of the patient-doctor relationship for a long time constituted the physician's main line of treatment. It remains an important variable in patient management, both as a form of treatment and as a means of determining true biological improvement from subjective improvement. The latter use is not adequately exploited, largely because it is time consuming, but it does help to avoid committing patients to potentially dangerous and possibly useless treatment. The background to this type of response has been discussed with reference to cancer patients undergoing trials of oral analgesics (MOERTEL et al., 1976): 50% of the patients gave a placebo response. Interestingly, patients responding to placebo also had an increased response to active drugs, were predominantly better educated, more independent and self sufficient. Although implying the use of an active treatment, a similar enhanced and spurious response is very easily obtained by the attitude, manner and status of the medical personnel. It is characteristic of the placebo response that it tends to wane unless reinforced. TRAUT and PASSARELL (1959) showed that the failing placebo response following oral therapy could be partially restored by placebo injections.

Finally, it must be mentioned that not only are there experienced trialists but, increasingly, experienced patients. A recent patient had previously taken four different drugs at different times all carefully camouflaged under code names. She now has no signs of inflammatory arthritis and the effective treatment remains a mystery.

Having decided upon the format of the trial, consideration of the circumstances under which it is performed is necessary. Thus, outpatients and inpatients may react quite differently. The time of day at which the tests are undertaken is also important since stiffness and grip strength may vary through the day.

V. Conclusions

Clinical trials are not easy to carry out and have often been badly conceived and run. They remain essential if management of patients is to improve.

The assessment of arthritic patients and the use of this to follow the progress of treatment has led to a better understanding of the diseases and a more rational approach to treatment. The simple methods used initially have become increasingly more complex. There are still those clinicians who feel that a combination of the ESR estimation and the question 'do you feel better' are the most appropriate assessments, and that occasionally the treatment is worse than the cure.

E. Treatment

Many standard reviews of treatment exist and reflect the many different objectives and situations of the authors. Hence only some points are discussed here.

In considering anti-inflammatory treatment, there are two courses open. The first is the conservative treatment of the patient by rest and general measures, followed by drug treatment for the remaining inflammation. Alternatively, treatment can be the immediate use of suppressive anti-rheumatic therapy by itself. Commonly, the practical course of combining the two therapies probably saves time but can also lead to the unnecessary use of drugs and, worse, to the increased risk of side-effects. The prime objective of all treatment is reduction of joint and tendon inflammation, the muscular improvement occurring as a secondary phenomenon. It must be emphasised that in spite of symptomatic relief there is no evidence that any drug protects the joint from further destruction. We again return to a clinical judgement; the risk of therapy may be regarded as too high in the early stages of the disease when spontaneous remission is still possible and again in the later stages when the possible benefits are too low because of the irreversible joint and tendon destruction present. Another difficult therapeutic problem concerns localised inflammatory arthritis when faced with the need to use potentially toxic drugs systemically. The alternative is to allow the disease to run its natural course in that joint, perhaps to complete destruction, rather than risk side-effects and/or the inconvenience of regular supervision. Factors other than the efficacy or otherwise of the therapy are important in deciding on a course of treatment. One of these, the age of the patient, has two distinct aspects. The elderly patient requires a satisfactory response simply and quickly without excessive monitoring and is not too concerned with complications that might occur in the unpredictable future. Corticosteroids fit this requirement well. The young patient with advancing crippledom is not too bothered with the future possibility of cancer or some other catastrophy 10–20 years later. The relative weighting put on the answers to these questions depends on the patient's and clinician's expectation and requirements. The variations possible are great and at the moment, in the author's view, both clinician and patient tend to have too pessimistic an outlook for the benefit of properly supervised therapy.

Where it is thought, and probably where the patient believes, that a line of treatment is beneficial, considerable self control is required to withhold treatment. The line of least resistance is to accept and use without analysis the treatments in general vogue.

Just as these diseases are infinitely variable in their clinical features so are the variations in therapy. During the course of chronic inflammatory disease there is a progressive change of function usually for the worse. Thus, the longer the disease continues the less likely is full function to be restored. It follows that at any point in time an assessment of the practical possibilities of benefit should be made and this will be continuously changing. In particular, the replacement of inflammatory causes of pain by mechanical causes during the course of chronic arthritis is common and requires a change in therapy. For the same reason, the part played in the total clinical picture by different facets of the inflammation must be analysed. Some will be untreatable or irreversible and prolonged therapy directed at these will give less benefit and be more liable to produce side-effects, perhaps from drug overdosage, than treatment of the more reversible features. Overtreatment is a frequent cause of side-effects and can be reduced if the different anti-inflammatory drugs are correctly given, reducing the need to search for ever better products.

In considering the claims of non-drug therapy (rest, heat, exercise etc.), animal models are not appropriate for extrapolation and even less firm data exists on which to base opinions than for drug therapy. Thus, dogmatic statements are at present baseless. SWEZEY (1974) has reviewed the subject.

I. Rest

Rest is the most satisfactory way to bring severe joint inflammation under control. Unfortunately, although initial benefit may be marked, further benefit may require prolonged rest and is associated with complications such as pressure sores and tissue wasting, especially of muscle and bone. These can be partly circumvented by resting parts of the body only, e.g. by splints, while the patients as a whole remains mobile. Benefit is frequently lost following mobilisation, 70% of the patients treated by LEE et al. (1974 b) deteriorated again within 18 months. Rest is positively contraindicated in the central arthritis associated with ankylosing spondylitis and similar syndromes where improvement seems to follow activity rather than rest and in which the subsequent symptomatic benefit is accompanied by reduction in acute phase reactants. This is one of the enigmas of clinical medicine for which there seems to be no satisfactory hypothesis. Emotional rest is hard to define and its value even harder to confirm, but it probably has a valuable part to play in treatment, particularly in aiding co-operation during management.

II. Heat

Subjective benefit follows local heat where the clinical activity is not great. Many of these patients with widespread inflammatory disease have a raised metabolic rate and if there is much inflammation then more generalised heat may make the patient feel much worse and the joints more painful. Heat does not appear to have any more beneficial effect on the disease other than as a means of easing pain and stiffness and allowing mobilising exercises to be undertaken.

III. Exercise

The value of exercise as distinct from rest (absolute) in the treatment of inflammatory arthritis is still debated. In the acute stages, absolute rest even for 2 weeks followed by gentle passive exercise to maintain the range of joint movement, will not lead to reduced joint movement.

In the less acute stages active exercises are necessary to restore muscle power. The stage of the disease at which one's approach changes varies with the clinician and the disease. Patients rarely over-exercise and the presence of increased and prolonged pain after exercise suggests the exercises are excessive. The inflammation of ankylosing spondylitis is quite distinct in being dramatically decreased by exercise, analgesia only being necessary to allow these exercises to be undertaken.

Hydrotherapy, in spite of the exaggerated claims for its benefits, has a part to play largely in relaxing joints and muscles and allowing *controlled* and supported movements to be undertaken.

Occupational therapists in their dual role of functional assessment and rehabilitation are slowly performing an increasingly useful service in patient management.

IV. Anti-Inflammatory Therapy

1. Non-Steroid Anti-Inflammatory Drugs

The early history of anti-inflammatory drug therapy belongs to analgesics and salicylates together with herbal remedies, many of which have never been properly evaluated. Later, antibiotics arrived and dramatically cured infection; they were in addition susceptible to in vitro testing. Gold was introduced in 1927 by LANDE but no formal controlled trial was undertaken until the EMPIRE RHEUMATISM COUNCIL (1960) report was published. It is interesting to note that by present standards, gold would not have been introduced into clinical practice because of its side-effects—slow excretion and the delay in onset of benefit (2 months)—which exceeds the length of trials normally performed up to a few years ago. Most of these therapies were discovered fortuitously and were subjected to haphazard trials. Part of the difficulty in evaluating therapy lay in the scarcity of trained rheumatologists and the lack of the controlled trial, a concept introduced by the above gold study and since improved. It was not until fenemates (1962) and indomethacin (1963) were introduced that any of these drugs were evolved by scientific experiment. In the last decade there has been a continuously increasing number of new non-steroid anti-inflammatory drugs introduced. They will be considered as a group since their relative advantages are not yet evaluated.

The non-steroid anti-inflammatory drugs seem to lie in the category of palliative rather than curative therapy. Although the clinical features of arthritis may be improved, there is *no* convincing evidence that prevention of joint or tendon destruction is occurring. However, in mild cases where the disease is not rapidly progressive, they may be sufficient to allow the patient to lead a normal life, although slow joint deterioration continues. Attempts to improve this inefficiency have not been very successful. One goal is to have the inactive compound carried to the site of inflammation before being released and then rendered active locally, thus avoiding systemic side-effects. While the search for better anti-inflammatory agents will obviously continue, more proficient use of those presently available is possible and some suggestions follow.

To obtain optimum results, the drugs must be used in adequate amounts; thus, aspirin is often prescribed in too small a dose and little benefit is shown. Random blood salicylate levels often show that some patients are not attaining adequate serum levels inspite of an apparently appropriate intake. Salicylate levels taken first thing in the morning following overnight lack of aspirin, may give a falsely low indication of the level of salicylate. The addition of further different non-steroid anti-inflammatory drugs does not help in improving responses, but there is no doubt that some patients feel better on one drug than another and that the addition of a second drug may increase the free levels of the first and thus its effectiveness, if it was being used in suboptimum amounts. More subtle changes may also account for the altered effect found by the addition of further similar drugs. The problems of protein binding and enzyme induction when more than one drug is used have already been mentioned. Larger doses of a drug may be taken if partly given by the rectal route as suppositories or by injection, thus avoiding gastric irritation. The correct timing of therapy may be important; short half-life drugs such as aspirin must be given frequently and where the patient suffers from morning stiffness this may be alleviated either by increasing the evening dose of non-steroid anti-inflammatory drug or by leaving a dose at the bedside to be taken on awakening in the night. Many patients find the frequent taking of tablets irksome and compliance is better with once daily therapy where possible (phenylbutazone, chloroquine). Finally, where a powerful anti-inflammatory agent, such as prednisone, is used there seems little point in using milder anti-inflammatory agents instead of analgesics.

2. Gold, Penicillamine, and Chloroquine

Without discussing the relative benefits or the largely unknown mode of action of these drugs, certain points about their use can be made. They are well known to have serious and even fatal side-effects and certainly in the case of gold, to be metabolised differently by different patients. Some of the side-effects may be due to idiosyncracy, others to induced hypersensitivity and yet others to straight toxicity from accumulation in tissues. Thus, care is needed in avoiding these complications and particularly in realising that different complications may occur at different times. For this reason, the use of 'courses' of treatment where each patient is given a set treatment schedule no matter what his response, seems rather less scientific than adjusting the treatment to the response, continuous monitoring for side-effects being maintained and not reduced until therapy is stabilised. This obviously commits large resources to continous follow up surveillance. With all these drugs it is suggested that the usual form of treatment is continued until clinical benefit, a fall in ESR (or other measure of acute phase reactants) or toxicity occurs. In the first two cases, the dose is stabilised, e.g. gold injections every 2 or 3 weeks instead of weekly, chloroquine daily or every odd calendar day, or the dose of penicillamine is not increased. If this tailoring of the dose to the patient's response instead of giving predetermined courses is observed, less toxicity probably occurs and prolonged treatment can be given. It must be emphasised that we do not at present know the value of prolonged treatment with any of these drugs. So far, no new side-effects have emerged with prolonged therapy, and where the treatment is carefully monitored there is a reduction in the incidence of the known side-effects. This is in contradiction to corticosteroid therapy where side-effects invariably increase with time.

One of the most radical changes has been in the use of penicillamine where the initial dose used for rheumatoid arthritis of some 1500 mg/day, which was taken from the treatment of Wilson's disease, has now been reduced to 500 mg/day and in a few cases to 125 mg/day.

The introduction of more graded increases in doses of penicillamine therapy have revealed one cause of discrepancy in the type of side-effect resulting from clinical trials. Starting with small doses and using slower increments, the incidence of blood dyscrasias and gastro-intestinal symptoms (Fig. 1 and Table 1) has been reduced, allowing more patients to continue on penicillamine for 6 months or longer when the late onset site-effects, presumably immunological, of kidney disease occur. Thus, different side-effects may be revealed by different trial proforma.

Clinically, the most striking benefit is found with these drugs. In practice, they are most effective in rheumatoid arthritis but in contradistinction to the non-steroid

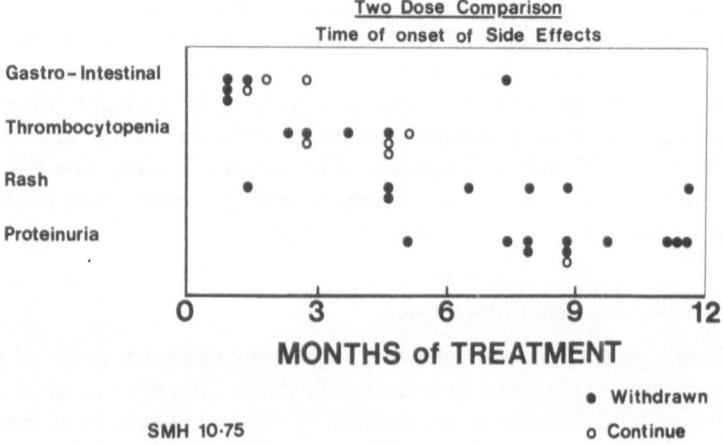

Fig. 1. Time related incidence of side-effects following penicillamine therapy in rheumatoid arthritis (courtesy HILL and HILL, 1975)

Table 1. Comparison of side effects following two dosage schedules "Go fast and high" 250 mg penicillamine increasing by 250 mg every fortnight to 1500 mg. "Go slow and low" 250 mg penicillamine increasing by 250 mg monthly to a maximum of 750 mg (courtesy HILL and HILL, 1975). Penicillamine in R.A. 2 dose comparison — 43 patients side-effects during first year

	Go fast and high (21)		Go slow and low (22)	
	Incidence	Withdrawn	Incidence	Withdrawn
Thrombocytopenia				
< 100,000	3	0	1	0
< 70,000	3	3	1	1
W.B.C. <4,000	1	1	0	0
Gastro-intestinal	7	5	1	0
Rash early	1	1	0	0
late	2	2	4	4
Proteinuria	2	2	9	8

S.M.H. 10.75.

anti-inflammatory drugs, there is a more all-or-none response. Thus, if benefit occurs it is good; alternatively there may be no benefit at all. The main problem is that of deciding in which cases and when to use this treatment and for how long to continue it. Prediction of the course of inflammatory arthritis is difficult both in terms of chronicity and of tissue damage. My own preference is to use these forms of therapy early, after 6 months of continuous rheumatoid disease of moderate severity, and continue for about 3 years.

3. Corticosteroids

Although undoubtedly rapidly effective, these drugs have many potential side-effects. The incidence of these and to what extent they are due to the therapy or to the underlying disease is not clear. Nor is it known the extent to which they may protect against the side-effects of the inflammation. Thus, in childhood both active disease and corticosteroids may reduce growth; however, treatment with steroids by reducing the inflammation could in fact increase growth. Similarly in the adult, osteoporosis for various reasons accompanies active inflammatory arthritis; again corticosteroids, by reducing the inflammation, may decrease the rate of bone loss. Neither of these questions has been satisfactorily answered and decisions concerning corticosteroids therapy are based on clinical judgement only.

The risk of the many side-effects may be justified if no other therapy is available or if a quick response is required for a specific purpose, such as mobilising a joint, or the patient is unable to attend the clinic and must continue at work. In the elderly, they may be used with advantage often in small doses.

In an attempt to reduce the growth-depressing effect in children, the corticosteroids are often given as the total daily dose in the morning to follow the normal circadian rhythm of corticosteroid secretion. To stimulate the patient's own secretion of corticosteroids, alternate day therapy with twice the normal daily dose may be used (ANSELL and BYWATERS, 1974).

4. Cytotoxic (Immunosuppressant) Therapy

The evidence that most of the drugs used, particularly in the dosage employed in treating chronic inflammatory arthritis, as distinct from the doses used in systemic lupus erythematosus etc., are significantly immunosuppressive, is unsatisfactory. They probably have a more important direct anti-inflammatory effect on the inflammatory reaction. This effect is clinically significant but may be gained at the expense of side effects, such as herpes zoster, blood dyscrasias and infection. Their role in treatment is undefined.

5. Local Anti-Inflammatory Therapy

Injections of corticosteroid either into tissue or into the synovial cavity can have a dramatic effect on the local inflammation but with reduced systemic side-effects. Still awaiting full evaluation is the use of intra-articular injections of radioactive compounds such as yttrium 99 or of anti-metabolites such as methotrexate. Experience with radioactive yttrium suggests that it reduces the inflammatory exudate. There is less experience with other compounds and published work suggests that they still need evaluation.

6. Lymphocyte Depletion

Apart from the use of cytotoxic drugs, including anti-lymphocytic globulin, the most popular techiques have been splenic irradiation and thoracic duct drainage. The latter is effective, even in diseases where inflammation is not marked as scleroderma, but of limited duration because the drainage system fails and the technique requires elaborate support facilities. It is thus a research model only.

7. Immune Potentiation

This is a poor term. In contradistinction to immunosuppression, the aim is to improve the immunity, in particular the regulatory mechanisms. This has been attempted by drugs (e.g. levamisole) (HUSKINSSON et al., 1976) or by the use of dialysable extract of normal lymphocytes (FROLAND et al., 1974; MAINI et al., 1976). Whether these treatments work and how they work has not been settled. Although changes in the immune response have been demonstrated, the reasons for this are not clear and may represent a local alteration in immunity rather than a central change.

8. Removal of Antibody

Recently, repeated plasmaphoresis has been used to remove circulating antibody and immune complexes in the hope that this will reduce the inflammation. Encouraging results have been reported (VERRIER-JONES et al., 1976), but this is again an extensive exercise and commits large resources. It is thus only applicable to extreme cases as a temporary expedient and as a research tool.

9. X-Ray Irradiation

External irradiation has been used in the treatment of the spine in ankylosing spondylitis; the effectiveness of this treatment is debated but it is probably beneficial. No benefit follows irradiation of peripheral joints either in ankylosing spondylitis or other inflammatory arthritis. The mode of action of this therapy is not clear; a local vasculitis may reduce inflammatory blood flow or, by a direct effect on the cell, inflammation may be reduced. Irradiation of local (focal) points of tenderness in ankylosing spondylitis can be dramatically effective and avoids the possibility of inducing leukaemia.

It cannot be stressed too often that the objective evidence that any form of drug therapy benefits the patient in the long term, is very poor. Where there is suggestive evidence of improvement there is also the problem of making a value judgment of the balance between clinical improvement and side-effects, both continuing and episodic.

The lack of consensus of opinion of the various treatment schemes is well demonstrated by the varying opinions held in different continents or even different parts of a country. Treatment implicitly believed in by their users (prescriber and consumer) are elsewhere unheard of, untried or discarded.

F. Summary

Marked improvements have occurred in anti-rheumatic therapy in recent years. Advances in the understanding of the underlying pathogenic mechanisms have resulted in improved diagnosis and management. However, the continuing search for more definitive therapy is being delayed by a lack of new and more appropriate models of inflammation and of knowledge of the aetiological factors concerned. Pending the discovery of these, disease in man remains the only satisfactory method of testing new treatments; hence the importance of a thorough understanding of techniques for assessment of inflammation and clinical status.

References

American Rheumatism Association: 1958 Revision of diagnostic criteria for rheumatoid arthritis. Arthr. and Rheum. **2**, 16—20 (1959)

Ansell, B. M., Bywaters, E. G. L.: Alternate day corticosteroid therapy in juvenile chronic polyarthritis. J. Rheum. **1**, 176—186 (1974)

Backlund, L., Tiselius, P.: Objective measurements of joint stiffness in rheumatoid arthritis. Acta. rheum. scand. **13**, 275—288 (1967)

Beck, F. J., Whitehouse, M. W.: Effect of adjuvant disease in rats on cyclophosphamide and iso-phosphamide metabolism. Biochem. Pharmacol. **22**, 2453—2468 (1973)

Boardman, P. J., Hart, F. D.: Clinical measurement of the anti-inflammatory effects of salicylates in rheumatoid arthritis. Brit. med. J. (1967) IV, 264—268

Chalmers, I. M., Bell, M. A., Buchanan, W. W.: Effect of flurbiprofen on the metabolism of antipyrine in man. Ann. rheum. Dis. **32**, 58—61 (1973)

Chen, W., Vrindten, P. A., Dayton, P. C., Burns, J. J.: Accelerated amidopyrine metabolism in human subjects pretreated with phenylbutazone. Life Sci. **I**, 35—42 (1962)

Cohen, A. S., Reynolds, W. E., Franklyn, E. C., Kulka, J. P., Roper, M. W., Shulman, L. E., Wallace, S. L.: Preliminary criteria for the classification of systemic lupus erythematosus. Bull. rheum. Dis. **21**, 643—647 (1971)

Collins, A. J., Ring, E. F. J., Cosh, J. A., Bacon, P. A.: Quantitation of thermography in arthritis using multi-isothermal analysis. Ann. rheum. Dis. **33**, 113—115 (1974)

Co-Operating Clinics Committee of American Rheumatism Association: A controlled trial of cyclophosphamide in rheumatoid arthritis. New Engl. J. Med. **283**, 883—889 (1970)

Dick, W. C.: The use of radioisotopes in normal and diseased joints. Semin. Arthr. Rheum. **1**, 301—325 (1972)

Dick, W. C., Fowler, P. F.: Personal Communication (1976)

Dickson, R. A., Nicolle, F. V.: The assessment of the rheumatoid hand. In: Holt, P. J. L. (Ed.): Current topics of Connective Tissue Diseases, pp. 95—114. London: Churchill Livingstone 1975

Duthie, J. J. R., Thompson, M., Weir, M., Fletcher, W. B.: Medical and social aspects of the treatment of rheumatoid arthritis. Ann. rheum. Dis. **14**, 133—149 (1955)

Empire Rheumatism Council: Gold therapy in rheumatoid arthritis—a report of a multicentre trial. Ann. rheum. Dis. **19**, 95—119 (1960)

Feinstein, A. R.: The need for humanised science in evaluating medication. Lancet **(1972)**II, 421—423

Feinstein, A. R.: Clinical biostatics. XIX. Ambiguity and abuse in the twelve different concepts of 'control'. Clin. Pharmacol. Ther. **14**, 112—122 (1973)

Froland, S. S., Natvig, J. B., Hoyeraal, H. M., Kass, E.: The principle of immunopotentation in rheumatoid arthritis treatment: effect of transfer factor. Scand. J. Immunol. **3**, 223—228 (1974)

Gelehrter, T. D.: Enzyme induction. New Engl. J. Med. **294**, 522—526, 588—595, 646—651 (1976)

Goldberg, M. A., Arnett, F. C., Bias, W. B., Shulman, L. E.: Histocompatibility antigens in systemic lupus erythematosus. Arthr. Rheum. **19**, 129—132 (1976)

Hawkins, C. F., Holt, P. J. L.: The Cuff dolorimeter. Proc. roy. Soc. Med. **59** (Suppl.), 95—96 (1966)

Haydu, G. G., Goldschmidt, L., Drymiotis, A. D.: Effect of imipramine on the rheumatoid factor titre of psychotic patients with depressive symptomatology. Ann. rheum. Dis. **33**, 273—275 (1974)

Holt, P. J. L., How, M. J., Long, V. J. W., Hawkins, C. F.: Mucopolysaccharides in synovial fluid: effect of aspirin and indomethacin on hyaluronic acid. Ann. rheum. Dis. **27**, 264—270 (1968).

Horvath, S. M., Hollander, J. L.: Intra-articular temperature as a measure of joint reaction. J. clin. Invest. **28**, 469—473 (1949)

Hughes, G. R. V.: Significance of anti DNA antibodies in systemic lupus erythematosus. Lancet **(1971)II**, 861—864

Huskisson, E. C.: Measurement of pain. Lancet **(1974)II**, 1127—1131

Huskisson, E. C., Dieppe, P. A., Scott, J., Trapnell, J., Balme, H. W., Milloughby, D. A.: Immunstimulant therapy with levamisole for rheumatoid arthritis. Lancet **(1976)I**, 393—395

Koch-Weser & Sellers, E. M.: Binding of drugs to serum albumin. New Engl. J. Med. **294**, 311—315, 526—531 (1976)

Lansbury, J.: Report of a three year study on the systemic and articular indices in rheumatoid arthritis. Arthr. Rheum. **1**, 505—522 (1958)

Lee, P., Baxter, A., Dick, W. C., Webb, J.: An assessment of grip strength measurements in rheumatoid arthritis. Scand. J. Rheum. **3**, 17—23 (1974 a)

Lee, P., Kennedy, A. C., Anderson, J., Buchanan, W. W.: The therapeutic benefits of hospital inpatient treatment in rheumatoid arthritis. Quart. J. Med. **43**, 203—214 (1974 b)

Levi, A. J., Sherlock, S., Walker, D.: Phenylbutazone and isoniazide metabolism in patients with liver disease in relation to previous drug therapy. Lancet **(1968)I**, 1275—1279

McCarty, D. J., Gatter, R. A., Steele, A. D.: A twenty pound dolorimeter for quantitation of articular tenderness. Arthr. Rheum. **11**, 696—697 (1968)

Mc Conkey, B., Crockson, R. A., Crockson, A. P., Williamson, A. R.: The effect of some anti-inflammatory drugs on the acute phase proteins in rheumatoid arthritis. Quart. J. Med. **42**, 785—791 (1973)

Maini, R. N., Scott, J. T., Roffe, L. M., Hamblin, A. S., Dumonde, D. C.: Preliminary experience of transfer factor in rheumatoid arthritis: clinical and immunological studies. In: Dumonde, D. C. (Ed.): Infection and Immunology in the Rheumatic Disease, pp. 579—589. London: Blackwell 1976

Medical Research Council and Nuffield Foundation: A comparison or cortisone and aspirin in the treatment of early cases of rheumatoid arthritis. Brit. med. J. **(1954)I**, 1223—1227

Moertel, C. G., Taylor, W. F., Roth, A., Tyce, F. A. J.: Who responds to sugar pills? Mayo Clin. Proc. **51**, 96—100 (1976)

Ritchie, D. M., Boyle, J. A., McInnes, J. H., Jasani, M. K., Dalakos, T. C., Grieveson, P., Buchanan, W. W.: Clinical studies with an articular index for assessment of joint tenderness in patients with rheumatoid arthritis. Quart. J. Med. **37**, 393—406 (1968)

Russell, A. S., Sturge, R. A., Smith, M. A.: Serum transaminases during salicylate therapy. Brit. med. J. **(1971)II**, 428—429

Savage, O.: Measurements in rheumatoid arthritis. Proc. roy. Soc. Med. **59** (Suppl.), 85—88 (1966)

Seaman, W. E., Ishak, K. C., Plotz, P. H.: Aspirin induced hepatoxicity in patients with systemic lupus erythematosus. Ann. intern. Med. **80**, 1—8 (1974)

Steinbrocker, O., Traeger, C. H., Batteman, R. C.: Therapeutic criteria in rheumatoid arthritis. J. Amer. med. Ass. **140**, 659—662 (1949)

Swezey, R. L.: Essentials of physical management and rehabilitation in arthritis. Semin. Arthr. Rheum. **3**, 349 (1974)

Talal, N.: Immunologic and viral factors in the pathogenesis of systemic lupus erythematosus. Arthr. Rheum. **13**, 887—894 (1970)

Traut, E. F., Passarell, E. W.: Placebos in the evaluation of treatment in rheumatic disease. Illinois med. J. **115**, 181—198 (1959)

Verrier-Jones, J., Cumming, R. H., Bucknall, R. C., Asplin, C. M., Fraser, I. D., Bothomley, J., Davis, P., Hamblin, T. J.: Plasmophoresis in the management of acute systemic lupus erythematosus? Lancet **(1976)I**, 709—711

Versey, J. M. B., Hobbs, J. R., Holt, P. J. L.: Complement metabolism in rheumatoid arthritis. 1. Longtudinal studies. Ann. rheum. Dis. **32**, 357—564 (1973)

Wright, V.: Some observations on diurnal variations of grip. Clin. Sci. **18**, 17—23 (1959)

Wright, V., Dowson, D., Longfield, M. D.: Joint stiffness—its characterisation and significance. Biomed. Engng **4**, 8 (1969)

Wright, V., Johns, R. J.: Physical factors concerned with the stiffness of normal and diseased joints. Bull. John Hopk. Hosp. **106**, 215—231 (1961)

Author Index

West, G.B., see Thomas, G. 154, *163*, 366, *396*, 669, *696*

West, L.A., see Dayton, P.G. 585, *592*

West, M., see Krupp, P. 331, *344*

Westerholm, B., see Moran, N.C. 498, *527*

Westermann, E., see Gjuris, V. 147, 155, *160*

Weston, W.L., Claman, H.N., Krueger, G.G. 633, 640, *659*

Weston, W.L., Mandel, M.J., Yeckley, J.A., Krueger, G.G., Claman, H.N. 633, *659*

Westra, J.G., see Steen, J. Van der 558, 559, *576*

Westwick, J., see Blackham, A. 119, 132, *136*, 230, 239, *246*, 363, 373, *384*

Westwick, W.J., Allsop, J., Watts, R.W.E. 9, *42*

Whaley, K., see Dick, C. 627, *650*

White, A., see Bach, J.F. 564, *567*

White, A., see Makman, M.H. 607, *655*

White, A.M., see Bullock, G.R. 613, 614, *650*

White, C.B., see Shriver, D.A. 294, *301*

White, F.R. 581, *597*

White, H.L., see Vinegar, R. 209, 211–214, 216, *222*

White, P., see Charache, P. 93, *104*

Whitehouse, G.H., see Tayler, R.T. 283, *302*

Whitehouse, M., see Bluestone, R. 579, *591*

Whitehouse, M.W. 3, 8, 9, *42*, 44, 61, *74*, 130, 131, *143*, 234, 239, 242, *254*, 285, *302*, 353, 379, *397*, 544, 556, 564, 565, *576*, 724, *739*

Whitehouse, M.W., Beck, F.W. 113, 124, *144*, 554, 558, 560, *577*

Whitehouse, M.W., Beck, F.W.J., Dröge, M.M., Struck, R.F. 544, 558, 559, *577*

Whitehouse, M.W., Beck, F.J., Kacena, A. 556, 558, *577*

Whitehouse, M.W., Famaey, J.P. 18, *42*

Whitehouse, M.W., Haslam, J.M. 9, 19, *42*

Whitehouse, M.W., Kippen, I., Klinenberg, J.R. 3, 4, 19, *42*

Whitehouse, M.W., Kippen, I., Klinenberg, J.R., Schlosstein, L., Campion, D.S., Bluestone, R. 585, *597*

Whitehouse, M.W., Orr, K.J., Beck, F.W., Pearson, C.M. 112, 113, *144*

Whitehouse, M.W., Skidmose, I.F. 3, 8, *42*

Whitehouse, M.W., see Baumgartner, W.A. 114, 115, 120, 121, 130, *136*

Whitehouse, M.W., see Beck, F.J. 130, 131, *136*, 536, 557, 559, 561, 563, *567*, 744, *765*

Whitehouse, M.W., see Denko, C.W. 725, *732*

Whitehouse, M.W., see Famaey, J.P. 4, 5, 9, *31*

Whitehouse, M.W., see Kippen, I. 584, *594*

Whitehouse, M.W., see Levy, J. 536, 563, *572*

Whitehouse, M.W., see Paulus, H.E. 108, 130, *141*, 156, *162*, 291, *300*, 540, *573*

Whitehouse, M.W., see Scherrer, R.A. 3, 8, 19, 26, 40, 108, *142*

Whitehouse, M.W., see Skidmose, I.F. 3, 4, 9, 19, *39*, 356, 360, *395*

Whitehouse, M.W., see Yu, D.T. 560, *577*

Whitelock, R.A.F., see Eakins, K.E. 382, *386*

Whittaker, V.P., see Braun, W. 586, *591*

Whittet, T.D., see Baker, J.A. 266, 267, *274*

Whittington, H., see Mawson, C. 426, 427, 429, 430, *462*

Whittle, B.A. 218, *222*

Whittle, B.A., see Atkinson, D.C. 676, *688*

Whittle, B.J.R. 614, *659*

Whittle, B.J.R., see Main, I.H.M. 377, *392*

Whorton, C.M., see Michael, M. 237, *250*

Widdicombe, J.G. 147, *163*

Widdicombe, J.G., see Mills, J. 153, *162*

Wiebelhaus, V.D., see Beyer, K.H. 586, *591*

Wieczorek, W., see Hanahoe, T.H.P. 500, *525*

Wied, D., de, Witter, A., Versteeg, D.H.G., Mulder, A.H. 686, *697*

Wiederman, G., see Weissmann, G. 133, *143*

Wiener, E., Marmary, Y. 611, *660*

Wiener, J., Lattes, R.G., Pearl, J.S. 635, *660*

Wiener, J., Loud, A.V., Kimberg, D.V., Saro, D. 613, *660*

Wiethold, G., Hellenbrecht, D., Lemmer, R., Palm, D. 6, *42*

Wiggan, G., see Sheppard, H. 510, *529*

Wiggins, L.F. 410, *414*

Wigley, R.D., see Caughey, D.E. 284, *297*

Wigzell, H., see Jondal, M. 535, *571*

Wijs, H., De, see Jollès, P. 112, *139*

Wilcox, W.R., Khalaf, A.R. 579, *597*

Wilcox, W.R., see Kippen, I. 579, *594*

Wilford, S., see Maling, H.M. 421, 430, 432, 444, 446, *461*

Wilhelm, D.L. 86, *90*, 209, *222*, 419, 432, *465*, 711, *739*

Wilhelm, D.L., Mason, B. 55, *74*, 84, *90*, 224, *254*, 421, 431, 434, 435, 439, 447, *465*

Wilhelm, D.L., see Baumgarten, A. 437, *457*

Wilhelm, D.L., see Graig, J.P. 436, *459*

Wilhelm, D.L., see Garcia Leme, J. 353, *388*

Wilhelm, D.L., see Logan, G. 44, 50, 52, 58, 72, 421, 435, 436, 440, 447, *461*

Wilhelm, D.L., see Miles, A.A. 420, 421, 432, *462*

Wilhelm, D.L., see Sparrow, E.M. 420, 434, 439, *464*

Wilhelmi, G. 44, 50, 60, 61, *74*, 229, 236, 238, *254*, 285, *302*

Wilhelmi, G., Domenjoz, R. 50, 62, *74*, 81, *91*, 365, *397*

Wilhelmi, G., Menassé-Gdynia, R. 292, *302*

Subject Index

Abscess
  PMN and   226
Acacetin
  anti-inflammatory activity   702, 704
  structure   700
Acetaminophen
  Aa bronchoconstriction inhibition   190
  Aa hypotension inhibition   190
  analgesic activity, assay   213—215, 219
  analgesic activity, mechanism of   215, 367,
    380
  antipyretic activity   190, 260, 261
  antipyretic activity, mechanism of   266, 369,
    380
  antipyretic activity, pyrogen fever and
    267—270
  ATP bronchoconstriction inhibition   191
  Bk bronchoconstriction inhibition   155,
    156, 191
  Bk hypotension inhibition   191
  carrageenin oedema inhibition   372
  endogenous pyrogen production and   261
  endotoxin shock and   189
  erythema inhibition and   61
  heat production and   263
  hypothalamic neurone receptor site
    antagonism   266
  PG biosynthesis inhibition in vivo   372
  PG synthetase inhibition, brain   15, 190,
    264, 369, 380
  PG synthetase inhibition in vitro   372
  PG synthetase inhibition, peripheral nerve
    380
  PG synthetase inhibition, platelet   190
  PG synthetase inhibition, spleen   369
  platelet aggregation inhibition   190
  RA therapy   399
  RCS synthesis inhibition   190
  SRS-C bronchoconstriction inhibition   191
  stretching response inhibition   219
Acetanilide
  antipyretic activity   260, 264
  erythema inhibition and   61
Acetic acid
  oedema formation and   85
  stretching assay   218, 219

Acetylcholine
  bronchoconstriction   155, 356
  fever and   272
  pain induction   367
  stretching assay   218
Acetylsalicylic acid
  Aa bronchoconstriction inhibition   174,
    175, 180
  Aa diarrhoea inhibition   218
  Aa fever inhibition   274
  Aa hypotension and   175, 177, 179, 180, 185
  adjuvant arthritis and   68, 77, 111, 118, 126
  ADP hypotension and   186
  adrenocortical stimulation   664
  adverse reaction   282, 283, 285, 286, 290, 664
  analgesic activity, assay   210, 211, 213, 214,
    218—220
  analgesic activity, clinical evaluation   219,
    220
  analgesic activity, mechanism of   210, 215,
    218, 220
  anti-Aa activity   175, 274
  anti-Bk activity   147, 155—157, 164, 167,
    194, 354
  anti-carrageenin activity   171, 195
  anti-inflammatory activity, mechanism of
    149, 315, 316, 336, 354, 357, 358, 368, 369,
    664
  anti-inflammatory assay   59, 60, 63, 77, 84,
    87, 101, 706
  anti-inflammatory assay in vitro   12, 13, 16,
    18
  antipyretic activity   260, 261, 267—270
  antipyretic activity, mechanism of   264, 265,
    369
  anti-thrombin activity   25, 168
  arthritis therapy   760, 761
  ATP bronchoconstriction inhibition   157
  Bk bronchoconstriction inhibition   147,
    155, 156
  Bk hypotension and   164, 165, 167
  Bk permeability response and   354
  cAMP elevation inhibition   150
  cAMP phosphodiesterase and   10
  carrageenin oedema inhibition   77, 83, 372,
    373, 664

Reviews of Physiology, Biochemistry and Pharmacology

formerly
Ergebnisse der Physiologie, biologischen
Chemie und experimentellen Pharmakologie

Editors: R. H. Adrian, E. Helmreich, H. Holzer,
R. Jung, K. Kramer, O. Krayer, R. J. Linden,
F. Lynen, P. A. Miescher, J. Piiper, H. Ras-
mussen, A. E. Renold, U. Trendelenburg,
K. Ullrich, W. Vogt, A. Weber

This series presents rapid and comprehensive
information on topical problems and research
in progress over the entire range of physiology, biochemistry, and pharmacology.
An international group of editors is responsible for inviting experts in these fields to
submit contributions. Every year three to four
volumes are published. The language of
publication is English.

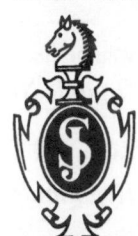

Springer-Verlag
Berlin
Heidelberg
New York

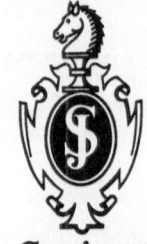

Springer-Verlag
Berlin
Heidelberg
New York